WJ 302 QUA £269

369 0299519

KU-067-203

MONKLANDS HOSPITAL
LIBRARY
MONKSCOURT AVENUE
AIRDRIE ML6 0JS
☎ 01236712005

WID

**FOR
REFERENCE ONLY**

WJ 302 QUA £269

# Medical Radiology

## Diagnostic Imaging

### Series Editors

A. L. Baert, Leuven
M. F. Reiser, München
H. Hricak, New York
M. Knauth, Göttingen

For further volumes:
http:/www.springer.com/series/4354

# Medical Radiology

## Diagnostic Imaging

### Editorial Board

Andy Adam, London
Fred Avni, Brussels
Richard L. Baron, Chicago
Carlo Bartolozzi, Pisa
George S. Bisset, Houston
A. Mark Davies, Birmingham
William P. Dillon, San Francisco
D. David Dershaw, New York
Sam Sanjiv Gambhir, Stanford
Nicolas Grenier, Bordeaux
Gertraud Heinz-Peer, Vienna
Robert Hermans, Leuven
Hans-Ulrich Kauczor, Heidelberg
Theresa McLoud, Boston
Konstantin Nikolaou, München
Caroline Reinhold, Montreal
Donald Resnick, San Diego
Rüdiger Schulz-Wendtland, Erlangen
Stephen Solomon, New York
Richard D. White, Columbus

Emilio Quaia (Ed.)

# Radiological Imaging of the Kidney

Foreword by

A. L. Baert

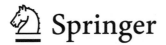 Springer

Prof. Emilio Quaia
Università Trieste
Ospedale di Cattinara
Ist. Radiologia
Strada di Fiume 447
34149 Trieste
Italy
equaia@yahoo.com

MONKLANDS HOSPITAL
LIBRARY
MONKSCOURT AVENUE
AIRDRIE ML60JS
☎01236712005

ISSN: 0942-5373

ISBN: 978-3-540-87596-3        e-ISBN: 978-3-540-87597-0

DOI: 10.1007/978-3-540-87597-0

Springer Heidelberg Dordrecht London New York

Library of Congress Control Number: 2010933084

© Springer-Verlag Berlin Heidelberg 2011

This work is subject to copyright. All rights are reserved, whether the whole or part of the material is concerned, specifically the rights of translation, reprinting, reuse of illustrations, recitation, broadcasting, reproduction on microfilm or in any other way, and storage in data banks. Duplication of this publication or parts thereof is permitted only under the provisions of the German Copyright Law of September 9, 1965, in its current version, and permission for use must always be obtained from Springer. Violations are liable to prosecution under the German Copyright Law.

The use of general descriptive names, registered names, trademarks, etc. in this publication does not imply, even in the absence of a specific statement, that such names are exempt from the relevant protective laws and regulations and therefore free for general use.

Product liability: The publishers cannot guarantee the accuracy of any information about dosage and application contained in this book. In every individual case the user must check such information by consulting the relevant literature.

*Cover design*: eStudio Calamar, Figueres/Berlin

Printed on acid-free paper

Springer is part of Springer Science+Business Media (www.springer.com)

*To my beloved Lorenza, Benedetta, Diletta, and Brigitta*

# Foreword

It is my great pleasure and privilege to introduce another volume, published in our book series "Medical Radiology–Diagnostic Imaging", which is devoted to Radiological Imaging of the kidney. It is edited by E.Quaia, widely known for his numerous original contributions to urogenital radiology, especially in the area of ultrasound, computed tomography and the role of ultrasound contrast media in the diagnostic management of diseases of the urogenital organs.

It covers in depth the complete spectrum of superb imaging modalities which are actually available to study the normal anatomy and the pathology of the kidney and upper urinary tract, including the latest technical advances in equipment design.

The clear and informative text, the numerous well-chosen illustrations of superb technical quality as well as the traditional Springer excellent standards of design and layout make this outstanding work a reference handbook for all certified general and urogenital radiologists. Also, radiologists in training will find it very useful for improving their knowledge and skills. Referring physicians such as urologists and nephrologists will benefit from it to improve the clinical management of their patients.

I am greatly indebted to the editor E.Quaia for his efficient and brilliant editorial work as well as for the judicious choice of the contributing authors, all well-known and internationally recognised experts in the field, who wrote the 36 excellent individual chapters of this outstanding volume.

Leuven                                                                    Albert L. Baert

# Preface

The aim of this book is to provide a comprehensive analysis of the embryology, normal anatomy, and of the pathology of the kidney and the upper urinary tract (renal pelvis and upper ureter) according to the modern diagnostic imaging techniques. The opportunity provided to me by Professor Albert Baert represents a wonderful occasion to present an up-to-date resume of what is possible to obtain nowadays by imaging in the evaluation of the normal and pathologic kidney.

Significant technical improvements have allowed the use of radiological techniques to play a growing role in the imaging of renal diseases. Several new imaging techniques and new technical improvements of the preexisting imaging techniques have been introduced in the recent years. Contrast-enhanced ultrasound is now considered a well-established imaging technique in the analysis of renal perfusion and tumors. Multidetector computed tomography (CT) is able to provide high spatial resolution images of the kidneys and renal arterial vessels (CT angiography) and urinary tract (CT urography). Magnetic resonance imaging (MRI) is now able to provide high signal-to-noise ratio and higher spatial and/or temporal resolution and to display both morphological information on renal parenchyma and vessels and functional data, such as perfusion, filtration, diffusion, or oxygenation. Molecular imaging techniques have recently been applied in the assessment of renal tumors and parenchymal perfusion. All these imaging modalities have now reached an extremely high level of accuracy in detecting renal abnormalities. This book also provides a complete insight in all these diagnostic fields with the aid of high-quality images obtained with state-of-the-art equipments, as well as by figures showing macroscopic and microscopic specimens to obtain an effective radiologic-pathologic correlation with diagnostic images.

Each chapter has been written by well-recognized experts in the field, and the principal effort of the editor was to provide excellent iconography and literature revision, besides text quality. This book is principally intended for the radiology community, from the resident to the expert radiologists, even though clinicians and academic persons could also find it useful for their daily clinical practice.

The imaging archive of the radiology department of Trieste, presenting a complete iconography of all renal pathologies collected through several years of intense clinical activity and research in this field, served as a gold mine for the preparation of the book.

My sincere gratitude to Professor Baert and to Miss Ursula Davis and Daniela Brandt from Springer for their continuous support and belief in this work. A note of thanks also to other staff of Springer for the editorial work.

Trieste                                                                 Emilio Quaia

# Contents

# Part I

# Embryology and Anatomy

# Embryology of the Kidney

Marina Zweyer

## Contents

M. Zweyer
Clinical Department of Biomedicine, University of Trieste,
via Manzoni 16, 34138 Trieste, Italy
e-mail: zweyer@units.it

## Abstract

> During the third week of pregnancy, the process of gastrulation results in the formation of trilaminar embryo in humans. This is the beginning of morphogenesis (development of body form). Three germ layers, ectoderm, mesoderm, and endoderm, are present. A specific part of mesoderm, the intermediate mesoderm, gives rise to urogenital system gradually. It starts to develop from nephrogenic cord, which divides in nephrotomes. They give rise to pronephroi and subsequently mesonephroi, the transitory kidneys. Finally, metanephroi appear as the permanent organs, from two different structures: the metanephrogenic blastema (mesenchimal component) that leads to nephrons, and ureteric bud (epithelial component) that gives rise to collecting tubules, calices, renal pelvis, and ureter. Following developmental steps depend on inductive signaling between metanephrogenic blastema and ureteric bud.

> Many genes, regulating proteins and pathways are involved in the physiological organogenesis. Cell proliferation and apoptosis keep the balance of the growth. Defects in these molecular and morphogenetic mechanisms may cause various congenital abnormalities of the kidney and urinary tract (CAKUT), which represent a family of diseases with a diverse anatomical spectrum.

## 1.1 Introduction

The morphological and functional complexity of the mammalian kidney arises from the highly coordinate series of events that lead to its development.

E. Quaia (ed.), *Radiological Imaging of the Kidney*,
Medical Radiology, DOI: 10.1007/978-3-540-87597-0_1, © Springer-Verlag Berlin Heidelberg 2011

The study of structural and molecular aspects of kidney formation has been carried out for a great part in humans. Nevertheless, the involvement of specific genes, proteins, and pathways in the patterning of kidney has been disclosed mainly by genetic ablation in experiments in mouse. The definition of early events that lead to kidney primordium has also been realized by investigating the processes in nonmammalian vertebrate species, like fish, frog, and chick embryos. These integrated studies have been possible for the conservation of many genes in the different vertebrates and for the common origin of their embryonic kidney.

For many decades, the researchers focused their attention on morphological aspects of the development. The first studies about cellular basis of embryogenesis have been carried out by Grobstein (1956). The inductive signals between the tissues and their effects on proliferation and differentiation were afterwards investigated by Saxén (1987), which have introduced the modern kidney embryology, using a mammalian in vitro organ culture system.

Recently, several authors excellently reviewed all the studies on the molecular basis of renal embryogenesis (Lehner and Dressler 1997; Davies and Bard 1998; Kuure et al. 2000; Dressler 2006; Rosenblum 2008).

Many investigations have, moreover, been focused on the congenital abnormalities of the kidney and urinary tract (CAKUT), and their origin from morphogenetic defects (Kuwajama et al. 2002; Miyazaki and Ichikawa 2003; Stahl et al. 2006; Schedl 2007).

Here we describe the basic structural events of kidney embryogenesis in the context of urinary system and provide a synthesis of the molecular basis of morphogenesis. Congenital anomalies of the kidney and urinary tract caused by an uncorrected development are finally presented.

## 1.2 Development of Urogenital System

During the third week of the development, the embryo is composed of three germ layers, ectoderm, mesoderm, and endoderm. Each of them gives rise to specific tissue and organs. Ectoderm is the source of the epidermis, the nervous system, and several other structures. Endoderm principally gives rise to epithelial component of the respiratory and digestive tracts, including associated glands. Mesoderm is the source of connective tissues, smooth and striated muscles, cardiovascular system and

blood, bone marrow, skeleton, and the reproductive and excretory systems. Mesoderm differentiates in three parts on each side of the embryo: beginning from the embryonic axis, the paraxial mesoderm, which gives rise to the somites, the intermediate mesoderm, and lateral mesoderm. In particular, the intermediate mesoderm plays a fundamental role in the development of urogenital apparatus.

The urogenital apparatus is functionally divided into the *urinary (excretory) system* and the *genital (reproductive) system*. During development, these two systems are tightly associated. Moreover, they are anatomically connected in adult males because both urine and semen pass through the urethra. In adult females, the urethra and vagina are separate, but open into a common cavity, the vestibule of the vagina (Moore 1992). The *suprarenal glands,* originated from lateral mesoderm and neural crests, are topographically associated to the superior poles of the kidneys, and its congenital hyperplasia causes anomalies both in female and male external genitalia. Intermediate mesoderm extends along the dorsal wall of the embryo.

During folding of the embryo in the horizontal plane, this mesoderm component is carried ventrally. A longitudinal elevation of the mesoderm called *urogenital ridge* forms on each side of the dorsal aorta. It gives rise to the urinary and genital systems. *Nephrogenic ridge* or *cord* (Fig. 1.1 a, b) is the urogenital ridge component, which gives rise to the urinary system. The part giving rise to the genital system is the *genital* or *gonadal ridge*. The urogenital ridge can be observed in Fig.1.2b. The urinary system begins to develop before the genital system.

## 1.3 Development of Urinary System

The urinary tract is composed of:

- The *kidneys*, the main filtrating organs in the mammalian organisms; the morphofunctional unit of the kidney is the nephron. It provides for blood filtration, reabsorption of water, salt, and other substances necessary for the organism. The nephrons modulate blood pressure and pH.
- The *ureters,* which convey urine from the kidneys to the bladder.
- The *urinary bladder*, which stores urine before elimination.
- The *urethra* which carries urine from the bladder to the exterior

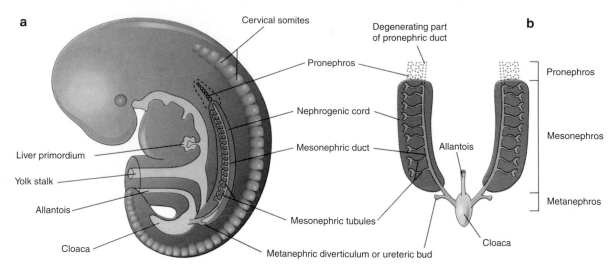

**Fig. 1.1** Diagrammatic sketches illustrating the three sets of excretory systems in an embryo during the fifth week. (**a**) Lateral view. (**b**) Ventral view. The mesonephric tubules have been pulled laterally; their normal position is shown in (**a**)

The intermediate mesoderm initially divides into metameric set of small cell masses called *nephrotomes* in the cervical and thoraco-lumbar regions. This division in segments does not occur in the lumbo-sacral region, which becomes a unique mesenchimal mass named *metanephric mass of intermediate mesoderm* or *metanephrogenic blastema.*

These structures represent three different excretory organs:

- The *pronephroi* (plural of pronephros), which are the first apparatuses that appear, are rudimentary and nonfunctional. They are analogous to the kidneys in primitive fishes.
- The *mesonephroi,* the second set of primitive kidneys, that are well developed and briefly function; they are analogous to the kidneys of amphibians.
- The *metanephroi,* the third set of kidneys which become the permanent kidneys.

## 1.3.1 Morphogenesis of Transient Kidney

### 1.3.1.1 Pronephroi

These structures appear in human embryos early in the fourth week from the seven most cephalic nephrotomes and are transitory and nonfunctional. They are represented by small cellular metameric masses, which give rise to many tortuous tubular structures in the cervical region (Fig. 1.1a). These pronephric ducts run caudally, connect one to the other in a longitudinal *pronephric*

*duct,* and open into the cloaca (Fig. 1.1a, b). The cloaca is the expanded terminal part of the hindgut. It ventrally receives allantois, a fingerlike diverticulum of the yolk sac. The rudimentary pronephroi soon degenerate in human development; in fact when the most caudal ducts appear, the cervical ducts have already been lost. The best observations on pronephros morphogenesis have been realized in animals, which utilize this organ like a definitive excretory organ, as the primitive fish lamprey.

### 1.3.1.2 Mesonephroi

During the second half of the fourth week, the mesonephroi develop from the nephrotomes from eighth cephalic somite to second lumbar somite, caudally to the rudimentary pronephroi (Fig. 1.1a, b). These large, elongated, excretory organs protrude into the celomic cavity. The mesonephroi are functional until the permanent kidneys develop (Fig. 1.1a, b). First of all, the nephrotomes undergo cavitation and become vesicles, then every vesicle gives rise to further vesicles.

Every vesicle grows laterally, bends caudally, and connects itself to the underlying vesicle. This process leads to the *mesonephric duct,* which was originally the pronephric duct. It also opens into the cloaca.

Mesonephric vesicles lengthen horizontally and change into small tortuous ducts. Medial ends of each duct expand and inflect itself to form a depression. This cavity is penetrated by a vascular ball produced by an arterial vessel coming from aorta. The structure just described is quite similar to the glomerulus typical of definitive kidney.

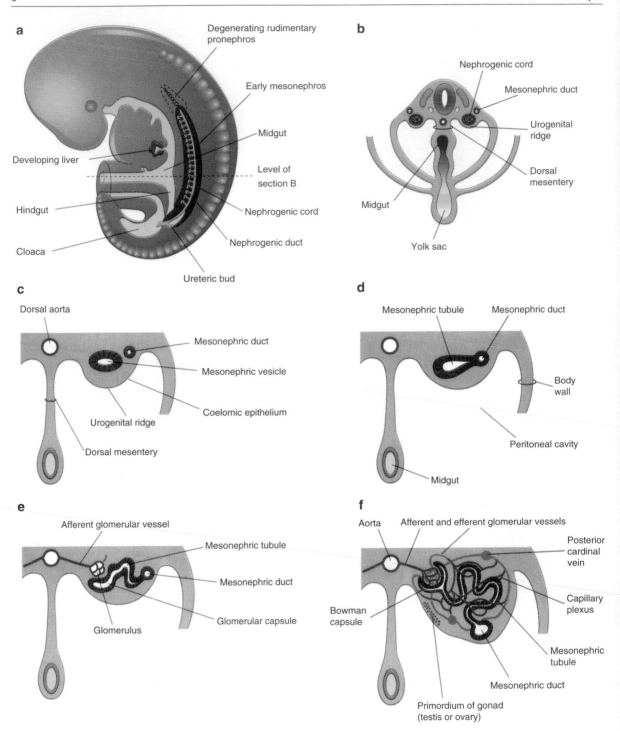

**Fig. 1.2** (**a**) Sketch of a lateral view of a 5-week embryo showing the extent of the mesonephros and the primordium of the metanephros or permanent kidney. (**b**) Transverse section of the embryo showing the nephrogenic cords from which the mesonephric tubules develop. Observe the position of the urogenital ridges and nephrogenic cords. (**c–f**) Sketches of transverse sections showing successive stages in the development of a mesonephric tubule between the fifth and eleventh weeks. Note that the mesenchymal cell cluster in the nephrogenic cord develops a lumen, thereby forming a mesonephric vesicle. The vesicle soon becomes an S-shaped mesonephric tubule and extends laterally to join the pronephric duct, now renamed the mesonephric duct. The expanded medial end of the mesonephric tubule is invaginated by blood vessels to form a glomerular capsule (Bowman capsule). The cluster of capillaries projecting into this capsule is the glomerulus

While mesonephric duct and glomeruli form, mesonephrus largely protrude into coeloma. In this step, it represents the so called *Walff body*. The *ureteric bud* derives from Walff body.

The two mesonephroi occupy almost completely the celomatic cavity in the seventh week of development.

The mesonephric kidneys consist of glomeruli and mesonephric tubules (Fig. 1.2). The mesonephroi disappear toward the ninth week; nevertheless, their tubules give rise to the efferent ductules of the testes and the epididymal duct and other derivatives in adult male. In the female the organs involve changing into a rudimentary structure called *Rosenmuller organ* or *epoophoron*.

### 1.3.2  Morphogenesis of Metanephros or Permanent Kidney

The third excretory system appears in the fifth week and becomes permanent. It begins to work during the 9–10th week (Behrman et al. 1996). Urine flows into the amniotic fluid and mixes with it. Amniotic fluid containing urine is swallowed by fetus and is absorbed by the intestine. During fetal life kidneys are not responsible for excretion. Catabolism derivatives are transferred into the maternal blood by placenta for elimination.

The metanephroi or permanent kidneys originate from:

1. The *metanephric mass of intermediate mesoderm, or metanephrogenic blastema*, which develops from intermediate mesoderm; their cells, derived from the caudal part of the nephrogenic cord, give rise to the *nephrons*, the morphofunctional units of the kidney.
2. The *metanephric diverticulum* or *ureteric bud*, derived from mesonephric duct, which gives rise to collecting tubules, calices, renal pelvis, and ureter (Fig. 1.3).

The ureteric bud appears as an outgrowth of the mesonephric duct close to the cloaca. It elongates and

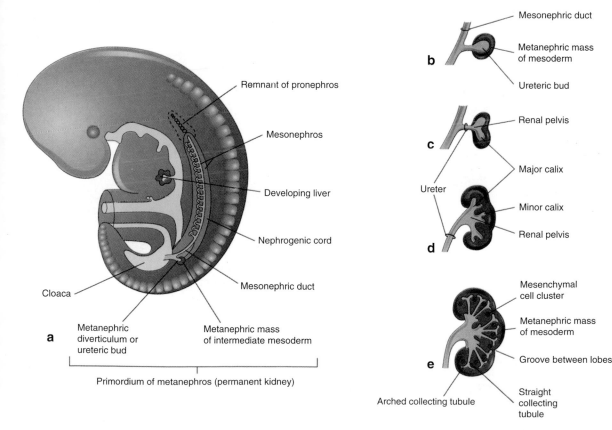

**Fig. 1.3** Development of the metanephros or permanent kidney. (**a**) Sketch of a lateral view of a 5-weeks embryo, showing the primordium of the metanephros. (**b**–**e**) Sketches showing successive stages in the development of the metanephric diverticulum or ureteric bud (5th–8th weeks). Observe the development of the ureter, renal pelvis, calices, and collecting tubules

penetrates the metanephrogenic blastema, inducing the evolution of the metanephric mass of mesoderm over its expanded end (Fig. 1.3a, b). The ureteric bud forms a peduncle, which gives rise to the *ureter*. Its expanded cranial end becomes the *renal pelvis*.

Straight collecting tubules appear, repeatedly branch, and then partially coalesce to form *minor* and *major calices*.

The remaining *collecting tubules* become arched. They induce the proliferation of clusters of mesenchymal cells in the metanephrogenic blastema to form small *metanephric vesicles* (Fig. 1.4a), which elongate and change into the *metanephric tubules* (Fig. 1.4b, c). The terminal end of every tubule initially takes the shape of comma (comma-shaped body), then develops in an S-shaped body and expands. A depression appears in this S terminal expanded end: this is the Bowman

capsule bud of the renal corpuscle. A group of mesenchimal cells accumulate in this cavity.

During this period, the surrounding tissue is rich in blood capillaries, but no vessel is present in this mesenchimal area and no basal lamina divides tubule cells from mesenchima.

Podocyte precursor cells secrete VEGF that attract endothelial cells (Eremina et al. 2003). These endothelial cells give rise to mesangial cell in response to induction by PDGF (platelet-derived growth factor) (Lindal et al. 1998). The endothelial cells and differentiating podocytes interact to lay down the glomerular basement membrane (GBM). The glomerulus basal lamina continues with the developing basal lamina of Bowman capsule parietal layer and remaining nephron tract. The basal lamina becomes very thicker close to podocytes than to the other parts of the nephron.

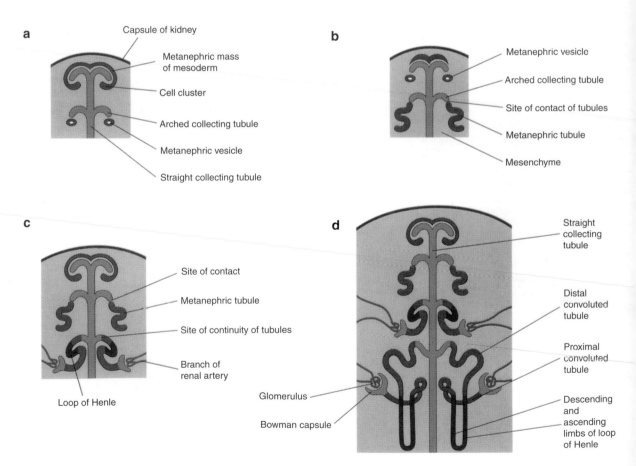

**Fig. 1.4** Diagrammatic sketches illustrating stages in nephrogenesis – the development of nephrons. (**a**) Nephrogenesis commences around the beginning of the eighth week. (**b**, **c**) Note that the metanephric tubules, the primordia of the nephrons, become continuous with the collecting tubules to form uriniferous tubules. (**d**) The number of the nephrons is more than double from 20 to 38 weeks. Observe that nephrons are derived from the metanephric mass of mesoderm and that the collecting tubules are derived from the metanephric diverticulum

Mesenchima actively proliferates and small spaces open among the cells. Erythrocytes appear in these cavities.

It is unknown if erythrocytes derive from the changing of local mesenchimal cells or of those arriving by migration from surrounding vessels.

Some of mesenchimal cells flatten and become endothelial elements of glomerular blood capillaries. Other theories maintain that the vascular glomerulus is produced by a branch of renal artery that penetrate into the Bowman cavity.

Other mesenchimal cells change into mesangial cells and at the same time, cells which will become podocytes swell and give out several elongations. Many roundish holes appear in endothelial cells and intercellular matrix accumulates around mesangial elements. Some smooth muscular fibers of arteriole afferent to glomerulus change into iuxta-glomerular cells. At the beginning of second month, groups of glomeruli develop in successive stages. They conclude their final maturation in about 1 month. The last generation of urinary tubules and glomeruli takes place in the external part of metanephroi during eighth/ninth month of fetal life.

The tubules evolve in a proximal convoluted part, a loop called *loop of Henle,* and a distal convoluted part. The *renal corpuscle* (Bowman capsule and glomerulus) and its *proximal convoluted tubule*, loop of Henle, and *distal convoluted tubule* represent a *nephron* (Fig. 1.4d), the morphofunctional unit of the kidney.

Finally, every distal convoluted tubule gets closed to an arched collecting tubule and coalesces with it.

The number of glomeruli increases slowly from the 10th to the 18th week, then abruptly from the 18th to the 32nd week, reaching an upper limit with nephrogenic blastema disappearance by the 32nd week (Gasser et al. 1993).

The *collecting tubule* and the *nephron* form the *uriniferous tubule*. It is derived from two embryologically different parts (Fig. 1.3), the first one from the metanephric diverticulum and the second one from the metanephric mass of mesoderm.

## 1.4 Migration of the Kidneys

At the beginning, the metanephric kidneys lie close to each other in the pelvis, at the dorsal-medial side of the mesonephros caudal end, ventrally to the sacrum (Fig. 1.5a). Afterwards, the kidneys progressively come to the abdominal posterior wall and move farther apart, while the abdomen and pelvis grow (Fig. 1.5b,c). At the end of the second month, the kidneys set themselves at the first four lumbar vertebras level, under suprarenal glands (Fig. 1.5d). This migration occurs mainly by the growth of the embryo's body caudal to the kidneys. Actually the caudal part of the body grows away from the kidneys, so that they gradually occupy a more cranial position. They may become retroperitoneal (external or

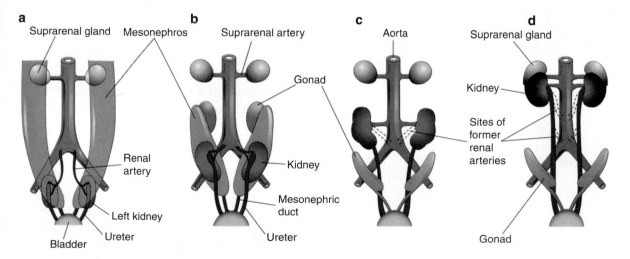

**Fig. 1.5** (**a–d**) Diagrammatic ventral views of the abdominopelvic region of embryos and fetuses (6th–9th weeks) showing medial rotation and "ascent" of the kidneys from the pelvis to the abdomen. (**a**) and (**b**) Observe also the size regression of the mesonephroi. (**c**) and (**d**) Note that as the kidneys "ascend," they are supplied by arteries at successively higher levels and that the hylum of the kidney (where the vessels and nerves enter) is eventually directed anteromedially

posterior to the peritoneum) on the posterior abdominal wall. The hylum of the kidney, which is crossed by vessels and nerves, faces ventrally before migration; it rotates medially almost 90° during the kidney rise. In the ninth week, the hylum is directed anteromedially (Fig. 1.5c, d).

## 1.5 Lobes of Kidney Surface

During fetal life human kidney surface is subdivided into polygonal lobes. This lobulation decreases at the end of pregnancy, but the lobes are still present in the kidneys of a newborn infant as involving structures. Lobulation disappears during infancy. It derives from the mechanism of kidney development.

The buds of minor calices penetrate into the metanephric blastema and give rise to 13 generations of branches and 13 trees of excretory ductules. Thousands of urinary tubules open into the excretory ductules. So every minor calyx gives rise to a big gland unit. This unit exhibits a medullar component named Malpighi pyramid and a cortical component which is separated from the others by interlobular sulci. This is the reason of lobulation. During pyramids development, metanephric tissue surrounds the collecting tubules system. Metanephric tissue penetrates between the pyramids going toward the kidney pelvis and giving rise to the Bertin columns.

At the pregnancy end, 800,000–1,000,000 nephrons are present in every kidney. The elongation of the proximal convoluted tubules, as well as an increase of interstitial tissue, causes the growth in kidney size after birth. The nephron development is complete at birth (Behrman et al. 1996), except in premature infants. After birth, the kidneys have further functional maturation. During ninth fetal week, glomerular filtration begins to work and the filtration activity increases after birth (Arant 1987; Behrman et al. 1996).

## 1.6 Vascular Variations

Initially, the common iliac arteries send branches to the kidneys (Fig. 1.5a, b), so the kidneys receive their blood supply from the distal end of the aorta. During migration at a higher level, they receive new branches from the aorta (Fig. 1.5c, d) and the iliac arteries undergo involution and disappear. Kidney migration stops in the ninth week, when kidneys take tight contact with the *suprarenal glands*. Finally, the kidneys receive the permanent renal arteries coming from the abdominal aorta.

## 1.7 Supernumerary Renal Arteries

We can find in adults some common variations in the blood supply to the kidneys. They depend on the changes of the urinary apparatus during development (Fig. 1.5). About 70% of people exhibit single renal artery to each kidney. On the other end, two to four renal arteries are present in 25% of adults (Moore 1992). The artery variations are about twice as common as vein variations.

Usually the supernumerary arteries come out from the abdominal aorta superior or inferior to the main renal artery and follow it through the hylum (Fig. 1.6a, c, d). They may enter the kidneys into the superior and/or the inferior poles. If a supernumerary artery enters the inferior pole, it may cross anterior the ureter and occlude it, leading to hydronephrosis. In this pathology, pelvis and calices swell by urine (Fig. 1.6b). The accessory arteries of inferior pole in right kidney usually cross anterior to the inferior vena cava and ureter. The supernumerary arteries may either be end arteries or not. If an accessory artery is damaged or ligated, the area of the kidney vascularized by it may undergo to ischemia.

## 1.8 Molecular Aspects of Kidney Development

### 1.8.1 Inductive Processes and Proliferation

Genetic ablation in experiments in rodents demonstrates the involvement of specific genes in the morphogenesis of related structures.
Early patterning of kidney deriving from intermediate mesoderm depends especially on Lim1, Pax2/8, ODD1, and other genes and their complex relationship (Dressler 2006).

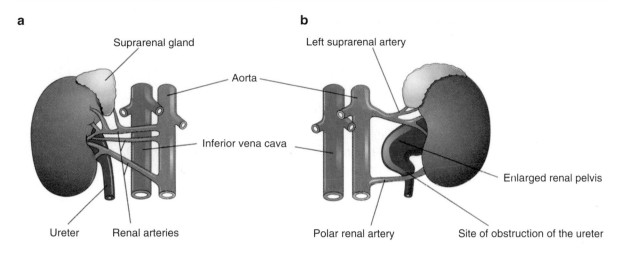

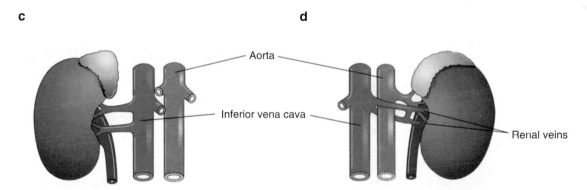

**Fig. 1.6** Drawings illustrating common variations of renal vessels. (**a**) and (**b**) Multiple renal arteries. Note the accessory vessels entering the poles of the kidney. The polar renal artery, illustrated in (**b**), has obstructed the ureter and produced an enlarged renal pelvis. (**c**) and (**d**) Multiple renal veins are less common than supernumerary arteries

Subsequent steps of renal development originate by the fundamental interactions between metanephric blastema (mesenchimal component) and ureteric bud (epithelial component).

At the beginning, GDNF (glial derived neurotrophic factor), released by metanephric blastema, is involved in the appearance of ureteric bud. It induces Wolff duct epithelial cells, presenting RETGIFRα1 (GDNF-family receptor α1), to proliferate. These cells give rise to the collecting ducts and their further branching. Metanephric blastema mesenchimal cells start to synthesize and secrete GDNF after expression activation of WT1 gene (Wilms tumor 1).

The GDNF expression must be precisely modulated. Transcription factors and extracellular signals participate in GDNF expression regulation. Extracellular signals are represented by WNT11 growth factor, which is produced and secreted by ureteric bud epithelial cells. This growth factor induces mesenchimal cells to release GDNF with positive continuous feedback mechanism (Maiumdar et al. 2003).

Also adhesion molecules, as α8β1 integrin of metanephric mesenchima, and its receptor nephronectin (expressed in ureteric bud and extracellular matrix) are involved in the induction of kidney development (Brandenberger et al. 2001).

Collecting system induces tubules and nephrons differentiation. At the beginning, ureteric bud secretes proteins of BMP family (bone morphogenetic protein) and FGF2 (fibroblast growth factor2), which inhibit apoptosis in mesenchimal cells, induce their condensation, and keep WT1 synthesis. In the further step, some factors secreted by collecting ducts epithelial cells induce WNT4 expression in adjacent mesenchimal cells. WNT4 exhibits an autocrine function, which induces mesenchimal cells to differentiate in epithelial cells. This is the unique conversion of mesenchyme to polarized epithelia (mesenchimal–to–epithelial transition), (Davies and Fisher 2002; Vainio 2003; Kispert et al. 1998).

Tubulogenesis starts to evolve from kidney vesicle and its elongated shape vs. S tubule, which give rise to the different nephron segments (Bowman capsule, proximal and distal convolute tubules, Henle loop).

Many other genes are responsible for nephrons development and different kidney components.

### 1.8.2 Apoptosis

Programmed cell death and mitosis keep the balance of the tissue growth during development. Apoptotic process has been well reviewed by many authors (Elmore 2007; Robertson et al. 2000).

Apoptosis actually plays a fundamental role in kidney embryogenesis, if 50% of the cells are fated to die (Camp and Martin 1996). Cells undergo the process even after inductive activity has taken place.

A first wave of programmed cell death occurs during early nephron formation (Koseki et al. 1992).

A second wave takes place in the S-shaped body step and the third wave occurs in the medullary epithelia, including the ureteric bud (Coles et al. 1993).

In p-53 overexpressing mice, excessive apoptosis takes place and small kidneys develop. In transgenic mice lacking bcl-2, a too early apoptosis appears. It is followed by hyperproliferation which causes epithelial cysts (Veis et al. 1993). Many other evidences confirm the importance of a correct ratio between proliferation and cell death in normal organogenesis.

### 1.9 Congenital Abnormalities of the Kidney and Urinary Tract

Figure 1.7 shows the various principal anomalies of the urinary system and illustrates the probable embryological basis of the anomaly. Congenital anomalies of the kidney are described in Chaps. 2 (anatomical

variants), 11 (renal malformations), and 12 (cystic congenital diseases).

### 1.9.1 Renal Agenesis (Fig. 1.7a)

An important cause might be a defect of metanephric blastema in inducing ureteric bud development by GDNF, or an anomaly of its RET receptor. The pathology does not originate by GDNF or RET mutation, but by defects of signaling (Schedl 2007). Otherwise, it is known that multicystic kidneys may undergo complete involution during pregnancy, leading to renal agenesis with a blind ending ureter on the same side (Mesrobian et al. 1993).

### 1.9.2 Hypoplastic Kidney

In this pathology an anomaly of renal mass seems to derive from an inadequate branching of ureteric bud/collecting ducts. In fact, nephrons number is tightly associated to the ureteric bud branches number. Environmental factors like hyponutrition may cause hypoplasia, but also genetic factors are involved, as a common allele of PAX2 (Quinlan et al. 2007).

### 1.9.3 Ectopic Kidney (Fig. 1.7b–e)

Sometimes the position of one or both kidneys may be abnormal. Often, they are more inferior than usual and the rotation has not been completed, so the hylum is in anterior position. Most frequently, ectopic kidneys are pelvic. When kidneys do not ascend, they stay positioned in the pelvic zone. Other ectopic/pelvic kidneys are close to each other and fuse to originate a discoid or *pancake kidney* (Fig. 1.7e). These kidneys receive the blood from internal or external iliac arteries and/or aorta. The *crossed renal ectopia* appears if a kidney crosses to the other side with or without fusion. Infrequently, *unilateral fused kidney* (Fig. 1.7d) develops. The kidneys fuse while they are in the pelvis, and when a kidney ascends to its final position, it brings the other one with it.

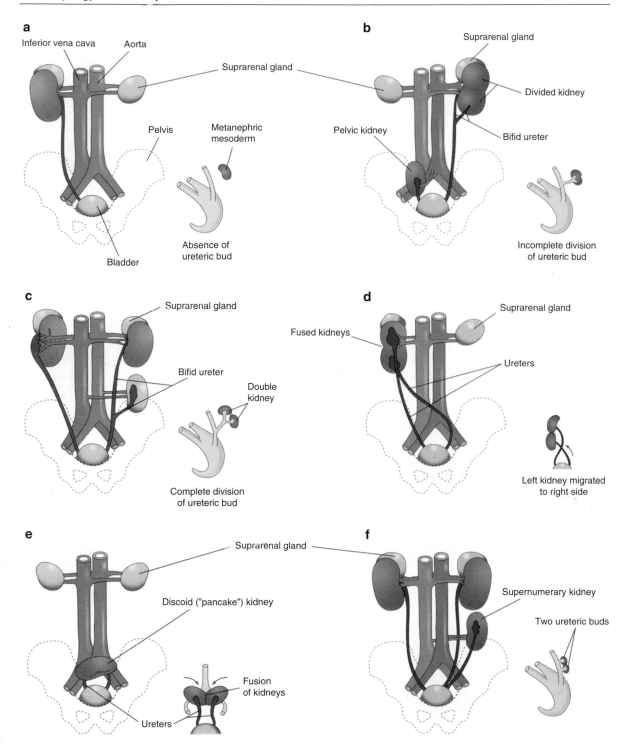

**Fig. 1.7** Drawings illustrating various anomalies of the urinary system. The small sketch to the lower right of each drawing illustrates the probable embryological basis of the anomaly. (**a**) Unilateral renal agenesis. (**b**) Right side, pelvic kidney; left side, divided kidney with a bifid ureter. (**c**) Right side, malrotation of the kidney; left side, bifid ureter and supernumerary kidney. (**d**) Crossed renal ectopia. The left kidney crossed to the right side and fused with the right kidney. (**e**) Discoid (named also pancake kidney) resulting from fusion of the kidneys while they were in the pelvis. (**f**) Supernumerary left kidney resulting from the development of two ureteric buds

### 1.9.4 Fused/Horseshoe Kidney

This renal abnormality is common in humans It is represented by fusion of kidney poles, usually inferior poles, and appears in about 1:500/1,000 patients. The fusion is carried out by a hystmus of renal or fibrous tissue. The cause might be defects in FOXD1 gene, responsible for correct renal capsule development (Levinson et al. 2005). Anomalies in capsule embryogenesis might lead to kidney fusion.

### 1.9.5 Ectopic Ureter

This abnormality may be present in several variations in male patients. Ectopic ureters may open into the bladder neck or into the prostatic component of the urethra (Moore 1992), into the ductus deferens, seminal vesicle, or prostatic utricle (Behrman et al. 1996). Also, in female patients ectopic ureters may appear. In females, they end in the bladder neck, urethra, vagina, or vestibule of the vagina. These anomalies prevent urine enter the bladder, so patients usually complain of incontinence. Urine constantly flows from the urethra in males and from the urethra and/or vagina in females. When the ureter is not fused with the posterior part of the urinary bladder, ureteric ectopia develops. The ureter is instead carried caudally and fuses with the caudal portion of the vesical part of the urogenital sinus.

### 1.9.6 Duplications of the Urinary Tract

Supernumerary kidney is rare (Fig. 1.7f). Duplications of the abdominal part of the ureter and the renal pelvis are on the contrary common. These abnormalities are caused by division of the metanephric diverticulum (ureteric bud). The extent of the duplication depends on how complete the diverticulum division is. If the ureteric primordium divides incompletely, a divided kidney with a bifid ureter forms. If the division is complete, a double kidney with a bifid ureter or separate ureters appears. When a supernumerary kidney with its own ureter is present, it probably develops from the appearance of two ureteric diverticula.

### 1.9.7 Wilms Tumor

Wilms tumor is the most common neoplasia in the human newborn (1:10,000) (Rivera and Haber 2005), but may also appear during fetal life. Wilms tumor exhibits a tight association with some congenital malformations, particularly with anirydia, hemipertrophia, genital male malformations like criptorchidysm, hypospadia, and pseudoermaphroditism. Less frequently, tumor is associated with nephroblastoma, trisomia 18, neurofibromatosis, and Beckwith-Wiedemann syndrome. This anomaly is characterized by nephrogenic embryonic remnants, derived from the failure of differentiation of metanephric blastema cells into nephrons. In 20% of patients WT1 gene on 11p13 chromosome (Wilms tumor 1) is mutated. Normally this is a multifunctional gene, because it controls several differentiative processes during kidney development. Mice with WT1 mutations may exhibit different anomalies, like the absence of kidneys and the kidney dysplasia. More recently mutations of WTX gene have also been observed in this pathology. WTX is a gene that codifies for a protein involved in signaling of factors inducing kidney tubules formation.

## 1.10 Conclusions

The study of kidney development is very important for deeper understanding of the genes and molecular pathways required, especially for the clinical aspects of organogenesis. Novel approaches may in fact be introduced in research to combat disease, as the use of stem cells in renal replacement therapy and the growth of artificial organs in vitro.

## Sitography

The GenitoUrinary Development Molecular Anatomy Project (GUDMAP) is a consortium of laboratories working to provide the scientific and medical community with tools to facilitate research. http://www.gudmap.org

European Renal Genome Project (EuRegene) is an integrated project funded by European Community, Framework Programme 6. http://www.euregene.org

## Permission

The illustrations have been copied from the text: "The Developing Human: Clinically Oriented Embryology," Moore et al. 1998, Saunders-Elsevier. The permission has been obtained from Elsevier, Permissions Department, Cambridge University Press.

## References

Arant BS Jr (1987) Postnatal development of renal function during the first year of life. Pediatr Nephrol 1:308–313

Behrman RE, Kliegman RM, Arvin AM (1996) Nelson textbook of pediatrics, 15th edn. WB Saunders, Philadelphia

Brandenberger R, Schmidt A, Linton J et al. (2001) Identification and characterization of a novel extracellular matrix protein nephronectin that is associated with integrin alpha8beta1 in embryonic kidney. J Cell Biol 154(2):447–458

Camp V, Martin P (1996) Programmed cell death and its clearance in the developing kidney. Exp Nephr 4:105–111

Coles HSR, Burne JF, Raff MC (1993) Large scale normal cell death in the developing rat kidney and its reduction by epidermal growth factor. Development (Cambridge, UK) 118:777–784

Davies JA, Bard JBL (1998) The development of the kidney. Curr Topics Devel Biol 39:245–301

Davies JA, Fisher CE (2002) Genes and proteins in renal development. Exp Nephrol 10:102–113

Dressler GR (2006) The cellular basis of kidney development. Annu Rev Cell Dev Biol 22:509–529

Elmore S (2007) Apoptosis: a review of programmed cell death. Toxicol Pathol 35(4):495–516

Eremina V, Sood M, Haigh J et al. (2003) Glomerular-specific alterations of VEGF-A expression lead to distinct congenital and acquired renal diseases. J Clin Invest 111:707–716

Gasser B, Mauss Y, Ghnassia JP et al. (1993) A quantitative study of normal nephrogenesis in the human fetus: its implication in the natural history of kidney changes due to low obstructive uropathies. Fetal Diagn Ther 8:371–384

Grobstein C (1956) Trans-filter induction of tubules in mouse metanephric mesenchyme. Exp Cell Res 10:424–440

Kispert A, Vainio S, McMahon AP (1998) Wnt-4 is a mesenchymal signal for epithelial transformation of metanephric mesenchyme in the developing kidney. Development 125:4225–4234

Koseki C, Herzlinger D, al-Awqati Q (1992) Apoptosis in metanephric development. J Cell Biol 119:1327–1333

Kuure S, Vuolteenaho R, Vainio S (2000) Kidney morphogenesis: cellular and molecular regulation. Mech Dev 92(1):31–45

Kuwajama F, Miyzaki Y, Ichikawa I (2002) Embriogenesis of the congenital anomalies of the kidney and urinary tract. Nephrol Dial Transplant 17 (suppl 9):45–47

Lehner MS, Dressler GR (1997) The molecular basis of embrionic kidney development. Mech Dev 62:105–120

Levinson RS, Batuorina E, Choi C et al. (2005) FOXD1-dependent signals control cellularity in the renal capsule, a structure required for normal renal development. Development 132:529–539

Lindal P, Hellstrom M, Kalen M et al. (1998) Paracrine PDGF-B/PDGF-Rβ signalling controls mesangial cell development in kidney development. Development 125:3313–3322

Maiumdar A, Vainio S, Kispert A et al. (2003) Wnt11 and Ret/Gdnf pathways cooperate in regulating ureteric branching during metanephric kidney development. Development 130(14):3175–3185

Mesrobian HG, Rushton HG, Bulas D (1993) Unilateral renal agenesis may result from in utero regression of multicystic renal dysplasia. J Urol 150:793–794

Miyazaki Y, Ichikawa I (2003) Ontogeny of congenital anomalies of the kidney and urinary tract, CAKUT. Pediatr Int 45(5):598–604

Moore KL (1992) Clinically oriented anatomy, 3rd edn. Williams & Wilkins, Baltimore

Quinlan J, Lemire M, Hudson T et al. (2007) A common variant of PAX2 gene is associated with reduced newborn kidney size. J Am Soc Nephrol 18:1915–1921

Rivera MN, Haber DA (2005) Wilms' tumor: connecting tumorigenesis and organ development in the kidney. Nature Rev Cancer 5:699–712

Robertson JD, Orrenius S, Zhivotovsky B (2000) Review: nuclear events in apoptosis. J Struct Biol 129(2–3):346–358

Rosenblum ND (2008) Developmental biology of the human kidney. Semin Fetal Neonatal Med 13:125–132

Saxén L., Sariola H (1987) Early organogenesis of the kidney. Pediatr Nephrol. Jul;1(3):385–392.

Schedl A (2007) Renal abnormalities and their developmental origin. Nat Rev Genet. Oct;8(10):791–802

Stahl DA, Koul HK, Chacko JK, Mingin GC (2006) Congenital anomalies of the kidney and urinary tract (CAKUT): a curren rewiev cell signalling processes in ureteral development. J Ped Urol 2:2–9

Vainio SJ (2003) Nephrogenesis regulated by Wnt signaling. J Nephrol 16(2)279–285. Review

Veis DJ, Sorenson CM, Shutter JR et al (1993) Bcl-2 deficient mice demonstrate fulminant lymphoid apoptosis and abnormal kidney development in Bcl-2 deficient mice. Am J Physiol 268: F73–F81

# Normal Radiological Anatomy and Anatomical Variants of the Kidney

**2**

Emilio Quaia, Paola Martingano, Marco Cavallaro, and Roberta Zappetti

## Contents

E. Quaia (✉), P. Martingano, M. Cavallaro, and R. Zappetti
Department of Radiology, Cattinara Hospital, University
of Trieste, Strada di Fiume 447, 34149 Trieste, Italy
e-mail: quaia@univ.trieste.it

## Abstract

> The kidneys are very vascularized organs. Each kidney receives the highest blood flow per gram of organ weight in the body (1.2 L/min corresponding to 20% of the cardiac output, and a perfusion value of 400 mL/min/100 g). The most employed indicator of the renal function is the glomerular filtration rate (GFR), which can be estimated according to different formulas. The calculation of the GFR is essential for a correct employment of iodinated and gadolinium-based contrast agents. The most widely used equations for estimating GFR are the Cockcroft–Gault and the Modification of Diet in Renal Disease Study Group (MDRD) formulas.

> The modern radiological imaging techniques allow a detailed depiction of the renal anatomy and of the anatomical variants. Ultrasound, computed tomography, and magnetic resonance imaging define accurately the anatomy and anatomical variants of the renal parenchyma, arteries, and intrarenal urinary tract.

## 2.1 Anatomy and Physiology of the Kidney

### 2.1.1 Normal Renal Anatomy

#### 2.1.1.1 Macroscopic Renal Anatomy

The kidneys are retroperitoneal organs that are located in the perirenal retroperitoneal space with a longitudinal diameter of 10–12 cm and a latero-lateral diameter of 3–5 cm and a weight of 250–270 g. The kidney initially develops opposite to the future S2 vertebra, but eventually comes to rest opposite the L1 or L2 vertebra (Federle 2006). In the supine position, the medial border of the normal kidney is much more anterior than the lateral border, so that the kidneys lie at an angle of about 30° from the horizontal (Nino-Murcia et al. 2000). The upper pole of each kidney is situated more posteriorly than the lower pole.

The right kidney, anteriorly, has a relation with the inferior surface of the liver with peritoneal interposition, and with the second portion of the duodenum without any peritoneal interposition since the second portion of the duodenum is retroperitoneal (Fig. 2.1a). The left kidney, anteriorly, has a relation with the pancreatic tail, the spleen, the stomach, the ligament of Treitz and small bowel, and with the left colic flexure and left colon (Fig. 2.1a). Over the left kidney, there are two important peritoneal reflections, one vertical corresponding to the spleno-renal ligament (connected to the gastro-diaphragmatic and gastrosplenic ligaments) and one horizontal corresponding to the transverse mesocolon. Posteriorly, both kidneys present a relationship with the diaphragm, with the lateral margin of the psoas muscle, with the aponevrosis of the transverse abdominis muscle, and with the lumbar muscle (Fig. 2.1b). Superiorly, both kidneys have a relation with the adrenal glands, while the right kidney is separated from the inferior surface of the liver by the interposition of a double peritoneal sheet which derives from the reflection of the peritoneum

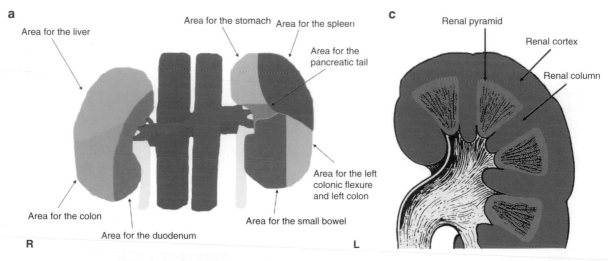

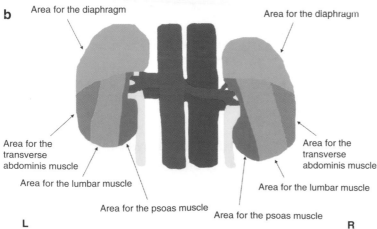

**Fig. 2.1** (**a**) Scheme of the anterior anatomical relations of the kidneys: *R* right; *L* left. (**b**) Scheme of the posterior anatomical relations of the kidneys: *R* right; *L* left. (**c**) Scheme of the main components of the renal parenchyma (renal cortex, renal columns, and renal medulla divided in multiple renal pyramids) overlied by the renal capsule (*black color*)

to the inferior limit of the coronary liver ligament that delimitates the hepatorenal space or Morrison pouch.

The renal parenchyma is composed of different components (Fig. 2.1c). The *renal capsule* is a tough fibrous layer surrounding the kidney (fibrous renal capsule) and covered by a thick layer of perinephric adipose tissue (fat renal capsule). The kidney is covered by the renal capsule formed by the fibrous and adipose renal capsule. The fibrous capsule represents the connective tissue investment of the kidney, continuous through the hilum to line the renal sinus. The adipose renal capsule represents the investment of fat surrounding the fibrous capsule of the kidney, continuous at the hilum with the fat in the renal sinus. The *renal cortex* is the outer portion of the kidney between the fibrous renal capsule and the renal medulla. In the adult, it forms a continuous smooth outer zone with a number of projections (cortical columns) that extend down between the pyramids. The renal cortex is the part of the kidney where ultrafiltration occurs. It contains the renal corpuscles and the renal tubules except for parts of the loop of Henle, which descend into the renal medulla. It also contains blood vessels and cortical collecting ducts. The renal column (or Bertin column, or column of Bertin) is a medullary extension of the renal cortex in between the renal pyramids, and it allows the cortex to be better anchored. Each column consists of lines of blood vessels and urinary tubes and a fibrous material.

The *renal medulla* is the innermost part of the kidney. The renal medulla is split up into a number of sections, known as the *renal pyramids* (Fig. 2.1c) about 8–18 in number. The broad *base* of each pyramid faces the renal cortex (outer medulla), and its apex, or papilla (inner medulla), points internally. The pyramids appear striped because they are formed by straight parallel segments of nephrons. Renal pyramids (or malpighian pyramids) are cone-shaped tissues of the kidney, and the *renal papilla* is the location where the medullary pyramids empty urine into the renal pelvis. Histologically, it is marked by medullary collecting ducts converging to channel the fluid.

Segmentation and duplications of the renal pelvis and/or ureters are secondary to segmentation of the wolffian duct, which forms the collecting system. The renal pelvis is generally triangular, and it tapers smoothly to its junction with the ureter defined as ureteropelvic junction. The pelvis exits from the kidney anteromedially. The right renal pelvis is usually located opposite to the L2 vertebra, and the left renal pelvis is

usually 0.5–1 cm higher (Friedenberg and Dunbar 1990). The *renal calyx* is a concave structure receiving the tip of the papilla of the renal medulla, and the fornices represent the side projections of the calyx surrounding the papilla. Two wide cup-shaped major renal calices are subdivided into 7–14 minor calices. Each single calyx or multiple minor calyces drain by means of an infundibulum into the renal pelvis. The renal sinus is the compartment that surrounds the pelvocalyceal system of the kidney, is filled by peripelvic fat, and communicates medially with the perinephric space. It contains the vascular and nervous structures that enter within the renal sinus, the lymphatics, the renal pelvis, and the surrounding fat. Cysts and sinus lipomatosis are the most common abnormalities in this space. The ureter also presents a restriction where it crosses the iliac vessels and enters the anatomical pelvis at the ureterovesical junction.

In each kidney, the *main renal artery* divides into the posterior and anterior branches that run posteriorly and anteriorly to the renal pelvis (Fig. 2.2). The anterior, superior, and inferior portions of the kidney are vascularized by the larger anterior branch. The posterior portion of the kidney are vascularized by the smaller posterior branch. The junction of the anterior and posterior branches of the main renal artery in the renal parenchyma creates a relatively avascular plane (Brodel's line), which is the preferred track of placing percutaneous nephrostomies and should be considered when performing biopsies of a native or transplanted kidney. The main renal artery divides into five segmental arteries near the renal hilum. The first division is typically the posterior branch, which arises just prior to the renal hilum and passes posterior to the renal pelvis to supply a large portion of blood flow to the posterior portion of the kidney.

The main renal artery then continues before dividing into four anterior branches at the renal hilum: the apical, superior, middle, posterior, and inferior segmental arteries (Fig. 2.2a), which subdivide into interlobar arteries (Fig. 2.2b). The apical and inferior arteries supply the anterior and posterior surfaces of the upper and lower poles, respectively; the upper and middle arteries supply the remainder of the anterior surface. Each interlobar artery penetrates the kidney through a column of Bertin and divides at the corticomedullary junction into arcuate arteries, which eventually run parallel to the surface (Fig. 2.2b). The arcuate arteries, in turn, supply interlobular arteries that penetrate the

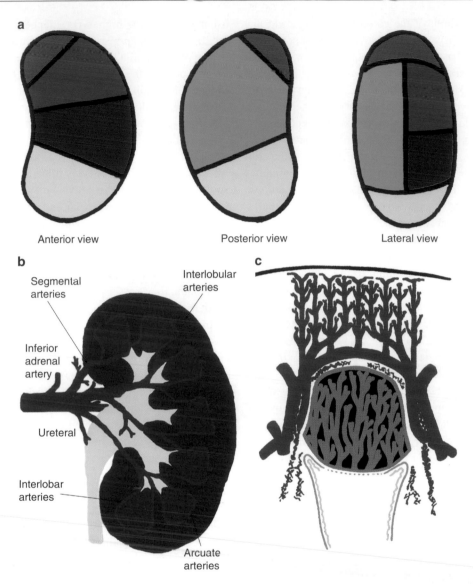

**Fig. 2.2** (**a–c**) Normal intrarenal arterial vessels. (**a**) Vascular areas of the renal parenchyma vascularized by the different segmental arteries and represented according to the anterior, posterior, and lateral views. The vascular areas are described as apical (*red*), superior (*blue*), posterior (*green*), middle (*violet*), and inferior (*yellow*). (**b**) Segmental, lobar, interlobular, and arcuate arteries represent the different intrarenal branches of the renal arteries. (**c**) The renal medulla presents a relationship with the lobar and arcuate arteries, while the interlobular arteries reach the renal cortical surface

cortex perpendicularly to the renal surface (Fig. 2.2c). Branching from each interlobular artery are numerous small arterioles, the afferent arteries. The fibers of the nervous renal plexus, including sympathetic nervous fibers triggering vasoconstriction, course along the renal artery to reach each kidney. The renal branches of the vagus nerve are small branches providing parasympathetic innervation to the kidney. Sensory input from the kidney travels to T10-11 levels of the spinal cord.

The renal lymphatics have not been fully documented in humans (Ischikawa et al. 2006). The distribution of the normal renal lymphatic system has been investigated in various animals using light microscopy by the ureteric occlusion technique, electron microscopy, and microradiography (Hogg et al 1992). In humans, microradiography has been performed to detect the renal lymphatics at autopsy (Cuttino et al. 1989). Lymphatic vessels are abundant

**Fig. 2.3** (**a**) Regional lymph nodes of the kidneys; (**b**) abdominal para-aortic (periaortic) lymph nodes including the interaortocaval (group 1), paracaval (group 2), precaval (group 3), retrocaval (group 4), preaortic (group 5), and retroaortic lymph nodes (group 6)

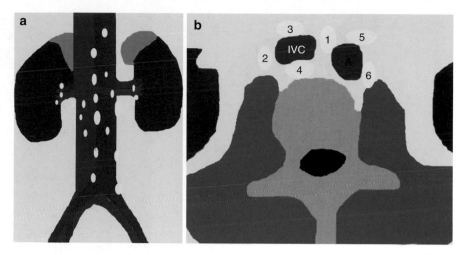

around the intrarenal arteries/veins, while they are scarce in the interstitium around the glomeruli or between the tubules (Ischikawa et al. 2006), since the lymphatic system begins in the cortical interstitium around the glomeruli or between the tubules. Lymph nodes for the kidneys include the renal hilar nodes and the abdominal para-aortic (periaortic) nodes including the interaortocaval, paracaval, precaval, retrocaval, preaortic, and retroaortic lymph nodes. The ureters are drained prevalently by the renal hilar and paracaval lymph node groups (Fig. 2.3).

### 2.1.1.2 Microscopic Renal Anatomy and Nephron Physiology

The cortex of each human kidney contains the glomeruli of 1–1.5 million nephrons. The afferent artery intimately interacts with the glomerular portion of the nephron, where the afferent artery breaks into a capillary network named the glomerular capillary tuft from which originate the efferent artery. The glomerular vessels are contained within the Bowman's capsule forming the Malpighian corpuscle (Fig. 2.4a). The Malpighian corpuscles represent small, round, deep red bodies in the cortex of the kidney, each communicating with a renal tubule. They average about 0.2 mm in diameter, with each capsule composed of two parts: a central glomerulus and a glomerular capsule, also called Bowman's capsule. The Bowman's capsule represents the glomerular portion of the nephron and is a double-walled, cup-shaped structure around the

glomerulus of each nephron and at the beginning of the tubular component of a nephron. The filtration barrier is composed of three layers corresponding to capillary endothelium, the basement membrane composed of glycoproteins, collagens, and mucopolysaccharides, and the epithelium of the Bowman's capsule. The basement membrane presents an average thickness in adults of 3,200 Å and contains three distinct areas: a central electron dense lamina densa and, on either side, a lamina rara externa and lamina rara interna (Fig. 2.4a). Thickening of the basement membrane is seen in a number of glomerular diseases.

The epithelial cells that surround the capillary tuft differ from those forming the rest of the Bowman's capsule, because they present numerous foot processes or pedicles which come into contact with the lamina rara externa of the basement membrane and are called podocytes (Fig. 2.4a). Between the foot processes is a space, named filtration split or split pore, 250–400 Å wide which is covered by a thin membrane, named the filtration slit diaphragm and located approximately 600 Å from the basement membrane. Interspread between the adjacent capillaries, the mesangium, containing mesangial cells and mesangial matrix, appears to provide support for the glomerular capillaries. Usually, the term glomerulus includes both the nephron and capillary components. At the glomerulus, the blood reaches a highly disfavorable pressure gradient and a large exchange surface area, which forces the serum portion of the blood out of the vessel into the renal tubules. About 20% of the water in plasma entering the afferent

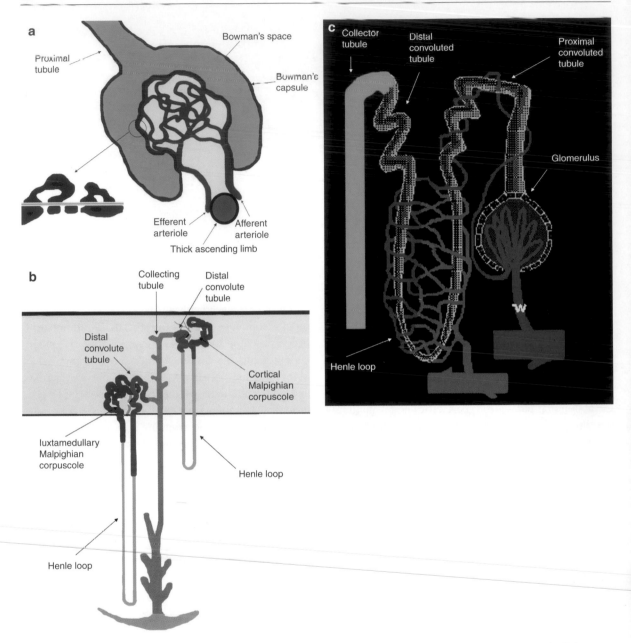

**Fig. 2.4** (**a**) Scheme of the Malpighian corpuscole. Mesangium with mesangial cells is represented in *dark yellow*. The filtration barrier is composed by three layers corresponding to capillary endothelium (*red*), the basement membrane, and the epithelium of the Bowman's capsule (*violet*). The basement contains three distinct areas, a central electron dense lamina densa (*green*) and a lamina rara externa and lamina rara interna (*light yellow*). The epithelial cells that surround the capillary tuft differ from those forming the rest of the Bowman's capsule, because they present numerous foot processes or pedicles which come into contact with the lamina rara externa of the basement membrane, and are called podocytes. (**b**) Scheme of cortical and juxtamedullary nephrons within the renal cortex (*gray color*), the proximal tubule (*red*), loop of Henle (thin descending limb, *light green*; thick ascending limb, *dark green*), the distal convoluted tubule (*blue*), and the connecting and collecting tubule (*gray*). The juxtaglomerular apparatus is represented in *black*. The loop of Henle begins at the end of the proximal straight tubule. In cortical nephrons the hairpin turn that forms the tip of the loop of Henle occurs not deeper than the junction between the outer and inner zones of the medulla, whereas in the juxtamedullary nephrons the hairpin turn may occur as deeply as the tip of papilla. (**c**) Scheme of the branches of the efferent arteries vascularizing the different regions of the nephrons forming the peritubular capillaries

artery filters out the glomerular capillary into the Bowman's space.

Fluids from blood in the glomerulus are collected in the Bowman's capsule forming the glomerular filtrate and further processed along the nephron to form urine. This process is known as ultrafiltration, which is performed by the glomerulus and then by the nephron (Fig. 2.4b). Flow continues through the renal tubules, including the proximal convoluted tubule, the loop of Henle with the thick ascending, and thin descending limb, and finally leaves the kidney by means of the collecting duct, leading to the renal ureter. The proximal tubule has traditionally been divided into the proximal convoluted tubule, which contorts itself in an apparently random fashion in the renal cortex, and the proximal straight tubule (or pars recta). The epithelial cells of the proximal tubule have a cuboidal shape (Laiken and Fanestil 1985). A layer of closely packed microvilli covers the luminal surface forming a brush border. The proximal tubule is responsible for the initial processing of the glomerular filtrate, and it both reabsorbs approximately two thirds of the filtered water and sodium (with bicarbonate instead of chloride) and almost all the filtered glucose and amino acids from the tubular fluid, and secretes organic acids (e.g., uric acid) and bases such as drugs (including diuretics) and drug metabolites into the tubular fluid. Sodium reabsorption in the proximal tubule occurs in cells and intercellular spaces. Entry of sodium across luminal membranes is passive and occurs by diffusion, coupled to the transport of other solutes (e.g., glucose, amino acids, phosphate), and in exchange with protons secreted from cell to lumen and reabsorption of bicarbonate. Sodium extrusion from cells into the intercellular spaces and across the basolateral membrane is an active process, which is accomplished by the sodium-potassium pump ($Na^+$-$K^+$-ATPase). Chloride is reabsorbed due to the diffusion gradient from the tubular lumen to the peritubular capillary.

The loop of Henle consists of a descending limb and as ascending limb. Most renal physiologists consider the loop of Henle to begin at the end of the proximal straight tubule (Laiken and Fanestil 1985) (Fig. 2.4b). Here the cuboidal epithelial cells of the proximal tubule are replaced by flat, squamous epithelial cells with a small number of short microvilli. This segment of the tubule is called the thin descending limb since the epithelial cell layer is very flat. The thin descending limb of the juxtamedullary nephrons is substantially longer

than that of cortical nephrons (Fig. 2.4b). In cortical nephrons the hairpin turn that forms the tip of the loop of Henle occurs not deeper than the junction between the outer and inner zones of the medulla, whereas in the juxtamedullary nephrons the hairpin turn may occur as deeply as the tip of papilla. In juxtamedullary nephrons the ascending limb begins with a segment of flat, squamous epithelial cells, termed the thin ascending limb. At the junction between the inner and outer zones of the renal medulla, the thick ascending limb begins (Laiken and Fanestil 1985). In this segment the epithelial cells are cuboidal and contain numerous mitochondria like the epithelial cells of the proximal tubule, even though these cells lack a luminal brush border. The thick ascending limb transverses the outer zone of the medulla (the medullary portion of the thick ascending limb) and then ascends through the renal cortex to the level of its nephron's glomerulus. In cortical nephrons, the ascending limb consists entirely of cuboidal epithelial cells, and cortical nephrons lack a thin ascending limb (Laiken and Fanestil 1985). The loop of Henle dissociates the absorption of sodium and water. The descending limb of Henle passively abstracts water into the hypertonic medullary interstitium, concentrating the tubular fluid, while the essentially water-impermeable thick ascending limb of Henle actively absorbs approximately 25% of filtered sodium chloride but little water (Andreoli 1992). In the thick ascending limb of the loop of Henle, sodium and potassium cross the luminal cell membrane together with two chlorides by a carrier-mediated uptake ($Na^+$/$K^+$/2Cl$^-$) under the energy of sodium-potassium ATPase on the basolateral membrane. The loop diuretics inhibit the apical cotransport system, thereby enhancing the sodium and chloride secretion.

In each nephron the thick ascending limb returns to the glomerulus of its own origin and contacts its originating glomerulus at the vascular pole, the region where the afferent and efferent arterioles, respectively, enter and leave the glomerulus (Fig. 2.4a, b). A specialized structure, the juxtaglomerular apparatus, is found at this contact point consisting of three components, the macula densa, the extraglomerular mesangial cells, and granular cells secreting renin. The juxtaglomerular apparatus is made up of specialized cells in the wall of the afferent arteriole and granular cells in the wall of the distal tubule (the macula densa). This area is innervated by adrenergic fibers and the granular cells carry renin in intracellular granules.

The distal nephron includes the distal convoluted tubule, the connecting tubule, and the collecting tubule (or duct) which can be subdivided into cortical collecting tubule, medullary collecting duct, and papillary collecting duct. The distal convoluted tubule primarily absorbs sodium by the sodium-potassium pump ($Na^+$-$K^+$-ATPase) under the influence of aldosterone and secretes protons, ammonia, and potassium in the tubular lumen. Aldosterone and other mineralcorticoids stimulate the rate of sodium absorption in the distal nephron. Aldosterone also increases the rate of net potassium secretion and net proton secretion (and consequently the rate of bicarbonate regeneration) by the distal nephron. The collecting tubule/duct develops from the ureteral bud, and the connecting tubule represents the connection between the embryonic nephron and the ureteral bud. The collecting duct system regulates the osmolality of the urine by absorbing water under the influence of the antidiuretic hormone (ADH) and tubular fluid equilibrates osmotically with the hypertonic medullary interstitium. ADH promotes the formation of a hypertonic urine both by increasing the rate of salt absorption in the thick ascending limb of Henle and by increasing the water permeability of the collecting duct system (Andreoli 1992).

The efferent artery disperses into a second capillary network that surrounds the tubular portion of the nephron (Fig. 2.4c), delivering substances for tubules to secrete into the tubular fluid and taking up water and solutes reabsorbed by the tubule. Most of the capillaries in this second network surround the tubules in the cortex and are termed peritubular capillaries. Some of these capillaries in the juxtamedullary nephrons, called vasa recta, descend to varying depths in the medulla before forming a capillary network and reunite while turning around and ascend back to the renal cortex. From the peritubular capillaries and vasa recta, blood flows into the peritubular veins and is drained by the renal veins.

## 2.1.2 Normal Renal Physiology

The principal function of the mammalian kidney is to maintain homeostasis or equilibrium between our internal volume and electrolyte status and that of the environment's influences, diet and intake. It functions to maintain our intra and extracellular fluid status at a constant, despite the wide variety of daily fluid and electrolyte intake. In man the kidneys consist of 2–3 million nephrons (Fig. 2.3) and weigh only 250 g. The kidneys' extraordinary excretory and regulatory objectives are achieved through the processes of glomerular ultrafiltration, tubular reabsorption, and tubular secretion. To a large extent, these excretory and regulatory processes depend on the blood supply to the kidneys.

The kidneys receive the highest blood flow per gram of organ weight in the body at 1 L/min. The renal blood flow is to consider the renal fraction, which corresponds to the fraction of the total cardiac output that flows through the kidneys. The kidneys are very vascularized parenchymas and a 70 kg man with a cardiac output of 6 L/min has a normal renal blood flow of about 1.2 L/min corresponding to 20% of the cardiac output. Considering the fact that each kidney in a normal 70 kg man weighs about 130–170 g, for a total weight of about 300 g of kidney, the average flow per gram of kidney weight (perfusion value) is about 400 mL/min/100 g. This is several times greater per unit weight of organ than the blood flow through most other organs. During various stress conditions or diseases, this renal fraction can vary considerably and be markedly affected. Blood flow to the kidneys will be dependent on a number of important systemic factors. Clearly, if there is a problem with volume (dehydration, hemorrhage) or cardiac output (congestive heart failure, myocardial infarct), blood flow is diminished. In less obvious ways, hypoalbuminemia (cirrhosis, nephrotic syndrome, and starvation) affects the intravascular volume so that the effective blood (volume) flow is diminished, despite many of these patients appearing with total body fluid overloaded. Finally, hypotension from severe vasodilatation (anaphylactic shock, sepsis) would also diminish blood flow to the kidneys.

Oxygen consumption by the kidneys is quite high and amounts to about 8% of the total oxygen consumption of the body. Oxygen delivery to any organ is directly dependent on hemoglobin content (blood) and cardiac output (blood flow). As in other tissues, an important function of blood flow is to provide adequate oxygenation and nutrition. Therefore, the relatively high blood flow to the kidneys exists to feed its metabolic demands as well as to allow ultrafiltration. In fact, the renal blood flow is so high that only a small percent of the available oxygen is extracted from the blood perfusing the kidneys.

The fundamental parameter to indicate the renal function is glomerular filtration rate (GFR) corresponding to the volume of water filtered out of the plasma through glomerular capillary walls into Bowman's capsules per unit of time. The normal value of the GFR is above 90 mL/min/1.73 m². The initial step in urine formation (ultrafiltration) occurs across the glomerular wall (Klahr 1992). The difference in hydrostatic pressure between the glomerular capillary pressure ($P_{GC}$) and Bowman's space ($P_{BS}$) favors filtration, whereas the colloid osmotic pressure inside the glomerular capillaries ($\Pi_{GC}$) opposes it.

$$ GFR = K_{uf}[(P_{GC} - P_{BS}) - \Pi_{GC}] \qquad (2.1) $$

$K_{uf}$ corresponds to the ultrafiltration coefficient and is a function of both total capillary surface and the permeability per unit of surface area. The Bowman's space ($P_{BS}$) pressure and the hydrostatic pressure ($P_{GC}$) remain relatively constant along glomerular capillaries, while the colloid osmotic pressure ($\Pi_{GC}$) undergoes a large progressive increase because the filtration of protein-free fluid results in an increase of protein concentration along the capillary lumen. Hence, the mean effective pressure for ultrafiltration decreases along the glomerular capillaries and becomes zero before the end of the capillary (Klahr 1992) with consequent end of filtration. Thus the GFR is highly dependent on the glomerular plasma flow rate because, at high flow rates, a slower rise in the colloid osmotic pressure occurs and glomerular filtration increases since it takes place across a greater length of the capillary (Klahr 1992).

The autoregulatory system accomplishes this by maintaining the glomerular capillary pressure around 60–70 mmHg. Renal blood flow and GFR are autoregulated within a wide range of renal arterial pressure. This ability to maintain renal perfusion pressure and $P_{GC}$ is impaired when mean arterial pressure drops below 70 mmHg. Unless cardiac output is severely reduced, however, GFR usually remains near normal. GFR is protected from reduced cardiac output and arterial pressure by autoregulation (Cohen 1991), which involves local activation of the rennin-angiotensin system in the juxtaglomerular apparatus via myogenic receptors in the wall of the afferent arteriole and granular cells carry renin in intracellular granules in the wall of the distal tubule (the macula densa). These sense blood pressure changes through stretch receptors and respond accordingly through relaxation or constriction. Renin, a glycoprotein of 340 amino acids, is produced in the granular cells as a precursor protein

(prorenin) that is cleaved to yield active rennin (Baxter 1992). The granular cells of the juxtaglomerular apparatus release rennin into the circulation where it has a half-life of around 15 min. Release of renin can be induced by altered sodium concentration at the macula densa of the distal tubule (tubuloglomerular feedback loop), by changes in the blood flow patterns of the afferent arteriole, or by adrenergic stimulation. Renin acts in the plasma and cleaves the rennin substrate angiotensinogen, secreted by the liver, to yield the decapeptide angiotensin I. Angiotensin I is not known to have a physiologically important action, while it serves as a substrate for the production of angiotensin II. The conversion of angiotensin I to the octapeptide angiotensin II is catalyzed by angiotensin converting enzyme that is present in a number of tissues and in high concentration in the lung. Angiotensin II is a potent vasoconstrictor and appears to constrict the efferent glomerular arteriole selectively (Cohen 1991). Angiotensin II is also a potent stimulator of aldosterone release from the adrenal glands. The afferent arteriole will respond to changes in renal perfusion pressure by either vasoconstriction or vasodilatation as a result of a direct myogenic response. The resultant increase in efferent arteriolar resistance maintains hydrostatic pressure within the glomerular capillaries and GFR (Cohen 1991).

As further endocrine functions of the kidney, besides the renin-angiotensin axis, the prostaglandin production, the operation of the kallikrein-kini system, and the degradation of low molecular weight proteins should be mentioned. The kidney is also the major site for the synthesis of erythropoietin, which is a glycoprotein produced by renal enzymatic action on a circulating precursor of hepatic origin (Andreoli 1992). The principal action of erythropoietin is to stimulate the rate of red blood cell production by the bone marrow.

### 2.1.3 Calculation of Glomerular Filtration Rate (GFR)

Unfortunately, blood urea nitrogen (BUN) and serum creatinine will not be raised above the normal range until 60% of total kidney function is lost. In particular, serum creatinine is known to be an unreliable indicator of GFR. Approximately 30% of elderly patients with normal serum creatinine (1.4 mg/dL or less) have chronic kidney disease based on an estimated GFR of less than 60 mL/min/1.73 m² (Lane et al. 2009). Thus the serum creatinine concentration may remain within the normal range, despite a substantial decrease in the GFR. Moreover, the creatinine concentration in the blood is affected by a number of factors other than creatinine filtration, including diet, muscle mass, and sex (Lameire et al. 2006). Older patients and women tend to have a lower muscle mass than younger men, and hence, the renal function, namely the GFR, may be lower than that expected from the serum creatinine.

GFR and creatinine clearance are the two indices that are usually employed to quantify the renal function. Recommendations for evaluating people at increased risk for chronic renal failure are to measure urine albumin to assess kidney damage and to estimate the GFR with an equation based on the level of serum creatinine (Stevens et al. 2006). Many studies support the similarity of creatinine clearance to GFR and its reciprocal relationship with the serum creatinine level. Creatinine clearance rate ($C_{Cr}$) is the volume of blood plasma that is cleared of creatinine per unit time and is a useful measure for approximating the GFR. Both GFR and $C_{Cr}$ may be accurately calculated by comparative measurements of substances in the blood and urine or estimated by formulas using just a blood test result. The results of these tests are important in assessing the excretory function of the kidneys, and the grading of chronic renal failure and dosage of drugs that are primarily excreted via urine are based on GFR (or $C_{Cr}$). GFR or its approximation of the creatinine clearance is measured whenever renal disease is suspected or careful dosing of nephrotoxic drugs is required. Creatinine is produced naturally by the body (creatinine is a metabolite of creatine in the muscle). It is freely filtered by the glomerulus, but also actively secreted by the renal tubules in very small amounts such that creatinine clearance overestimates actual GFR by 10–20%. This margin of error is acceptable considering the ease with which creatinine clearance is measured and the steady-state concentration in the blood.

Creatinine is an amino acid derivative with a molecular mass of 113 Da that is freely filtered by the glomerulus and secreted by the proximal tubule cells. Consequently, the creatinine clearance exceeds the GFR (Stevens et al. 2006). Tubular secretion of creatinine varies among and within individual persons and

is influenced by some drugs, including trimethoprim and cimetidine, which inhibit creatinine secretion, thereby reducing creatinine clearance and elevating the serum creatinine level without affecting the GFR. The generation of creatinine is determined primarily by muscle mass and dietary intake, which probably accounts for the variations in the level of serum creatinine observed among different age, geographic, ethnic, and racial groups. Extrarenal elimination of creatinine may be increased at low levels of GFR; this increase is mainly related to the degradation of creatinine by intestinal bacteria and can be affected by the use of antibiotics.

GFR can be calculated by measuring any chemical that has a steady level in the blood and is freely filtered, but neither reabsorbed nor secreted by the kidneys. The rate measured, therefore, is the quantity of the substance in the urine that originated from a calculable volume of blood.

$$\text{GFR} = \frac{\text{urine concentration} \times \text{urine flow}}{\text{plasma concentration}} \quad (2.2)$$

The GFR can be determined by injecting inulin into the plasma. Since inulin is neither reabsorbed nor secreted by the kidney after glomerular filtration, its rate of excretion is directly proportional to the rate of filtration of water and solutes across the glomerular filter. Cystatin C, a nonglycosylated basic protein with a low molecular mass (13 kD) that is freely filtered by the glomerulus, is currently under investigation as a replacement for serum creatinine in estimating the GFR since its concentration is independent of muscle mass and does not seem to be correlated with age and sex. After filtration, cystatin C is reabsorbed and catabolized by the tubular epithelial cells; only small amounts are excreted in the urine. Consequently, although cystatin C is cleared by the kidneys, its urinary clearance cannot be measured, which makes the study of the factors affecting its clearance and generation difficult.

In practice, the GFR is often estimated from the serum creatinine level (estimated GFR, eGFR). Creatinine clearance ($C_{Cr}$) can be calculated if values for creatinine's urine concentration ($U_{Cr}$), urine flow rate ($V$), and creatinine's plasma concentration ($P_{Cr}$) are known. Since the product of urine concentration and urine flow rate yields creatinine's excretion rate, creatinine clearance is also said to be its excretion rate

$(U_{Cr} \times V)$ divided by its plasma concentration. This is commonly represented mathematically as

$$GFR = \frac{U_{Cr} \times V}{P_{Cr}}. \tag{2.3}$$

Commonly a 24 h urine collection is undertaken, from empty-bladder one morning to the contents of the bladder the following morning, with a comparative blood test then taken. The urinary flow rate is still calculated per minute, hence:

$$GFR = \frac{U_{Cr} \times 24 - \text{h urine volume}}{P_{Cr} \times 24 \times 60 \, \text{min}} \tag{2.4}$$

To allow comparison of results between people of different sizes, the $C_{Cr}$ is often corrected for the body surface area (BSA) and expressed compared to the average sized man as mL/min/1.73 m². While most adults have a BSA that approaches 1.7 m² (1.6–1.9 m²), extremely obese or slim patients should have their $C_{Cr}$ corrected for their *actual* BSA, which can be calculated on the basis of the weight and height.

$$C_{Cr\text{-}corrected} = \frac{C_{Cr} \times 1.73}{BSA} \tag{2.5}$$

The National Kidney Foundation (2002) Kidney Disease Outcome Quality Initiative (K/DOQI; 2002) recommends that clinicians should use an estimated creatinine clearance rate (e$C_{Cr}$) calculated from the serum creatinine as an index of renal function, rather than serum creatinine alone. A number of formulae have been devised to estimate GFR or $C_{Cr}$ values on the basis of serum creatinine levels. The most widely used equations for estimating GFR are the *Cockcroft–Gault* (Cockcroft and Gault 1976) and the *Modification of Diet in Renal Disease Study Group*, MDRD (Levey et al. 1999) formulas.

*Cockcroft–Gault* (1976) formula may be used to calculate e$C_{Cr}$, which in turn estimates GFR:

$$eC_{cr} \, (\text{mL} / \text{min}) = \frac{(140 - \text{age}) \times \text{weight (kg)} \times 1.23}{\text{Serum creatinine} \, (\mu\text{mol/L})} \tag{2.6}$$

the resulting value must be multiplicated by 1.04 for women.

The most recently advocated formula for calculating the GFR is the one that was developed by the MDRD study. The most commonly used formula is the "four-variable MDRD," which estimates GFR using four variables: serum creatinine, age, race, and gender. According to this formula, for creatinine in mg/dL:

$$\begin{aligned} eGFR \, (\text{mL} / \text{min}/ 1.73 \, \text{m}^2) = {} & 186 \times \text{Serum creatinine}^{-1.154} \\ & \times \text{Age}^{-0.203} \times [1.212 \, \text{if black}] \\ & \times [0.742 \, \text{if female}]. \end{aligned} \tag{2.7}$$

For creatinine in µmol/L:

$$\begin{aligned} eGFR \, (\text{mL} / \text{min} / 1.73 \, \text{m}^2) = {} & 186 \times (\text{Serum creatinine} / 88.4)^{-1.154} \\ & \times \text{Age}^{-0.203} \times [1.212 \, \text{if black}] \\ & \times [0.742 \, \text{if female}] \end{aligned} \tag{2.8}$$

Creatinine levels in µmol/L can be converted to mg/dL by dividing them by 88.4. The equations have been validated in patients with chronic kidney disease. Both equation versions underestimate the GFR in healthy patients with GFRs over 60 mL/min, while the equations have not been validated in acute renal failure.

In the equation used in MDRD, the factors of age, sex, and race are surrogates for muscle mass (Stevens and Levey 2005). Many chronic illnesses, including cardiovascular disease, affect muscle mass through malnutrition, inflammation, and deconditioning. Thus people with chronic illness are more likely to have lower levels of serum creatinine than are healthy people, even for the same level of GFR and the same age, sex, and race. In such persons, estimating equations based on serum creatinine may overestimate GFR. It must be emphasized that both the *Cockcroft–Gault* and *MDRD* equations can only provide estimates of GFR and, where there is doubt about renal function, direct GFR measurement is preferable (Lameire et al. 2006).

In children, the *Schwartz formula* (1984) is used (Schwartz et al. 1984). This employs the serum creatinine (mg/dL), the child's height (cm), and a constant to estimate the GFR:

$$eGFR = \frac{k \times \text{height}}{\text{serum creatinine (mg/dL)}}, \tag{2.9}$$

where $k$ is a constant that depends on muscle mass, which itself varies with a child's age. In the first year of life, for preterm babies $K = 0.33$, and for full-term infants $K = 0.45$. For infants between 1 and 12 years of age, $K = 0.55$. The method of selection of the $K$-constant value has been questioned as being dependent upon the gold-standard of renal function used (i.e., creatinine clearance, inulin clearance, etc.) and also may be dependent upon the urinary flow rate at the time of measurement.

For most patients, a GFR over 60 mL/min is adequate. But, if the GFR has significantly declined from a previous test result, this can be an early indicator of kidney disease requiring medical intervention. The sooner the kidney dysfunction is diagnosed and treated, the greater the odds of preserving remaining nephrons and preventing the need for dialysis. The normal ranges of GFR, adjusted for BSA, are $70 \pm 14$ mL/min/m$^2$ for males and $60 \pm 10$ mL/min/m$^2$ for females.

## 2.1.4 Calculation of Glomerular Filtration Rate (GFR) in Acute Renal Failure

Measurement and estimation of GFR in acute renal failure present numerous challenges (Dagher et al. 2003). Serum creatinine concentration alone will provide inaccurate information of eGFR when the GFR is rapidly changing or before it is reaching an equilibrium value. Thus equations to estimate creatinine clearance from serum creatinine cannot be used. In addition, clearance also inaccurately estimates true GFR because of tubular secretion of creatinine.

Oral cimetidine, a blocker of tubular creatinine secretion, improves the accuracy of measuring creatinine clearance, but requires a pretreatment period (Dagher et al. 2003). In addition, the GFR measurements after cimetidine administration have not been validated in patients with acute renal failure. Urinary clearance of GFR markers may provide better information. Thus, if a bolus of a marker such as inulin was administered intravenously and its urinary clearance measured, an estimate of GFR can be obtained (Dagher et al. 2003).

The choice of the GFR marker such as inulin, 125-I iothalamate, and others has been validated in patients with stable renal function. These measurements presume the marker is filtered, not metabolized, neither reabsorbed nor secreted by the tubule, and can be reliably measured in the blood and urine. However, with tubular obstruction and backleak, these assumptions may not hold true. Leakage of substances filtered at the glomerulus, but which leak back across the tubular epithelium, may underestimate GFR in ARF. The permeability to those substances most commonly used for filtration rate determination, such as inulin, may be the principal cause of this phenomenon. Distal recovery of inulin is reduced by only 15% in kidneys showing severely restricted renal function in animal models (Olbricht et al. 1977). Thus the reduction in whole kidney inulin clearance reflects primarily a reduction in GFR.

GFR is commonly measured using plasma or renal clearance of marker solutes administered as a bolus or continuous infusion. The reference standard is renal inulin clearance, but other solutes commonly used include radioactive ($^{125}$I-iothalamate [Glofil], 51Cr-EDTA) or nonradioactive markers (iothalamate, iohexol, polyfructosan). Paramagnetic agents (gadolinium DTPA) are rarely used.

GFR can be measured by various methods in patients with acute renal failure, including the continuous infusion method, the standard clearance method, or the plasma clearance method. The infusion method consists in the infusion at a constant rate, usually following a bolus-loading dose, of a known concentration of GFR marker. Since the GFR is often unstable in patients with ARF, a steady state may not be achieved, a major assumption underlying this method. Therefore, this method is not suitable for use in patients with ARF.

In calculating GFR by the standard clearance method, bolus and infusion of a GFR marker is carried out in a manner identical to the above. In addition, urine is collected at three to six timed intervals of 20–30 min each in a water-loaded state (Dagher et al. 2003). The urine flow rate ($V$) and urinary iothalamate concentration ($U$) are recorded. Peripheral venous blood is drawn immediately before and after the urine collection period for measurement of plasma maker concentration ($P$). $P$ represents the logarithmic average of the marker concentration before and after the collection period. The renal clearance is calculated by the formula:

$$GFR = \frac{U \times V}{P}$$

This method lends itself well to estimation of GFR in ARF when hemodynamic changes can be rapid. By collecting urine and plasma at timed intervals, rapid changes in GFR can be detected.

## 2.2 Normal Radiological Anatomy of the Renal Parenchyma, Intrarenal Vasculature, and Anatomical Variants

### 2.2.1 Conventional Radiography

The longitudinal (Fig. 2.5a) and transverse (Fig. 2.5b) represent the two fundamental planes employed for renal imaging. The conventional plain radiography of the abdomen, or kidney-ureter-bladder (KUB) radiograph, is a first-line imaging technique in the assessment of the kidney. It is performed in the antero-posterior projection with the patient in the upright or supine position. It is indicated to evaluate the renal shape, margins, dimensions, and location, and to identify renal calcifications, stones, or transparencies due to fat or gas.

On the abdomen plain radiography, both kidneys are clearly visible due to the natural contrast provided by the perirenal fat (Fig. 2.6) and can be assessed regarding their position, morphology, margins, and dimensions. Both kidneys present a longitudinal diameter of 10–12 cm, and a latero-lateral diameter of 3–5 cm should not have a difference in the largest longitudinal diameter higher than 1.5 cm. In the long body

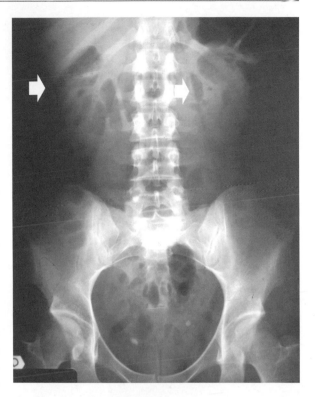

**Fig. 2.6** Conventional plain radiograph of the abdomen. The kidneys (*arrows*) are easily identified due to the natural contrast provided by the perirenal fat which allows the differentiation between the kidneys and the psoas muscle

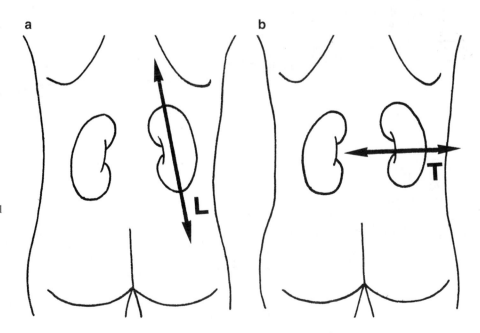

**Fig. 2.5** (**a**, **b**) Fundamental planes employed for renal imaging. The longitudinal axis (**a**) is parallel to the major diameter of each kidney. The transverse axis (**b**) is perpendicular to the major diameter of each kidney

habitus subjects, the longitudinal diameter may exceed the highest range, while in the short body habitus subjects, the normal 15–20° inclination of the renal longitudinal diameter on the frontal plane may be much higher with an apparent reduction of the longitudinal diameter on the antero-posterior projection. The psoas muscle profile is another important parameter to evaluate since it is canceled by the intestinal methorismor by retroperitoneal effusions.

The fundamental radiopacities that should be detected at the conventional plain radiograph of the abdomen (Fig. 2.7) correspond to renal stones, or calcifications due to vascular structures, chronic inflammations (e.g., tuberculosis), traumatic lesions (e.g., hematoma), or solid or cystic neoplasms.

The fundamental radiolucencies visible on plain radiography are determined by gas (e.g., emphysematous pyelonephritis, Fig. 2.8) or fat (e.g., angiomyolipomas, lyposarcomas, renal sinus lypomatosis).

## 2.2.2 Gray-Scale and Doppler Ultrasound

Gray-scale US is a reliable technique for renal dimension assessment, even though renal volume is influenced by patient age and hydration. In a newborn's kidneys (Fig. 2.9), renal cortex is iso or hyperechoic to liver and spleen parenchyma (Kasap et al. 2006), whereas pyramids are more prominent than in adults. The renal cortex hyperechogenicity compared to the liver is more evident in premature infants. This is because in a newborn, during the first 2 months of life, the kidney loops of Henle are still within the cortex in

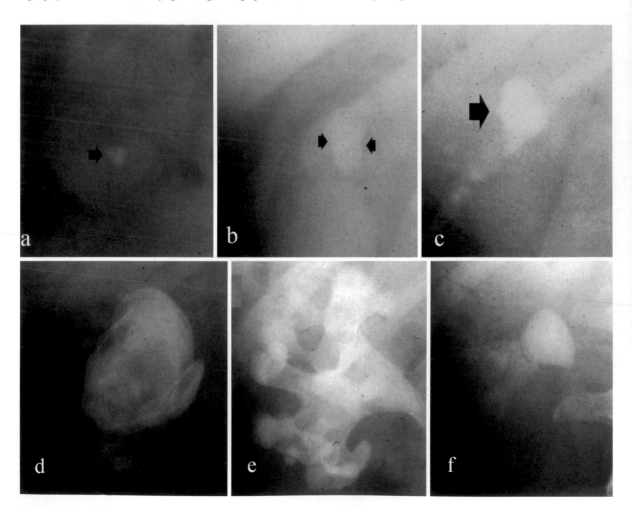

**Fig. 2.7** (**a–f**) Plain radiograph. Different type of high-density opacities (*arrows*) projecting on the renal anatomical site. (**a**) Stone; (**b–e**) different type of staghorn stone; (**f**) putty kidney

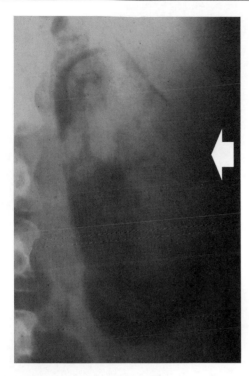

**Fig. 2.8** Plain radiograph. Radiolucency (*arrow*) in the kidney region due to emphysematous pyelonephritis

(Chiara et al. 1990). Compound calyces and associated compound pyramids are present in the upper and lower renal poles in newborns and may appear as large irregular hypoechoic areas, mimicking an obstructed pole of a duplex collecting system, focal caliectasis, hydrocalyx, a cyst, or a hypoechoic mass. Neonatal kidneys also show a paucity of renal sinus echoes due to a minimal renal sinus fat. Within 2–6 months, the kidneys become progressively less echogenic than the liver and assume the features of the adult kidney between 6 and 24 months of life.

In a normal adult, the length of both kidneys is considered normal when it is comprised between 9 and 13 cm. Normally, renal margins are smooth, except in some normal anatomical variants such as functional parenchymal defects and renal fetal lobations. Mean normal value of renal cortical thickness (distance between the renal capsule and the outer margin of the pyramid) is 1–1.5 cm, while the normal value of renal parenchyma thickness (distance between the renal capsule and the margin of the sinus echo avoiding renal columns) is 1.4–1.8 cm, avoiding renal medulla, and measured in the cortical tract interposed between the renal columns. Renal cortical echogenicity is normally lower than the echogenicity of liver, spleen, and renal sinus (Fig. 2.10). When liver parenchyma appears hyperechoic on US, spleen echogenicity is used as a standard reference; however, kidneys may be isoechoic to the liver even when no clinical or laboratory evidence of renal disease are documented. Renal cortical echogenicity is correlated to severity of histological changes in renal parenchymal diseases such as

large percentage while glomeruli occupy proportionately a greater volume of the renal cortex than in adults and an increased number of acoustical interfaces results (Hricak et al. 1983). However, an unusually increased renal echogenicity in newborns may be observed in infantile polycystic kidney disease, hemolytic-uremic syndrome, and renal vein thrombosis

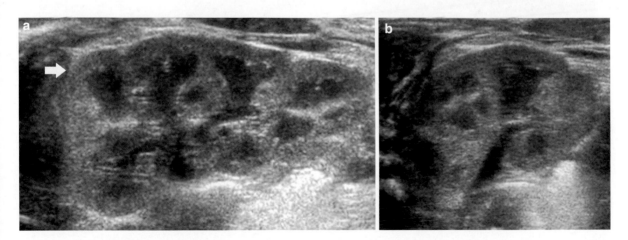

**Fig. 2.9** (**a**, **b**) Ultrasound. Longitudinal (**a**) and transverse scan (**b**). Normal neonatal kidney. The renal cortex (*arrow*) appears hyperechoic with evident hypoechoic medulla. On the upper renal pole the adrenal gland (**a**) is evident

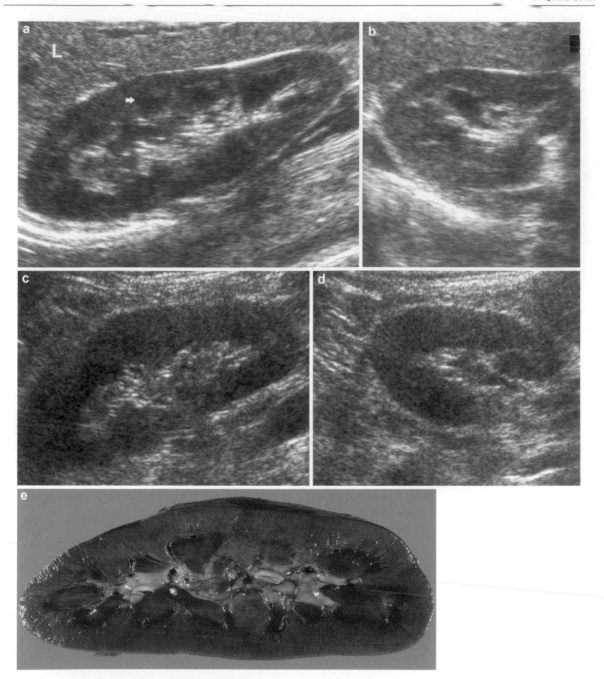

**Fig. 2.10** (**a–e**) Normal anatomy of the adult kidney at ultrasound (**a**) Longitudinal scan. On US renal pyramids (*arrows*) appear hypoechoic in comparison with renal cortex, which appears normally hypoechoic or isoechoic to the adjacent liver parenchyma (*L*), whereas renal sinus is hyperechoic. (**b**) Transverse scan. The renal pelvis appears hyperechoic due to sinusal fat. (**c**, **d**) Longitudinal and transverse scan of a normal kidney with a lower corticomedullary differentiation if compared with the previous example. (**e**) Gross specimen of a cadaveric kidney from a young adult

global sclerosis, focal tubular atrophy, and hyaline casts per glomerulus. On US, renal pyramids appear triangular and hypoechoic and may be differentiated from renal cortex in approximately 50% of adult patients (Fig. 2.10), being more conspicuous in slim patients and children and with hydration and diuresis. Renal sinus appears hyperechoic if compared with renal parenchyma, for the presence of hilar adipose tissue with fibrous septae, blood vessels, and lymphatics. Renal sinus may appear inhomogeneous, less echogenic, and poorly differentiated from renal parenchyma when edema, fibrosis, or cellular infiltration are present. With increasing age, amount of renal parenchyma decreases and renal sinus fat increases with the evidence of renal contour irregularities due to vascular scars or nephrosclerosis (Fig. 2.11). Renal sinus fat tissue may also be increased in renal sinus lipomatosis, which can be determined by obesity, parenchymal atrophy, and normal variants.

Color and power Doppler US accurately depict renal vessels (Fig. 2.12) with possible assessment of single vessel flows by pulsed Doppler interrogation (Fig. 2.13). Renal parenchymal arterial and venous vessels have to be evaluated by color and power Doppler by using low wall filter, flow optimization for slow flows with low-pulse repetition frequency, and by appropriate gain setting with the lowest possible level of noise.

Assessment of renal vascular resistances is obtained by Doppler waveform analysis (Fig. 2.13), obtaining resistive indices (RIs) which correspond to peak systolic velocity minus end diastolic velocity divided by peak systolic velocity. Increased sensitivity of color Doppler and power Doppler provided by latest digital US equipment allows depiction and Doppler interrogation of the renal parenchymal vessels up to the interlobular arteries. The RIs measured on segmental, interlobar, and arcuate renal parenchymal arteries are normally below 0.70 and decrease progressively from segmental to interlobular vessels. RIs are significantly higher in elderly subjects. Studies that correlate RIs values with biopsy findings in various renal parenchymal diseases have revealed that kidneys with active disease in tubulo-interstitial or vascular compartment present elevated RIs (>0.80), whereas kidneys with glomerular diseases present more often normal RIs values.

### 2.2.3 Computed Tomography

Current generation multidetector helical computed tomography (CT) scanners allow for the acquisition of volumetric data. Such data can be used to generate both bubmillimetric transverse images and thicker reconstructed transverse sections with increased signal-to-noise ratio (SNR). CT is the ideal technique to scan the retroperitoneal organs. Both kidneys are placed in the perirenal retroperitoneal space, which is delimited by the anterior para-renal fascia (Gerota's fascia) and posterior para-renal fascia (Zuckerkandl's

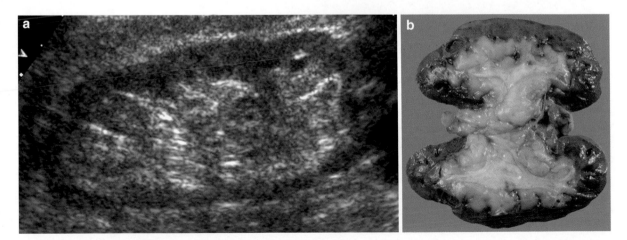

**Fig. 2.11** (**a**) Gray-scale ultrasound. Longitudinal scan of a kidney of an 80-year-old patient. Reduction of the renal parenchyma thickness and increase in the renal sinus fat with the evidence of renal contour irregularities due to vascular scars or nephrosclerosis. (**b**) Gross specimen of a cadaveric kidney from a elderly patient

**Fig. 2.12** (**a**, **b**) Normal renal parenchymal vascularization may be effectively revealed by color Doppler (**a**) and power Doppler (**b**), by setting correctly color gain and by using a low-pulse repetition frequency (slow flows setting optimization). Power Doppler is superior to color Doppler in delineating renal parenchymal blood flows, particularly at the renal poles and superficial cortex

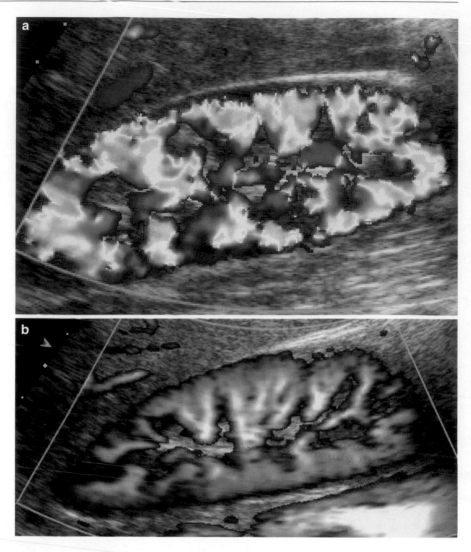

fascia). Kidneys are connected to the para-renal fasciae by the reno-fascial fibrotic septa, which rely on the perirenal fat.

The renal parenchyma is homogeneous on unenhanced CT with a density ranging from 30 to 60 HU, which increases up to 80–120 HU after iodinated contrast agent administration. Iohexol (Omnipaque), iopamidol (Isovue or Iopamiro), iopromide (Ultravist), iomeprol (Iomeron), iobitridol (Xenetix), and ioversol (Optiray) are all nonionic monomers, whereas ioxaglate (Hebabrix) is the only ionic dimer available for the clinical use (Davidson et al. 2006). These compounds are all classified as low-osmolar contrast media. Nonionic dimers with a lower osmolality include iodixanol (Visipaque), which is iso-osmolar to blood and is classified as isomolar contrast medium.

Renal sinus and perinephric fat provide intrinsic contrast for the renal parenchyma appearing hypodense in comparison to the renal parenchyma. Different phases of contrast uptake (Fig. 2.14) can be differentiated (arterial, corticomedullary, nephrographic, and excretory phase) after iodinated contrast agent administration. The arterial CT phase is reached about 20–30 s after commencement of intravenous contrast media injection (for renal arteriography, a contrast bolus of 3.5 mL/s is desirable). The corticomedullary CT phase (about 30–70 s after i.v. contrast according to the patient time of circulation) shows high contrast in the renal cortex. Early opacification of renal veins is also detectable. The renal medulla demonstrates with low contrast. The corticomedullary phase is suitable for depiction of normalvascularrenal anatomy and

**Fig. 2.13** Intrarenal arteries may be interrogated by pulsed Doppler. In particular, segmental arteries are well suitable for this task. The resistive index may be calculated by measuring the peak systolic and the end diastolic velocity

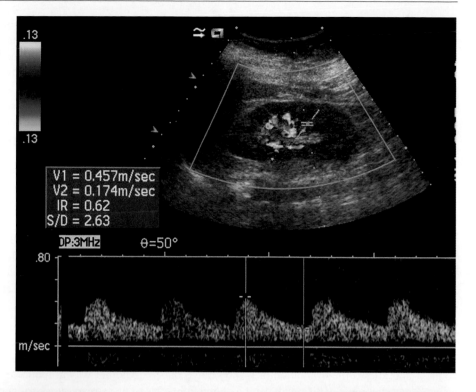

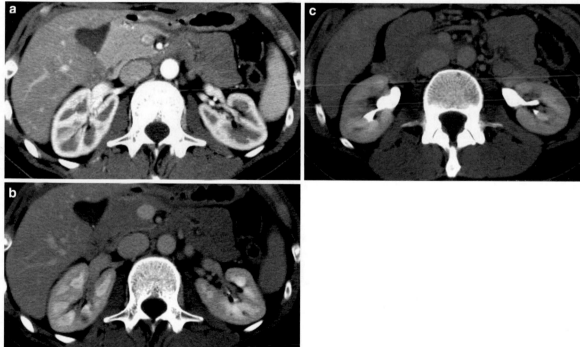

**Fig. 2.14** (**a–c**) Normal computed tomography (CT) dynamic phases evident on renal parenchyma after iodinated contrast agent injection. (**a**) The corticomedullary phase begins about 30–70 s after intravenous contrast agent injection shows high contrast in the renal cortex. (**b**) The nephrographic CT phase (80–120 s after contrast agent injection) shows renal cortex and medulla with equal enhancement. (**c**) The excretory CT phase (more than 180 s after intravenous contrast media administration) shows the opacified renal pelvis, ureter, and urinary bladder

alterations of vascular anatomy (aneurysms, arteriovenous malformations, fistulas, etc.). The nephrographic CT phase (80–120 s) shows renal cortex and medulla with equal enhancement and it is considered the optimal phase for renal tumor detection (see Chap. 5). The excretory CT phase (more than 180 s after intravenous contrast media administration) shows the opacified renal pelvis, ureter, and urinary bladder (complete filling of the urinary bladder with contrast media usually takes about 20 min).

### 2.2.4 Magnetic Resonance Imaging

Nowadays, magnetic resonance (MR) imaging produces a image quality of the kidney, which is comparable to CT. MR sequences provide information about tissues, including T1 and T2 relaxation times, lipid or fat content, and enhancement characteristics of tissues. MR imaging provides versatile and unique soft tissue contrast and allows the evaluation of a wide range of urinary tract disorders. This result can be obtained by the intensity of the static magnetic field, gradient quality and intensity, multichannel phased-array coils, parallel imaging, fast sequences, and gadolinium-based contrast agents. Currently, 1- to 1.5-T systems are generally used for abdominal imaging, but the advent of 3-T MRI systems brings a twofold increase in the SNR. The increase in SNR can be spent on higher resolution or on even faster imaging. When combined with parallel imaging techniques such as sensitivity encoding (SENSE), the speed of any sequence can be increased by up to a factor of 4 or higher.

Kidneys are optimally represented in the different acquisition planes, transverse, coronal, and sagittal. The coronal plane allows the good visualization of both kidneys and of their spatial relation with the adjacent anatomical structures. Usually, the MRI scanning of the kidneys is obtained on the axial and coronal planes with breath-hold sequences including T2-weighted half-Fourier single-shot fast (or turbo) spin echo sequence (SSFSE, GE Healthcare; HASTE, Siemens Medical Solutions), T2-weighted turbo spin echo sequence with fat suppression including spectral fat saturation inversion recovery (SPIR), or spectral presaturation with inversion recovery (SPAIR), or short-tau inversion recovery (STIR) sequences, axial dual-echo in-phase and opposed-

phase gradient echo T1-weighted sequence, and axial or coronal three-dimensional (3D) frequency-selective fat-suppressed fast spoiled gradient echo (SPGR) T1-weighted sequence obtained before and after the intravenousadministration of gadolinium-based contrast agents (0.1 mmol/kg of body weight) at a rate of 2 mL/s by using a power injector followed by a 20-mL saline flush. Gadopentetate dimeglumine (Gd-DTPA, Magnevist), gadobenate dimeglumine (Gd-BOPTA, Multihance), gadoxetate disodium (Gd-EOB-DTPA, Primovist), and gadofosveset trisodium (Vasovist) are linear ionic agents, while gadoterate meglumine (Gd-DOTA, Dotarem) is a macrocyclic ionic agent. Gadodiamide (Gd-DTPA-BMA, Omniscan) and gadoversetamide (Gd-DTPA-BMEA, Optimark) are linear nonionic agents, while gadobutrol (Gd-DO3A-butrol, Gadovist) and gadoteridol (Gd-HP-DO3A, Prohance) are macrocyclic nonionic agents. Their effect in T1 and T2 is similar, but since tissue T1 is much higher than T2, the predominant effect at low doses is that of T1 shortening.

Another way to reduce respiratory motion artifacts is to use a respiratory triggering technique. This technique allows one to use shorter echo train length, more signal averaging, and higher spatial resolution, without being restricted by breath-hold time. This approach can result in a higher SNR in comparison with breath-hold approaches.

The renal parenchyma is composed of two distinct zones, the cortex and medulla. Since renal cortex presents lower T1 and T2 relaxation times in comparison to renal medulla, the two zones can be easily distinguished. Anyway, renal corticomedullary image contrast is usually more conspicuous on T1-weighted images. On T1-weighted sequences, the renal cortex appears much brighter than renal medulla, while on T2-weighted sequences, the renal cortex appears slightly less intense than renal medulla (Fig. 2.15). The renal pelvis containing fat appears hyperintense on T1- and T2-weighted sequences. When fat-suppressed MRI sequences are employed, the fat appears hypointense. After the intravenous administration of gadolinium-based contrast agents, the vascular corticomedullary phase begins immediately after the contrast medium reaches the kidneys (Fig. 2.16). The nephrographic phase begins 60–90 s after contrast administration (Fig. 2.16). The excretory phase begins 2 min after contrast administration with evidence of contrast excretion in the collecting system.

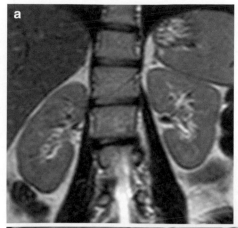

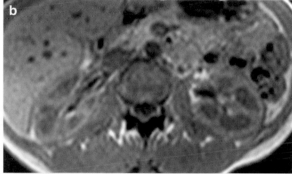

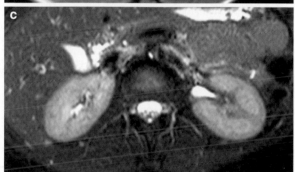

**Fig. 2.15** (**a–c**) Normal kidney on magnetic resonance (MR) imaging. On T1-weighted sequences (**a, b**) the renal cortex appears much brighter than renal medulla, while on T2-weighted sequences (**c**) the renal cortex appears slightly less intense than renal medulla

## 2.2.5 Anatomical Variants of Renal Morphology

Renal cortical defects, hypertrophied column of Bertin, the dromedary or splenic hump, and persistence of fetal lobation, represent frequent anatomical variations of the renal parenchyma which can simulate renal tumors. For this reason, they are also included in the renal pseudotumor category.

- Junctional parenchymal defects. Junctional parenchymal defect results from the incomplete fusion of the two embryonic parenchymatous masses with normal renal sinus fat extending into a groove of renal cortical surface. On US, it appears as a peripheral triangular or round echogenic area located in the anterior surface of upper renal pole or, less frequently, in the posterior surface of the lower renal pole and must be differentiated by renal scars for its continuity with renal sinus. The connection between the intrarenal sinusal fat and the perirenal fat determines a cortical defect, presenting variable evidence between patients, corresponding to a hyperechoic triangular fat on gray-scale US (Fig. 2.17a). Some cortical defects containing fat may mimic a small subcapsular hyperechoic tumor on US. Differential criteria include the evidence of a junctional hyperechoic line associated with the parenchymal notch (Fig. 2.17b). Some fatty tissue arising from the renal sinus fat may branch inside the renal parenchyma up to the corticomedullary junction and can mimic a hyperechoic renal tumor within the renal cortex. On the other hand, the intrasinusal growth of a hyperechoic solid tumor may prevent tumor identification while mimicking renal sinus lipomatosis.
- Column of Bertin. Column of Bertin corresponds to normal renal cortex projecting into renal sinus, more frequently at the junction of the upper and middle third of the left kidney. It is visible in 47% of healthy subjects, and in 18%, it is bilateral, whereas in 4% two columns are visible in one kidney (Fig. 2.18). The US appearance of two or more pyelocalyceal elements is often similar to that of a column of Bertin and consists of a portion of normal renal parenchyma extending from the renal cortex to divide the renal sinus (Fig. 2.19).
- The hypertrophied column of Bertin represents an invagination of the renal cortex toward the renal sinus. Hypertrophied column of Bertin is considered as renal pseudomass, which can be differentiated from renal tumors by power Doppler US revealing normal parenchymal vessels in the pseudomass (Fig. 2.20). Hypertrophied column of Bertin is bilateral in 60% of patients with this variant, which can be identified also on CT (Fig. 2.21). Differently from the hypertrophied column of Bertin, lobar dismorphism (Fig. 2.22) corresponds to a well-defined hypertrophic deep renal parenchyma region appearing isoechoic to the renal cortex and with the

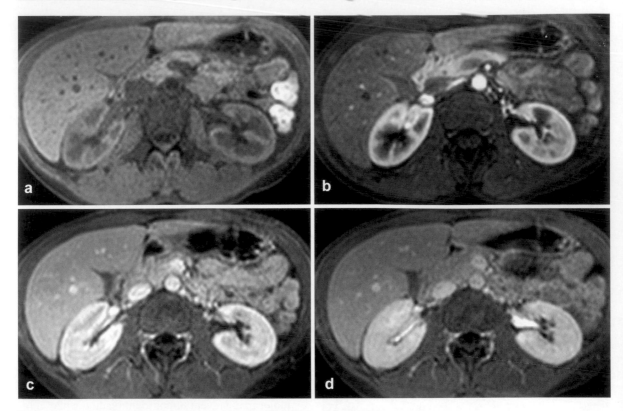

**Fig. 2.16** (**a–d**) Normal MR dynamic phases evident on renal parenchyma before (**a**) and after gadolinium-based contrast agent injection (**b–d**). (**b**) The corticomedullary phase begins immediately after the contrast medium reaches the kidneys (25–30 seconds after injection). The nephrographic phase (**c**) begins 60–90 s after contrast administration, which progresses toward the medullary papillae. The excretory phase (**d**) begins 2 min after contrast administration with evidence of contrast excretion in the collecting system

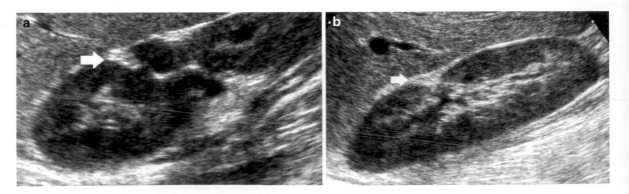

**Fig. 2.17** (**a, b**) Renal cortical defect. Ultrasound. Longitudinal scan. (**a**) The hyperechoic triangular fat (*arrow*) corresponding to a cortical defect through which there is a connection between the intrarenal sinusal and perirenal fat. (**b**) Evidence of a junctional parenchymal hyperechoic line associated with the parenchymal notch

evidence of a hypoechoic Malpighi's pyramid (Yeh et al. 1992).

- Dromedary or splenic hump. The dromedary or splenic hump corresponds to a prominent bulge on the superolateral border of the left kidney. The abnor-

mality is best appreciated as an alteration in left renal contour at US renal contour at Fig. 2.23. It is believed to arise secondary to molding of the upper pole of the left kidney by the spleen during development. The normal nature of this finding is confirmed by the

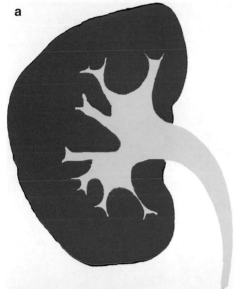

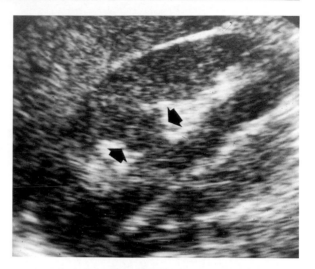

**Fig. 2.19** Duplication of the renal pelvis. Longitudinal scan. A portion of normal renal parenchyma (*arrows*) extends from the renal cortex to divide the renal sinus

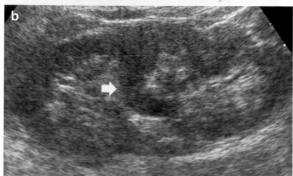

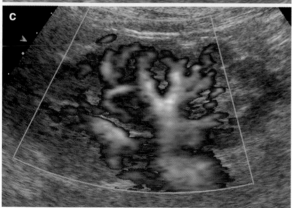

**Fig. 2.18** (**a–c**) Column of Bertin. (**a**) Scheme. (**b**) Longitudinal scan. Mesorenal column (*arrow*). (**c**) Power Doppler ultrasound. The mesorenal column presents a regular vascularization

4–5 years. Renal fetal lobations represent single or multiple notches of renal profile. Persistent fetal lobations can be identified in approximately 5% of adult patients undergoing renal imaging. A key finding in fetal lobation is a normal thickness of the renal parenchyma (≥14 mm) with the indentation occurring so that calyces are centered between indentations and normal vascularization of the renal cortex at color Doppler ultrasound (Fig. 2.24), which differentiates fetal lobations from renal scars, reflux nephropathy, and papillary necrosis where the renal cortex indentations overlie, respectively, the claviform, calyx, and the necrotic renal papilla.

### 2.2.6 Anatomical Variants of Renal Parenchyma

20–30% of all congenital anomalies are represented by kidneys and ureters malformations, and about 1:500 of all newborn infants present these anomalies (Schedl 2007). These abnormalities may be identified also in utero through prenatal US examination.

- Anomalies of number. Unilateral renal agenesis (Fig. 2.25) occurs about once in every 5,000 subjects and results from the failure of the ureteric bud to reach the metanephric blastema since it fails to form or degenerates prematurely. This phenomenon appears more frequently in males then in females,

uniform thickness of the bulging renal parenchyma over the underlying renal calyces.
- Persistent fetal lobations. The fetal lobation represents a vestige of the lobar development of the kidney, and lobar anatomy is usually lost by the age of

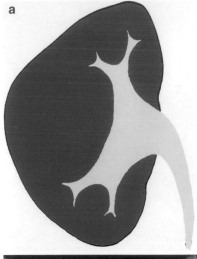

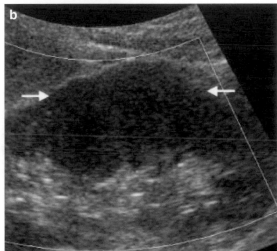

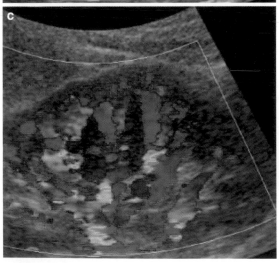

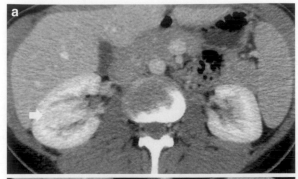

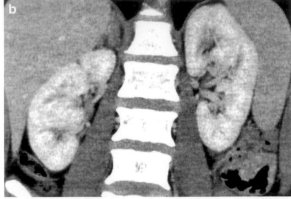

**Fig. 2.21** (**a**, **b**) Renal pseudomass due to hypertrophied column of Bertin. (**a**) Contrast-enhanced CT, nephrographic phase. Transverse plane (**a**) and coronal reformation (**b**). Hypertrophied column of Bertin (*arrows*)

**Fig. 2.20** (**a**) Hypertrophied column of Bertin. (**b**) Gray-scale ultrasound. Renal pseudomass (*arrows*) due to hypertrophied column of Bertin; (**c**) color Doppler ultrasound which reveals normal parenchymal vessels in the pseudomass

and the absence usually regards the left kidney. The infants with this pathology have the following morphological features: an increased distance between the eyes and the presence of epicanthic folds, a low position of the ears, a broad and flat nose, a receding chin, and defects of the limb. Fetal electrolyte balance is kept by exchange through the placental membrane. Renal unilateral or bilateral agenesis probably has multifactorial etiology.

- Unilateral absence of a kidney usually causes no symptoms and is not discovered during infancy because the other kidney undergoes compensatory hypertrophy and performs the function of the absent kidney. Unilateral agenesis is often identified during investigations in other congenital anomalies, or because some urinary tract symptoms appear (Twining 1994). In 20% of the male individuals with renal agenesis, there is an absence of the ipsilateral epididymis, vas deferens, or seminal vesicle, or presence of an associated ipsilateral seminal vesicle cyst. In 70% of women with unilateral renal agenesis, associated genital anomalies are present.

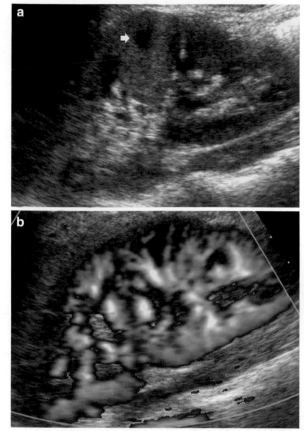

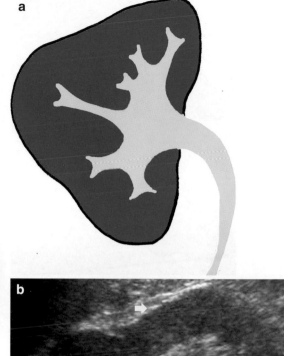

**Fig. 2.22** (**a, b**) Lobar dismorphism. (**a**) Gray-scale ultrasound. A well-defined mass arising from the deep renal parenchyma and isoechoic to the renal cortex projects inside the renal sinus with the evidence of a hypoechoic Malpighi's pyramid (*arrow*). (**b**) Power Doppler ultrasound which reveals normal parenchymal vessels in the pseudomass

**Fig. 2.23** (**a, b**) Dromedary or splenic hump. (**a**) Renal pseudomass due to dromedary hump of the left kidney. (**b**) Gray-scale ultrasound. Longitudinal scan. Prominent bulge on the superolateral border of the left kidney (*arrow*)

- Bilateral renal agenesis is rare 1/3000-4000 deliveries live births) and is incompatible with life. Most infants with bilateral renal agenesis die after birth if the death has not occurred in the fetal life. Associated ureteral abnormalities are universally present including absence of the ipsilateral ureter or presence of a blind-ending ureteral stump. Bilateral agenesis is often associated with oligohydramnios because urine is not excreted into the amniotic fluid (Peipert and Donnenfeld 1991). If the amniotic fluid volume is abnormally decreased, in the absence of other causes, such as rupture of fetal membranes, it must induce to investigate about escretory system anomalies (Mahony 1994).

- Supernumerary kidneys are very rare and result from the formation of two ureteral buds on one side. Usually, the supernumerary kidney occurs on the left side inferior to the normal kidney and is hypoplasic. Supernumerary kidneys may be drained by a bifid ureter draining the second ipsilateral kidney, or by an independent ureter.

- Anomalies of rotation. The fetal kidneys undergo a 90° rotation around the longitudinal axis during their ascent from the pelvis before they reach their final position by the end of the eighth week of fetal life. Malrotation and nonrotation of the kidneys are common anomalies. These anomalies consist in a normal position of the kidney in the flank region, but the long axis is rotated due to the absent 90° rotation of the kidney during proximal migration with the entire process completed by the end of the ninth week (Fig. 2.26). Malrotation is most commonly associated with an ectopic (Fig. 2.27) or

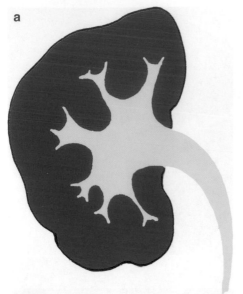

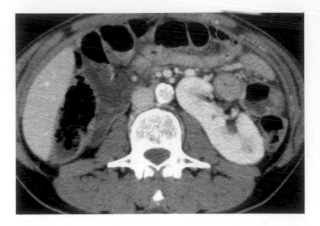

**Fig. 2.25** Contrast-enhanced CT. Nephrographic phase. Agenesia of the right kidney, with the right renal region occupied by the bowel loops. The left kidney presents malrotation

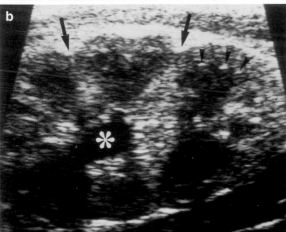

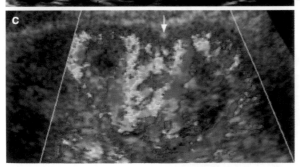

**Fig. 2.24** (**a**) Renal fetal lobations. (**b**) Ultrasound, longitudinal scan. Two notches (*arrows*) on renal profile are visualized, with no reduction of renal cortical thickness with respect to renal medulla (*arrowheads*). (**c**) Normal parenchymal vascularization is visualized by color Doppler in the renal parenchyma between the notch (*arrow*)

fused kidney, but may also occur in kidneys that undergo complete ascent, and may be unilateral or bilateral. Incomplete rotation or nonrotation represents the most common types of rotation anomalies. In this condition, the renal pelvis is in the anterior position or in an intermediate position between the anterior and the normal medial position. In reversed rotation the renal pelvis rotates laterally and the renal vessels are twisted anteriorly around the kidney. In the hyperrotation the kidneys rotate more than 180° but less than 360°, the renal pelvis faces laterally, and the renal vessels are carried posteriorly to the kidney. On intravenous excretory urography (Fig. 2.26) or computed tomography urography (CTU) (Fig. 2.27), renal malrotation is identified as the renal pelvis, instead of arising from the kidney medially, appears to arise centrally. The renal calyces appear often distorted, even without any association with urinary tract obstruction. Some calyces are located medially to the renal pelvis and seem to arise on either side of the pelvis, a hallmark of rotational anomalies. Anomalies of rotation may produce partial ureteropelvic junction obstruction.

- Renal ectopia. Renal ectopia describes the arrest or exaggeration of normal caudal-to-cranial ascent of the kidneys. The autopsy incidence of renal ectopia is about 5.9% (Barakat and Drougas 1991). Renal ectopia is an abnormal location of the kidney or axis orientation or position of renal pelvis due to developmental anomaly (Barakat and Drougas 1991) with kidneys lower or higher than the normal site. Underascent is far more common than

**Fig. 2.26** (**a**, **b**) Intravenous excretory urography. Malrotation of the right kidney. The right renal pelvis appears to arise centrally instead of arising from the kidney medially. Some calyces are located medially to the renal pelvis and seem to arise on either side of the pelvis

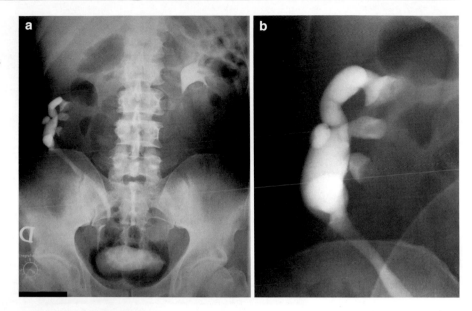

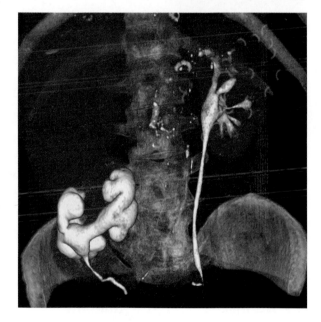

**Fig. 2.27** Computed tomography urography (CTU). Malrotation and ectopia of the right kidney. Color-coded three-dimensional (3D) volume rendering. The right kidney appears on the right pelvic region and its pelvis appearing malrotated with the renal pelvis faces anteriorly and with a short ureter. The right renal kidney appearing ectopic with the ureter length is appropriate for the kidney position

overascent of the kidney. An ectopic kidney undergoes an incomplete rotation around its axis and is malrotated, and the renal pelvis faces anteriorly. Ectopic kidneys tend to be dysplastic and are often associated with contralateral renal anomalies including malrotation, or ectopia of the contralateral kidney. Anomalous blood supply to the kidney, deriving from adjacent vessels, is always present in renal ectopia. In renal ectopia the ureter length is appropriate for the kidney position (Fig. 2.27). The renal collecting system does not drain as readily as in the normal kidney. This results in urinary stasis and in an increased prevalence of stone formation. Bilateral ectopic kidney may fuse. Renal ectopia may also be associated with anomalies of fusion or lateral crossed anomalies. Crosses-fused ectopia is an uncommon congenital anomaly in which one kidney crosses the midline and fuses with the opposite kidney. The ectopic kidney is malrotated and the ureter from the ectopic lower kidney crosses the midline and usually inserts in its normal position. Incrossed renal ectopia both kidneys are on one side of the abdomen. Both kidneys lie to one side of the spine and the ureter of the crossed kidney extends across the midline to enter the bladder on the site opposite to the fused kidney. Pelvic kidney. In the case of a pelvic kidney (1/1,000 live births), also known as renal ptosis, the vascular supply, beside from renal arteries, could come also from branches of the lower abdominal aorta or of the iliac arteries. Pelvic kidneys are usually relatively small and irregular in shape, have a veriable degree of rotation, and may fuse to form a discoid or pancake kidney. Pelvic kidneys are associated with an increased incidence of ureteropelvic junction obstruction. The length of the ureter, which appears tortuous, and the

**Fig. 2.28** (**a**, **b**) Pelvic kidney. (**a**) Computed tomography angiography (CTA) with CTU. 3D volume rendering images maximum intensity projection (MIP) reconstruction, and (**b**) color-coded volume rendering. The renal artery (*arrows*) presents a length appropriate for the kidney position

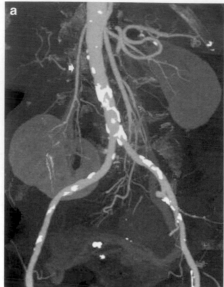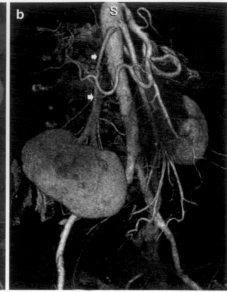

length of the renal artery are not appropriate to the position of the kidney (Fig. 2.28), and it represents an important point in the differentiation from renal ectopia. The principal differential diagnosis are renal allograft (transplanted kidney in iliac fossa), renal autotransplantation (surgical repositioning patient's own kidney), horseshoe kidney, and acquired renal displacement due to large liver, spleen, or any retroperitoneal tumor. Other pelvic kidneys are close to each other and fuse to originate a *discoid* or *pancake kidney*. These kidneys receive the blood from internal or external iliac arteries and/or aorta.

- Fusion anomalies and horseshoe kidney. The horseshoe kidney represents a congenital anomaly of the kidney where two kidneys are fused by isthmus at the lower pole. The horseshoe kidney represents the prototype of abnormalities of renal fusion, a male-to-female predominance (2:1), and is the most common renal anatomical anomaly (1/400 live births). Wilms' tumors are two to eight times more frequent in children with horseshoe kidney than in the general population. If Turner syndrome is present, about 7% of this people have horseshoe kidneys (Behrman et al. 1996). The horseshoe kidney (Fig. 2.29) develops after a midline connection between the two metanephric mass tissues. The midline connection, or isthmus, may consist of a fibrotic band or functional renal parenchyma. The

horseshoe kidney is usually positioned low in the abdomen as a result of the arrest of normal ascent, which is hampered by the origin of the inferior mesenteric artery. The horseshoe kidney is related to an increased incidence of vascular anomalies, ureteropelvic junction obstruction, duplication anomalies, stone formation, and urinary tract infections. The *crossed renal ectopia* (see Chap. 12) appears if a kidney crosses to the other side with or without fusion. Infrequently, *unilateral fused kidney* develops. The kidneys fuse while they are in the pelvis, and when a kidney ascends to its final position, it brings the other one with it.

## 2.3 Normal Radiological Anatomy of Renal Vessels and Anatomical Variants

Traditionally, the evaluation of renal vascular abnormalities was performed with conventional angiography. Cross-sectional imaging now plays an important and increasing role in evaluating renal vascular abnormalities in both the native and transplant kidneys.

The renal arteries originate directly from the aorta and course posteriorly and laterally to the renal parenchyma. Single renal arteries to each kidney most

**Fig. 2.29** (**a–c**) ) Horseshoe kidney with the two kidneys fused by isthmus at the lower pole. (**a**) CTU; (**b, c**) 3D maximum intensity projection with evidence of the horseshoe kidney (*arrow*)

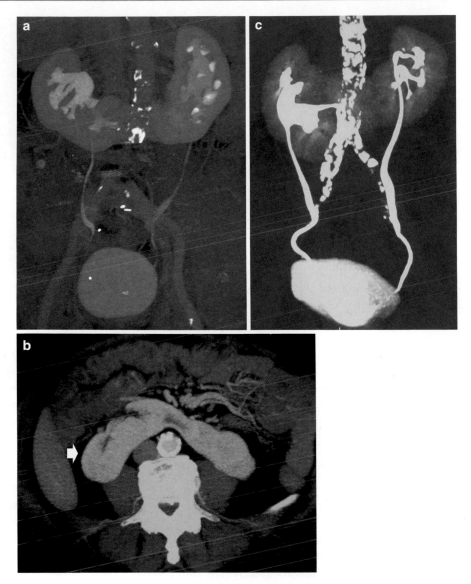

commonly arise from the abdominal aorta near the L1–2 level. The right renal artery usually originates from the anterolateral aspect of the aorta, while the left renal artery usually originates from a posterolateral aspect of the aorta. The renal arteries assume a dorso-infero-lateral course until they enter the kidney at the renal hilum. Renal arteries originate 1–2 cm below the level of origin of the superior mesenteric artery. Normally, each kidney is supplied by a single renal artery and a single renal vein, arising from the abdominal aorta and the inferior vena cava, respectively. These vessels typically originate off the aorta, at the level of L1–L2, below the takeoff of the superior

mesenteric artery (SMA), with the vein anterior to the artery. Both vessels then course anterior to the renal pelvis before entering the medial aspect of the renal hilum. The right renal artery typically demonstrates a long downward course to the relatively inferior right kidney, traversing behind the inferior vena cava. Conversely, the left renal artery, which arises below the right renal artery and has a more horizontal orientation, has a rather direct upward course to the more superiorly positioned left kidney. In addition, both renal arteries course in a slightly posterior direction because of the position of the kidneys. Depiction of the relatively avascular plane between the anterior and posterior arterial divisions of the kidney is of importance to the surgeon, because it allows for a clean incision toward the renal pelvis at the time of surgery. This is usually located one third of the distance between the posterior and anterior surfaces of the kidney. A similar avascular transverse plane exists between the posterior renal segment and the polar renal segments.

The renal venous anatomy parallels the arterial anatomy. The renal cortex is drained sequentially by the interlobular veins, arcuate veins, interlobar veins, and lobar veins. The lobar veins join to form the main renal vein. The renal vein usually lies anterior to the renal artery at the renal hilum. The left renal vein is longer than the right renal vein. The left renal vein averages 6–10 cm in length and will normally course anteriorly between the SMA and the aorta before emptying into the medial aspect of the inferior vena cava. The right renal vein averages 2–4 cm in length and joins the lateral aspect of inferior vena cava (IVC). Unlike the right renal vein, the left renal vein receives several tributaries before joining the inferior vena cava. It receives the left adrenal vein superiorly, the left gonadal vein inferiorly, and a lumbar vein posteriorly.

### 2.3.1 Gray-Scale and Doppler Ultrasound

The principal renal arteries may be clearly identified at their origin from the abdominal aorta (Fig. 2.30). Doppler US evaluation of the main renal arteries is highly related to operator experience, especially in situations such as patient obesity, intervening bowel gas, or deep renal arteries location. The principal renal artery is often difficult to be detected at baseline color Doppler US for the perpendicular position to the ultrasound beam direction and for the depth position. Since accessory renal arteries occur in up to 25% of patients and may contain stenoses determining renovascular hypertension (Grant and Melany 2001), the visibility of these vessels is very important for a complete diagnostic work-up of the patient. The velocitometric analysis of Doppler trace derived from renal arteries is of primary importance to identify renal artery stenosis. Direct Doppler criteria have been proposed for the detection of renal arterial stenosis, including an increased peak systolic velocity (>150–180 cm/s) and end diastolic velocity at the

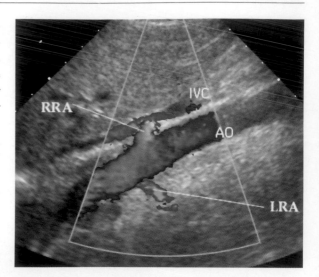

**Fig. 2.30** Color Doppler ultrasound longitudinal scan. Normal anatomy of the main renal arteries at the origin from the aorta (*AO* aorta; *IVC* inferior vena cava; *RRA* right renal artery; *LRA* left renal artery)

level of the stenosis (Correas et al. 1999; Grant and Melany 2001), poststenotic flow disturbance resulting in spectral broadening and reversed flow (Correas et al. 1999), increased ratio (≥3.5) of peak systolic velocity in renal artery and aorta (renal-aortic ratio), and the presence of turbulence within the renal artery (Desberg et al. 1990; Helenon et al. 1995). Although this technique is easy to perform, its accuracy is questionable because the lack of an early systolic peak has a low sensitivity for moderate stenoses and the waveform is dependent on the maintenance of vessel compliance, which limits its effectiveness in elderly patients and patients with atherosclerosis (Bude et al. 1994; Bude and Rubin 1995).

### 2.3.2 CT Angiography

Computed tomography angiography (CTA) is now considered a fundamental technique in the assessment of the renal arteries (Fig. 2.31). 3D volume-rendered (CTA) provides a fast, noninvasive modality for the evaluation of the renal vessels. CTA can reliably and accurately depict the renal arteries and veins as conventional angiography in the assessment of most vascular abnormalities. The number, size, course, and relationship of the renal vasculature are easily

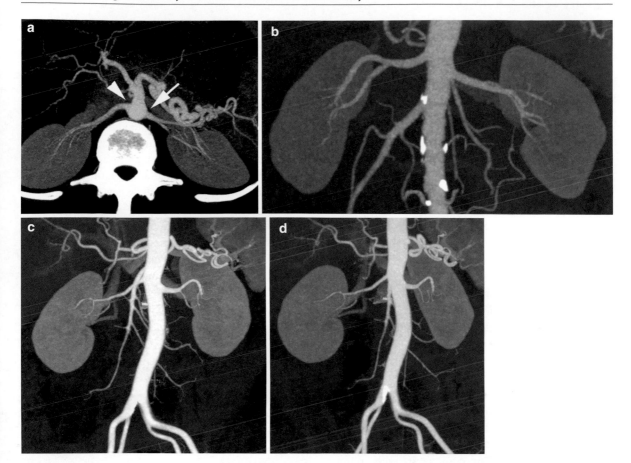

**Fig. 2.31** (**a**–**d**) Normal anatomy of the renal arteries (*arrows*) as seen on contrast-enhanced angio-CT. Maximum intensity projection. (**a**) Transverse plane. Maximum intensity projection reconstruction shows the posterolateral origin of the left renal artery (*arrow*) and anterolateral origin of the right (*arrowhead*). (courtesy of Dr. Therese M. Weber, Department of Radiology, University of Alabama at Birmingham.) (**b**) Coronal reformation of renal arteries and abdominal aorta. (**c**, **d**) Rotation of the 3D data set allows the accurate assessment of the origin of both renal arteries

appreciated utilizing real-time interactive editing. The CTA protocol requests a double scout view and the following scanning parameters for 64-row CT: beam collimation, 0.5 mm × 64; normalized pitch, 0.828; revolution time, 0.4 s; bolus tracking. Of the many 3D reconstruction algorithms available for performing CTA, volume rendering has emerged as the rendering technique of choice. With volume rendering, the user can actively interact with the dataset, editing and modifying the position, orientation, opacity, and brightness of the image in real-time. For CTA, volume rendering is commonly preformed with a window/level transfer function that results in high-density material (for example, enhanced vessels or vascular calcifications) to appear bright and opaque, while less-dense structures appear dim and translucent. Overlying structures are easily removed with an interactive clip-plane, and the vessels of interest are easily rotated into the best orientation for depiction of the region of interest. For evaluation of the renal hilum, axial, coronal, and sagittal views are often used in conjunction with optimal evaluation of the number, caliber, and course of the renal arteries and veins. Perspective rendering allows the user to view the dataset from within the vessel, producing angioscopic views which are also helpful for identifying a vascular orifice and stenosis. Volume-rendered CTA can very quickly and accurately determine the location and course of the renal vascular anatomy. Angioscopic and maximum intensity projection (MIP) views provide additional information on the renal vascular anatomy and compliment conventional volume-rendered images. Typically, arterial branches can be confidently identified to at least the segmental level. Limitation for detection occurs with vessels smaller than 2 mm in size. Sensitivity for the demonstration and location of main renal arteries, however, approaches 100%. Surgical and CT findings correlate in over 95% of cases. The renal venous anatomy is also well demonstrated with CTA and is especially important to document for patients undergoing evaluation for laparoscopic donor nephrectomy. The left renal anatomy is especially critical, and this is the preferred side for donation. Tributaries into the left renal vein, especially posterior lumbar branches, are confidently displayed and are of potential surgical importance if noted to be enlarged. MIP represents the other common reconstruction algorithm commonly employed when evaluating the renal vasculature. The MIP technique evaluates each voxel from the viewers' eye through the dataset and selects the maximal voxel value as the value of the corresponding displayed pixel. The image produced lacks depth orientation, but a 3D effect can be produced with rotational viewing of multiple projections. MIP images can provide useful information regarding atherosclerotic burden, vascular stents, and vascular stenoses and are often reconstructed and interpreted in conjunction with volume-rendered images.

## 2.3.3 MR Angiography

Magnetic resonance arteriography (MRA) provides an alternative to intra-arterial digital subtraction angiography in the detection and staging of structural abnormalities of the aorta and its branches. It uses no ionizing radiation and does not require arterial access. A number of imaging techniques have been developed to visualize the circulation using MR imaging, including "black blood" techniques, two-dimensional (2D) and 3D time of flight (TOF) methods, phase contrast (PC) techniques, and 3D contrast-enhanced methods using gadolinium compounds and other paramagnetic or superparamagnetic agents. The most commonly used are 2D-TOF MRA and 3D-contrast-enhanced methods (Grist 2000). For the evaluation of renal artery stenosis, both 2D-TOF MRA and PC methods are generally limited to the assessment of the proximal portion of the renal artery because the long acquisition times preclude breath-hold imaging. 3D contrast-enhanced methods, which require the intravenous administration of a contrast agent, overcome many of the limitations of 2D-TOF MRA.

Contrast-enhanced 3D MR angiography (Fig. 2.32) has become the standard technique for renal artery MR angiography due to its speed, high SNR, minimal artifacts, and relatively high spatial resolution. In particular, the use of an MR contrast agent is reported to reduce artifacts in the image and allow images to be acquired more rapidly, both of which should result in an improvement in overall accuracy of the techniqu e. Clinical practice today usually uses a double dose (≈0.2 mmol/kg bw) of contrast agent for CE-MRAs. Lowering the dose would result in considerably lower costs and lower risk for nephrogenic systemic fibrosis induction.

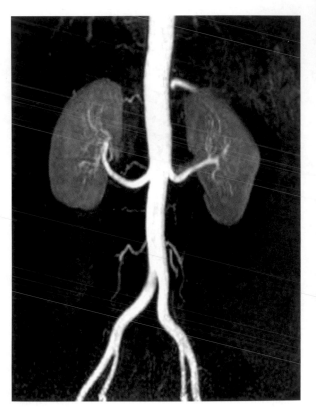

**Fig. 2.32** Normal anatomy of the renal arteries as seen on angio-MR, after Gd-based agent injection

## 2.3.4 Anatomical Variants of Renal Vessels

Knowledge of the variations in renal vascular anatomy is important for renal transplantation surgery and before laparoscopic donor or partial nephrectomy and vascular reconstruction for renal artery stenosis or abdominal aortic aneurysm. Recently, multidetector CTA has become a principal imaging investigation for the assessment of the renal vasculature and has challenged the role of conventional angiography (Türkvatan et al. 2009). It is an excellent imaging technique because it is a fast and noninvasive tool that provides highly accurate and detailed evaluation of normal renal vascular anatomy and variants. The number, size, and course of the renal arteries and veins are easily identified by CTA. In about one third of the general population, there are variations in number, location, and branching patterns of the renal arteries, with over 30% of subjects having one or more accessory renal arteries. Familiarity with anatomic variants and their associations contributes to the safety and success of both open and minimally invasive renal surgery.

- Early branching of renal artery. The main renal artery originates at a more or less constant position opposite the renal hilus, from the abdominal aorta, and continues undivided in its straight course to the renal hilum except for small branches including the inferior adrenal, the perirenal, and the ureteral arteries (Fig. 2.2a). Frequently, the renal artery presents early branching and this may have important implications in renal surgery. Prehilar arterial branching is a common variant necessary for the detection of patients undergoing evaluation for donor nephrectomy (Fig. 2.33). A person with early branching of the renal artery might be considered a poor candidate as a potential living renal donor.

- Hilar and extrahilar accessory renal arteries. An accessory renal artery, other than the main renal artery, is one that arises from the aorta and terminates in the kidney (Satyapall et al. 2001). Accessory renal arteries have also been described as additional, supernumerary, or supplementary. Accessory renal arteries arise from the aorta anywhere from the level of T11 to the level of L4, but may rarely originate from the iliac arteries or superior mesenteric artery. Accessory renal arter- ies are the sole renal arteries which supply a portion of the renal parenchyma (Fig. 2.34). They are seen in up to 25–28% of patients (Satyapall et al. 2001). In healthy adults, the mean maximum diameter of the renal artery lumen is about 5–6 mm. The diameter of accessory renal arteries is highly variable, but it is generally equal to or smaller than the main renal artery. Frequently the accessory artery is visualized coursing into the renal hilum to vascularize the lower renal pole (Fig. 2.35). Accessory renal arteries may be a contraindication to laparoscopic donor nephrectomy, and injury of a crossing vessel during endopyelotomy for ure- teropelvic junction obstruction may result in severe hemorrhage (Yeh et al. 2004). The polar or extrahilar arteries may be ligated or transacted unintentionally during renal, aortic, or other retro- peritoneal abdominal surgeries. Accessory renal arteries usually arise inferior to the main renal artery, but occasionally will supply the upper pole of the kidney. Renal anomalies such as horseshoe or pelvic kidney almost always have multiple renal arteries that arise from the aorta or iliac arteries. Accessory renal arteries are now routinely seen on CTA or MRA, but are frequently not noted on renal Doppler.

- Right renal artery passing anteriorly to the inferior vena cava. Right renal arteries are traditionally described as passing posterior to the inferior vena cava, although dominant and accessory right renal arteries that pass anteriorly to the inferior vena cava (Fig. 2.36) have been described in about 5% of patients and the anterior rotation of the lower pole of the right kidney should prompt a search for pre- caval renal arteries (Yeh et al. 2004). A right renal artery that passes anterior to the inferior vena cava is of particular importance for presurgical plan- ning, because it may be injured inadvertently, espe- cially during the retroperitoneal approach when only the right gonadal vein is expected to lie in the precaval area.

- Renal vein anomalies. Anomalies of the renal veins are less common than those of the arteries, but are encountered in clinical practice and may have important implications. All anomalies are variations of the embryological development and represent a persistence of portions of the paired longitudinal channels, the subcardinal and supracardinal veins,

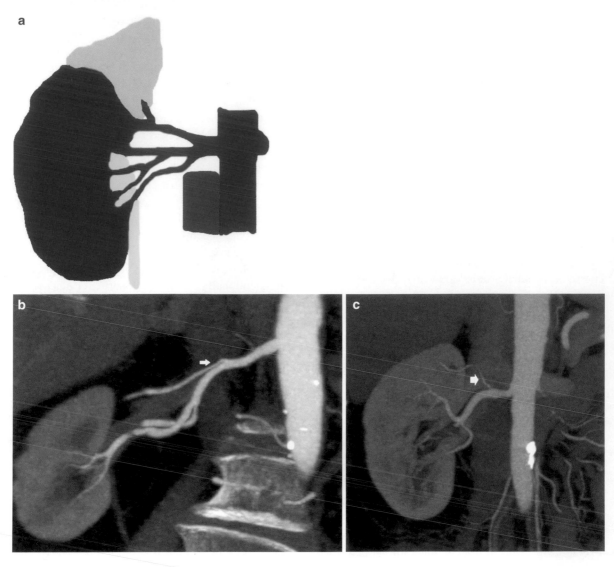

**Fig. 2.33** (**a–c**) Early branchings of right renal artery (*arrows*). (**a**) Scheme; (**b, c**) CTA, coronal reformations

which form a ladderlike collar around the aorta. Normally, only the anterior components persist, becoming the renal veins, which course anterior to the aorta. Accessory renal veins are less frequent than accessory renal arteries and are more common on the right than the left. Left renal vein variants include the circumaortic and retroaortic renal veins. Knowledge of these anomalies becomes important in surgical planning, IVC filter placement, and collection of renal or adrenal vein samples. The most common anomaly of the left renal venous system is the circumaortic renal vein (Fig. 2.37). The circumaortic renal vein represents persistence of the

posteriorly located left supracardinal vein and a midline supracardinal anastomosis between right and left vessels. This anomaly has been reported in 2–16% of patients, based on anatomic and angiographic studies. Persistence of the whole collar results in a circumaortic renal vein, which is a more common anomaly than an isolated retroaortic renal vein. In this anomaly, the left renal vein bifurcates into ventral and dorsal limb, which encircles the abdominal aorta. Less common is the retroaortic renal vein (Fig. 2.38), seen in up to 4% of patients. Here, the single left renal vein courses posterior to the aorta and drains into the lower lumbar

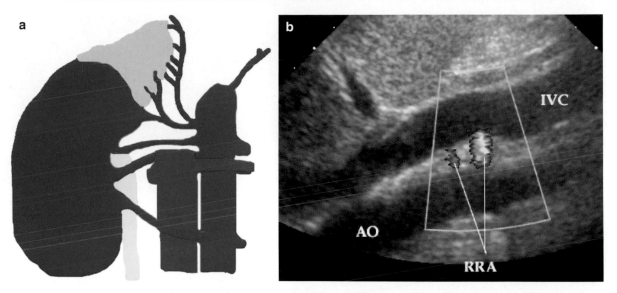

**Fig. 2.34** (**a**) Scheme representing both hilar and extrahilar accessory renal arteries. (**b**) Color Doppler US. The main and accessory renal arteries at their origin from the abdominal aorta

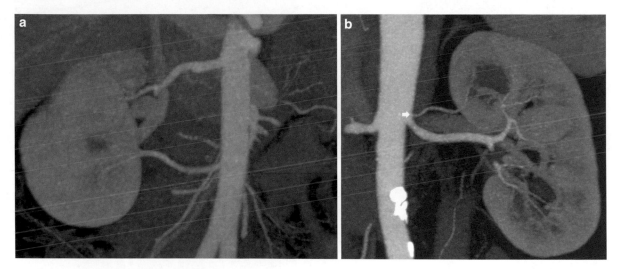

**Fig. 2.35** (**a–d**) Hilar (**a**), and extrahilar (**b**) accessory renal arteries perfusing the upper renal pole. (**b**) The extrahilar accessory renal artery vascularizes the upper renal pole (*white arrow*) originates immediately above the origin of the main renal artery and it appears hypoplasic in comparison with the main renal artery. (**c, d**) The accessory renal artery vascularizing the lower renal pole (*white arrow*) may originate immediately above (**c**) or below (**d**) the origin of the main renal artery (*black arrow*) and it may appear hypoplasic in comparison with the main renal artery (**c**) or with a diameter similar to the main renal artery (**d**). A renal carcinoma is also evident in the lower renal pole on the (**d**) image

portion of the IVC. In addition, multiple renal veins are seen in approximately 15% of the patients. Supernumerary renal veins often are retroaortic when present on the left. The retroaortic left renal vein occurs less frequently. Reed et al. (1982) reported from a CT series that 1.8% of patients have a single retroaortic renal vein. In a recent study by Karazincir et al. (2007), the incidence of retroaortic left renal vein was found to be significantly higher in patients with varicocele compared with control patients. The left renal vein receives drainage from the inferior phrenic, capsular, ureteric, adrenal, and gonadal veins. In patients with a left-sided IVC, the left common iliac vein continues cranially as the

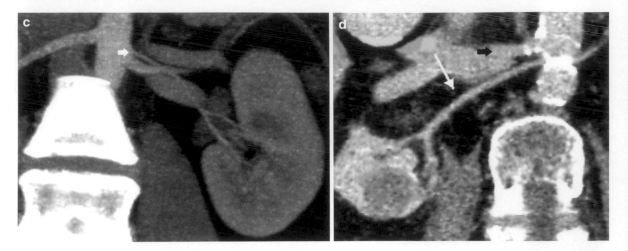

**Fig. 2.35** (continued)

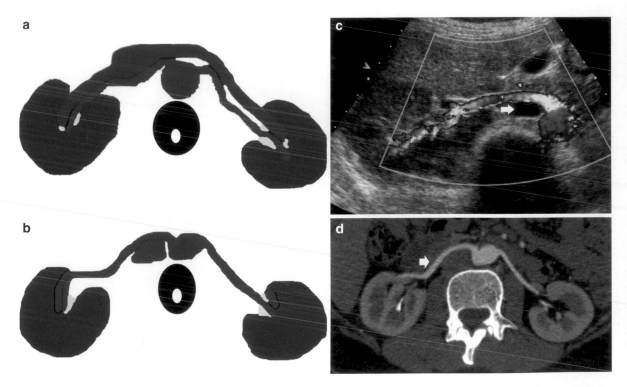

**Fig. 2.36** (a) Scheme. Normal anatomy of the renal vessels on the transverse plane. (b) Scheme. Precaval right renal artery. (c) Color Doppler US. Transverse plane. Precaval right renal artery (*arrow*). (d) CTA. Precaval renal artery (*arrow*)

left IVC and drains into the inferior aspect of the left renal vein. The right renal vein is shorter than the left and courses obliquely into the IVC. The right renal vein receives capsular and ureteric veins; however, the right inferior phrenic and gonadal veins enter directly into the IVC. Valves may be present within the renal veins with marked variation in the reported incidence. Renal vein varices may be secondary to renal vein thrombosis or portal hypertension, or may be idiopathic. Like varicoceles, renal varices are more common on the left than on the right. The "nutcracker" phenomenon results from

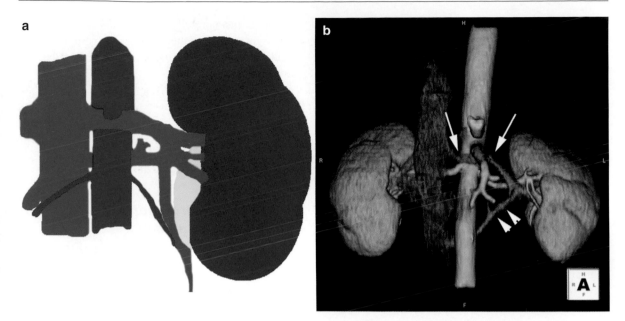

**Fig. 2.37** (**a, b**) Anatomical variants of renal veins. (**a**) The left renal vein bifurcates into ventral and dorsal limb which encircle the abdominal aorta. (**b**) Coronal volume reconstructed image of CTA shows the preaortic venous component (*arrows*) at the level of the renal arteries and retroaortic component more caudally located (*arrowheads*). (courtesy of Dr. Therese M. Weber; Dept of Radiology; University of Alabama at Birmingham)

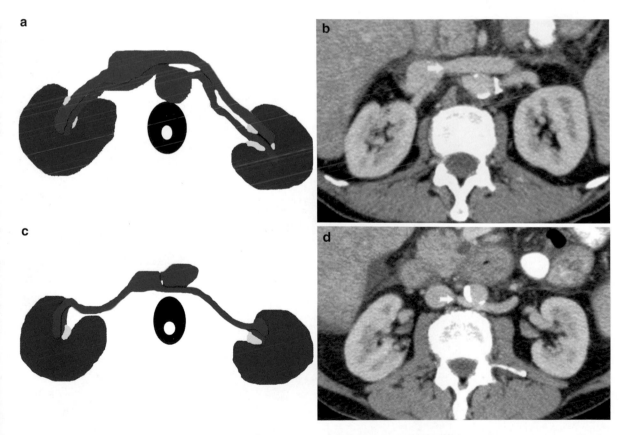

**Fig. 2.38** (**a**) Scheme. Normal anatomy of the renal vessels on the transverse plane. (**b**) Contrast-enhanced CT. Transverse plane. Normal anatomy of the left renal vein (*arrow*) passing anteriorly to the aorta. (**c**) Scheme. Retroaortic left renal vein. (**d**) Retroaortic left renal vein (*arrow*)

compression of the left renal vein between the superior mesenteric artery and the aorta and may lead to left renal vein hypertension, hematuria, and varix formation. It is important to remember that a distended left renal vein may be seen in 51–72% of the normal population by CT, MR, or ultrasound (Buschi et al. 1980). Therefore, measurement of a pressure gradient between the IVC and the left renal vein needs to be done before renal vein compression diagnosis. Color Doppler may provide noninvasive evidence of renal vein compression when collateral veins are demonstrated. In cases of renal vein thrombosis, collateral pathways through the inferior phrenic, adrenal, gonadal, and ureteric veins may be involved with left renal vein thrombosis, while only the ureteric vein forms collaterals with the right renal vein.

- Venous anomalies may also affect the ureter, such as a circumcaval or retrocaval ureter, which are very rare. A circumcaval ureter occurs more commonly in men than women and is usually an incidental finding. Persistence of the right subcardinal vein traps the ureter behind the IVC. The ureter passes posterior to the IVC, then crosses anteriorly around the medial border of the cava to partially encircle the IVC. On CT, the IVC will have a more lateral location than normally seen, usually lying lateral to the right pedicle of the third lumbar vertebral body, and the course of the opacified ureter can be followed around the IVC.

## 2.4 Normal Radiological Anatomy of the Urinary Tract and Anatomical Variants

### 2.4.1 Excretory Urography and Anterograde and Retrograde Pyelography

Intravenous urography is the examination traditionally employed to assess the urinary tract pathology (Fig. 2.39), and it was used for a large variety of clinical indications. Its utilization decreased when each of these indications was shown not to be clinically valid and cross-sectional imaging techniques have since proved superior to intravenous urography for most, if not all, remaining indications (Silverman et al. 2009). Even until the late 1990s, intravenous urography, because of its superior spatial resolution, was still

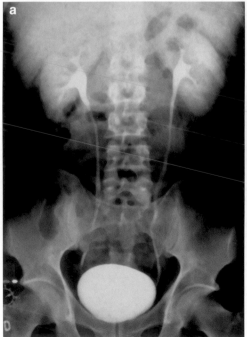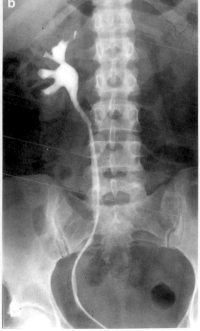

**Fig. 2.39** (**a**, **b**) Normal anatomy of the intrarenal urinary tract. (**a**) Intravenous excretory urography; (**b**) retrograde pyelography

considered the examination of choice for evaluating the urothelium (Silverman et al. 2009). When unenhanced CT was shown to reliably detect urolithiasis, intravenous urography was pronounced dead in 1999 with the caveat that there might remain rare instances in which it is an appropriate examination (Amis 1999).

The usual examination protocol employed in the intravenous urography is variable between the different imaging departments. The fundamental examination included a preliminary plain radiograph of the abdomen and nephrotomograms from 60 to 90 s after iodinated contrast agent injection to assess cortical nephrogram representing contrast material within the tubules. Then a radiograph on the renal urinary tract is obtained 5–7 min after contrast injection, and under balloon ureteral compression, while a panoramic radiograph of the whole urinary tract is obtained 15 min after contrast injection after removal of the balloon compression employed to assess the whole urinary tract. Finally, 20–30 min after contract injection, radiographs were performed on the bladder.

When depicted frontally (Fig. 2.40), a minor calyx appears circular, while when depicted in profile, the minor calyx is concave connected to two well-defined, sharp forniceal angles (Fig. 2.41). All branches from the pelvis, whether single or multiple, are defined infundibula. The infundibulum is also known as major calyx.

Anterograde pyelography is the evaluation of the urinary tract after the injection of the iodinated contrast agent in the renal pelvis after a nephrostomy procedure. The principal indication is the assessment of hydro-ureteronephrosis to identify the nature and the level of the obstruction in a functionally excluded kidney (absence of contrast excretion after 24 h from i.v. contrast administration) or to assess the correct position of a nephrostomy drainage. Retrograde pyelography (Fig. 2.39b) is performed after incannulation of the interior ureteral meatus, and its principal indication is the assessment of opacification defects of the urinary tract. It is invasive and rarely performed.

## 2.4.2 CT Urography

Nowadays, the development of CT urography (CTU) (Fig. 2.42) has completely covered all the clinical indications previously addressed by intravenous urography. The term CTU is often used in clinical practice for a multitude of multidetector computed tomography (MDCT) techniques for the evaluation of the urinary tract. CTU became conceptually possible with the advent of MDCT, the final technologic advance needed to image the urothelium in detail (Silverman et al. 2009). MDCT provides the ability to obtain thin (submillimeter) collimated data of the entire urinary tract during a short, single breath-hold (Van Der Molen et al. 2008). The resulting thin-section images provided higher spatial resolution relative to that of single-detector CT scans (although not as high as with intravenous urography). Also, isotropic voxels allowed images of equal spatial resolution to be obtained in any plane. The term CTU is often used in clinical practice for a multitude of MDCT techniques for the evaluation of the urinary tract. The indications for CT were expanded to include hematuria (Joffe et al. 2003), and CTU has essentially replaced intravenous urography in most imaging practices. Symptomatic hematuria in patients younger than 40 years should be evaluated by unenhanced CT for the identification of calculi, while asymptomatic hematuria in patients older than 40 years should be evaluated by CTU. Even though urinary tract calculi, bladder tumors, and prostate-related process are the most common causes of hematuria, upper urinary tract urothelial neoplasms must be excluded frequently. Other indications for CTU are the identification of congenital malformations of the intrarenal excretory tract (e.g., in patients in whom a lithotripsy procedure is scheduled), renal infections, renal tuberculosis, suspected papillary necrosis, identification and staging of renal tumors, renal traumas, characterization of complicated (e.g., hemorrhagic cysts) or complex renal masses (e.g., renal tumors with a solid and cystic component), renal colic and acute flank pain, and ureteral pathology.

## 2.4.3 Magnetic Resonance Imaging and MR Urography

MR urography has received a relatively lower attention than MDCT urography, being hampered by the low spatial resolution, which is crucial for calyceal evaluation and by the requirement of updated MR units. However, excellent contrast resolution and lack

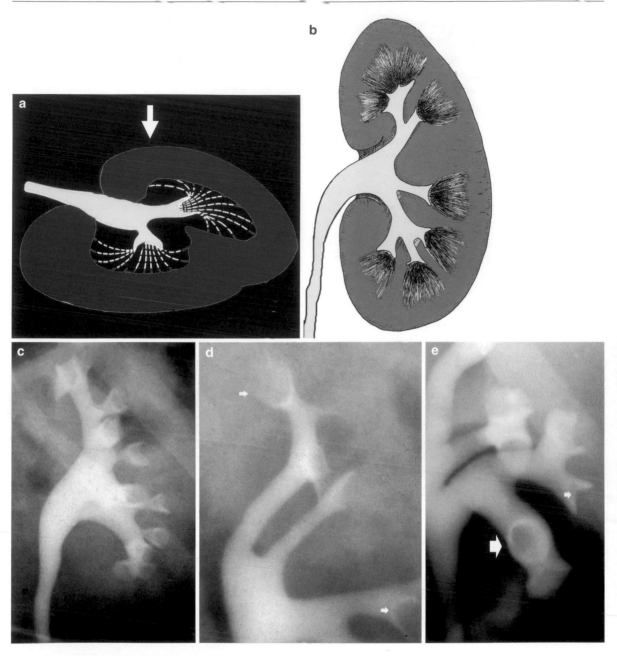

**Fig. 2.40** (**a–e**) Normal appearance of the intrarenal urinary tract as seen on intravenous urography according to the X-ray beam incidence (*arrow*). (**a–c**) Normal 5-min urogram with orthogonal incidence of the X-ray beam. The renal pelvis branches to form infundibula. (**c**) The calyx is formed by the impression of the papilla, and the fornix is the side of the calyx. The calyx is a concave structure receiving the tip of the papilla of the renal medulla, and the fornices represent the side projections of the calyx surrounding the papilla. (**d, e**) When depicted frontally a minor calyx appears circular (*large arrow*), while when depicted in profile (*small arrows*) the minor calyx is concave connected to two well-defined, sharp forniceal angles

of ionizing radiation make MR urography a useful technique for noninvasively evaluating the entire urinary tract, especially when ionizing radiation is to be avoided, such as in pediatric or pregnant patients. The MR urographic techniques can be divided into two categories: static-fluid MR urography and excretory MR urography.

The static-fluid MR urography (Fig. 2.43) utilizes unenhanced, heavily T2-weighted pulse sequences to image the urinary tract. On the heavily T2 weighted

**Fig. 2.41** (**a–d**) Normal appearance of the intrarenal urinary tract as seen on intravenous urography according to the X-ray beam incidence (arrow). (**a, b**) Schemes representing the incidence of the X-ray beam (**a**) and the resulting image (**b**). (**c, d**) Normal 5-min excretory urogram with a progressive increasing obliquity of the incidence of the X-ray beam  The minor calyx is concave (*small arrows*) connected to well-defined, sharp forniceal angles

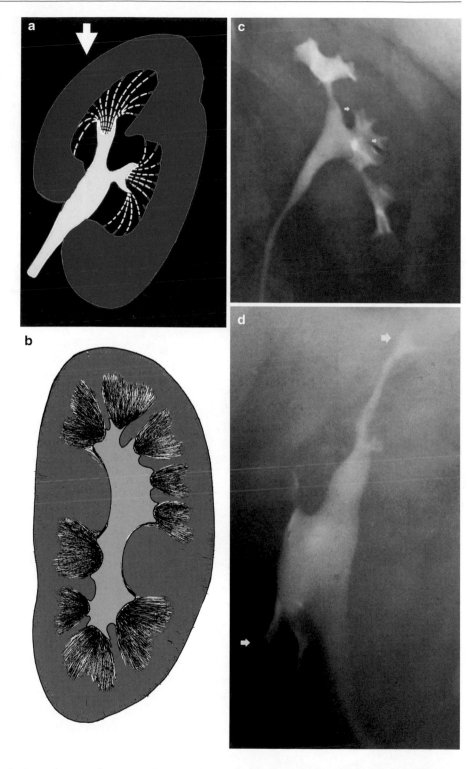

images, the urinary tract is hyperintense because of its long relaxation time, independent of the excretory renal function. This technique is ideally suited for patients with dilated or obstructed collecting system. In excretory MR urography (Fig. 2.44), intravenous gadolinium is combined with a T1-weighted 3D gradient echo (GRE) sequence. The practicability of excretory MR urography depends on the ability of the kidneys to excrete the intravenously administered gadolinium agent. Administration of low-dose furosemide

**Fig. 2.42** (**a**, **b**) Normal
anatomy and anatomical
variants of the renal calices
and pelvis as seen on CTU.
(**a**) 3D maximum intensity
projection; (**b**) 3D color-
coded volume rendering

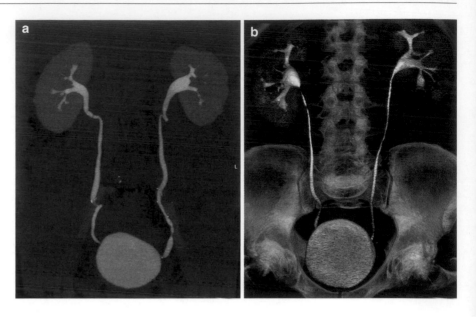

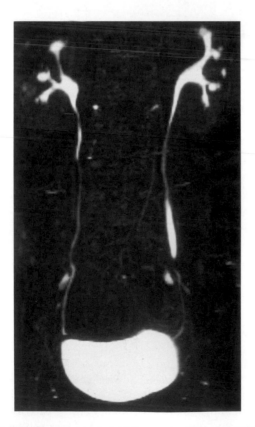

**Fig. 2.43** Normal anatomy of the renal calices and pelvis as
seen on static-fluid MR urography

can improve the quality of excretory MR urography
by enhancing urine flow, and therefore, providing a
uniform distribution of the contrast material inside the
entire urinary tract. Excretory MR urography provides
high-quality images of both nondilated and obstructed
collecting systems.

Early practitioners of MR urography used
T2-weighted techniques alone, such as rapid acquisition with relaxation enhancement (RARE) and
half-Fourier acquisition single-shot turbo spin echo
(HASTE), to image the renal collecting systems, ureters, and bladder, essentially treating the urinary tract
as a static collection of fluid. T2-weighted MR techniques rely on the intrinsically high-signal intensity of
urine for image contrast, and therefore, do not require
the administration of intravenous contrast material.
Coronal T2-weighted images of the entire urinary tract
were particularly attractive since they mimicked the
images obtained with intravenous urography. The main
appeal of these techniques was that they could be performed quickly and in any image plane. Furthermore,
because T2-weighted MR urography techniques could
be performed without ionizing radiation or intravenous contrast material, they were considered to have
their greatest utility in children, pregnant women, or
other patients in whom intravenous contrast material
was contraindicated. However, the clinical utility of
MR urography performed with T2-weighted imaging

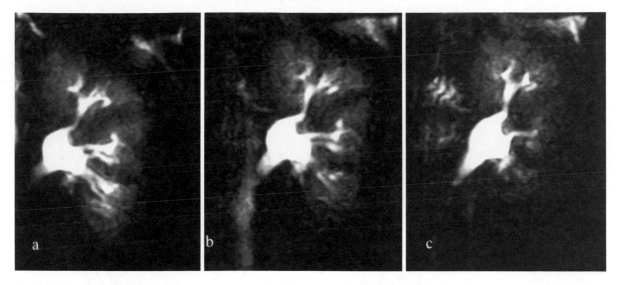

**Fig. 2.44** (**a–c**) Normal MR excretory urography after Gd-based contrast agent injection

alone is limited in patients with nondistended urinary collecting systems. For urinary tracts that are not distended, imaging with a full urinary bladder can improve upper tract visualization, but additional techniques are needed often.

The challenge of MR urography is to obtain diagnostic quality images of the KUB within a reasonable amount of time while limiting the effects of respiratory motion, ureteral peristalsis, and flowing urine. Impediments to addressing this challenge satisfactorily include a finite SNR for a given MR system and the limited breath-holding capacity of patients. Because SNR constrains the maximum interpretable resolution achievable with MR imaging, MR urography is best performed with a phased-array surface coil; these coils increase SNR. Exceptions include some gravid patients in the latter stages of pregnancy and large patients whom the imager bore cannot accommodate with a surface coil in place. Depending on the MR imaging system, some surface coils limit the field of view to less than that required to encompass the kidneys and bladder in a single acquisition. In such cases, the urinary tract is imaged in segments, repositioning the surface coil as necessary.

Further increases in SNR can be achieved by imaging patients with higher field strength, 3.0-T MR systems. The SNR gained when moving from 1.5 to 3.0 T can be used to improve spatial or temporal resolution. Theoretically, improvements in spatial resolution could improve detection of small urothelial lesions, although this has not been systematically studied to date. Additionally, there is evidence to suggest that the conspicuity of enhancement related to gadolinium chelates increases at 3.0 T relative to 1.5 T, although the impact of this difference is unknown for MR urography. The potential benefits of 3.0-T MR imaging must be weighed against the limitations inherent to higher field strength imaging, such as increased specific absorption rate, prolonged T1 relaxation times, and worsening of some artifacts.

The principal indications for the MR urography are the evaluation of urothelial tumors, anomalies of the urinary tract, and the assessment of urinary tract dilatation and obstructive disease.

### 2.4.4 Anatomical Variants of the Urinary Tract

Intravenous excretory urography and CTU provide a reliable depiction of the intrarenal urinary tract, which presents an extremely variable morphology (Figs. 2.45–2.47). Congenital variants of the pelvocalyceal system are common and may be observed in about 4% of the general population. The renal pelvis may present a

**Fig. 2.45** (**a–i**) Scheme. Different morphologies of the upper urinary tract including calyces, infundibula, and pelvis which can be identified on intravenous excretory urography or CT urography.

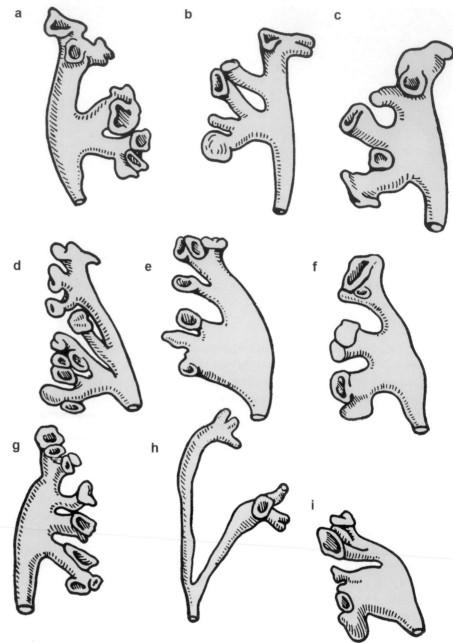

**Fig. 2.46** (**a–d**) Intravenous excretory urography. Different morphologies of the upper urinary tract

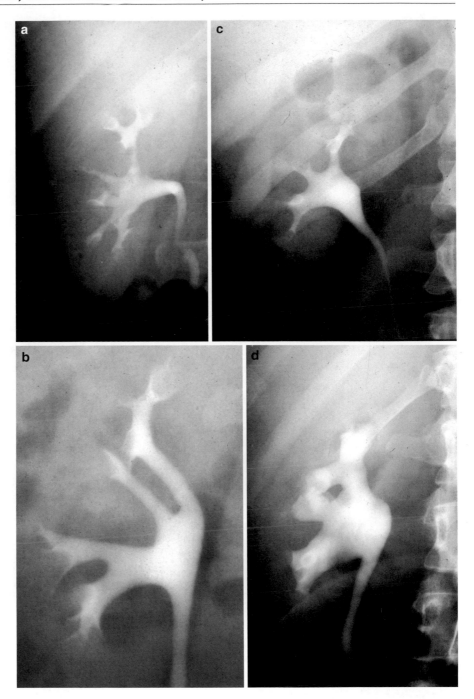

**Fig. 2.47** (**a–d**) CT urography. Different morphologies of the upper urinary tract. (**a**, **b**) Usual morphology of the renal calyces and renal pelvis with a progressive more clear division between the upper and lower group calyces; (**c**, **d**) bifid renal pelvis

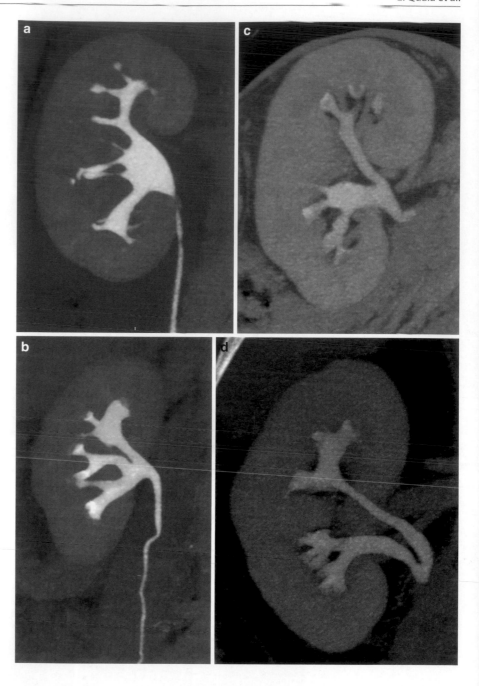

progressively increasing separation between the upper and lower group renal calyces (Figure 2.47), and it may be completely intrarenal, completely extrarenal, or a combination of both (Figure 2.48) (Friedenberg and Dunbar 1990).

The renal calyx is a concave structure receiving the tip of the papilla of the renal medulla, and the fornices represent the side projections of the calyx surrounding the papilla (Fig. 2.40). Frequently, multiple single calyces fail to completely divide and form a larger compound calyx, which is normally seen in the upper and lower poles of the kidney (Figs. 2.49 and 2.50). Compound calyces present a distorted shape and the circular shape of the minor calyx is frequently not present. Multiple papillae (two or more) draining into a single calyx are defined as a compound calyx. The average number of

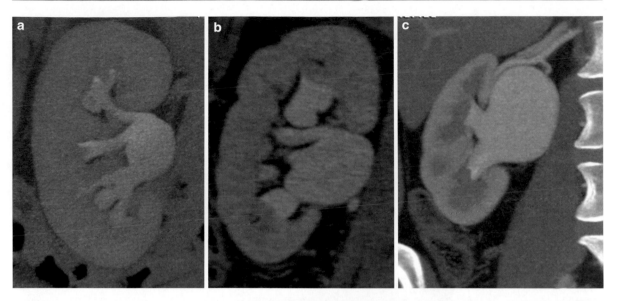

**Fig. 2.48** (**a–c**) CTU. Normal appearance of renal pelvis and renal calyces, and anatomical variants. (**a**) Distended pelvis; intrarenal (**b**) and extrarenal (**c**) ampullary pelvis in which calyces open in a common dilated pelvis

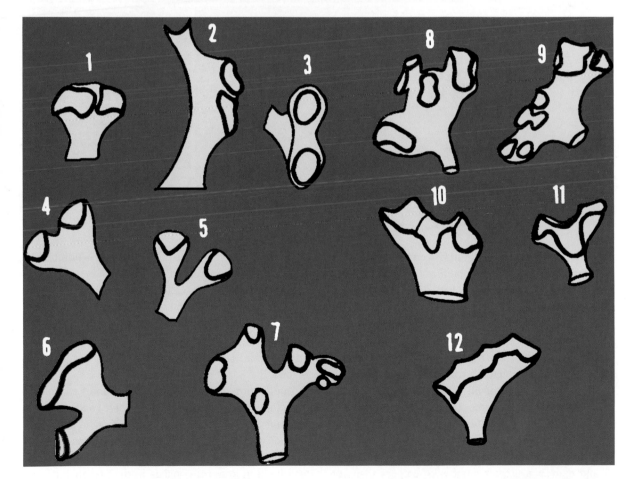

**Fig. 2.49** Scheme. Normal morphology of the kidney and upper urinary tract. Different morphology of renal papillae. *1* Two duplex papillae with a single calyx; *2* Two duplex papillae draining into an upper pole calicine system; *3–4* Two separated papil- lae with a single calyx; *5* Separated papillae with separate calyces; *6* One separate and one duplex papilla; *7–9* Multiple separate single or duplex papillae draining into one complex calyx; *10–12* Multiple fused papillae draining into one calyx

**Fig. 2.50** (**a–c**) Intravenous excretory urography. (**d**) Multidetector CTU. Various appearances of complex renal papillae (*arrow* in **d**).

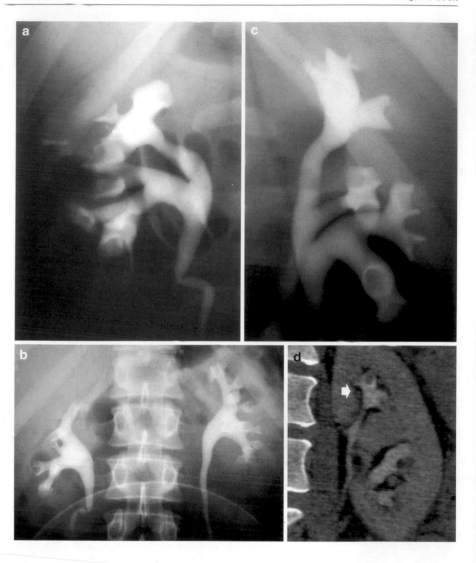

calyces is seven to nine per kidney, even though it may be as low as four or five, or as high as 18 or 19, or more (polycalycosis). Many fetal urinary apparatus modifications can be identified during pregnancy by US.

- Complex renal calyces and megacalycosis. Megacalycosis (Fig. 2.51a, b) represents a nonobstructive asymptomatic congenital disorder manifesting as dilatation of some or all renal calyces and normal renal pelvis and ureter. It may be associated to megaureter. Renal calyces present a blunted morphology as in renal papillary necrosis. Typically, megacalycosis involves all of the calyces uniformly and there is a greater number of calyces than normal (i.e., >15). Papillary necrosis tends to be dis-

similar from calyx to calyx, and the number of calyces is not increased.
- Calyceal diverticula. Calyceal diverticula represent a focal extrinsic dilatation of a renal calyx (Fig. 2.51c). Typically, calyceal diverticula connect to the calyceal fornix and project into the renal cortex (including a column of interlobar cortex) and not into the medulla.
- Duplication anomalies. Duplication anomalies include bifid renal pelvis (Fig. 2.47c) and complete or incomplete ureteral duplication, which develop when two or more ureteral buds form from the mesonephric duct. Ureteropelvic duplication (duplex collecting system) consists in the presence of two separate pyelocalyceal collecting system in one

**Fig. 2.51** (**a, b**) Intravenous excretory urography. Megacalycosis (*arrow*) involving one (**a**) or multiple renal calyces (**b**). (**c**) Intravenous excretory urography. Calyceal diverticulum (*arrow*). (**d**) CTU. Calyceal diverticulum with a renal stone (*arrow*)

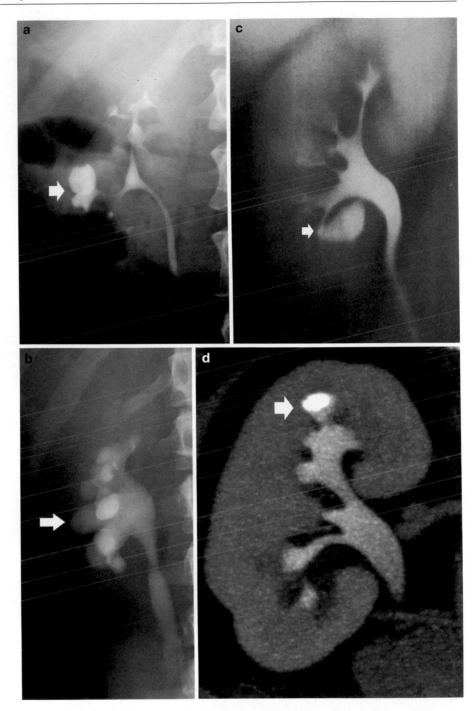

kidney extending from a bifid pelvis to a bifid ureter. Two draining ureters may join above the bladder (partial duplication) or insert into the bladder separately (complete duplication). Duplication anomalies result from the development of a second ureteric bud (complete duplication) or redundant duplication of the single ureteric bud. Complete ureteral duplication (Fig. 2.52), with a common or ectopic entry of the upper pole moiety, is less common than incomplete duplication. The ureter draining the upper segment of the kidney prevalently inserts in the bladder inferior and medial to the ureter draining

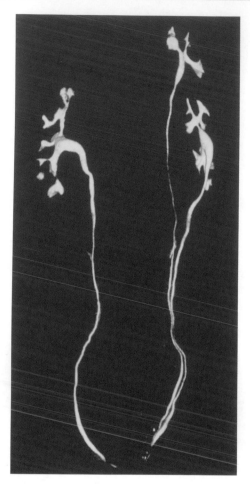

**Fig. 2.52** CTU. 3D volume-rendered images. Complete urinary tract duplication on the left side

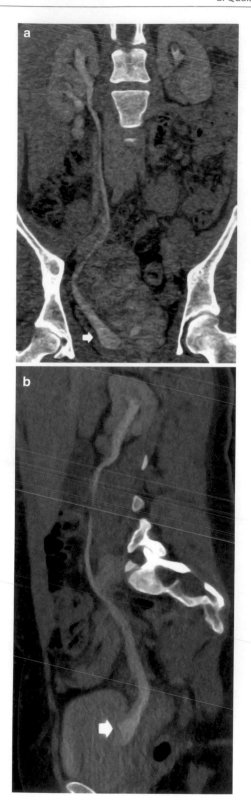

the lower segment of the kidney (Weigert-Meyer rule) representing the truly ectopic ureter in a complete duplication which is prone to ureteroceles (Fig. 2.53) and extravesical insertion or vesicoureteral reflux. The lower moiety of the completely duplicated system is generally normal. Ureteral duplication may also be bilateral (Fig. 2.54). Triple moiety may also be observed (Fig. 2.55).

• The anatomical variants of the renal urinary tract must be differentiated from the morphologic changes visible on renal calyces, infundibula, and renal pelvis on intravenous excretory urography, CTU, or MR urography due to specific renal pathologies (see Appendix).

**Fig. 2.53** (**a**, **b**) CTU. (**a**) Coronal and (**b**) curvilinear reformation. Urinary tract duplication with ureterocele (*arrow*).

**Fig. 2.54** (**a, b**) Bilateral urinary tract duplication. CTU. The duplication involved incompletely the ureter on the right side, and exclusively the renal pelvis on the left side

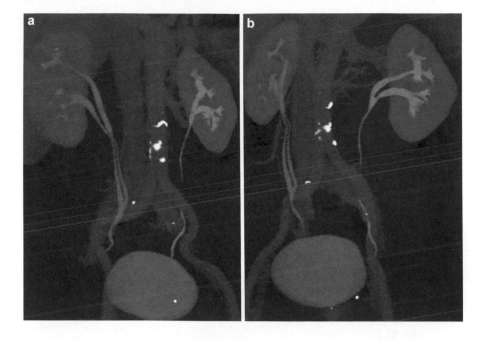

**Fig. 2.55** (**a, b**) Color-coded CTU. Triple division of the urinary tract on the right kidney (*arrow*)

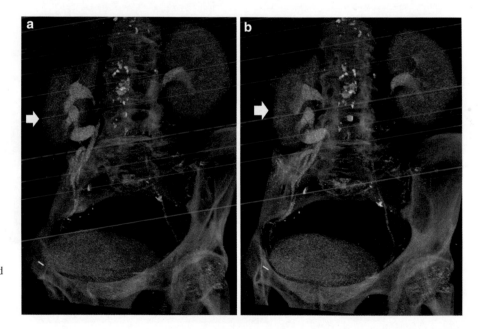

## 2.5 Appendix: Basic Morphological Changes of the Intrarenal Urinary Tract Visible on Intravenous Excretory Urography and Multidetector CT Urography

The anatomical variants (see chapter) of the normal renal urinary tract (see Fig. 2.56) must be differentiated from the pathologic morphological changes visible on renal calyces, infundibula, and renal pelvis on intravenous excretory urography, multidetector computed tomography urography (CTU), or MR urography due to specific renal pathologies.

Essentially, two fundamental pathologic morphological changes of the renal calices may be identified by intravenous excretory urography or multidetector CTU corresponding to plus (contrast agent projecting outside the renal calyx profile) and minus (contrast filling defects within the renal calyx or pelvis profile) images. To identify the fundamental alterations of the renal urinary tract, and particularly of the renal calyces, it is useful to consider an ideal line connecting the external renal calyx profiles (Hodson's line). Plus images include calyceal deformities and cavitations (Fig. 2.57), calyceal deformities due to parenchymal scarring (Fig. 2.58), urinary tract dilatation (Fig. 2.59), and calyceal deformities due to papillary atrophy (Fig. 2.60).

Minus images include calyceal defects or amputations (Fig. 2.61), changes of the infundibulum or calyceal profile (Fig. 2.62), or renal pelvis or calyceal displacement (Fig. 2.63).

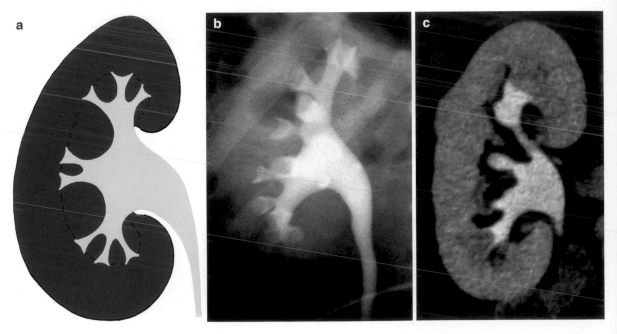

**Fig. 2.56** (**a–c**) Normal intrarenal urinary tract. (**a**) Scheme with the evidence of the ideal line (Hodson's line) connecting the external renal calyx profiles; (**b**) intravenous excretory urography; (**c**) multidetector computed tomography urography (CTU)

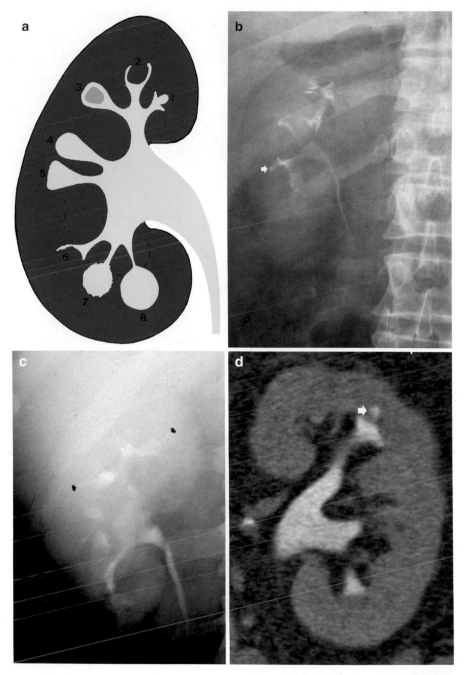

**Fig. 2.57** (**a–h**) Appearances of plus images of the renal calyces manifesting as calyceal deformities or cavitations. (**a**) Scheme with the evidence of the ideal line connecting the external renal calyx profiles – Hodson's line: *1* renal medullary necrosis; *2–3* renal papillary necrosis from initial detachment of necrotic papillae to the triangular filling defect due to the sloughing of the necrotic papilla; *4* calyceal deformity and clubbing due to parenchymal scarring in chronic renal infection; *5* calyceal deformity with convexity of the calyceal profile in initial renal hydronephrosis; *6* calyceal ulceration; *7* cavitation; *8* hydrocalyx. (**b**) Intravenous excretory urography. Calyceal diverticulum (*arrow*) connect to the calyceal fornix

and projecting into the renal cortex. (**c, d**) Intravenous excretory urography (**c**) and CT urography (**d**). Renal medullary necrosis at the tip of the papilla appearing as microcavities (*arrows*) surrounded by the papilla fornices. (**e, f**) Intravenous excretory urography (**e**) and CT urography (**f**). Renal papillary necrosis (*arrow*) with blunted calyx and preservation of the renal profile. On image (**f**) there is also evidence of hypodense blood coagula at the level of the pyelo-ureteral junction. (**g**) Intravenous excretory urography. Ulcerations (*arrows*) of the upper renal calyces due to renal tuberculosis. (**h**) Intravenous excretory urography. Hydrocalycosis (*arrow*) due to tubercular infundibolar stenosis

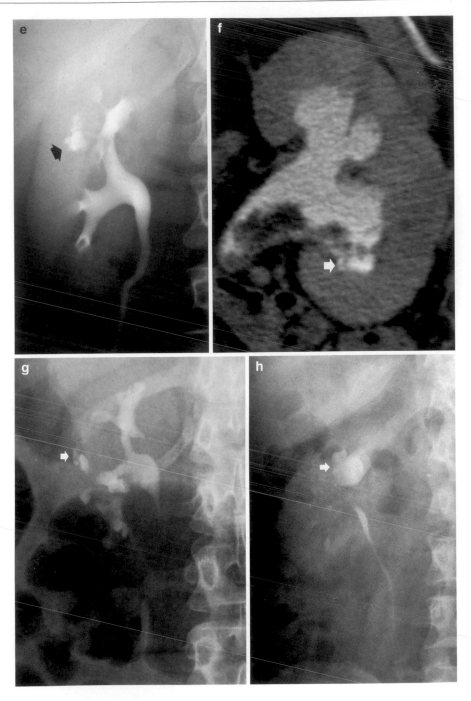

**Fig. 2.57** (continued)

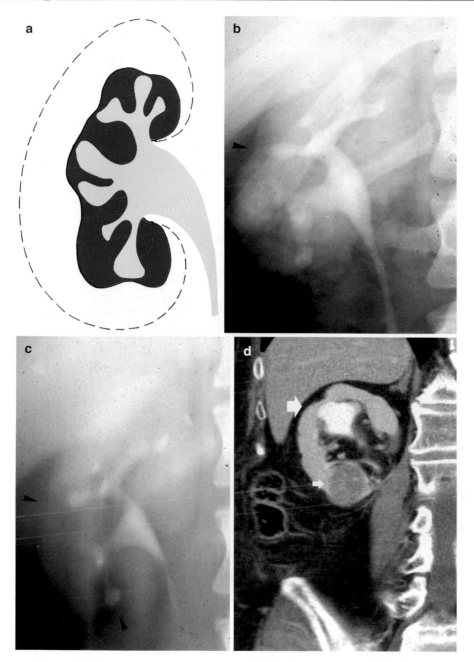

**Fig. 2.58** (**a–d**) Appearances of plus images manifesting as pelvis, or calyceal deformities. (**a**) Scheme with the evidence of the ideal line representing the normal renal profile. Calyceal deformities due to reflux nephropathy with cortical loss over dilated deformed calyx with a calviform shape. (**b**, **c**) Intravenous excretory urography. Reflux nephropathy with typical calyceal deformities (*arrowheads*) and alteration of the renal profile. (**d**) CT urography. Reflux nephropathy with clubbing deformation of the renal calyces and parenchymal scarring with alteration of the renal profile (*large arrow*). A solid renal tumor (*small arrow*) is also identified on the lower renal pole

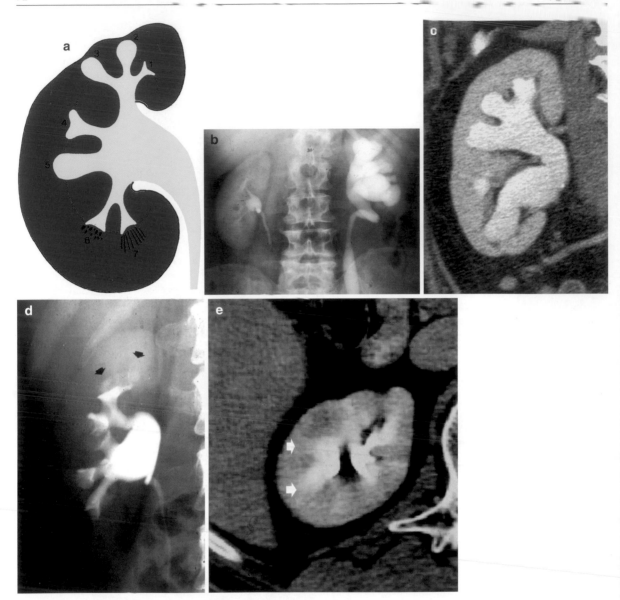

**Fig. 2.59** (a–e) Appearances of plus images due to dilatation of the urinary tract. (**a**) Scheme with the evidence of the ideal line connecting the external renal calyx profiles: *1* normal calyx; *2–3* reflux nephropathy; *4–5* hydronephrosis; *6–7* sponge kidney with linear striations (*6*) and small round contrast collections (*7*). (**b**) Intravenous excretory urography. Hydronephrosis of the left urinary tract. (**c**) CTU. Hydronephrosis of the right urinary tract. (**d**) Intravenous excretory urography. Medullary sponge kidney with the evidence of linear striations and small round contrast collections (*arrows*). (**e**) CT urography. Medullary sponge kidney. Linear striations at the level of renal papillae (*arrows*)

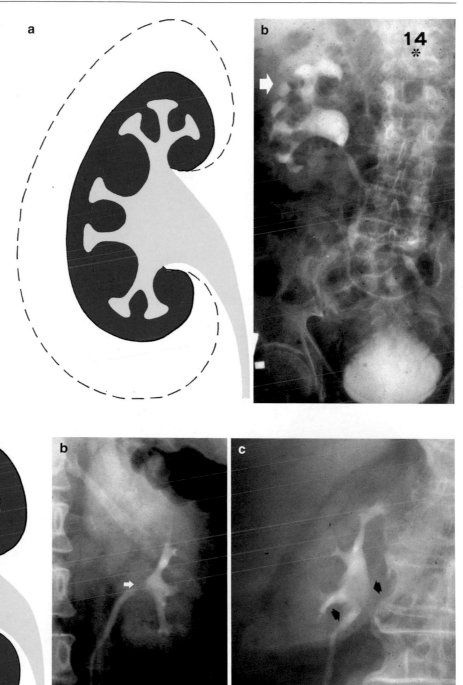

**Fig. 2.60** (**a**, **b**) Appearances of plus images manifesting as calyceal deformities due to papillary atrophy. (**a**) Scheme with the evidence of the ideal line representing the normal renal parenchyma profile; (**b**) intravenous excretory urography. Papillary atrophy with the absence of the normal concave calyceal profile and the evidence of convex calyceal profile (*arrow*) due to benign prostatic hypertrophy

**Fig. 2.61** (**a–e**) Appearances of minus images corresponding to renal pelvis or calyceal defects or amputations. (**a**) Scheme with the evidence of the ideal line connecting the external renal calyx profiles: *1* vascular notching; *2* filling defect due to a tumor, stone, or clot; *3* calyceal erosion due to tumor; *4* normal calyx; *5* calyceal deformity due to tumor; *6* calyceal amputation due to tumor; *7* calyceal amputation due to tuberculosis; (**b**) intravenous excretory urography. Vascular notching (*arrow*) on one of the infundibula of the upper renal pole. Vascular notches may determine minus images with alteration of the calyx morphology. (**c**, **d**) Filling defects (*arrows*) of the renal pelvis or renal calyces due to urothelial carcinoma. (**e**) Multidetector CTU. Coronal reformation. Filling defect on the renal pelvis with infundibula amputation due to renal lymphoma (*arrow*). (**f**) intravenous excretory urography-nephrotomography. Upper calyceal amputation (*arrow*) due to renal fibrosclerosing tuberculosis

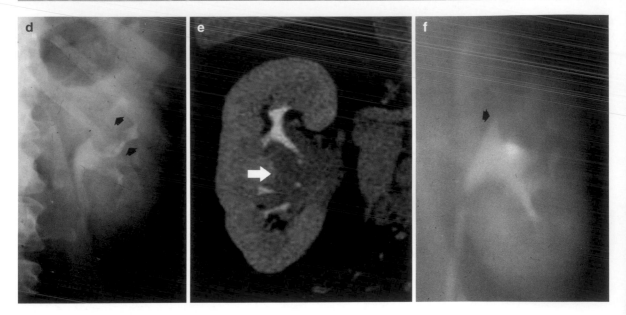

**Fig. 2.61** (continued)

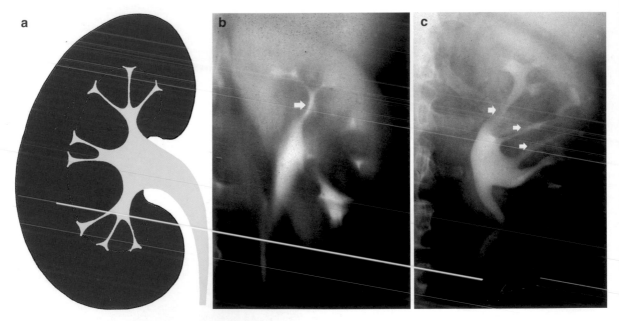

**Fig. 2.62** (**a**, **b**) Appearances of minus images corresponding to changes of the infundibulum or calyceal profile. (**a**) Scheme with evidence of the ideal line connecting the external renal calyx profiles; (**b**, **c**) intravenous excretory urography. Urography-nephrotomography (**b**) and intravenous urography (**c**). Narrowing of the renal calyces (*arrow* in **c**, and *arrows* in **d**) due to renal sinus lipomatosis. (**d**) CT urography. Narrowing of the renal due to renal sinus lipomatosis in a 65-year-old man. Renal sinus lipomatosis may determine minus images with the alteration of the calyx morphology with the elongation of the infundibulum profile. (**e**) CT urography. Narrowing of the renal calyces (*arrow*) due to parapyelic cysts

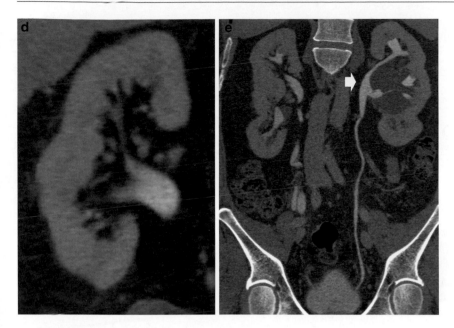

**Fig. 2.62** (continued)

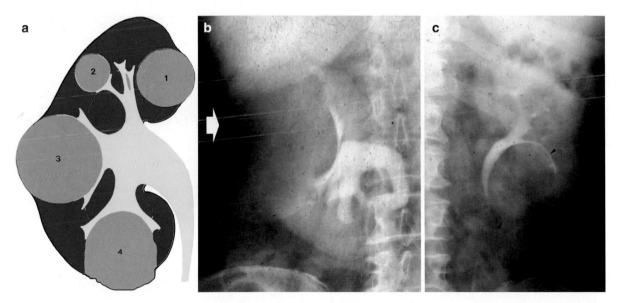

**Fig. 2.63** (**a**) Appearances of minus images corresponding to renal pelvis or calyceal displacement due to renal cyst or solid mass of different size (numbered from 1 to 4). (**a**) Scheme with the evidence of the ideal line connecting the external renal calyx profiles; (**b**) intravenous excretory urography. Calyceal displace-ment (*arrow*) due to renal cysts; (**c**) intravenous excretory urography. Calyceal displacement (*arrowheads*) due to a solid renal mass; (**d**, **e**) multidetector CTU. Calyceal displacement (*arrow*) due to renal cysts

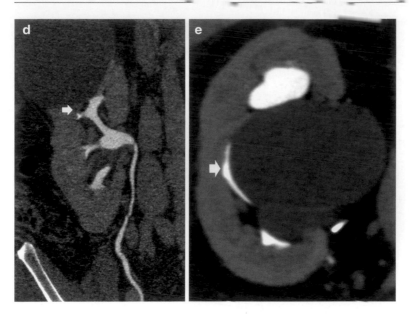

**Fig. 2.63** (continued)

# References

Amis ES Jr (1999) Epitaph for the urogram. Radiology 213: 639–640

Andreoli TE (1992) Approach to the patient with renal disease. In: Wyngaarden JB, Smith LH, Bennett JC (eds) Cecil textbook of medicine. Saunders, Philadelphia, pp 477–482

Barakat AJ, Drougas JG (1991) Occurrence of congenital abnormalities of kidney and urinary tract in 13775 autopsies. Urology 38:347–350

Baxter JD (1992) Regulation of adrenal steroid production. In: Wyngaarden JB, Smith LH, Bennett JC (eds) Cecil textbook of medicine. Saunders, Philadelphia, pp 1275–1277

Behrman RE, Kliegman RM, Arvin AM (1996) Nelson textbook of pediatrics, 15th edn. WB Saunders, Philadelphia, PA

Bude RO, Rubin JM, Adler RS (1994) Power versus conventional color Doppler sonography: comparison in the depiction of normal intrarenal vasculature. Radiology 192(3): 777–780

Bude RO, Rubin JM (1995) Detection of renal artery stenosis with Doppler sonography: it is more complicated than originally thought (editorial). Radiology 196:612–613

Buschi AJ, Harrison RB, Norman A et al. (1980) Distended left renal vein: CT/sonographic normal variant. AJR Am J Roentgenol 135:339–342

Chiara A, Chirico G, Comelli L et al (1990) Increased renal echogenicity in the neonate. Early Hum Dev 22:29–37

Cockcroft DW, Gault MH (1976) Prediction of creatinine clearance from serum creatinine. Nephron 16(1):31–41

Cohen AJ (1991) Use of diuretics in the intensive care units. In: Rippe JM, Irwin RS, Alpert JS et al. (eds) Intensive care medicine. Little, Brown and Company, Boston, pp 733–742

Correas JM, Helenon O, Moreau JF (1999) Contrast enhanced ultrasonography of native and transplant kidney diseases. Eur Radiol 9(suppl 3):394–400

Cuttino JT Jr, Clark RL, Jennette JC (1989) Microradiographic demonstration of human intrarenal microlymphatic pathways. Urol Radiol 11:83–87

Dagher PR, Herget-Rosenthal S, Ruehm SG et al. (2003) Newly developed techniques to study and diagnose acute renal failure. J Am Soc Nephrol 14:2188–2198

Davidson C, Stacul F, McCullough PA et al. (2006) Contrast medium use. Am J Cardiol 98(suppl):42K–58K

Desberg AL, Paushter DM, Lammert GK et al (1990) Renal artery stenosis: evaluation with color Doppler flow imaging. Radiology 177:749–753

Federle MP (2006) Embryology of the abdomen. In: Federle MP, Rosado-de-Christenson ML, Woodward PJ et al. (eds) Diagnostic and surgical imaging anatomy. Chest, abdomen, pelvis. Amirsys, Altona, Canada, pp 446–483

Friedenberg RM, Dunbar JS (1990) Excretory urography. In: Pollack HM (ed) Clinical urography. Saunders, Philadelphia, pp 101–243

Grant EG, Melany ML (2001) Ultrasound contrast agents in the evaluation of the renal arteries. In: Goldberg BB, Raichlen JS, Forsberg F (eds) Ultrasound contrast agents. Basic principles and clinical applications, 2nd edn. Martin Dunitz, London, pp 289–295

Grist TM (2000) MRA of the abdominal aorta and lower extremities. J Magn Reson Imaging 11:32–43

Helenon O, Rody EL, Correas JM et al (1995) Color Doppler US of renovascular disease in native kidneys. Radiographics 15: 833–854

Hogg CM, Reid O, Scothorne RJ (1982) Studies on hemolymph nodes. III. Renal lymph as a major source of erythrocytes in the renal hemolymph node of the rat. J Anat 135:291–299

Hricak H, Slovis TL, Callen CW et al. (1983) Neonatal kidneys: sonographic anatomic correlation. Radiology 147:699

Ischikawa Y, Akasaka Y, Kiguchi H et al. (2006) The human renal lymphatics under normal and pathological conditions. Histopathology 49(3):265–273

Joffe SA, Servaes S, Okon S et al. (2003) Multi-detector row CT urography in the evaluation of hematuria. RadioGraphics 23:1441–1455

Karazincir S, Balci A, Gorur S et al. (2007) Incidence of the retroaortic left renal vein in patients with varicocele. J Ultrasound Med 26:601–604

Kasap B, Soylu A, Türkmen M et al. (2006) Relationship of increased renal cortical echogenicity with clinical and laboratory findings in pediatric renal disease. J Clin Ultrasound 34:339–342

Klahr S (1992) Structure and function of the kidneys. In: Wyngaarden JB, Smith LH, Bennett JC (eds) Cecil textbook of medicine. Saunders, Philadelphia, PA, pp 482–492

Laiken ND, Fanestil DD (1985) Anatomy of the kidneys. In: West JB (ed) Best and Taylor's physiology basis of medical practice. Williams & Wilkins, Baltimore, MA, pp 451–460

Lameire N, Adam A, Becker CR et al. (2006) Baseline renal function screening. Am J Cardiol 98(suppl):21K–26K

Lane BR, Poggio ED, Herts BR et al. (2009) Renal function assessment in the era of chronic kidney disease: renewed emphasis on renal function centered patient care. J Urol 182(2):435–443

Levey AS, Bosch JP, Lewis JB et al. (1999) A more accurate method to estimate glomerular filtration rate from serum creatinine: a new prediction equation. Modification of diet in Renal Disease Study Group. Ann Intern Med 130(6): 461–470

National Kidney Foundation (2002) K/DOQI clinical practice guidelines for chronic kidney disease: evaluation, classification, and stratification. Am J Kidney Dis 39(suppl 1): S1–S266

Nino-Murcia M, de Vries PA, Friedland GW (2000) Congenital anomalies of the kidney. In: Pollack HM, Mc Clennan BI (eds) Clinical urography. Saunders, Philadelphia, PA, pp 690–763

Olbricht C, Mason J, Takabatake T et al. (1977) The early phase of experimental acute renal failure. II. Tubular leakage and the reliability of glomerular markers. Pflugers Arch 372:251–258

Peipert JF, Donnenfeld AE (1991) Oligohydramnios: a review. Obstet Gynecol Surv 46(6):325–39.

Reed MD, Friedman AC, Nealey P (1982) Anomalies of the left renal vein: analysis of 433 CT scans. J Comput Assist Tomogr 6:1124–1126

Satyapal KS, Haffejee AA, Singh B, et al. (2001) Additional renal arteries: incidence and morphometry. Surg Radiol Anat 23(1):33–38.

Schedl A (2007) Renal abnormalities and their developmental origin. Nat Rev Genet 8(10):791–802

Schwartz GJ, Feld LG, Langford DJ (1984) A simple estimate of glomerular filtration rate in full-term infants during the first year of life. J Pediatr 104(6):849–854

Silverman SG, Leyendecker JR, Amis SE (2009) What is the current role of CT urography and MR urography in the evaluation of the urinary tract. Radiology 250:309–323

Stevens LA, Coresh J, Greene T et al. (2006) Assessing kidney function – measured and estimated glomerular filtration rate. N Engl J Med 354:2473–2483

Stevens LA, Levey AS (2005) Chronic kidney disease in the elderly – how to assess risk. N Engl J Med 352:2122–2124

Türkvatan A, Özdemir M, Cumhur T et al. (2009) Multidetector CT angiography of renal vasculature: normal anatomy and variants. Eur Radiol 19(1):236–244. doi: 10.1007/s00330-008-1126-3

Twining P (1994) Genitourinary malformations. In: Diagnostic Imaging of fetal anomalies. Nyberg AD, McGahan JP, Pretorius DH, Pilu G (eds). Lippincott Williams and Wilkins, Philadelphia, PA, pp 603–659

Van Der Molen AJ, Cowan NJ, Mueller-Lisse UG et al. (2008) CT urography: definition, indications and techniques. A guideline for clinical practice. Eur Radiol 18:4–17

Yeh BM, Coakley FV, Meng MV et al. (2004) Precaval right renal arteries: prevalence and morphologic associations at spiral CT. Radiology 230:429–433

Yeh HS, Halton KP, Shapiro RS et al. (1992) Junctional parenchyma: revised definition of the hypertrophic column of Bertin. Radiology 185:725–732

# Normal Radiological Anatomy of the Retroperitoneum

**3**

Emilio Quaia

## Contents

**Abstract**

> This chapter describes the normal anatomy of the retroperitoneal space according to cross-sectional imaging techniques. The retroperitoneal space is divided into three fundamental spaces by the anterior and posterior renal fasciae, namely the pararenal anterior, the perirenal and the pararenal posterior spaces. The fat contained in the retroperitoneal space communicates with the fat contained in the abdominal space since the anterior pararenal space communicates with the mesentery and mesocolon through the connective tissue involved in the peritoneal foldings. Inferiorly, the different retroperitoneal spaces communicate also with the perirenal space where the kidneys are located.

## 3.1 Normal Anatomy of Retroperitoneum

The retroperitoneum is a complex compartment, the anatomy of which has yet to be fully validated (Burkill and Healy 2000). The currently accepted model of the retroperitoneum anatomy has been proposed by Meyers (1974, 1994) who led to an enhanced understanding of retroperitoneal anatomy and pathology.

The retroperitoneum is limited anteriorly by the posterior parietal peritoneum and posteriorly by the fascia trasversalis. The fascia trasversalis fuses anteriorly with the parietal peritoneum, and posteriorly with the muscular fasciae of the psoas and quadratum lomborum muscles.

E. Quaia
Department of Radiology, Cattinara Hospital, University of Trieste, Strada di Fiume 447, 34149 Trieste, Italy
e-mail: quaia@univ.trieste.it

E. Quaia (ed.), *Radiological Imaging of the Kidney*,
Medical Radiology, DOI: 10.1007/978-3-540-87597-0_3, © Springer-Verlag Berlin Heidelberg 2011

The retroperitoneal space is divided into three fundamental spaces: the pararenal anterior, the perirenal and the pararenal posterior (Fig. 3.1). This classical division of the retroperitoneal space has been extensively revised in the recent years. In particular, it has been underlined that the retroperitoneum, namely the anterior pararenal space, communicates with the mesentery and mesocolon through the connective tissue involved in the peritoneal foldings (Molmenti et al. 1996). The rapidly collecting fluid collections tend to escape the retroperitoneal site of origin into planes, whose distribution strongly suggests that these represent sites of fusion of peritoneal planes during embryologic development (Molmenti et al. 1996). Dodds et al. (1986), using embryologic considerations to explain clinical observations discordant with the simple three-compartment model, suggested that pancreatic fluid escapes the pancreatic portion of the anterior pararenal space into planes created by fusion of the dorsal mesentery during embryologic development.

The renal fasciae, namely the anterior and posterior renal fasciae, represent the fundamental anatomical structures for the division of the retroperitoneal space, and they are clearly visible on computed tomography (Fig. 3.2) and in magnetic resonance imaging (Fig. 3.3). The renal fasciae are usually not thicker than 3 mm. If renal fasciae appear thicker than 3 mm, this is often due to a retroperitoneal space disease, corresponding mainly to acute pancreatitis (Fig. 3.4), renal pathologies and abdominal aorta aneurysm rupture. The

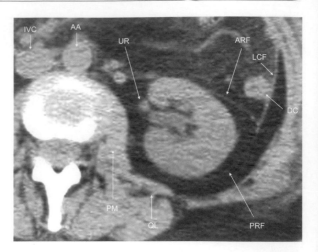

**Fig. 3.2** Computed tomography. Anatomy of the retroperitoneal space. *AA* abdominal aorta; *ARF* anterior renal fascia; *DC* descending colon; *IVC* inferior vena cava; *LCF* lateroconal fascia; *PRF* posterior renal fascia; *PM* psoas muscle; *QL* quadratus lomborum muscle; *UR* ureter

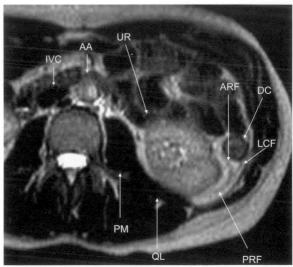

**Fig. 3.3** Magnetic resonance imaging, T2-weighted sequence. Anatomy of the retroperitoneal space. *AA* abdominal aorta; *ARF* anterior renal fascia; *DC* descending colon; *IVC* inferior vena cava; *LCF* lateroconal fascia; *PRF* posterior renal fascia; *PM* psoas muscle; *QL* quadratus lomborum muscle; *UR* ureter

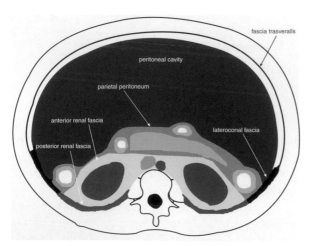

**Fig. 3.1** Scheme. Anatomy of the different retroperitoneal spaces, the anterior pararenal space (*brown*), the perirenal space (*yellow*), the posterior pararenal space (*violet*) and the properitoneal compartment (*dark violet*)

anterior pararenal space is limited anteriorly by the posterior sheet of the parietal peritoneum and posteriorly by the anterior renal fascia known also as Gerota's fascia. Superiorly, it extends to the dome of the diaphragm and hence to the mediastinum, and inferiorly, communicates with the pelvis and the posterior pararenal space (Burkill and Healy 2000). It contains the pancreas, the second (descending), third (transverse), and

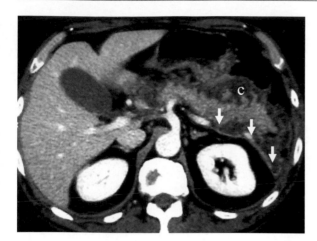

Fig. 3.4 Computed tomography. Transverse plane. Diffuse thickening of the anterior renal fascia (*arrows*) due to a collection located in the anterior pararenal space (c) due to a necrotic-haemorrhaic pancreatitis

fourth (ascending) loops of the duodenum, and the descending and ascending colon tracts. The ascending and descending colon are retroperitoneal and not abdominal organs because they do not have a meso formed by the peritoneal folds. The right and left sides of the anterior pararenal space communicate across the midline.

The perirenal space (Figs. 3.5 and 3.6) is a retroperitoneal space that is limited anteriorly by the anterior renal fascia and posteriorly by the posterior renal fascia (Zuckerkandl's fascia). Raptopoulos et al. (1986), using clinical observations supported by dissection of prepared cadavers, showed that the posterior renal fascia is an expandable potential space and a pathway for extension of fluid that arises in the perirenal or anterior pararenal space. The two renal fasciae fuse to form the lateroconal fascia laterally and blend loosely with the periureteric

Fig. 3.5 (a, b) Perirenal space, coronal plane. (a) Scheme. Anatomy of the perirenal spaces. (b) Contrast-enhanced CT. Coronal plane. The cone-like morphology of the perirenal space (*arrow*) due to the superior fusion of the renal anterior and posterior fasciae which are fixed to the diaphragmatic fascia above the adrenal glands

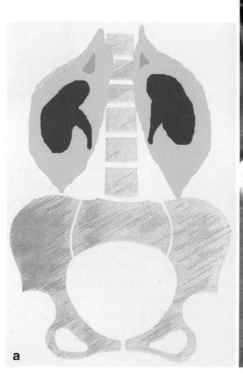

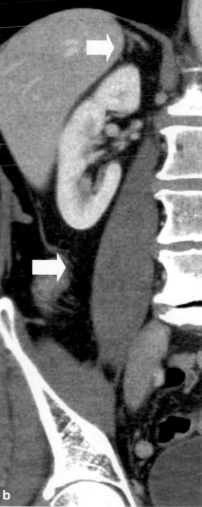

**Fig. 3.6** (**a**, **b**) Perirenal space, sagittal plane. (**a**) Scheme. Anatomy of the perirenal space (*yellow*) and relationship with the other retroperitoneal spaces, the anterior pararenal space (*brown*), and the posterior pararenal space (*violet*). (**b**) Contrast-enhanced CT. Sagittal plane. The cone-like morphology of the perirenal space (*large arrow*) due to the superior fusion of the renal anterior and posterior fasciae (*curved arrow*) which are fixed to the diaphragmatic fascia above the adrenal glands. *L* liver; *k* kidney

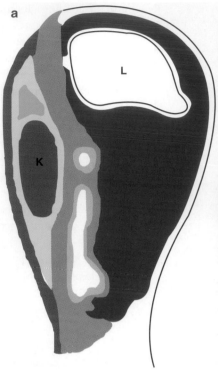

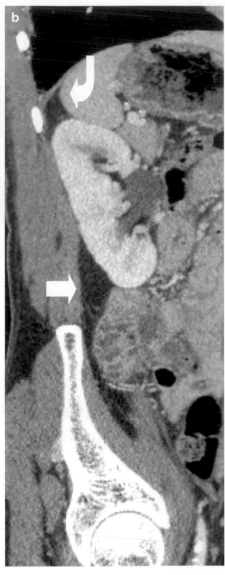

connective tissue medially. Actually, the lateroconal fascia represents the lateral continuation of the posterior renal fascia, while the posterior and anterior renal fasciae may be detached by a collection in the anterior pararenal space. The anterior renal fascia anteriorly fuses with the fibrous tissue surrounding the main vascular vessels, namely inferior vena cava and abdominal aorta, so that the right perirenal space does not communicate with the left perirenal space above the iliac region.

The perirenal space abuts the bare area of the liver on the right and the subphrenic space on the left and communicates with mediastinum via the diaphragmatic hiatae. The anterior and posterior renal fasciae

enclose a gradually tapering cone-like space produced by the embryologic ascent of the kidneys from the pelvis to the adult retroperitoneal position (Figs. 3.5 and 3.6). Superiorly, the two renal fasciae are fixed to the diaphragmatic fascia above the adrenal glands, while inferiorly, they blend with the iliac fascia and do not fuse and determine a free communication between the anterior and posterior pararenal space and the perirenal space (Fig. 3.6). In the other regions, the renal fasciae do not fuse and a collection in the anterior or posterior pararenal space does not extend directly to the perirenal space (Fig. 3.7). Sometimes, the anterior renal fascia, which overlies the upper portion of the right kidney

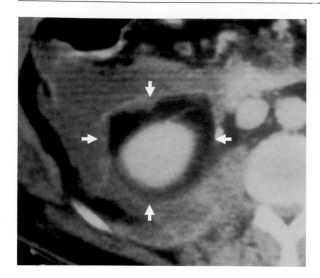

**Fig. 3.7** Computed tomography. Transverse plane. The retroperitoneal collection extending in the anterior and posterior pararenal space does not extend in the perirenal space (*arrows*) due to limit of pararenal fasciae

and adrenal gland, may be deficient and allow communication of the perirenal space with the hepatic bare area. The perirenal space contains the kidneys, adrenal glands, proximal ureters, perirenal fat, lymphatic vessels, and blood vessels. Within the fat surrounding the kidney in the perirenal space there is a network of thin fibrous septae and bridging septa (Kunin septa) that connect the renal capsule with the anterior and posterior renal fasciae. The left and right perirenal spaces communicate with each other across the midline and with the pelvic peritoneal spaces below the iliac fossa (Thornton et al. 2001).

The posterior pararenal space (Figs. 3.1–3.3) is a retroperitoneal space that is limited anteriorly by the posterior renal fascia and posteriorly by the fascia trasversalis. Laterally, it continues with the properitoneal compartment containing fat. It is potentially in continuity anteriorly with the properitoneal fat of the anterior abdominal wall; it contains only fat and does not contain any parenchymal organ. It is open toward the pelvis inferiorly, but limited superiorly by the fusion of the posterior renal fascia with the fascia of the quadratus lumborum and psoas muscles.

# References

Burkill GJC, Healy JC (2000) Anatomy of retroperitoneum. Imaging 12:10–20

Dodds WJ, Darweesh RMA, Lawson TL et al. (1986) The retroperitoneal spaces revisited. AJR Am J Roentgenol 147:1155–1161

Meyers MA (1974) Radiologic features of the spread and localization of extraperitoneal gas and their relationship to its source: an anatomical approach. Radiology 111:7–26

Meyers M (1994) Dynamic radiology of the abdomen: normal and pathology anatomy, 4th edn. Springer, Berlin Heidelberg New York.

Molmenti EP, Balfe DM, Kanterman RY et al. (1996) Anatomy of the retroperitoneum: observations of the distribution of pathologic fluid collections. Radiology 200:95–103

Raptopoulos V, Kleinman P, Marks S et al. (1986) Renal fascial pathway: posterior extension of pancreatic effusions within the anterior pararenal space. Radiology 158:367–374

Thornton FJ, Kandiah SS, Monkhouse WS et al. (2001) Helical CT evaluation of the perirenal space and its boundaries: a cadaveric study. Radiology 218:659–663

# Ultrasound of the Kidney

## Emilio Quaia

4

## Contents

**Abstract**

> Ultrasound (US) represents the first-line imaging technique in the assessment of the kidney. US image quality has greatly improved in recent years with advances in the transducer and beam-former technology. Gray-scale US, with the addition of harmonic and compound speckle-reduction modes, and color Doppler US may provide a diagnostic clue in most renal abnormalities. US artifacts are extremely important in the US assessment of the kidney because they must be differentiated by true images and may be extremely useful in the renal assessment. Nowadays, contrast-enhanced US with dedicated contrast-specific techniques and microbubble contrast agents further improves the sensitivity of US in depicting renal vasculature.

Ultrasound (US) represents a first-line imaging technique in the assessment of the kidney, and it presents several advantages over the other imaging techniques including low financial cost, portability, availability, lack of restrictions in performing frequent serial examinations at short intervals, and absence of exposure to radiation or nuclear tracers.

Doppler US analysis of renal vessels has to be performed after conventional gray-scale US examination since it allows functional evaluation of the kidneys. Doppler US sensitivity has considerably increased in the latest US equipments, but Doppler US is even more dependent on patient compliance than conventional

E. Quaia
Department of Radiology, Cattinara Hospital,
University of Trieste, Strada di Fiume 447, 34149 Trieste, Italy
e-mail: quaia@univ.trieste.it

E. Quaia (ed.), *Radiological Imaging of the Kidney*,
Medical Radiology, DOI: 10.1007/978-3-540-87597-0_4, © Springer-Verlag Berlin Heidelberg 2011

US. Gray-scale US, with the addition of harmonic and compound speckle-reduction modes, and color Doppler US may provide a diagnostic clue in most renal abnormalities.

## 4.1 Technology

In the last decade, the image quality in US had important improvements due to technology advancements particularly in the new array transducers with a high number of elements, in the US systems with numerous focus lines, and in the computer processing power corresponding to a powerful beamformer with higher resolution and higher dynamic range in the images. The most important technological advances in the US field were introduced in the signal transmission and reception processes, compounding and equalization, color and power Doppler, and the 3D and elastographic imaging (Claudon et al. 2002).

- Signal transmission. In the signal transmission process, the transducer arrays, formed by ceramic polymer composite elements of variable shape and thickness, and the multilayered technology led to a more accurate shaping of the US pulses in terms of frequency, amplitude, phase, and length (Whittingham 1999a, b). The development of piezo-electric crystals with a lower acoustic impedance and greater electromechanical coupling coefficients, the improvement of the physical characteristics of the absorbing backing layers, and the quarter-wave impedance matching layers represent the most significant results of the US transducer research (Claudon et al. 2002).
  - Increased bandwidth of the transducers allows a better spatial and contrast resolution with a consequent improvement of the axial resolution due to shorter pulse length. Shorter transmission pulses used in a broadband emission generates shorter echo pulses that can be faithfully converted into electric signals (Whittingham 1999b). Since short pulses are attenuated to a greater extent and are characterized by less penetration than long pulses, specific techniques have been introduced by different manufacturers to allow a more accurate shaping of the US pulse in terms

of the control of the transmission frequency, amplitude, phase, and pulse length. Phase can be determined only by the comparison with a reference waveform or another pulse. This can be achieved by using multiple beamformers that allow the direct integration of the phase information from the signal received from the adjacent lines (Claudon et al. 2002). Another way to improve penetration is by increasing the output power (Pedersen et al. 2003), even though it is limited by safety limits, or by utilizing excitation signals much more sophisticated than the single-carrier short pulses currently used in the US scanners. These signals are usually defined coded excitation and increase the signal-to-noise ratio and the frame rate. In coded-emission mode, the scanner transmits not a single pulse, but a sequence of 8–22 short, high-frequency transmission pulses that may have different phases and are modulated in a code sequence. Comparison between transmitted pulses and received signal shapes using matched filtering (decoding) is subsequently performed with a very high sampling rate (Claudon et al. 2002). In chirp encoding, a long specially shaped pulse is transmitted with progressively varied frequency and amplitude. The matched filtering process involves comparing the echoes with a stored reference version of the transmitted chirp. When the two waveforms present identical shape but different amplitude, they are out of alignment, and the output of the process is low. The filter output is a large amplitude compressed pulse for every match between a genuine chirp echo and the reference chirp.

- Electronic focusing, obtained by activating a series of elements in the array with appropriate delay, can easily be used to regulate the focal depth. The higher the number of channels involved to activate the array elements in a combined mode and with the appropriate delays, the more accurately the US beam can be focused. In the dynamic transmit focusing modality, edge crystal elements have a longer pulse excitation than center elements, making the US beam focus at two different points in the insonated field, improving lateral resolution. As the resulting wavefront has the characteristics of a short excitation pulse, the axial resolution is preserved (Claudon et al. 2002). The spatial and contrast resolution of the US image had a further improvement due to matrix transducers which allow a further reduction in the thickness of the US beam with better spatial resolution.

- Signal reception. Tissue harmonic imaging has allowed a further improvement in the signal-to-noise ratio and image quality due to the improved contrast resolution and speckle and artifact reduction even in patients with a limited explorability including obese patients. Harmonic imaging requires large transducer bandwidth, and that the system is configured to preferentially receive harmonics components produced by tissues, hence at double the transmitted frequency, by a high-pass filter, and to cancel out the fundamental echo signals generated directly from the transmitted acoustic energy. Such filtering is successful in eliminating echoes from solid stationary tissues which present prevalently linear properties, even though the effect is to reduce the range of frequencies (or bandwidth) contained in the received echoes, causing a low spatial axial resolution of the resulting image. Harmonic imaging and speckle-reduction techniques have improved signal-to-noise ratio and also image quality in patients who are difficult to explore by US, such as obese or large body habitus subjects.

- Compound imaging and equalization. Compound imaging may be obtained by spatial (transmit compounding) or frequency compound. In spatial compound imaging, the same insonated slice is interrogated according to different insonation angles, while in frequency compound imaging, the same slice is insonated more number of times with different frequencies. The resulting images are managed by subtracting all echoes step-by-step, which appears incoherently in the different acquired images, corresponding essentially to noise. Compound imaging allows a reduction of speckles, clutter, and noise, without compromising other beneficial image characteristics such as spatial resolution, and improves contrast-to-noise ratio and better depiction of the curved surface such as the renal poles. Compounding also reduces shadowing from strongly reflecting interfaces such as organ boundaries, fascial planes, and vessel walls. Tissue equalization is based on regional and adaptive methods to analyze, using regional speckle statistics and thermal noise identification, and apply an algorithm to perform region-by-region adjustment to lateral gain, depth gain, and overall gain (Claudon et al. 2002).

- Color and power Doppler. The color and power Doppler techniques have become highly sensitive for the renal parenchymal flows. In particular, the introduction of wide-band Doppler technology, making use of short pulses, has led to some advantages in imaging subtle blood flows due to the improved frame rate and axial resolution. In contrast to color Doppler, the sensitivity of power Doppler for the renal flows is not dependent on the angle of insonation. Moreover, power Doppler has a higher sensitivity than color Doppler for the renal parenchyma flow in particular at renal poles. The introduction of wide-band color Doppler (e.g., advanced dynamic flow) has improved the sensitivity and contrast resolution for the flow signal of the renal parenchymal vessels up to the interlobular vessels which can be imaged with a 2–5 MHz convex US transducer.

- 3D and elastographic imaging. 3D US acquisition is obtained by using multidimensional matrix transducers with parallel processing of the signal. Digitally stored volume data can then be displayed in a multiplanar array that simultaneously shows three perpendicular planes throughout the volume: axial; sagittal; and reconstructed coronal views. The volume can be explored by scrolling through parallel planes in any of the three views, and by rotating the volume to obtain an optimal view of the structure of interest (Claudon et al. 2002). Data can also be displayed as true 3D images using various rendering algorithm, including maximum intensity projections and transparent and surface renderings. Elastographic imaging is based on the different mechanical and acoustic properties of soft tissues according to their stiffness. It has been used to provide a flexible and real-time exploration of different tissues (Claudon et al. 2002). The acquisition of RF signals during compression allows the strain of the tissue, which is related to the stiffness of the tissue, to be imaged. Both 3D US and elastographic imaging have limited applications in the kidneys.

## 4.2 Ultrasound Scanning Technique of the Kidneys

### 4.2.1 Gray-Scale Ultrasound

#### 4.2.1.1 Normal Anatomy

Convex-array US transducers (frequency band of 2–5 MHz in adults, and 5–8 MHz in pediatric patients) are usually employed in the US scanning of the kidney. The kidney is examined with the patient in the supine position with both the upper extremities raised over the head. The scanning of the kidney with the patient lying on one side is often necessary to eliminate the intestinal gas interposition, while the breath-hold technique is frequently necessary to obtain a complete examination of the renal parenchyma.

There are different possible acoustic views for the examination of the kidney by US including the anterior, lateral, and the posterior views with longitudinal or transverse scanning planes (Figs. 4.1 and 4.2). The lateral acoustic views employ the acoustic window through the liver parenchyma. The posterior acoustic view is usually employed in the pediatric patient, while the lateral acoustic view allows also an intercostal acoustic window which is often necessary to eliminate the bowel gas interposition in ancient or noncompliant patients.

When the kidney is scanned on the longitudinal plane, the operator should remember that the kidney has an ovoidal shape and that both the renal poles should also be contemporarily visualized (Fig. 4.3) by using breathold or patient lying on one side (Fig. 4.4). The normal longitudinal diameter of the kidney is between 9 and 12 cm. The length of both the kidneys is considered normal when it is between 9 and 13 cm. Normally, renal margins are smooth, except in some normal anatomical variants such as functional parenchymal defects and renal fetal locations. The mean normal value of renal cortical thickness (distance between the renal capsule and the outer margin of the pyramid) is 1–1.5 cm, while the normal value of renal parenchyma thickness (distance between the renal

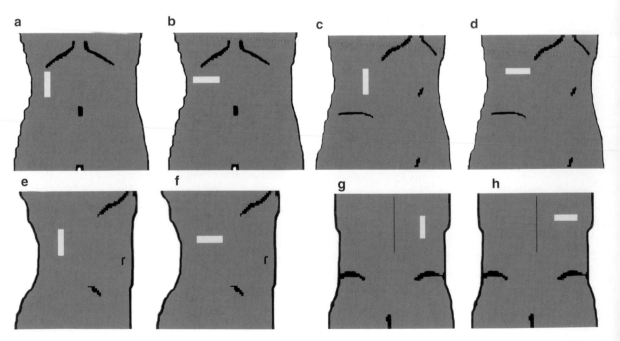

**Fig. 4.1** The schemes represent the different possible acoustic views for the US examination of the kidney. (**a, b**) Anterior acoustic window at the level of the anterior axillary line: longitudinal (**a**) and transverse scanning plane (**b**). (**c, d**) Lateral acoustic window between the anterior and posterior axillary line: longitudinal (**c**) and transverse scanning plane (**d**). (**e, f**) Lateral acoustic window on the posterior axillary line: longitudinal (**e**) and transverse scanning plane (**f**). (**g, h**) Posterior acoustic windows behind the posterior axillary line: longitudinal (**g**) and transverse scanning plane (**h**). The anterior axillary line is defined as the vertical line extending inferiorly from the anterior axillary fold; the posterior axillary line is defined as the vertical line extending inferiorly from the posterior axillary fold; while the midaxillary line refers to a vertical line intersecting a point midway between the anterior and posterior axillary folds

**Fig. 4.2** The different appearance of the kidney scanned through the different acoustic views. The resulting ultrasound (US) image is represented in gray-scale level. (**a–c**) Longitudinal scanning planes of the kidney obtained through different directions of the acoustic beam according to anterior acoustic view (**a**), lateral acoustic window between the anterior and posterior axillary line (**b**), and lateral acoustic window on the posterior axillary line (**c**). (**d**) Transverse scan of the kidney. The resulting US image is represented in gray-scale level

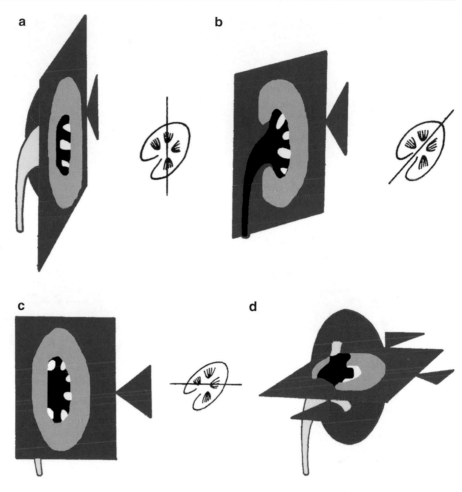

capsule and the margin of the sinus echo avoiding renal columns) is 1.4–1.8 cm. A renal parenchyma thickness < 1 cm is associated with irreversible changes. The renal cortical echogenicity is normally lower than the echogenicity of the liver, spleen, and renal sinus. When the liver parenchyma appears hyperechoic on US, spleen echogenicity is used as a standard reference; however, kidneys may be isoechoic to the liver even when no clinical or laboratory evidence of renal disease are documented. The renal cortical echogenicity is correlated to the severity of histological changes in renal parenchymal diseases such as global sclerosis, focal tubular atrophy, and hyaline casts per glomerulus. On US, the renal pyramids appear triangular and hypoechoic and may be differentiated from the renal cortex in approximately 50% of adult patients, being more conspicuous with hydration and diuresis. The renal sinus appears hyperechoic when compared with renal parenchyma, for the presence of hilar adipose tissue with fibrous septae, blood vessels, and lymphatics.

The renal sinus may appear inhomogeneous, less echogenic, and poorly differentiated from renal parenchyma when edema, fibrosis, or cellular infiltration are present. With increasing age, the amount of renal parenchyma decreases and the renal sinus fat increases. The renal sinus fat tissue may be increased also in renal sinus lipomatosis which can be determined by obesity, parenchymal atrophy, and normal variants. Tissue harmonic and compound imaging (Fig. 4.5) allow a better definition of the kidney profiles, the better identification of renal calculi and parenchymal calcifications, the better depiction of the intracystic septa in the complex cystic renal masses, the better characterization of the content in the dilated excretory tract, and the more accurate evaluation of the parenchyma echotexture.

Only dilated ureters may be identified by gray-scale US, even though the presence of interposing bowel gas often masks the dilated ureter. The employment of the posterior acoustic view through the ipsilateral psoas muscle is fundamental in the assessment of the dilated ureter.

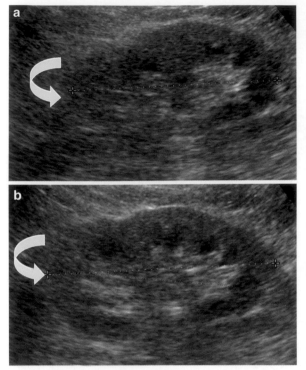

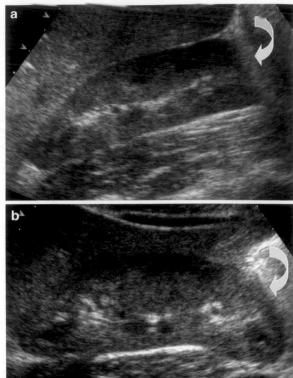

**Fig. 4.3** Gray-scale US. Longitudinal scan. Optimal scanning technique to identify the upper renal pole (*arrow*). (**a**) An irregular US scan does not allow a correct insonation of the upper renal pole. (**b**) A regular US scan allows the correct insonation of the upper renal pole

**Fig. 4.4** Gray-scale US. Longitudinal scan. Optimal scanning technique to identify the lower renal pole (*arrow*). (**a**) An irregular US scan does not allow a correct insonation of the lower renal pole due to the interposing bowel gas. (**b**) A regular US scan, obtained with the patient lying on one side, allows the correct insonation of the lower renal pole

#### 4.2.1.2 Fundamental Alterations of Renal Echogenicity

The alterations in the echogenicity on gray-scale US are always compared to the surrounding tissues and may involve the renal parenchyma or the renal sinus. Diffuse renal parenchyma diseases, including acute glomerulonephritis (Fig. 4.6a), vasculitides, and acute tubular necrosis, determine the increased echogenicity of the renal cortex with an increased cortico-medullary differentiation. Autosomal recessive polycystic kidney disease manifests with enlarged and hyperechoic kidneys (Fig. 4.6b) due to the unresolved 1–2 mm cystic dilatation of the collecting tubules that increases the number of acoustic interfaces.

Calcium determines the focal or diffuse hyperechogenicity often with posterior acoustic shadowing. Focal parenchymal calcifications are due to Randall's plaque characterized by comet-tail artifact (Fig. 4.7a), a reverberation type of artifact (Thickman et al. 1983) consisting of dense tapering trail of echoes just distal to a

strongly reflecting structure, or papillary calcifications (Fig. 4.7b) in the medullary sponge kidney. Randall's plaques correspond to the focal deposition of interstitial crystal at or near the papilla tip (Randall 1937) prevalently composed of apatite or calcium oxalate which may have a potential pathogenetic role as a precursor for calcium oxalate nephrolithiasis (Sakhaee 2009). Focal papillary calcifications appear as focal hyperechoic spots within or at the tip of renal papillae, and they can be observed in sarcoidosis, primary hyperparathyroidism, diabetes mellitus, medullary sponge kidney, drug nephropathy and in long dialysis treatment. Medullary hyperechogenicity (Fig. 4.7c) is due to medullary nephrocalcinosis which is characterized by diffuse calcium deposition within the renal medulla. Underlying causes include medullary sponge kidney, distal renal tubular acidosis, hyperparathyroidism, milk-alkali syndrome, hypervitaminosis D,

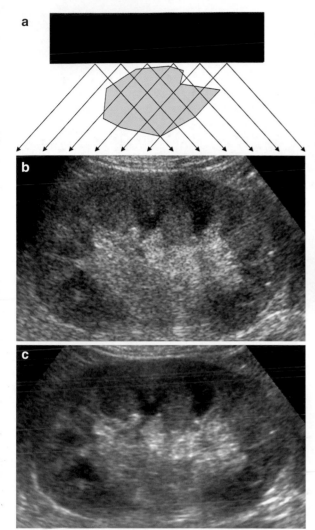

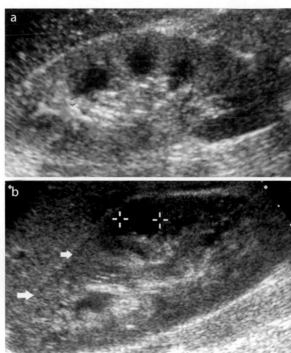

**Fig. 4.6** Gray-scale US. Longitudinal scan. (**a**) Increased renal cortical echogenicity and cortico-medullary differentiation in a patient with acute glomerulonephritis. (**b**) Autosomal recessive polycystic kidney disease manifesting with enlarged and hyperechoic kidneys due to the unresolved small cystic dilatation of the collecting tubules that increases the number of acoustic interfaces

**Fig. 4.5** Compound imaging in the depiction of the renal margins. (**a**) In spatial compound imaging, the same insonated slice is interrogated according to different insonation angles. The resulting images are managed by subtracting all echoes step-by-step which appears incoherently in the different acquired images, corresponding essentially to noise. (**b**) Conventional gray-scale US. (**c**) Tissue harmonic imaging and compound imaging allow speckle reduction with better depiction of the renal echotexture and profiles

chronic pyelonephritis, chronic glomerulonephritis, sarcoidosis, glycogen storage disease, Wilson's disease, sickle cell anemia, infections of the renal medulla, and in hyperuricemic (gout, Lesch–Nyhan syndrome) or hypokalemic conditions (primary hyperaldosteronism, long-term furosemide therapy, and Bartter's syndrome due to an inherited defect in the thick ascending limb of the loop of Henle) (Kim and Kim 1990). Frequently, hyperechogenicity is determined by renal stones which

present a posterior acoustic shadowing if larger than 3 mm (Fig. 4.7d). The calcifications in the cyst wall (Fig. 4.7e) may determine a diffuse posterior acoustic shadowing with the impossibility to visualize the cystic content (Fig. 4.7f).

### 4.2.1.3 Solid and Cystic Renal Tumors

US is considered the first choice imaging modality when a renal mass is suspected. Due to the high diagnostic quality of today's state-of-the-art US equipment, a constantly increasing number of both benign and malign focal renal lesions are detected. Baseline grayscale US presents a low accuracy in the characterization of renal masses, especially if smaller than 3 cm in diameter, since benign and malignant tumors frequently present similar appearance (Correas et al. 1999). Also benign and malignant renal masses >4 cm

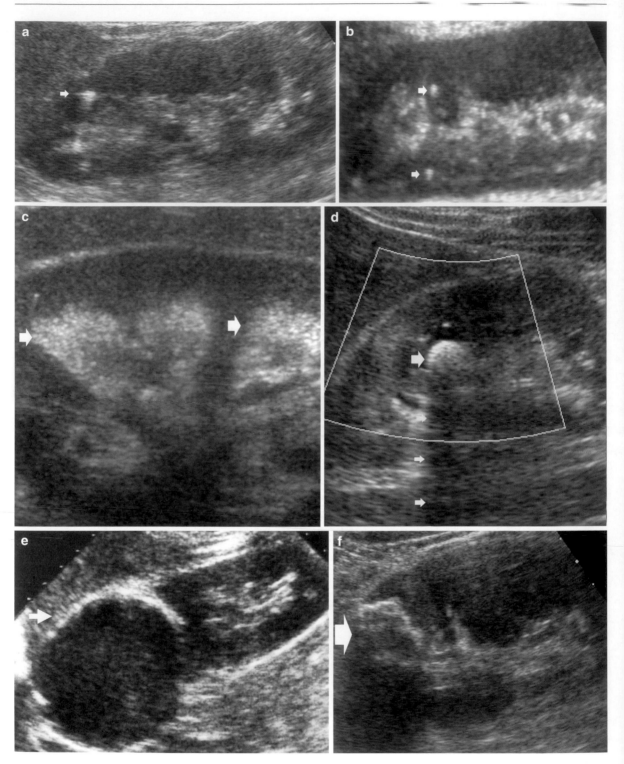

**Fig. 4.7** Hyperechogenicity. (**a**) Gray-scale US. Longitudinal scan. Randall's plaque (*arrow*) with comet-tail artifact. (**b**) Longitudinal scan. Focal papillary calcifications (*arrows*) in a medullary sponge kidney. (**c**) Diffuse hyperechogenicity of the renal medulla (*arrows*) due to medullary nephrocalcinosis in a patient with medullary sponge kidney. (**d**) Transverse scan. Hyperechogenicity with posterior acoustic shadowing (*small arrows*) due to a renal stone (*large arrow*). (**e**) Longitudinal scan. Hyperechogenicity due to diffuse wall calcifications (*arrow*) in a renal cyst. (**f**) Longitudinal scan. The calcifications of a cystic wall (*arrow*) do not allow the assessment of the cystic content due to diffuse acoustic shadowing

may present similar appearance, and large renal cell carcinomas prevalently reveal heterogeneous appearance due to intratumoral necrosis, calcifications, and hemorrhage similar to large angiomyolipomas which may reveal heterogeneous appearance due to solid, adipose, and hemorrhagic components. In daily routine work, the most useful one may be the widely accepted approach to do an initial differentiation between solid and cystic lesions by gray-scale US. In case malignancy is suspected based on the US appearance, further diagnostic workup with CT or MRI is recommended. The reverse sequence of imaging studies, that is, an equivocal lesion diagnosed on CT or MRI, is referred for further evaluation by US, or contrast-enhanced US (CEUS) may occur in an institution where high level US expertise is available or if percutaneous ablation is considered.

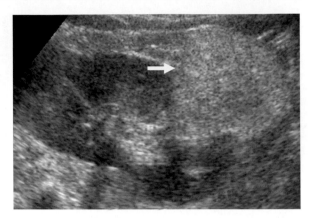

**Fig. 4.8** Hyperechoic homogenous solid renal lesion (*arrow*). Large renal angiomyolipoma (*arrow*) with a prevalently extrinsic development appearing as a homogeneously bright renal mass with wedge-shaped connection with the renal parenchyma resulting in a parenchyma defect

• Solid renal tumors. Solid renal tumors may present all the possible degrees of echogenicity. The most typical pattern is the homogeneous hyperechogenicity of renal angiomyolipoma (Fig. 4.8) which presents a homogeneously bright appearance and a wedge-shaped connection with the renal parenchyma resulting in a parenchyma defect, also with evidence of posterior acoustic shadowing (Yamashita et al. 1992; Helenon et al. 1997, 2001; Jinzaki et al. 1997). Atypical iso-hypoechoic and slightly hyperechoic angiomyolipoma accounts respectively for 6 and 29% (Helenon et al. 2001) Among small renal cell carcinomas (3 cm or less in diameter), 23–46% of solid tumors are iso- or hypoechoic compared with normal renal parenchyma (Helenon et al. 2001). Approximately, 30% of solid renal cell carcinomas smaller than 3 cm appear as hyperechoic masses (Forman et al. 1993). Tumors of papillary architecture are prevalently hyperechoic at US (Fig. 4.9a, b). There is no correlation of cell differentiation and cell architecture with echogenicity or tumor vascularity (Yamashita et al. 1992). The hypoechoic appearance, sometimes with evidence of an anechoic rim (Fig. 4.9c) or small intratumoral cysts (Fig. 4.9d), is frequently observed in renal cell carcinoma. Histologically, homogeneous tumors of solid architecture are usually isoechoic (Fig. 4.10) or hypoechoic at gray-scale US (Fig. 4.11) (Yamashita et al. 1993; Siegel et al. 1996). Solid renal cell carcinomas larger than 3 cm appears prevalently heterogeneous at baseline US due to intratumoral necrosis, calcifications (Helenon et al. 2001),

and hemorrhage. Some typical US patterns were described also for renal oncocytoma, as the presence of a central scar appearing as a stellate hypoechoic area and the absence of hemorrhage and necrosis (Helenon et al. 2001). Tissue harmonic imaging is useful in complicated solid renal masses to identify intratumoral necrosis or hemorrhagic perirenal collection from tumoral rupture (Fig. 4.12).

• Cystic renal tumors. Renal cysts are common incidental findings during the clinical diagnostic workup of patients (Helenon et al 2001), and the simple renal cyst is the most common renal lesion encountered. Renal cysts frequently present an obvious simple cystic pattern at US and/or CT and such cysts do not deserve any further imaging assessment or surgical procedure. In some cases, however, renal cysts show a complex pattern and vary in their malignant potential according to the number and thickness of intracystic septations, and the presence of mural nodules and peripheral calcifications.

Well-established characteristics of a simple renal cyst include sharp borders and particularly, sharply defined back wall, thin wall, anechoic contents, and strong enhancement of through sound transmission (Fig. 4.13a, b). The content of renal cysts typically appears more complex at US than at CT, owing to the greater accuracy of US in depicting thin intracystic septations and the corpuscular content due to hemorrhage or tumor debris. Varying degrees of cyst complexity are often shown at US, such as single or multiple septations (Fig. 4.13c–e), low-level echoes (due to hemorrhagic

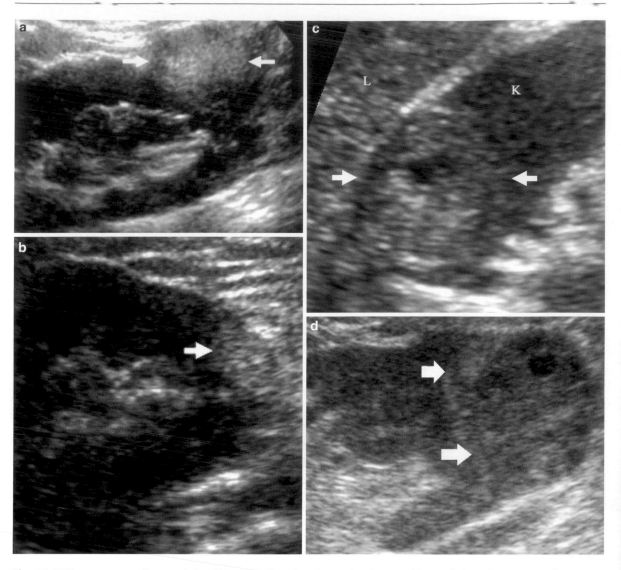

**Fig. 4.9** Different patterns of hyperechoic solid renal cell carcinoma. (**a**) Large papillary cell-type renal cell carcinoma. (**b**) Small papillary cell-type renal cell carcinoma. (**c**) Hyperechoic clear cell-type renal carcinoma with peripheral hypoechoic rim (*arrows*) and a central hypoechoic region corresponding to central necrosis (*L* liver; *K* kidney). (**d**) Hyperechoic clear cell-type renal carcinoma (*arrows*) with intratumoral hypoechoic cysts (*small arrows*)

or proteinaceous debris – Fig. 4.13f), thick walls, calcifications, and mural nodularity (Fig. 4.13g). Renal cyst content may be easily characterized by using tissue harmonic imaging and compound imaging which allows speckle reduction and improved contrast-to-noise ratio with an increased diagnostic confidence in the differentiation between simple and complicated renal cysts (Figs. 4.14–4.18).

The Bosniak (1986, 1991) classification categorizes the renal cysts according to their CT features: category I, simple benign fluid-containing cysts with the attenuation of water and thin walls without septa or calcification; category II, minimally complicated benign cysts with hairline-thin septa, fine calcifications in the walls or septa or segmental slightly thickened calcifications, with or without minimal septal or mural enhancement (high-attenuation, sharply marginated, completely intrarenal, and not enhancing cystic masses ≤3 cm are also included in this category); category IIF (F indicates follow-up), more complex cystic lesions that cannot be classified as category II nor are complex enough to be characterized as category III since they

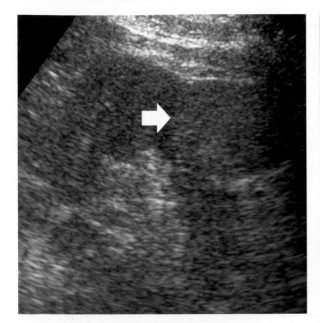

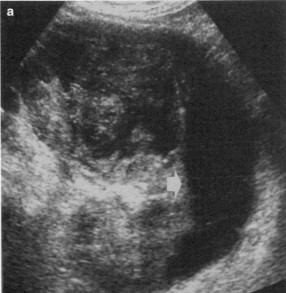

**Fig. 4.10** Solid renal lesion isoechoic to the adjacent renal parenchyma with bulging of the renal profile. Clear cell-type renal carcinoma (*arrow*)

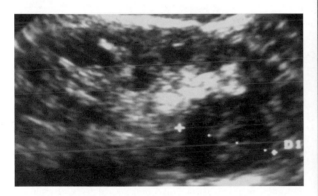

**Fig. 4.11** Hypoechoic solid renal lesion. Papillary cell-type renal carcinoma (callipers)

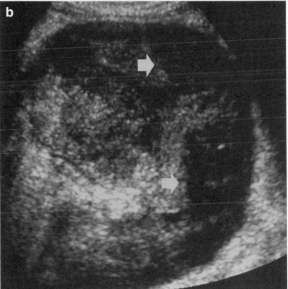

**Fig. 4.12** Usefulness of tissue harmonic imaging in complicated solid renal masses. Rupture of a solid renal tumor with hemorrhagic perirenal collection. (**a**) Conventional gray-scale US. A perirenal hypoechoic collection (*arrow*) is identified; (**b**) tissue harmonic imaging allows a better characterization of the perirenal collection (*arrows*) by depicting a corpuscular pattern typical of the hemorrhagic collection

may contain an increased number of septa and an increased amount of calcifications in the walls or septa, which may be thicker and nodular (high-attenuation, sharply marginated, completely intrarenal, and not enhancing cystic masses >3 cm are also included in this category); category III, indeterminate cystic masses whose benign or malignant nature cannot be determined with imaging studies, with thickened (>2 mm) irregular walls or septa, which may appear hyperdense on unenhanced CT and may contain either small or large amounts of calcification with septal and/or mural contrast enhancement; category IV, cysts showing either small or large amounts of calcifications within a thickened, enhancing irregular wall or septum and presenting enhancing soft-tissue nodular components adjacent to or extending from the wall or septum.

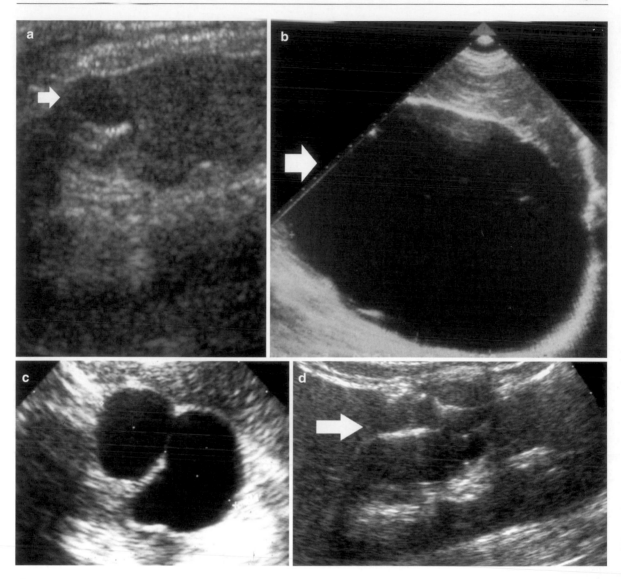

**Fig. 4.13** Different appearances of renal cysts on gray-scale US. (**a**) Simple small renal cyst with posterior acoustic shadowing; (**b**) large renal cyst with diffuse posterior acoustic shadowing; (**c**) renal cyst with a single septation; (**d**) renal cyst with multiple septations (*arrow*); (**e**) complex renal cyst with multiple septations corresponding to a multilocular cystic nephroma; (**f**) hemorrhagic renal cyst with hyperechoic content; (**g**) complex renal cyst with mural nodularity (*arrow*) and echoic content

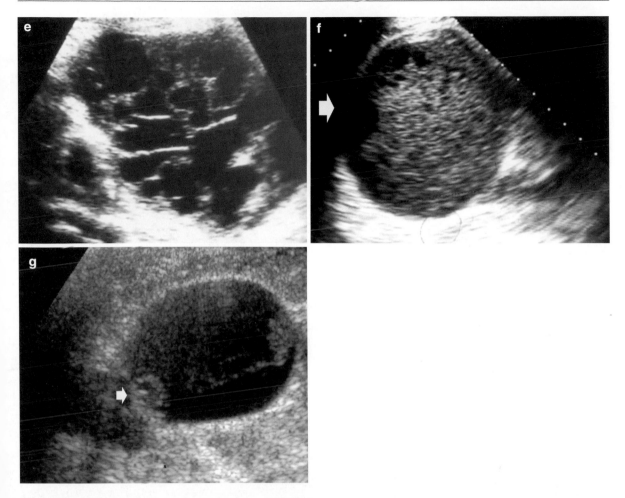

**Fig. 4.13** (continued)

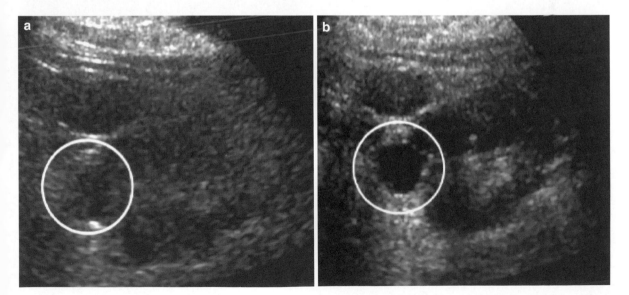

**Fig. 4.14** Tissue harmonic imaging. Simple renal cyst with anechoic appearance (*circle*). (**a**) Conventional gray-scale US. Doubtful content of the lesion. (**b**) Tissue harmonic imaging allowing a better characterization of the anechoic liquid content of the renal cyst with evidence of posterior acoustic enhancement

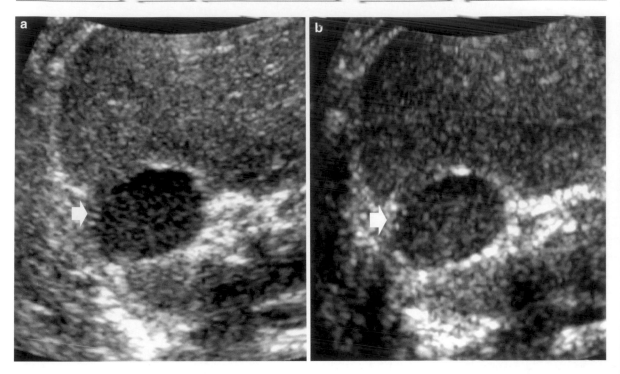

**Fig. 4.15** Tissue harmonic imaging. Hemorrhagic renal cyst with hyperechoic corpuscular content. (**a**) Conventional gray-scale US. The renal cyst reveals a corpuscular content. (**b**) Tissue harmonic imaging confirms the corpuscular content of the renal cyst

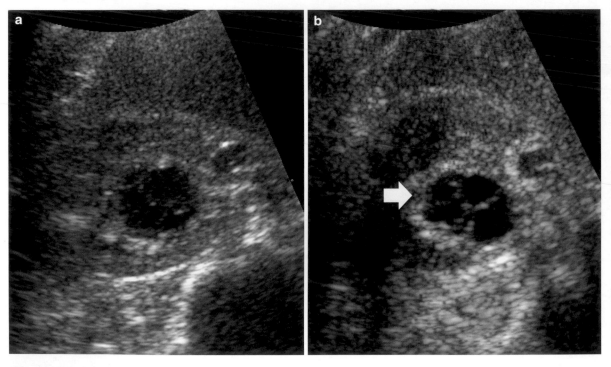

**Fig. 4.16** Tissue harmonic imaging. Complex renal cyst with septations. (**a**) Conventional gray-scale US reveals indistinct content of the cyst; (**b**) tissue harmonic imaging allows speckle reduction with a better depiction of the intracystic septations and a better characterization of the liquid content (*arrow*)

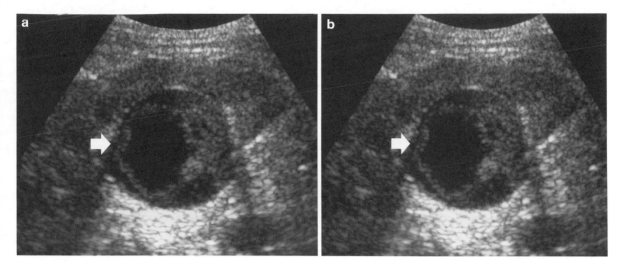

**Fig. 4.17** Tissue harmonic imaging. Complex renal cyst with peripheral wall thickening (*arrow*). (**a**) Conventional gray-scale US reveals a cystic pattern with peripheral wall thickening; (**b**) tissue harmonic imaging allows speckle reduction with a better characterization of the liquid content (*arrow*) and a better depiction with peripheral wall thickening

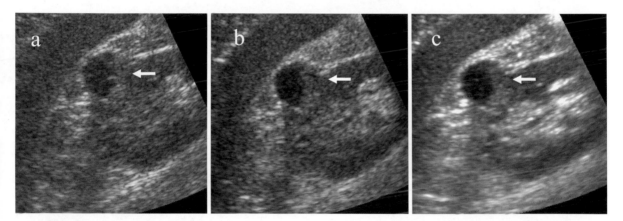

**Fig. 4.18** Tissue harmonic imaging and compound imaging. Complex renal cyst with peripheral wall thickening. (**a**) Hypoechoic renal mass (*arrow*) on the upper pole of the right kidney; (**b**) harmonic imaging reveals the cystic nature of the lesion with a peripheral wall thickening; (**c**) compound imaging combined to harmonic imaging confirms the cystic nature of the lesions with the addition of a better depiction of the lesion margins with respect to the adjacent renal parenchyma

### 4.2.2 Color and Power Doppler Ultrasound

#### 4.2.2.1 Normal Anatomy

Beside the evaluation of both the kidneys by gray-scale US (which should be extended to the bladder in every patient), color/power Doppler analysis of renal parenchyma vascularity should be performed in every patient to identify global or partial renal cortical perfusion defects. Color Doppler is a Doppler technique in which a color map displays the mean Doppler frequency shift of Doppler signal, giving information relative to the presence and direction of flows in renal vessels. Color Doppler presents some technical limitations, including US beam attenuation with depth, insonation angle dependence, and motion artifacts.

The peripheral vasculature of the renal cortex distal to the arcuate level is abundant and is made of a dense series of small interlobular vessels (Martinoli et al. 1999). Nowadays, the US equipments allow the depiction of the renal parenchyma vessels up to arciform and interlobular arteries and veins and of the capsular vessels (Fig. 4.19a), while the renal medulla appears hypovascular at color Doppler. The depiction of the renal parenchymal vessels by color Doppler US is reduced with an insonation angle close to 90° (renal poles) and is dependent on the kidney depth and the frequency of the US transducer. Moreover, the depiction of the renal parenchyma flows is reduced in the elderly patient. To increase the visualization of the renal parenchyma vessels, it is important to employ a low wall filter, a low pulse repetition frequency, and an appropriate signal gain with the lowest level of the noise and clutter. The renal medulla is avascular at color/power Doppler analysis since those renal vessels present a slow-flow velocity.

Power Doppler is a Doppler technique in which a color map displays the integrated amplitude of Doppler signal. Power Doppler is not dependent on insonating angle and is superior to color Doppler in delineating renal parenchymal blood flows, particularly at the renal poles and the superficial renal cortex (Fig. 4.19b). Power Doppler reveals a diffuse, homogeneous, low-amplitude color blush of the entire renal cortex generated from the sum of the numerous weak signals from interlobular vessels and their distal branches, and by high-frequency transducers, Power Doppler is able to solve color blush into the series of interlobular vessels also with the possibility of tissue background suppression by using colored masks (Fig. 4.19c). Failure of power Doppler to produce the cortical blush in normal native kidneys may occur either selectively in the far renal cortex due to the attenuation of the signal with depth, or diffusely as a result of obesity or inability of the patient to breath-hold adequately (Martinoli et al. 1999).

Occasionally, flow signals may be visible in the medullary regions. It is possible to obtain a 3D visualization of renal vessels by using matrix US transducers. Wideband color Doppler US (Fig. 4.19d), employing different color

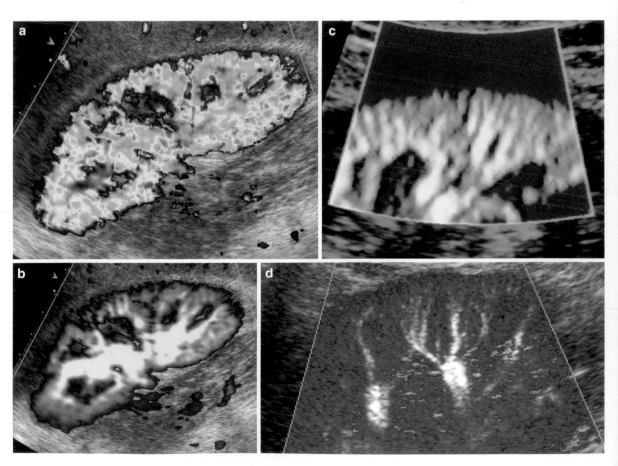

**Fig. 4.19** Color and power Doppler of the renal vasculature. (**a**) Color Doppler, (**b**) power Doppler, (**c**) power Doppler with tissue background suppression by a colored mask, and (**d**) wideband color Doppler allow an accurate depiction of the renal vessels up to the arcuate arteries

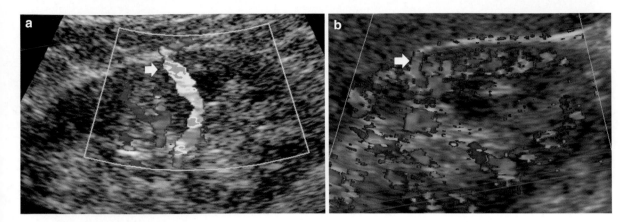

**Fig. 4.20** Renal perforating arterial (**a**) and venous (**b**) vessels. Color Doppler. (**a**) Renal perforating arterial vessel (*arrow*) in a patient with chronic renal failure. (**b**) Renal perforating venous vessel (*arrow*) in a young individual visualized during diastole

maps according to the US equipment, allows obtaining a better spatial resolution with an improved differentiation of the single vessels in the renal cortex.

The renal perforating vessels, traveling through the renal capsule, are recognizable using color Doppler, both in healthy subjects and in patients with renal failure (Bertolotto et al. 2000). Renal perforating arterial vessels (Fig. 4.20a) are occasionally identified in normal individuals, while renal perforating venous vessels (Fig. 4.20b) are frequently identified, especially in the young patient, and present a flow visible during diastole. Generally, the prevalence and flow characteristics of renal perforating vessels differ between healthy subjects, patients with mild and with severe chronic renal failure, and those with chronic renal failure complicated by acute renal insufficiency caused by renal artery stenosis (Bertolotto et al. 2000). The renal perforating arteries in healthy and hypertensive patients present various resistance indices and flow toward the capsule. Renal perforating arteries with a lower mean resistance index than the mean interlobar resistance index and flow toward the capsule are detected in the majority of kidneys in the patients with mild chronic renal failure (Fig. 4.20a) and in some patients with severe chronic renal failure. On the other hand, only a few perforating renal veins are visible in patients with chronic renal failure (Bertolotto et al. 2000). In kidneys with renal artery stenosis, detected in the patients with chronic renal failure complicated by acute renal insufficiency, some renal perforating arteries are detectable with flow toward the kidney and a mean resistance index higher than the mean interlobar resistance index (Bertolotto et al. 2000).

### 4.2.2.2 Fundamental Alterations of Renal Parenchyma Vascularity

The renal parenchyma vascularity is reduced on color and power Doppler analysis in nephrosclerosis (Fig. 4.21) and in renal parenchyma diseases. The fundamental alterations of renal parenchyma visible at color and power Doppler US include perirenal hematoma (Fig. 4.22) and renal perfusion defects or infarctions (Fig. 4.23). The principal limitation of color Doppler US is the limited sensitivity in the detection of renal perfusion defects which is much improved by contrast-enhanced US (Robbin et al. 2003).

One peculiar employment of color and power Doppler US is the renal stone detection and characterization through the color comet-tail artifact. The color comet-tail artifact (or twinkling sign) is a rapidly alternating color Doppler signal that occurs immediately deep in relation to the object causing it. It is typically observed behind a renal stone (Fig. 4.24). Because of the normal echogenic background of the renal sinus, small kidney stones are often difficult or impossible to detect or differentiate from small echogenic foci that are not caused by calcification (Tchelepi and Ralls 2009). The color comet-tail artifact is of value in identifying such stones. The artifact appears on images as a linear aliased band of color (Tchelepi and Ralls 2009) and depends both on the roughness of the surface of the object imaged (Rahmouni et al. 1996) and on machine settings, color gain, color-write priority, pulse repetition frequency, and gray-scale gain (Kamaya et al. 2003). Sometimes, the artifact is enhanced by an increase in color gain and moving the transmit zones deep in relation to the object causing the

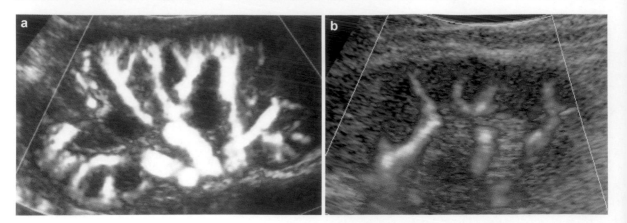

**Fig. 4.21** Renal nephrosclerosis. Power Doppler US. (**a**) Normal distribution of renal vessels. (**b**) Renal vessel distribution in nephrosclerosis

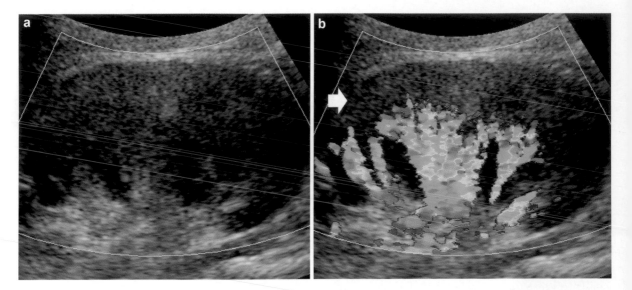

**Fig. 4.22** Renal subcapsular hematoma. (**a**) Conventional US. A diffuse cortical thickening of the right kidney. (**b**) Color Doppler allows the identification of a sucapsular renal hematoma (*arrow*)

artifact. Lower color Doppler frequency seems to produce a more prominent color comet-tail artifact than does a higher frequency (Tchelepi and Ralls 2009).

### 4.2.2.3 Renal Tumors

Color and power Doppler US are usually employed for the characterization of renal solid masses. Each renal tumor must be preliminary scanned by baseline gray-scale and color Doppler US, also with the employment of speckle-reducing technique such as tissue harmonic imaging and compound imaging (Claudon et al.

2002). Baseline color Doppler US is performed by using slow-flow settings (pulse repetition frequency 800–1,500 Hz, wall filter of 50 Hz, high levels of color vs. echo priority and color persistence). Color gain should be varied dynamically during the examination to enhance color signals and avoid excessive noise, with the size of the color box adjusted to include the entire lesion in the field of view. Spectral analysis of central and peripheral tumoral vessels is performed by pulsed Doppler to reveal continuous venous or pulsatile arterial flows. The intratumoral or penetrating vessel pattern is considered most frequent in angiomyolipomas (Fig. 4.25). The peripheral (Fig. 4.26) or mixed

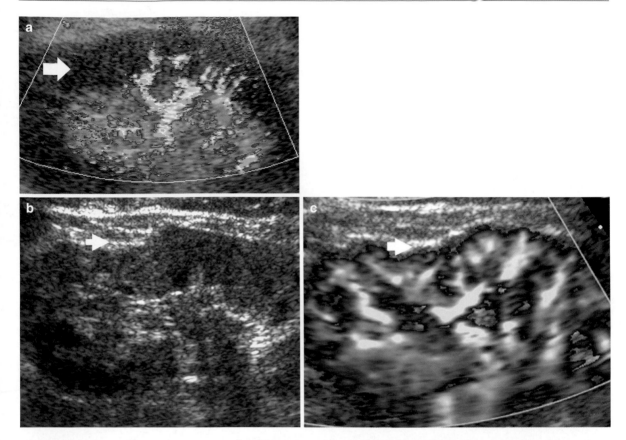

**Fig. 4.23** Different appearance of renal vascular alterations. (**a**) Color Doppler US. Renal perfusion defect (*arrow*) in a 60-year-old male patient with lack of renal cortical vessels in the upper pole of the right kidney due to acute renal infarction. (**b**, **c**) Renal vascular scar due to previous renal infarction. Clear parenchymal scar (*arrows*) on gray-scale US (**b**) which appears as a vascular defect on power Doppler (**c**)

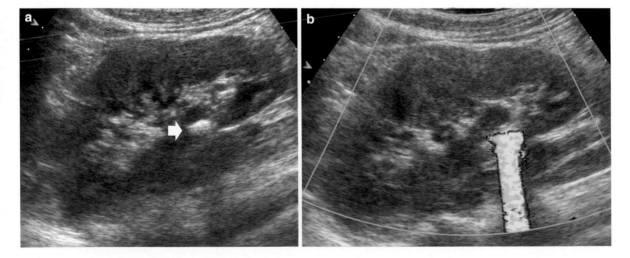

**Fig. 4.24** Twinkling artifact due to renal stone. (**a**) Conventional US identifies a renal stone (*arrow*) with posterior acoustic shadowing. (**b**) Color Doppler allows a correct characterization of renal stone through the visualization of the twinkling artifact

penetrating and peripheral tumoral vessel distribution (Fig. 4.27) may be observed in renal cell carcinomas (Jinzaki et al. 1998).

#### 4.2.2.4 Assessment of Renal Vessels

Color Doppler US is a fundamental technique in the screening of renal artery stenosis (Havey et al. 1985). For the evaluation of the main renal artery by Doppler US (Berland et al. 1990), the patient should follow a diet similar to that employed for intravenous urography during the 3 days before the examination to reduce the

intestinal metheorism also with rectal enema on the day of examination. For color Doppler examination, coronal plane must be employed to visualize the flow in the main renal arteries with an insonation angle lower than 60° (Figs. 4.28 and 4.29). An insonation angle close to 0° allows obtaining a cosine value close to 1 which allows an accurate calculation of the frequency shift which is equal to $2vf_i\cos\Phi/c$, with $v=$ blood velocity; $f_i=$ US frequency; $\cos\Phi=$ cosine of the angle between the blood flow direction and the US beam direction; $c=$ US beam velocity in the medium. The velocitometric analysis of Doppler trace derived from renal (Fig. 4.30) and intrarenal arterial vessels is of primary

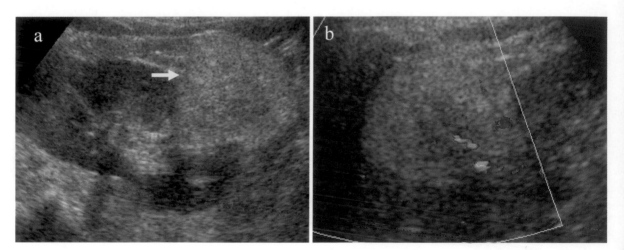

**Fig. 4.25** Vessel distribution pattern at color Doppler. Renal angiomyolipoma. (**a**) Hyperechoic renal solid mass (*arrow*). (**b**) Penetrating vessel distribution at color Doppler

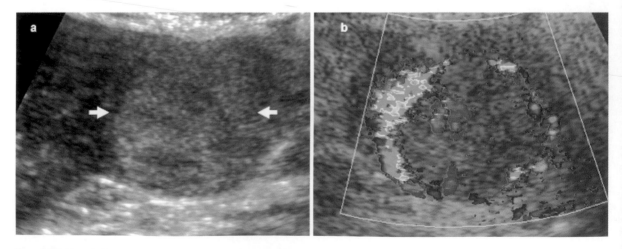

**Fig. 4.26** Vessel distribution pattern at color Doppler. Renal cell carcinoma. (**a**) Hyperechoic renal solid mass (*arrows*). (**b**) Prevalently peripheral vessel distribution at color Doppler

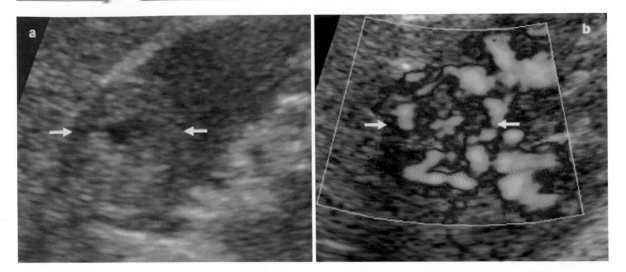

**Fig. 4.27** Vessel distribution pattern at color Doppler. Renal cell carcinoma. (**a**) Hyperechoic renal solid mass (*arrows*) with a hypoechoic peripheral rim. (**b**) Peripheral and intratumoral vessel distribution at color Doppler (*blue color map*)

importance (Fig. 4.31). The renal vein flow should also be analyzed by pulsed Doppler, and reveals a typical biphasic pattern (Fig. 4.32).

Assessment of renal vascular resistances is obtained by Doppler waveform analysis, obtaining the renal Resistive Index (RI) which corresponds to the peak systolic velocity minus the end-diastolic velocity divided by the peak systolic velocity. Increased sensitivity of color Doppler and power Doppler provided by the latest digital US equipment allows depiction and Doppler interrogation of the renal parenchymal vessels up to the interlobular arteries. The renal RI is considered a reflection of renal parenchymal resistance (Jensen et al. 1994; Bude and Rubin 1999; Tublin et al. 1999, 2003) and has been widely used to support diagnostic and therapeutic procedures. The glomerular circle presents a low influence in the RI value which is principally determined by the systemic cortical and medullary vascular circle in the kidney. The mean reference value for normal RI in adults was determined to be 0.60 ± 0.10, with 0.70 as the upper limit of normal (Platt et al. 1989, 1990; Kim et al. 1992; Keogan et al. 1996; Rivolta et al. 2000; Radermacher et al. 2002). The RIs measured on segmental, interlobar, and arcuate renal parenchymal arteries are normally below 0.70, and decrease progressively from segmental to interlobular vessels. RIs are usually higher than 0.7 in the children younger than 4 years, while RIs are similar to adults after 4 years of age. RIs are significantly higher in the elderly subjects. Studies that correlate

RIs values with biopsy findings in various renal parenchymal diseases have revealed that kidneys with active disease in tubulo-interstitial or vascular compartment present elevated RIs (>0.80), whereas kidneys with glomerular diseases more often present normal RIs values. A further important index is the Pulsatility Index (PI) which is calculated through the analysis of the Doppler trace registered at the level of the renal parenchyma vessels and is equal to systolic peak minus the end diastole velocity up to the mean velocity.

The velocitometric analysis of Doppler trace derived from renal arteries (Fig. 4.33) is of primary importance to identify renal artery stenosis. Direct Doppler criteria have been proposed for the detection of renal arterial stenosis, including an increased peak systolic velocity (>150–180 cm/s) and end-diastolic velocity at the level of the stenosis (Correas et al. 1999; Grant and Melany 2001), poststenotic flow disturbance resulting in spectral broadening (Fig. 4.33) and reversed flow (Correas et al. 1999, 2003), increased ratio (≥3.5) of peak systolic velocity in renal artery and aorta (renal/aortic ratio), and the presence of turbulence within the renal artery (Desberg et al. 1990; Helenon et al. 1995, 1998). The maximal systolic velocity measured in the main renal artery ($V_{max}$ renal artery) should be compared to the maximal systolic velocity measured in the abdominal aorta at the level of the renal arteries ($V_{max}$ aorta) to calculate the renal/aortic ratio ($V_{max}$ renal artery/$V_{max}$ aorta). Although this technique is easy to perform, its accuracy is questionable, because the lack

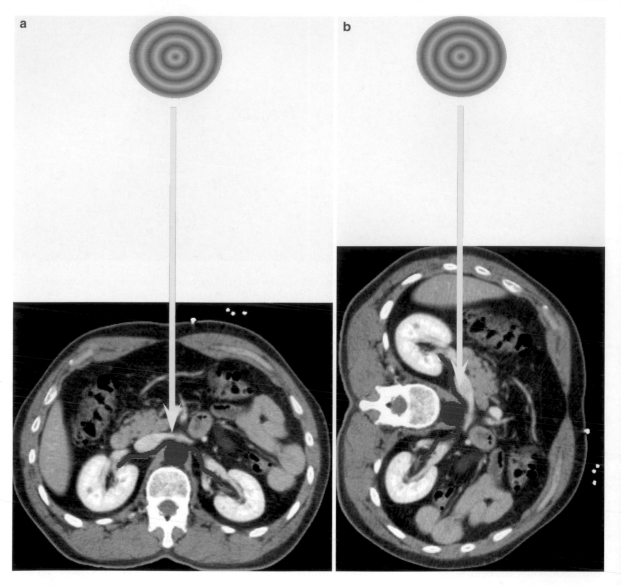

**Fig. 4.28** Insonation angle to image renal arteries by color Doppler (**a**) Incorrect insonation angle between the US beam and the renal artery close to 90° (**b**) Correct insonation angle between the US beam and the renal artery close to 0°

of an early systolic peak has a low sensitivity for moderate stenoses, and the waveform is dependent on the maintenance of vessel compliance, which limits its effectiveness in elderly patients and patients with atherosclerosis (Bude et al. 1994; Bude and Rubin 1995). Downstream hemodynamic repercussions of renal artery stenosis in the distal intrarenal arterial bed may be identified by Doppler US and may provide an indirect diagnosis of renal artery stenosis. Numerous parameters are still debated (Correas et al. 1999) except in cases of critical stenosis (>80%). In fact, even though the intraparenchymal arteries examination is technically easier than the evaluation of the main renal artery, Doppler US findings in interlobar-arcuate renal cortical arteries are less reliable than Doppler US findings on stenotic site, since downstream repercussions are absent in 20% of the principal renal artery tight stenosis (>80%), for a well-developed collateral blood supply. The assessment of the morphology of the Doppler trace, since, in the presence of an hemodynamically significant renal artery stenosis, the Doppler trace measured at poststenotic or intrarenal tract of renal artery reveals a "tardus et parvus" (Stavros et al. 1992; Bude et al. 1994) profile (Fig. 4.33), consisted of an increased time to reach the peak of the trace (acceleration time >70 ms) with loss of early systolic

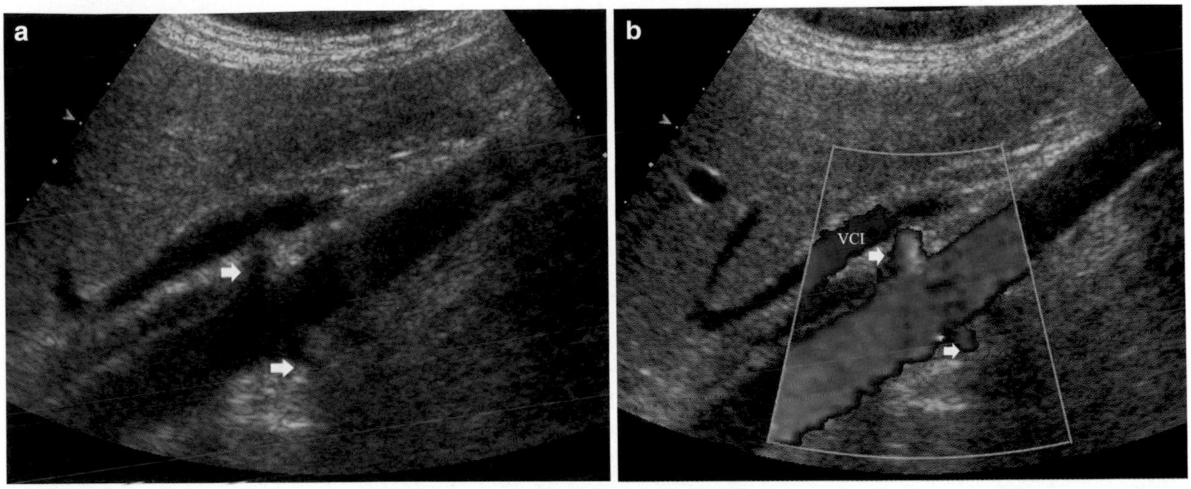

Fig. 4.29 Optimal visibility of renal arteries (*arrows*) at color Doppler US. (**a**) Conventional US. (**b**) Color Doppler. *VCI* Inferior Vena Cava

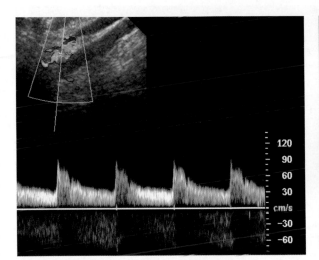

Fig. 4.30 Color Doppler US with Doppler interrogation of the main renal artery. The normal Doppler trace of the main renal artery

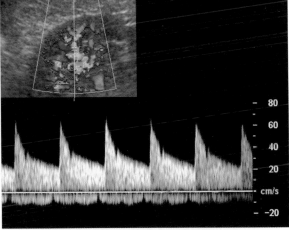

Fig. 4.31 Color Doppler US with Doppler interrogation of the intrarenal segmentary renal artery. The normal Doppler trace of the renal segmental artery

peak and decreased acceleration index – Doppler frequency/sec – (<300 cm/sec$^2$). Acceleration time should be measured at the level of the initial increase in the systolic velocity up to peak systolic velocity or to the highest velocity value of the spectral Doppler trace according to the Doppler trace morphology. Poststenotic pulsus tardus is caused by the compliance of the poststenotic vessel wall in conjunction with the stenosis, which produces the tardus effect by damping the high-frequency components of the arterial waveform. This information allows the identification of those conditions which may produce false-positive or false-negative results when the tardus phenomenon is used to predict hemodynamically significant upstream stenosis (Bude et al. 1994). This is the case of the loss of vascular compliance in severe diffuse atherosclerosis which may prevent the tardus-parvus phenomenon, decreasing the sensitivity of color Doppler US (Grant and Melany 2001). Other findings which may be observed in the intraparenchymal arteries in the presence of renal artery stenosis are decreased resistive indices in interlobar-arcuate renal cortical arteries with increased side difference higher than 10% (Correas et al. 1999). In patients suspected of having renal

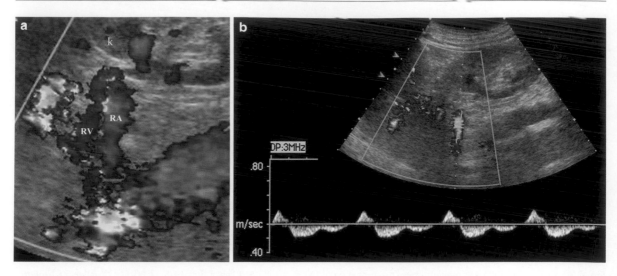

**Fig. 4.32** Normal renal veins on color Doppler. The renal vein is represented in blue color since the blood is moving away from the transducer (**a**). (**b**) Normal biphasic Doppler trace of the renal vein. *RA* renal artery; *RV* renal vein; *k* left kidney

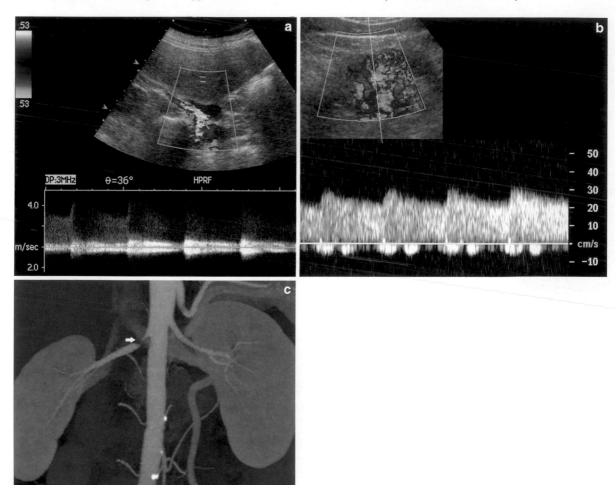

**Fig. 4.33** Right renal artery stenosis. (**a**) Increase of the peak systolic velocity with aliasing (*arrow*) and spectral broadening of the Doppler trace at the level of the proximal right renal artery. (**b**) Tardus-and-parvus flow is identified in a segmental intrarenal artery. (**c**) Contrast-enhanced angio-CT examination confirms a tight stenosis on the right renal artery

arterial stenosis and with a poor acoustic window, microbubble contrast agents increased the number of diagnostic renal arterial Doppler studies (Correas et al. 1998; Claudon et al. 2000; Grant and Melany 2001) in a "color Doppler rescue" setting.

## 4.3 Clinical Indications for Renal Ultrasound Examination

The indications for the US examination of the kidneys and urinary tract correspond almost to all clinical situations which could be related to a renal pathology. The principal indications of gray-scale US are the assessment of renal morphology and dimensions; renal colic or acute flank pain; identification and assessment of hydronephrosis; assessment of the renal parenchyma in renal parenchyma diseases; acute and chronic renal failure; identification and characterization of solid and cystic renal tumors; identification of intrarenal urinary tract tumors; differential diagnosis between intrarenal urinary tract tumors, calculi, and coaguli; renal trauma; guidance for interventional procedures including renal biopsy and nephrostomy. The diagnostic workup of patients with renal colic, the detection of renal hydronephrosis, detection of renal tumors, and hematuria are probably the most important indications for renal US examination. The other fields of application of renal US are extensively described in the dedicated chapters.

In patients with acute flank pain, US is the first choice imaging modality. US is employed to detect hydronephrosis in urinary track obstruction, to identify the renal stone in patients with renal colic, to assess the renal size and renal parenchyma thickness if clinical causes other than urinary stones (renal hemorrhage, renal infections, or renal ischemia) are suspected, and to detect complications. US is the most sensitive imaging technique in detecting renal hydronephrosis. In nonhydrated patients, US presents a sensitivity of 35–73% and a specificity of 74%, while the sensitivity becomes 85–100% and the specificity 83–100% in hydrated patients (Svedström et al. 1990; Haddad et al. 1992; Dalla Palma et al. 1993). In the detection of renal stones, US has a low sensitivity (20–30%) and high specificity (90%), while in the detection of ureteral stones, US presents a moderate sensitivity (60–70%) and high specificity (90–95%) (Fowler et al. 2002). The main variables affecting the US sensitivity in detecting urinary stone are the stone size and position, and the patient body habitus, while the stone composition does not affect the diagnostic sensitivity and specificity of US. US allows the evaluation of the kidney and pelvis provided the bladders are distended. The US findings in a patient with renal colic are the direct identification of the stone, increased echogenicity of renal parenchyma, pelvicalyceal and ureteric dilatation, and subcapsular collections (urinomas) (Fig. 4.34). The detection of urinary stones and the clarity of posterior shadowing are significantly improved by harmonic imaging (Fig. 4.35) (Ozdemir et al. 2008). Duplex Doppler sonography has been reported to be a useful noninvasive imaging method for the diagnosis of renal obstruction. A mean RI >0.7, a difference >0.08–0.1 between the mean RI of the two kidneys, and a progressive increase in RI following fluid administration and diuretics have been considered diagnostic of obstruction (Platt 1992; Platt et al. 1993). The evaluation of renal parenchyma RIs presents a controversial role in the acute renal colic with a sensitivity from 19 to 92% and a specificity from 88 to 98% according to the different series (Platt et al. 1989; Tublin et al. 1994; Lee et al. 1996).

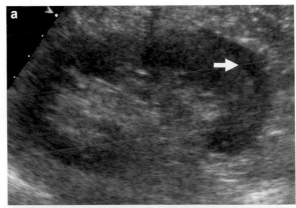

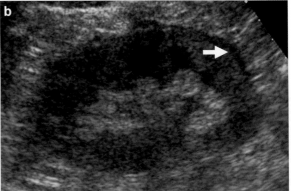

**Fig. 4.34** Patient with acute renal colic. (**a**) Gray-scale US. Longitudinal scan of the right kidney. Slight pelvicalyceal dilatation with subcapsular urinoma (*arrows*) visualized by tissue harmonic imaging (**b**)

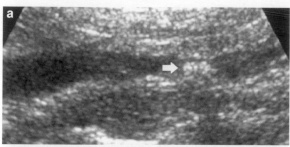

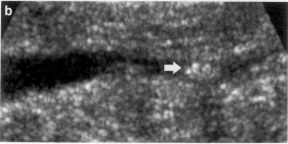

**Fig. 4.35** Patient with acute renal colic. Gray-scale US. Renal stone (*arrow*) located in the distal tract of the ureter. (**a**) Gray-scale US. (**b**) Tissue harmonic imaging. The detection of urinary stones and the clarity of posterior shadowing are significantly improved by harmonic imaging

Gray-scale US has an essential role in the detection of renal tumors even though the sensitivity is inferior to CT. Since US is routinely used for the examination of the abdomen, the detection rate of renal tumors in asymptomatic patients has increased dramatically. Baseline gray-scale US, also with the addition of speckles and noise reducing techniques such as tissue harmonic imaging and compound imaging (Claudon et al. 2002), is a reliable imaging technique for the early diagnosis of renal tumors (Helenon et al. 2001). In addition to some technical and anatomical factors that may alter US performance, the detectability of renal tumors depends mainly on the size, location, and echogenicity of the lesion with increased visibility of hyperechoic renal tumors. In particular, the main limitations of baseline US in the detection of renal tumors are related to small isoechoic intraparenchymal tumors and tumors of polar origin with extrarenal growth that may be obscured by bowel gas. Gray-scale US has a sensitivity of 85% in detecting renal masses >3 cm. Anyway, baseline gray-scale US is less accurate than contrast material-enhanced CT in revealing small renal masses <3 cm in diameter (Zagoria 2000) with a sensitivity of 26% for CT-confirmed renal masses <1 cm (Warshauer et al. 1988). Baseline color Doppler does not seem to significantly increase the detection rate of small tumors,

even though the absence of intratumoral vessels due to signal filtration improves the tumoral visibility (Fig. 4.36) (Helenon et al. 2001). Thus, gray-scale US is inadequate for screening for renal tumors, especially in patients with hereditary renal cancer (von Hippel–Lindau disease, hereditary papillary renal cell carcinoma), and contrast-enhanced CT is indicated in such cases.

Hematuria is the most common clinical indication for renal US. Hematuria represents a common urologic problem that accounts for 4–20% of all urologic visits (O'Connor et al. 2008). The prevalence of asymptomatic microscopic hematuria varies between 0.6–21% and is among the most important clinical signs of a urologic malignancy. A cause for asymptomatic microscopic hematuria can be found in 32–100% of patients undergoing a full urologic evaluation, with 3.4–56% of these patients having either moderately or highly clinically significant diagnoses (O'Connor et al. 2008). The wide variability in percentage is mainly due to the population studied, but in total, presents a conundrum regarding how best to evaluate these patients. Nevertheless, a full urologic evaluation is recommended in many patients with asymptomatic microscopic hematuria. On the other hand, hematuria (particularly when microscopic) may not always signal the presence of serious disease, and therefore, it has long been debated as to how aggressively these patients should be evaluated.

In addition to the evaluation of hematuria, US is the first imaging technique to be employed in patients with acute flank pain, and patients with obstructive uropathy to identify urinary tract dilatation with different grades of hydronephrosis and hydroureter. Other fields of applications include the surveillance of patients with a history of urothelial or renal cell cancers, or any time a comprehensive evaluation of the urinary tract is warranted including renal trauma, and renal vascular diseases. Moreover, US represents the most employed imaging technique to guide the interventional procedures such as renal biopsy and renal nephrostomy.

## 4.4 Microbubble Contrast Agents and Contrast-Specific Ultrasound Techniques

US microbubble contrast agents have gained an increasing interest in the recent years, and contrast-enhanced US (CEUS) represents a rapidly evolving

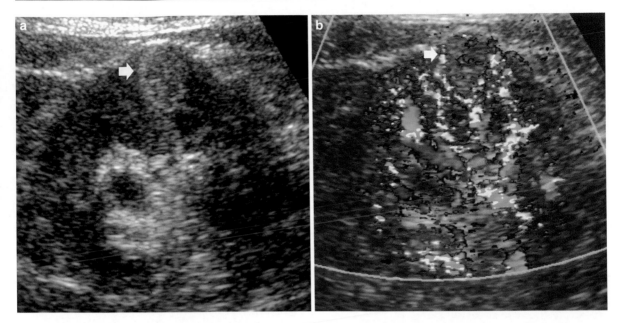

**Fig. 4.36** Improved tumoral visibility with color Doppler US. (**a**) Gray-scale US. Transverse scan. Small renal parenchyma solid tumor (*arrow*); (**b**) color Doppler US. The tumor visibility is improved due to the prevalence of normal parenchymal vessels surrounding the lesion with absent intratumoral vessels on color Doppler US. The absence of intratumoral vessels is due to signal filtration to eliminate the clutter produced by stationary or slow moving tissues which eliminates also the slow flows from small intratumoral vessels

technique with many clinical applications (Quaia 2007a, b). Innovative US techniques namely contrast-specific were introduced to selectively register the harmonic signal produced by the nonlinear physical behavior of microbubbles. This was determined by the impossibility of traditional color and power Doppler to manage the harmonic signals produced by microbubble insonation, since they are limited by the strong presence of artifacts including the blooming and jail bar artifacts.

## 4.4.1 Chemical Composition of Microbubble Contrast Agents

Microbubble contrast agents are now approved in most European countries, and are largely employed also in Asia and Canada. The Food and Drug Administration in United States has not yet approved microbubble contrast agents for noncardiac use. The recently introduced sulfur hexafluoride or perfluorocarbon-filled microbubbles offer both an excellent safety profile, and a longer persistence in the peripheral circle than air-filled microbubbles. Microbubble contrast agents are composed of a shell of biocompatible material such as a proteins, lipids, or biopolymers. Microbubble contrast agents are injectable intravenously and can pass through the pulmonary capillary bed after a peripheral injection, since their diameter (3–10 µm) is below that of red blood cells.

Two principal strategies were developed to increase microbubble stability and persistence in the bloodstream: the stability of the external microbubble encapsulation in the peripheral bloodstream and the selection of filling gases with a low diffusion coefficient. The peripheral shell presents a thickness ranging from 10 to 200 nm, and may be stiff (e.g., denaturated albumin or biopolymers) or more flexible (phospholipids). Low-solubility low-diffusibility gases, such as perfluorocarbons and sulfur hexafluoride gas, are employed to improve the persistence of microbubbles in the peripheral bloodstream. The physical properties of microbubble contrast agents are closely related not only to their gas content and to the peripheral shell chemical composition, but also to the frequency of the US beam, the pulse repetition frequency, and overall, to the acoustic power employed for insonation. The different microbubble contrast agents are reported in Table 4.1.

**Table 4.1** Microbubble contrast agents classified according to the filling gas

| Air (nitrogen) | Perfluorocarbon | Sulfur hexafluoride |
| --- | --- | --- |
| Albunex (Mallinckrodt)[a] | BR14 (Bracco) | SonoVue (Bracco) |
| Echovist (Shering)[b] | Definity (Bristol–Myers Squibb Medical Imaging) | |
| Levovist (Shering)[b] | Echogen (Sonus Pharmaceuticals)[d] | |
| Myomap (Quadrant)[a] | Imagent – Imavist (Alliance) | |
| Quantison (Quadrant)[a] | Optison (GE Healthcare)[a] | |
| Sonavist (Shering)[c] | Sonazoid (GE Healthcare) | |

*Note*. Echovist, Levovist, Optison, and SonoVue are currently approved and marketed within European countries. Definity, Imagent, and Optison are approved in USA for cardiologyIn perfluorocarbon-filled agents, the filling gas is perfluorobutane (BR14, Optison, and Sonazoid), octafluoropropane (Definity), or perfluorohexane (Imagent)

Levovist, Sonavist, Imagent, and Sonazoid present a late hepato and spleno-specific phase. All the agents present a phospholipid shell except for:

[a] Albumin shell

[b] Galactose shell

[c] Cyanoacrylate shell

[d] Phase shift agent. A perflenapent liquid-in-liquid emulsion which contains dodecafluoropentane liquid in the dispersed phase which shifts to a gas phase at body temperature forming microbubbles of 3–8 μm of diameter

## 4.4.2 Safety

The safety of diagnostic microbubbles is somewhat complex because not only must their safety as drugs be studied, as with other contrast agents, but additionally, the effects of sonication need to be taken into account. The safety of US contrast media is the subject of recent reports by the World Federation of Ultrasound in Medicine and Biology (Barnett et al. 2007). The adverse reactions in humans are rare, usually transient, and of mild intensity (Correas et al. 2001; Quaia et al. 2007b) and include tissue irritation in the vicinity of the injection site, dyspnea, chest pain, hypo or hypertension, nausea and vomiting, taste alterations, headache, vertigo, warm facial sensation, cutaneous eruptions, and asymptomatic premature ventricular contractions. However, serious allergic reactions have been observed at a very low incidence (estimated to be 1:10,000).

In 2004, the European Agency for the Evaluation of Medical Products (EMEA) temporarily withdrew the approval for SonoVue for cardiac applications due to three deaths reported in temporal relation with the application of SonoVue. All the patients did not present any allergic reaction, but all of them had unstable ischemic heart disease. Nineteen cases of severe, nonfatal adverse events (0.002%) were reported, and most of the cases were considered to be allergic reactions. The EMEA committee recognized a favorable risk/benefit ratio for SonoVue when patients with acute coronary

syndromes and unstable heart disease were excluded, and the committee otherwise restored the approval for cardiac indications. Even more recently, the FDA issued a black-box warning for Definity in October 2007 due to postmarketing reports of deaths in 4 patients with significant underlying progressive cardiovascular disease that were temporally related to contrast agent use. On 12 May 2008 and 6 June 2008, revised labeling changes were again implemented for Definity and Optison, respectively, following mounting evidence of safety and unequivocally favorable risk–benefit profile in the acute setting. The present FDA documents state that Definity and Optison are not to be administered to patients in whom right-to-left, bidirectional, or transient right-to-left cardiac shunts, hypersensitivity to perflutren, or to blood products, or albumin are known or suspected (Mulvagh et al. 2008). Except for SonoVue, both Definity and Optison may be used in acute coronary syndromes (Senior et al. 2009). It is hoped that EMEA will follow for SonoVue, the FDA statement for Definity and Optison, since SonoVue has a similar safety profile to Definity and Optison. At present, SonoVue may be used 7 days after acute coronary syndrome. The intrarterial injection of US contrast agents is also contraindicated.

Experimental studies on small animals and cell preparation have shown that potential adverse bioeffects from microbubble-based contrast agents under an US field, including hemolysis, platelet aggregation, disruption of cell membrane, rupture of small vessels, and induction of ectopic heart beats, can be induced under extreme conditions (exteriorized heart preparation, no or minimal attenuation, low-frequency high-acoustic pressures, and long pulse durations). The phenomenon of inertial cavitation – the rapid formation, growth, and collapse of a gas cavity in a fluid as a result of US exposure – is considered the cause of most of the microbubble side effects observed in animals in experimental studies, and no evidence of bioeffects from a clinically comparable US exposure and microbubble concentration has been reported in humans. These experimental findings cannot be extrapolated to the clinical setting where the attenuation of US significantly reduces patient exposure, even though these conditions could be reproduced also in the clinical setting during lithotripsy, and focused US ablation.

### 4.4.3 Insonation Power

To obtain a useful harmonic signal for imaging, the microbubbles have to be insonated at their specific fundamental frequency, defined also as resonance frequency, which corresponds to the frequency range of 3 to 3.7 MHz, usually employed for the abdominal US examination. The acoustic power employed to insonate the microbubbles is usually expressed by the mechanical index. It is defined as: mechanical index $= p-/\sqrt{fc}$, where $p-$ is the largest peak negative (rarefactional) pressure that the transmitted US pulse achieves during its travel through a medium of specified attenuation coefficient, and $fc$ is the center frequency of the pulse. The mechanical index is actually a safety index indicating the potential for nonthermal bioeffects during intonation. Anyway, it presents the disadvantage to be poorly reproducible between the different US equipments. A more correct and reproducible manner is to express the insonation transmit power as MPa (mega Pascal) which is mentioned in the operative screen of some US equipments.

There are two quite different approaches to insonate microbubbles. One group of methods, commonly known as high transmit power insonation, use large pulse amplitudes (about 1 MPa) and produce microbubble destruction with the emission of an irregular wide band harmonic signal, similar to an explosion, named stimulated acoustic emission (SAE). The threshold for

destruction is variable and depends on a number of different factors such as the size, the shell material, and the filling gas of microbubble, and the attenuation of the US beam power from the overlaying tissues. These methods are generally employed to insonate air-filled microbubble contrast agents with a soft shell presenting a low harmonic behavior at low transmit power insonation, and are limited by the transiency of the signal which persists only for 2–3 frames. Intermittent imaging at low frame rates (one image every 2–3 s) may overcome this problem by limiting the destruction of microbubbles.

The other group of methods consists in the low transmit power insonation (30–70 kPa). This technique reduces the microbubble destruction and the magnitude of harmonic signals produced by stationary tissues, and employs the nonlinear physical behavior of microbubbles. When the microbubbles are insonated at the fundamental (resonance) frequency with a low acoustic power, the microbubbles present a non linear physical behavior and become relatively more resistant to compression than to expansion. This leads to asymmetric or nonlinear oscillations which contain both fundamental and harmonic frequencies multiple of the fundamental frequency. This insonation method is employed with sulfur hexafluoride or perfluorocarbon-filled microbubbles, and allows a real-time scanning due to the long persistence of the signal.

### 4.4.4 Contrast-Specific Ultrasound Techniques

The different contrast-specific US techniques may be differentiated from their basic principles in pseudo-Doppler, harmonic, phase modulation, amplitude modulation, and phase and amplitude modulation techniques (Quaia 2005; Whittingham 2005; Qin et al. 2009) (Table 4.2).

(a) Pseudo-Doppler techniques. These are multipulse high transmit power techniques. Pseudo-Doppler techniques employ the SAE effect which corresponds to the emission of a wide band signal when microbubbles are destroyed by a high transmit power insonation. These techniques are limited by the presence of motion artifacts and by the

**Table 4.2** Contrast-specific ultrasound techniques

| Pseudo-Doppler | Harmonic imaging | Coded imaging | Phase modulation | Amplitude modulation | Phase and amplitude modulation |
|---|---|---|---|---|---|
| – Stimulated acoustic emission (SAE)<br>– Cadence agent detection imaging (ADI)<br>– Advanced dynamic flow (ADF)<br>– Tissue signature imaging (TSI) | Gray-scale techniques<br>– Second harmonic imaging<br>– cCube<br>– Flash echo imaging<br>– Extended pure harmonic detection (ePHD)<br>– Contrast tuned imaging (CnTI)<br>– Ultraharmonic imaging<br>– Subharmonic imaging<br>– 1.5 Harmonic imaging<br>Doppler technique<br>– Harmonic power Doppler | – Coded Harmonic angio<br>– Chirp excitation | Gray-scale techniques<br>– Pulse inversion<br>– Microflow imaging[a]<br>– Contrast tissue discriminator (CTD)<br>– Coherent contrast imaging (CCI)<br><br>Doppler techniques:<br>– Power pulse inversion<br>– Vascular recognition imaging (VRI)<br>– Low MI color flow contrast | – Power modulation | – Cadence contrast pulse sequencing (CPS) |

*Note.* General classification of specialized contrast-specific US techniques according to the pulse transmission and signal processing
[a]*Microflow imaging* is based on the summation of multiple consecutive frames and represents a multiintensity projection algorithm of data obtained by a phase-inversion technique. It improves the visualization of slowly perfused organs (e.g., breast) by monitoring the tracks of single microbubbles. Further discrimination of microbubbles with respect to the stationary tissues is achieved by comparing consecutive frames with each other, pixel for pixel. If the content of a pixel has not changed from one frame to the next, it is rejected, leaving, ideally, only echoes from moving microbubbles

transiency of the signal. The stationary tissues and contrast information can be displayed separately or simultaneously by an electronic system which measures the Doppler power in each pixel and represents a pixel as a color pixel if the Doppler power exceeds a threshold value (priority) or as a gray-scale pixel if the Doppler power is lower according to the B-mode echo amplitude for that pixel. This Doppler threshold value is easily exceeded if microbubble contrast agents are employed resulting in the presence of artifacts as blooming (presence of Doppler signal not determined by the mean frequency shift) and clutter (low-frequency Doppler signal produced by stationary tissues overlapping the real Doppler signal). To limit the blooming artifact and clutter, the B-mode and Doppler power for a pixel are compared and the larger one is used to set the pixel gray level. This avoids blooming and clutter since a pixel will not display a power Doppler signal if the B-mode signal for that pixel is large, while the pixels with a strong clutter will merge relatively inconspicuously with those showing strong B-mode stationary tissue signals.

(b) Harmonic imaging techniques. These are multipulse techniques that employ the nonlinear physical properties of microbubbles to suppress the stationary tissue background. These techniques employ a high or low transmit power insonation. Since the second harmonic (double of the insonating frequency) has the highest

amplitude among the harmonics, it is therefore the most relevant harmonic frequency for the contrast-specific US imaging even though the signal may be persistent or transient according to the employed acoustic power. Moreover, these techniques are limited by the presence of tissue harmonic components which are present at high transmit power insonation which leads to a relative production of harmonics frequency and to the consequent poorer contrast resolution of the technique. In *tissue harmonic imaging* mode, the system is configured to preferentially receive second harmonic echoes produced by microbubbles, hence at double the transmitted frequency, by a high-pass filter. This technique presents several limitations. Even though such filtering is successful in eliminating echoes from solid stationary tissues which present prevalently linear properties, the effect is to reduce the range of frequencies (or bandwidth) contained in the received echoes, causing a low spatial axial resolution of the resulting image. Moreover, if the transmit pulse bandwidth (centered at the fundamental frequency $f_o$) and the receive bandwidth (centered at $2f_o$) overlap, then a portion of the echo from linear scattering will contaminate the harmonic receive signal, reducing the difference between microbubble agent and stationary tissue and, consequently, the contrast resolution of the technique.

– *Ultraharmonic imaging* employs a wide-band frequency transducer. Ultraharmonics ($3f_o/2$, $5f_o/2$, $7f_o/2$, …) refer to radiofrequency signals that occur between higher harmonics ($2f_o$, $3f_o$, $4f_o$, ...). Very little ultraharmonic signals arise from nonlinear propagation of US through tissue, while ultraharmonics are effectively produced by microbubbles both by high and low transmit power intonation. With ultraharmonic imaging, a combination of high and low pass filters can be used to selectively display only ultraharmonic frequencies where the signal-to-noise ratio is intrinsically greater. Subharmonic imaging is a further harmonic imaging technique. When microbubbles are insonated at one frequency, some return echoes with a frequency component at half the insonation frequency, as well as at the fundamental frequency and the second, third, and higher integer harmonics mentioned previously. Two causes have been identified for the subharmonic signal. One is certainly the nonlinear response of a microbubble to an incident pulse. The other is ringing (continuing oscillations) at the natural frequency of the bubble after the forced oscillation due to the incident pulse has stopped. Both the effects are greater for transmitted pulses containing a larger number of cycles, and for the more flexible microbubbles. The strength of the subharmonic component in the scatter spectrum of microbubbles is greater than that of the second harmonic. This, combined with the fact that nonlinear propagation of US in tissue does not generate a subharmonic component, suggests that subharmonic detection might offer an imaging method with greater contrast between microbubble and tissue echoes. Moreover, the lower frequency of the subharmonic means that attenuation is less. Against these advantages must be set the fact that pulses containing more cycles generate stronger subharmonic signals and such long pulses would not give good spatial axial resolution.

(c)   Phase modulation techniques. Nowadays, low transmit power contrast-specific techniques are employed. The newer modalities also share a common feature – namely the transmission of multiple pulses of US per scan line, followed by the processing of the received radiofrequency signals from each line. The purpose of these techniques is to remove linear or predominantly tissue signal, from nonlinear microbubble signals to

improve the contrast resolution and the signal / noise ratio. These techniques employ a low transmit power and allows a long persistence of the signal produced by microbubbles with the possibility of continuous and real-time scanning.

– *Pulse inversion harmonic imaging* was developed to address two important limitations of harmonic imaging – to provide better discrimination between tissue and microbubble contrast agents, and to overcome the requirement of the use of a narrow-band signal for harmonic imaging with the consequently reduced spatial axial resolution. In Pulse Inversion, two sequential US waves that are inverted replicas of each other are transmitted into tissue, and the resulting echoes are summed. For a linear medium, the echoes from the two waves are inverted copies of each other, and the resulting sum is zero. For nonlinear media such as microbubbles, the echoes will not be inverted copies, the sum is not zero. If a high acoustic power of insonation is employed for imaging, however, tissue harmonics are not eliminated by pulse inversion, but are incompletely canceled, and tissue and microbubble second harmonics may still overlap. The advantage of the pulse inversion method over the harmonic techniques is that overlap between the fundamental and second harmonic spectra does not matter, and there is no need to restrict the transmission spectrum to the lower half of the transducer frequency range. This allows short (large bandwidth) pulses to be used and hence good axial spatial resolution to be achieved. The disadvantage of the method, however, is a reduction in frame rate due to the need to interrogate each scan line twice. The tissue-contrast discrimination that can be achieved by pulse inversion is limited by any tissue movement between the two transmissions. Where there is tissue movement, the positions of the tissue interfaces in the second echo sequence will not match those in the first, and the cancelation of the linear signal will not be perfect.

– *Vascular recognition imaging* combines the nonlinear detection performance of pulse inversion imaging with the motion discrimination capabilities of color and power Doppler. It is the first contrast-specific technique that discriminates moving from stationary microbubbles. It involves transmitting four pulses, alternately inverted, along each scan line. The echoes from the first three are summed with weights (1, 2, 1) to give one fundamental-free signal, and the echoes from the last three are summed the same way to give a second fundamental-free signal. The phase difference between these two principally second harmonic signals gives a velocity estimate and their mean magnitude gives a power estimate. Stationary bubbles are shown in green, while moving bubbles are either red or blue, depending on their flow direction. A disadvantage of using only a few transmission/receive sequences for each scan line is that the accuracy of Doppler frequency measurement is much less than in conventional color flow imaging.

(d) Amplitude modulation techniques. Power modulation represents the paradigm of amplitude modulation contrast-specific technique. At low acoustic power insonation, the tissue signal may also be suppressed online by alternating acoustic power rather than phase. For power modulation, a train of three low power US pulses are transmitted per image line. The pulses are transmitted at two power levels, where the first and third pulses are half-height amplitude relative to the second pulse. Since all the pulses are transmitted at a low acoustic power, little nonlinear tissue backscatter is generated. Subsequently, the received echoes from the half-height transmitted pulses are scaled and subtracted from the full-height signal, which results in effective removal of tissue clutter. On the other hand, microbubbles continue to respond nonlinearly to all three pulses, resulting in residual microbubble signal even after subtraction.

(e) Amplitude and phase modulation technique. The contrast pulse sequencing (CPS) technique works by interrogating each scan lines a number of times with pulses having various amplitudes and phases. Three pulses are employed with a typical sequence of pulse as ½, −1, ½, which means that each line is interrogated three times, with the first and last transmitted pulses having amplitudes half that of the central pulse which is inverted. A processor first amplifies the echo sequence from each transmission by a particular weighting factor (for example ×2 or ×−1) and then sums all the weighted echo sequences. It registers and represents both harmonic and nonlinear fundamental

signals from microbubbles in a gray-scale or color map. By suitable choice of transmission pulses and weighting factors, it is possible to isolate or suppress the linear fundamental echoes from stationary tissues.

## 4.5 Dynamic Phases After Microbubble Injection in the Kidney

### 4.5.1 Dynamic Phases

The renal cortex rapidly enhances from 15 to 20 s after microbubble injection, while the vessels of the renal medulla are progressively filled from 30 to 35 s and completely filled from 40 to 50 s after microbubble injection. This is because the renal medulla presents a lower global perfusion than the renal cortex (about 400 vs. 190 mL/min/100 g of renal tissue). For these reasons, it is correct to identify, after microbubbles injection, an early arterial cortico-medullary phase (from 20 to 40 s) with cortico-medullary differentiation, and a late cortico-medullary phase (from 45 s up to 120 s) with homogeneous renal enhancement in both the renal cortex and medulla (Fig. 4.37).

### 4.5.2 Microbubble Artifacts

Most microbubble–specific artifacts are found with color and power Doppler modes, because the settings of US equipments become inappropriate following a strong increase of the backscattered signals and the need to be recognized to avoid interpretative errors (Forsberg et al. 1994).

- High-intensity transient signals. This artifact is determined by microbubble collapse or by the aggregates of macrobubbles producing sharp spikes on the Doppler spectral tracing, heard as crackling on the audio output. These spikes are easily recognized since they cover the entire frequency spectrum. This artifact may also be detected with color and power Doppler imaging appearing as color pixels of higher intensity within the more uniform signal of the vessel.
- Pseudoacceleration of the systolic peak velocity. An increase in the systolic peak velocity of up to 50% can be found at peak enhancement. This artifact is

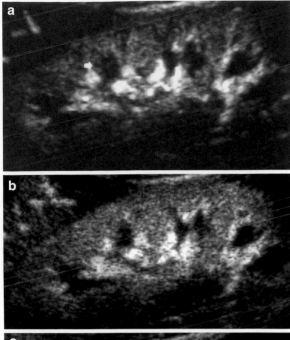

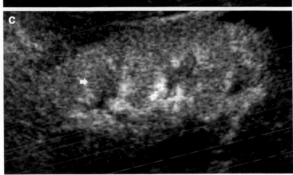

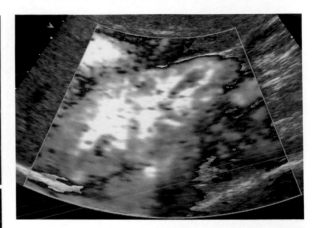

**Fig. 4.38** Artifacts after microbubble injection. Blooming artifact at power Doppler. Diffuse signal outside the renal vessels

**Fig. 4.37** Dynamic phases after microbubble injection at low acoustic power insonation. Renal cortex rapidly enhances from 20 s after microbubble injection (**a**), with echo-signal intensity, increases up to 40 s after microbubble injection (**b**), while the vessels of renal medulla (*arrow*) are completely filled from 45 s after microbubble injection (**c**)

probably the result of signals that were too weak to be detected before microbubble injection and it may be almost completely canceled by reducing the Doppler gain or by employing slow infusion of microbubbles. The increase in systolic peak velocity may produce an error in grading the stenotic lesions of the vessels.

• Blooming artifact. In Doppler tracing only the mean frequency shift is displayed, while the Doppler signal intensity is increased after microbubble injection since the increase in backscattering echo-signal intensity determines the appearance also of the lowest velocities that were too weak to be registered

before microbubble injection. When color or power Doppler is turned on, the overload of the Doppler signal registration apparatus is determined by the strong signals and multiple rereflections between adjacent microbubbles (Fig. 4.38). Such artifact can be limited by reducing the color gain and persistence and the MI or by increasing the wall filter and the pulse repetition frequency, resulting in a decreased sensitivity of the system. The slow infusion of microbubbles limits this artifact because of a decrease in the peak signal intensity. Dedicated US contrast-specific modes were introduced principally to avoid this artifact.

• Jail bar artifact. The jail bar artifact is prevalently observed with power Doppler mode. It is determined by an error in image interpolation when the management of the backscattering signal intensity from the US system approaches the saturation. Since each frame is reconstructed from an interpolation mathematical procedure of the image view lines, the saturation of signal determines a lack of color along the interpolating view (Fig. 4.39).

## 4.6 Clinical Applications of Microbubble Contrast Agents in the Kidney

After the heart and the liver, the kidneys are the next most useful organs for the application of microbubble contrast agents for diagnosis, especially of vascular abnormalities (Cosgrove and Harvey 2009). CEUS allows real-time observation of tissue enhancement associated with real-time identification of blood flow,

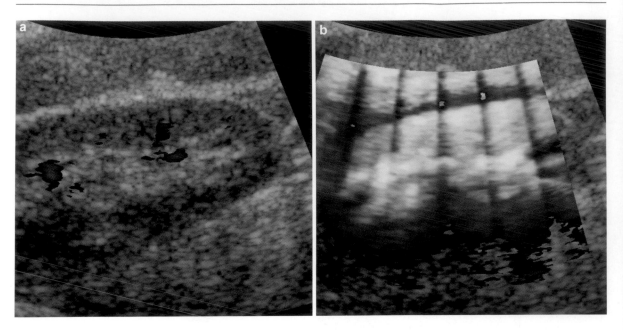

**Fig. 4.39** Artifacts after microbubble injection. Jail bar artifact due to signal saturation. (**a**) Image without the power Doppler mask. (**b**) Power Doppler after microbubble injection reveals the existence of a jail bar artifact

and provides excellent spatial resolution and a higher temporal resolution than all other imaging modalities. The principal applications of microbubble contrast agents are quantification of renal parenchyma (Lucidarme et al. 2003a, b; Quaia et al. 2009), detection of renal perfusion defects (Quaia et al. 2006; Bertolotto et al. 2008), and the characterization of solid and cystic renal masses (Quaia et al. 2003, 2008).

Microbubbles may be used as tracers for the functional assessment of renal vascularity. Renal perfusion may be calculated by analyzing the replenishment kinetics of the volume from microbubbles after their destruction by initial high transmit power insonation (Cosgrove et al. 2001). The video-intensity of a digital cine-clip may be quantified by positioning the ROI in a region of the parenchyma and by correlating the time with the video-intensity measured in a linear or logarithmic scale. The fundamental assumption is that the relation between microbubble concentration and video-intensity is linear up to the achievement of a plateau phase (Correas et al. 2000). Software packages produced by the US scanner manufacturers access the raw data before the application of nonlinear modifications and allow proper quantification. Different mathematical functions have been proposed to analyze the replenishment kinetics of microbubbles (Wei et al. 1998;

Lucidarme et al. 2003a, b; Quaia et al. 2009). The slope of the first ascending curve (~blood flow velocity) and the maximum amplitude of the refilling curve (~fractional blood volume) are calculated to quantify organ perfusion (Fig. 4.40). CEUS should be considered an additional imaging tool for the noninvasive quantization of solid organ perfusion even though nuclear medicine techniques, SPECT and PET, are still considered the reference imaging modalities.

Microbubble-based contrast agents and contrast-specific imaging techniques significantly improved the diagnostic confidence level in identifying nonperfused renal parenchymal zones (Quaia et al. 2006; Bertolotto et al. 200), especially in renal infarction, with a reliable depiction of renal perfusion defects. Renal perfusion defects appear as regional or, in the case of renal artery occlusion, complete filling defects. Regional renal infarctions appear as single or multiple focal wedge-shaped areas of absent, diminished, or delayed contrast enhancement (Fig. 4.41) in comparison to the adjacent renal parenchyma after microbubble injection. This is particularly useful for renal transplants, especially as microbubbles are not nephrotoxic (Schwenger et al. 2006; Cosgrove and Harvey 2009).

Solid renal cell carcinomas smaller than 3 cm reveal diffuse, homogeneous, or heterogeneous contrast

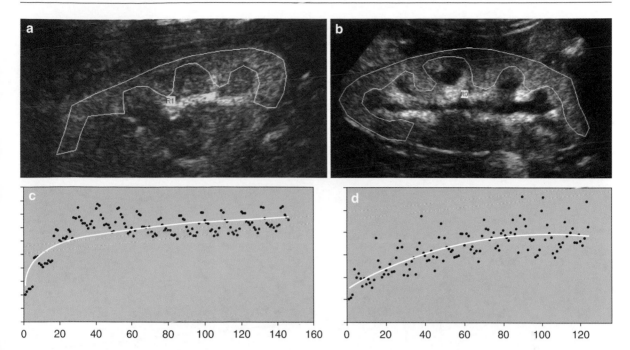

**Fig. 4.40** Reduced renal parenchyma perfusion due to nephroangiosclerosis in patients without any pharmacologic treatment and quantified by contrast-enhanced US (CEUS). Progressive refilling kinetics of renal cortex after microbubble destruction. The echo-signal intensity may be quantified by a manually-defined ROI positioned in a region of renal parenchyma excluding renal medulla. Data were fitted by a negative exponential function (*white curve*). The kidney of a 25-year-old volunteer (**a**, **c**) presents an higher slope of the first ascending tract of the curve, expressing a higher blood flow velocity, in comparison to the curve obtained from a 65-year-old volunteer (**b**, **d**)

enhancement (Fig. 4.42) after microbubble injection during the early cortico-medullary phase, limited to the solid viable regions (Xu et al. 2009), sparing intratumoral avascular necrotic, hemorrhagic, or cystic components which increased their conspicuity (Fig. 4.43) with contrast washout during the late cortico-medullary phase (Fig. 4.44). Renal cell carcinomas appear isoechoic or slightly hypoechoic to the adjacent renal parenchyma, with a progressive reduction of contrast enhancement at late cortico-medullary phase. If tumoral thrombus is present in the renal vein or inferior vena cava, it may reveal contrast enhancement (Correas et al. 1999, 2003). CEUS may be even more sensitive than contrast material-enhanced CT in revealing contrast enhancement in solid renal tumors, due to the high sensitivity of US contrast-specific modes to the harmonic signal produced by microbubbles insonation.

CEUS is a valuable tool to identify contrast enhancement in the intratumoral septa (Fig. 4.45), peripheral wall, or septal or mural nodules (Fig. 4.46) of cystic renal tumors. This is due to the high sensitivity of contrast-specific mode to the harmonic signals produced by microbubbles which probably makes CEUS even more effective that contrast material-enhanced CT and MR in the detection of contrast enhancement in cystic renal tumors.

Microbubble-based contrast agents were shown to improve renal cysts and atypical cystic renal masses characterization (Kim et al. 1999; Quaia et al. 2003, 2008) by revealing different enhancement patterns. After microbubble injection, a variety of contrast enhancement patterns may be observed in cystic renal tumors: (a) absent, no difference before and after microbubble injection; (b) continuous or (c) discontinuous, peripheral rim-like enhancement in a cystic lesion with or without intratumoral septa; (d) peripheral nodular enhancement limited to the peripheral wall and to the nodular papillary endocystic components; (e) peripheral wall and septal enhancement or (f) diffuse nodular and septal enhancement with nodular components both in the peripheral wall and in the intratumoral septa. CEUS was shown to improve the sonographic detection of vascularity within the septations and peripheral wall of complex cystic renal masses (Kim et al. 1999).

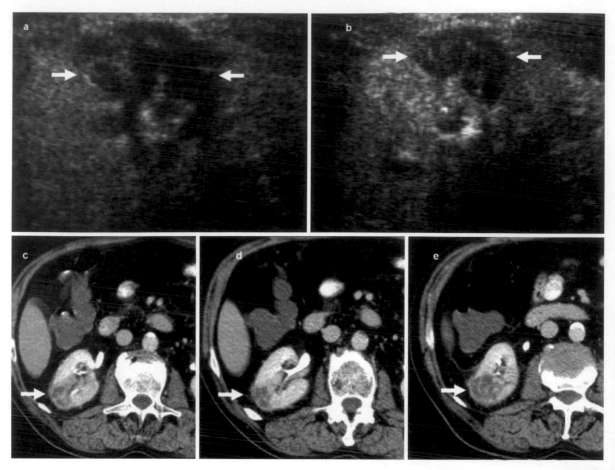

**Fig. 4.41** Focal renal perfusion defect in a 75-year-old male patient. (**a, b**) Contrast-enhanced US after microbubble-based agent injection (contrast-specific mode: pulse inversion mode). CEUS allows a reliable depiction of renal perfusion defect (*arrows*). The same renal perfusion defect (*arrow*) is confirmed at contrast material-enhanced CT (**c–e**) after iodinated agent injection

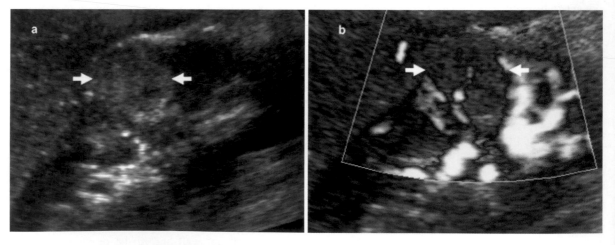

**Fig. 4.42** Clear cell-type Solid renal tumor after microbubble contrast agent injection. (**a**) The renal tumor (*arrows*) appear hyperechoic on gray-scale US, with peripheral and penetrating vessels on power Doppler US (**b**). (**c, d**) CEUS. Pulse inversion contrast-specific mode. The renal tumor reveals diffuse contrast enhancement after microbubble injection during the arterial phase (**c**) with contrast washout during the late phase (**d**)

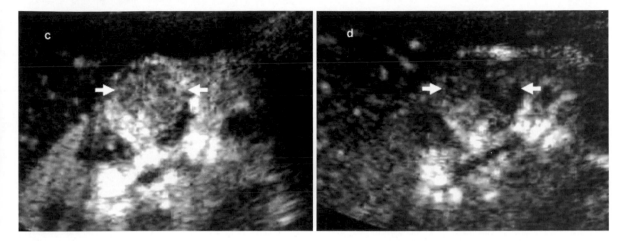

**Fig. 4.42** (continued)

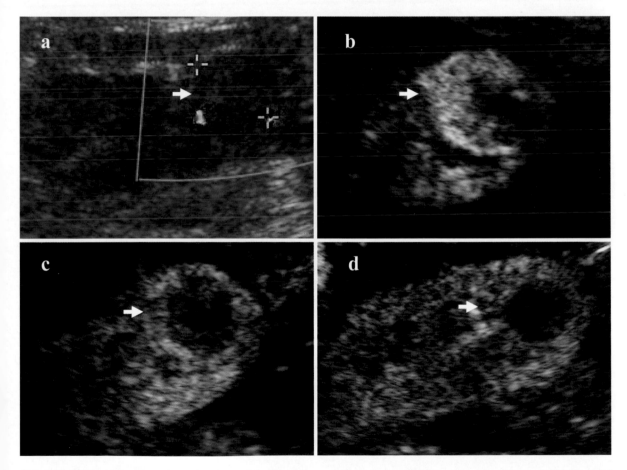

**Fig. 4.43** Solid renal tumor after microbubble injection. (**a**) Unenhanced gray-scale US reveals a hypoechoic solid renal tumor on the lower pole of the left kidney. (**b**–**d**) CEUS after sulfur-hexafluoride microbubble injection. Cadence contrast pulse sequencing (CPS) as contrast-specific mode. (**b**) The renal tumor reveals diffuse contrast enhancement sparing an intratumoral necrotic component which appears hypovascular. (**c, d**) A peripheral pseudocapsule is revealed in the following seconds

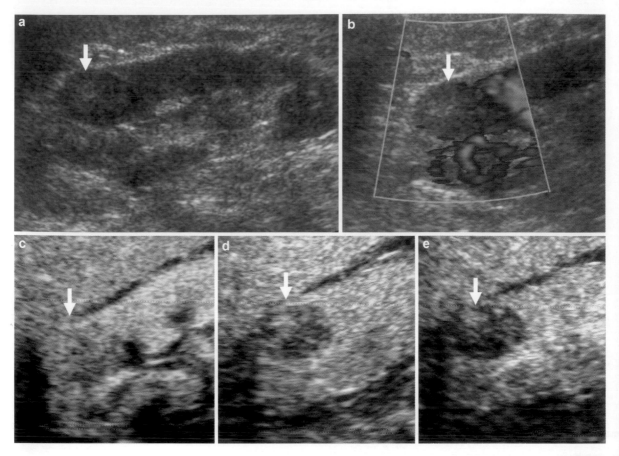

**Fig. 4.44** Solid renal tumor (*arrow*) after microbubble injection. (**a**) Unenhanced gray-scale US reveals a hypoechoic solid renal tumor on the lower pole of the left kidney. (**b**) Power Doppler US does not reveal any tumoral vessels. (**c–e**) CEUS after sulfur-hexafluoride microbubble injection. Cadence CPS as contrast-specific mode. The renal tumor reveals diffuse contrast enhancement with progressive washout

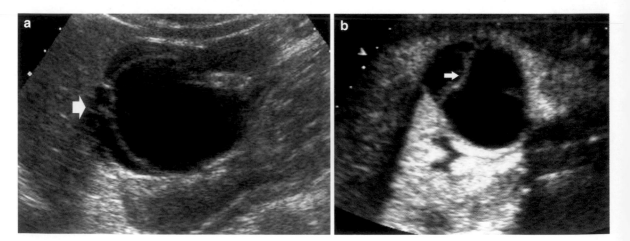

**Fig. 4.45** Cystic renal tumor of the right kidney. (**a**) Unenhanced gray-scale US reveals a cystic renal mass with a septation on the upper pole of the right kidney. (**b**) Contrast-enhanced US after sulfur-hexafluoride microbubble injection. Cadence CPS as contrast-specific mode. The intratumoral sep- tations reveal enhancement after microbubble injection without evidence of mural or septal nodules. The patient with complex renal cyst underwent simple 3–6 months follow-up by US examination which revealed constant dimensions and morphol- ogy of the cyst

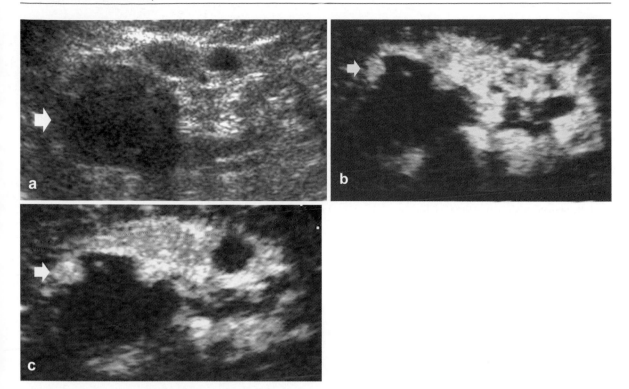

**Fig. 4.46** Cystic renal tumor of the right kidney. (**a**) Unenhanced gray-scale US reveals a hypoechoic complex renal mass on the upper pole of the right kidney. (**b, c**) Contrast-enhanced US after sulfur-hexafluoride microbubble injection. Cadence CPS as contrast-specific media. The renal tumor reveals contrast enhancement on peripheral mural nodules (*arrow*)

Bosniak classification (1986, 1991) of renal cysts is considered as an accurate and efficient method for treatment planning. Although the Bosniak classification scheme is very useful for the clinical management of cystic renal masses, interreader variation in distinguishing between category II, IIF, and III lesions does exist (Siegel et al. 1997) and may present problems in recommending surgical vs. conservative management in some cases. Moreover, CT may not reveal thin intracystic septations due to volume averaging which limits the identification of those renal cysts which deserve further assessment by follow-up. Magnetic resonance (MR) and CT reveals similar findings in the majority of cystic renal masses, even though MRI may depict additional septa, thickening of the wall and/or septa, or enhancement, which may lead to an upgraded Bosniak cyst classification and can affect case management (Israel et al. 2004).

Recently, a classification and diagnostic workup scheme for cystic renal lesions has been proposed that uses CEUS as the reference technique (Robbin et al. 2003), and a classification and workup scheme based on CEUS as the reference technique has recently been proposed for renal cystic lesion in which the absence of enhancement after microbubble injection implies no further workup, whereas evidence of thickened septations or mural nodules with contrast enhancement after microbubble injection is considered a reliable criterion of malignancy. CEUS is appropriate in the Bosniak classification of renal cysts (Ascenti et al. 2007), and was found to be superior to CT in detecting additional septa, thickening of the wall and/or septa, and solid components.

## References

Ascenti G, Mazziotti S, Zimbaro G et al. (2007) Complex cystic renal masses: characterization with contrast-enhanced US. Radiology 24(1):158–165

Barnett SB, Duck F, Ziskin M (2007) WFUMB symposium on safety of ultrasound in medicine: conclusions and recommendations on biological effects and safety of ultrasound contrast agents, 2006. Ultrasound Med Biol 33:233–234

Berland LL, Koslin DB, Routh WD et al. (1990) Renal artery stenosis : prospective evaluation of diagnosis with color duplex US compared with angiography. Radiology 174:421–423

Bertolotto M, Martegani A, Aiani L et al. (2008) Value of contrast-enhanced ultrasonography for detecting renal infarcts proven by contrast-enhanced CT. A feasibility study. Eur Radiol 18(2):376–383

Bertolotto M, Quaia E, Galli G et al. (2000) Color Doppler sonographic appearance of renal perforating vessels in subjects with normal and impaired renal function. J Clin Ultrasound 28(6):267–276

Bosniak MA (1986) The current radiological approach to renal cyst. Radiology 158:1–10

Bosniak MA (1991) Difficulties in classifying cystic lesions of the kidney. Urol Radiol 13:91–93

Bude RO, Rubin JM (1995) Detection of renal artery stenosis with Doppler sonography: it is more complicated than originally thought (editorial). Radiology 196:612–613

Bude RO, Rubin JM (1999) Relationship between the resistive index and vascular compliance and resistance. Radiology 211:411–417

Bude RO, Rubin JM, Platt JF et al. (1994) Pulsus tardus: its cause and potential limitations in detection of arterial stenosis. Radiology 190:779–784

Claudon M, Plouin PF, Baxter GM et al. (2000) Renal arteries in patients at risk of renal arterial stenosis: multicenter evaluation of the echo-enhancer SH U 508A at color and spectral Doppler US. Radiology 214:739–746

Claudon M, Tranquart F, Evans DH et al. (2002) Advances in ultrasound. Eur Radiol 12:7–18

Correas JM, Bridal L, Lesavre A et al. (2001) Ultrasound contrast agents: properties, principles of action, tolerance, and artifacts. Eur Radiol 11:1316–1328

Correas JM, Burns PN, Lai X et al. (2000) Infusion versus bolus of an ultrasound contrast agent: in vivo dose-response measurements of BR1. Invest Radiol 35:72–79

Correas JM, Claudon M, Tranquart F et al. (2003) Contrast-enhanced ultrasonography: renal applications. J Radiol 84:2041–2054

Correas JM, Helenon O, Moreau JF (1999) Contrast enhanced ultrasonography of native and transplant kidney diseases. Eur Radiol 9(suppl 3):394–400

Correas JM, Menassa L, Helenon O et al. (1998) Diagnostic improvement of renal ultrasonography in humans after IV injections of Perflenapent emulsion. Acad Radiol 5:S185–S188

Cosgrove D, Harvey C (2009) Clinical uses of microbubbles in diagnosis and treatment. Med Biol Eng Comput 47:813–826

Cosgrove DO, Eckersley R, Blomley M et al. (2001) Quantification of blood flow. Eur Radiol 11:1338–1344

Dalla Palma L, Stacul F, Bazzocchi M et al. (1993) Ultrasonography and plain film versus intravenous urography in ureteric colic. Clin Radiol 47(5):333–336

Desberg AL, Paushter DM, Lammert GK et al. (1990) Renal artery stenosis: evaluation with color Doppler flow imaging. Radiology 177:749–753

Forman HP, Middleton WD, Melson GL et al. (1993) Hyperechoic renal cell carcinoma: increase in detection at US. Radiology 188:431–434

Forsberg F, Liu JB, Burns PN et al. (1994) Artifacts in ultrasonic contrast agent studies. J Ultrasound Med 13(5):357–365

Fowler KAB, Locken JA, Duchesse JH et al. (2002) US for detecting renal calculi with nonenhanced CT as a reference standard. Radiology 222:109–113

Grant EG, Melany ML (2001) Ultrasound contrast agents in the evaluation of the renal arteries. In: Goldberg BB, Raichlen JS, Forsberg F (eds) Ultrasound contrast agents. Basic principles and clinical applications, 2nd edn. Martin Dunitz, London, pp 289–295

Haddad MC, Sharif HS, Shahed MS et al. (1992) Renal colic: diagnosis and outcome. Radiology 184:83–88

Havey RJ, Krumlowsky F, deGreco F et al. (1985) Screening for renovascular hypertension. JAMA 254:388–393

Helenon O, Correas JM, Balleyguier C et al. (2001) Ultrasound of renal tumors. Eur Radiol 11:1890–1901

Helenon O, Correas JM, Chabriais J et al. (1998) Renal vascular Doppler imaging: clinical benefits of power mode. Radiographics 18:1441–1454

Helenon O, Merran S, Paraf F et al. (1997) Unusual fat-containing tumors of the kidney: a diagnostic dilemma. Radiographics 17:129–144

Helenon O, Rody EL, Correas JM et al. (1995) Color Doppler US of renovascular disease in native kidneys. Radiographics 15:833–854

Israel G, Hindman N, Bosniak MA (2004) Evaluation of cystic renal masses: comparison of CT and MR imaging by using the Bosniak classification system. Radiology 231:365–371

Jensen G, Bardelli M, Volkmann R et al. (1994). Renovascular resistance in primary hypertension: experimental variations detected by means of Doppler ultrasound. J Hypertens 12:959–964

Jinzaki M, Ohkuma K, Tanimoto A et al. (1998) Small solid renal lesions: usefulness of power Doppler US. Radiology 209(2):543–550

Jinzaki M, Tanimoto A, Narimatsu Y et al. (1997) Angiomyolipoma: imaging findings in lesions with minimal fat. Radiology 205:497–502

Kamaya A, Tuthill T, Rubin JM (2003) Twinkling artifact on color Doppler sonography: dependence on machine parameters and underlying cause. AJR Am J Roentgenol 180:215–222

Keogan MT, Kliewer MA, Hertzberg BS et al. (1996) Renal resistive indexes: variability in Doppler US measurement in a healthy population. Radiology 199:165–169

Kim AY, Kim SH, Kim YJ et al. (1999) Contrast-enhanced power Doppler sonography for the differentiation of cystic renal lesions: preliminary study. J Ultrasound Med 18:581–588

Kim SH, Kim B (1990) Renal parenchyma disease. In: Pollack HM, McClennan BL, Dyer R, Kenney PJ (eds) Clinical urography. Saunders, Philadelphia, pp 2652–2687

Kim SH, Kim WH, Choi BL et al. (1992) Duplex Doppler US in patients with medical renal disease: resistive index vs. serum creatinine level. Clin Radiol 45:85–87

Lee HJ, Kim SH, Jeong YK et al. (1996) Doppler sonographic resistive index in obstructed kidneys. J Ultrasound Med 15(9):613–618

Lucidarme O, Franchi-Abella S, Correas JM et al. (2003a) Blood flow quantification with contrast-enhanced US: "entrance in the section" phenomenon – phantom and rabbit study. Radiology 228:473–479

Lucidarme O, Kono Y, Corbeil J et al. (2003b) Validation of ultrasound contrast destruction imaging for flow quantification. Ultrasound Med Biol 29:1697–1704

Martinoli C, Bertolotto M, Pretolesi F et al. (1999) Kidney: normal anatomy. Eur Radiol 9(suppl 3):S389–S393

Mulvagh SL, Vannan MA, Becher H et al. (2008) American Society of Echocardiography consensus statement on the clinical applications of ultrasonic contrast agents in echocardiography. J Am Soc Echocardiogr 21(11):1179–1201

O'Connor OJ, McSweeney SE, Maher MM (2008) Imaging of hematuria. Radiol Clin North Am 46:113–132

Ozdemir H, Demir MK, Temizöz O et al. (2008) Phase inversion harmonic imaging improves assessment of renal calculi: a comparison with fundamental gray-scale sonography. J Clin Ultrasound 36(1):16–19

Pedersen MH, Misaridis TX, Jensen JA (2003) Clinical evaluation of chirp coded excitation in medical ultrasound. Ultrasound Med Biol 29(6):895–905

Platt JF (1992) Duplex Doppler evaluation of native kidney dysfunction. Obstructive and nonobstructive disease. AJR Am J Roentgenol 158:1035–1042

Platt JF, Ellis JH, Rubin JM et al. (1990) Intrarenal arterial Doppler sonography in patients with nonobstructive renal disease: correlation of resistive index with biopsy findings. AJR Am J Roentgenol 154:1223–1227

Platt JF, Rubin JM, Ellis JH (1993) Acute renal obstruction: evaluation with intrarenal duplex Doppler and conventional US. Radiology 186:685–688

Platt JF, Rubin JM, Ellis JH et al. (1989) Duplex Doppler US of the kidney: differentiation of obstructive and nonobstructive dilatation. Radiology 171:515–517

Qin S, Caskey CF, Ferrara KW (2009) Ultrasound contrast microbubbles in imaging and therapy: physical principles and engineering. Phys Med Biol 54:R27–R57

Quaia E (2005) Physical basis and principles of action of microbubble-based contrast agents. In: Quaia E (ed) Contrast media in ultrasonography: basic principles and clinical applications. Springer, Berlin, pp 15–30

Quaia E (2007a) Contrast-specific ultrasound techniques. Radiol Med 112:473–490

Quaia E (2007b) Microbubble ultrasound contrast agents: an update. Eur Radiol 17(8):1995–2008

Quaia E, Bertolotto M, Cioffi V et al. (2008) Evaluation of contrast – enhanced ultrasound in the malignancy diagnosis in complex cystic renal masses: comparison with unenhanced ultrasound and contrast-enhanced computed tomography. AJR Am J Roentgenol 191:1239–1249

Quaia E, Nocentini A, Torelli L (2009) Assessment of a new mathematical model for the computation of numerical parameters related to renal cortical blood flow and fractional blood volume by contrast-enhanced ultrasound. Ultrasound Med Biol 35(4):616–627

Quaia E, Siracusano S, Bertolotto M et al. (2003) Characterization of renal tumours with pulse inversion harmonic imaging by intermittent high mechanical index technique. Preliminary results. Eur Radiol 13:1402–1412

Quaia E, Siracusano S, Palumbo A et al. (2006) Detection of focal renal perfusion defects in rabbits after sulphur hexafluoride – filled microbubble injection at low transmission power ultrasound insonation. Eur Radiol 16:166–172

Radermacher J, Ellis S, Haller H (2002) Renal resistance index and progression of renal disease. Hypertension 39:699–703

Rahmouni A, Bargoin R, Herment A et al. (1996) Color Doppler twinkling artifact in hyperechoic regions. Radiology 199:269–271

Randall A (1937) The origin and growth of renal calculi. Ann Surg 105:1009–1027

Rivolta R, Cardinale L, Lovaria A et al. (2000) Variability of renal echo-Doppler measurements in healthy adults. J Nephrol 13:110–115

Robbin ML, Lockhart ME, Barr RG (2003) Renal imaging with ultrasound contrast: current status. Radiol Clin North Am 41:963–978

Sakhaee K (2009) Recent advances in the pathophysiology of nephrolithiasis. Kidney Int 75(6):585–595

Schwenger V, Hinkel UP, Nahm AM et al. (2006) Real-time contrast-enhanced sonography in renal transplant recipients. Clin Transplant 20(suppl 17):51–54

Senior R, Becher H, Monaghan M et al. (2009) Contrast echocardiography: evidence-based recommendations by European Association of echocardiography. Eur J Echocardiogr 10:194–212

Siegel CL, McFarland EG, Brink JA et al. (1997) CT of cystic renal masses: analysis of diagnostic performance and interobserver variation. AJR Am J Roentgenol 169:813–818

Siegel CL, Middleton WD, Teefey SA et al. (1996) Angiomyolipoma and renal cell carcinoma: US differentiation. Radiology 198(3):789–793

Stavros AT, Parker SH, Yakes WF et al. (1992) Segmental stenosis of the renal artery: pattern recognition of tardus and parvus abnormalities with duplex sonography. Radiology 184:487–492

Svedström E, Alanen A, Nurmi M (1990) Radiologic diagnosis of renal colic: the role of plain film, excretory urography and sonography. Eur J Radiol 11(3):180–183

Tchelepi H, Ralls PW (2009) Color comet-tail artefact: clinical applications. AJR Am J Roentgenol 192:11–18

Thickman DI, Ziskin MC, Goldenberg NC et al. (1983) Clinical manifestations of the comet tail artifact. J Ultrasound Med 2(5):225–230

Tublin ME, Bude RO, Platt JF (2003) The resistive index in renal Doppler sonography: where do we stand? AJR Am J Roentgenol 180:885–892

Tublin ME, Dodd GD, Verdile VP (1994) Acute renal colic: diagnosis with duplex Doppler US. Radiology 193(3):697–701

Tublin ME, Tessler FN, Murphy ME (1999) Correlation between renal vascular resistance, pulse pressure, and the resistive index in isolated perfused rabbit kidneys. Radiology 213:258–264

Warshauer DM, McCarthy SM, Street L et al. (1988) Detection of renal masses: sensitivities and specificities of excretory urography/linear tomography, US, and CT. Radiology 169:363–365

Wei K, Jayaweera AR, Firoozan S et al. (1998) Quantification of myocardial blood flow with ultrasound-induced destruction of microbubbles administered as a constant infusion. Circulation 97:473–483

Whittingham T (2005) Contrast-specific imaging techniques: technical perspective. In: Quaia E (ed) Contrast media in ultrasonography: basic principles and clinical applications. Springer, Berlin, pp 43–70

Whittingham TA (1999a) An overview of digital technology in ultrasonic imaging. Eur Radiol 9(suppl 3):S307–S311

Whittingham TA (1999b) Broadband transducers. Eur Radiol 9(suppl 3):S298–S303

Xu ZF, Xu XZ, Xie XY, Liu GJ, Zheng YL, Liang JY, Lu MD (2009) Renal cell carcinoma: real-time contrast-enhanced ultrasound findings. Abdom Imaging DOI: 10.1007/s00261-009-9583-y

Yamashita Y, Takahashi M, Watanabe O et al. (1992) Small renal cell carcinoma: pathologic and radiologic correlation. Radiology 184(2):493–498

Yamashita Y, Ueno S, Makita O et al. (1993) Hyperechoic renal tumors: anechoic rim and intratumoral cysts in US differentiation of renal cell carcinoma from angiomyolipoma. Radiology 188(1):179–182

Zagoria RJ (2000) Imaging of small renal masses. A medical success story. Am J Roentgenol 175:945–955

# Computed Tomography

**5**

Emilio Quaia, Paola Martingano, Marco Cavallaro,
Roberto Pozzi-Mucelli, Giulia Zamboni,
Livia Bernardin, and Alberto Contro

## Contents

### Abstract

> The recent technological development of Computed Tomography (CT) imaging technique, mainly the multidetector CT (MDCT), allows the possibility of obtaining larger volume coverage in shorter scan times, sumillimetric slice thickness with an improved longitudinal resolution along the $z$-axis represents, and higher contrast resolution. These capabilities are well suited for the assessment of the kidney. CT provides high spatial and contrast resolution with the possibility of obtaining multiplanar reformats and volumetric reconstructions. Unenhanced CT is principally employed in the detection of urinary stones, to detect hemorrhage and calcifications, and as the precontrast scan to quantify contrast enhancement in renal tumors. Multiphasic CT is employed in the detection and characterization of renal tumors. CT angiography represents the first-line imaging technique in the assessment of renal vasculature. CT urography has now replaced excretory urography in the assessment of the renal and extrarenal urinary tract.

E. Quaia (✉), P. Martingano and M. Cavallaro
Department of Radiology, Cattinara Hospital, University
of Trieste, Strada di Fiume 447, 34149 Trieste, Italy
e-mail: quaia@univ.trieste.it

R. Pozzi-Mucelli, G. Zamboni, L. Bernardin and A. Contro
Department of Radiology, G. B. Rossi Hospital, University
of Verona, Piazzale L. A. Scuro 10, 37134 Verona, Italy

## 5.1 General Concepts

(*Emilio Quaia, Paola Martingano, and Marco Cavallaro*)

Computed tomography (CT) is an extremely valid modality for the study of the kidneys and the urinary tract. The kidneys, the renal vessels, the pelvis, calyces

E. Quaia (ed.), *Radiological Imaging of the Kidney*,
Medical Radiology, DOI: 10.1007/978-3-540 87597-0_5, © Springer-Verlag Berlin Heidelberg 2011

and ureter, the peri and pararenal spaces, and the surrounding organs are visualized in a single examination in great detail. For all these structures, CT allows to accurately assess the anatomy and the pathology, defining its presence, site, and extension. CT has evolved, during the years, from conventional to spiral and, nowadays, to multidetector technology.

Multidetector computed tomography (MDCT) has further increased the efficacy of this technique and expanded its applications in the urinary tract. Among these new applications, the evaluation of the urinary tract – the so-called MDCT urography – is the most innovative. In general, all the structures can be examined and visualized in great detail due to the high contrast and spatial resolution of CT images and multiplanar reconstructions, including 3D renderings. CT technology has developed rapidly over the past years with single-slice, and 4-, 8-, 16-, 32-, and 40-row detector scanners. The main drawbacks of single-slice spiral CT are the insufficient volume coverage within one breathhold time of the patient or missing spatial resolution in the $z$-axis due to wide collimation. With single-slice spiral CT, the ideal isotropic resolution, that is, of equal resolution in all three spatial axes, can only be achieved for very limited scan ranges. The technological development of MDCT offers new possibilities for better imaging of organic structures that can be used in the diagnosis of the kidney. Narrow collimation results in isotropic voxels in 64-channel MDCT scanners of recent release, and images in arbitrarily reconstructed planes come close to the image quality in the original scan plane. Small slice thickness improves the detection of small structures and allows better discrimination of solid and cystic structures as partial volume effects diminish. Slice fusion options improve contrast and contrast-to-noise ratio. Due to short scan times, the kidneys can be depicted in well-defined (dynamic) phases of contrast enhancement, so that lesions can be characterized more precisely. In practice, it is advisable to choose a reconstruction thickness of 3–5 mm as a compromise between spatial resolution and contrast-to-noise ratio. Depending on radiological findings, reconstructions in other planes and slice thickness down to the submillimeter range can be added (depending on scanner type and number of detector rows available).

MDCT represents an advance in CT technology that involves the use of a multiple-row detector array instead of the traditional single-row detector array used in spiral CT (Coppenrath and Mueller-Lisse 2006). MDCT allows a larger volume coverage in shorter scan times and thinner slices with an improved longitudinal resolution along the $z$-axis (patient axis). Subsecond gantry rotation and large detector size allow rapid volume coverage that not only facilitates multiphase scanning with short breath-holds, but also minimizes respiratory motion artifacts. On multidetector-row CT scanners, each individual detector is segmented in the $z$-axis direction. Retrospective thin-section data reconstruction permits routine acquisition of isotropic data that can be displayed in a multitude of multiplanar and 3D formats with minimal artifacts (Prasad et al. 2008). The thinner slices allow a better spatial resolution, and slice fusion allows improved contrast resolution. The isotropic voxel has been realized in the latest 64-channel scanners providing the same spatial resolution in all imaging planes and the image quality of arbitrarily reconstructed planes has arrived at the image quality of the scan plane. Faster scanning allows studies in different contrast phases, which is helpful for better discrimination of benign or malignant lesions, especially in the highly vascularized kidney.

With a single-slice CT detector, different collimated slice widths are obtained by prepatient collimation of the X-ray beam. For a very elementary model of a two-slice CT detector consisting of $M=2$ detector rows, different slice widths can be obtained by prepatient collimation if the detector is separated midway along the $z$-extent of the X-ray beam. For $M>2$, this simple design principle must be replaced by more flexible concepts requiring more than $M$ detector rows to simultaneously acquire $M$ slices. Different manufacturers of MDCT scanners have introduced different detector designs. In order to be able to select different slice widths, all scanners combine several detector rows electronically to a smaller number of slices according to the selected beam collimation and the desired slice width. The fixed array detector consists of detector elements with equal size in the longitudinal direction, and different slice widths may be obtained by electronically combining several detector rows to a smaller number of slices. The adaptive array detector comprises detector rows with different sizes in the longitudinal direction, and the different slice widths may be obtained by appropriate combinations of the detector rows. Images are usually reconstructed in the transversal plane.

CT has been used to effectively evaluate many urinary tract disorders including renal masses (Bosniak 1991; Curry 1995; Silverman et al. 2008), urinary tract calculi (Fielding et al. 1998; Smith et al. 1996), genitourinary trauma (Herschorn et al. 1991), and renal infection (Dalla Palma et al. 1997). Indications for CT investigation of the kidney include urolithiasis, tumor diagnosis and staging, renal trauma, and vascular disease. Even in children, special indications for CT of the kidney remain in polytrauma and tumor staging. MDCT of the kidney has become a very valuable tool in urology, but a careful protocol strategy is mandatory.

### 5.1.1 Technical Parameters

#### 5.1.1.1 Imaging

The technique of examination of the kidney and the urinary tract has progressively changed during the years with the advances in CT technology. State-of-the-art X-ray CT tube/generator (Fig. 5.1a, b) combinations provide a peak power of 60–120 kW, usually at various user-selectable voltages, for example, 80, 100, 120, and 140 kV. The spatial resolution of the CT images may achieve 24 lp/cm with an image matrix size of $512 \times 512$, $768 \times 768$, or $1,024 \times 1,024$ pixels. Modern MDCT systems use solid-state detectors (Fig. 5.1c, d) consisting of a radiation-sensitive solid-state material (cadmium tungstate, gadolinium-oxide, or gadolinium oxi-sulfide with suitable dopings), which converts the absorbed X-rays into visible light. The light is then detected by a Si photodiode. The resulting electrical current is amplified and converted into a digital signal. CT detectors must provide different slice widths to adjust the optimum scan speed, longitudinal resolution, and image noise for each application.

Once the scans have been performed, CT images are available for the evaluation. Nowadays, the visualization at the workstation is supported by simple

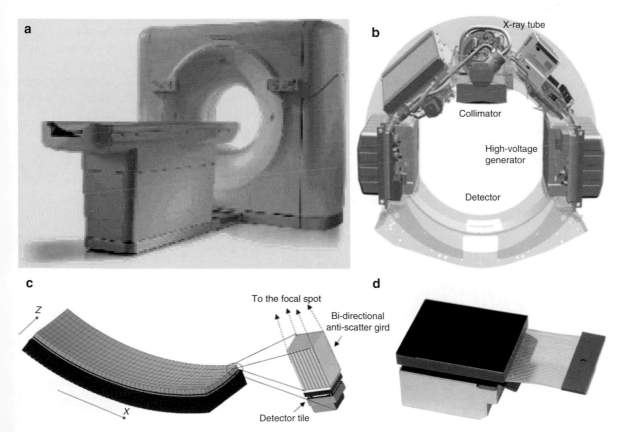

**Fig. 5.1** (a–d) Geometry of X-ray tube scanning in the multidetector CT (MDCT). (a, b) Modern 256-rows MDCT scanner (a); basic system components of a modern MDCT scanner (b). (c) MDCT detector array with evidence of a single detector structure with bidirectional anti-scatter grid; x corresponds to the rotating axis; z corresponds to the patient long axis. (d) A last generation detector with bidirectional anti-scatter grid (courtesy of Philips)

visualization interfaces so that the radiologist can review the images on axial, coronal, and sagittal multiplanar reformation (MPR) images. In the case of the kidney, coronal images are useful because they depict the kidneys in one single image rather than in multiple axial sections, and thus the images are easier to understand, especially for the urologist. This is true also for the images of the urinary tract, although normal MPR coronal images cannot depict the entire ureter in a single image. Maximum intensity projection (MIP) images are more indicated for this purpose, when the urinary tract is opacified with contrast media. The coronal plane is suitable for reconstruction of an "in situ" perspective that resembles the view of the abdominal or urologic surgeon. The MPR describes the option of arbitrary plane reconstruction from voxel data sets. These planes can be chosen in an orthogonal plane (sagittal, coronal), oblique plane, or even in a curved-planar reconstruction (e.g., for course of vessels). Best reconstruction results are obtained in a pseudo-2D display with isotropic voxels. MIP depicts the structures of highest CT density within a volume of interest. Volume rendering technique (VRT) is an image-processing option that emphasizes regions of selected CT density range, thereby accentuating specific tissues or organs.

The best attainable image quality of any given CT system is determined by a number of scanning parameters that the user can modify: (a) collimation, (b) pitch (Fig. 5.2), (c) reconstruction interval, and (d) timing of scanning after contrast injection. Optimizing these parameters to achieve the best possible image quality

for a specific MDCT examination requires a thorough understanding of their interrelationships. *Collimation* is related to spatial resolution, image noise, and length of coverage. Spatial resolution may be increased by means of a decrease in the collimator width, but decreased collimator width also results in increased image noise and decreased length of coverage. The reduced coverage encountered with narrow collimation, however, can potentially be overcome with an increase in pitch. The *effective detector row thickness* is simply the sum of the widths of the contributing detector rows for each channel. In multidetector row CT scan acquisitions, the effective detector row thickness of all channels must be identical. Effective detector row thickness is an important parameter because the reconstructed section thickness cannot be smaller than the effective detector row thickness. The term *detector configuration* succinctly describes a given scan acquisition mode in terms of the number of $z$-axis data channels being used and the effective detector row thickness of each data channel (Saini 2004). *The beam collimation* is simply the product of the number of data channels being used and the effective detector row thickness (Saini 2004).

In single-slice helical CT, pitch ($p$) is defined as the table feed during a 360° rotation of the tube-detector apparatus (mm/rotation) divided by the collimator width in millimeter (collimated beam width). It shows whether data acquisition occurs with gaps ($p > 1$) or with overlap ($p < 1$) in the longitudinal direction. In MDCT the beam collimation is different from the slice collimation, and the beam collimation depends on the

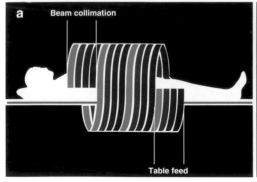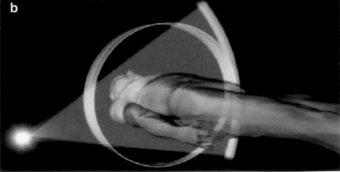

**Fig. 5.2** (**a**) Scanning geometry of the fan beam produced by the MDCT scanner (courtesy of Toshiba). (**b**) The concept of pitch that corresponds to the table feed during a 360° rotation of the tube-detector apparatus divided by the collimator width. For single detector computed tomography (CT) scanners, the pitch corresponds to the table feed/collimation. For MDCT, there are two distinct versions of pitch, depending on whether the detector collimation (i.e., beam/4 in 4 detector row multislice CT) or the entire beam collimation is considered

number of detector rows. In particular, in MDCT there are two distinct versions of pitch, depending on whether the entire beam collimation is considered or the "detector" collimation (Fig. 5.2) (i.e., beam/4 in 4 detector row MDCT) is used. The selection of pitch for MDCT is affected by such factors as the required length of coverage, reconstructed section thickness, and image noise. For a given duration of scanning, minimization of collimation (thus, an increase in pitch) will allow a narrow reconstructed section thickness and potentially improve spatial resolution, particularly in nonaxial planes. However, maximization of pitch may also result in a decrease in contrast resolution. Thus, the most appropriate choice of scanning parameters is dependent on the imaging problem under consideration. For example, because CT angiography (CTA) allows imaging of structures with very high attenuation against a background of much lower attenuation (i.e., high inherent contrast), the loss of contrast resolution caused by maximization of pitch can be disregarded. The smaller the reconstruction interval, the greater the longitudinal ($z$-axis) resolution, with a resultant loss in $z$-axis coverage. If it is expected that multiplanar reconstructions will be required, a small reconstruction interval with overlapping sections is advantageous. With the evolution of CT from single-slice spiral CT to MDCT, the collimation has been reduced from 3–5 mm to 0.5–1 mm of the most recent 64 row MDCT scanners (0.5–0.625 mm). A decrease in pitch from 1–1.5 to 0.75–0.80 has also been achieved. As a consequence, the thickness of the reconstructed images has been decreased from 5 to 1–2 mm. The final result is the "isotropic voxel," which allows to obtain coronal, sagittal, and oblique multiplanar reformats with the same resolution of the original axial CT sections. A further advantage of state-of-the-art MDCT is the short scan time which varies from 0.33 to 0.5 s for a single 360° rotation.

MDCT examination is performed before and after intravenous contrast administration. Breath-hold images that are essentially free from motion artifact and respiratory misregistration can be quickly obtained during multiple phases of renal enhancement. The preliminary scan without intravenous contrast administration should be performed also without administration of hyperdense oral contrast agents (e.g., Gastrografin), because these might impair visualization of the kidneys or the ureters in MIP images. The timing of peak aortic and hepatic contrast enhancement is primarily dependent

on the rate of injection. Rapid or low-volume (shorter-duration) injections produce earlier peak enhancement, whereas slow or high-volume (longer-duration) injections result in later peak enhancement. These factors must be taken into account before a fixed scanning delay is instituted. A preliminary minibolus (5 mL/s for 4 s), with scanning every 2 s beginning 10 s after the injection is started, can be used. The time to peak aortic enhancement is determined from the resultant time attenuation curve and is used to calculate the scanning delay. The scanning delay can also be accurately timed with a bolus tracking software program.

### 5.1.1.2 Artifacts

- Beam hardening: An X-ray beam is composed of individual photons with a range of energies. As the beam passes through an object, it becomes "harder," that is to say its mean energy increases, because the lower-energy photons are absorbed more rapidly than the higher-energy photons (Barrett and Keat 2004). Cupping artifact manifests when the X-rays passing through the middle portion of a uniform cylindrical phantom are hardened more than those passing though the edges because they are passing though more material. As the beam becomes harder, the rate at which it is attenuated decreases, so the beam is more intense when it reaches the detectors than would be expected if it had not been hardened. Therefore, the resultant attenuation profile differs from the ideal profile that would be obtained without beam hardening. In very heterogeneous cross sections, dark bands or streaks can appear between two dense objects in an image. They occur because the portion of the beam that passes through one of the objects at certain tube positions is hardened less than when it passes through both objects at other tube positions. This type of artifact can occur both in bony regions of the body and in scans where a contrast medium has been used (Barrett and Keat 2004).
- Renal cyst pseudoenhancement: Renal cyst pseudoenhancement refers to the artifactual increase in the attenuation ( >10 HU) of simple intrarenal renal cysts surrounded by normally enhancing renal parenchyma following contrast material administration, even when the effects of partial volume averaging have been removed (Prasad et al. 2008).

Pseudoenhancement is believed to be a consequence of overcorrection for beam-hardening effects of the enhanced renal parenchyma combined with artifact introduced by the CT image reconstruction algorithm (Abdulla et al. 2002; Coulam et al. 2000). This effect is more pronounced with smaller, predominantly intrarenal lesions, because volume averaging and beam hardening have a higher statistical impact on the measurement within small renal lesions, particularly those less than 2 cm. Pseudoenhancement is most problematic for small cysts (usually <1.5 cm in diameter) and at high levels of renal parenchymal enhancement (Fig. 5.3). This problem is magnified by the fact that renal cysts are present in 20–40% of the population and that certain renal cell carcinomas, such as the papillary subtype, typically enhance in a weak and homogeneous manner. Pseudoenhancement may, therefore, lead to mischaracterization of a small renal cyst as an enhancing neoplasm and unnecessary intervention. Pseudoenhancement may be solved by US, which presents the highest accuracy in the characterization of solid vs. cystic renal masses.

A recent report suggests that pseudoenhancement is worse with newer-generation MDCT scanners than with earlier scanners (Wang et al. 2008). Given the increasing prevalence of 16- and 64-detector scanners in clinical practice, confirmation of these findings, as well as improved understanding of the means to reduce pseudoenhancement, is clearly needed. While it is known that peak tube voltage settings affect CT image contrast and attenuation measurement, the influence of peak tube voltage on pseudoenhancement is not well studied. Therefore, we undertook this study to determine the effect of the number of detectors and peak tube voltage on renal cyst pseudoenhancement in a phantom model.

Partial volume: The partial volume effect represents a separate problem from partial volume averaging, which yields a CT number representative of the average attenuation of the materials within a voxel. The partial volume effect manifests mainly in small cystic renal lesions with a diameter smaller than 1 cm. The thin slices of MDCT represent an advantage in the kidney since cysts are the most common focal lesions in the kidney, and frequently, they are small in size.

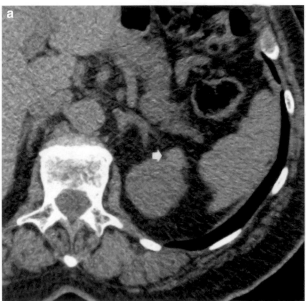
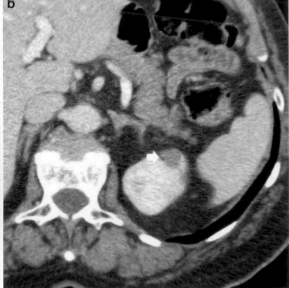

**Fig. 5.3** (**a**, **b**) Pseudoenhancement in a small cyst (*arrow*) of the upper renal pole of the left kidney. Seventy-year-old woman with incidental renal lesion. (**a**) Unenhanced CT image (collimation, 0.5 mm) shows a 1-cm lesion isodense partially intraparenchymal lesion measuring 20 HU. (**b**) Nephrographic phase (collimation 0.5 mm, beam pitch 1) of the same lesion in (**a**). Enhanced attenuation was 50 HU (pseudoenhancement 30 HU). Lesion revealed a cystic pattern on US and was stable for more than 3 years on CT follow-up (not shown)

Therefore, the exact density measurement in Hounsfield units (HU) may be prevented by partial volume effect (or artifact). In some cases, the differential diagnosis with a small renal tumor cannot be established. Thin slices (0.5–1 mm) minimize the partial volume effect and allow to measure the exact density in most cases. The distinction between solid and cystic renal lesions seen at CT is determined primarily on the evaluation of whether the lesion enhances after the intravenous administration of iodinated contrast material. While this approach is generally robust, the assessment of enhancement in small renal cystic lesions may be unreliable. This is because attenuation measurements for such small lesions may erroneously suggest enhancement even though the lesion is truly cystic because of partial volume averaging. There are a number of ways (Fig. 5.4) in which the partial volume effect can lead to image artifacts. One type of partial volume artifact occurs when an object (Fig. 5.4C) lying off-center protrudes partway into the width of the X-ray beam and

may create the false impression of contrast enhancement. Another type of partial volume artifact occurs when a small cystic renal mass has a diameter smaller than the CT section thickness (Fig. 5.4D) and is represented with an attenuation between the liquid and renal parenchyma.

- Photon starvation: A potential source of serious streaking artifacts is photon starvation, which can occur in highly attenuating areas such as the shoulders or when the patient arms are lying along the body. When the X-ray beam is traveling horizontally, the attenuation is greatest and insufficient photons reach the detectors. The result is that very noisy projections are produced at these tube angulations. The reconstruction process has the effect of greatly magnifying the noise, resulting in horizontal streaks in the image. On some scanner models, the tube current is automatically varied during the course of each rotation, a process known as *milli-amperage modulation*. This allows sufficient photons to pass through the widest parts of the patient without unnecessary dose to the narrower parts.
- Cone beam effect (artifact): As the number of sections acquired per rotation increases, as in the MDCT scanner, a wider collimation is required and the X-ray beam becomes cone-shaped rather than fan-shaped. As the tube and detectors rotate around the patient (in a plane perpendicular to the diagram), the data collected by each detector correspond to a volume contained between two cones, instead of the ideal flat plane. This leads to artifacts similar to those caused by partial volume around off-axis objects. The cone beam artifacts are more pronounced for the outer detector rows than for the inner ones where the data collected correspond more closely to a plane (Barrett and Keat 2004) and increase with the increase in the number of detector rows. With 4-slice scanners, the total X-ray beam width was sufficiently narrow (e.g., 5 mm wide for four 1.25-mm slices) or else the slices were sufficiently thick (four 5-mm slices) so that the cone beam effects were tolerable and conventional filtered backprojection reconstruction was still usable. However, MSCT scanners of later generations, which collected more and thinner slices, required the development of alternate cone beam reconstruction algorithms (Goldman 2008).

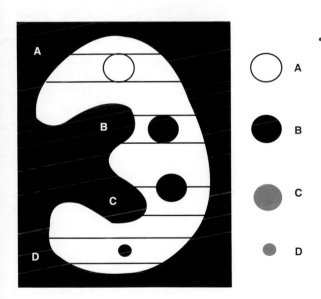

**Fig. 5.4** Scheme showing the partial volume effect on small renal masses. (**A**) Solid mass completely filling the CT section thickness appearing hyper or isodense in comparison to the adjacent renal parenchyma; (**B**) Cystic renal mass completely filling the CT section thickness correctly represented with liquid attenuation; (**C**) Partial volume effect. Cystic renal mass partly crossing the CT section limits and incorrectly represented with a supraliquid attenuation. (**D**) Partial volume effect. Cystic renal mass with a diameter smaller than the CT section thickness and represented with an attenuation between the liquid and renal parenchyma

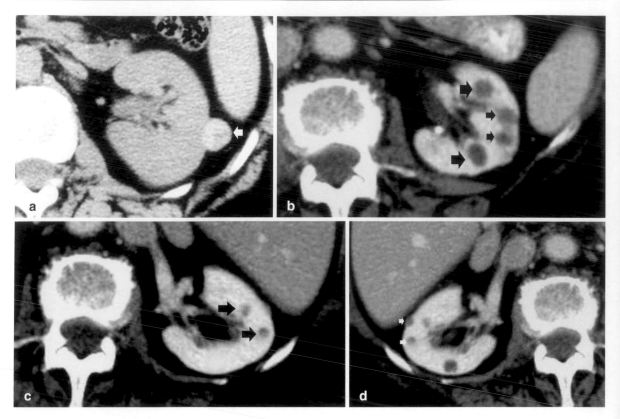

**Fig. 5.5** (**a–d**) Partial volume effect on the renal lesions density. (**a**) Solid renal mass with hyperdense appearance (*arrow*); (**b**) Multiple cystic renal lesions correctly represented with a liquid attenuation (*arrows*); (**c**) Cystic renal lesions (*arrows*) partly crossing the CT section limits with equivocal density due to partial volume artifact. (**d**) Small renal cystic lesions (*arrows*) with a diameter smaller than the CT section thickness with equivocal density due to partial volume artifact

### 5.1.1.3 Radiation Dose

CT scanning is capable of providing high-quality diagnostic information, but it is also usually described as being a high-dose procedure (Cohnen et al. 2003). With the introduction of MDCT scanners, the performance capability of the scanners has increased dramatically and a wider range of examinations can now be performed. Shorter scan times, multiphase protocols, and much thinner slices are now possible. Factors that may contribute to the delivery of high radiation dose from CT evaluation of the urinary tract include the replacement of conventional radiography by CT, the need for multiple follow-up CT studies, and the need for multiphase CT protocols (Kalra and Singh 2008).

*Absorbed dose* is the energy absorbed per unit mass and is measured in Gray (Gy) and its subunit the milliGray (mGy). The *effective dose* is defined by the International Commission on Radiological Protection (ICRP 2007) as a single dose quantity reflecting the overall risk to a reference person from any radiation exposure, where the risk is averaged over all ages and both sexes. *Effective dose* is calculated by summing the absorbed dose in individual organs, weighted by the radiation sensitivity. It is useful for comparing the risks to a reference patient from different imaging techniques and procedures, even though it should not be used for individual patients or detailed risk assessment. The *equivalent dose*, measured in sieverts (Sv), accounts for differences in the sensitivity of target organs to radiation damage and is calculated by multiplying the absorbed dose to a specific tissue with the radiation weighting factor, which is equal to 1 for X-rays.

Noise has an important influence on image quality and it is inversely related to the radiation dose and represents a limiting factor in the improvement in spatial resolution. CT image noise generally depends on the number of X-ray photons interacting with the detector array (quantum noise), the electronic noise of the detector system, and the reconstruction kernel (sharper kernels give noisier images). The level of noise can be quantified easily from images by positioning a standard region of interest in an anatomical structure of known density and measuring the standard deviation of the HUs values. Noise is also dependent on the patient's individual attenuation, convolution filters, slice thickness, pixel dimension, and radiation dose. Reduced dose should, therefore, always be weighed against diagnostic image quality. Also, the detriment from radiation dose is different for different clinical populations.

Scanning parameters – tube current (mAs), tube potential (peak kV – pkV), and scan length – affect significantly the radiation dose received by the patient. Recently, the effective milliampere-seconds (mAs) parameter (mA × time/pitch) has been proposed as the fundamental parameter related to the MDCT dose. In particular, dose is directly dependent on milliampere-seconds and the 2.5 power of the kVp. Dose is also dependent on scanner-specific design factors, e.g., multislice scanners allow higher milliampere-seconds values and provide a higher dose to the patient. Dose limitation is possible with the application of dose modulation software, also named automatic exposure control (AEC) software (Fig. 5.6). The aim of dose modulation is to adjust radiation dose according to the patient's attenuation. Dose modulation is based on the principle that decrease in body diameter (i.e., the anteroposterior diameter when compared to the lateral diameter) translates into decrease in radiation necessary to obtain a certain contrast-to-noise ratio in the resulting CT image data. Dose management technology in CT has led to the optimization of CT protocols using in-plane ($xy$-axes), longitudinal ($z$-axis), or combined ($xyz$-axes) modulation of the dose through dedicated automated dose modulation algorithms. It is important to realize that AEC reduces dose in small patients, even though the dose may actually increase in large patients to compensate for the increase in image noise.

MDCT radiation dose and image quality are also affected by helical pitch (table feed/X-ray beam collimation) and radiation dose is inversely related to the pitch value. The radiation dose decreases proportionally with increasing pitch in CT systems with a single detector row, as the tube voltage and current are kept constant, while for multislice CT scanners the relationship between pitch and radiation dose is nonlinear in ECG-gated acquisition and linear in noncardiac mode. MDCT increases dose as a result of thinner collimation, overbeaming, and overranging effects. For example, in four-row scanners, effective dose is about 30% higher with a collimation of 1 mm than with a collimation of 2.5 mm.

In current MDCT scanners with more than four rows that allow for two different collimations (millimeter and submillimeter), radiation dose increases only by about 10% when the smaller collimation is chosen. In spiral technique, additional tube rotations have to be performed at the beginning and at the end of the scan range because adjacent data from both sides are necessary for image reconstruction (interpolation). Therefore, the scanned volume exceeds the reconstructed volume. The number of additional rotations depends on pitch, cone beam correction, and scanner type. The relative effect is high with short scan lengths or when a large collimation and high pitch are combined. The overranging effect (Fig. 5.7a) may cause considerable increase of dose resulting from the difference between the total table feed (table feed × (scan time/rotation time)) and the scan length as planned. A further problem of MDCT is the width of the fan beam in $z$-axis direction. As four or more detector chambers have to be exposed, a broader X-ray beam is used

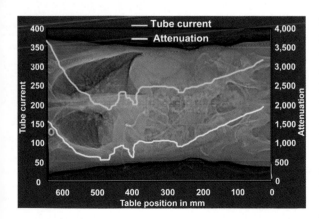

**Fig. 5.6** Automatic exposure control (AEC). Dose modulation is based on the principle that decrease in body diameter (i.e., the anteroposterior diameter when compared to the lateral diameter) translates into decrease in radiation necessary to obtain a certain contrast-to-noise ratio in the resulting CT image data. Tube current is in milliampere; attenuation is expressed as the ratio between the incident intensity over the transmitted radiation intensity through a layer of material

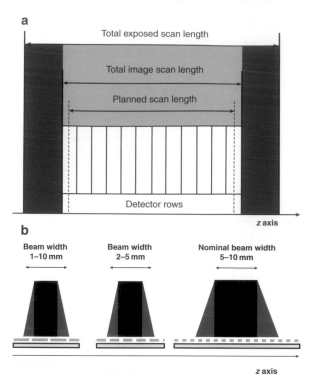

**Fig. 5.7** (**a**) Overranging effect. In current MDCT scanners with more than four rows, additional tube rotations have to be performed at the beginning and at the end of the scan range because adjacent data from both sides are necessary for image reconstruction (interpolation). Therefore, the scanned volume (*red*) exceeds the reconstructed volume (*blue*). The number of additional rotations depends on pitch, cone beam correction, and scanner type. (**b**) Overbeaming effect. The width of the fan beam in *z*-axis direction is broader in MDCT scanner with four or more detector rows and overbeaming reduces the portion of the beam that is captured by the detector array (beam efficiency). In order to avoid penumbral effects in the outer portions of the detector array (detector area covered by the red area of the fan beam), the primary collimation must be made wider than necessary to expose only the detector array. The wider the incident beam, the smaller the percentage of "wasted" radiation due to overbeaming. Since unused radiation is delivered to the patient owing to overbeaming, when the beam collimation is consequently reduced, for a given *z*-axis coverage at a constant pitch, the number of rotations will need to be increased, contributing "wasted" radiation

compared with the fan beam in single-slice CT. In order to avoid penumbral effects in the outer portions of the detector array, the primary collimation must be made wider than necessary to expose only the detector array.

Overbeaming or "penumbra" effect (Fig. 5.7b) is a specific characteristic of MDCT, which reduces the

portion of the beam that is captured by the detector array (beam efficiency) with a consequent increase in noise and decrease in the contrast-to-noise ratio. Even when the incident X-ray beam is collimated to the targeted detector rows, the beam is always slightly wider than the rows. At multidetector row CT, the incident X-ray beam is about 2 mm wider than the selected detector configuration (Saini 2004). Hence, the wider the incident beam, the smaller the percentage of "wasted" radiation due to overbeaming. Since unused radiation is delivered to the patient owing to overbeaming, when the beam collimation is consequently reduced, for a given *z*-axis coverage at a constant pitch, the number of rotations will need to be increased, contributing "wasted" radiation. Thus, for example, a $16 \times 0.625$-mm acquisition will require twice as many rotations as a $16 \times 1.25$-mm acquisition, and therefore, an approximately 3% higher radiation dose will be delivered (Saini 2004).

Moreover, the bowtie filters are commonly employed in CT scanners to minimize radiation dose by reducing intensity variations across detector elements in the presence of patient anatomy. This filtration modifies a number of X-ray beam properties (effective energy, flux, first and second order statistics), making them nonuniform across the fan beam field of view.

Tube load parameters are very scanner-specific, and *CT dose index* (CTDI) and *dose-length product* (DLP) are better usable entities to indicate the absorbed dose for protocol comparison and optimization. The fundamental parameter of radiation dose is the *CTDI* measured by a dose phantom in rays (Gy) and represents the integrated dose along the *z*-axis from a single rotation of the X-ray tube. CTDI can be measured in air or in a perspex phantom of 16 cm (representing head) or 32 cm (representing body) diameter. All of these values are the CTDI, but serve different purposes. Within perspex phantoms, measurements are commonly made at both the center and the periphery (1 cm from the surface). The weighted sum of central and peripheral CTDI values is known as the weighted CTDI ($\text{CTDI}_w$) and represents the mean dose in the *x–y* plane. However, the CTDI does not indicate the precise dose for any individual patient, but is rather an index of the dose as measured and calculated in a phantom, and it does not take into account patient-associated parameters such as size, shape, and inhomogeneous composition (Lee et al. 2008). In helical scanning the pitch must be taken into account to give the mean dose within a scanned volume, and the *volume CTDI* ($CTDI_{vol}$) corresponds to the weighted CTDI corrected by the pitch factor (dose index divided by pitch). The $CTDI_{vol}$ can be used to express the average dose delivered to the scan volume for a specific examination. This is the mean dose within a scanned medium. Normalized weighted CTDI ($_nCTDI_w$) in air is 0.070 mGy/mAs. $CTDI_w$ multiplied to a conversion factor (1/0.38) is converted to $_nCTDI_w$.

Another parameter used is the DLP, which is related to the total radiation exposure (mGy×cm) and gives an approximation of radiation risk, but it cannot give a direct assessment of the patient dose since it does not take specific organs into account. DLP is calculated from $CTDI_w$ as:

$$DLP(mGy \times cm) = CTDI_w \times n\ N \times h,$$

where $CTDI_w$ is effective weighted CTDI (mGy); $n$ is tube rotations; $N$ is the number of detectors; and $h$ is slice thickness (in centimeters). DLP may be calculated also from $CTDI_{vol}$ multiplied by the length of the volume scanned.

$$DLP(mGy \times cm) = CTDI_{vol} \times L$$

After CT examination, the patient effective dose may be calculated by multiplying DLP for a specific coefficient representing typical adult and pediatric patients. This provides sufficiently precise estimates of effective dose for standard protocols and reference patients (Deak et al. 2008; Huda 2007; Shrimpton 1997).

## 5.1.2 Unenhanced and Contrast-Enhanced CT

Recent advances in MDCT technology allow fast, multiphase, and high-resolution imaging of the kidney. In particular, thin-section 1-mm-collimation with a low pitch is possible in MDCT imaging of the urinary tract. After acquisition of a digital projection radiograph (topogram), examinations are usually performed from the superior aspect of the kidneys to the pubic symphysis comprising the adrenal glands and the bladder by using 120 kVp tube voltage, and 16 (detector rows)×0.75-mm (section thickness), 64×0.5 mm, or 32×1-mm-collimation, and 2-mm interval reconstruction. The tube current (100–330 mA, with a mean of 150 mA) is adjusted for each examination according to patient body habitus by using automated dose modulation algorithm. Breath-hold scanning through the entire kidney is possible in less than 10 s, allowing for acquisition of thin-section images of the kidney during the corticomedullary, nephrographic, and excretory phases with little or no respiratory or patient-motion artifacts (Prasad et al. 2008).

### 5.1.2.1 Patient Preparation

To guarantee optimal excretion of contrast media during renal CT, sufficient hydration of the patient is essential. This can be achieved by oral or intravenous administration of fluid volume. However, concomitant disease, such as cardiac or renal insufficiency, has to be considered. Hydration may also minimize nephrotoxic effects of intravenous contrast media. Simultaneous filling of the gastrointestinal tract with oral contrast media may be useful. Interfering effects may occur with CT arteriography or CT urography and the application of positive oral contrast media.

### 5.1.2.2 Unenhanced CT

Precontrast Scan

In CT protocols the unenhanced CT scans are obtained initially to locate the kidneys and visualize morphological anomalies and to detect renal or urinary stones (Fig. 5.8) or calcifications in the renal parenchyma (Fig. 5.9), or in a complex renal mass (usually previously detected at US) (Fig. 5.10). Unenhanced CT scan is also mandatory to detect hemorrhage in the renal and perirenal collections (Fig. 5.11a, b) or in solid renal masses (Fig. 5.11c), the macroscopic fat component in a solid renal mass (Fig. 5.12a), and to scan patients with acute or chronic renal failure. The unenhanced CT scan of the kidney should be part of every protocol for the evaluation of a suspected renal mass since it provides a baseline from which to measure the enhancement within the lesion after the administration of intravenous contrast material and to obtain

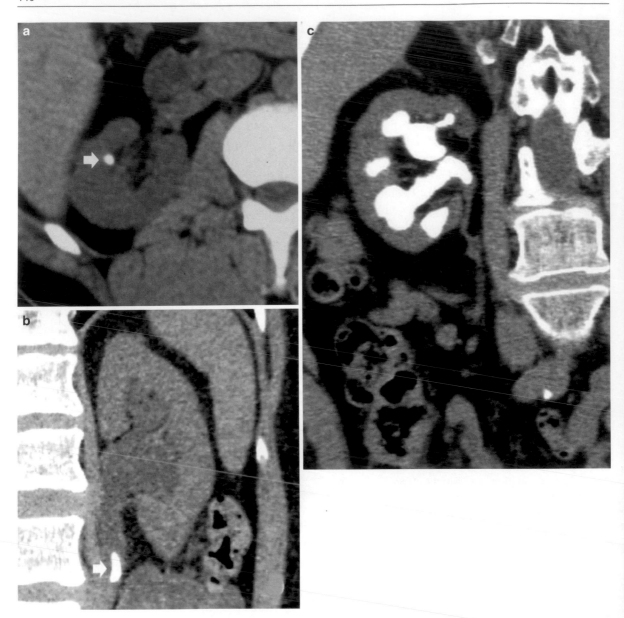

**Fig. 5.8** (a–c) Unenhanced CT. Calcifications due to renal or urinary stones. (**a**) Transverse plane. Renal stone (*arrow*). (**b, c**) Coronal reformation. (**b**) Urinary stone (*arrow*). (**c**) Staghorn renal calculosis

the baseline attenuation value of renal masses (Sheth et al. 2001). The air (Fig. 5.12b) (e.g., in emphysematous pyelonephritis) is the further component which may be detected on unenhanced CT.

## Renal Colic (Acute Flank Pain)

The principal indication for unenhanced CT is the detection of renal stones within the urinary tract in

patients with renal colic. Unenhanced spiral or multi-detector-row CT is now considered the reference imaging techniques for urolithiasis. In contrast to standard radiography, excretory urography, ultrasonography, and nephrotomography, CT enables to accurately assess location, size, and chemical composition of urinary calculi and to differentiate between urinary calculi and other pathologic processes, such as blood clots and tumors (Boll et al. 2009). Unenhanced CT is more effective than intravenous urography (IVU) – now

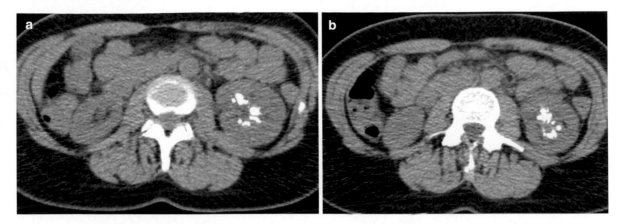

**Fig. 5.9** (**a**, **b**) Unenhanced CT. Calcifications in the renal parenchyma. Medullary nephrocalcinosis with diffuse calcium deposition within the renal medulla of the left kidney

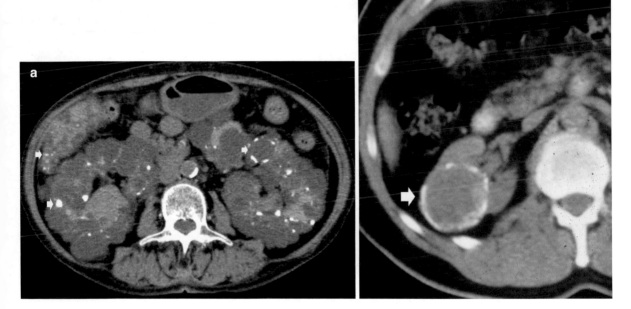

**Fig. 5.10** (**a**, **b**) Unenhanced CT. Calcific density. (**a**) Diffuse pericystic calcifications (*arrows*) in a polycystic adult kidney involving also the liver (*arrow*). (**b**) Peripheral calcific hyper- density due to tumoral calcifications in a solid clear cell type renal carcinoma (*arrow*)

replaced by MDCT urography - in precisely identifying ureteric stones and is equally effective as IVU in the determination of the presence or absence of ureteric obstruction (Smith et al. 1995). Nowadays, thin-section 1-mm-collimation with a low pitch is possible in MDCT imaging of the urinary tract. Table 5.1 shows the value of the technical parameters for unenhanced CT for renal colic. The main determinants in the clinical care of patients with urolithiasis are the location, size, and chemical composition of calculi. Especially, if extracorporeal shock wave lithotripsy is considered, the size and location of the urinary

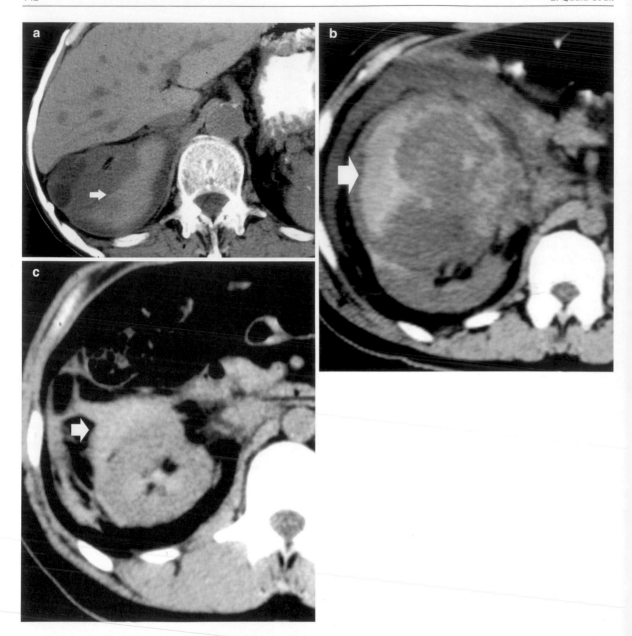

**Fig. 5.11** (**a**–**c**) Unenhanced CT. Hyperdensity from hemorrhage. (**a**) Perirenal hyperdense hemorrhagic collection (*arrow*) due to renal parenchyma laceration following motor bike accident. (**b**) Perirenal and renal spontaneous hematoma (*arrow*) in a patient under anticoagulant treatment. (**c**) Intratumoral hemorrhagic component (*arrow*) in a large solid renal tumor of the right kidney

stones and the anatomy of the urinary tract are of great importance to ensure smooth passage of the fragmented calculi. A low-dose technique may be applied for this indication.

Unenhanced CT shows direct and indirect findings of colic pain due to stone. The direct finding is the visualization of the calculus itself. Multiplanar reconstruction is indicated in the study of the entire ureter course to identify the exact site of the calcification for the urologist to perform an evaluation similar to that obtained by urography. Multiplanar reconstruction is indicated in the study of the entire ureter course to

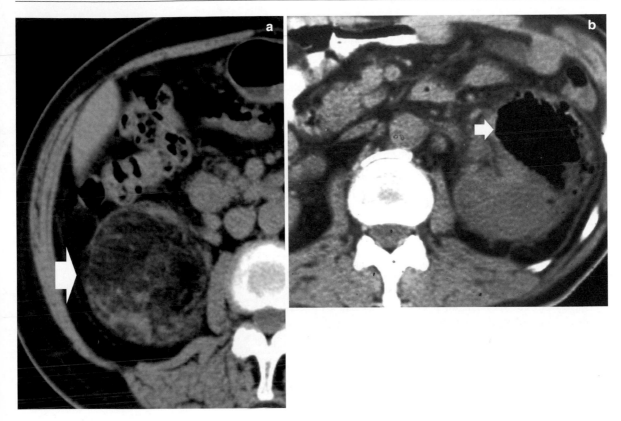

**Fig. 5.12** (**a**, **b**) Unenhanced CT, fat and air component. (**a**) Macroscopic fat component in a renal angiomyolipoma (*arrow*). (**b**) Intrarenal air component (*arrow*) due to emphysematous pyelonephritis in a diabetic patient

**Table 5.1** Low- and ultra low-dose unenhanced CT protocol

| CT systems | 1-slice | 4-slices | 16-slices | 64-slices |
|---|---|---|---|---|
| Peak voltage (kVp) | 120 | 120 | 120 | 120 |
| Exposure[a] | 160 | 70<br>30–40[b] | 70<br>30–40[b] | 80<br>30–40[b] |
| Collimation[c] | 3 | 4×1 | 16×0.75 | 64×0.5<br>32×0.1 |
| Table feed per rotation (mm/rotation) | 5 | 5 | 24 | 32 |
| Gantry rotation time (s/rotation) | 0.8 | 0.5 | 0.5 | 0.3 |
| Helical pitch[d,e] | 1.4 | 1.25 | 1–1.4 | 0.9 |
| Reconstruction interval (mm) | 3 | 1 | 1 | 0.5–1 |
| Reconstruction section thickness[f] (mm) | 3 | 3 | 2 | |

Note. The principal parameters employed in the unenhanced CT for urinary stone detection. Scan is performed from the superior aspect of the kidneys to the pubic symphysis
[a]Data are in milliampere-seconds
[b]Ultra low-dose CT
[c]Detector configuration. Number of detector rows (channels)×mm
[d]Equal to table feed per 360° rotation/single section collimation for single-slice CT scanners
[e]Equal to table increment per 360° rotation/total beam width for multislice CT scanners
[f]Corresponding to increment

identify the exact site of the calcification for the urologist to perform an evaluation similar to that obtained by urography. Regardless of composition, almost all renal stones are detected at unenhanced CT because the attenuation of stones is higher than that of surrounding tissue, even though the attenuation of uric stones is lower than the attenuation of calcium stones (Taourel et al. 2008). Indirect signs include hydronephrosis (Fig. 5.9) and ureteral dilatation (frequency: 65–90%), perinephric and periureteral stranding (36–82%), rim sign around the ureter (frequency 50–77%), renal enlargement (frequency 36–71%), renal sinus fat blurring, and reduced attenuation (>5 HU) of the renal parenchyma (Smith et al. 1996; Niall et al. 1999; Sourtzis et al. 1999). It has to be underlined that the reduced attenuation of the renal parenchyma is not specific for the renal colic since it may be caused also by interstitial edema in acute pyelonephritis and by venous congestion in renal vein thrombosis. Dual-energy MDCT may simultaneously acquire low- and high-energy attenuation profiles, thereby allowing the development and implementation of pixel-by-pixel postprocessing algorithms. Renal stone characterization with spectral analysis consisting in the assessment of tissue-specific attenuation values at distinct X-ray voltages is now possible by dual-energy MDCT (Boll et al. 2009). Another important task of unenhanced CT is the differentiation of renal colic from other causes of acute flank pain including renal hemorrhage (bleeding from an underlying renal mass, vascular abnormality or renal ischemia, anticoagulation or blood disorders – Fig. 5.11b), renal infections, large renal tumors, diverticulitis or appendicitis, pelvic masses, bowel obstruction, and aortic aneurysm. Most of these pathologic entities may be characterized by unenhanced CT. The addition of intravenous contrast agent can confirm the diagnosis.

Since the radiation exposure from standard radiography is 0.5–0.9 mSv, from IVU is 1.33–3.5 mSv, and from regular dose CT is 4.3–16.1 mSv, the employment of low-dose unenhanced CT is advocated. In single-slice CT the higher the pitch, the lower the corresponding dose, while in MDCT the lower the current tube (mAs), the lower the corresponding dose (Mahesh et al. 2001). With the most recent low-dose CT protocols (Table 5.1), it is possible to achieve a dose of 0.97–1.35 mSv (Knöpfle et al. 2003), while with ultra low-dose CT (20 mAs) a dose of 0.5–0.7 mSv (Kluner et al. 2006).

### 5.1.2.3 Contrast-Enhanced CT

Table 5.2 shows the value of the technical parameters for contrast-enhanced CT for renal parenchyma examination. Different phases of contrast uptake can be differentiated (arterial, corticomedullary, nephrographic, and excretory phase) after contrast material

**Table 5.2** Contrast-enhanced CT protocol for renal parenchyma

| CT systems | 1-slice | 4-slices | 16-slices | 64-slices |
|---|---|---|---|---|
| Peak voltage (kVp) | 120 | 120 | 120 | 120 |
| Exposure[a] | 160 | 180 | 200 | 200–250 |
| Collimation[b] | 5 | 4×1 | 16×0.75 | 64×0.5<br>32×1 |
| Table feed per rotation (mm/rotation) | 5 | 5 | 24 | 32 |
| Gantry rotation time (s/rotation) | 0.8 | 0.5 | 0.5 | 0.3 |
| Helical pitch[c,d] | 1.4 | 1.25 | 1–1.4 | 0.9 |
| Reconstruction interval (mm) | 5 | 5 | 3 | 0.5–1 |

Note. The principal parameters employed in the unenhanced CT for urinary stone detection. Scan is performed from the superior aspect of the kidneys to the pubic symphysis
[a]Data are in milliampere-seconds
[b]Detector configuration. Number of detector rows (channels)×mm
[c]Equal to table feed per 360° rotation/single section collimation for single-slice CT scanners
[d]Equal to table increment per 360° rotation/total beam width for multislice CT scanners

injection. Usually, 80–120 mL (350–370 mg/I) of nonionic contrast medium are administered through an 18–20 G catheter in an antecubital vein at 4 mL/s, followed by 30–40 mL of saline solution at the same injection rate.

Contrast-enhanced CT scans are acquired in different contrast-enhancement phases: the cortical or arterial phase, the nephrographic phase, and the urographic phase. Not all phases have to be acquired in every examination, and it is important to avoid unnecessary acquisitions to reduce the radiation dose. Imaging of the kidneys in different phases after intravenous contrast injection depends on sequential arrival of blood carrying contrast media in different parts of the renal parenchyma (Fig. 5.13). With normal renal function, iodinated intravascular contrast medium is excreted by passive glomerular filtration. The amount of a substance undergoing glomerular excretion is determined by the product of its "freely filterable" serum concentration and glomerular filtration rate (GFR). GFR varies on the basis of weight, age, and gender. GFR decreases in systemic hypotension, renal

vasoconstriction, or glomerulonephrytis (decreased number of functional nephrons). Different phases are easily recognizable within the kidney during contrast medium administration. Their relative onset times depend on methods of contrast medium administration and patient characteristics.

Imaging phases have to be selected carefully in accordance with clinical indication. The comprehensive evaluation of renal masses by CT requires a dedicated renal CT protocol including unenhanced, arterial, corticomedullary, nephrographic, and excretory phases. Unenhanced CT scans are used to detect calcifications and allow quantification of tumoral enhancement on the postcontrast scans (Prasad et al. 2008).

The arterial CT phase is reached about 15–25 s after commencement of intravenous contrast media injection (for renal arteriography, a contrast bolus of 3.5 mL/s is desirable). When performing a contrast-enhanced CT of the kidney, it is critical, mainly for the arterial phase, to scan at the peak of contrast enhancement in the renal cortex: nowadays, this is easily achieved with the "bolus

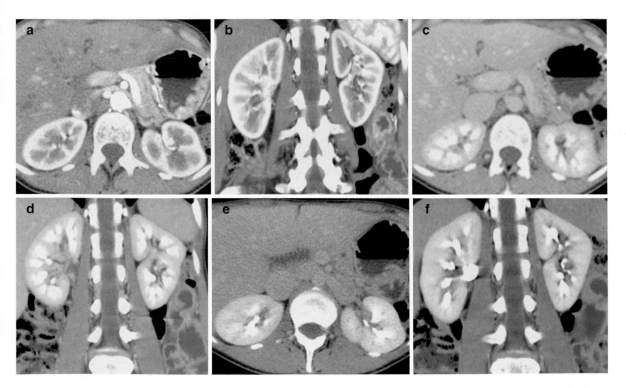

**Fig. 5.13** (**a–f**) Transverse images and coronal reformations of the arterial cortico-medullary phase (**a, b**), the late venous nephrographic phase (**c, d**), and the delayed excretory phase (**e, f**), after a split-bolus contrast administration protocol (from Professor Roberto Pozzi Mucelli, University of Verona, Italy)

tracking" technique, which has replaced the simple "test bolus" technique. The use of empirical fixed delays (i.e., 25–30 s), with small variations depending upon patient age or body habitus, should be abandoned because with state-of-the-art MDCT the temporal window to perform the acquisition of the examination is very narrow (Bae et al. 2008; Erturk et al. 2008; Kock et al. 2007; Schoellnast et al. 2005; Stacul et al. 2008). Alternatively, a test bolus scan or a bolus tracking program can be applied for optimal start of the arterial scan. In the arterial phase, renal arterial stenosis or evaluation of stent implantation can be judged, and acute bleeding can be detected or ruled out.

The corticomedullary CT phase (about 25–70 s after i.v. contrast) shows high contrast in the renal cortex (Fig. 5.13a, b). During the corticomedullary phase, the contrast resides in the capillaries of the renal cortex and peritubular cells, the proximal convoluted tubules, and columns of Bertin (Schreyer et al. 2002). During this phase, renal cortex is clearly distinguishable from the medulla due to greater cortical vascularity and because contrast material fills only the more proximal tubular structures. Peak enhancement of the renal vessels during the early corticomedullary phase also provides information on vascular anatomy and patency. Early opacification of renal veins is also detectable. The renal medulla demonstrates with low contrast. The optimal delay time for the corticomedullary phase depends on the rate of contrast injection, the amount of contrast material administered, and the patient's cardiac output (Prasad et al. 2008). The cortical phase gives a perfect visualization of the cortex (hyperdense) and medulla (hypodense), and therefore, of the morphology of the kidney. This is the best phase to evaluate the vascularity of a mass: as most renal tumors are hypervascular, this phase is useful in the characterization of renal masses. This phase is also fundamental when evaluating the renal arteries, for example, in patients with hypertension of suspected renovascular origin. The corticomedullary phase is also suitable for the depiction of vascular renal anatomy (aneurysm, arteriovenous malformation, fistula) and the assessment of vessel patency.

The nephrographic (parenchymal) CT phase (80–180 s delay) shows renal cortex and medulla with equal enhancement due to contrast medium equilibrating between vascular and interstitial compartments entering loops of Henle and collecting tubules. During the nephrographic phase, the renal parenchyma enhances, homogeneously allowing the best opportunity for discrimination between the normal renal medulla and

masses. Nephrographic phase may be divided into an early phase and a late phase (Fig. 5.13c, d), with the latter overlapping the excretory phase. This is the best phase to detect renal masses since all lesions appear hypodense compared to the renal parenchyma. This phase is also useful for the evaluation of the renal veins and inferior vena cava. Mostly, CT examination includes a noncontrast phase followed by the arterial and nephrographic phases. This technique is suggested for the diagnosis of renal tumors, complex renal masses, trauma, and infections. For the last two indications, an additional delayed scan in the urographic phase or later (3-h delayed scans) may be added.

The excretory CT phase (Fig. 5.13e, f) begins 3 min after intravenous contrast media administration and shows the opacified renal pelvis, ureter, and urinary bladder (complete filling of the urinary bladder with contrast media usually takes about 20 min). The excretory phase may be part of a CT examination of the kidney, added to the previous phases at 5–10 min from the injection (Fig. 5.1), or performed as a separate protocol known as MDCT urography. During this phase, the nephrogram remains homogeneous, but its attenuation is diminished. It should be emphasized that a CT urogram, as defined here, is not needed to evaluate many urinary problems. Indeed, specific portions of a CT urogram are not only sufficient to address many clinical questions, but also are preferred since they result in less radiation exposure. For benign indications where only the excretory phase will be relevant (variant urinary tract anatomy, congenital anomalies of the urinary tract, ureteral pseudodiverticulosis, and iatrogenic ureter trauma), single-phase CT urography can suffice. For lower-risk groups, CT urography can be used as a problem-solving test if traditional work-up remains negative and significant undiagnosed symptoms persist. Patients with more complex benign diseases and those with chronic symptomatic urolithiasis (complex infections, percutaneous nephrolithotomy (PCNL) planning) may benefit from adding an unenhanced phase to the excretory phase. In chronic urolithiasis without complete obstruction, furosemide-assisted CT urography can demonstrate most ureteral stones within the enhanced urine. So for the evaluation of hydronephrosis due to obstruction by stones, the unenhanced phase may be safely deleted, whereas diagnosis of small nonobstructing stones may be done by an unenhanced phase limited to the kidneys. For example, an unenhanced CT scan is the test of choice in patients who present with flank pain and a high probability of an obstructing stone. Often, an excretory phase CT scan alone is adequate when a congenital anomaly or a postoperative complication (e.g., urinary extravasation) is suspected. Also, in the setting of urinary tract trauma, simply using nephrographic and excretory phase CT scans is sufficient in most patients. According to the patient history and clinical presentation, different CT protocols are employed. In the acute flank pain, optimized low-dose unenhanced CT scan is usually performed.

## CT Examination of Renal Masses

Contrast-enhanced CT is regarded as the method of choice for detection and characterization of renal lesions, even though there are still some limitations, e.g., nephrotoxicity of contrast media and the obvious lack of clear discrimination between benign and malignant tumors. Most renal masses are neoplastic in nature, while infectious, inflammatory, and nonneoplastic renal masses are more rare. Comprehensive evaluation of a renal mass requires a dedicated renal CT protocol including unenhanced scan, and contrast-enhanced scans during corticomedullary, nephrographic, and excretory phases are usually requested. The preliminary unenhanced CT scan is used to detect intratumoral calcification, fat, or hemorrhage or also to quantify contrast enhancement on the postcontrast scan. The corticomedullary phase scan allows the differentiation of normal variants of renal parenchyma from renal masses and the better depiction of tumoral hypervascularity due to contrast enhancement. The nephrographic phase is considered the optimal phase for the detection and characterization of small renal masses (Szolar et al. 1997; Prasad et al. 2008), even though it may miss transient lesion enhancement. The excretory phase defines the relationship of the renal mass with the collecting system, especially for planning nephron-sparing surgery. Nephrographic or excretory phase images appear to be similar to one another, but superior to corticomedullary phase images in the ability to both detect and characterize renal masses. The corticomedullary phase should also be included for staging (Kopka et al. 1997; Zagoria 2000).

Detection of renal masses: Small renal tumors or complex cysts detected by US need confirmation and characterization by CT. CT is more sensitive than US in the detection of small renal tumors above all when <1.5 cm. Contrast material-enhanced CT is considered a reliable technique in the detection of renal tumors (Jamis-Dow et al. 1996; Szolar et al. 1997; Zagoria 2000). All renal masses can be detected by CT and approximately 15% of all renal masses detected on CT are benign, while the remaining 85% are malignant renal tumors (Zagoria 2000). Nevertheless, the corticomedullary phase is not mandatory for the tumor protocol, since the nephrographic phase is more sensitive for tumor detection (Cohan et al. 1995) (Fig. 5.14).

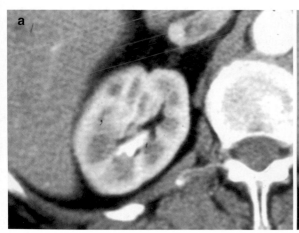
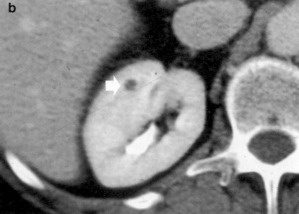
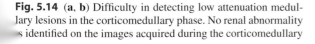

**Fig. 5.14** (**a**, **b**) Difficulty in detecting low attenuation medullary lesions in the corticomedullary phase. No renal abnormality s identified on the images acquired during the corticomedullary phase (**a**) A small simple cyst (*arrow*) is easily identified in the medullary region during the nephrographic phase (**b**)

In fact, the two main disadvantages of the corticomedullary phase are the difficulty in detecting small hypovascular lesions of the renal medulla, which appears hypoattenuating during this phase, and detecting small hypervascular tumors of the renal cortex, which may enhance to the same degree of the renal cortex.

Some diagnostic pitfalls were described for contrast material-enhanced CT (Kopka et al. 1997; Szolar et al. 1997). The principal diagnostic pitfalls are small hypervascular renal cell carcinomas with similar contrast enhancement to renal cortex, which may be mistaken for normal parenchyma at the corticomedullary phase, and centrally located tumors which are mistaken for the normal hypoattenuating renal medulla (Yuh and Cohan 1999). Most studies indicate that MR imaging is comparable to CT for the detection of small renal masses (Semelka et al. 1992; Zagoria 2000), but it requires more time at a greater expense. In order to characterize a solid renal mass, the CT examination should be biphasic including the corticomedullary phase to recognize the vascularization of the tumor and the tubular phase to recognize the enhancement level and all the outline of the lesion.

Characterization of renal masses: Any mass detected initially on US or evaluated with US after detection with another imaging technique that does not meet the strict US criteria for a simple cyst should be further evaluated with CT or MR imaging of the kidneys (Zagoria 2000). Based on imaging findings, renal masses may be classified into predominant soft tissue, adipose tissue, or cystic masses (Prasad et al. 2008). Most renal cell carcinomas are solid lesions with attenuation values of 20 HU or greater at nonenhanced CT. Renal cell carcinoma is the most common soft tissue mass in the kidney. However, renal cell carcinomas may demonstrate different intratumoral components and may appear entirely cystic or show a small proportion of macroscopic fat. Benign renal tumors, including oncocytoma, metanephric adenomas, and mesenchymal neoplasms, usually manifest as a soft tissue renal mass. Cystic renal lesions include simple or hemorrhagic or proteinaceous cysts, abscesses, and cystic neoplasms including multilocular cystic renal cell carcinoma, cystic nephroma, and mixed epithelial and stomal tumors. Most angiomyolipomas contain macroscopic fat and account for most renal masses with detectable adipose tissue.

The unenhanced CT scan provides a baseline from which to measure the enhancement within the lesion after the administration of intravenous contrast material. The demonstration of enhancement is considered a reliable sign of vascular renal tumor, even though it is not considered a sign of malignancy. Renal mass enhancement is dependent on multiple factors, including the amount and rate of the contrast material injection, the imaging delay, and the nature of the tissue within the mass (Israel and Bosniak 2005, 2008). This enhancement characteristic is important in distinguishing hyperdense cysts from solid tumors. When a cystic renal mass presents entirely a fluid attenuation (0–20 HU) surrounded by a hairline-thin smooth wall and does not enhance, the mass is benign. When a cystic renal mass contains fluid that is of higher attenuation than simple fluid, has calcification within its walls or septa, has a thickened wall or septa, or contains an enhancing soft-tissue component, the mass may be benign or malignant according to the degree of thickness and irregularity and enhancement of the wall septa classified by the Bosniak classification (1986).

Most renal cell carcinomas are solid lesions with attenuation values of 20 HU or greater at unenhanced CT (Silverman et al. 1994). Even though there is no universally agreed upon specific number that can be used as definitive and unequivocal evidence of enhancement within a renal mass, an increase of 20 HU attenuation (Maki et al. 1999; Israel and Bosniak 2005; Silverman et al. 2008) within a renal lesion after the intravenous administration of contrast agent has been generally accepted as a threshold for contrast enhancement. If a solid lesion measuring at least 2 cm appears hyperdense with a change in lesion density >20 HU compared to baseline, it has to be considered to be a solid enhancing malignant mass as a first hypothesis because renal cell carcinoma is often hypervascularized. If the change in lesion density is between 10 and 20 HU (equivocal enhancement) or if the change in lesion density is <10 HU (absent enhancement), the lesion may be a solid benign or malignant (typically papillary-cell carcinoma) or cystic (Siegel et al. 1999; Israel and Bosniak 2005). In this case the renal lesion should be considered indeterminate and further evaluation with contrast-enhanced US or MR imaging with image subtraction technique (Hecht et al. 2004) should be performed.

In renal cell carcinoma contrast enhancement at CT is usually diffuse and intense sparing necrotic intratumoral areas (Soyer et al. 1997), except for papillary-cell subtype which appears hypovascula on contrast material-enhanced CT or MR imaging (Choyke et al. 1997, 2003). Distinct areas of fat may be present as well. Cystic areas may be prevalently present so that tumor presents a frank cystic appearance. Anyway, the enhancement patterns of neoplastic renal masses are variable and mainly depend on tumoral vascularity and histotype. Clear cell renal cell carcinomas show hypervascularity on contrast-enhanced CT during the corticomedullary phase. In many cases, the enhancement degree within a renal neoplasm is dense and heterogeneous (Fig. 5.15). Even if the enhancement degree is not particularly high at visual analysis but appears irregular or nodular within the renal mass (Fig. 5.16), the mass is most likely neoplastic. Multiplanar and 3D reformations may allow a better assessment of contrast enhancement within a solid renal mass and its relationships with the adjacent anatomical structures (Fig. 5.17). However, some hypovascular renal masses may present more subtle and uniform enhancement (Figs. 5.18–5.20), and there are instances when it is difficult to confidently characterize a mass as enhancing, specifically in the case of hyperattenuating cysts or minimally enhancing renal cell carcinoma. For these reasons, the current standard practice in genitourinary radiology is to compare attenuation measurements between the unenhanced CT scan

and each of the postcontrast phases. In particular, papillary renal cell carcinomas are more often multicentric than clear cell renal cell carcinomas and commonly appear as homogeneous soft tissue cortical masses with foci of calcifications, hemorrhage, or necrosis. Papillary renal cell carcinomas are often hypovascular on contrast-enhanced CT (Figs. 5.18 and 5.19) and typically show a lesser degree of contrast enhancement than clear cell renal cell carcinomas. Chromophobe renal cell carcinomas typically appear as homogeneous renal mass with a cortical epicenter and show a uniform, or slightly heterogeneous, and lesser degree of contrast enhancement (Fig. 5.20). Renal oncocytomas are typically hypervascular at contrast-enhanced CT.

The contrast washout during the nephrographic phase can be useful as the initial enhancement for the renal mass characterization. Moreover, the evidence of contrast washout may be useful if only a single-phase contrast-enhanced CT scan of the abdomen was performed (e.g., 25–35 s after contrast administration in CTA, or 70–90 s after contrast administration in abdominal tumor staging or follow-up) and the renal mass is incidentally detected before the patient left the imaging suite (Prasad et al. 2008). In this case, rescanning the kidneys permits the assessment of "de-enhancement" (Macari and Bosniak 1999), and if the

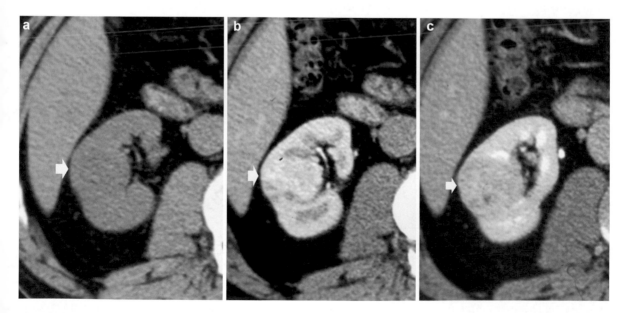

**Fig. 5.15** (**a–c**) Soft tissue density renal mass. Clear cell cell carcinoma. Hyperdensity after contrast administration. (**a**) Unenhanced CT. The solid renal tumor (*arrow*) appears isodense to the adjacent renal parenchyma. (**b**, **c**) Contrast-enhanced CT. The solid renal tumor (*arrow*) appears hyperdense in comparison to the adjacent renal parenchyma during the corticomedullary phase (**b**) and hypodense due to contrast washout during the nephrographic phase (**c**)

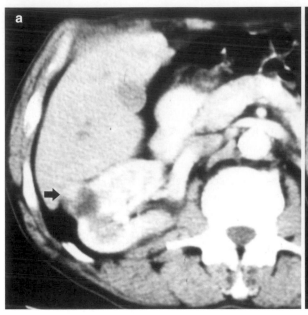 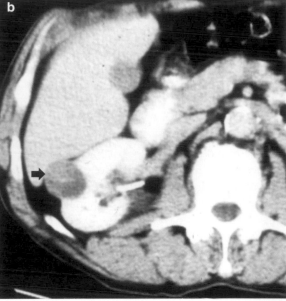

**Fig. 5.16** (**a**, **b**) Hyperdensity after contrast administration. Clear cell renal cell carcinoma. (**a**) Contrast-enhanced CT. Corticomedullary phase. Nodular appearance of tumoral con-trast enhancement (*arrow*) after iodinated contrast agent admin-istration. (**b**) Contrast-enhanced CT. Nephrographic phase. Tumoral contrast washout (*arrow*)

area of enhancement decreases visually or quantita-tively (at least of 10 HU), neoplasm is suspected. Recently, dual-energy CT (DECT) was shown to be highly effective in the differentiation of enhancing renal masses from hyperdense cysts in a phantom model (Brown et al. 2009) by taking advantage of the unique capability of DECT to classify iodine-contain-ing voxels in the area of interest, and therefore, charac-terizing the lesion as an enhancing tumor.

Renal angiomyolipoma represents the most fre-quent renal mass with predominant macroscopic fat (Fig. 5.21), which is readily identified on unenhanced CT. However, the intratumoral fat content may be vari-able and angiomyolipomas with minimal fat cannot be distinguished by other renal tumors by imaging criteria (see Chap. 20).

Most cystic renal lesions are benign (Fig. 5.22). Renal cystic lesions that require interventional or sur-gical management include abscesses and cystic neo-plasms. Hemorrhagic (Fig. 5.23) or proteinaceous (Fig. 5.24) hyperdense renal cysts with nonsignificant contrast enhancement after iodinated contrast agent

injection often present difficult or impossible differ-ential diagnosis from solid renal tumor by CT. In these cases, US may help the differential diagnosis by depicting the cystic or solid nature of the lesion. CT scans of the kidneys obtained approximately 3 h after contrast administration often reveal useful information in patients with renal abscesses (Dalla Palma et al. 1997) by revealing a focal staining or a hyperdense rim surrounding micro and macroabscesses (Fig. 5.25). Contrast-enhanced CT shows intratumoral septations (Fig. 5.26) and allows a correct assessment of the cyst wall with the possibility to indentify mural nodules (Fig. 5.27).

## CT Examination of Renal Traumas

Renal trauma, blunt or penetrating, usually requests a multiphase protocol including a preliminary unen-hanced CT scan to identify renal parenchyma hemor-rhage (Fig. 5.11), the nephrographic (Fig. 5.28), and the excretory phase to detect contrast extravasation

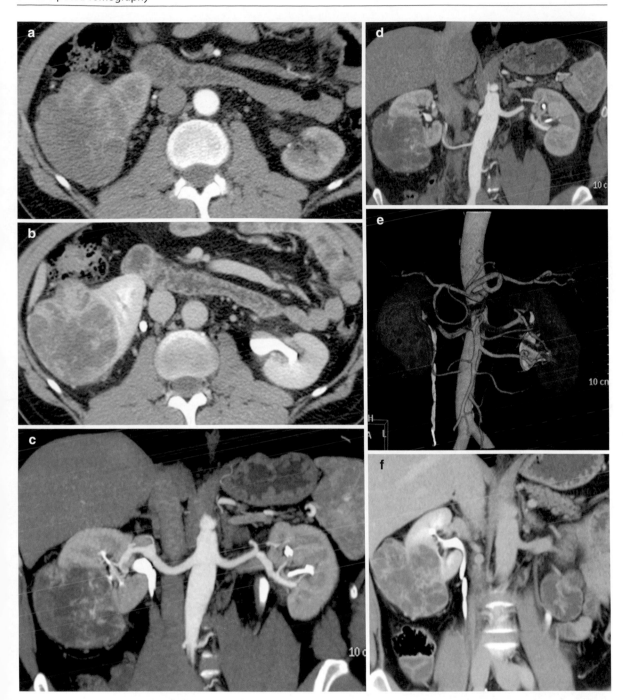

**Fig. 5.17** (**a–f**) Soft tissue density renal mass. Hyperdensity after contrast administration. Large renal cell carcinoma at the lower pole of the right kidney: transverse images in the arterial (**a**) and nephrographic phase (**b**) after bolus contrast medium administration. Curved maximum intensity projection (MIP) images showing the renal arteries (**c**) and the polar artery for the lower pole of the right kidney (**d**). Volume rendering image depicting the renal arteries and the right inferior polar artery (**e**). Coronal 5-mm multiplanar reformation (MPR) shows the relationship between the tumor and the collecting system (**f**) (from Professor Roberto Pozzi Mucelli, University of Verona, Italy)

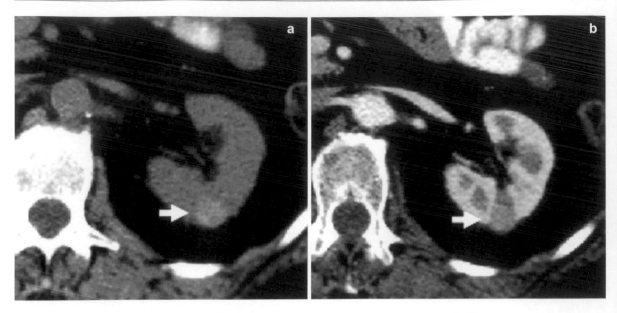

**Fig. 5.18** (**a**, **b**) Soft tissue density renal mass. Hypodensity after contrast administration. (**a**) Hypodense solid renal tumor (*arrow*) corresponding to a papillary-cell type renal carcinoma.

(**b**) The tumor shows no significant contrast enhancement (*arrow*) after iodinated contrast agent injection (50 vs. 57 HU)

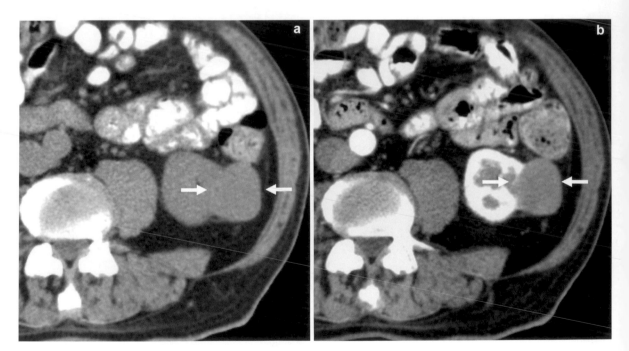

**Fig. 5.19** (**a**, **b**) Soft tissue density renal mass. Solid papillary-cell type renal carcinoma (*arrows*) on the left kidney. (**a**) Unenhanced CT. Hyperdense renal mass (*arrows*) with 55 HU density. (**b**) Contrast-enhanced CT after iodinated contrast agent

injection. Corticomedullary phase. The renal mass (*arrows*) shows 60 HU density with a nonsignificant contrast enhancement if compared to unenhanced CT scan

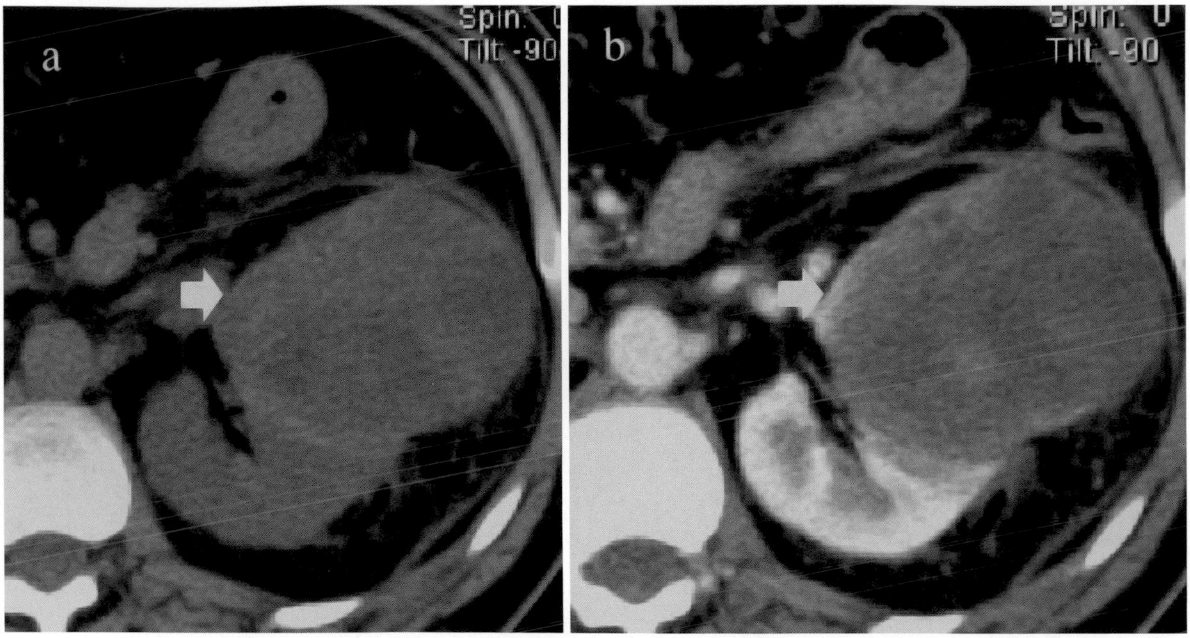

**Fig. 5.20** (**a**, **b**) Soft tissue density renal mass. Solid chromophobe cell type renal carcinoma (*arrow*) on the left kidney. (**a**) Unenhanced CT. Heterogenous renal mass (*arrow*). (**b**) Contrast-enhanced CT after iodinated contrast agent injection. Corticomedullary phase. The renal mass (*arrow*) shows slightly heterogenous contrast enhancement distributed throughout the lesion

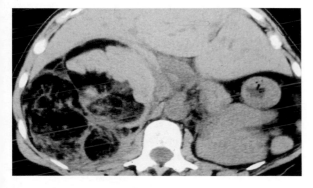

**Fig. 5.21** Fat tissue density renal mass. Giant angiomyolipoma with predominant fat component

due to renal pelvis rupture. If active bleeding is suspected, arterial or corticomedullary phase should be added. In iatrogenic renal traumas (e.g., biopsy, percutaneous nephrostomy, or postextracorporeal shock wave lithotripsy – Fig. 5.29), the same protocol is used (see Chap. 19).

## CT Examination of the Postoperative Kidney

The assessment of the kidney immediately after surgery or interventional procedures is usually performed by a multiphase protocol including the corticomedullary phase, nephrotomographic phase, and the excretory phase to assess lesions of the urinary tract (see Chap. 32).

### 5.1.3  CT Nephrogram Alterations

The CT nephrogram alterations are expressions of impaired contrast medium delivery, transit, and excretion by the kidney and are strictly related to the inner pathophysiological mechanisms underlying each condition associated with alteration of the renal function.

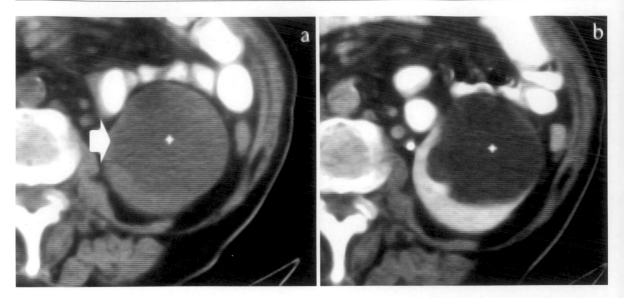

**Fig. 5.22** Simple renal cyst (*arrow*). (**a**) Unenhanced CT. Hypodense homogeneous renal lesion (*arrow*) with the typical cyst density. (**b**) Contrast-enhanced CT after iodinated contrast agent injection. Nephrographic phase. Absence of contrast enhancement

### 5.1.3.1 Delayed CT Nephrogram

The CT nephrogram is delayed (Fig. 5.30) when it appears more than 120 s after contrast medium injection. The principal causes are as follows: (1) Prerenal vascular causes (i.e., renal artery stenosis). Reduced renal perfusion causes delayed contrast material delivery to the kidney, while GFR also decreases, determining a low density nephrogram; (2) Hypotension or abnormality in renal function (always bilateral) results in reduced GFR. Furthermore, concurrent tubular stasis causes increased water reabsorption and tubular concentration of contrast medium; (3) Venous obstruction; (4) Urinary tract obstruction. The delayed parenchymogram is caused by increased intrarenal resistance against renal artery flow. In the renal vein or urinary tract obstruction, the CT nephrogram density also appears persistent due to increased intrarenal resistance (often unilateral) which can reduce tubular transit rate, resulting in contrast material persisting in the kidney.

### 5.1.3.2 Increased Density of CT Nephrogram

The CT nephrogram density increases in: (1) high dose of iodinated contrast medium or high infusion rate (always bilateral) due to increased contrast medium volume and iodinate concentration; (2) high transit time (also unilateral) increased sodium and water absorption and consequently increased preurine concentration due to tubular stasis.

Increased pyelogram density is due to: (1) low osmolarity contrast medium (always bilateral): reduced osmolar effect with reduced urine volume and dehydration (always bilateral); (2) urinary tract obstruction (see Chap. 14). Pyelogram density depends on the urine iodinate concentration and volume. The pyelogram presents a progressive increase in density with a clear delay (1–3 h) in comparison to the controlateral kidney.

### 5.1.3.3 Decreased Density or Absence of CT Nephrogram

The CT nephrogram density decreases homogeneously in: (1) renal artery occlusion resulting in reduced perfusion in the territory of the occluded artery; (2) renal diseases reducing GFR (always bilateral) such as glomerulonephritis due to the reduced number of functioning nephrons or reduced renal perfusion; (3) renal obstructive disease (more often unilateral). Reduced GFR and renal blood flow due to vasoconstrictors (acute obstruction) or increased intrarenal resistance due to vessel compression by a dilated excretory system (chronic obstruction). In the renal obstructive disease the nephrogram may also be delayed (more than 180 s).

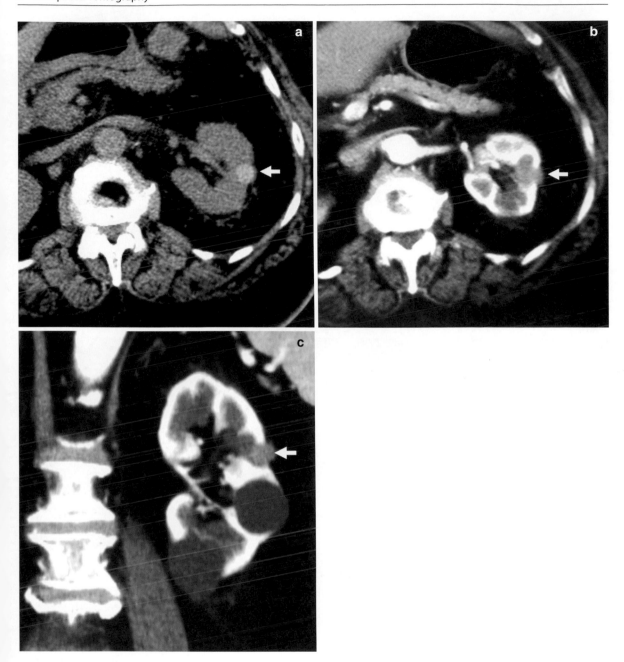

**Fig. 5.23** (**a**, **b**) Hyperdense hemorrhagic renal cyst. Hemorrhagic renal cyst (*arrow*) on the right kidney. (**a**) Unenhanced CT. Hyperdense renal mass (*arrow*) with 95 HU density on the left kidney. (**b**, **c**) Contrast-enhanced CT after iodinated contrast agent injection. Corticomedullary phase, transverse plane (**b**), and coronal reformation (**c**). The hyperdense renal mass (*arrow*) shows 97 HU density with a nonsignificant contrast enhancement if compared to unenhanced CT scan

The CT nephrogram density decrease is more often expressed by wedge-shaped areas of decreased attenuation radiating from the papilla in the medulla to the cortical surface featuring alternating linear bands of high and low attenuation oriented parallel to the axis of the tubules and collecting ducts. This pattern can be sustained by: (a) acute pyelonephritis in which striations are due to alternating normal tubules and obstructed ones by inflammatory cell and debris. This first results in decreased enhancement due partially to increased

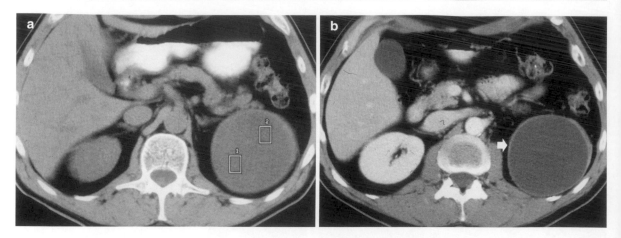

**Fig. 5.24** (**a**, **b**) Infected renal cyst with proteinaceuous content (40 - 45 HU density measured by the regions of interest 1 and 2). (**a**) Unenhanced CT reveals a large homogenous lesion on the left kidney. (**b**) Contrast-enhanced CT, nephrographic phase. The lesion reveals its cystic nature with peripheral wall thickening

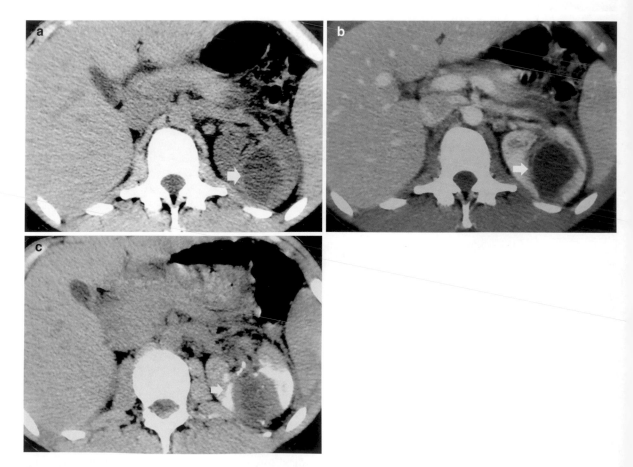

**Fig. 5.25** (**a–c**) Renal abscess. (**a**) Unenhanced CT. Hypodense renal lesion (*arrow*) is identified on the left kidney. (**b**) Contrast-enhanced CT. Nephrographic phase. The renal lesion presents a cystic density (*arrow*) with a peripheral dense rim corresponding to the pyogenic wall. (**c**) CT scans of the kidneys obtained approximately 3 h after contrast administration reveal a hyperdense rim (*arrow*) surrounding the abscess

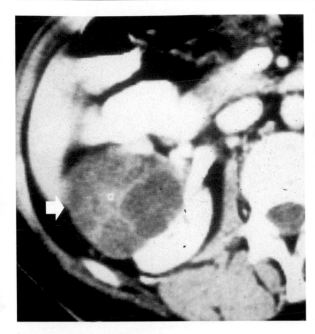

**Fig. 5.26** Contrast-enhanced CT, nephrographic phase. A complex renal cyst (*arrow*) with multiple renal septations corresponding to multicystic nephroma

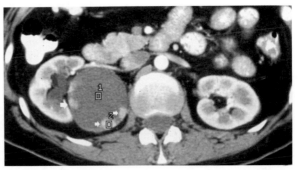

**Fig. 5.27** Cystic clear cell renal carcinoma. Contrast-enhanced CT, corticomedullary phase. Multiple enhancing (as shown by the region of interest 2, if compared to the region of interest 1 placed in the liquid component) mural nodules (*arrows*) are visualized

interstitial edema, then in increased density due to contrast medium hyperconcentration in delayed phases in the edematous areas; (b) urinary tract obstruction with contrast medium hyperconcentration within dilated medullary rays; (c) renal contusion; (d) Renal vein thrombosis; (e) Renal lymphoma: striations are due to the intrarenal diffusion of the disease.

In arterial occlusion nephrogram appears segmentally decreased with segmental disappearance of the nephrogram in the territory of the occluded artery(ies) (Fig. 5.31). In acute pyelonephritis (Figs. 5.32 and 5.33) hypodense striations are due to alternating normal tubules and obstructed ones by inflammatory cell and debris. CT scans of the kidneys obtained approximately 3 h after contrast administration often reveal useful information in patients with renal infections (Dalla Palma et al. 1997) by revealing a nephrogram replacing a variable portion of the low density areas present in the early enhanced phase (Dalla Palma et al. 1997). In renal vein thrombosis the nephrogram may be absent or heterogeneous (Fig. 5.34).

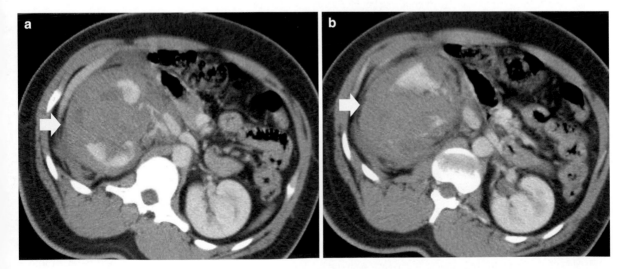

**Fig. 5.28** (**a**, **b**) Renal fracture (*arrow*) due to a motorbike accident. Contrast-enhanced CT. Nephrographic phase

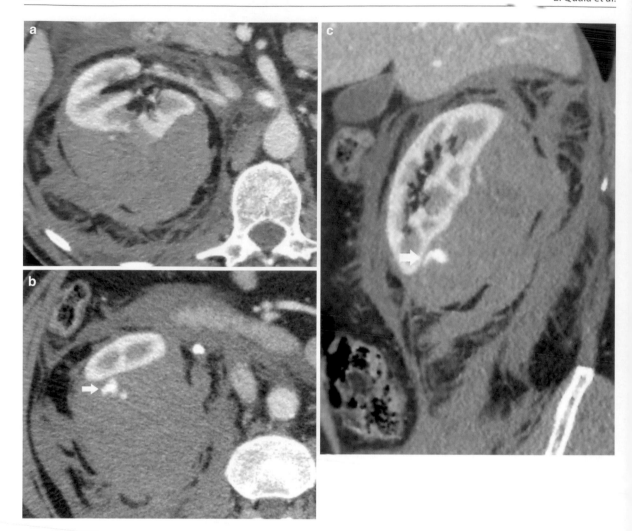

**Fig. 5.29** (**a–c**) Contrast-enhanced CT. Corticomedullary phase. (**a**, **b**) Transverse plane; (**c**) sagittal reformation. Perirenal hematoma after extracorporeal shock wave lithotripsy. Contrast extravasation (*arrow*) is visible on the right perinephric space

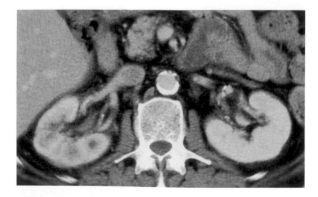

**Fig. 5.30** Contrast-enhanced CT. Nephrographic phase. Delayed nephrogram on the right kidney in a patient with right pyelonephritis

### 5.1.3.4 Cortical (Rim) Nephrogram

Cortical or "rim" nephrogram consists in the opacification only of a peripheral rim of the renal cortex with prolonged persistence of corticomedullary differentiation. The findings have been described in a variety of situation: (1) *renal artery occlusion:* the cortical rim sign (Fig. 5.35) represents peripheral cortex spared from the ischemic damage through collateral capsular, peripelvic, and periureteric arteries. It may be considered the best differential CT feature in distinguishing renal infarction from pyelonephritis (Wong et al. 1984); (2) *renal vein thrombosis:* altered perfusion gradient due to the interstitial pressure increased by venous

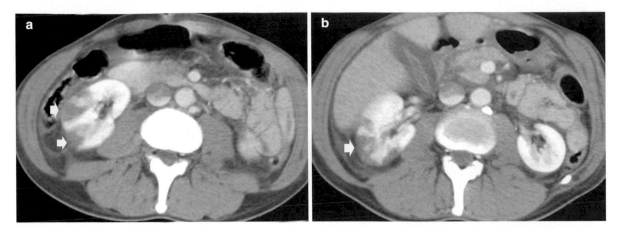

**Fig. 5.31** (**a, b**) CT nephrogram alteration. Contrast-enhanced CT. Nephrographic phase. Segmentally altered nephrogram in the right kidney due to multiple renal perfusion defects (*arrows*) due to embolic parenchymal infarctions

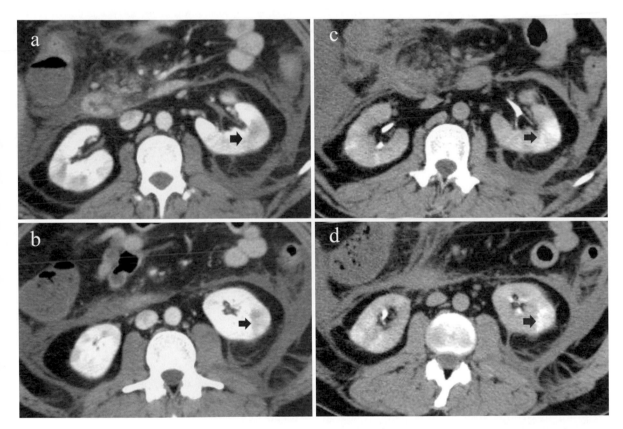

**Fig. 5.32** (**a–d**) CT nephrogram alteration. Contrast-enhanced CT. Nephrographic (**a, b**) and delayed phase scan at 3 h (**c, d**). (**a, b**) Altered nephrogram in the left kidney (*arrows*) due to parenchymal perfusion defects due to acute pyelonephritis. (**c, d**) Delayed scan reveals contrast enhancement (*arrows*) replacing the low density areas evident on the nephrographic phase

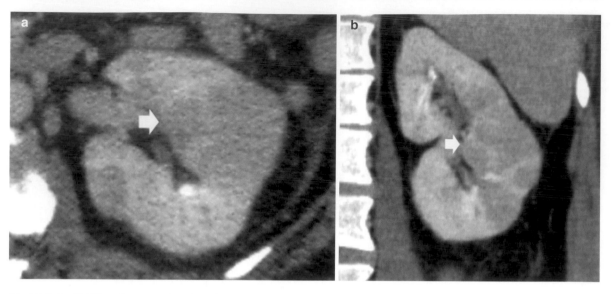

**Fig. 5.33** (**a**, **b**) CT nephrogram alteration. Contrast-enhanced CT. Nephrographic phase. Altered nephrogram in the left kidney (*arrow*) due to focal hypodensity corresponding to focal pyelonephritis

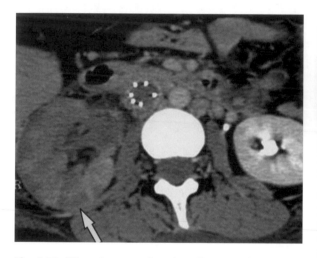

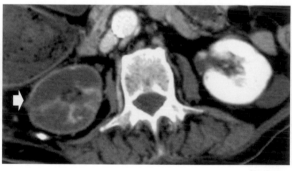

**Fig. 5.35** CT nephrogram alteration. Contrast-enhanced CT. Nephrographic phase. Complete renal infarction with evidence of cortical rim sign (*arrow*) due to right renal artery occlusion determining peripheral cortical enhancement due to peripheral revascularization

**Fig. 5.34** CT nephrogram alteration. Contrast-enhanced CT. Nephrographic phase. Reduced and heterogenous nephrogram in the right kidney (*arrow*) due to right renal vein thrombosis

occlusion, with preserved renal cortex; (3) *acute ureteral obstruction*: increased tubular pressure transmitted in a retrograde manner to the nephron results in impaired arterial perfusion gradient. Outer cortex is spared probably by contribution of collateral vessels. Furthermore, increased tubular pressure due to stasis causes reduced or absent progression of contrast medium into the tubules. Anyway, during acute obstruction, the presence of contrast medium in the renal pelvis without opacification of renal medulla is noted. This is probably due to substitution of glomerular filtration by tubular active secretion, thereby explaining contrast medium accumulation in the collecting system with no significant medullar opacification.

## 5.2 Multidetector CT Urography and CT Angiography

(*Roberto Pozzi Mucelli, Giulia Zamboni, Livia Bernardin, Alberto Contro*)

## 5.2.1 Multidetector CT Urography

MDCT scanners allow a high spatial resolution due to the narrow collimation, which results in isotropic voxels in 64-channel MDCT scanners. Small slice thickness improves the detection of small structures and minimizes partial volume effects, while slice fusion options improve contrast and contrast-to-noise ratio. These features make MDCT the ideal diagnostic tool to evaluate the urinary tract. Intravenous excretory urography was used in the past for a large variety of clinical indications in the diagnostic assessment of the urinary tract, and its utilization decreased when cross-sectional imaging techniques have since proved superior to excretory urography for most, if not all, remaining indications (Silverman et al. 2009). When unenhanced CT was shown to reliably detect urolithiasis, excretory urography was pronounced dead in 1999 with the caveat that there might remain rare instances in which it is an appropriate examination (Amis 1999). MDCT excretory phase imaging of the urinary tract was initially described by several groups (Perlman et al. 1996; McNicholas et al. 1998). MDCT provided the ability to obtain thin (submillimeter) collimated data of the entire urinary tract during a short, single breath-hold.

Nowadays, the development of MDCT urography has completely covered all the clinical indications previously addressed by excretory urography. As suggested by the CT Urography Working Group of the European Society of Urogenital Radiology (Stacul et al. 2008), MDCT urography is a dedicated multiphasic CT scanning technique optimized for imaging the urinary tract in which intravascular contrast medium is used and in which high-resolution images of the renal parenchyma and urinary tract (including the bladder) are obtained. The use of this definition means that CT exams performed for many of the current indications for CT of the urinary tract, such as characterization of complex renal masses, staging of renal cell carcinoma, acute flank pain, renal infection. and evaluation of renal arteries for possible renovascular hypertension, should not be labeled MDCT urography (Stacul et al. 2008). In fact, this procedure is optimized for evaluating both the renal parenchyma and the entire excretory pathway.

Dalla Palma (2001) summarized the residual roles of IVU, which then was indicated for asymptomatic hematuria (where it complemented ultrasound, plain film of the abdomen and cystoscopy), congenital anomalies of the urinary tract, prior to endourological procedures, possible fistulas, renal transplantation, urinary tuberculosis, and suspected ureteral pathology. Five years later, Nolte-Ernsting and Cowan (2006) reported the most frequent indications for multidetector computed tomography urography (MDCTU): suspected urothelial tumor (hematuria or unexplained hydronephrosis), urinary tract trauma, pre and postoperative urinary tract assessment, 3D planning for difficult cases of PCNL, and complex cases of urinary tract infection, including tuberculosis. There is considerable overlap between these indications and those listed in 2001 as residual roles of IVU. Morcos (2007) was even more determined, stating that MDCTU has the same applications as IVU. Nolte-Ernsting and Cowan (2006), on the other hand, observed that no consensus had yet been reached on the indications for MDCTU (Morcos 2007). An analysis of the results of comparative studies of MDCTU and IVU is required in order to compare the diagnostic accuracy of the two techniques.

### 5.2.1.1 Technique

The radiological literature describes several technical variants for performing MDCTU (Caoili et al. 2005b; Chow and Sommer 2001; Heneghan et al. 2001; Huang et al. 2006; Kemper et al. 2005); the differences mainly concern contrast-agent administration, number of phases, examination technique (supine or prone patient position, use of ureteral compression, saline infusion, oral hydration, or use diuretics such as furosemide), and acquisition timing.

The MDCTU study does not require any special preparation. No bowel preparation is needed. The use of positive contrast medium for bowel should be avoided as it interferes with subsequent evaluation of 3D images. Oral hydration (900 mL) with water, instead of contrast, is without any additional cost. It avoids dehydration, promotes diuresis, and acts as a negative contrast medium for the gastrointestinal tract. Up to 1,000 mL of water in 20–60 min before CT has been used. It can improve delineation of ureteral segments and may facilitate the diagnosis of incidental findings. If patients cannot tolerate the oral intake of water, diuresis may be promoted somewhat by a slow intravenous drip-infusion of 0.9% saline (to a maximum of 500 mL) before and during the CT urography.

Patients are asked to void immediately prior to the examination, and bladder catheters must be clamped before CT urography.

Supine positioning is the standard practice for MDCTU. Prone imaging may be advantageous in the unenhanced phase to discriminate ureterovesical junction stones from stones passed into the bladder. Prone positioning for improved depiction of the upper urinary tract during excretory phase has shown mixed results. An early study showed better opacification of the collecting system to midureter by prone positioning, but more recent studies could not show any benefit and other factors than positioning play a greater role. Given the more cumbersome position for the patients, prone imaging is not advocated for routine use. However, turning the patient several times before excretory phase imaging can avoid layering effects of the contrast medium, especially when the renal collecting system is dilated.

Typically, CT urography consists of a multiphasic helical CT protocol (Browne et al. 2005). A preliminary unenhanced CT scan is obtained from the upper pole of the kidney to the lower edge of the symphysis pubis to detect calculi, reveal the unenhanced appearance of masses (throughout the urinary tract), and provide a baseline attenuation value to calculate enhancement of masses and other abnormalities. Unenhanced images are also useful for evaluating masses for fat or calcium (Silverman

et al. 2009). The acquisition protocols for the most commonly acquired phases in MDCTU are detailed in Table 5.3. Traditionally, CTU studies have been examined in the transverse plane. Thicker sections are easier to review than thinner ones, because there are fewer images (Dillman et al. 2007a). Thinner slices can be used for better characterization of lesions, although these images can be grainy due to a lower signal-to-noise ratio.

The most frequently used contrast medium concentrations contain 300–350 mg of iodine per milliliter (mgI/mL). However, ideally the volume of contrast medium should be adapted to the contrast medium concentration and the patient's weight (e.g., 1.7–2.0 mL/kg of 300 mgI/mL CM or 1.4–1.6 mL/kg of 370 mgI/mL contrast medium), while adaptation of the injection rate to the patient's weight (e.g., 0.04 mL/s/kg) ensures a constant injection duration, which is optimal for MDCT. Two major approaches have been followed: (1) a single bolus of contrast medium, combined with a three- to four-phase study using unenhanced, nephrographic, and excretory phase series, vs. (2) a split-bolus contrast medium injection, combined with a two- to three-phase study using unenhanced and a combined nephrographic-excretory phase series.

The number of CT urography phases in the single-bolus technique generally varies between two and four: (1) an unenhanced phase of the abdomen and pelvis, (2) a nephrographic phase of the kidney, and (3) an

**Table 5.3** CT urography protocol

| MDCT parameters 4-row/16-row/64-row | Unenhanced 4-row/16-row/64-row | Nephrographic 4-row/16-row/64-row | Excretory 4-row/16-row/64-row |
|---|---|---|---|
| Scan delay | – | 120 | 8 min |
| Scout | A-P abdomen and pelvis | | |
| Patient position | Supine | Supine | Supine |
| Scan interval | Kidneys–bladder | Diaphragm–kidneys | Kidneys–bladder |
| Tube voltage (kVp) | 120 | 120 | 120 |
| Tube current (mA) | 80–180 | 80–180 | 80–180 |
| Collimation | $4 \times 2.5/16 \times 1.5/64 \times 0.6$ | $4 \times 2.5/16 \times 1.5/64 \times 0.6$ | $4 \times 2.5/16 \times 1.5/64 \times 0.6$ |
| Pitch | 1 | 1 | 1 |
| Table feed | 10 | 10 | 10 |
| Slice thickness (mm) | 3 | 3 | 3 |
| Reconstruction interval (mm) | 3 | 3 | 3 |

Note. The principal parameters employed in the CT urography according to the CT equipment
*A-P* anteroposterior

excretory phase of the abdomen and pelvis. Only a few groups employ the use of a corticomedullary phase since the arterial phase information is not needed routinely. Some extend the nephrographic phase to the pelvis, especially when the patient is at increased risk of malignancy. Such a nephrographic phase facilitates complete tumor staging or evaluation of associated findings. Because of the high radiation dose of CT urography, the number of phases should be kept to a minimum.

The so-called "split bolus" technique is the one which has probably the largest consensus, also because it limits the radiation exposure to the patient. Instead of obtaining two (nephrographic and excretory phase) separate scans after intravenous contrast material administration, a "split-bolus" technique has been described to reduce the total number of scans from three to two, and therefore, decrease radiation exposure (Chow et al. 2007). A split-bolus technique allows a two-phase CT urography with a synchronous nephrographic and pyelographic excretory phase (Chow et al. 2007; Dillman et al. 2007b) (Fig. 5.36). The split-bolus technique is summarized in Table 5.4. Once the patient is positioned on the table, furosemide is administered i.v. (0.1 mg/kg), and an unenhanced scan is acquired from the upper pole of the kidneys to the bladder base. The contrast agent is then injected in two boluses, for a total patient dose of 600 mgI/kg. A first bolus of 400 mgI/kg is injected, followed by a second bolus of

200 mgI/kg after a 6-min delay and a saline flush. Two minutes after the second bolus, a second scan is acquired of the entire abdomen and pelvis, which affords both an effective nephrographic-phase image (thanks to the second bolus of contrast material) and good opacification and distension of the urinary tract (thanks to the time delay after the first bolus) (Fig. 5.37).

The advantage of split-bolus administration is to obtain a combined nephro-pyelographic phase, instead of two separate phases, with a relatively reduced radiation exposure. Anyway, radiation exposure is a critical issue and further optimization is achieved by using low-dose protocols and tube current modulation. The main drawbacks of slit-bolus technique is the reduced contrast effect due to contrast fractionation with ureters and bladder not imaged appropriately, the evidence of beam hardening artifacts in the kidney if furosemide is not provided, and limited reduction of dose (about 15%) if compared with the standard single bolus technique with three-phase CT urography.

### 5.2.1.2 Optimizing Excretory Phase

The goal in MDCTU, derived from the experience with IVU, is to obtain the maximum distension and opacification of the urinary tract. For optimal timing of the contrast enhancement during the excretory phase,

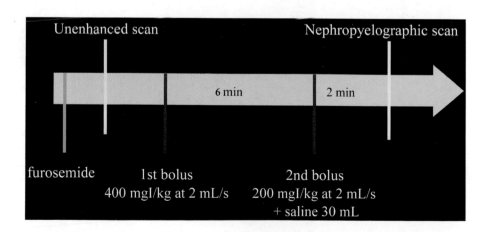

**Fig. 5.36** CT urography. Scheme of the split-bolus technique (see text)

**Table 5.4** Split-bolus technique

| Contrast medium (400 mgI/kg) 2 mL/s | 6 min | Contrast medium (200 mgI/kg) 2 mL/s | 2 min |
|---|---|---|---|
| Unenhanced scan | | | Nephrograhic-excretory scan |

**Fig. 5.37** (**a**) Transverse unenhanced image shows a large hyperattenuating stone in the distal left ureter. (**b**) Transverse image in the contrast-enhanced phase after split-bolus contrast medium administration shows reduced parenchymal enhancement in the left kidney, which shows dilated calyces and pelvis, as compared to the right normal kidney. (**c**, **d**) Coronal MIP images in the contrast-enhanced phase depict the right ureter, while the left ureter is nonopacified. (**e**) Coronal 5-mm MPR shows the asymmetric enhancement of the kidneys and the nonopacified left collecting system. (**f**) Coronal oblique 5-mm MPR shows the nonopacified left collecting system and ureter

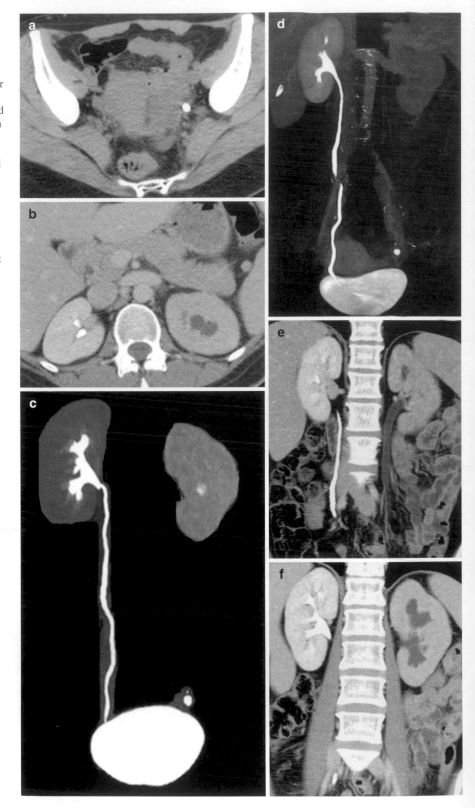

the individual delay time in each patient may be determined exactly using single-slice test-images obtained at different intervals after injection of the contrast agent bolus (Silverman et al. 2009).

A number of ancillary maneuvers have been proposed to improve the quality of the MDCTU examination. Compression devices, also used during the IVU era, can be applied during CT urography to distend the upper tracts, and when removed, the distal ureters frequently fill due to flushing from above (Heneghan et al. 2001). External compression was first proposed by McNicholas et al. (1998) based on the experience with IVU: the authors concluded that it improved opacification of the renal collecting system and the ureters. Caoili et al. (2005b), however, observed that external compression did not significantly improve urinary tract distension or opacification. However, compression devices are cumbersome, necessitate imaging the upper and lower tracts separately, and are often ineffective (Caoili et al. 2005b), particularly in large body habitus patients. Furthermore, these devices, as in the IVU era, are relatively contraindicated in patients with abdominal aortic aneurysms, acute obstruction, or abdominal stomas and in patients who have undergone recent abdominal surgery.

Several authors have attempted intravenous hydration prior to excretory CTU imaging, based on the assumption that an increased intravascular volume would result in increased renal excretion and thus in improved upper urinary tract distension and opacification; moreover, dilution of the hyperdense urine could improve disease identification reducing the risk of artifacts. McTavish et al. (2002) noticed improved distal ureter opacification after i.v. hydration with saline prior to excretory imaging. Caoili observed that i.v. administration of 250 mL of saline solution prior to excretory phase imaging improves dilatation of the intrarenal collecting system and the proximal ureter in a small, though significant, extent Caoili et al. (2005b).

Other authors, however, observed different results. Sudakoff et al. (2006) did not observe any significant improvement in collecting system opacification after administration of a saline bolus prior to excretory imaging. Similarly, Silverman et al. (2006) observed that administration of i.v. saline prior to excretory imaging does not add additional benefit in the setting of furosemide administration. Kawamoto et al. (2006) have proposed oral hydration before performing CTU: if an adequate volume of water is ingested enough time before the exam, the effect is similar to that of i.v. hydration.

Furosemide (5–10 mg i.v.) use provides improved opacification and distension of the middle and distal ureters compared with use of i.v. saline alone (Nolte-Ernsting et al. 2001) and improves the enhancement of the entire urinary tract. Furosemide belongs to the class of loop diuretics. Furosemide is secreted by the organic acid transport route into the proximal tubule, and its main site of action is the thick ascending limb of the loop of Henle by inhibiting the $Na^+$–$K^+$–$2Cl^-$ cotransport mechanism, thereby enhancing the sodium and chloride secretion. This determines an overwhelming solute and fluid load to the distal tubule and collecting system. The use of intravenous furosemide is now standard in most institutions because it increases the urinary flow rate: its diuresis is predominantly due to NaCl reabsorption in the thick ascending limb of Henle. Furosemide has been demonstrated to have a greater effect on ureteral opacification than saline (Silverman et al. 2006). Sanyal et al. (2007) observed that the use of furosemide yielded a 93% of completely opacified ureters. Contraindications to furosemide include allergy to sulfa, hypokalemia, exposure to cytotoxic medications, use of cardiac amynoglicosides, and systolic blood pressure <90 mmHg. Furosemide maximizes the urinary tract and ureteral opacification and distension (Silverman et al. 2006) with a greater effect than saline by increasing the urinary flow rate and the delivery of contrast medium to the middle and distal ureter. Another advantage provided by furosemide is the elimination of beam hardening artifacts in the kidney due to contrast medium dilution. An additional logistic benefit is that the delay of the excretory phase can be shortened when furosemide is used. In patients with normal renal function a median delay of the excretory phase of 420 s (mean $450 \pm 120$ s) was seen. Furosemide administration allows a good bladder distension during the excretory phase necessary to assess masses and wall thickening. The urine opacification maximizes the contrast-to-noise ratio and helps to detect bladder masses. Good mixing of contrast media (no contrast media-urine level) and urine provides homogeneous background from which bladder lesion can be detected. Furosemide injection also provides some drawbacks. First, sometimes contrast medium in the urine is too dilute reducing the contrast-to-noise ratio and potentially masking some TCC. Second, some type of stone, for example, urate calculi (400 HU), may be isodense to the urine and become not detectable.

### 5.2.1.3 Reconstruction Algorithms

MPR can be used to characterize lesions, especially in the longitudinal axis, and to assess more easily the anatomy. McTavish et al. (2002) used 3-mm thick coronal sliced, with a 3 mm increment. Thinner slices can also be used, as suggested by Dillman et al. (2007a) (Fig. 5.38a).

Metser et al. (2009) demonstrated that, with 64-MDCT, the use of a coronal plane improves conspicuity and detection rate of stones smaller than 5 mm; for all stones, stone size estimation was improved in the coronal plane, especially for vertically oriented stones, which can be underestimated in the axial plane by more than 20%. Evaluation of the coronal plane may be clinically valuable if the axial plane is negative for stones or if a stone is not confidently diagnosed on the axial plane.

The creation of coronal and curved-planar reformatted images (Figs. 5.38b, c and 5.39a–d) comes at no additional radiation cost and provides an increase in the depiction of renal pathologies. The use of curved-planar reformatted images has been proposed, because these images can project the entire length of the upper urinary tract in one single image. The disadvantages include the increased effort and time required to create these images and the distortion of the anatomy and pathology.

Dillman et al. (2008) analyzed the sensitivity of 16-row MDCTU axial, coronal reformatted, and curved-planar reformatted images in the detection of urothelial neoplasms of the upper tract and observed that axial, coronal reformatted, and curved-planar reformatted image have similar sensitivities; the authors conclude that reviewing multiple image-types increases sensitivity.

3D images are created interactively by radiologists on a 3D workstation. Thin-slab volume rendering (VR) (Fig. 5.38d, e), average intensity projections (AIP) (Fig. 5.38f), or maximum intensity projection (MIP) 3D images (Figs. 5.38g–i and 5.39e) can be used for interactive image evaluation. McNicholas et al. (1998) first described the use of MIP and AIP images in CTU: these techniques allow to display a 3D dataset in a single coronal plane (Fig. 5.38g–i).

### 5.2.1.4 Radiation Dose

Higher radiation doses are associated with MDCT urography than with stone unenhanced CT protocol. The relatively high radiation dose of multiphase CT urography is a significant limitation of the widespread acceptance of this technique. Radiation dose with MDCT urography significantly exceeds excretory urography (Nolte-Ernsting and Cowan 2006). Current multiphase CT urography protocols can be associated with effective doses as high as 25–35 mSv, depending upon the number of phases included. Substantial dose reduction currently cannot be recommended in cases of intrinsic urinary tract lesions. If the excretory CT phase is performed additionally in the tumor-staging protocol when obstruction of the urinary tract from the outside is suspected, substantial dose reduction may be reasonable. In a population with a high suspicion for or with known malignant disease, radiation dose plays only a relatively small role. However, for patients with benign diseases or for susceptible patient populations, such as children and young or pregnant women, dose is an issue. Strict indications for multiphase CTU and reduction of the number of phases are important tools to manage this relatively high-dose examination.

In consideration of five possible phases of renal CT (unenhanced, arterial, corticomedullary, nephrographic, and excretory phases), a selection has to be made for clinical indications to avoid accumulation of dose. Effective dose was measured about 15 mSv for CT urography. Effective dose can vary depending on the number of abdominal scans. In split-bolus technique, intravenous contrast media is applied at two different time points (e.g., with an interval of 10 min) before a single CT scan of the kidneys and urinary tract is obtained. The urinary tract is opacified with excreted contrast media from the first bolus when the scan commences after the second bolus of contrast media. If the scan is started such that there is a delay of 80–120 s after commencement of the second bolus, the kidneys are depicted in the nephrographic phase, while the renal collecting systems and the ureters are depicted in the excretory phase. Therefore, only one scan is necessary for investigating two contrast media phases. For investigation of children, MRI appears more suitable in most cases. However, there are rare indications that require rapid action, such as polytrauma. In this case, dose reduction can be adjusted to noise or body weight. Tumor staging of nephroblastoma by means of CT has been proven to be reasonable in children.

In some modern systems this can also be combined with 3D adaptive noise filtration. Data on radiation dose optimization or optimal levels of noise indices using these 3D dose modulation or 3D noise filtering techniques for CTU applications are currently lacking,

**Fig. 5.38** (**a–h**) Image visualization modalities: (**a**) Five millimeter thick coronal MPRs; (**b**, **c**) curved reformations; (**d**, **e**) coronal volume rendering (VR) images with different presets; (**f**) average intensity projection (AIP); thick MIP images (**g**, **h**) coronal, and coronal oblique (**i**)

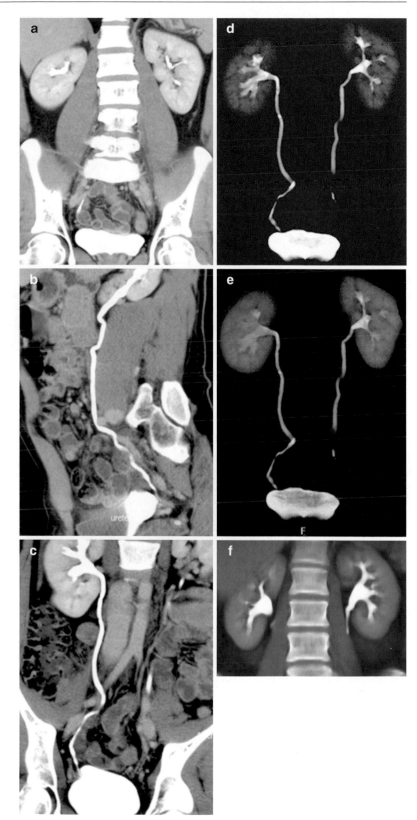

**Fig. 5.38** (continued)

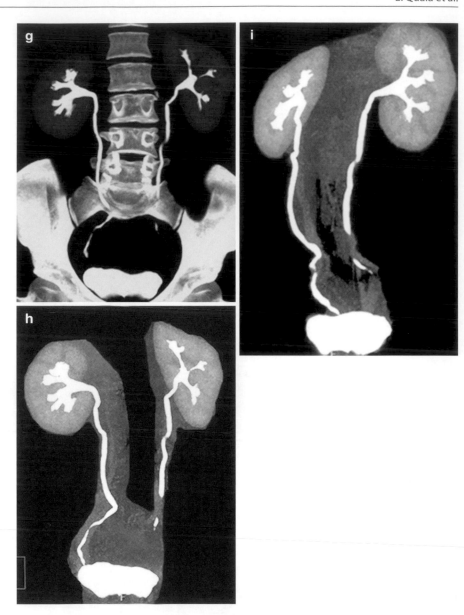

but these techniques may lead to dose reductions of 20–30%, compared with currently published fixed milliampere-seconds protocols, without significant loss in diagnostic image quality.

Radiation dose has been one of the most important driving factors in the optimization of CT urography techniques and in the selection of justified indications. The increased patient dose of CT urography is justified by its increased performance, especially in populations at increased risk for GU malignancy. Few data on CT urography radiation doses have been presented. Four- and 16-slice scanners employing three- to four-phase protocols are usually associated with effective dose levels of 23–35 mSv (McTavish et al. 2002).

For the unenhanced scan, the abdomen and pelvis are imaged by using a maximum collimation of 2.5 mm. Given these preliminary data, we suggest that in average-sized patients (60–80 kg) excretory phase imaging with thin collimation may well be performed at a $CTDI_{vol}$ of 5–6 mGy. The nephrographic phase

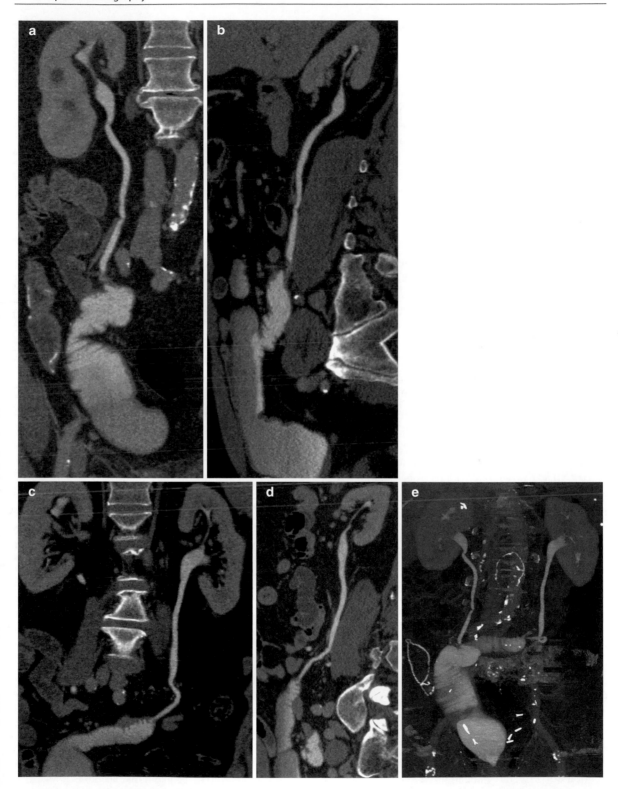

**Fig. 5.39** (**a–e**) CT urography in a patient with orthotopic neobladder. Coronal and sagittal reformatted images of the right (**a**, **b**) and the left kidney (**c**, **d**). (**e**) MIP 3D image (courtesy of Prof. Quaia)

may require a slightly higher dose for more optimal diagnosis in the liver ($CTDI_{vol}$ in the order of 7–8 mGy). Even lower doses for unenhanced CT ($CTDI_{vol}$ in the order of 2–3 mGy) are acceptable, and even doses comparable with one abdominal plain film ($CTDI_{vol}$ 0.9 mGy) may suffice. With such optimization, even three-phase protocols with effective doses below 7 mSv can be realized with the limitation of the scan coverage (summed over all scan phases) and efficient selection of scanning acquisition parameters (detector configuration, pitch, tube current–time product).

The use of a low-dose unenhanced scan can further reduce the minimum dose to 20.1 mSv. Furthermore, using the lowest-effective-dose CT urography protocol, filling defects of 0.25 mm could be reliably detected using the newest level of scanner technology, equivalent to the performance using CR. The heterogeneous 4-MDCT protocols represent the oldest level of CT urography technique, which is being rapidly replaced by 16- and 64-MDCT techniques. The trend toward increased dose efficiency is consistent with increased attention to dose reduction by the radiology community. However, for practices where 4-MDCT is still in use, the results presented here can be used to optimize scanning protocols.

The mean effective dose for patients undergoing three phases MDCT urography with the four-section MDCT scanner and a three-scan protocol has been reported to be 14.8 mSv ± 3.1 (Nawfel et al. 2004), or 1.5 times that of IVU with full nephrotomography. These data, however, were obtained without dose modulation at a single institution and cannot be generalized (Silverman et al. 2009). A comprehensive evaluation of hematuria and suspected transitional cell carcinoma can be performed at an effective dose of approximately 20.1 mSv, which is 8.2 mSv (≈70%) higher than that of a traditional excretory urography examination (11.9 mSv) consisting of five KUBs (anteroposterior), one KUB (prone), three kidney radiographs, and eight kidney tomograms (Vrtiska et al. 2009).

A very low-dose protocol using a $CTDI_{vol}$ of 2.1 mGy is unlikely to be sufficient to depict intraluminal lower ureter lesions, but may allow biphasic excretory imaging with improved distal ureteral opacification for selected indications. Other studies indicated that image quality of excretory phase CTU is adequate at a $CTDI_{vol}$ of 5.0–7.1 mGy, which is currently used in clinical practice. These data were further substantiated by low-dose simulation experiments in which image quality was negligibly degraded with a dose reduction to a $CTDI_{vol}$ of 6.1–6.7 mGy. Furthermore, lower tube voltages of 90–100 kV have favorable effects on image quality (contrast-to-noise ratio) in the low-dose range.

### 5.2.1.5 Indications

MDCT urography is currently considered the most sensitive and comprehensive imaging modality for the evaluation of the entire urinary tract (Caoili et al. 2002) by providing a comprehensive examination of the kidneys, collecting systems, ureters, and bladder. CT urography is now accepted as the primary diagnostic investigation for the detailed anatomy of the pelvicaliceal system and ureters. Most frequent present-day indications for CT urography include the investigation of hematuria, patients at increased risk for having upper or lower tract urothelial neoplasms, urinary diversion procedures following cystectomy, hydronephrosis, chronic symptomatic urolithiasis including planning of percutaneous nephrolithotomy, traumatic and iatrogenic ureteral injury, and complex urinary tract infections. In renal urolithiasis CT urography is indicated after unenhanced CT when the urologist requests a map of the urinary tract for percutaneous or endoureteral or also surgical procedures, when a urothelial tumor is suspected given the need to evaluate the entire urinary tract, and when the renal colic arises in a diabetic patient in whom no stone is detected and papillary necrosis is suspected. The use of CT urography for other indications is largely anecdotal. CT urography may be useful in guiding PCNL procedures, to depict abnormal postoperative findings in patients after urinary diversions, or to effectively diagnose medullary and papillary necrosis in an early stage when treatment can reverse the ischemic process. Also, during CT urography significant extraurinary findings may be found. However, additional imaging was needed in few patients and the per-patient incremental costs were minimal.

The first indication for MDCT urography is hematuria (Joffe et al. 2003; Silverman et al. 2009). Hematuria is a common urologic problem that accounts for 4–20% of all urologic visits. Microscopic hematuria corresponds to >3 red blood cells/high power microscopic field, and it is present in 9–18% of normal patients. The prevalence of asymptomatic microscopic hematuria varies 0.6–21% and is among the most important clinical signs of a urologic malignancy. A cause for asymptomatic microscopic hematuria can be found in 32–100% of patients undergoing a full urologic evaluation, with 3.4–56% of these patients having either moderately or highly clinically significant diagnoses. On the other hand, hematuria (particularly when microscopic) may not always signal the presence of serious disease, and therefore, it has long been debated how aggressively these patients can be evaluated. It must be underlined that hematuria may be determined by plenty of causes, many of which are insignificant (renal cyst, exercise, polyps, urethritis, urethrigonitis), others are significant and require observation (benign prostatic hyperplasia, papillary necrosis, trauma, arteriovenous fistula), some others are significant and require treatment (urolithiasis, vesicoureteral reflux, ureteropelvic junction obstruction, renal artery stenosis, renal vein thrombosis, renal infections), while the rest are life-threatening (malignancies, abdominal aortic aneurysm).

The American Urological Association Best Practice Policy guidelines for asymptomatic microscopic hematuria were published in 2001 and included either IVU or CT urography as the initial imaging test (Grossfeld et al. 2001a, b). CT urography had a better diagnostic yield when compared with IVU (Gray Sears et al. 2002), even though both IVU and CT urography have been rated equally (score 8) in the hematuria diagnostic work-up by the American College of Radiology on 2005. Patients with hematuria younger than 40 years represent the low-risk group for urologic disease, while patients with hematuria older than 40 years, or smokers, or patients with gross hematuria or irritating voiding symptoms, urinary tract infections, or exposure to carcinogens (pelvic irradiation, analgesic abuse, cyclophosphamide, chemicals/dyes) represent the high-risk group (Grossfeld et al. 2001a, b). High-risk patients with one positive urine sediment (>3 red blood cells/high power microscopic field) should undergo urinary upper tracy imaging, cytology, and cystoscopy. If these examinations are negative, they should undergo further work-up every year for 3 year. Low-risk patients with two of three positive urine sediments should undergo upper tracy imaging, cytology, and cystoscopy. If these examinations are negative, further work-up is considered optional (Grossfeld et al. 2001a, b). Symptomatic hematuria in patients younger than 40 years should be evaluated by unenhanced CT for the identification of calculi, while asymptomatic hematuria in patients older than 40 years should be evaluated by CT urography. In addition, relative to IVU, CT urography can be used to depict structures outside the urinary tract and thus is useful in detecting unsuspected extraurinary disease. Nevertheless, a full urologic evaluation is recommended in many patients with asymptomatic microscopic hematuria.

Studies focusing on CT urography in patients with microscopic hematuria show that causes for hematuria are identified in 33.0–42.6% with overall CT urography sensitivity for identification of the cause of hematuria of 92.4–100% and specificity of 89.0–97.4% (Van Der Molen et al. 2008). In studies on microscopic or unselected hematuria, upper tract TCC was present in 0.9–7.3%. In these populations, CT urography detection of upper tract TCC is high and significantly better than IVU. When applied to selected high-risk groups of macroscopic hematuria, TCC tumor prevalence may increase to 25–30% and it has been shown that CT urography of the upper tract is equivalent to retrograde pyelography (Van Der Molen et al. 2008). CT may still have problems of correctly staging advanced tumors. Thin-section ($\leq$3 mm) MDCT images can be used to depict urothelial abnormalities just as well, if not better than, contrast material-enhanced radiographs (Caoili et al. 2005a; Silverman et al. 2009). Although radiographs have higher spatial resolution (Kawashima et al. 2004), the higher contrast resolution and other inherent advantages of cross-sectional imaging outweigh the advantages of conventional radiography in IVU. Radiography is a projectional imaging technique, and therefore, overlapping structures can obscure important findings (Silverman et al. 2009). Hence, there is a sound rationale for believing that thin-section axial images obtained in the excretory phase are more sensitive than contrast-enhanced radiographs for the detection of urothelial abnormalities. As a result, it is now generally accepted that CT urography is best performed with MDCT alone (Silverman et al. 2009). CT urography can also be powerful in the diagnosis of bladder tumors, but results differ depending on the specific population studied. In a population of patients with microscopic hematuria, CT urography sensitivity in comparison with cystoscopy was only 40%, while in a high-risk group with macroscopic hematuria, unequivocal CT urography results were 93% sensitive and 99% specific for the detection of bladder cancer, which may obviate the need for many flexible (diagnostic) cystoscopies.

In addition to the evaluation of hematuria, CT urography can be useful in the surveillance of patients with suspected urothelial cancer (positive urine cytology), follow-up of urothelial cancers (Silverman et al. 2009), patients with obstructive uropathy (e.g., hydronephrosis, hydroureter of unknown etiology), or any time, a comprehensive evaluation of the urinary tract is warranted. Given the relatively high radiation doses associated with multiphase technique, pretest probabilities for cancer should be taken into consideration. CT urography can be justified as a first-line test for the upper and lower urinary tract in hematuria patients with a high pretest probability for TCC. Important risk factors include age >40 years, macroscopic hematuria, smoking, history of GU malignancy, and occupational exposure. The risk from the use of radiation is relatively less important in such high-risk groups and any comprehensive two- or three-phase CT urography protocol can be performed. Effective for cost management in such patients could be the replacement of the traditional work-up of ultrasound + IVU + cystoscopy by a faster CT urography + cystoscopy work-up.

### 5.2.2 CT Angiography

Multidetector CTA is replacing conventional angiography in the evaluation of renal vascular anatomy (Fig. 5.40) and pathology. The indications for renal CTA include renovascular hypertension work-up and posttreatment assessment, renal donor transplant evaluation, oncologic preoperative staging, and renal anomaly and variant work-up (Beregi et al. 1999; Fraioli et al 2006; Kawamoto et al. 2003; Namasivayam et al. 2006; Turkvatan et al. 2009). MDCT has a high accuracy for the identification of accessory renal arteries (Kawamoto et al. 2003; Namasivayam et al. 2006) and for the assessment of renal artery stenosis (Beregi et al. 1999).

MDCTA angiography of the renal arteries can be performed with any MDCT scanner with submillimeter collimation; scan parameters for 64-row MDCT scanners are reported in Table 5.5. The scan region should include from the diaphragm to the iliac arteries (Fraioli et al 2006; Turkvatan et al. 2009) to cover all the potential origins of the accessory renal arteries.

The patient is instructed before the scan in the breath-hold technique. The CTA protocol requests a double scout view. The arterial CT phase is reached about 15–25 s after the commencement of intravenous contrast media injection (for renal arteriography, a contrast bolus of 3.5 mL/s is desirable). Alternatively, a test bolus scan or a bolus tracking program after iodinated contrast agent administration (350–400 mgI/mL; 100–120 mL of contrast volume; 4 mL/s) can be applied for optimal start of the arterial scan. The extent covered includes the whole abdomen. A delayed phase CT of the abdomen may be performed to assess parenchymal or urinary tract abnormalities. The number, size, course, and relationship of the renal vasculature are easily appreciated utilizing real-time interactive editing. Multiplanar or curvilinear reformations and different postprocessing 3D reconstruction algorithms with multiple 3D images rotated in 10° steps are employed. VR has emerged as the rendering technique of choice. With VR, the user can actively interact with the dataset, editing and modifying the position, orientation, opacity, and brightness of the image in real-time. For CTA, VR is commonly performed with a window/level transfer function that results in high-density material (for example, enhanced vessels or vascular calcifications) to appear bright and opaque, while less-dense structures appear dim and translucent. Overlying structures are easily removed with an interactive clip-plane, and the vessels of interest are easily rotated into the best orientation for the depiction of the region of interest. For evaluation of the renal hilum, axial, coronal, and sagittal views are often used in conjunction for optimal evaluation of the number, caliber, and course of the renal arteries and veins. MIP represents the other common reconstruction algorithm commonly employed when evaluating the renal vasculature. The MIP technique evaluates each voxel from the viewer's eye through the dataset and selects the maximal voxel value as the value of the corresponding displayed pixel. The image produced lacks depth orientation, but a 3D effect can be produced with rotational viewing of multiple projections. MIP images can provide useful information regarding atherosclerotic burden, vascular stents, and vascular stenoses and are often reconstructed and interpreted in conjunction with volume-rendered images.

CTA has many documented applications in the renal pedicle, including the evaluation of renal artery stenosis and fibromuscolar hyperplasia, renal arterial disease related to aortic diseases, preoperative evaluation of renal donors, and preoperative evaluation of renal anatomy prior to surgery. CTA provides an accurate assessment of the renal vasculature in a fast and efficient manner without the risks of conventional angiography.

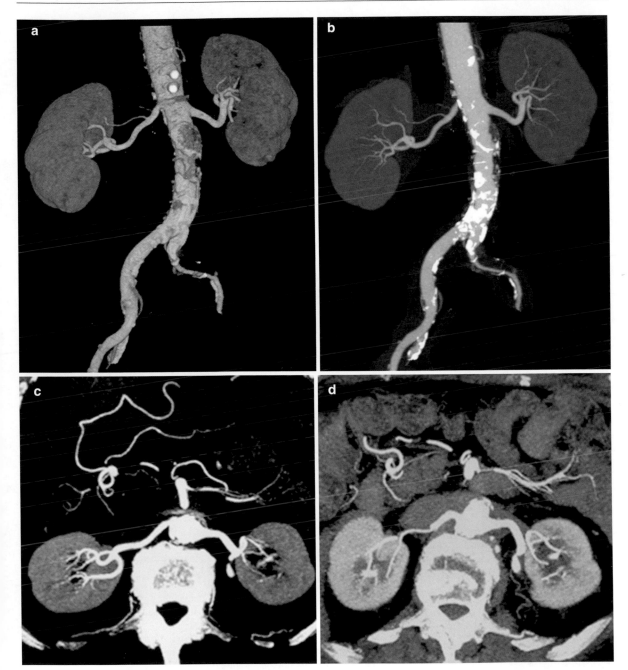

**Fig. 5.40** (**a–d**) Coronal VR (**a**) and MIP (**b**) images and transverse thick MIP images (**c, d**) show the bilateral single renal arteries and depict clearly the right renal artery's early branching to the upper pole

### 5.2.3 Dual-Energy CT

In the past, different dual-energy approaches have been tested for renal stones characterization, with promising results in vitro using data from consecutive CT examinations performed with different X-ray energies (Deveci et al. 2004; Mitcheson et al. 1983; Sheir et al. 2005). However, this approach is not feasible clinically because of the exposure to higher radiation doses and the possible motion artifacts complicating the alignment of the two CT scans. The recently introduced dual-source CT system (Somatom Definition, Siemens

**Table 5.5** CT angiography (CTA) protocol

| 64-row MDCT | Unenhanced | Arterial/corticomedullary | Nephrographic |
|---|---|---|---|
| Scan delay | – | bolus tracking | 90–100 |
| Scout | A–P abdomen and pelvis | | |
| Patient position | Supine | Supine | Supine |
| Scan interval | Kidneys–bladder | Kidneys to iliac arteries | Diaphragm–kidneys |
| Tube voltage (kVp) | 120 | 120 | 120 |
| Tube current (mA) | (180–250); modulated | (180–250); modulated | (180–250); modulated |
| Collimation | 64×0.6 | 64×0.6 | 64×0.6 |
| Pitch | 0.9 | 0.9 | 0.9 |
| Table feed (mm/rotation) | 17.28 | 17.28 | 17.28 |
| Slice thickness (mm) | 3 | 3 | 3 |
| Reconstruction interval (mm) | 3 | 3 | 3 |

Note. The principal parameters employed in the CTA according to the CT equipment

Medical Solutions, Forchheim, Germany) allows simultaneous dual-energy acquisitions, with immediate semiautomatic postprocessing. The material decomposition algorithm has recently been tested in vitro and in vivo, showing high accuracy for the discrimination between uric acid calculi and other calculus types (Graser et al. 2008; Grosjean et al. 2008; Primak et al. 2007; Stolzmann et al. 2008). Thomas et al. (2009) evaluated a low-dose dual-energy protocol and observed that dual-energy analysis was able to distinguish between calcified and noncalcified calculi in all cases.

Brown et al. (2009) have investigated the ability of DECT to classify phantom renal lesions as cysts or enhancing masses and observed that the DECT iodine overlay technique is highly sensitive in detecting enhancing renal masses and differentiating a renal cyst from a solid, enhancing lesion in a phantom model. Graser et al. (2009) have demonstrated that virtual nonenhanced datasets obtained with DECT are a reasonable approximation to true nonenhanced datasets, and that integration of dual-energy scanning into a renal mass protocol could lower radiation exposure by 35%.

# References

Abdulla C, Kalra MK, Saini S (2002) Pseudoenhancement of simulated renal cysts in a phantom using different multidetector CT scanners. AJR Am J Roentgenol 179:1473–1476

Amis ES Jr (1999) Epitaph for the urogram. Radiology 213: 639–640

Bae KT, Seeck BA, Hildebolt CF et al. (2008) Contrast enhancement in cardiovascular MDCT: effect of body weight, height, body surface area, body mass index, and obesity. AJR Am J Roentgenol 190(3):777–784

Barrett JF, Keat N (2004) Artifacts in CT: recognition and avoidance. Radiographics 24:1679–1691

Beregi JP, Louvegny S, Gautier C et al. (1999) Fibromuscular dysplasia of the renal arteries: comparison of helical CT angiography and arteriography. AJR Am J Roentgenol 172(1):27–34

Boll DT, Patil NA, Paulson EK et al. (2009) Renal stone assessment with dual-energy multidetector CT and advanced postprocessing techniques: improved characterization of renal stone composition – pilot study. Radiology 250:813–820

Bosniak MA (1986) The current radiological approach to renal cysts. Radiology 158:1–10

Bosniak MA (1991) The small (less than or equal to 3.0 cm) renal parenchymal tumor: detection, diagnosis, and controversies. Radiology 179:307–317

Brown CL, Hartman RP, Dzyubak OP et al. (2009) Dual-energy CT iodine overlay technique for characterization of renal masses as cyst or solid: a phantom feasibility study. Eur Radiol 19:1289–1295

Browne RF, Meehan CP, Colville J et al. (2005) Transitional cell carcinoma of the upper urinary tract: spectrum of imaging findings. Radiographics 25:1609–1627

Caoili EM, Cohan RH, Inampudi P et al. (2005a) MDCT urography of upper tract urothelial neoplasms. AJR Am J Roentgenol 184:1873–1881

Caoili EM, Cohan RH, Korobkin M et al. (2002) Urinary tract abnormalities: initial experience with multi-detector row CT urography. Radiology 222:353–360

Caoili EM, Inampudi P, Cohan RH et al. (2005b) Optimization of multi-detector row CT urography: effect of compression, saline administration, and prolongation of acquisition delay. Radiology 235:116–123

Chow LC, Kwan SW, Olcott EW et al. (2007) Split-bolus MDCT urography with synchronous nephrographic and excretory phase enhancement. AJR Am J Roentgenol 189:314–322

Chow LC, Sommer FG (2001) Multidetector CT urography with abdominal compression and three-dimensional reconstruction. AJR Am J Roentgenol 177(4):849–855

Choyke PL, Glenn GM, Walther MM et al. (2003) Hereditary renal cancers. Radiology 226:33–46

Choyke PL, Walther MM, Glenn GM et al. (1997) Imaging features of hereditary papillary renal cancers. J Comput Assist Tomogr 21:737–741

Cohan RH, Sherman LS, Korobkin M et al. (1995) Renal masses: assessment of corticomedullary-phase and nephrographic-phase CT scans. Radiology 196:445–451

Cohnen M, Poll LW, Puettmann C et al. (2003) Effective doses in standard protocols for multi-slice CT scanning. Eur Radiol 13(5):1148–1153

Coppenrath EM, Mueller-Lisse UG (2006) Multidetector CT of the kidney. Eur Radiol 16:2603–2611

Coulam CH, Sheafor DH, Leder RA et al. (2000) Evaluation of pseudoenhancement of renal cysts during contrast enhanced CT. AJR Am J Roentgenol 174:493–498

Curry NS (1995) Small renal masses (lesions smaller than 3 cm): imaging evaluation and management. AJR Am J Roentgenol 164:355–362

Dalla Palma L (2001) What is left of i.v. urography? Eur Radiol 11(6):931–939

Dalla Palma L, Pozzi Mucelli R, Pozzi Mucelli F (1997) Delayed CT in acute renal infections. Semin Ultrasound CT MR 18(2):122–128

Deak P, van Straten M, Shrimpton PC et al. (2008) Validation of a Monte Carlo tool for patient-specific dose simulations in multi-slice computed tomography. Eur Radiol 18(4):759–772

Deveci S, Coskun M, Tekin MI et al. (2004) Spiral computed tomography: role in determination of chemical compositions of pure and mixed urinary stones – an in vitro study. Urology 64(2):237–240

Dillman JR, Caoili EM, Cohan RH (2007a) Multi-detector CT urography: a one-stop renal and urinary tract imaging modality. Abdom Imaging 32(4):519–552

Dillman JR, Caoili EM, Cohan RH et al. (2007b) Comparison of urinary tract distension and opacification using single-bolus 3-phase vs. split-bolus 2-phase multidetector row CT urography. J Comput Assist Tomogr 31(5):750–757

Dillman JR, Caoili EM, Cohan RH et al. (2008) Detection of upper tract urothelial neoplasms: sensitivity of axial, coronal reformatted, and curved-planar reformatted image-types utilizing 16-row multi-detector CT urography. Abdom Imaging 33(6):707–716

Erturk SM, Ichikawa T, Sou H et al. (2008) Effect of duration of contrast material injection on peak enhancement times and values of the aorta, main portal vein, and liver at dynamic MDCT with the dose of contrast medium tailored to patient weight. Clin Radiol 63(3):263–271

Fielding JR, Silverman SG, Samuel S et al. (1998) Unenhanced helical CT of ureteral stones: a replacement for excretory urography in planning treatment. AJR Am J Roentgenol 171:1051–1053

Fraioli F, Catalano C, Bertoletti L et al. (2006) Multidetector-row CT angiography of renal artery stenosis in 50 consecutive patients: prospective interobserver comparison with DSA. Radiol Med 111(3):459–468

Goldman LW (2008) Principles of CT: multislice CT. J Nucl Med Technol 36:57–68

Graser A, Johnson TR, Bader M et al. (2008) Dual energy CT characterization of urinary calculi: initial in vitro and clinical experience. Invest Radiol 43(2):112–119

Graser A, Johnson TR, Hecht EM et al. (2009) Dual-energy CT in patients suspected of having renal masses: can virtual nonenhanced images replace true nonenhanced images? Radiology 252(2):433–440

Gray Sears CL, Ward JF, Sears ST et al. (2002) Prospective comparison of computerized tomography and excretory urography in the initial evaluation of asymptomatic microhematuria. J Urol 168:2457–2460

Grosjean R, Sauer B, Guerra RM et al. (2008) Characterization of human renal stones with MDCT: advantage of dual energy and limitations due to respiratory motion. AJR Am J Roentgenol 190(3):720–728

Grossfeld GD, Litwin MS, Wolf JS et al. (2001a) Evaluation of asymptomatic microscopic hematuria in adults: the American Urological Association best practice policy panel – part I. Definition, detection, prevalence, and etiology. Urology 57:599–603

Grossfeld GD, Litwin MS, Wolf JS et al. (2001b) Evaluation of asymptomatic microscopic hematuria in adults: the American Urological Association best practice policy panel – part II. Patient evaluation, cytology, voided markers, imaging, cystoscopy, nephrology evaluation, and follow-up. Urology 57:604–610

Hecht EM, Israel GM, Krinsky GA et al. (2004) Renal masses: quantitative analysis of enhancement with signal intensity measurements versus qualitative analysis of enhancement with image subtraction for diagnosing malignancy at MR imaging. Radiology 232:373–378

Heneghan JP, Kim DH, Leder RA et al. (2001) Compression CT urography: a comparison with IVU in the opacification of the collecting system and ureters. J Comput Assist Tomogr 25:343–347

Herschorn S, Radomski SB, Shoskes DA et al. (1991) Evaluation and treatment of blunt renal trauma. J Urol 146:274–276

Huang J, Kim YH, Shankar S et al. (2006) Multidetector CT urography: comparison of two different scanning protocols for improved visualization of the urinary tract. J Comput Assist Tomogr 30(1):33–36

Huda W (2007) Radiation doses and risks in chest computed tomography examination. Proc Am Thorac Soc 4:316–320

ICRP (2007) The 2007 recommendations of the International Commission on Radiological Protection: ICRP publication 103. Ann ICRP 37(2–4):1–332

Israel GM, Bosniak MA (2005) How I do it: evaluating renal masses. Radiology 236:441–450

Israel GM, Bosniak MA (2008) Pitfalls in renal mass evaluation and how to avoid them. AJR Am J Roentgenol 28:1325–1338

Jamis-Dow CA, Choyke PL, Jennings SB et al. (1996) Small (< 3-cm) renal masses: detection with CT versus US and pathologic correlation. Radiology 198:785–788

Joffe SA, Servaes S, Okon S et al. (2003) Multi-detector row CT urography in the evaluation of hematuria. Radiographics 23:1441–1455

Kalra MK, Singh S (2008) CT of the urinary tract: turning attention to radiation dose. Radiol Clin North Am 46:1–9

Kawamoto S, Horton KM, Fishman EK (2006) Opacification of the collecting system and ureters on excretory-phase CT using oral water as contrast medium. AJR Am J Roentgenol 186(1):136–140

Kawamoto S, Montgomery R, Lawler L et al. (2003) Multi-detector CT angiography for preoperative evaluation of living laparoscopic kidney donors. Am J Roentgenol 180: 1633–1638

Kawashima A, Vrtiska TJ, LeRoy AJ et al. (2004) CT urography. Radiographics 24:S35–S54

Kemper J, Adam G, Nolte-Ernsting C (2005) Multislice CT urography aspects for technical management and clinical application. Radiologe 45(10):905–914

Kluner C, Hein PA, Gralla O et al. (2006) Does ultra-low-dose CT with a radiation dose equivalent to that of KUB suffice to detect renal and ureteral calculi? J Comput Assist Tomogr 30(1):44–50

Knöpfle E, Hamm M, Wartenberg S et al. (2003) CT in uretero-lithiasis with a radiation dose equal to intravenous urography: results in 209 patients. Rofo 175(12):1667–1672

Kock MC, Dijkshoorn ML, Pattynama PM et al. (2007) Multi-detector row computed tomography angiography of periph-eral arterial disease. Eur Radiol 17(12):3208–3222

Kopka L, Fischer U, Zoeller G et al. (1997) Dual-phase helical CT of the kidney: value of the corticomedullary and nephro-graphic phase for evaluation of renal lesions and preopera-tive staging of renal cell carcinoma. Am J Roentgenol 169:1573–1578

Lee CH, Goo JM, Lee HJ et al. (2008) Radiation dose modula-tion techniques in the multidetector CT era: from basics to practice. Radiographics 28:1451–1459

Macari M, Bosniak MA (1999) Delayed CT to evaluate renal mass incidentally discovered at contrast-enhanced CT: dem-onstration of vascularity with deenhancement. Radiology 213:674–680

Mahesh M, Scatarige JC, Cooper J et al. (2001) Dose and pitch relationship for a particular multislice CT scanner. AJR Am J Roentgenol 177(6):1273–1275

Maki DD, Birnbaum BA, Chakraborty DP et al. (1999) Renal cyst pseudoenhancement: beam-hardening effects on CT numbers. Radiology 213:468–472

McNicholas MM, Raptopoulos VD, Schwartz RK et al. (1998) Excretory phase CT urography for opacification of the urinary collecting system. AJR Am J Roentgenol 170: 1261–1267

McTavish JD, Jinzaki M, Zou KH et al. (2002) Multi-detector row CT urography: comparison of strategies for depicting the normal urinary collecting system. Radiology 225:783–790

Metser U, Ghai S, Ong YY et al. (2009) Assessment of urinary tract calculi with 64-MDCT: the axial versus coronal plane. AJR Am J Roentgenol 192(6):1509–1513

Mitcheson HD, Zamenhof RG, Bankoff MS et al. (1983) Determination of the chemical composition of urinary cal-culi by computerized tomography. J Urol 130(4):814–819

Morcos SK (2007) Computed tomography urography technique, indications and limitations. Curr Opin Urol 17(1):56-64

Namasivayam S, Kalra M, Waldrop S et al. (2006) Multidetector row CT angiography of living related renal donors: is there a need for venous phase imaging? Eur J Radiol 59:442–452

Nawfel RD, Judy PF, Schleipman AR et al. (2004) Patient radia-tion dose at CT urography and conventional urography. Radiology 232:126–132

Niall O, Russell J, MacGregor R et al. (1999) A comparison of noncontrast computerized tomography with excretory urography in the assessment of acute flank pain. J Urol 161(2):534–537

Nolte-Ernsting CC, Cowan N (2006) Understanding multislice CT urography techniques: many roads lead to Rome. Eur Radiol 16:2670–2686

Nolte-Ernsting CC, Wildberger JE, Borchers H et al. (2001) Multi-slice CT urography after diuretic injection: initial results. Rofo 173:176–180

Perlman ES, Rosenfield AT, Wexler JS et al. (1996) CT urogra-phy in the evaluation of urinary tract disease. J Comput Assist Tomogr 20:620–626

Prasad SR, Dalrymple NC, Surabhi VR (2008) Cross-sectional imaging evaluation of renal masses. Radiol Clin North Am 46:95–111

Primak AN, Fletcher JG, Vrtiska TJ et al. (2007) Noninvasive differentiation of uric acid versus non-uric acid kidney stones using dual-energy CT. Acad Radiol 14(12):1441–1447

Saini S (2004) Multi-detector row CT: principles and practice for abdominal applications. Radiology 233:323–327

Sanyal R, Deshmukh A, Singh Sheorain V et al. (2007) CT urography: a comparison of strategies for upper urinary tract opacification. Eur Radiol 17(5):1262–1266

Schoellnast H, Brader P, Oberdabernig B et al. (2005) High-concentration contrast media in multiphasic abdominal mul-tidetector-row computed tomography: effect of increased iodine flow rate on parenchymal and vascular enhancement. J Comput Assist Tomogr 29(5):582–587

Schreyer HH, Uggowitzer MM, Ruppert-Kohlmayr A (2002) Helical CT of the urinary organs. Eur Radiol 12:575–591

Semelka RC, Shoenut JP, Kroeker MA et al. (1992) Renal lesions: controlled comparison between CT and 1.5-T MR imaging with nonenhanced and gadolinium-enhanced fat suppressed spin-echo and breath-hold FLASH techniques. Radiology 182:425–430

Sheir KZ, Mansour O, Madbouly K et al. (2005) Determination of the chemical composition of urinary calculi by noncon-trast spiral computerized tomography. Urol Res 33(2): 99–104

Sheth S, Scatarige JC, Horton KM et al. (2001) Current concepts in the diagnosis and management of renal cell carcinoma: role of multidetector CT and three-dimensional CT. Radiographics 21(spec issue):S237–S254

Shrimpton P (1997) Reference doses for computed tomography. Radiological protection bulletin 193. National Radiological Protection Board, Chilton, England, pp 16–19

Siegel CL, Fisher AJ, Bennett HF (1999) Interobserver variabil-ity in determining enhancement of renal masses on helical CT. AJR Am J Roentgenol 1725:1207–1212

Silverman SG, Akbar SA, Mortele KJ et al. (2006) Multi-detector row CT urography of normal urinary collecting sys-tem: furosemide versus saline as adjunct to contrast medium. Radiology 240:749–755

Silverman SG, Israel GM, Herts BR et al. (2008) Management of the incidental renal mass. Radiology 249:16–31

Silverman SG, Lee BY, Seltzer SE et al. (1994) Small (<3-cm) renal masses: correlation of spiral CT features and patho-logic findings. AJR Am J Roentgenol 163:597–605

Silverman SG, Leyendecker JR, Amis SE (2009) What is the current role of CT urography and MR urography in the eval-uation of the urinary tract. Radiology 250:309–323

Smith RC, Rosenfield AT, Choe KA et al. (1995) Acute flank pain: comparison of non-contrast-enhanced CT and intravenous urography. Radiology 194(3):789–794

Smith RC, Verga M, McCarthy S et al. (1996) Diagnosis of acute flank pain: value of unenhanced helical CT. AJR Am J Roentgenol 166:97–101

Sourtzis S, Thibeau JF, Damry N et al. (1999) Radiologic investigation of renal colic: unenhanced helical CT compared with excretory urography. AJR Am J Roentgenol 172(6): 1491–1494

Soyer P, Dufresne AC, Klein I et al. (1997) Renal cell carcinoma of clear cell type: correlation of CT features with tumor size, architectual patterns and pathologic staging. Eur Radiol 7:224–229

Stacul F, Rossi A, Cova MA (2008) CT urography: the end of IVU? Radiol Med 113(5):658–669

Stolzmann P, Scheffel H, Rentsch K et al. (2008) Dual-energy computed tomography for the differentiation of uric acid stones: ex vivo performance evaluation. Urol Res 36(3–4): 133–138

Sudakoff GS, Dunn DP, Hellman RS et al. (2006) Opacification of the genitourinary collecting system during MDCT urography with enhanced CT digital radiography: nonsaline versus saline bolus. AJR Am J Roentgenol 186(1):122–129

Szolar DH, Kammerhuber F, Altziebler S et al. (1997) Multiphasic helical CT of the kidney: increased conspicuity for detection and characterization of small (<3 cm) renal masses. Radiology 202:211–217

Taourel P, Thuret R, Hoquet MD et al. (2008) Computed tomography in the nontraumatic renal causes of acute flank pain. Semin Ultrasound CT MRI 29:341–352

Thomas C, Patschan O, Ketelsen D et al. (2009) Dual-energy CT for the characterization of urinary calculi: in vitro and in vivo evaluation of a low-dose scanning protocol. Eur Radiol 19(6):1553–1559

Turkvatan A, Ozdemir M, Cumhur T et al. (2009) Multidetector CT angiography of renal vasculature: normal anatomy and variants. Eur Radiol 19(1):236–244

Van Der Molen AJ, Cowan NJ, Mueller-Lisse UG et al. (2008) CT urography: definition, indications and techniques. A guideline for clinical practice. Eur Radiol 18:4–17

Vrtiska TJ, Hartman RP, Kofler JM et al. (2009) Spatial resolution and radiation dose of a 64-MDCT scanner compared with published CT urography protocols. AJR 192:941–948

Wang ZJ, Coakley FV, Fu Y et al. (2008) Renal cyst pseudoenhancement at multidetector CT: what are the effects of number of detectors and peak tube voltage? Radiology 248(3)910–916. doi:10.1148/radiol.2482071583

Wong WS, Moss AA, Federle MP et al. (1984) Renal infarction: CT diagnosis and correlation between CT findings and etiologies. Radiology 150:201–205

Yuh BI, Cohan RH (1999) Different phases of renal enhancement: role in detecting and characterizing renal masses during helical CT. Am J Roentgenol 173:747–755

Zagoria RJ (2000) Imaging of small renal masses. A medical success story. Am J Roentgenol 175:945–955

# Magnetic Resonance Imaging of the Kidney

**6**

Maria Assunta Cova, Marco Cavallaro, Paola Martingano, and Maja Ukmar

## Contents

## Abstract

> This chapter describes the correct imaging technique for the magnetic resonance (MR) examination of the kidney, from the fundamental morphologic sequences to the MR urography sequences up to diffusion sequences. The basic MR features of vascular and infectious renal diseases and solid benign and malignant renal tumors up to the cystic renal tumors are described. The advanced applications of the MR technique in the kidney are described as a general introduction to the following chapters describing the different renal pathologies.

> Cross-sectional imaging plays a critical role in the detection and work-up of renal pathologies. Even if computed tomography (CT) is still playing the leader, the role of magnetic resonance imaging (MRI) is ever increasing, thanks to its better tissue contrast resolution and the absence of radiation exposure; furthermore, it can be used as a problem-solving modality when CT findings are nondiagnostic (Radiol Clin North Am 41(5):877–907, 2003). Although the nephrogenic systemic fibrosis was recently recognized, the gadolinium-based contrast agents used in MRI, are still safe and can be used even in atopic patients and in patients with moderate impairment of renal function (estimated glomerular filtration rate >30 mL/min/1.73 m$^2$) (Perez-Rodrigue et al. 2009).

M.A. Cova (✉), M. Cavallaro, P. Martingano, and M. Ukmar
Department of Radiology, Cattinara Hospital, University
of Trieste, Strada di Fiume 447, 34149 Trieste, Italy
e-mail: cova@gnbts.univ.trieste.it

E. Quaia (ed.), *Radiological Imaging of the Kidney*,
Medical Radiology, DOI: 10.1007/978-3-540-87597-0_6, © Springer-Verlag Berlin Heidelberg 2011

> While MRI has been shown to be useful in the detection and characterization of renal masses, in the staging of cancers, and in the evaluation of urinary tract anomalies and obstructive disease, attempts are being made to use it for assessment of renal function, such as perfusion, glomerular filtration rate, or intrarenal oxygen measurement (Eur Radiol 11(3):355–372, 2001; Eur Radiol 17(11):2780–2793, 2007; Radiology 250(2):309–323, 2009).

## 6.1 Technique

### 6.1.1 Equipment

MRI of the kidney and, in particular, MR urography (MRU) is most commonly performed at 1.5 T. Even if some investigators have performed these studies at low and mild-field strength magnets, better performance in terms of signal-to-noise ratio (SNR) are obtained at higher fields with ultra fast gradients (Nolte-Ernsting et al. 2001a, b). Different surface coils may be employed, and the body coil alone could also offer good images. However, the use of phased array coils is important to increase augment SNR and especially to obtain rapid imaging to avoid breathing motion artifacts. Parallel imaging or partially parallel imaging techniques, such as sensitivity encoding, simultaneous acquisition of spatial harmonics, and array spatial sensitivity encoding technique, can be used to accelerate fast imaging sequences without increasing gradient switching rates of radiofrequency power deposition. 3T systems also make imaging without phased array coils feasible and extend capabilities of parallel imaging, with a better SNR but at the cost of more magnetic susceptibility artifacts (Zhang et al. 2003).

### 6.1.2 Patient Positioning

The patient has to lie supine upon the scanner table, keeping arms raised above the head. If it is not possible to avoid aliasing in coronal imaging, arms may be supported along the body on cushions to keep them anterior to coronal plane of interest (Nikken and Krestin 2007).

### 6.1.3 Breath Holding

Respiratory motion of the kidneys dramatically decreases image quality, and for this reason, it is important to perform scan with rapid sequences within a breath-hold.

Even a short period of hyperventilation helps to maintain a longer breath-hold. When subtraction postprocessing is needed or the single breath-hold is shorter than the needed sequence, it is better to use endexpiratory breath-hold, since it is more reproducible, in particular if preceded by a brief coaching session.

In noncooperative patients, very fast sequences, such as single-shot imaging, Half-Fourier technique, or magnetization-prepared gradient-echo imaging, are mandatory. The placement of a saturation band over subcutaneous fat of the anterior abdominal wall could reduce respiratory artifacts in the abdominal cavity.

A variety of techniques are used to compensate inplane motion artifacts, but acquisition becomes much more longer: respiratory gating limits data acquisition to end-expiration, respiratory triggering initiates the acquisition at a fixed point of the respiratory cycle. Motion correction may also be obtained with the use of a navigator, recording diaphragmatic motion, but these approaches are impractical for dynamic contrastenhanced imaging (Zhang et al. 2003).

### 6.1.4 Sequences

On T2 weighted (T2W) sequences, normal kidney is hyperintense compared to liver and shows a similar signal intensity to spleen. Renal cortex is hypointense to renal medulla. A standard renal study protocol has to contain a T2W sequence to differentiate cyst from solid masses and to show the caliber and contour of excretory tracts. Renal cysts are homogenously hyperintense, while the presence of hypointense nodularity, septations, or variable degrees of hypointense content are possible signs of malignancy. Conventional spin echo sequences have long acquisition time, exceeding possible breath-hold, and so motion artifacts can reduce image quality. To avoid this problem, echotrain imaging, named differently by vendors (e.g., turbo spin echo, fast spin echo), is used, but on these sequences fat tissue shows high-signal intensity and so a fat suppression is needed. In patients with limited breath-hold capacity, the use of respiratory triggering could reduce respiratory artifacts in the abdomen. To further decrease acquisition time in patients without breathing control, Half-Fourier reconstruction (e.g. HASTE, SSFSE) could be added to echo-train sequences. These sequences last less than a second on a per-slice base, acquiring only one half of the k space, while other data are mathematically reconstructed. They offer a rapid survey of abdominal structures, particularly cysts and excretory system, but with a low signal to noise and contrast to noise ratio and a blurring effect that render them less sensitive for small, low-contrast lesions (Zhang et al. 2003).

On T1 weighted (T1W) sequences, normal renal cortex is slightly higher in signal intensity than medulla and medulla has a similar signal intensity compared with muscle. T1W sequences are needed for a complete lesion characterization. Most cysts have a long signal intensity on T1W, appearing hypointense upon renal parenchyma, while hemorrhagic, proteinaceous, melanin, or fat content ones have a short signal intensity on T1W, appearing hyperintense. Multishot gradient-echo techniques are most commonly used; a repetition time (TR) of 120–200 ms can provide full coverage of the kidney in a single breath-hold, allowing even dynamic contrast-enhanced imaging also when fat suppression is applied. T1W spoiled gradient-echo imaging performed before, during, and after intravenous gadolinium-based contrast agent administration is essential for contrast enhancement pattern demonstration; comparison between pre and postcontrast image, obtained in corticomedullary and nephrographic phases, permits differentiation of solid masses from complicated cystic lesions, while delayed postcontrast imaging depicts tumor extension in the perinephric fat and in venous structures. The use of a three-dimensional (3D) acquisition allows the generation of multiplanar reformations, greatly enhancing the multiplanar assessment of renal lesions, while with 2D gradient-echo sequences, smaller lesions can be missed or insufficiently characterized (Sun and Pedrosa 2009; Zhang et al. 2003).

Sometimes lesional enhancement detection could be difficult, especially if precontrast T1W signal intensity is high or intermediate, and so subtraction technique is necessary. It is possible to subtract nonenhanced image set from contrast-enhanced ones, using each contrast phase as a template. A misregistration of data set, with hyperintense rim in the direction of motion artifact, can result in areas of apparent enhancement (Sun and Pedrosa 2009).

Frequency selected fat suppression technique is a useful tool to depict fat component within lesions, typical of angiomyolipoma.

On gradient-echo sequences, performed with specific echo time (TE) values, images in which water and fat are either in-phase or opposed-phase with one another can be obtained with a signal loss in the second one, when in the same voxel both coexist, like in intracellular lipids of some clear cell renal carcinoma. On opposed-phase sequences, a chemical-shift artifact (India ink artifact) appears as a black line between renal parenchyma and retroperitoneal fat and disappears when a mass is extending beyond renal capsule, even if it does not involve adjacent structures, helping cancer staging. The same artifact appears at the periphery of bulk fat content area, highlighting the presence of gross intralesional fat like in angiomyolipoma (Zhang et al. 2003; Prasad et al. 2008a).

Diffusion weighted imaging (DWI) is used to show Brownian motion of water molecules within tissues using sequential application of strong gradients. This sequence has been long used in neuroradiology, but abdominal application has been hampered by motion of intraabdominal structures. New fast imaging techniques, like Half-Fourier reconstruction and motion compensation, allow DWI even in kidney study. It has been shown that Brownian motions are inversely proportional to cellular density and extracellular viscosity, according to interstitial water diffusion reduction. When water diffusion is restricted, DWI shows a high-signal area, but it can be altered by shine trough effect of water since it is a T2W image; so assessment of water molecules motion is better obtained using an apparent coefficient diffusion (ADC) map, calculated by a workstation software from two images acquired with different gradient duration and amplitude ($b$-values). ADC reduction may occur in tumor and high viscosity fluids (e.g., abscesses, pyonephrosis), while simple cysts and hydronephrosis are characterized by high ADC values. ADC values seem to be useful even in renal masses characterization, since renal cell carcinomas (RCCs) show significantly lower ADCs than simple and mild complicated cysts or oncocytomas.

Actually, these ADC values differ a lot considering various imaging parameters and so, at present time, it is not possible to provide an ADC scale with threshold values for the correct renal masses differentiation (Taouli et al. 2009).

Furthermore, it has been found that ADC values correlate with renal function both in native and transplanted kidney (Zangh et al. 2008).

Magnetic resonance angiography (MRA) is performed when a diagnostic evaluation of the renal vasculature is requested. At present time, MRA replaces invasive examination in many circumstances thanks to gradient hardware improvements and parallel imaging introduction, which have reduced acquisition times and improved spatial resolution.

Early studies emphasized noncontrast sequences, such as time-of-flight or phase contrast (Glockner and Vrtiska 2007); the image quality of these flow-sensitive techniques is limited by diminished flow in patients with vascular stenosis or parenchymal disease and by motion artifacts due to respiration during acquisition times that are too long for breath-hold.

Today, the dominant technique is 3D contrast-enhanced magnetic resonance angiography (3D CE MRA). This consists of a 3D fast spoiled gradient-echo sequence performed in conjunction with intravenous bolus injection of contrast medium. Perfect bolus timing is essential to get maximum arterial gadolinium concentration during the center of k space. There are several techniques available for determining contrast flow time from intra venous site to renal arteries; in order to correctly coordinate the initiation of bolus injection with the initiation of scanning, the most widely used is an automatic pulse sequence. This technique, named Bolus track, Care bolus, and Fluoroscopic triggering depending on vendors, allows direct visualization of contrast arrival in the aorta with a real-time 2D acquisition, typically updated every second. The CE MRA acquisition can then be triggered manually or automatically with the visualization of contrast arrival.

The typical 3D CE MRA sequence also has the effect of suppressing background tissue not exposed to gadolinium through relatively high flip angles and short repetition times. Additional background suppression can be achieved by adding fat suppression pulses to the sequence, little elongating imaging time, or by subtracting the contrast-enhanced sequence from a precontrast mask acquisition, with the limits of misregistration artifacts in patients whose breath holding is not similar enough in the two acquisitions.

CE MRA produces 3D data set that can be reconstructed into an unlimited number of projections using different slab thickness, orientations, and rendering methods. Maximum Intensity Projection, Multi Planar Reconstructions, and 3D Volume Rendering are the most commonly postprocessing techniques (Zhang and Prince 2004; Glockner and Vrtiska 2007).

Magnetic resonance urography (MRU) allows urinary tract evaluation. It is recommended in pregnant, pediatric, and young patients, but some intrinsic limitations, such as insensitivity in renal calcification detection, long imaging time, motion sensitivity, and low spatial resolution, limit its clinical applications. MRU may be performed with a static fluid or an excretory technique.

Static-fluid MRU is performed on T2W sequences, exploiting the long T2 relaxation time of urine, without contrast material administration (Fig. 6.1). Thick-slab single-shot fast spin echo is optimal for obtaining heavily T2W images in a short time. For urinary tract peristalsis evaluation and stenosis confirmation, multiple images can be obtained and played as a cine-loop. Single acquisitions have to be separated by 5–10 s to prevent radiofrequency saturation of the tissue and to avoid progressive signal loss. The signal intensity of soft tissue can be adjusted by modifying the echo time or using fat suppression. Three-dimensional respirator-triggered sequences can be used too, obtaining VR or MIP images. Static-fluid MRU is helpful to evaluate the urinary tract course and diameter, even in cases of obstructed or poorly excreting kidney. Oral negative contrast agent administration could be requested to avoid bowel contents' signal intensity visualization.

Excretory MRU is performed by T1W sequences obtained after gadolinium-based contrast agent administration during the excretory phase (Fig. 6.1). For excretory MRU, the thinnest partitions that maintain acceptable SNR and anatomic coverage should be prescribed. Breath holding is essential for excretory phase imaging, as acquisition times of 20–30 s are typical with most widely available 3D gradient-echo sequences. A through-plane resolution of 2–3 mm is usually achievable with currently available MR systems operating at 1.5–3.0 T. The use of parallel imaging techniques reduces acquisition times with a modest penalty in SNR. For patients with limited breath-holding capacity, the urinary tract can be imaged in segments.

Coronal 3D gradient-echo fat suppression sequences are used. Using a standard dose of contrast material (0.1 mmol/kg), gadolinium quickly becomes concentrated in the urine and can give $T2^*$ effects, reducing

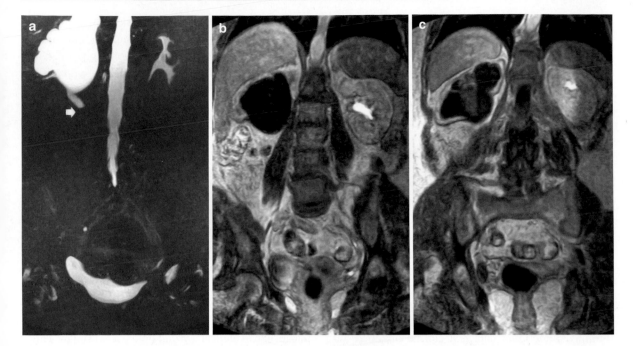

**Fig. 6.1** (**a–c**) MR urography (MRU) in a patient with right ureteral carcinoma. (**a**) Static-fluid MRU. Dilatation of the right upper urinary tract with the evidence of obstruction at the level of the upper right ureter (arrow) (**b, c**) Excretory MRU after Gd-based contrast agent injection. Absent contrast excretion on the right kidney which reveals third-grade hydronephrosis, and regular contrast excretion on the left urinary tract

the signal intensity of urine. To avoid this artifact, a low dose of gadolinium-based contrast material (0.05 mmol/kg) is advisable. Diuretic administration (0.1 mg/kg of furosemide) can improve the quality of excretory MRU by enhancing urine flow and give a better dilution and uniform distribution of the contrast agent through urinary tract. Before examination starts, the patient is to be invited to void to prevent discomfort and possible exam interruption. Excretory MRU requires the excretion of contrast medium into the collecting system and so it does not have a role in the evaluation of patients with obstructed or poorly excreting kidney (Nolte-Ernsting et al. 2001a, b). Furthermore, contrast medium administration is not possible in patients with severely compromised renal function for the risk of nephrogenic systemic fibrosis (Leyendecker et al. 2008).

A number of studies have shown that MRU is a useful examination for investigating the causes of urinary tract dilatation and diagnosing urinary tract obstruction in adult and pediatric populations. Because MR is relatively insensitive for the detection of calcification, the diagnosis of ureteral calculi often relies on detecting secondary signs of obstruction such as ureteral

dilatation and perinephric fluid; sometimes a persistent filling defect can be identified. The sensitivity of MRU for ureteral calculi is technique-dependent, with higher sensitivities for excretory MRU than for static-fluid T2-weighted techniques. MRU is more sensitive for diagnosing the cause of urinary tract obstruction due to causes other than urolithiasis compared with unenhanced CT. Although urothelial neoplasms can be detected with MRU, its sensitivity remains to be determined and probably is lower than CT urography. MRU has been shown to be as effective as US, intravenous urography, and nuclear scintigraphy for the assessment of many pediatric.

MRU has been used to depict a wide range of congenital abnormalities, including an abnormally positioned, rotated, duplicated, dysplastic, or absent kidney, as well as ectopic ureter, retrocaval ureter, primary megaureter, and ureteropelvic junction obstruction. Because of the excellent diagnostic performance of CT for the diagnosis of many problems of the urinary tract (e.g., patients with flank pain or hematuria), MRU, to date, has been reserved for patients who cannot receive iodinated contrast material or for whom exposure to ionizing radiation is particularly undesirable. Even in this population, MRU has had relatively limited application due to limited availability of expertise and the technical rigors of producing a high-quality examination. Furthermore, MRU will require further clinical validation before it can be considered the initial test for the evaluation of hematuria and exclusion of urothelial neoplasms. Currently, MRU is most commonly indicated in children and pregnant patients with dilated collecting systems. This stems primarily from the desire to avoid ionizing radiation in these patients. In the former group, indications for MRU include preoperative anatomic imaging for the assessment of vascular anatomy, evaluation of duplex systems, and distinction between pelvicalyceal dilatation and cystic disease. Both anatomic and functional information about the urinary tract can be obtained in a single examination, potentially eliminating the need for other diagnostic examinations such as nuclear scintigraphy. Functional data that can be obtained with MRU include renal transit time, differential renal function, and estimated GFR. Static-fluid and excretory MRU techniques have been shown to be complementary when evaluating children. In pregnant patients, physiologic dilatation of the right ureter can be distinguished from an obstructive uropathy caused by a calculus without intravenous contrast material. Because most static-fluid MRU techniques are quick and relatively easy to perform, the examination is well tolerated, even in the advanced stages of pregnancy. To avoid potentially nephrotoxic iodinated contrast material, MRU can be used also to evaluate potential renal transplant donors and assess for urologic complications following renal transplantation.

## 6.2 Magnetic Resonance Appearance of Renal Diseases

### 6.2.1 Renal Cell Carcinoma

RCC is the most common neoplasm of the kidney. RCC is composed of different histologic subtypes with variable histology, tumor biology, and prognosis, and consequently, it can have various imaging appearance.

In general, RCC appears as a variegated solid cortical mass of intermediate signal intensity on T1W and mild hyperintensity to renal cortex on T2W, with enhancement after contrast medium administration (Fig. 6.2). Different grades of hemorrhage or necrosis change signal intensity. Central necrosis areas typically manifest as foci of low-signal intensity on T1W and high signal on T2W, without contrast enhancement. Hemorrhagic aspects vary along with the age of blood products. Although MR is insensitive for calcifications, they may be recognized as signal loss spots within the lesion in all sequences. On DWI sequences, RCC shows restricted diffusion with hyperintense signal. Some authors (Cova et al. 2004; Squillaci et al. 2004) have proposed ADC values evaluation to differentiate various histologic subtypes, but at the present time, it is not possible to propose threshold values of ADC, since they change depending on MR unit and sequence's technical parameter setting (Taouli et al. 2008).

The most common subtype is clear cell RCC (ccRCC). It is characterized by cell with clear cytoplasm, due to cholesterol and lipids dissolved in. Those intracellular lipids cause a signal loss in opposed-phase images in comparison to in-phase ones at dual-echo gradient-echo imaging.

ccRCC typically has a rich vasculature, so it shows intense enhancement after contrast administration and a propensity to hemorrhage. A true capsule of fibrotic tissue or, more often, a pseudo capsule of compressed parenchyma could be present at the periphery of the mass, appearing as a thin line of hypointensity both on T1W and T2W sequences. These tumors show a propensity to vein invasion, so it is important to perform a careful evaluation of renal vein and inferior vena cava, even with the use of gadolinium-based contrast agent, to differentiate bland from tumor thrombus. The ccRCC could appear as a predominantly cystic mass with thick septa and septal nodularity.

Papillary carcinoma (pRCC), characterized by papillary or tubulopapillary histologic architecture, is the second most common subtype of RCC. It may be multifocal in 20–40% of patients. Frequently, it appears on T2W as a low-signal intensity peripheral mass with a low and progressive enhancement. Subtraction images may help in the demonstration of really low grade enhancement, differentiating pRCC from hemorrhagic cysts. Papillary carcinoma often presents hemorrhage and necrosis, and in rare cases, it may show a focus of macroscopic fat, seen as a hyperintensity area on T1W becoming hypointense on fat saturate sequences; this possibility has to be well known to perform a correct

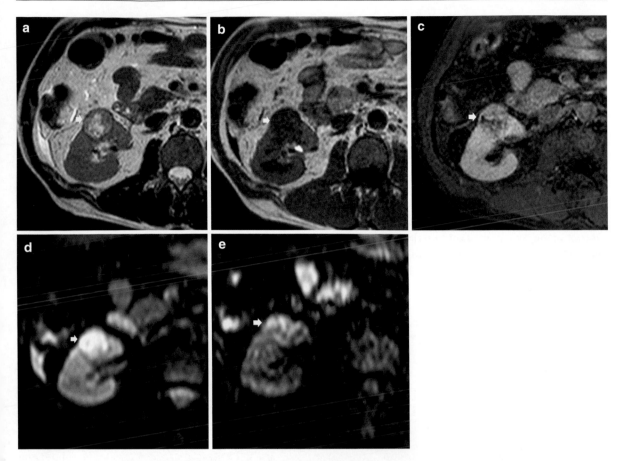

**Fig. 6.2** (**a–e**) Clear cell renal cell carcinoma in a 65-year-old man. Axial TSE T2W (**a**) and GE T1W (**b**) images show hyperintensity and hypointensity of the renal parenchyma mass (*arrow*), respectively. Axial GE T1W image obtained after gadolinium-based contrast agent administration, during nephrographic phase (**c**), demonstrates heterogeneous mass enhancement. Axial single-shot echo-planar DWI shows hyperintensity of the mass at $b=0$ s/mm$^2$ (**d**), remaining hyperintense at $b=500$ s/mm$^2$ (**e**) indicating restricted diffusion

differential diagnosis with angiomyolipoma (AML). In most of the reported cases, fat containing pRCC also presents calcifications, very rare in AML, but nevertheless, a solid mass, in which fat component is not predominant, must be suspected and carefully investigated before considering it a benign AML.

Cromophobe RCC (cRCC) contains variable proportions of cells with clear or eosinophic cytoplasm arranged in sheet-like architecture along vascular septae. The prognosis for cRCC is better than in other subtypes of RCC. It typically appears as a well-circumscribed, homogenous renal mass with a cortical epicenter. Differently from ccRCC, its enhancement pattern is moderate and necrotic areas may not be present, even in large tumors.

Multilocular cystic RCC is a well-circumscribed mass, with fibrous wall and multiple cysts with thin smooth enhancing septae; it has an excellent prognosis.

Medullary carcinoma is a rare form that develops almost exclusively in patients with sickle cell trait. It is an infiltrative mass centered in renal medulla with frequent hemorrhage.

Collecting duct carcinoma is a very rare tumor with a poor prognosis. This tumor typically presents as an infiltrating central mass and sometimes it may not be differentiated from an invasive urothelial tumors.

Other histological subtypes are rare (Pedrosa et al. 2008a; Prasad et al. 2008b; Sun and Pedrosa 2009).

### 6.2.2 Urothelial Carcinoma

Transitional cell carcinoma (TCC) is the most common urothelial tumor. Although it rises more frequently from bladder, it occurs even in upper urinary tract. Since at the moment no direct comparison between MRU and CT urography sensitivity in urothelial tumors detection exists, CT, with its higher spatial resolution, has to be considered the technique of choice. On the other hand, MRU and particularly static-fluid MRU, offering a high intrinsic contrast resolution, could visualize collecting system without contrast medium administration. So it may be a useful tool in patients with renal function impairment or with a contrast excretion too limited to allow tumor detection. TCC appearance differs along with dimension and degree of invasion. Small TCC appears as filling defect, hypointense inside hyperintense urine on T2W, isointense to renal parenchyma on T1W, and with mild enhancement after contrast medium administration. Subtracted images may help in demonstrating enhancement to differentiate TCC from other small filling defects, like clots, but have to be considered carefully to detect mild enhancement and not mistake a misregistration artifact for enhancement. TCC may appear as a focal enhancing urothelial thickening and in this case differential diagnosis with inflammatory disease is difficult. Larger infiltrative masses may obliterate renal sinus or invade renal parenchyma, preserving renal shape, or may present extension along the collecting system. In this case TCC is typically hypointense-isointense to renal parenchyma on T2W with a low grade of enhancement on postgadolinium T1W, but larger masses could heterogeneously enhance. DWI shows hyperintense signal, indicating restricted diffusion (Fig. 6.3).

Squamous cell carcinoma of the urothelium is much less common than TCC and it may develop in stone disease or other chronic urothelial irritations.

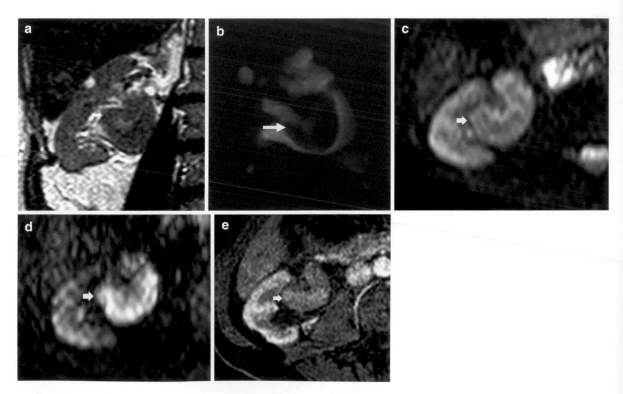

**Fig. 6.3** (**a–e**) Transitional cell carcinoma in 81-year-old man. Coronal TSE T2W (**a**) image shows a pelvic mass (*arrow*) isointense to renal cortex. Static-fluid MRU image shows renal pelvis defect (*arrow*) (**b**). Axial single-shot echo-planar DWI shows mild hyperintensity at $b=0$ s/mm$^2$ (**c**) and marked hyperintensity at $b=500$ s/mm$^2$ (**d**) indicating restricted diffusion. Axial GE T1W image obtained after gadulinium-based contrast administration shows mass (*arrow*) enhancement (**e**)

It appears as a large and infiltrative mass that may obliterate renal sinus and enlarge kidney. Sometimes it is indistinguishable from xanthogranulomatous pyelonephritis (Nikken and Krestin 2007; Pedrosa et al. 2008b).

### 6.2.3 Lymphoma

Renal lymphoma is usually a secondary involvement of a systemic disease, more often with non-Hodgkin's disease, but also solitary renal lymphomas are documented. The most common pattern is bilateral, multiple homogenous renal masses, iso-hypointense to renal cortex both on T1W and T2W, and with mild heterogeneous enhancement after gadolinium-based contrast agent administration. Occasionally, it appears as a solitary mass, with a direct invasion from lymphadenopathy, or as a perirenal rind of soft tissue. Perinephric invasion, appearing as a homogeneous mass enveloping but not distorting the kidney or stranding in the Gerota's fascia, is nearly pathognomonic for lymphoma. Primary or secondary involvement of renal sinus is seen as wall thickening of the collecting system, hypointense on T1W and T2W images, and with low-level enhancement (Fig. 6.4) (Pedrosa et al. 2008b).

### 6.2.4 Metastasis

Renal metastasis is not a common aspect, although kidneys may be involved either from hematogenous or lymphangitic dissemination. Lung cancers may spread with both path of dissemination and even a perirenal mass may be seen. Also breast, melanoma, and gastrointestinal tract malignancy could develop renal metastasis. Usually multiple low enhancing masses are seen, but lung, breast, and colon carcinomas may also determine a single mass, difficult to distinguish from RCC (Sun and Pedrosa 2009).

### 6.2.5 Angiomyolipoma

AML is a benign hamartomatous tumor containing fat, smooth muscle, and blood vessels in varying proportion. A predominant component of macroscopic fat is considered pathognomonic of AML. Macroscopic fat appears as a hyperintense signal area on T1W, showing a signal drop in spectral fat suppression sequences.

In-phase and opposed-phase imaging could help in the differentiation between macroscopic fat of AML and intracellular fat component of some ccRCC. AML is hyperintense on in-phase images and shows a signal

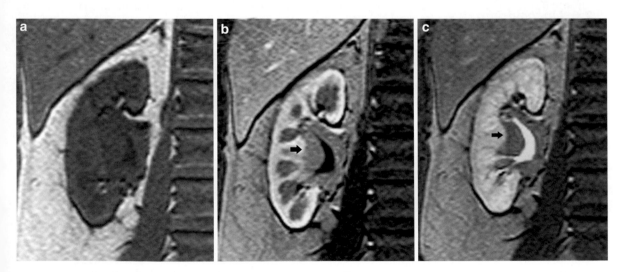

**Fig. 6.4** (**a–c**) Non-Hodgkin follicular B-cell lymphoma in a 64-year-old man. Coronal GE T1W images obtained before (**a**) and after gadolinium-based contrast agent administration, during nephrographic (**b**) and excretory (**c**) phase, show soft enhancing tissue (*arrow*) occupying renal sinus without collecting system distortion

loss only at the interface between macroscopic fat and surrounding tissue on opposed-phase ones (India ink artifact – see Chap. 20), while ccRCC is hyper-isointense on in-phased images and shows a drop of signal in the entire fatty area on opposed-phased ones. Unfortunately, also pRCC may show a small area of macroscopic fat and so differential diagnosis to AML is very difficult. The presence of central necrosis or calcifications may be helpful to suggest pRCC diagnosis, since they are rare even in larger AML. In case of poor fat, AML enhancement pattern determination seems to help, since AML shows a more homogeneous and prolonged enhancement compared to RCC in CT and, likely but not proven, in MR. Nevertheless, differential diagnosis is still difficult because enhancement pattern changes depend on the amount of vascular tissue components.

AML with a large predominantly exophtyic mass may be confused with a perirenal liposarcoma; differential diagnosis may be helped by two AML characteristics. First, AML arises from the kidney, so a small defect will be present in renal parenchyma at its origin, while a well-differentiated liposarcoma compresses, displaces, and distorts the kidney but not invades it. Second, typical AML feature is the presence of aneurismal vessels, while liposarcoma is relatively hypovascular (Nikken and Krestin 2007; Prasad et al. 2008a, b; Sun and Pedrosa 2009).

### 6.2.6 Oncocytoma

Oncocytoma is a benign renal tumor composed of uniform round or polygonal eosinophilic cells (oncocytes). The MRI appearance of oncocytoma is variable and nonspecific: low-signal intensity on T1W and heterogeneous high-signal intensity on T2W. In 33–54% of them, a central low T1W and T2W intensity scar is recognizable. After gadolinium-based contrast agent administration, a spoke-wheel-like enhancement may be seen on dynamic sequences. Oncocytoma may have a pseudo capsule, which appears as a low T1W and T2W intensity rim. Those characteristics present an important overlap to RCC and so therapy is usually nephron-sparing surgery.

Taouli et al. (2008) studied renal masses differentiation using DWI in alternative to contrast medium administration. They found significantly lower ADC values in RCC, indicating restricted diffusion, than in

oncocytoma, but at the present time, it is not possible to propose threshold value of ADC, since they change depending on MR unit and sequence's technical parameter setting (e.g., $b$-value) (Nikken and Krestin 2007; Prasad et al. 2008a, b; Sun and Pedrosa 2009).

### 6.2.7 Other Benign Renal Masses

Metanephric adenoma is a rare tumor composed of very small epithelial cells. It appears as a well-circumscribed solid mass, homogenously hypointense on T1W and iso-hyperintense on T2W in case of small tumors or with heterogeneous intensity due to hemorrhage, necrosis, and calcifications in larger ones. It shows low delayed enhancement.

Renal leiomyomas and solitary fibrous tumors arise from renal capsule; they appear as expansile, exophytic, well-defined solid peripheral masses, ipointense on T2W and isointense to renal cortex on T1W, with mild enhancement in the corticomedullary phase and heterogeneous enhancement in the delayed phases.

Juxtaglomerular cell tumor (reninoma) is a benign tumor derived from juxtaglomerular cells, causing renin hypersecretion and tough hypertension with hypokalemia, typically in women in the third or fourth decade. On MRI it appears as small (<3 cm) mass, hypointense on T1W and T2W, with low-level enhancement.

Hemangioma is a rare mesenchymal neoplasm consisting in blood fill vascular spaces. It is a solitary tumor, without capsule, arising from renal pyramids or renal pelvis. It is hyperintense on T2W and may show an early and persisting enhancement on delayed images (Prasad et al. 2008a, b).

### 6.2.8 Cystic Lesions

Cystic lesions are very common findings in the cross-sectional imaging of the kidney and can present various appearances. Since a variety of cystic lesion exists, it is fundamental to differentiate benign from malignant ones. Bosniak introduced a classification (Bosniak 1986; Israel and Bosniak 2003) to categorize cystic lesions in benign (class I and II), benign but needing a follow-up to prove it (class IIF), and those needing surgery because probably or certainly malignant (class III and IV). This classification was first based on CT features, but is now commonly applied also to contrast-enhanced ultrasound and MRI (Israel et al. 2004) – see Chap. 26.

According to Bosniak classification, category I represents simple benign cyst with thin smooth wall and homogeneous strong hyperintensity on T2W images and homogeneous hypointensity on T1W and DWI images (Fig. 6.5). Category II cysts could appear as hyperintense masses on T1W, T2W, and DWI images (Fig. 6.6) or, sometimes, like category I cysts but with a few hairline thin septa, perceivable enhancement, or calcifications. Category IIF cysts appear like category II ones, but larger than 3 cm or with multiple hairline thin septa or minimal smooth thickening of the wall or septa.

Category III indicates an indeterminate cystic mass with thickened wall or septa in which measurable enhancement is present. In this case image subtraction could be very useful to assess even mild enhancement, especially in high-signal T1W lesions. Category IV indicates an obviously malignant lesion, which contains enhancing soft-tissue components (Fig. 6.7).

Sometimes, a cluster of simple benign cysts produces a localized cystic disease of the kidney and it is essential to differentiate it from a multilocular cystic RCC or a benign multilocular cystic nephroma. Both multilocular cystic RCC and multilocular cystic nephroma are surrounded by a fibrous capsule, appearing hypointense on T1W and T2W images, while a localized cystic disease is not encapsulated. After contrast material administration, both multilocular cystic nephroma and multilocular cystic RCC present enhancement of thick septa, but the former usually does not show nodularity. Multiplanar evaluation of 3D fat-saturated T1W spoiled gradient-echo images permits to differentiate renal parenchyma intervening among a cluster of cysts, with enhancement identical to the rest of renal parenchyma, from enhancing septa (Sun and Pedrosa 2009; Israel and Bosniak 2008).

Also, DWI could be useful in differential diagnosis between benign and malignant cystic lesions.

Zangh et al. (2008) found that tumors show a significantly higher signal on DWI, with lower ADC values, than benign cysts. Furthermore, areas of solid enhancing tumor showed lower ADCs than nonenhancing necrotic or cystic components. Cystic components of tumors, even if with similar characteristics at conventional MRI, had lower ADCs than benign cyst. On the other hand, these ADC values, thought to be significantly different, also showed a nonnegligible overlap, particularly as regard T1 hyperintense lesions. Moreover, the study did not include truly cystic tumors, such as multilocular cystic RCC and multilocular cystic nephroma. Furthermore, at the

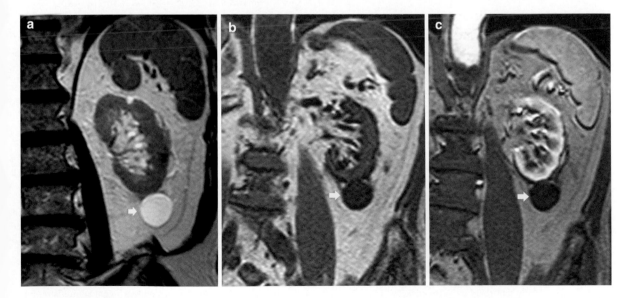

**Fig. 6.5** (**a–c**) MRI appearance of simple cyst (*arrow*): hyperintense on T2W (**a**), hypointense on T1W before (**b**) and after gadolinium-based agent administration (**c**)

**Fig. 6.6** (**a–d**) MRI appearance of hemorrhagic cyst (*arrow*): hyperintense both on T1W (**a**) and T2W (**b**) images. Axial single-shot echo-planar DWI shows hyperintense signal at $b = 0$ s/mm$^2$ (**b**), remaining hyperintense at $b = 500$ s/mm$^2$ (**c**) indicating restricted diffusion

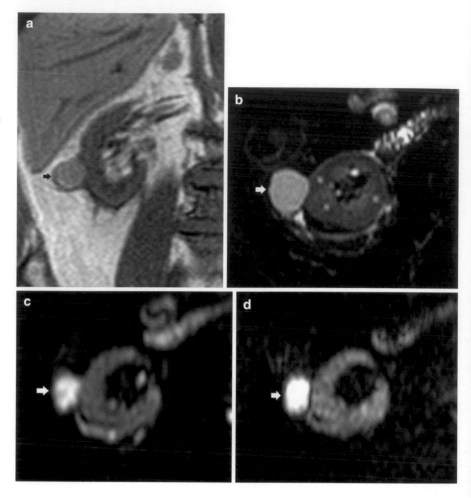

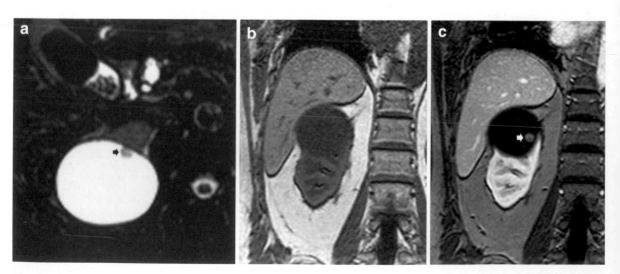

**Fig. 6.7** (**a–c**) Malignant renal cyst (Bosniak IV) in a 41-year-old man. (**a**) Axial TSE T2W image shows a hypointense mural nodule (*arrow*). Coronal GE T1W images, obtained before (**b**) and after (**c**) gadolinium-based contrast agent administration, demonstrate mural nodule enhancement

present time, it is not possible to propose threshold value of ADC , since they change depending on MR unit and sequence's technical parameter setting (e.g., $b$-value) (Taouili et al. 2009).

### 6.2.9  Renal Infections

Renal infection diagnosis is usually based on clinical and laboratory findings, while imaging evaluation has to be reserved to nonresponder patients or to patients at high risk for complications, like diabetics and immune-deficient ones. MRI in acute pyelonephritis is not routinely used in clinical practice, but it has to be considered as an alternative study when imaging evaluation is requested in young patients. MRI can show lesions and their intrarenal and perinephric extension. Parenchymal edema shows a low T1W signal and a high T2W signal, with reduced differentiation between cortex and medulla. Static-fluid MRU may show urinary tract dilatation in case of urinary tract obstruction. After gadolinium-based contrast agent administration, involved regions are hypointense on T1W with an inflammatory stranding. Other renal infection signs are perinephric and renal sinus fat blurring, Gerota's fascia thickening, renal parenchyma enlargement or renal pelvis, and caliceal wall thickening (Stunnel et al. 2007).

Furthermore, MRI has shown a high diagnostic accuracy in the differentiation between simple hydronephrosis and pyonephrosis, the second one showing a low T2W signal and, sometimes, debris floating inside renal pelvis; DWI is helping, showing a high signal with low ADC values due to restricted diffusion of water molecule in the high viscosity fluid (Fig. 6.8) (Chan et al. 2001).

Renal abscess may appear as a homogeneous low T1W and high T2W signal region or as a complex cystic lesion. On the base of debris' entity, even a fluid–fluid level may be seen inside. MRI is particularly helpful in determining lesion dimension and diffusion to perinephric fat (Browne et al. 2004; Prasad et al. 2008b).

Xanthogranulomatous pyelonephritis is a rare chronic pyelonephritis that develops secondary to a urinary tract obstruction, typically a stone. Proteus and E. coli species are involved in this infection. Lipid-laden macrophages extensively replace renal parenchyma in a focal or diffused pattern. Focal xanthogranulomatous pyelonephritis may be mistaken for a RCC. Depending on fatty macrophages concentration, T1W signal could be from isointense to highly hyperintense, similar to perinephric fat. T2W signal is isointense to normal parenchyma and this feature could help in the differential diagnosis with hyperintense RCC. Inside the lesion, fluid cavity with high T2W and low T1W signal is recognizable. Xanthogranulomatous tissue does not enhance, but inflammatory surrounding tissue and thickened fascia do (Verswijvel et al. 2000).

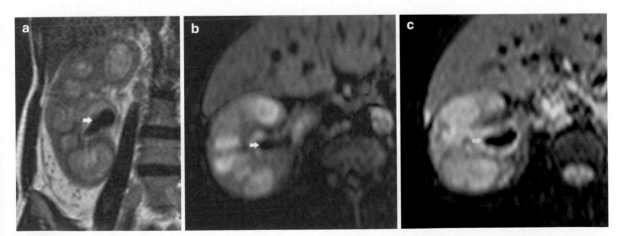

**Fig. 6.8** (**a–c**) Right pyonephrosis in a 35-year-old women with stone disease. Coronal SE T2W image (**a**) shows right hydroneprosis with low-signal intensity. The signal void on the renal pelvis corresponds to a renal stone (*arrows*). Axial single-shot echoplanar DWI shows slightly hyperintense material in the renal pelvis at $b = 0$ s/mm² (**b**), becoming strongly hyperintense at $b = 500$ s/mm²

### 6.2.10 Renal Artery Stenosis

Atherosclerosis is the most common cause of renal artery stenosis and consequent secondary hypertension. In addition, renovascular disease is the primary cause of renal insufficiency in approximately 15% of patients >50 years of age who develop end-stage renal disease.

Most of the studies have concluded that renal MRA is highly accurate in most cases in detecting arterial stenosis, up to sensitivity and specificity of gadolinium-enhanced MRA of 97% and 85%, respectively, so renal CE MRA could replace conventional angiography in most patients with suspected atherosclerotic renal artery stenosis (Fig. 6.9).

Data analysis is an important aspect of renal MRA that can affect accuracy and reliability. Severity of disease could be assessed by measuring the percent of stenosis i.e., one minus the ratio of the stenotic and normal renal artery diameters; and also cross-sectional area measurements of stenotic arteries could routinely be obtained to eliminate interobserver variability.

MRI offers a number of information to assess the functional status of the kidneys as well as to evaluate the functional severity of the stenosis, including loss of cortical-medullary differentiation on T1W precontrast images, renal atrophy, and poststenotic dilatation. The most important drawback in MRA is insensibility to calcium components in atherosclerosis plaques, a useful information in interventional therapy planning.

Fibromuscolar dysplasia is the second most common cause of renal artery stenosis. It is more frequent in young patients and women, and in contrast to atherosclerotic stenosis, it tends to affect mild and distal renal artery. If spatial resolution used is sufficient, MRA permits visualization of the pathology affecting the proximal as well as the distal renal arteries, but none of the intrarenal segmental renal arteries (Zhang and Prince 2004; Glockner and Vrtiska 2007).

## 6.3 Renal Transplant

Deterioration of renal function in renal transplant, especially if there is associated new onset or severe hypertension, could be caused by the transplant renal artery stenosis. Early diagnosis of this entity is essential to save a failing renal allograft – see Chap. 30.

The transplant renal artery examination is performed in a manner similar to native renal artery imaging, but shifted lower into the pelvis to cover the transplant kidney and in-flow from iliac arteries (Fig. 6.10). Three-dimensional CE MRA is performed in coronal plane encompassing the lower abdominal aorta and extending down to below the femoral heads. Postcontrast T1W images within 5–10 min of intravenous gadolinium-based contrast agent administration should be acquired to asses renal excretory function and so demonstrate perfusion defects, masses, or infarctions. Vascular clips in the surgical bed may produce metallic

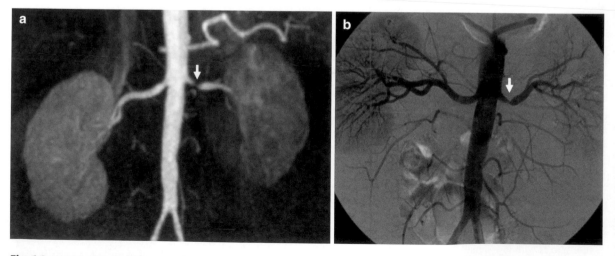

**Fig. 6.9** (**a, b**) Left renal artery stenosis in a 41-year-old man. (**a**) Subvolume MIP image from contrast-enhanced MR angiography reveals proximal left renal artery severe stenosis (*arrow*) with an excellent correlation with the conventional angiogram (**b**)

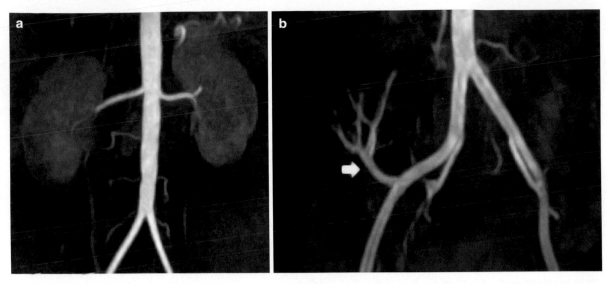

**Fig. 6.10** Subvolume MIP image from contrast-enhanced MR angiography shows normal appearance of renal arteries (**a**) and of transplanted right renal artery (*arrow*) (**b**)

artifacts on MRA. Contrast-enhanced MR nephrography (see below) could help in differential diagnosis between acute tubulare necrosis and acute rejection.

Living renal donors and laparoscopic nephrectomy need an accurate description of the number, length, and location of renal arteries for proper surgical planning. It is also important to identify anatomic variations in the renal venous and parenchymal anatomy. CE MRA is an ideal technique for assessing renal vessels and parenchyma without the associated risk of ionizing radiation (Zhang and Prince 2004; Glockner and Vrtiska 2007).

## 6.4   Advanced Applications

### 6.4.1   Magnetic Resonance Angiography Without Gadolinium-Based Contrast Administration

The nephrogenic systemic fibrosis risk in patients with severely compromised renal function, estimated glomerular filtration rate <30 mL/min/1.73 m², has given a new boost in MRI without the use of gadolinium-based contrast agent.

On *3D Phase Contrast sequences,* flow is encoded in all three axes and image intensity corresponds to blood flowing velocity. Flowing blood is bright while stationary tissues are dark. Signal drop-out is related to intravoxel dephasing caused by disordered and chaotic flow in the region of severe stenosis (>70%). An in vitro study shows that the degree of this spin dephasing is directly correlated with the trans-stenotic pressure gradient. Probably in the future, one would be able to use the information on spin dephasing to estimate pressure gradients: more dephasing indicates a more significant stenosis.

*2D Cine Phase Contrast sequences* can noninvasively measure renal artery blood flow. Cardiac gating and breath holding are needed to improve spatial and temporal resolution. Flow volume data per unit time as well as a velocity-time curve for a region of interest can be derived from phase contrast images and so analyzed. On these curves, delayed systolic peaks with reduction in renal capillary resistance are signs of significant renal artery stenosis (Glockner and Vrtiska 2007).

### 6.4.2   Contrast-Enhanced Magnetic Resonance Renography

There is no consensus on MR renography technique, but most of proposed techniques include the following steps: acquisition of dynamic images before, during, and after gadolinium-based contrast agent administration, conversion of the signal intensity of the renal tissue to gadolinium concentration, and generation of functional curves plotting gadolinium concentration variation in time.

This procedure gives important information about renal blood flow, GFR, and cortical and medullary blood flow for each kidney. Total acquisition time goes from 3 up to 10 min. The highest GFR precision achievable is 0.02–0.025 mmol/kg.

This technique proved useful in assessing perfusion parameters in renal artery stenosis, particularly sensitive if implemented with angiotensin-converting enzyme inhibitor in detecting emodynamically significant stenosis.

When an allograft dysfunction appears in the early postoperative period, MR renography may differentiate acute tubular necrosis, in which cortical and medullary perfusion is maintained, from perfusion reduction of acute rejection.

Although these optimistic results are obtained, MR nephrography has not spread in the clinical practice mainly for the difficulties found in calculating gadolinium concentration from signal intensity and in post-processing (Chandarana and Lee 2009).

### 6.4.3  Diffusion MRI and Renal Function

Single-shot echo-planar imaging with different diffusion gradients ($b$-values) application is the most frequently used technique for DWI and ADC maps calculation. It has been found to be a good linear correlation between serum creatinine level and ADC value of the renal cortex, so DWI has the possibility to investigate the function of each kidney separately in case of renal insufficiency and to assess if a hydronephrotic kidney still maintains or has already lost its function.

Although at high $b$-values ADC is dominated by diffusion effects, at lower $b$-values there is an influence by perfusion in the microvasculature, and some investigators have tried to exploit the perfusion information of DWI to diagnose renal artery stenosis without contrast-enhanced MRA. Unfortunately, the lack of consensus regarding $b$-values selection for renal imaging makes it difficult to compare different studies and generate standardized ADC values for disease and health (Chandarana and Lee 2009).

### 6.4.4  BOLD MRI

In animal models renal failure has been found to be subsequent to renal medulla hypoxia, a possible consequence of hypertension and diabetes. BOLD MRI exploits paramagnetic effect of deoxyhemoglobin to image medullary oxygenation. A 2D multiple gradient-recalled echo technique, with eight to sixteen echoes acquired after each excitation pulse, with maximum TE of 50 ms at 1.5T and 25 ms at 3T, equal to renal T2* value, is used. If deoxyhemoglobin concentration increases, there is more dephasing and a decrease in T2* relaxation time of protons in the surrounding tissues, so higher tissue oxygenation results in increased T2* relaxation time and a shorter T2* value. The T2* value can be obtained by measuring the slope of the line fit of natural log of signal intensity vs. TE, generating a map on a per-voxel basis. The major limit in this technique is that we actually do not know if BOLD signal intensity is a mirror of oxygen supply or of oxygen consumption; furthermore, even hematocrit, plasma oxygen, and blood flow influence BOLD signal (Chandarana and Lee 2009).

### 6.4.5  USPIO Particles

The lymph node metastasis detection using conventional gadolinium-based contrast agents relies mainly on size and shape of the lymph nodes. Ultra-small superparamagnetic iron oxide particles are ingested by macrophages and accumulate in healthy lymph nodes, determining a signal intensity decrease on T2W and T2*W images. Metastatic cells displace normal macrophages from lymph node, so pathologic lymph nodes do not show signal intensity loss after USPIO injection. The use of USPIOs seems to improve diagnostic accuracy for several type of metastasis, but it is not yet entered in clinical practice (Nikken and Krestin 2007).

# References

Bosniak MA (1986) The current radiological approach to renal cysts. Radiology 158:1–10

Browne RFJ, Zwirewich C, Torreggiani WC (2004) Imaging of urinary tract infection in the adult. Eur Radiol 14 (suppl 3): 168–183

Chan JH, Tsui EY, Luk SH et al. (2001) MR diffusion-weighted imaging of kidney: differentiation between hydronephrosis and pyonephrosis. Clin Imaging 25:110–113

Chandarana H and Lee VS (2009) Renal functional MRI: are we ready for clinical application? AJR Am J Roentgenol 192:1550–1557

Cova M, Squillaci E, Stacul F et al. (2004) Diffusion-weighted MRI in the evaluation of renal lesions: preliminary results. Br J Radiol 77:851–857

Glockner JF, Vrtiska TJ (2007) Renal MR and CT angiography: current concepts. Abdom Imaging 32:407–420

Israel GM, Bosniak MA (2003) Renal imaging for diagnosis and staging of renal cell carcinoma. Urol Clin North Am 30:499–514.

Israel GM, Bosniak MA (2008) Pitfalls in renal mass evaluation and how to avoid them. Radiographics 28:1325–1338

Leyendecker JR, Barnes CE, Zagoria RJ (2008) MR urography: techniques and clinical applications. Radiographics 28:23–46

Nikken JJ, Krestin GP (2007) MRI of the kidney-state of the art. Eur Radiol 17:2780–2793

Nolte-Ernsting CC, Adam GB et al. (2001a) MR urography: examination techniques and clinical applications. Eur Radiol 11:355–372

Nolte-Ernsting, CC, Tacke J et al. (2001b) Diuretic-enhanced gadolinium excretory MR urography: comparison of conventional gradient-echo sequences and echo-planar imaging. Eur Radiol 11:18–27

Pedrosa I, Sun MR, Spencer M et al. (2008a) MR imaging of renal masses: correlation with findings at surgery and pathologic analysis. Radiographics 28:985–1003

Pedrosa I, Chou MT, Ngo L (2008b) MR classification of renal masses with pathologic correlation. Eur Radiol 18: 365–375

Perez-Rodriguez J, Lai S et al. (2009) Nephrogenic systemic fibrosis: incidence, associations, and effect of risk factor assessment–report of 33 cases. Radiology 250: 371–377

Prasad SR, Surabhi VR, Menias CO et al. (2008a) Benign renal neoplasm in adults: cross-sectional imaging findings. AJR Am J Roentgenol 190:158–164

Prasad SR, Dalrymple NC, Surabhi VR (2008b) Cross-sectional imaging evaluation of renal masses. Radiol Clin North Am 46:95–111

Silverman SG, Leyendecker JR et al. (2009) What is the current role of CT urography and MR urography in the evaluation of the urinary tract? Radiology 250:309–323

Squillaci E, Manenti G, Cova M et al. (2004) Correlation of diffusion-weighted MR imaging with cellularity of renal tumors. Anticancer Res 24:4175–4479

Stunnel H, Buckley O, Feeney J et al. (2007) Imaging of acute pyelonephritis in adult. Eur Radiol 17:1820–1828

Taouili B, Thakur R, Mannelli L et al. (2009) Renal lesions: characteristics with diffusion-weighted imaging versus contrast-enhanced MR imaging. Radiology 251:398–407

Verswijvel G, Oyen R, Van Poppel H et al. (2000) Xanthogranulomatous pyelonephritis: MRI findings in the diffuse and the focal type. Eur Radiol 10:586–589

Zhang H, Prince MR (2004) Renal MR angiography. Magn Reson Imaging Clin North Am 12:487–503

Zhang J, Pedrosa I et al. (2003) MR techniques for renal imaging. Radiol Clin North Am 41:877–907

Zangh J, Teherani YM, Wang L et al. (2008) Renal masses: characterization with diffusion-weighted MR imaging – a preliminary experience. Radiology 247:458–464

# Renal Angiography and Vascular Interventional Radiology

**7**

Fabio Pozzi-Mucelli and Andrea Pellegrin

## Contents

## Abstract

> A brief introduction is given about the diagnostic role of angiography, which, at present, is significantly reduced compared to the other noninvasive techniques such as color Doppler ultrasound, multidetector CT angiography, and magnetic resonance angiography. Then, there is a focus on technical aspects in diagnostic angiography, discussing materials and imaging parameters; subsequently, the technical aspects of interventional vascular procedures are considered. Anatomy is then reviewed as is apparent on angiographic studies.

> The rest of the chapter describes angiographical appearance and interventional management of the pathologies of the kidney amenable of an endovascular approach, starting with occlusive vascular disease due to atherosclerosis, fibromuscular dysplasia, or other causes. Then, less common vascular conditions are discussed, such as renal ischemia, aneurysms, A-V fistulas, trauma, and complications of transplant surgery.

> Final part of the chapter concentrates on renal neoplasm, both benign and malignant, with special emphasis on the endovascular management by means of the different techniques of embolization.

F. Pozzi-Mucelli (✉) and A. Pellegrin
Department of Radiology, Cattinara Hospital,
University of Trieste, Strada di Fiume 447,
34149 Trieste, Italy
e-mail: fabio.pozzimucelli@alice.it

## 7.1 Introduction

For imaging of renal pathology, a broad spectrum of radiologic diagnostic procedures is available, competing among each other, in their diagnostic performance and

E. Quaia (ed.), *Radiological Imaging of the Kidney*,
Medical Radiology, DOI: 10.1007/978-3-540-87597-0_7, © Springer-Verlag Berlin Heidelberg 2011

relevance. Nowadays, in the work-up of neoplastic lesions, ultrasound (US), computed tomography (CT), or magnetic resonance imaging (MRI) is performed predominantly, while on the other hand, the contribution of diagnostic angiography is no longer required. Digital subtraction angiography (DSA) maintains a limited role, especially in the evaluation of renal arteries, and until recently, catheter-based DSA has been considered as gold standard. However, noninvasive techniques such as CT-angiography (CTA) and MR-angiography (MRA) are evolving parallel to their quantum leap of resolutions and readiness to use. Nevertheless, shared consensus for quality assessment of these new modalities is still lacking; more comparison studies are urgently warranted. US color Doppler is a cheap and readily available technology, but it requires great experience and training for effectively assessing renal vessels, and even in that case, a substantial percentage of patients are not properly examinable. CTA is an extremely promising technique, but still has to prove itself, because its intrinsic spatial resolution could not be sufficient in pathologies like vasculitides, or in some cases, in fibromuscular dysplasia (FMD). With regard to MRI, despite the availability of ultrashort pulse sequences applying the T1 relaxation reduction effect of gadolinium-enhanced MR techniques, overestimation of renal artery stenosis still poses a substantial problem. There is also need to address that, in the past few years, nephrogenic systemic fibrosis has been recognized as a clinical entity related to the administration of gadolinium chelates to patients with renal failure. Therefore, the use of gadolinium-based contrast is under a growing concern, and it is no more considered as a harmless alternative to iodinated contrast as it has been in the past. Nevertheless, a recent study has suggested the possibility to use a lower dose of gadobenate dimeglumine to achieve signal intensity enhancement similar to that achieved with a double dose of a conventional gadolinium-based contrast agent, with excellent specificity (Soulez et al. 2008).

On the contrary, the field of renal intervention is growing, as is implied by a variety of procedures such as percutaneous transluminal angioplasty (PTA), stent placement, and embolization of both trauma and benign or malignant tumors. These methods have emerged over the last two decades, starting from an experimental setting up to a fully accepted treatment option. When renal artery angioplasty is embedded in an aggressive approach including stenting as an adjunct for more complex cases (like renal ostial lesions) and a well-organized follow-up

regimen is scheduled, the therapeutic potential of organ preservation appears promisingly high. Providing an adequate perinterventional drug regimen, restenosis rates may be as low as 10%.

Endovascular interventions also include, in selected cases, capillary embolization that might be used as an alternative to nephrectomy with a similar clinical outcome. Specifically, the development of superselective small caliber embolization catheters in synergy with further refinement of embolization materials has aided to realize superselective occlusion techniques in benign vascular lesions and renal trauma.

## 7.2 Technique

### 7.2.1 Diagnostic Angiography

Angiography in the evaluation of kidney must be done by an intra-arterial approach generally using the femoral route; brachial or radial approaches are also feasible (Scheinert et al. 2001). The former is frequently used by cardiologists, performing peripheral interventions as a primary choice. However, brachial or radial approaches are the only options in cases of bilateral iliac occlusion or infrarenal aortic occlusion. It is also the most favorable in cases of extremely tortuous iliac axes or in patients with femoral surgical grafts.

The technique has been explained in the following: after the infiltration of the skin and subcutaneous tissue with a small amount of local anesthetic, a 19-gauge hollow core needle (single wall puncture needle is preferable) is inserted through the femoral (or brachial or radial) artery, and after the advancement of a short 0.035" guide wire, a 4 or 5 French (Fr) sheath is introduced. In case of femoral approach and the lack of significant stenosis or tortuosity, a standard 0.035" teflon-coated metallic guide wire can be advanced in the abdominal aorta. While in the presence of iliac axes with multiple atheromatous or calcific plaques, a 0.035" hydrophilic-coated guide wire is preferred to the standard guide wire. Sometimes, a selective diagnostic catheter (with a Cobra or multipurpose configuration) is used in association with a guide wire in order to increase the support and obtain a more easy advancement in the iliac artery.

Once reached the abdominal aorta, a 4 or 5 Fr high-flow catheter with a pig-tail or straight tip configuration is advanced over the guide wire. The tip of the catheter is positioned at the level of L1 body. After a preliminary test hand injection, which confirms the intraluminal position of the catheter, a connection to a power injector pump is established. Generally, when angiography is performed with injection from the catheter positioned in the aortic lumen, a total amount of 25–30 mL at 15–20 mL/s of iodinated nonionic contrast media are used. We prefer high concentration contrast media (320–370 mgI/mL), which may be prewarmed before injection in order to reduce the viscosity, and therefore, resistance. For selective angiography, a wide variety of catheters can be used, but the basic ones used to gain access to the renal artery are curved catheters such as the "Cobra 2" or the "Renal Double curve" or the "Simmons 1" or the "Simmons 2." The flow rate for selective injection must be reduced to 6–8 mL at 3/4 mL/s (Figs. 7.1 and 7.2).

For acceptable diagnostic results, the equipment must be of high quality with x-ray tube and generator able to give good results in terms of spatial and contrast resolution also in large patients. Modern DSA

systems are based on digital fluoroscopy/fluorography systems and are equipped with special software and display facilities. The mask and the serial images are obtained from the television camera in analog form or from the charge-coupled device (CCD) television camera in digital form. Using a conventional TV camera with the image intensifier will require that the images are digitized in an analog-to-digital converter, which converts the TV line image (525/625 or 1,023/1,249 lines) to an image matrix, commonly with 512×512, 1,024×1,024, or 2,048×2,048 pixels. From a CCD camera, the images are digitized already in the electronics close to the light-sensitive CCD chip.

The last evolution of digital angiography systems is the introduction of flat-panel technology. This allows direct digital imaging without the intermediate step of analog-to-digital conversion with significant improvement of efficiency of the system. The dominating method is based on an indirect X-ray conversion process, using cesium iodide scintillators. It offers considerable advantages in radiography, angiography, and fluoroscopy. The

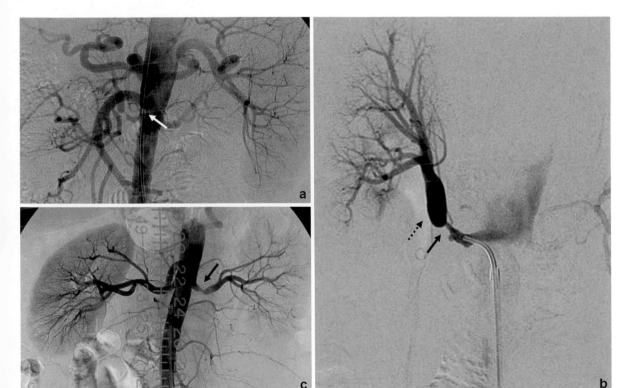

**Fig. 7.1** (**a**) Catheter tip (*arrow*) seems correctly positioned, but renal artery opacification is faint for the prevalent opacification of celiac trunk and superior mesenteric artery, which overlays right renal artery. (**b**) Selective renal angiography, a stenosis is present (*arrow*), as well as a postenotic dilatation (*dashed arrow*). (**c**) Renal arteries, correct visualization with a 20° LAO projection, a stenosis of the proximal left renal artery is evident (*arrow*)

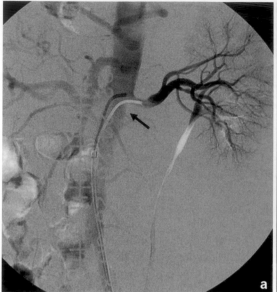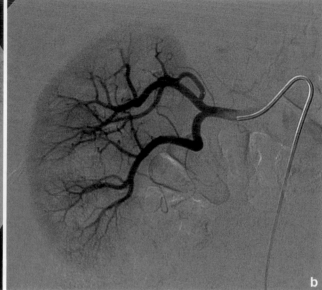

**Fig. 7.2** (**a**) Selective renal angiography: an unstable catheter for shape and position can become dislodged (*arrow*) for the high flow during power injection. (**b**) If the catheter is positioned too distal in the main renal artery, the first part of the lumen is not visualized, an ostial stenosis could, therefore, go unnoticed

other method employs a direct converter such as selenium, which is particularly suitable for mammography. Both flat detector technologies are based on amorphous silicon active pixel matrices. Flat detectors facilitate the clinical workflow in radiographic rooms, with improved image quality, and provide the potential to reduce dose. This added value is based on their large dynamic range, their high sensitivity to X-rays, and the instant availability of the image. Advanced image processing is instrumental in these improvements and expand the range of conventional diagnostic methods. In angiography and fluoroscopy, the transition from image intensifiers to flat detectors is facilitated by ample advantages they offer, such as distortion-free images, excellent coarse contrast, large dynamic range, and high X-ray sensitivity. Furthermore, another major advantage of flat-panel technology is that, although the tube is essentially unchanged, the image intensifier is eliminated. The image-receiving component of the unit, the flat panel itself, is smaller and more compact, allowing easier access to the patient during interventional procedures.

Another important facility in DSA systems is postprocessing of images. The radiologist can use many processing options such as windowing, filtering, and quantitative measurements of distance and density. Sometimes, the anatomical structures move after the

mask has been acquired, and for perfect subtraction, the mask has to be moved a few pixels or perhaps just a fraction of a pixel (pixel shift). Such functions are available in most DSA systems. The frame rate of acquisition must be quite high (at least 3 frames/s) in the first 3–5 s (arterial phase), then it can be decreased at 2 frames/s (parenchymal phase). In cases of prolonged acquisitions, when also a venous phase is acquired, the frame rate can be further reduced to 1 frame/s. Generally, when the diagnostic problem is focused on the arterial bed, only arterial and parenchymal phases are performed.

Concerning the position of the tip of the catheter, it should not be placed too cranial in order to avoid the filling of the celiac trunk and the superior mesenteric artery with contrast media, and therefore, cause problems of overmatching of these arteries on the renal arteries (Fig. 7.1).

Considering the correct projections, it must be underlined that it is crucial to visualize the ostium of renal arteries, since it is the most frequent site of atheromatous lesions; their detection depends not only on their position, but also on the size of the aorta, which once filled with contrast media can hide the origin of the renal arteries. In the second half of the nineties, some papers were published on the contribution of CT elucidating this topic, based on the fact that CT is very effective in a precise evaluation of the position of the renal artery origin and their relationship with the aorta (Verschuyl et al. 1997a, b). These papers have shown that left renal artery can be well depicted in the antero-posterior view because in 80% of cases its origin is between 90 and 120° in respect to aorta axes, but it is useful to add a left anterior oblique (LAO) projection of 20°. Right renal artery shows a variable degree of origin and in 85% of cases it is between −85 and −45°. For this side, the projection that better shows the right renal ostium is always the LAO at 20°, but sometimes a LAO at 40° is useful. In Verschujl et al.'s experience (Verschuyl et al. 1997b), the routine use of AP and LAO projections at 20 and 40° gave a correct evaluation of 92% of 400 renal arteries considered. In detail, the first projection to be done is the LAO at 20°, and if this one is not sufficient, the AP projection can be performed followed by the LAO at 40° in selected cases. Other authors suggest to do only a LAO at 15° (Harrington et al. 1983).

Another alternative solution for renal artery evaluation is to proceed at selective angiography: this modality has the advantage to better define the distal branches of the main trunk; however, often it is unable to correctly evaluate the ostium because the tip of the catheter is placed distally with respect to the ostium Fig. 7.2).

It must be underlined that this type of maneuver is not totally risk-free, particularly in the case of atheromatous stenosis of the ostium for the risk of colesterinic embolization (Morita et al. 1989).

Another problematic issue is the detection of accessory or polar renal arteries, which are not an unusual event due to an incidence of 32% in the monolateral form and 12% in the bilateral form and may represent a cause of clinical problems and also technical problems (Verschuyl et al. 1997a). In some cases these accessory arteries may originate on the same plane of the main trunk, and for this reason, reduce the detection of this vessel (Fig. 7.3). In these cases, oblique cranio-caudal or caudo-cranial projections are useful to distinguish overlapping vessels or proceed to selective catheterization (Fig. 7.3b).

## 7.3 Interventional Renal Vascular Procedures

### 7.3.1 Vascular Interventions

Since its introduction in 1978, percutaneous transluminal renal angioplasty (PTRA) has emerged as a highly effective technique for the correction of renal artery stenoses. Renal angioplasty has notable physiologic, psychological, and economic advantages over other treatment modalities, and it should now be considered the therapy of choice for renovascular hypertension.

The indications of renal angioplasty are still evolving. The common indications are as follows (Kidney and Deutsch 1996):

- Sudden onset of hypertension.
- Hypertension in a patient without a positive family history.
- Hypertension in a patient without a medical history of factors known to cause hypertension.

**Fig. 7.3** (**a**) In the AP projection the origin of the two accessory renal arteries (*arrow*) is on the same plane, main trunk is more cranial (*dashed arrow*). (**b**) After cranio-caudal projection, the origins of the two accessory renal arteries (*arrows*) are better defined

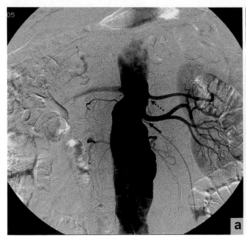
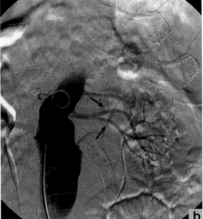

- Malignant hypertension.
- Hypertension refractory to pharmacotherapy.
- Patient noncompliance with medications.
- Hypertension in a patient with abdominal bruit suggestive of renal artery narrowing.
- Hypertension in a patient who develops renal failure while taking captopril.
- Sudden onset of hypertension in a young woman not taking oral contraceptives (for patients in this group, the likelihood of FMD is increased).

From a technical point of view, different modalities to perform endovascular treatment of renal artery stenosis are available as follows:

- Simple balloon transluminal renal angioplasty, with selective stenting in case of suboptimal result at PTA.
- Primary renal artery stenting.
- Renal artery stenting with distal protection device.

Regarding evolution of material employed in this type of intervention, the "trend" is to use materials derived from coronary intervention experience, and significant improvements have been introduced for diagnostic catheters, guidewires, PTA catheters, and stents.

Diagnostic catheters: in the past, 4 or 5 French preshaped diagnostic catheters (Cobra, Renal Double Curve, Simmons, etc.) were used to catheterize a stenotic renal artery, and in association with hydrophilic guide wires, the stenosis was negotiated (Fig. 7.4a). Frequently, catheters were advanced beyond the stenosis and hydrophilic guidewires were changed with stiff Teflon-coated stainless steel wires (such as 0.035"Rosen Heavy Duty), and standard profile PTA balloon catheters and premounted stent were advanced over this wire. In the last years, many centers have adopted the use of guiding catheters specifically designed for renal interventions. These guiding catheters, derived from coronary intervention experience, are larger in caliber (6–8 Fr) and have a large lumen. Usually they give a superior support compared to conventional diagnostic catheters and are advanced close to the ostium of the renal artery. At this point, the stenosis is negotiated with a 0.014" or 0.018" guidewire avoiding fragmentation of the atheromatous plaque. Then low-profile balloon catheter or premounted stent are advanced (Fig. 7.4b). This technique has been also defined "Do not touch technique" because it avoids, as much as possible, passages of materials and devices at the level of the atheromatous plaque.

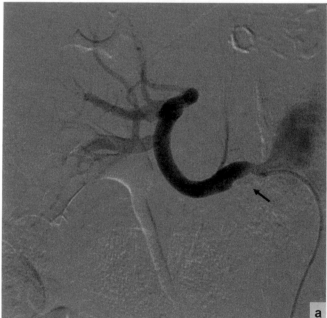 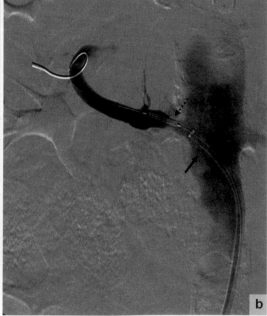

**Fig. 7.4** (a) Selective renal angiography with a 5 French diagnostic catheter, a stenotic plaque (*arrow*) is present at the ostium. (b) Same patient, but angiography is now performed through the guiding catheter (*arrow*), during stent placement (*dashed arrow*). The advantage of guiding catheter is that it enables to check every moment of the different steps of the procedure

Guide wires: while negotiation of renal stenosis was done with 0.035" guide wire in the past, several cath lab adopt the rule to negotiate stenosis with 0.014" or 0.018" guidewires in the last years, in order to decrease trauma to arterial plaques, and therefore, reduce distal embolization. Both stainless steel and nitinol guide wires are used, generally with a short soft tip, and still able to give a support to the advancement of low-profile PTA balloon catheters or stents.

Balloon catheters: for many years, standard balloon catheters were employed for dilatation of renal artery stenosis. These catheters have the following characteristics:

- Shaft corresponding to a 5 F catheter.
- "Over the wire" construction: this means that the entire catheter runs on the guide wire.
- Short tip (shorter then 5 mm): this can be useful in the case of distal stenosis near the proximal division of the main trunk.
- Balloon can be noncompliant or with low-compliance structure: in the first case, once reached the nominal pressure of the balloon (i.e., 8 atm), further increment of pressure will not lead to further increase in the diameter of the balloon. In the second case, once reached the nominal pressure of the balloon, further increment of pressure will cause further smooth increase in the nominal diameter of the balloon till 10% of the nominal diameter. The choice of the type of balloon is operator-dependent and well-defined guidelines do not exist.

In the last years, many centers have adopted the use of low-profile PTA balloon catheters derived from coronary interventions. These differ significantly from standard PTA catheters for the following reasons:

- Very low-profile tip: the tip has a diameter of 2.6 F (0.66 mm) or lower compared to 1.65 mm of standard PTA balloon, and for this reason, an atraumatic advancement of the catheter through the stenosis is warranted.
- Generally, this catheter is provided of a hydrophilic coating on the surface of the balloon and on the distal part of the shaft, which enables advancement.
- Monorail or rapid exchange construction: this term defines a particular way of construction of the catheter for which only the last 30–40 cm of the catheters run over the wire. This gives the significant advantage to the following:

- Avoid changes of guidewires.
- Avoid the use of long guidewires.
- Reduces procedural times.

Stents: also in the field of stent, significant evolutions have been introduced moving from balloon expandable stent to be crimped over standard PTA balloon catheter to premounted balloon expandable stent on standard PTA catheter to the very last generation of low-profile premounted stent over rapid exchange or monorail balloon catheter. This last type of material as microguidewires and low-profile balloon catheters reduce the risk of traumatism to the atheromatous plaques responsible for distal embolization. Although in the past some authors treated renal artery stenosis with self-expandable stent (Raynaud et al. 1994), there is a general agreement that balloon expandable stents are much more preferable because their deployment is more precise and these stents have superior radial force. Until few years ago, only stainless steel stents were available, while in the recent years new materials such as chromocobalt alloy has been introduced. This alloy has similar strength of stainless steel, but inferior weight and superior long-term results are expected, even if not proven currently. Few data are available on the use of drugeluting stents in the treatment of renal artery stenosis. One recent multicenter trial in which a Sirolimuseluting stent was compared to a bare-metal stent shows that the angiographic outcome at 6 months did not reveal any significant difference between the two stents. Renal artery stenting with both stents significantly improved blood pressure. The paper concludes that only further studies with larger patient population and longer angiographic follow-up will be able to determine if there is a significant benefit of drug-eluting stents in treating ostial renal artery stenosis (Zahringer et al. 2007). Stents are mounted over no-compliant or lowcompliant balloon catheters. In the first case, manufacturers offer stents with intermediate diameters such as 4.5, 5.5, 6.5 mm. While in the case of stents premounted on low-compliant balloon, no intermediate measures are available due to the possibility of overdilatation of these types of balloons. Generally, the length of the stents are 10, 12, 15, 18 until 24 mm. In addition, stents with a "flaring effect" are also available. This option allows the possibility to oversize the proximal diameter of the stent at the level of the ostium.

Postprocedural imaging has been used for follow up and, to assess the effectiveness of percutaneous revascularization, clinical criteria, and laboratory findings together. Serial Doppler ultrasound (US) is a ready available technique and able to diagnose residual stenosis or restenosis (Akan et al. 2003). Anyway, Doppler US is known to be challenging; even for the evaluation of native RAs owing to patient-related factors, its diagnostic performance in patients with implanted stents is additionally hampered by metal-induced waveform distortion (Sharafuddin et al. 2001; Parenti et al. 2008; Rocha-Singh et al. 2008). Magnetic resonance angiography after stent placement is limited by the ferromagnetic artifacts caused by most stents (Tello et al. 1998). More recently, technical advances with multidector CT have pointed out with prospective studies (Steinwender et al. 2009) how CT angiography can provide excellent noninvasive technique to detect and evaluate intra-stent restenosis, in comparison with invasive DSA.

Distal embolic protection devices: this device was firstly designed for carotid endovascular interventions as carotid artery stenting. It is a sort of microguidewire which mounts on the distal part a conic shaped filter made of a membranous material as polyurethane or nylon or a windsock-like nitinol basket, 2–3 cm distal to a floppy tip (Fig. 7.5). Distal protection devices work by interrupting or filtering blood flow in the internal carotid artery. Its use in renal interventions is still under investigation. Some centers have evaluated this tool on significant number of cases (Henry et al. 2003). The most important characteristics are the ability to cross stenotic lesions and the "capture capability." Generally, they are able to entrap embolic debris from medium to large size, generally particles more than 100 μm in long diameter. The aim of distal filter is to reduce embolization during the different phases of the maneuver. Some limitations in this filter exist due to the fact that they are not specifically designed for renal arteries, but for carotid arteries. The main limitation is that the "landing zone" of the filter may end distally to the main division of the main renal trunk and so only part of the kidney parenchyma is protected by the risk of debris embolization.

### 7.3.2 Other Endovascular Interventions

Arterial embolization: renal conditions eligible to be occluded by means of an embolization procedure of a renal artery consist mainly of kidney tumors (both benign as angiomyolipomas (AML) or malignant as advanced renal cell carcinomas), the other common setting of embolic therapy is renal trauma.

From a technical point of view, this procedure needs confidence with the use of embolic materials such as:

- Coils: these are mechanical devices with a helical shape variable in diameter and length. Frequently, nylon filaments are added on their surface. Coils can be pushable or detachable: the first ones, once released from the catheter cannot be retrieved, while the detachable coils, if the final position is not correct, can be reintroduced in the catheter and changed with another coil. A recent evolution of coils are the so called "vascular plugs." They are mechanical devices made of nitinol mesh with different shapes, self-expandable and able to achieve rapid occlusion of the target vessel. Once released in the vessel, if the deployment is not correct, the device can be recaptured and repositioned. When the plug is in the right position, it can be easily detached. Compared with the coils, it has the significant advantage that occlusion of the target vessel is obtained with a single device instead of several coils.

- Particulate agents: most of them are based on polyvinyl alcohol (PVA) particles of different size from 50 to 1,200 μm. Usually, embolization with PVA particles causes a permanent occlusion of vessels of the size of the particles used. Recent evolution consists in new types of microspheres consisting of a biocompatible, acrylamido PVA macromer, which shows deformable capability, lower tendency to aggregate inside the catheter during injection with lower body reactions. An alternative are gelatine or fibrine sponge. These materials are manually reduced to small fragments by operator and then mixed with contrast media and slowly injected under fluoroscopic control. They are quite easy to use, but the main limitation is that the effect of this type of embolization is limited to a short period, and after 10–20 days, many of the vessels may be reopened.

- Liquid embolic agents: N-butyl-cyanoacrylate (NBCA) was the first liquid embolic agent applied in the clinical practice. It is a monomer acrylic glue which rapidly polymerizes when in contact with ionic media such as blood and causes a permanent occlusion. To avoid adherence to the tissue of the thin catheters required for the superselective embolization, NBCA has to be injected through a catheter washed with a 5% dextrose solution and the catheter has to be withdrawn promptly after injection. The technique requires considerable expertise; there is also the risk of undesired embolizations. Moreover,

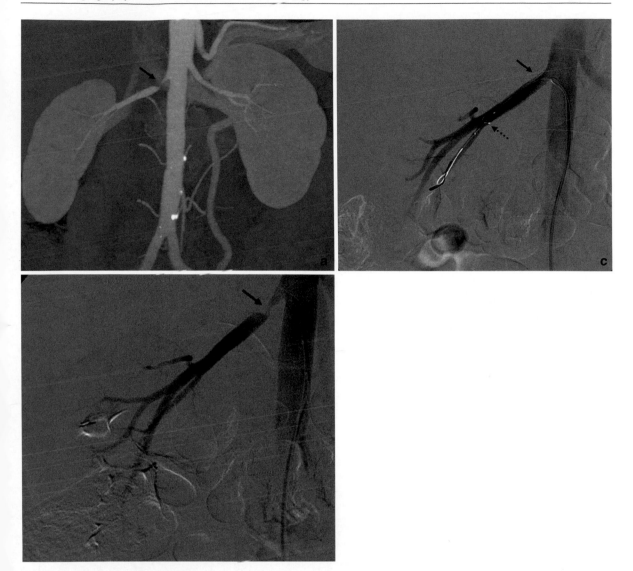

**Fig. 7.5** (**a**) 3D MIP CT-angio shows a high-grade short stenosis of the proximal right renal artery (*arrow*). (**b**) Preprocedural selective angiography confirms the lesion. (**c**) Postprocedural, a stent (*arrow*) has been placed and normal caliber has been restored. Note the embolic protection device in the distal segment of the main trunk (*dashed arrow*)

NBCA polymerizes with an exothermic reaction, causing pain to the patient. Its use was mainly diffused in neuroradiologic embolization procedures, but in the last years, this product was abandoned also because it does not have the regular mark approval for an endovascular use (CE Mark). Glubran 2 is an acrylic glue bearing a CE mark authorized for surgical and endovascular use in neuroradiology and interventional radiology. The comonomer of Glubran 2 comprises a monomer of NBCA and a monomer of Metacryloxysulpholane (MS) (owned by GEM Srl). MS allows the monomer of NBCA to polymerize with a lower exothermic reaction (45°C) and a slightly longer polymerization time (Leonardi et al. 2002). Compared to the monomer NBCA, the Glubran 2 causes less pain to the patient and is associated with a lower risk of adherence of the catheter to the tissue, hence showing a greater ease of use. Differently, acrylic glues, once deposited into the nidus, determine its permanent occlusion and prevent its replenishment through feeding branches.

### 7.3.3 Renal Phlebography

From the diagnostic point, the only role left for renal phlebography is the sampling of the blood from the renal veins in patient with renal hypertension to clarify which kidney is responsible for an increased production of the hormone renin. In these cases no particular imaging documentation of veins is required, unless anatomic significant variants are found. It is, however, important to obtain blood samples from each renal vein and from the inferior vena cava above and below the renal veins. Samples need not be simultaneous; however, it is better if they are closely spaced temporally. Renin levels from one kidney, which are >1.5 times of the contralateral kidney, are indicative of renovascular hypertension. An increased renin value in the suprarenal inferior vena cava compared to the infrarenal vena cava is also suggestive of renovascular hypertension.

## 7.4 Anatomy and Variants

### 7.4.1 Arteries

In the majority of patients, main renal arteries originate between the upper margin of L1 and the lower margin of L2 vertebrae and frequently the origin of the right renal artery is higher than left renal artery. The ostium of both renal arteries is located laterally; however, the ostium of the right renal artery tends to be located on the ventral aspect of the abdominal aorta, and as previously said and well shown on CT studies (Verschuyl et al. 1997a), there is a significant variation in its position.

The ostium of the left renal artery more frequently originates on the lateral aspect of the abdominal aorta; however, in a significant number of cases, it tends to be located on the dorsal wall of the aorta. The right renal artery in the first 1–2 cm has an anterior course and then turns posteriorly with a cranio-caudal obliquity. The left renal artery has a more linear and horizontal course. The caliber of the artery in the proximal part generally is 6 mm. The main renal artery divides into segmental arteries near the renal hilum (Kadir and Brothers 1991). The first division is typically the posterior branch, which arises just before the renal hilum and passes posterior to the renal pelvis to supply a

large portion of the blood flow to the posterior portion of the kidney. The main renal artery then continues before dividing into four anterior branches at the renal hilum: the apical, upper, middle, and lower anterior segmental arteries. The apical and lower anterior segmental arteries supply the anterior and posterior surfaces of the upper and lower renal poles, respectively; the upper and middle segmental arteries supply the remainder of the anterior surface. The segmental arteries then course through the renal sinus and branch into the lobar arteries. Further divisions include the interlobar, arcuate, and interlobular arteries (Fig. 7.6).

Renal artery variations are divided into two groups: early division and extrarenal arteries. Branching of the main renal arteries into segmental branches more proximally than the renal hilus level is defined early division (Fig. 7.7), while with the term of "extrarenal artery" two groups are defined: hilar (accessory) and polar (aberrant) arteries. Hilar arteries enter kidneys from the hilus with the main renal artery, whereas polar arteries enter kidneys directly from the capsule outside the hilus. The origin of these extra renal arteries is quite variable and

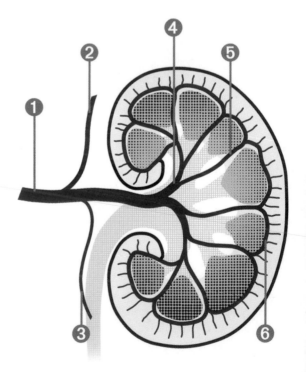

**Fig. 7.6** Schematic anatomy of the renal arteries and branching. *1* main trunk, *2* adrenal artery, *3* gonadal artery, *4* segmentary artery, *5* lobar artery, *6* arcuate artery

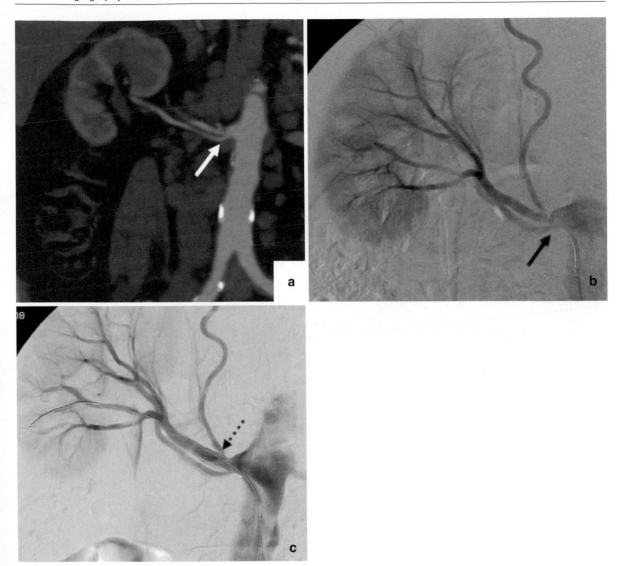

**Fig. 7.7** (**a**) CT-angio shows an early division (*arrow*) from the main renal trunk, with an eccentric stenosis of the superior artery. (**b**) Same patient, selective angiography confirms the finding. (**c**) Angiography poststent deployment

majority of them arise from the abdominal aorta over or below the main trunk. Infrequently, they may arise from the common iliac arteries. Renal artery origins arising above the superior mesenteric artery are extremely rare. Congenital anomalies of renal position and conformation are often associated with aberrant location of renal artery origins and supernumerary vessels. In particular, horseshoe kidney has a 100% incidence of multiple renal arteries (Fig. 7.8). The renal pelvis and proximal ureters are supplied by small branches of the interlobular, arcuate, and distal main renal arteries. The middle portion of the

ureters is supplied by the gonadal arteries (Fig. 7.6). The distal ureters are supplied by terminal branches of the internal iliac arteries, most notably the cystic artery.

In several anatomic and angiographic studies, it was stated that the rate of bilateral extrarenal arteries is to be 10–15% (Kadir and Brothers 1991; Talovic et al. 2004), that the rate of early division in the general population is 15%, that aberrant renal arteries are observed twice as often as accessory renal arteries and the frequency rate of extrarenal arteries is the same on the right and left sides, and that in 12% of the general population

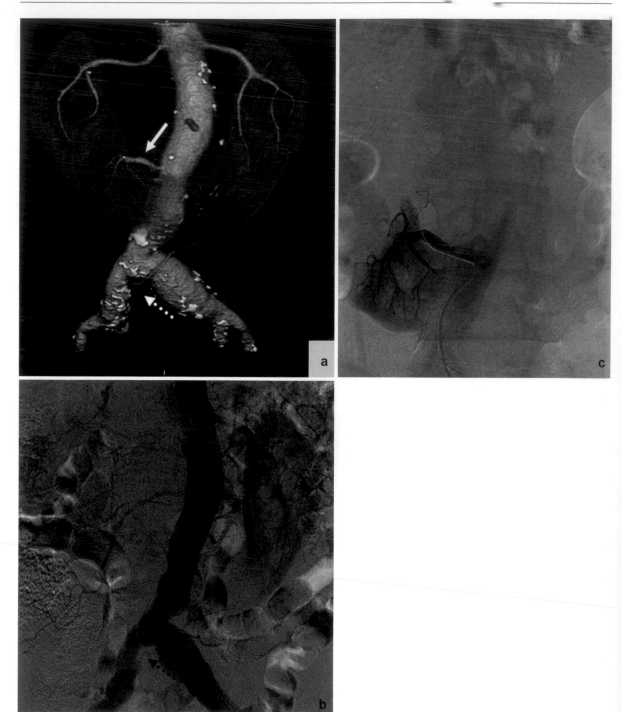

**Fig. 7.8** (**a**) CT-angio shows a horseshoe kidney in a patient with an abdominal aortic aneurysm involving both iliac arteries. Note the two polar arteries, the first (*arrow*) arising from the abdominal aorta and supplying the right inferior renal pole, and the second (*dashed arrow*) arising from the proximal tract of the right common iliac artery and supplying the left lower renal pole. (**b**) Diagnostic aortography failed to show the polar arteries, only the second (*dashed arrow*) is barely visible. (**c**) The first polar artery is later shown after selective catheterism

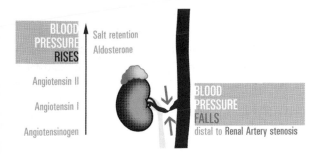

**Fig. 7.9** Shows RAS cascade. Critical stenosis at the main renal artery reduces flow and pressure distal to it. Kidney releases renin (not shown) that converts angiotensinogen to angiotensin-I (AT-I), then metabolized into the lungs to angiotensin-II, the effect is constricting arterioles and rising the aldosterone level. The final outcome is rise in systemic blood pressure

extrarenal arteries are bilateral. In a recent series (Ozkan et al. 2006), the frequency rate of early division and bilateral extrarenal arteries was 8 and 5%, respectively, which is low when compared to other major series. In this series, no statistically significant differences were detected between the frequency rates of ERA on the right and left sides, and this finding was compatible with other studies.

The renal arteries are end arteries. In contrast to other districts (i.e., the colonic and hepatic), the intrarenal collateral pathways are poorly developed. In the presence of slowly progressive proximal renal artery stenosis, renal capsular, ureteral, adrenal, and other retroperitoneal arteries may enlarge sufficiently to provide a collateral blood supply to keep kidney perfusion, but with a compromised function. Acute proximal occlusion of a previously normal renal artery results in profound ischemia due to insufficient preexisting collateral supply.

the inferior vena cava. Unlike the right renal vein, the left renal vein receives several tributaries before joining the inferior vena cava. It receives the left adrenal vein superiorly, the left gonadal vein inferiorly, and a lumbar vein posteriorly.

While anatomic variants of the renal veins are commonly visible in CT, their demonstration during renal phlebography is not so obvious and easy. Multiple renal veins constitute the most common venous variant and are seen in approximately 15–30% of patients (Kadir and Brothers 1991). Multiple right renal veins occur in up to 30% of individuals, and sometimes a single vein may divide before joining the inferior vena cava (Beckmann and Abrams 1980).

The most common anomaly of the left renal venous system is the circumaortic renal vein, seen in up to 17% of patients (Kahn 1973; Ferris 1969). In this anomaly, the left renal vein bifurcates into ventral and dorsal limbs that encircle the abdominal aorta. The posterior limb is usually the smaller of the two, although this is certainly variable. There are two common variants of the circumaortic vein: in the most frequent (approximately 75% of cases), one renal vein at the renal hilum subsequently divides before entering the inferior vena cava; in the less common variant, two distinct veins originate from the renal hilum (Beckmann and Abrams 1979, 1980). In the presence of a circumaortic renal vein, the gonadal vein will typically join the retroaortic limb and the adrenal vein will join the preaortic limb (Kadir and Brothers 1991). A less common venous anomaly is the completely retroaortic renal vein, seen in 3% of patients. Here, the single left renal vein courses posterior to the aorta and drains into the lower lumbar portion of the inferior vena cava. Alternatively, the retroaortic renal vein can drain into the iliac vein (Satyapal et al. 1999).

## 7.4.2 Veins

The renal cortex is drained sequentially by the arcuate veins and interlobar veins. The lobar veins join to form the main renal vein. The renal vein usually lies anterior to the renal artery at the renal hilum. The left renal vein is almost three times longer than the right renal vein. The left renal vein averages 6–10 cm in length and normally courses anteriorly between the superior mesenteric artery and the aorta before emptying into the medial aspect of the inferior vena cava. The right renal vein averages 2–4 cm in length and joins the lateral aspect of

## 7.5 Occlusive Disease

The majority of renal occlusive disease (>90%) is due to atherosclerosis and FMD. These pathologies can be present as clinical asymptomatic or with symptoms and signs, consisting of arterial hypertension or renal failure. Less common causes of stenosis of the renal artery are dissection, vasculitis, neurofibromatosis (NF), compression from mass effect (i.e., neoplasia, haematoma), and developmental.

The majority of hypertensive patients (95%) are affected from what is defined as primary hypertension;

in other terms, there is no structural abnormality that can be isolated as cause of the condition. In only 1–5% of the hypertensive population, the condition can be attributed to the stenosis of renal arteries, in that case it is then defined as secondary.

The mechanisms of arterial hypertension due to stenotic disease of the renal artery are based on the activation of the renin-angiotensin-aldosterone system (RAAS) (Fig. 7.9).

In the human physiology the most important mechanism to control circulatory volume on the long term is the renal-body fluid feedback system. If the arterial pressure is too high, the kidney excretes increased quantities of sodium and water, and on the other hand, when arterial pressure falls, the kidney reduces the rate of sodium and water excretion until pressure returns to normal levels. This mechanism acts over the period of several days.

The kidneys control pressure through the renin-angiotensin system (RAS). When the arterial pressure falls too low, the kidney releases a small protein (renin) that activates the RAS. This helps to raise arterial pressure in several ways, and by doing so, corrects the initial fall of pressure. Angiotensin-II (AT-II) is the end product of this chain and acts constricting arterioles and veins throughout the body, raising total peripheral resistances and decreasing vascular capacity (Guyton and Hall 2006).

This consideration explains how stenosis of renal arteries causes hypertension. This behavior has been described in the "Two-kidney one clip" hypertension model by Goldblatt (Goldblatt 1934; Glodny and Glodny 2006). In this experiment a constrictor is placed on a renal artery of an animal, thus the reduced blood flow to the kidney induces production of large amounts of renin from the cells of the juxtaglomerular apparatus. During several days, there is a steady increase in blood pressure until arterial pressure rises to a level that allows return to normal renal perfusion. Same happens in clinical renovascular hypertension.

About clinical presentation, there are some signs that are characteristics of renovascular hypertension compared to the primary form. Generally, renovascular hypertension is hard to control with drug therapy; moreover, the onset and the increase in blood pressure are usually sudden, in addition, at physical examination, a high-pitched epigastric bruit can be present. As previously stated, patients are poorly responsive to drug therapy; moreover, if treated with ACE-inhibitors or AT-II blockers, acute renal failure may appear, with consequent rise in serum creatinine.

Further manifestations of renal hypertension are left ventricular dysfunction and renal dysfunction. The first is due to left ventricular hypertrophy as a consequence of myocardial fibrosis and leads to diastolic and later systolic dysfunction with significant morbidity and mortality. The second one, renal dysfunction, may be caused by severe bilateral renal artery stenosis or functional single kidney. An important role may have been the contemporary presence of diabetes mellitus causing nephrosclerosis.

Duplex Doppler ultrasonography is a good screening test in many patients, but it has limitations in larger persons and can overlook small accessory arteries. For patients with normal renal function but a high clinical index of suspicion for renovascular disease, contrast-enhanced magnetic resonance angiography and computed tomographic angiography are the most accurate imaging tests (Hartman and Kawashima 2009) (Table 7.1).

### 7.5.1 Atherosclerotic Renal Artery

Most of the patients with a positive imaging for renal artery stenosis are asymptomatic. At angiography, atherosclerotic plaques are usually localized within 1 cm to the ostium, most often consisting of stenosis at the origin, since less than 10% of the stenosis are distal than 1 cm. On that basis, lesions can be classified as ostial stenosis or proximal stenosism, and on the other hand, intrarenal branches are affected on a variable degree. Frequently, plaque formation begins in the aorta wall with progression into the renal artery lumen, inducing the typical appearance of the ostial, usually eccentric location of the atherosclerotic renal artery stenosis.

Epidemiology of atherosclerotic plaques is focused on male rather than female gender, affecting especially individuals older than 60 years. In a large autopsy series, stenosis producing more than >50% of reduction in

**Table 7.1** Clinical presentation of vascular ischemic renal disease

| Acute renal failure (ARF) |
| --- |
| Progressive azotemia in a patient diagnosed with renovascular hypertension |
| New onset of azotemia in a patient without a history of renal hypertension |
| Hypertension and azotemia in a renal transplant patient |

caliber was found in 18% of those between 65 and 74 years and in 42% of those older than 75 years (Fauci and Harrison 2009). The quantification of a renal stenosis on angiography is based on the degree of luminal narrowing: some authors consider significant a narrowing superior or equal to 50%, while other authors tend to set a 70% degree of stenosis as threshold (Olin et al. 1995) (Fig. 7.10). During angiography, sometimes anterior or posterior plaques may be underestimated or even undetected on AP and oblique views (Cam et al. 2010). Other indirect signs suggesting a stenosis of the renal artery are the poststenotic dilatation (Fig. 7.11), the slow flow distal to the lesion, the presence of collateral circulation, and the reduced size of the renal parenchyma. Sometimes angiography may detect irregularities such as dissections or ulcerations (Fig. 7.12) of the surface of the plaque responsible for the stenosis. Calcifications of the

plaque are underestimated in DSA due to automatic subtraction of calcium; however, they can be visualized as linear artifacts at the site of the plaque (Fig. 7.13). A useful sign of the severity for a renal artery stenosis is a systolic pressure gradient >10 mmHg between the aorta and the renal artery distal to the lesion. However, it must be underlined that sometimes a catheter placed through a moderate lesion to measure pressure may further decrease the cross-sectional area of the lumen and then overestimate the gradient (Kaufman 2003).

Atherosclerotic renal artery stenosis is a progressive disease, even in initially unaffected arteries with

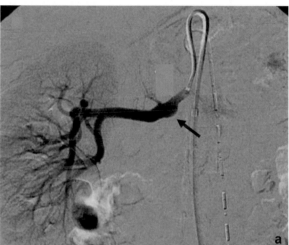

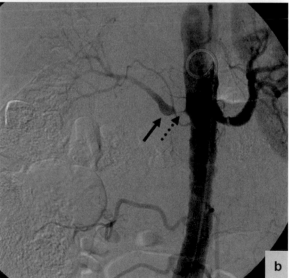

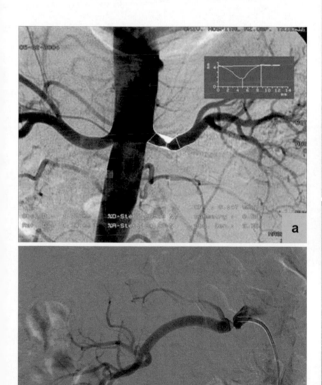

**Fig. 7.10** (**a**) Typical proximal stenosis of the left renal artery, diameter analysis. (**b**) Short high-grade stenosis of the right renal artery (selective catheterism)

**Fig. 7.11** (**a**) Vessel ectasia (*arrow*) after a moderate stenosis. (**b**) postenotic dilatation (*arrow*) after a high-grade stenosis (*dashed arrow*)

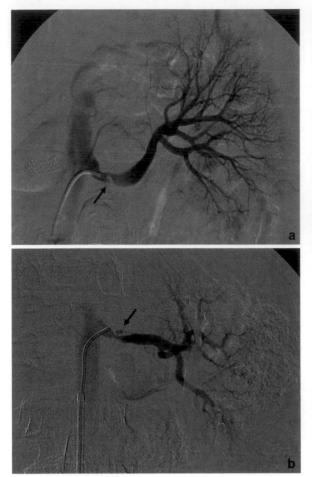

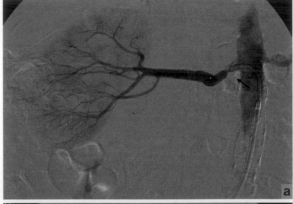

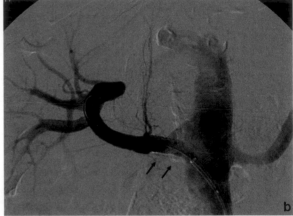

**Fig. 7.13** (**a**) Calcified plaques are commonly underestimated at angiography, but can often be diagnosed as subtraction artifacts (*arrow*). (**b**) Different patient, a calcified plaque is dislocated at margin of the lumen (*arrows*) after stent deployment

**Fig. 7.12** (**a**) Stenosis with dissected appearance of the plaque (*arrow*). (**b**) Ulcerated plaque (*arrow*) in a young boy with fibromuscular dysplasia (FMD)

up to 18% occlusion rate over 5 years (Tollefson and Ernst 1991; Schreiber et al. 1984).

In time, a stenosis can progress into renal insufficiency, especially if it is bilateral. As a matter of fact, 10% of all the patients requiring haemodialysis are related to an evolution of a bilateral renal artery stenosis. Restenosis, due to intimal hyperplasia after stenting, develops in a subset of patients and repeat intervention may be required. The incidence of restenosis after angioplasty and stenting using color Doppler has been recently assessed with result that restenosis occurs in a substantial number of patients treated. Preoperative statin medication use and increased preoperative diastolic blood pressure are associated with reduced risk of restenosis (Corriere et al. 2009).

However, no general agreement on the efficacy of endovascular treatment of renal artery stenosis by angioplasty or stenting compared to medical therapy is available. The last largest trial (ASTRAL trial) conducted mainly in United Kingdom and completed in the beginnings of 2008 in which 806 renal failure patients (serum creatinine approximately 2 mg/dL) with atherosclerotic renal artery stenosis were randomized to receive either catheter-based intervention and medical therapy or medical therapy alone failed to show an advantage of endovascular treatment over medical therapy alone. On an average, the percentage of stenosis in the renal artery was 75% and no significant difference in the baseline characteristics between the intervention group and the medical therapy group were observed. The procedure was successful in 88% of patients with a residual renal artery stenosis <50%. At 1 year, there was no difference in the change in serum creatinine between the two groups (serum creatinine increased by 0.2 mg/dL in both groups).

At 1-year follow-up, there was no statistically significant difference in the rates of myocardial infarction, cerebrovascular events, or hospitalization due to angina, heart failure, the need for percutaneous coronary intervention, or bypass surgery between the intervention and medical therapy groups (66% vs. 59%, HR 0.9 (0.66–1.15), $p=0.3$). Risk-adjusted mortality was also the same in the two treatment arms (HR 0.92 (0.68–1.26), $p=0.6$). The investigators concluded that there is "currently no evidence of benefit from catheter-based revascularisation on renal function in the ARVD patients entered into the ASTRAL study" (The Astral Investigators 2009).

Some observations to these not very encouraging results have been recently reported (Weinberg 2010). The first is the absence of a quantitative angiography which could grade the stenosis. The second observation regards the inclusion criteria and the end point: the study was finalized to evaluate improvement in renal function in patients which underwent renal artery stenting or medical therapy. However many patients had unilateral disease and 41% had a stenosis less than 70%. It has been argued that these are patients whose condition would not be expected to worsen with medical therapy nor to improve with stenting. The third limitation concerns the long period of recruitment started in 2000 and lasted at the end of 2008 and the high number of centers enrolled with a very low number of patients for some centers (two patient/year) with a superior rate of adverse events in comparison to other trials. Furthermore in this "long" period of recruitment significant advances in materials were introduced and many of the procedures were performed without "state of art" materials.

### 7.5.1.1 Endovascular Treatment of Atherosclerotic Renal Artery Stenosis

The preliminary experiences at the beginning of the 1990s obtained with conventional balloon angioplasty for the treatment of renal artery stenosis proved to be effective in atherosclerotic stenosis of the main renal trunk and in FMD with procedural success rate of 82–100% and restenosis rate of about 10% (Safian and Textor 2001; Canzanello et al. 1989; Plouin et al. 1998). However, the simple balloon angioplasty of ostial atherosclerotic lesions showed a low beneficial effect due to inferior technical success and higher restenosis rate of up to 47% over the long term and explained with the elastic recoil and rigidity of the lesion and potential dissection

(Blum et al. 1997; Van de Ven et al. 1995). The introduction of stenting has revolutionized endovascular renal revascularization and two randomized trials proved the superiority of stenting over conventional balloon angioplasty, particularly in the treatment of atherosclerotic ostial lesions. With the new low-profile premounted stents, the success rate of treatment is obtained in about 100% of cases with restenosis rates ranging from 0 to 23% (Dorros et al. 1998; Zeller 2005; Jokhi et al. 2009). The procedure, however, is not always successful and deterioration of renal function following stenting has been reported (Safian and Textor 2001; Zeller et al. 2003). Main causes are embolism and contrast-induced nephropathy. The first may be reduced by an accurate technique of manipulation of different devices and by cleaning the tip of the guiding catheter from debris collected during the engagement of the renal artery by aspiration of blood through the catheter. The use of distal protection device may be useful; however, as previously mentioned, it is limited by the anatomy of the renal artery.

## 7.5.2 Fibromuscular Dysplasia (FMD)

FMD consists of a heterogeneous group of lesions affecting the arterial wall, characterized by nonatherosclerotic intimal, medial, or adventitial thickening (periarterial fibromuscular dysplasia). It accounts for less than 10% of cases of renal artery stenosis, and 90% of the cases involve the media.

As previously stated, FMD, most of the time, consists of medial fibrodysplasia, in this conditions weblike tissue reduces the lumen of the vessel (Kumar 2009). More forms of FMD exist especially in young patients, where the distinction between neurofibromatosis and arteritis is challenging or not possible at all.

Imaging features of FMD on angiography are the typical beaded, aneurismal appearance of the middle to distal main renal artery. This pattern is valid for medial FMD, other angiographical patterns appear for less common entities (Olin 2007).

### 7.5.2.1 FMD, Variants, and Appearance on Angiography

- Medial FMD: string of beads. Most common. The beading is larger than the normal caliber. Localized medial-distal renal artery and its branches.

Seventy-five to eighty percent of the total. Some areas of thinning may develop aneurysm in a minority of patients (Fig. 7.14a, b). Infrequently, FMD may affect other districts as carotid arteries or iliac arteries as well (Fig. 7.14c, d).

- Perimedial: it occurs in young girls 5–15 years old; fewer beads of smaller diameter; collateral arteries often form around area of stenosis. It accounts for 10%.
- Medial hyperplasia: it appears as a concentric focal band; it resemble intimal fibroplasia.

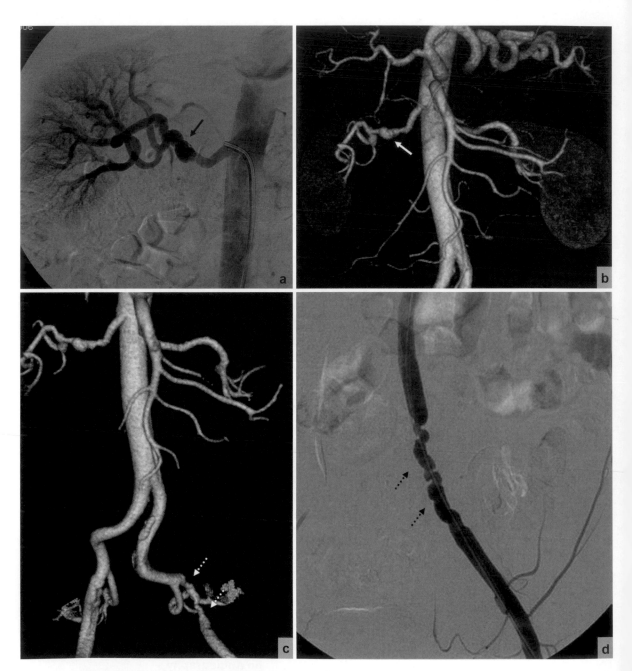

**Fig. 7.14** (**a**) Selective angiography of the right renal artery, classical appearance of the "string of beads" pattern (*arrow*) in medial fibromuscular dysplasia. (**b**) CT-angio shows the same finding: proximal tract of the main renal trunk is unaffected. (**c**) same patient, complete CT-angio shows left iliac artery is affected as well, stenosed with a beaded pattern (*dashed arrows*). (**d**) Selective angiography of the left iliac artery (*dashed arrows*), confirms

- Intimal FMD: a focal, concentric stenosis; a long smooth narrowing (that could be confused for Takayasu arteritis or giant cell arteritis) or a focal band-like narrowing. Around 10% of the cases (Fig. 7.15).
- Adventitial: a perimedial collar of focal stenosis: occasionally multiple, robust collateral network, lesser number of beads than in medial FMD. Rare.

Multidetector CT seems to be a promising technique for imaging of FMD, still some complex case could require the superior spatial resolution of catheter-based angiography for a definitive assessment (Blondin et al. 2009).

The location of FMD is typically in the distal portion of the renal artery (Fig. 7.14), but sometimes extends to the distal branches (Cluzel et al. 1994). In more or less half of the patients, the condition is bilateral. However, the degree of involvement is extremely

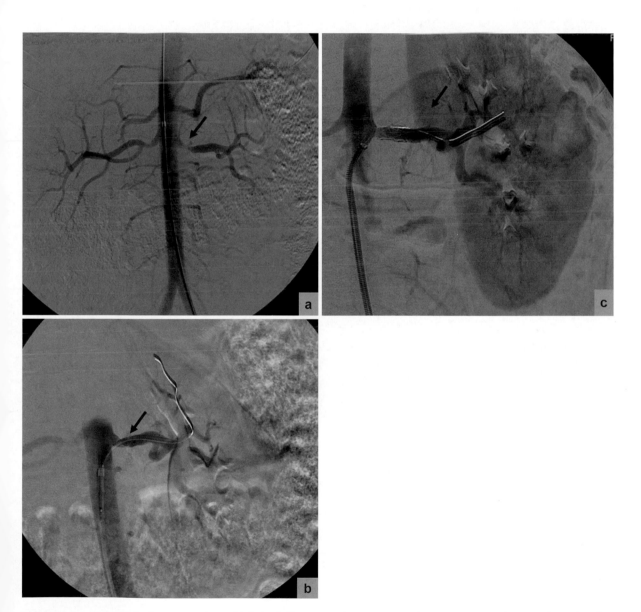

**Fig. 7.15** (**a**) Aortography in a young boy with intimal fibromuscular dysplasia shows a band-like stenosis of the left renal artery (*arrow*). (**b**) Treated with angioplasty (*arrow*), with partial results. (**c**) Later, for recurrence of hypertension after few months, a stent (*arrow*) has been placed

variable also in the same kidney in the case of multiple arteries (Fig. 7.16).

FMD can rarely produce secondary acute dissections with signs on CT scans such as a hypodense wedge (infarcts), iperdense mass (hemorrhage), and clinically with hematuria and flank pain. Intimal and periarterial fibromuscular dysplasia is more commonly associated with progressive dissection and thrombosis: anyway, macroaneurysms and dissections are complications of FMD and do not represent distinct histopathological changes (Slovut and Olin 2004).

In contrast with atherosclerotic renal artery stenosis, FMD typically affects relatively young patients: close to 30 year-old and is more common in the female sex (girls and women between 15 and 50 years of age) (Safian and Textor 2001).

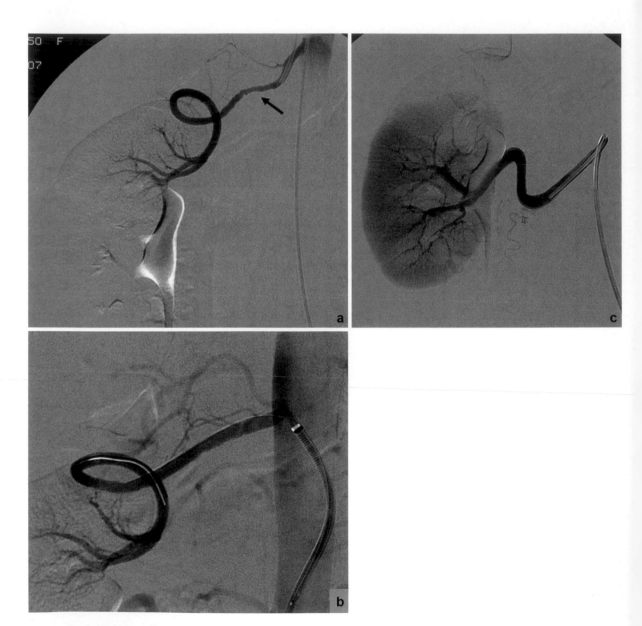

**Fig. 7.16** (a) Selective catheterism, a polar artery (*arrow*) is affected by a mild form of fibromuscolar dysplasia. (b) The lesion is treated with angioplasty. (c) Same patient, selective catheterism of the main renal trunk delineates the vessel as unremarkable

Contrary to atherosclerotic stenosis, FMD rarely leads to renal artery occlusion, and at the same time, also renal failure secondary from FMD is very rare.

The cause of fibromuscular dysplasya in unknown, even if many theories have been proposed, such as smoking, genetic predisposition, or hormonal factors.

Sometimes it could be difficult to differentiate FMD from vasculitis; anyway, the former is by a noninflammatory process, and therefore by definition, it is not associated with inflammatory acute phase reactants, anemia, or thrombocytopenia.

### 7.5.2.2 Endovascular Treatment of FMD

Before the advent of endovascular treatment, surgical revascularization was the primary alternative for patients with refractory hypertension. Technical rate of success was variable from 89 to 97% with hypertension cured in 33–66% of patients; a long-standing hypertension, high-grade atheromasic lesions, or the need for complex branch-vessel repair have lowered the change of success.

Compared to surgery, percutaneous revascularization by angioplasty technique (Fig. 7.16) is less costly, less invasive, associated with a lower morbidity, and could be proposed as an outpatient procedure; moreover, if it fails, the surgical option is still feasible.

Placement of a stent, which is a common procedure for atherosclerotic stenosis, is not advised in FMD and has been reserved for cases with complications with suboptimal results on angioplasty or especially when renal artery dissection or restenosis or persistent hypertension occurs (Fig. 7.15).

The success of angioplasty results in the reduction of blood pressure in few weeks, which represents the reduced excretion of plasma renin: technical success ranges from 85 to 100%, depending on the cases series examined. The rate of restenosis ranges from 7 to 27% over follow-up period of 6 month to 2 years.

After the intervention, there is imaging to assess the technical result of the procedure; moreover, the patients are candidates for yearly follow-up with color Doppler ultrasonography to assess the progression of disease, restenosis, or reduction in kidney volume.

As a final note, even if it lies beyond the aims of this book, we ought to remind that FMD is often a multifocal disease, affecting the extracranial cerebrovascular circulation (carotid or vertebral arteries), in association with the presence of intracranial aneurysm. More rarely, other arterial beds could be affected, such as popliteal, iliac, splanchnic, or coronary.

### 7.5.3 Other Causes

These causes are much less common and include compressive lesions on the lumen of the renal artery or other conditions that alter the wall of the vessel. It can be due to extension of an aortic dissection or iatrogenic events such as unintentional ostium coverage by aortic stent-graft or by a vasculitis. Compressions are most commonly caused by a subcapsular hematoma (from a tumor or trauma).

## 7.6 Acute Renal Ischemia

Thrombosis of the main renal artery and their branches, especially in the elder population, is a significant cause of reduction in glomerular filtration rate (GFR), and therefore, renal function.

When acute renal occlusion in otherwise normal renal artery presents, infarct of the entire organ is prone to happen within 1 h since the collateral blood supply, mostly from capsular arteries, is unable to provide enough flow. In the setting of a chronic renal artery stenosis, a complete occlusion can result in an incomplete infarct of the kidney, since the gradual development of collaterals can provide some perfusion.

Acute ischemia is secondary due to a number of conditions, from intrinsic pathology of the renal vessels (posttraumatic, atherosclerotic, inflammatory), as a complication of an aortic dissection (Fig. 7.17), or resulting from distant emboli: fat emboli, emboli from the left heart (mural thrombi, bacterial endocarditis), or paradoxical emboli (in the presence of patent foramen ovale or atrial-septal defect).

Short-warm ischemia time means that only a limited amount of cases are amenable of treatment with endovascular therapy or surgical revascularization.

Clinical presentation is variable and linked to the speed of onset: if sudden, symptoms such as flank pain, fever, hematuria, and nausea may be present. More gradual occlusions (i.e., with a renal stenosis already in place) can go undetected.

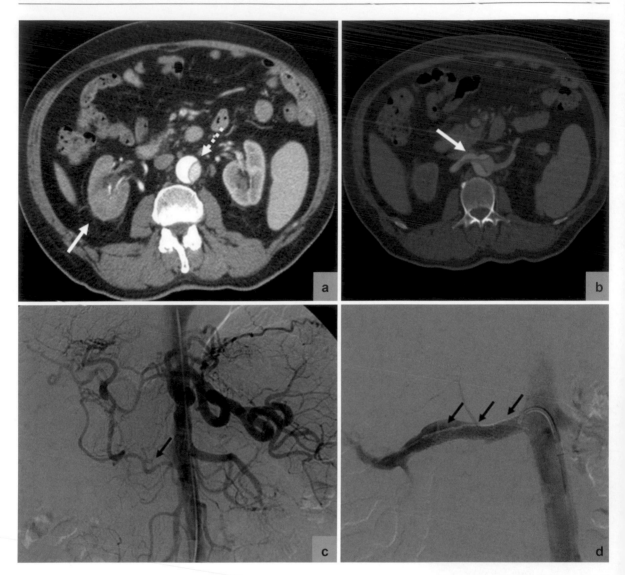

**Fig. 7.17** (**a**) CT-angio shows aortic dissection (*dashed arrow*): left kidney is vascularized while right kidney is under perfused (*arrow*). (**b**) The dissection flap enters in the right renal artery (*arrow*). (**c**) Same patient, aortography confirms the right kidney (*arrow*) is underperfused. (**d**) The right renal artery is patent after placement of three sequential stents (*arrows*)

### 7.6.1 Renal Vein Thrombosis

The thrombosis of one or both renal veins has a number of different predisposing conditions, like trauma, extrinsic compression, invasion by renal tumors, pregnancy, oral contraceptives, dehydratation, nephrotic syndrome, etc.

As in arterial occlusion, clinical symptoms are dependent from the onset; if the thrombosis is fast or abrupt, significant pain is expected, while in gradual

thrombosis the only symptoms may consist in recurrent pulmonary emboli.

## 7.7 Renal Artery Aneurysms

It can be atheromatous or manifestation of fybromuscular dysplasia. Their incidence is quite low, about 0.3–0.7 of autopsies and up to 1% of renal arteriographic procedures (Tham et al. 1983). Most of renal artery aneurysms are localized at the first or second order branches of the renal arteries and have a saccular and noncalcified appearance. Frequently, they are observed in patient with FMD, and for this reason, a female predilection is observed. On the other hand, when secondary to some sort of vasculitis, they are often distributed to the distal, intraparenchimal, branches. Mycotic or traumatic pseudoaneurysms are a differential diagnosis, but could require similar treatment.

Renal artery aneurysms are frequently clinically silent; however, association with hypertension is reported in significant percentage (Canzanello et al. 1989). Hypotheses regarding the causes of hypertension are the contemporary presence of a renal artery stenosis, microembolization from the aneurysm sac, compression or kinking of the renal artery or of its branches, and turbulent flow.

The risk of rupture is very low and decisions regarding management should be based on patient age and gender, severity of hypertension, anticipated pregnancy, and anatomic features of the aneurysm. Although size greater than 2 cm is considered a threshold for surgical treatment, rupture of aneurysms less than 2 cm has been reported (English et al. 2004). Clinical picture during this phase includes flank pain, hematuria, and shock.

The diagnosis of large aneurysms can be done with CT-angio or MR-angio techniques, but small (usually intraparenchimal) aneurysms still require angiography for a confident identification and subsequent characterization.

There are different papers concerning endovascular treatment of renal artery aneurysms and different options are suggested (Klein et al. 1997; Schneidereit et al. 2003). Until few years ago, "coiling" of the aneurysmatic sac with "free" or "detachable" coils (Fig. 7.18), with a typical neuroradiologic fashion, was the only adopted technique and it is particularly useful in the case of aneurysm located on the branch division. In the last years, with the availability of covered stent, this way

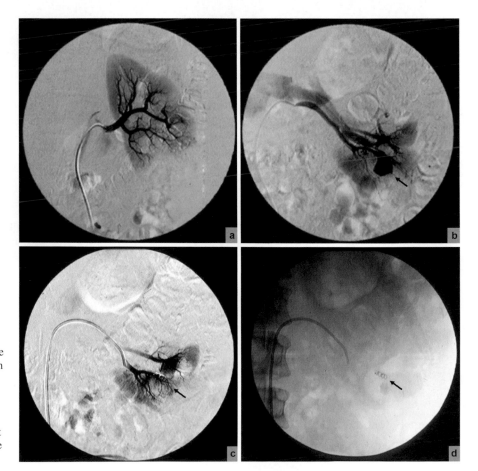

**Fig. 7.18** (**a**) Left kidney, selective angiography, the patient underwent a renal biopsy, and few days after, sudden hematuria appeared with decreased hemoglobin level. (**b**) Selective angiography of a polar artery shows the presence of a pseudoaneurysm (*arrow*). (**c**) Postprocedural, the feeding artery to the pseudoaneurysm was filled with coils (*arrow*) and lesion is no longer visible. (**d**) Direct image shows the coils in place (*arrow*)

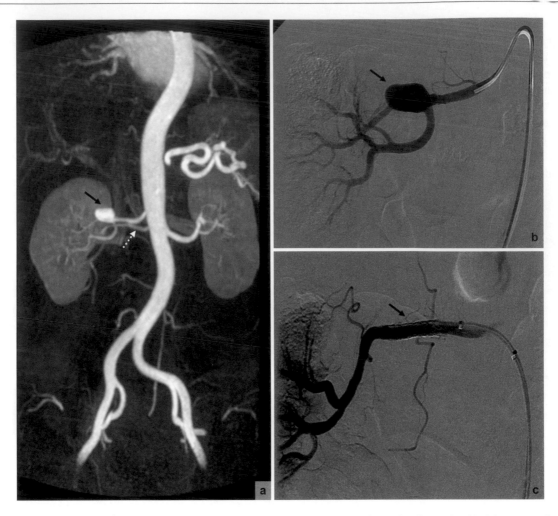

**Fig. 7.19** (**a**) Contrast-enhanced MR shows right renal artery aneurysm (*arrow*), localized on the main trunk, a polar artery is also present (*dashed arrow*). (**b**) Same patient, selective angiography confirms the diagnosis. (**c**) After covered stent deployment (*arrow*), angiography shows complete exclusion of the aneurysmal sac

of treatment was frequently reported and it is preferred when the aneurysm arises in the main trunk (Bruce and Kuan 2002; Liguori et al. 2002) (Fig. 7.19).

The possibility to use uncovered stent together with detachable coils in the case of wide-necked renal artery bifurcation aneurysms has also been reported (Manninen et al. 2008).

## 7.8 Arteriovenous Fistulas

Renal arteriovenous fistulas (RAVF) are a rare condition that can be acquired, congenital, or idiopathic. It usually affects patients who underwent a trauma or

iatrogenic accidents. Iatrogenic RAVF are the most common and are usually asymptomatic, many regress spontaneously over time. However, symptoms due to high-output heart failure are reported. Imaging with CT or MR can be difficult, especially for the detection of the site of the fistula, and angiography is required for a definitive diagnosis using a selective catheterization. However, indirect signs may be easily detected on CTA as fast and high opacification of the renal vein and increase of its caliber. Traditionally, these arteriovenous fistulae were treated by surgery, but the mainstay of treatment has shifted to an endovascular approach by coil embolization (Sendi et al. 2005; Bozgeyik et al. 2008; Klein et al. 1996), (Fig. 7.20). Embolization procedures are often difficult secondary

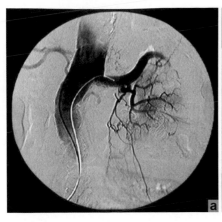
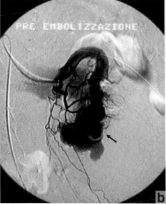
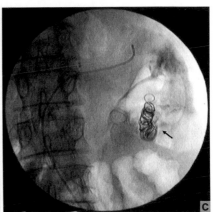

**Fig. 7.20** (**a**) Left kidney, selective angiography shows massive A-V fistula, from the main renal artery. (**b**) Later phase shows a dilated renal vein (*arrow*). (**c**) Postprocedural, the dilated feeding artery has been filled with several coils (*arrow*) and the A-V fistula is no longer visible

to problems due to "high flow" with a nonnegligible risk of distal embolization of coils. In these cases balloon occlusion angiography could be necessary (Mansueto et al. 2001). Recently, vascular plugs were also proposed (Campbell et al. 2009).

## 7.9 Trauma

Renal artery can be injured both in penetrating and nonpenetrating traumas. Moreover, iatrogenic accidents can be source of lesions affecting the main renal artery and distal branches.

Closed trauma consists mostly of renal contusions or small cortico-medullary tears: vascular pedicle of the kidney is injured only in fraction of cases, with thrombosis or dissection of the renal artery. More often than a nonpenetrating one, penetrating trauma can result in transection of the main renal artery. With the evolution of diagnostic imaging, mainly CT, there is always a more frequent possibility to detect bleeding lesions from the kidney caused by blunt traumas.

Angiography is required to assess if the lesion is amenable of treatment. Aortography is used to evaluate the basic anatomy and then selective renal angiography will be performed. From a diagnostic point of view, traumatic lesions appear as abnormal area of perfusion of the kidney with interrupted vessels or pseudoaneurysms or extravasation of contrast media and filling of the pyelocaliceal system. Angiography will

also determine if the treatment could be endovascular or surgical (Fig. 7.21).

Iatrogenic lesions happen usually during a percutaneous drainage, biopsies, nephron sparing surgery, pyelostomies, and extra corporeal shock wave litotripsy and present clinically with fresh hemorrhage in the drainage tube and may involve the renal parenchyma or the collecting system or both. More rarely, the event could result in retroperitoneal hematoma.

In selected cases, the option to manage these lesions with an endovascular approach may be considered (Dinkel et al. 2002; Brewer et al 2009).

## 7.10 Renal Transplantation

Evaluation of transplanted kidneys as a standard of care is performed with cross-sectional imaging, and most often, with ultrasonography (Bankier and Antretter 2008).

Angiography is used to provide a definitive diagnosis of renal artery stenosis and it should only be performed when percutaneous revascularization is already planned. To preserve renal function, it should be done with the lowest amount of iodine contrast agent or using protective agents as carbon dioxide ($CO_2$).

Understanding the postoperative anatomy is useful to select the correct approach for diagnostic catheter placement. The first year after transplantation is special, as it is characterized by the highest rates of acute rejection and opportunistic infections. During the first month

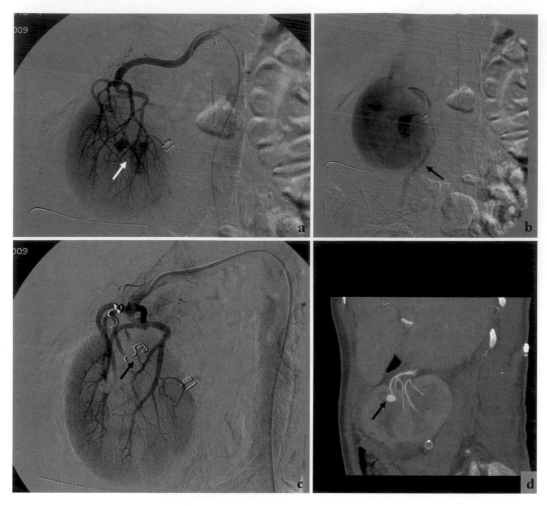

**Fig. 7.21** (**a**) Right kidney, selective angiography: multiple iatrogenic pseudoaneurysms of the distal branches (*arrow*), secondary to nephron sparing nephrectomy, are present. (**b**) Early filling of the caliceal system (*arrow*) confirms bleeding in direct connection with the urinary system. (**c**) Postprocedural: embolization with metallic coils (*arrow*) shows there is no more filling of the aneurysmal lesions. (**d**) A CT-angio was done before the catheter angiography, but it was able to show just a single (*arrow*) psuedoaneurysmal lesion

in more than 10% of transplanted kidney, a vascular complication occurs. When there is an acute thrombosis, loss of the kidney can be expected in most of the cases, due to the lack of collateral supply in the transplanted organ. Thrombosis can present early (surgical complications, acute rejection) or late due to rejection or artery stenosis. The stenosis can appear in any point of the inflow artery or usually localize far from the anastomosis, occurring predominantly in the distal segments of the donor artery. Transplant renal artery stenosis is the most frequent vascular complication following transplantation and is a potential curable cause of resistant hypertension, allograft dysfunction, and graft loss. Percutaneous angioplasty is the treatment of choice, but

the incidence of restenosis may be as high as 35%. Alternative treatment option combines the angioplastic procedure with the placement of a stent. In the experience of Valpreda and Rabbia (Valpreda et al. 2008) of the 30 allograft that underwent stent placement with a mean follow-up time of 7.1 years, all were patent at the last follow-up, with five restenosis (15.6%) of which only one needed to be retreated endoluminally.

In a similar fashion, venous thrombosis occurs early (more common, 4% of transplants) or late, the kidney can then be compromised as in arterial thrombosis.

Close to the anastomosis, pseudoaneurysms can develop, commonly caused by infection. When pseudoanerysms appear in the renal parenchyma, they are usually subsequent from a postbioptic infection. Another complication of percutaneous biopsies is the formation of A-V fistulas.

## 7.11 Neoplasms

A variety of productive lesions can affect the kidney, malignant or benign in nature. Nowadays, the role of angiography in the diagnosis of renal masses is limited and cross-sectional imaging is currently used for diagnosis and staging. Still, some angiographic details are useful to understand and manage these lesions.

Signs exist that there are always strong predictors for malignant processes, the most reliable is the venous invasion or invasion of nearby structures by the tumor.

### 7.11.1 Benign Tumors

#### 7.11.1.1 Angiomyolipoma (AML)

Renal AML are benign tumors composed by smooth muscle cells, adipose cells and have a rich vasculature. They may be solitary tumors or multiple and be associated to other manifestations (Bourneville disease). When small in size, they are asymptomatic, but if they grow over 4–5 cm in size, the risk of spontaneous bleeding significantly increase. At angiography AML is characterized by notable neoangiogenesis, sometimes associated with small asymmetrical aneurysms, and absence of shunting.

There are many reports in the literature about endovascular management of bleeding AML (Chang et al. 2007; Unlu et al. 2006; Van Baal et al. 1990) and also some reports about preventive embolization treatment in larger than 4 cm AML to avoid the risk of shock (Soulen et al. 1994; Kothary et al. 2005).

#### 7.11.1.2 Oncocytoma

Oncocytoma are uncommon benign tumors usually seen in middle and old aged people, with man more commonly affected than women (1.7:1). Angiography shows a hypervascular mass with a spoke-wheel arrangement

of tumor vessels and a typically central scar. Other signs are the absence of encasement, the detection of vascular occlusions, arteriovenous shunts, and contrast lakes. Frequently, a homogeneous tumor contrast during the capillary phase, a sharp demarcation from the kidney and surroundings, and a peritumoral halo are observed. Also, CT scan is characteristic when able to demonstrate the central scar, which shows low attenuation values compared to the rest of the lesion generally showing homogeneous high attenuation value. This tumor has a slow growth and is generally asymptomatic, and no reports about endovascular management of this lesion are reported.

### 7.11.2 Malignant Tumors

#### 7.11.2.1 Advanced Renal Cell Carcinomas

Progress in the diagnosis of early stages of renal carcinomas as well as the improvement of both surgical techniques and anesthetic procedures has lead to a change in the selection of patients for embolization. The main indications for kidney embolization of advanced renal cell carcinomas are tumors with thrombus into the vena cava or T4 tumors. Other indications are bleeding from inoperable kidney tumor or symptomatic inoperable kidney tumor causing flank pain or paraneoplastic syndromes, but asymptomatic inoperable kidney tumor can also be treated if this is the patient's wish (Hallscheidt et al. 2006). Other indications are patients with poor general conditions or with advanced metastatic disease. The complete occlusion of the vascular bed of the tumors leads to a considerable reduction in intraoperative blood loss and to simplification of the surgical preparation. By using particulate embolic agents derived from PVA or metallic coils (Fig. 7.22) or absolute alcohol or glue, palliation of a hemorrhage or of tumor-related pain in inoperable patients is usually successful in about 90% of patients (Hallscheidt et al. 2006). Although local control of the tumor disease, including complete tumor ablation, is achieved by embolization, the median survival rate of palliatively embolized patients is low (Hansmann et al. 1999). Complications of the procedure are pain due to renal infarction, which sometimes need to be treated with analgesics and transitory fever (Guy et al. 2007).

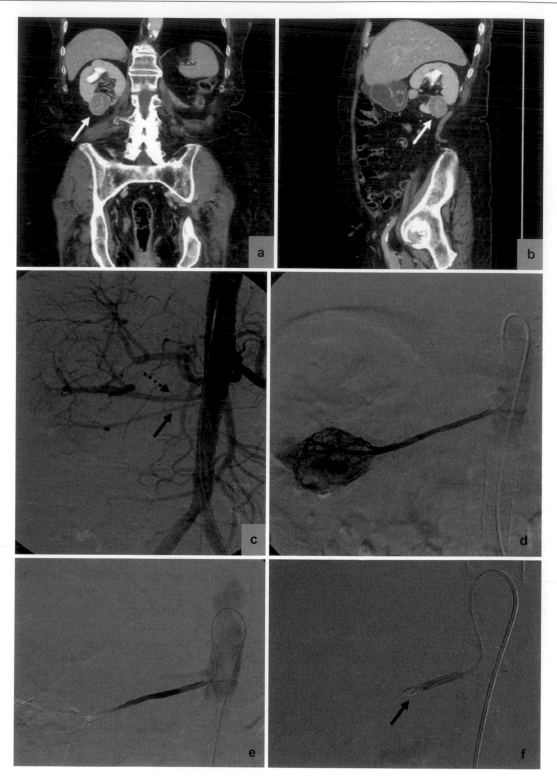

**Fig. 7.22** (**a**, **b**) CT-angio, coronal and sagittal reformats, show a renal tumor in a solitary malrotated kidney (*arrow*). (**c**) Aortography shows a main right renal artery (*dashed arrow*) and a polar artery (*arrow*). (**d**) Selective catheterism of this polar artery shows a highly vascularized tumor. (**e**, **f**) Angiography after embolization with particles and coils (*arrow*)

Kidney tumor embolization was proposed also in patients with solitary kidney (Deutz et al. 1988; Kozak et al. 1987).

### 7.11.2.2 Malignant Lesions

Renal cell carcinoma has a variable, but usually prominent degree of neoangiogenesis; it is hypervascular, with mass effect on nearby parenchima; shunting is present.

Preoperative embolization may be helpful in patients undergoing laparoscopic "nephron-sparing surgery" with the aim to reduce intraoperative bleeding.

Transitional cell carcinoma usually presents neoangiogenesis; it is slightly hypervascular and can encase nearby structures; shunting is not an usual feature.

Lymphoma is predominantly avascular, with mass effects on normal surrounding renal vasculature.

Metastatic carcinoma, depending on the primary cancer, can present as avascular (breast, lung, gastrointestinal) or hypervascular (melanoma, sarcoma).

# References

Akan H, Arik N, Saglam S et al. (2003) Evaluation of the patients with renovascular hypertension after percutaneous revascularization by doppler ultrasonography. Eur J Radiol 46(2): 124–129

Bankier AA, Antretter H (2008) Imaging in transplantation. Springer, Berlin

Beckmann CF, Abrams HL (1979) Circumaortic venous ring: incidence and significance. AJR Am J Roentgenol 132(4): 561–565

Beckmann CF, Abrams HL (1980) Renal venography: anatomy, technique, applications, analysis of 132 venograms, and a review of the literature. Cardiovasc Intervent Radiol 3(1): 45–70

Blondin D, Lanzman R, Schellhammer F et al. (2009) Fibromuscular dysplasia in living renal donors: still a challenge to computed tomographic angiography. Eur J Radiol. [Epub ahead of print]

Blum U, Krumme B, Flugel P et al. (1997) Treatment of ostial renal-artery stenoses with vascular endoprostheses after unsuccessful balloon angioplasty. N Engl J Med 336(7):459–465

Bozgeyik Z, Ozdemir H, Orhan I et al. (2008) Pseudoaneurysm and renal arteriovenous fistula after nephrectomy: two cases treated by transcatheter coil embolization. Emerg Radiol 15(2):119–122

Brewer ME Jr, Strnad BT, Daley BJ et al. (2009) Percutaneous embolization for the management of grade 5 renal trauma in hemodynamically unstable patients: Initial experience. J Urol 181(4):1737–1741

Bruce M, Kuan YM (2002) Endoluminal stent-graft repair of a renal artery aneurysm. J Endovasc Ther 9(3):359–362

Cam A, Chhatriwalla AK, Kapadia SR (2010) Limitations of angiography for the assessment of renal artery stenosis and treatment implications. Catheter Cardiovasc Interv 75:38–42

Campbell JE, Davis C, Defade BP et al. (2009) Use of an amplatzer vascular plug for transcatheter embolization of a renal arteriovenous fistula. Vascular 17(1):40–43

Canzanello VJ, Millan VG, Spiegel JE et al. (1989) Percutaneous transluminal renal angioplasty in management of atherosclerotic renovascular hypertension: results in 100 patients. Hypertension 13(2):163–172

Chang YH, Wang LJ, Chuang CK et al. (2007) The efficacy and outcomes of urgent superselective transcatheter arterial embolization of patients with ruptured renal angiomyolipomas. J Trauma 62(6):1487–1490

Cluzel P, Raynaud A, Beyssen B et al. (1994) Stenoses of renal branch arteries in fibromuscular dysplasia: results of percutaneous transluminal angioplasty. Radiology 193(1):227–232

Corriere MA, Edwards MS, Pearce JD et al. (2009) Restenosis after renal artery angioplasty and stenting: incidence and risk factors. J Vasc Surg 50:813–819

Deutz FJ, Rubben H, Vorwerk D et al. (1988) Superselective embolization of inoperable renal carcinoma in patients with solitary kidney. Eur Urol 15(1–2):134–138

Dinkel HP, Danuser H, Triller J (2002) Blunt renal trauma: minimally invasive management with microcatheter embolization experience in nine patients. Radiology 223(3):723–730

Dorros G, Jaff M, Mathiak L et al. (1998) Four-year follow-up of palmaz-schatz stent revascularization as treatment for atherosclerotic renal artery stenosis. Circulation 98(7):642–647

English WP, Pearce JD, Craven TE et al. (2004) Surgical management of renal artery aneurysms. J Vasc Surg 40(1):53–60

Fauci AS, Harrison TR (2009) Harrison's manual of medicine, 17th edn. McGraw-Hill, New York

Ferris EJ (1969) Venography of the inferior vena cava and its branches. Williams & Wilkins, Baltimore

Glodny B, Glodny DE (2006) John loesch, discoverer of renovascular hypertension, and harry goldblatt: Two great pioneers i Weinberg MD (2010) Stenting for atherosclerotic renal artery stenosis: one poorly designed trial after another. Cleveland Clinic Journal of Medicine 77(3); 164-171 n circulation research. Ann Intern Med 144(4):286–295

Goldblatt H (1934) The production of persistent elevation of sistolic blood pressure by means of renal ischemia. J Exp Med 59:347–379

Guy L, Alfidja AT, Chabrot P et al. (2007) Palliative transarterial embolization of renal tumors in 20 patients. Int Urol Nephrol 39(1):47–50

Guyton AC, Hall JE (2006) Textbook of medical physiology, 11th edn. Elsevier Saunders, Philadelphia

Hallscheidt P, Besharati S, Noeldge G et al. (2006) Preoperative and palliative embolization of renal cell carcinomas: follow-up of 49 patients. Rofo 178(4):391–399

Hansmann HJ, Hallscheidt P, Aretz K et al (1999) [Renal tumor embolization]. Radiologe 39(9):783–789

Harrington DP, Levin DC, Garnic JD et al. (1983) Compound angulation for the angiographic evaluation of renal artery stenosis. Radiology 146(3):829–831

Hartman RP, Kawashima A (2009) Radiologic evaluation of suspected renovascular hypertension. Am Fam Physician 80(3): 273–279

Henry M, Henry I, Klonaris C et al. (2003) Renal angioplasty and stenting under protection: the way for the future? Catheter Cardiovasc Interv 60(3):299–312

Jokhi PP, Ramanathan K, Walsh S et al. (2009) Experience of stenting for atherosclerotic renal artery stenosis in a cardiac catheterization laboratory: technical considerations and complications. Can J Cardiol 25(8):e273–e278

Kadir S, Brothers MF (1991) Atlas of normal and variant angiographic anatomy, 1st edn. Saunders, Philadelphia

Kahn (1973) Selective venography of the branches. In: Krieger (ed) Venography of the inferior vena cava and its branches. Huntington, NY, 154–224

Kaufman JA (2003) Vascular and interventional radiology. Mosby, St. Louis

Kidney DD, Deutsch LS (1996) The indications and results of percutaneous transluminal angioplasty and stenting in renal artery stenosis. Semin Vasc Surg 9(3):188–197

Klein GE, Szolar DH, Breinl E et al. (1997) Endovascular treatment of renal artery aneurysms with conventional non-detachable microcoils and guglielmi detachable coils. Br J Urol 79(6):852–860

Klein GE, Szolar DH, Karaic R et al. (1996) Extracranial aneurysm and arteriovenous fistula: embolization with the guglielmi detachable coil. Radiology 201(2):489–494

Kothary N, Soulen MC, Clark TW et al. (2005) Renal angiomyolipoma: long-term results after arterial embolization. J Vasc Interv Radiol 16(1):45–50

Kozak BE, Keller FS, Rosch J et al. (1987) Selective therapeutic embolization of renal cell carcinoma in solitary kidneys. J Urol 137(6):1223–1225

Kumar V (2009) Robbins and cotran pathologic basis of disease, 8th edn. Saunders, Philadelphia

Liguori G, Trombetta C, Bucci S et al. (2002) Percutaneous management of renal artery aneurysm with a stent-graft. J Urol 167(6):2518–2519

Leonardi M, Barbara C, Simonetti L et al. (2002) Glubran 2: a new acrylic glue for neuroradiological endovascular use experimental study on animals. Interv Neuroradiol 8:245–250

Manninen HI, Berg M, Vanninen RL (2008) Stent-assisted coil embolization of wide-necked renal artery bifurcation aneurysms. J Vasc Interv Radiol 19(4):487–492

Mansueto G, D'onofrio M, Minniti S et al. (2001) Therapeutic embolization of idiopathic renal arteriovenous fistula using the "Stop-flow" technique. J Endovasc Ther 8(2):210–215

Morita T, Uekado Y, Kyoku I et al. (1989) [Transcatheter arterial embolization in patients with renal arteriovenous malformation: a report of two cases]. Hinyokika Kiyo 35(10): 1761–1765

Olin JW (2007) Recognizing and managing fibromuscular dysplasia. Cleve Clin J Med 74(4):273–274, 277–282

Olin JW, Piedmonte M, Young JR et al. (1995) The utility of duplex ultrasound scanning of the renal arteries for diagnosing significant renal artery stenosis. Ann Intern Med 122:833–836

Ozkan U, Oguzkurt L, Tercan F et al. (2006) Renal artery origins and variations: angiographic evaluation of 855 consecutive patients. Diagn Interv Radiol 12(4):183–186

Parenti GC, Palmarini D, Bilzoni M et al. (2008) Role of color-doppler sonography in the follow-up of renal artery stenting. Radiol Med 113(2):242–248

Plouin PF, Chatellier G, Darne B et al. (1998) Blood pressure outcome of angioplasty in atherosclerotic renal artery stenosis: a randomized trial. Essai multicentrique medicaments vs angioplastie (emma) study group. Hypertension 31(3): 823–829

Raynaud AC, Beyssen BM, Turmel-Rodrigues LE et al. (1994) Renal artery stent placement: Immediate and midterm technical and clinical results. J Vasc Interv Radiol 5(6):849–858

Rocha-Singh K, Jaff MR, Lynne Kelley E (2008) Renal artery stenting with noninvasive duplex ultrasound follow-up: 3-year results from the renaissance renal stent trial. Catheter Cardiovasc Interv 72(6):853–862

Safian RD, Textor SC (2001) Renal-artery stenosis. N Engl J Med 344(6):431–442

Satyapal KS, Kalideen JM, Haffejee AA et al. (1999) Left renal vein variations. Surg Radiol Anat 21(1):77–81

Scheinert D, Braunlich S, Nonnast-Daniel B et al. (2001) Transradial approach for renal artery stenting. Catheter Cardiovasc Interv 54(4):442–447

Schneidereit NP, Lee S, Morris DC et al. (2003) Endovascular repair of a ruptured renal artery aneurysm. J Endovasc Ther 10(1):71–74

Schreiber MJ, Pohl MA, Novick AC (1984) The natural history of atherosclerotic and fibrous renal artery disease. Urol Clin North Am 11(3):383–392

Sendi P, Toia D, Nussbaumer P (2005) Percutaneous embolization of renal arteriovenous fistula. Vasa 34(3):207–210

Sharafuddin MJ, Raboi CA, Abu-Yousef M et al. (2001) Renal artery stenosis: duplex us after angioplasty and stent placement. Radiology 220(1):168–173

Slovut DP, Olin JW (2004) Fibromuscular dysplasia. N Engl J Med 350(18):1862–1871

Soulen MC, Faykus MH Jr, Shlansky-Goldberg RD et al. (1994) Elective embolization for prevention of hemorrhage from renal angiomyolipomas. J Vasc Interv Radiol 5(4): 587–591

Soulez G, Pasowicz M, Benea G et al. (2008) Renal artery stenosis evaluation: Diagnostic performance of gadobenate dimeglumine-enhanced mr angiography—comparison with dsa. Radiology 247(1):273–285

Steinwender C, Schutzenberger W, Fellner F et al. (2009) 64-detector ct angiography in renal artery stent evaluation: prospective comparison with selective catheter angiography. Radiology 252(1):299–305

Talovic E, Kulenovic A, Voljevica A et al. (2004) Angiographic imaging of supernumerary kidney arteries by nonselective angiography. Med Arh 58(5):263–267

Tello R, Thomson KR, Witte D et al. (1998) Standard dose Gd-DTPA dynamic MR of renal arteries. J Magn Reson Imaging 8(2):421–426

Tham G, Ekelund L, Herrlin K et al. (1983) Renal artery aneurysms. Natural history and prognosis. Ann Surg 197(3): 348–352

The Astral Investigators (2009) Revascularization versus medical therapy for renal artery stenosis. N Eng J Med 361; 1953–1962

Tollefson DF, Ernst CB (1991) Natural history of atherosclerotic renal artery stenosis associated with aortic disease. J Vasc Surg 14(3):327–331

Unlu C, Lamme B, Nass P et al. (2006) Retroperitoneal haemorrhage caused by a renal angiomyolipoma. Emerg Med J 23(6):464–465

Valpreda S, Messina M, Rabbia C (2008) Stenting of transplant renal artery stenosis: outcome in a single center study. J Cardiovasc Surg (Torino) 49(5):565–570

Van Baal JG, Lips P, Luth W et al. (1990) Percutaneous transcatheter embolization of symptomatic renal angiomyolipomas: a report of four cases. Neth J Surg 42(3):72–77

Van De Ven PJ, Beutler JJ, Kaatee R et al. (1995) Transluminal vascular stent for ostial atherosclerotic renal artery stenosis. Lancet 346(8976):672–674

Verschuyl EJ, Kaatee R, Beek FJ et al. (1997a) Renal artery origins: location and distribution in the transverse plane at ct. Radiology 203(1):71–75

Verschuyl EJ, Kaatee R, Beek FJ et al. (1997b) Renal artery origins: best angiographic projection angles. Radiology 205(1): 115–120

Weinberg MD (2010) Stenting for atherosclerotic renal artery stenosis: one poorly designed trial after another. Cleveland Clinic Journal of Medicine 77(3); 164–171

Zahringer M, Sapoval M, Pattynama PM et al. (2007) Sirolimus-eluting versus bare-metal low-profile stent for renal artery treatment (great trial): angiographic follow-up after 6 months and clinical outcome up to 2 years. J Endovasc Ther 14(4): 460–468

Zeller T (2005) Renal artery stenosis: epidemiology, clinical manifestation, and percutaneous endovascular therapy. J Interv Cardiol 18(6):497–506

Zeller T, Frank U, Muller C et al. (2003) Technological advances in the design of catheters and devices used in renal artery interventions: Impact on complications. J Endovasc Ther 10(5):1006–1014

# Nuclear Medicine

**8**

Egesta Lopci and Stefano Fanti

## Contents

## Abstract

> In the era of multimodality imaging techniques, functional information represents a remarkable aspect in medical imaging and nuclear medicine is the technique par excellence for functional information. One of the first applications of radioactive substances in clinical practice is represented by renal disorders, nowadays largely investigated by nuclear medicine examinations. Among the different physiologic processes in which kidneys take part, the excretory process is the main renal function undergoing study, basically in keeping with the characteristics of the tracers utilized in renal nuclear medicine. Investigations utilized are variegated, ranging from radioassays to challenging tests, and match with the diagnostic gap left by the other imaging modalities, by becoming in some cases mandatory.

> The aim of this chapter is to give a summarized overview of renal nuclear medicine and its principal clinical indications that clinicians must be aware of.

## 8.1 Introduction

Medical imaging is undoubtedly a vast discipline with unreplaceable applications in the modern medicine. Among the conventional imaging techniques, there is a special place for nuclear medicine, which represents a very specialized area of medical imaging concerning diagnosis by the means of radioactive materials. Unlike

S. Fanti (✉) and E. Lopci
Nuclear Medicine Department, S.Orsola-Malpighi Hospital,
Via Massarenti 9, Bologna, Italy
e-mail: stefano.fanti@aosp.bo.it

E. Quaia (ed.), *Radiological Imaging of the Kidney*,
Medical Radiology, DOI: 10.1007/978-3-540-87597-0_8, © Springer-Verlag Berlin Heidelberg 2011

radiology, whose imaging is based on transmitted radiations originating outside the patient, in nuclear medicine the radiations derive directly from the patient, who has previously been administered a radioactive tracer. This fact draws the implicit deduction that the administered substance must either enter the physiological pathways or be safely processed by the organism without interfering with the natural ongoing mechanisms. The final result comes out as visual representation of specific functional characteristics concerning the physiological pathway the physician is interested in. In this overview, nuclear medicine, therefore, can be essentially defined as a functional imaging technique.

As a scientific branch, nuclear medicine involves different disciplines, including chemistry, physics, mathematics, computer technology and medicine, whose final goal is the study of different organs and tissues through their functional characteristics.

One of the first applications of radioactive substances in physiological measurements has been represented by renal pathologies, although the effective use in clinical practice was introduced only after the Second World War (Christiansen et al. 1924; Taplin et al. 1956). Nowadays, renal disorders represent one of the main areas of clinical applications , concerning a definite branch of medical imaging, which is renal nuclear medicine.

The fundamental principles and some of the most important clinical applications of renal nuclear medicine are dealt with in this chapter and will subsequently be discussed in the following paragraphs.

## 8.2 Renal Nuclear Medicine Principles

Renal nuclear medicine, in agreement with the rest of nuclear medicine, reckons on the administration of radioactive tracers, which cover specific courses in the organism. Since its initial introduction by Von Hevesy (Brucer 1990), in the twentieth century, we recognize it as radioactive tracer, or radiotracer, a marker to a physiologic pathway, which does not interfere with the pathway and can be followed in its distribution thanks to a radioactive nuclide to which the label of tracer has been applied.. The radionuclide is represented by a prevalently gamma ray emitter isotope and the technology, permitting the

recognition of the tracer distribution, is based on gamma camera.

Gamma camera was conceived in 1957 by Anger (1957) and has eventually become the principal instrument for nuclear medicine imaging. Essentially, it is a compound of one or more detectors, mounted on a gantry, which is connected to a computer system. The detectors are substantially flat crystal planes, with the capability to "scintillate", or more precisely to flash a visible light, in response to the incident gamma rays deriving from the patient. This initial glitter is amplified and transformed in an electrical signal, which can be elaborated by the computer and displayed as a 2D image. The reconstructed image portrays a visual representation of the distribution and the relative concentration of radioactive tracer in the different organs and tissues imaged.

In renal nuclear medicine, the structures undergoing examination are the kidneys and the urinary tract with their specific functions. Among the different physiologic activities representing renal function, nuclear medicine is selectively concerned with the excretory process. It is a relatively complex activity which starts in the intravascular compartment and ends in the urinary tract with the final urine formation and the accomplishment requires a good integrity of the different anatomic components. The acquired knowledge on the renal function and on the mechanisms controlling the excretory process has led to the development of dedicated nuclear medicine examinations, which rely on the discovery of specific tracers promptly extracted and excreted by the kidneys.

The modalities utilized in renal imaging with radiotracers are variegated, but all comprise the intravenous (IV) injection of the specific radiopharmaceutical and the subsequent acquisition of the images derived from its uptake and distribution in the kidney and excretory system. In synthesis, renal nuclear medicine mainly gives information on excretory function by estimating three of the main features in this renal process, which are represented by renal plasma flow (RPF), glomerular filtration rate (GFR) and functional renal mass.

In recent years, there has been a significant advancement in nuclear medicine imaging of cancers with positron emission tomography (PET), which has been successfully used for several indications in oncology. However, in kidney tumours, PET failed to achieve widespread acceptance due to the lack of accurate tracers.

As the substances injected are radioactive, it is important for all nuclear medicine operators to optimize the relation between diagnostic quality images and minimal radiation doses. This principle is known as ALARA (as low as reasonably achievable).

## 8.2.1 Radiopharmaceuticals

Selection of the radiopharmaceutical in renal imaging is crucial and depends largely on the disorder to be investigated, as each tracer has special characteristics suitable for dedicated examinations. Broadly, the radiopharmaceuticals utilized in clinical practice can be initially categorized in two main groups. The first group includes radiotracers that are rapidly eliminated by the kidneys and can be used in the evaluation of renal function and urinary drainage. The second group comprises those tracers that are in someway retained by the renal parenchyma (cortical agents) and permit a good approximation of the functioning renal mass distribution. When considering the intrinsic features prevalently characterizing the radiopharmaceutical behaviour, it is possible to make a further division of the first group of renal tracers in glomerular-filtered agents and tubular excreted agents.

### 8.2.1.1 Glomerular-Filtered Agents

Glomerular-filtered agents are those radiopharmaceuticals that are almost exclusively or prevalently extracted by the kidneys through glomerular filtration, thereby permitting a good approximation to the GFR. The characteristics required for agents suitable for this purpose were described by Smith (1956) and are nowadays introduced in specific guidelines (EANM procedure guidelines). More precisely, the agent must be: (a) a substance filtered through the glomerular capillary membrane and not protein bound or fractioned in the filtration process; (b) a substance biologically inert, therefore neither reabsorbed, nor secreted, nor metabolized in the kidney; (c) a substance without any effect on the renal function when infused in the organism; (d) a substance quantifiable in both urine and plasma; (e) a substance radiochemically stable (Müller-Suur 1994). The perfect agent for GFR estimation is inulin, or other surrogates, but they

are not easily obtained and are usually managed in small amounts for radioassays without any imaging function.

One of these agents is EDTA (ethylene diamine tetracetidate) labelled with 51Cr. It was first used in the 1966 by Stacy and Thornburn (1966) for GFR determination. 51Cr-EDTA is a stable radiotracer commercially available, with a very low plasma protein binding, which is freely filtrated by the kidney and presents no renal tubular handling. The 51Cr-EDTA clearance has a very high degree correlation with real GFR, as it estimates values which are only 5% lower than those established by inulin (Bianchi 1972). Despite these advantages, the tracer can be used only in blood sampling with the injection of very small amounts, as a consequence of its unfavourable radiation exposure and unsuitable imaging qualities.

Another glomerular-filtered agent, largely utilized in renal imaging for decades, is DTPA (diethylene triamino pentacetic acid) marked with 99mTc. As a tracer in renal nuclear medicine, it was introduced in 1970, years after the acknowledgment that chelating agents, usually administered in toxic metal poisoning, were eliminated by glomerular filtration without undergoing metabolic alteration (Eckelman and Richards 1970; Stevens et al. 1962). 99mTc-DTPA fulfils most of the requirements necessary for agents suitable for measuring GFR (Smith 1956), with the advantage of being the least expensive renal radiopharmaceutical,

After IV injection, 99mTc-DTPA enters the extracellular fluid, without diffusing into cells because of its lipid insolubility and negative charge (Ikeda et al. 1982; Kempi and Persson 1975). It binds for around 10% to the plasma proteins (Russell et al. 1983) and is almost exclusively removed from the circulation through glomerular filtration, with negligible extrarenal excretion (McAfee et al. 1979). A maximum of 5% in each kidney is achieved 2–3 min after injection (Treves et al. 2007). 99mTc-DTPA has no tubular reabsorption or secretion, with an excellent linear correlation to clearance of other glomerular markers and GFR (Klopper et al. 1972). Despite its slightly lower GFR values when compared to references, DTPA gives some excellent renal imaging, offers simplicity of kit preparation, and has a good commercial availability (Müller-Suur 1994).

Main drawback in clinical application is its low extraction fraction (ER), conceived as the percentage of the agent extracted with each pass through the kidney, which is approximately 20%. 99mTc-DTPA, therefore, is not the tracer of choice in patients with impaired renal function (Taylor and Nally 1995).

### 8.2.1.2 Tubular Excreted Agents

The tubular excreted agents are radiopharmaceuticals prevalently eliminated through tubular excretion. This characteristic determines a high ER, conceived as the ratio between the arteriovenous concentration differences of those agents, leading to the possibility of a good approximation of RPF. The ideal extraction should be 100%, but no substance is totally extracted by the kidneys. The agent with the most effective tubular excretion known is PAH (para amino hippurate), with a clearance of only 10% lower than real RPF, which is therefore called effective renal plasma flow (ERPF). A substance, suitable for ERPF estimation, must be: (a) a substance not metabolized in the kidney; (b) a substance that dissociates from the plasma protein during transit through the kidney; (c) a substance with a high and well-known renal ER; (d) a substance that can be easily analyzed in the plasma and urine by radioassay (Müller-Suur 1994).

The ERPF has usually a good proportion with RPF in normal kidneys, but may lack accuracy especially in renal vascular diseases (Taylor and Eshima 1994). Despite that, PAH is still the standard of reference for ERPF.

Much similar to PAH is OIH (orthoiodo hippurate), which is marked either with 131I or 123I and has been largely used in renal nuclear medicine as a tubular agent. It has an ER of 85%, with an ERPF round 500–600 mL/min (Taylor and Nally 1995). When labelled with 131I, OIH has significant limitations concerned with the high gamma ray energy and the beta particle emission, which lead to suboptimal imaging characteristics and high radiation exposure, especially in patients with impaired renal function. On the other hand, 123I-OIH is an excellent renal radiopharmaceutical, but its use is limited by the unfavourable long half-time of the isotope (13 h), its high cost, and the relatively difficult availability, as a cyclotron is necessary for the production of 123I (Taylor and Nally 1995).

The radiotracer more largely applied in clinical practice for the approximate estimation of RPF is MAG3 (mercapto acetyl triglycine) marked with 99mTc. More precisely, when using MAG3, we refer to TER (tubular extraction rate) rather than to ERPF.

As a tracer, it was first introduced in 1986 by Fritzberg et al. (1986), as a result of the necessity to get around the known drawbacks of the other renal agents. 99mTc-MAG3 has nowadays replaced many of them, by becoming the principal radiopharmaceutical in renal scintigraphy.

Most MAG3 excretion occurs via tubular secretion (90%), more precisely in the late part of the proximal tubule, with an ER of 40–50% (Bubeck et al. 1990; Despopoulus 1965), more than twice that of DTPA. MAG3 is highly protein bound and only 10% of the injected tracer is filtered by the kidneys. A part of the tracer presents a hepatobiliary elimination thanks to its lipophilic characteristics. Approximately 0.5% of the injected dose of MAG3 may accumulate in the gallbladder within 30–60 min after the injection, proportionally with the degree of renal impairment and kit impurity (Taylor et al. 1988; Eshima and Taylor 1992).

MAG3 renal clearance ranges from 300 to 350 mL/min (50–60% that of OIH) and after 3 h, 90% of the injected dose is present in the urine (Treves et al. 2007), with a high kidney to background ratio. There seems to be a linear correlation between MAG3 and OIH. The former is more highly protein bound and tends to remain in the intravascular compartment (Bubeck et al. 1990). The greater proportion of MAG3 in the plasma and the increased plasma concentration compensate for the lower ER, leading to an essentially similar behaviour with OIH. The results present with almost identical renogram curves (Taylor and Nally 1995). By knowing MAG3 clearance (TER), it is possible to calculate OIH clearance (ERPF) by dividing the former with 0.56 (Taylor et al. 1988; Russell et al. 1988)

Moreover, being the MAG3 extraction 2–3 times superior to DTPA, its imaging permits a more accurate estimation of renal function even in patients with renal impairment.

### 8.2.1.3 Cortical Agents

Cortical agents are those radiopharmaceuticals that when injected get stably fixed to the tubular cells, which are mostly located in the renal cortex (cortical agents). Renal imaging this way is principally focused on the estimation of the distribution of renal parenchyma and on the evaluation of the functional renal mass. The two main tracers utilized in renal imaging are GHA (glucoheptonate) and DMSA (dimercapto-succinic acid), both labelled with 99mTc (Taylor and Nally 1995).

99mTc-GHA was first suggested as a tracer for renal imaging in the 1970s (Boyd et al. 1973), although it was till then utilized as a brain scanning agent (Waxman et al. 1975). The principal injected quote is rapidly eliminated by the kidneys, mainly through tubular transport and less via glomerular filtration. Almost 1 h post-injection, 40% of the tracer leaves the urinary tract, while 8–15% is still present in the kidneys (Arnold et al. 1975; Taylor and Nally 1995). These characteristics make GHA a tracer capable both for dynamic scintigraphy or delayed static imaging (after 2 h). The main drawbacks of static scintigraphy are related to the immediately excreted quote. In case of obstruction, the retained tracer in the collecting system may determine false interpretations of the parenchymal distribution, while in case of renal impairment the tracer tends to follow an alternative pathway, the hepatobiliary route, leading to relevant presence of GHA in the bowel after few hours post-injection (Treves et al. 2007).

At the present, the most widely used cortical agent is DMSA. It was originally utilized as an in vivo chelating agent for the treatment of heavy metal poisoning (Wang et al. 1965), and later on, was introduced in renal imaging as a parenchymal tracer (Müller-Suur 1994).

99mTc-DMSA does not have a well-defined excreting process, but is rather eliminated by a complex interaction of glomerular filtration, peritubular uptake and tubular excretion (Blaufox et al. 1996).

There seems to be a correlation between DMSA uptake and renal blood flow (Treves et al. 2007). After the injection, 90% of the tracer is bound to the plasma proteins and up to 5% is associated with red cells (Enlander et al. 1974). After each cardiac circulation, 5% of the tracer is extracted and fixed in the renal parenchyma. DMSA gets principally localized in the cortex, while only some negligible activity is seen in the papilla and medulla, with a cortex-to-medullary ratio of 22:1 and glomerular-to-interstitial ratio of 1:27 (Hosokawa et al. 1978). The unbound quote is then progressively filtered by the glomerula up to 2–3 h post-injection. Renal uptake is round 50% of the injected dose at 1 h post-injection and up to 70% at 24 h (Enlander et al. 1974).

Only occasionally, in case of severe urinary stasis in the collecting system, there is still some unfixed tracer in cycle, requiring a delayed acquisition beyond 3 h.

### 8.2.1.4 Oncological Tracers

At present, the large majority of nuclear medicine studies in oncology are based on PET–CT. PET studies provide functional information using radiolabelled tracers, with fluoro-dexoxy-glucose (FDG) being the most commonly used. PET applications in oncology have covered several indications: a) detection and staging of tumours at presentation; b) evaluation of response to treatment; c) evaluation of residual disease after therapy completion; and d) detection of recurrent disease during follow-up. For these purposes, FDG-PET has been successfully used in several clinical situations, but FDG has limitations in kidney tumours, mainly as a consequence of the fact that excreted FDG present in the urinary tract interferes with image reading and the generally moderate FDG uptake by primary renal tumours (Ramdave et al. 2001). In the literature, different authors investigated a possible added role of PET in the detection of the primary renal tumour, but in all cases PET did not offer advantages over CT (Bachor et al. 1996; Montravers et al. 2000; Aide et al. 2003).

For this reason, alternative tracers have been suggested, in particular radiopharmaceuticals directed toward tumour-associated antigens. Promising results have been obtained using Iodine labelled cG250, an antibody extensively studied in clear cell kidney cancer. The antibody showed very good specificity for renal cancer and can be conveniently labelled with 131- and 124-Iodide (Perini et al. 2008).

## 8.2.2 Principal Investigations

### 8.2.2.1 Blood Sampling

One of the most representative parameters of renal function is GFR. In clinical practice, the commonest index used to assess GFR is serum creatinine, which unfortunately gives only a very rough estimation. A patient in fact may lose more than 50% of renal function before showing an abnormal serum creatinine (Levey et al. 1991).

The technique considered as reference for the measurement of GFR is the direct assessment of inulin clearance, which is based on the constant infusion of the substance followed by serial plasma and urine samples. The main drawbacks are related to the inherent complexity of the technique and the relative invasiveness.

An accurate measurement of GFR can be obtained also with radioactive tracers, such as 99mTc-DTPA and 51Cr-EDTA (Hilson et al. 1976; Fleming et al. 1991), by the means of camera-based techniques (former one) as well as with blood sampling.

The most accurate method in the assessment of absolute GFR is blood sampling with 51Cr-EDTA, based on the calculation of the plasma disappearance of a glomerular-filtered agent previously injected in a single bolus. The clearance of the tracer is then given by the rapport between the injected dose and the area under the time/activity curve, which expresses the trend of the tracer concentration with respect to time.

For a full accuracy of the method, it is necessary to obtain nine blood samples over 4–6 h (Hilson 2003). However, a good GFR estimation can also be done with three samples taken at 2, 3, and 4 h, and in case of severe impairment, another sample at 24 h (Chantler et al. 1969). At present, the easiest method is the one described by Christensen and Groth (1986). The method requires only a single blood sample taken 4 h after tracer injection, and in case of an expected GFR of more than 30 mL/min, the technique is at least as accurate as the above-mentioned ones. When the expected GFR is <30 mL/min, three blood samples are required, and if GFR is <15 mL/min, an additional 24 h sampling is necessary.

Blood sampling is approved as the gold standard in GFR estimation, whose determination should be considered each time renal impairment is suspected, even when plasma creatinine is within the normal range.

Apart from GFR, other approved indications for blood sampling (EANM procedure guidelines) include the evaluation and the follow-up of renal function in chronic glomerulopathies, in single kidney, in chemotherapy regimen and nephrotoxic drugs administration, or before and after surgical intervention. However, in some cases, a concomitant camera-based uptake determination is required.

### 8.2.2.2 Dynamic Renal Scintigraphy

Dynamic renal scintigraphy refers to the acquisition of serial imaging after the administration of rapidly excreted agents, such as 99mTc-DTPA and 99mTc-MAG3. The examination permits the visualization of

all the different passages of the tracer from the vascular compartment, through renal parenchyma, via the excretory process, till the final urine formation. These passages can be divided into three main phases: the perfusional phase, corresponding to the blood flow (first minute), followed by the functional phase, corresponding to the renal extraction (2–3 min), and at last the drainage phase, corresponding to the urinary outflow. Dynamic scintigraphy can give a qualitative evaluation of the overall renal function and split renal function, by examining, in addition, the performance of the urinary tract.

Images are acquired generally in the posterior view with the patient in the supine position, although in particular cases orthostatic images as well as anterior views may be necessary. The acquisition starts from the injection of the tracer, which must be done in a single bolus, and continues for 20–30 min, according to the pathology of interest.

The number and duration of the images (or frames) depend on the phase of the scintigraphy. For a proper visualization of the perfusional phase, frames should be acquired for 1–3 s for the first minute. For the functional phase, 10–15 s frames are required for about 4 min, and then for the drainage phase, 10–30 s frames are sufficient to assess the urinary system (Inoue et al. 2004). However, if the evaluation of renal blood flow is not needed, the study can be performed without the first phase.

During the functional phase, there is the visualization of the renal parenchyma, mainly determined by renal clearance, which reflects GFR for DTPA and TER for MAG3. On a visual point of view, a good renal function presents with an intense uptake in the perfusional phase, while a weak visualization reflects a low renal function. The maximum tracer uptake, or activity peak, is reached 2–3 min after the injection, according to the radiopharmaceutical utilized (Boubaker et al. 2006). After the peak, the collecting system appears and there is a rapid weakening of the parenchymal visualization. In case of low renal function, there is a higher tracer concentration in the plasma, determining a less apparent parenchymal visualization and the lower vis a tergo would determine a slower excretion phase. Urinary stasis is instead seen in case of drainage problems.

After the acquisition, quantitative analyses are performed through computer-generated renogram curves and quantitative indexes are calculated from the curves.

Renograms offer an overview of the time course of renal radioactivity. For this purpose, a region of interest (ROI) is drawn for each kidney to estimate the radioactivity in the renal area, as well as background ROIs are selected for the subtraction of the activity derived from the overlapping extrarenal tissues. The background-subtracted attenuation-corrected renal activity is normalized to the injected dose, and the activity attenuation is determined via empiric equations on the basis of the patients' height and weight (Inoue et al. 2000, 2004). In normal subjects renograms are symmetric and present a rapid increase in uptake during the perfusional and the functional phases till the curve reaches the maximum activity peak (3–4 min), then the curve presents a progressive decline during the excretion phase, visible as a concave line (Fig. 8.1).

Dynamic scintigraphy can be performed either as described above or as a challenging test. The provocative substance can be a diuretic agent, usually furosemide, or an ACEi, principally captopril. In the first case, the dynamic study is called diuretic scintigraphy and is performed in case of dilated collecting system, query obstruction. The ACEi challenging test is performed in case of high blood pressure, when an underlying renovascular cause is suspected.

## Diuretic Scintigraphy

A special mention must be made for diuretic renal scintigraphy. The method comprises a dynamic study performed under diuretic challenging conditions. The aim is the creation of an acute stress to the collecting

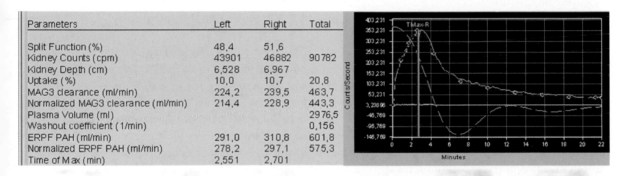

| Parameters | Left | Right | Total |
|---|---|---|---|
| Split Function (%) | 48,4 | 51,6 | |
| Kidney Counts (cpm) | 43901 | 46882 | 90782 |
| Kidney Depth (cm) | 6,528 | 6,967 | |
| Uptake (%) | 10,0 | 10,7 | 20,8 |
| MAG3 clearance (ml/min) | 224,2 | 239,5 | 463,7 |
| Normalized MAG3 clearance (ml/min) | 214,4 | 228,9 | 443,3 |
| Plasma Volume (ml) | | | 2976,5 |
| Washout coefficient (1/min) | | | 0,156 |
| ERPF PAH (ml/min) | 291,0 | 310,8 | 601,8 |
| Normalized ERPF PAH (ml/min) | 278,2 | 297,1 | 575,3 |
| Time of Max (min) | 2,551 | 2,701 | |

**Fig. 8.1** 99m-TC MAG3 dynamic scintigraphy in an adult patient. Images are compound by three different views: functional parameters on the upper left view; renogram curves (*red line* for the right kidney; *green line* for the left kidney) on the upper right view; sequential dynamic images on the lower view, acquired with a 3 s frame for the first 3 min, followed by 10 s frames for the remaining time. The study represents a normal dynamic scintigraphy, with a good split renal function (renogram curves are symmetric). The first images visualize the perfusional phase (up to 1 min), reflecting a rapid increase of the renogram curve. The collecting system and bladder appear in the third to fourth minute, after the activity peak ($T_{max}$). The excretory phase presents with rapid disappearance of the tracer from the renal parenchyma and drainage through the urinary tract, in keeping with the decreasing part of the renogram (*concave line*)

system, which should help in differing between obstructed and non-obstructed urinary tract. Published guidelines (EANM procedure guidelines) and reported recommendations suggest the use of furosemide as principal diuretic agent at the dose of 1 mg/kg in infants (<1 year of age), 0.5 mg/kg in children (up to 20 mg), and 40 mg in adults. The furosemide action generally starts 2–4 min after the administration, with maximal effect on diuresis within 15 min (Taylor and Nally 1995).

The validated timing for furosemide can be either 20 min after tracer administration (F+20), when the maximal tracer retention occurs, or 15 min prior to the injection (F-15), for a maximal diuretic effect during the examination (Hilson 2003).

F+20 method allows the observation of both unmodified renal handling of the tracer as well as the effect of an acute diuretic stress, determined by a rapidly increasing urinary flow.

F-15 method (English et al. 1987) includes the administration of furosemide 15 min before the tracer and allows the observation of the urinary tract behaviour under a maximal diuretic effect. The last method to be introduced is F+0 (Adeyoju et al. 2001). This procedure can be safely performed, as the diuretic does not interfere with the detection of the renal function (Boubaker et al. 2006), and in children, it is preferred for the unique advantage of permitting a single simultaneous injection of tracer and furosemide.

All different methods are interchangeable, because in 90% of the cases there is no significant difference in results in between the various timings of furosemide administration (O'Reilly 2003).

## Quantitative Methods

Although the "gold standard" for absolute renal function is based on blood sampling, the gamma camera-based methods are sufficiently reliable, even in infants (Piepsz et al. 2005). Dynamic scintigraphy, through a camera-based method, permits the calculation of renal clearance thanks to the fact that early renal uptake is directly related to the renal function. It is also possible to have an estimation of the split renal function (separate renal function) of the kidneys, by calculating the area under the renogram curve, in the initial part of the study, or by calculating the ratio of the slopes over a short period in the uptake phase (Hilson 2003).

There are other accurate and reproducible methods for the renogram analysis (Blaufox et al. 1996), such as the Patlak–Rutland plot (Peters 1994), the deconvolution analysis for parenchymal transit time (Cosgriff and Berry 1982; Lupton et al. 1984), the renal output efficiency (Chaiwatanarat et al. 1993), the pelvic excretion efficiency (Anderson et al. 1997), the normalized residual activity (Piepsz et al. 2000), etc.

Nevertheless, it is worth saying that all known methods used for quantitative evaluation lack accuracy in case of poor renal function (Piepsz et al. 1996).

An overview of the general indications to dynamic scintigraphy includes: (a) estimation of renal function through GFR, ERPF and split renal function; (b) urinary tract dilatation/obstruction, (c) renovascular disease; (d) congenital abnormalities; (e) renal transplantation; (f) pre- and post-operative follow up; (g) renal trauma.

### 8.2.2.3 Static Renal Scintigraphy

The principle of static renal scintigraphy is based on the stable fixation of the radiotracer to the renal parenchyma, permitting the visualization of a distribution map of the functional renal mass, with the possibility to calculate the differential renal function (DRF). Static scintigraphy conceives the acquisition of a single frame image (2–3 h post-injection), usually on the posterior view, but also in other views when necessary, such as anterior or posterior oblique images. Renal and background ROIs are drawn and DRF is estimated by arithmetic or geometric mean on the basis of the revealed radioactivity expressed in k counts.

A possible completion to static scintigraphy is the acquisition of tomographic images through the single photon emission tomography (SPET) technique. The reconstruction of the data gives way to visual representation of the images in the transaxial, coronal and sagittal planes, but despite special cases, when the 3D vision of the kidneys is necessary, the SPET images do not find a routine utilization in renal nuclear medicine.

Static scintigraphy permits a proper evaluation of the kidneys, by revealing their localization, number, morphology and dimension. This is the case of detection of any possible abnormality, including renal ectopia, displasia, hypoplasia, agenesia or any other congenital condition (horse shoe kidneys, cross fused kidneys, etc.). On the basis of tracer distribution, which should be generally homogeneously fixed in the renal parenchyma, it is possible to detect renal damage visible as areas of abnormal or irregular uptake. This is the case of acute pyelonephritis, renal scars, renal infarction, or other pathologies. Lesions usually present as hypoactive or cold areas, with regional reduction of tracer uptake, mainly located in the renal profile. In extreme cases, parenchymal damage can present with generalized hypofixation and reduced renal volume, up to a shrinked kidney (Figs. 8.2–8.6).

An overview of the principal indications for static scintigraphy includes: (a) acute pyelonephritis; (b) estimation of renal scarring; (c) determination of functional renal mass and DRF; (d) congenital abnormalities; (e) post-renal transplantation.

### 8.2.2.4 Radionuclide Cystography

Radionuclide cystography (RNC) is the nuclear medicine alternative to voiding cystourethrography (VCUG). As its radiological relative, RNC focuses on the detection and qualification of physiologic and anatomic abnormalities of the genitourinary system by producing images of diagnostic quality.

The technique contemplates two possible approaches. The first is the direct radionuclide cystography (DRC), which similarly to VCUG, requires cathetcrization of the bladder and instillation of radionuclide and fluids for a maximal distension of the bladder. Images are then acquired from the filling of the bladder to the voiding and post-voiding phases. The tracer utilized can be 99mTc-sodium pertechnetate, sulphur colloid, or DTPA, with a very low administered activity (round 37 MBq). The amount of liquids to introduce in the bladder is usually calculated through age-related formulas, which differ whether the patient is an adult or a child (EANM procedure guidelines).

Main drawbacks of DRC are related to invasiveness, similar to VCUG, and non-physiologic setting, as the bladder is forcedly filled and the urinary flow does not follow natural course.

The other alternative for RNC is called indirect radionuclide cystography (IRC), which does not require bladder catheterization, but generally follows a dynamic scintigraphy, with an IV injection of the radiopharmaceutical (mainly MAG3 or DTPA). The main limitation of IRC is the necessity of toilet trained patients. Principally, RNC is used to evaluate vesicoureteral reflux, with comparable sensitivity, but with less gonadal

radiation, when compared with conventional radiological technique (VCUG). RNC, however, does not provide the same anatomic details, and this is the reason why it is not the first-line investigation in males.

In both cases images are acquired in the posterior view, with a framing rate of 10–30 s per frame. Specific ROIs are drawn over the bladder and in the renal regions, for the elaboration of time/activity curves. Post-mincturition residual volumes are quantified with a delayed image post-voiding.

Common indications for a RNC, as reported by approved guidelines (EANM procedure guidelines), include initial evaluation of females with urinary tract infection (UTI) for reflux, diagnosis of familial reflux, evaluation of vesicoureteral reflux after medical management, assessment of the results of antireflux surgery, and serial evaluation of bladder dysfunction for reflux.

## 8.3 Clinical Applications

Nuclear medicine investigations hold a significant diagnostic role in clinical practice thanks to the remarkable information they provide. These information include the possibility to study the entire excretory system, including kidneys and urinary tract, to obtain functional data and quantify them, and at last, the possibility to perform challenging tests.

An integrated and optimal diagnostic approach must also take into account other potentialities and peculiarities, which render functional investigation generally advantageous. First of all, they are easily feasible, relatively cheap and non-invasive procedures, conceiving generally IV injections. The maximum invasiveness is represented by bladder catheterization in case of DRC. Nuclear medicine investigations utilize radioactive substances, but the radiation burden to whom patients are submitted is objectively low. An overview of the effective doses during the main examinations performed documents 0.5–0.7 mSv for a static 99mTc-DMSA scintigraphy and 0.3–0.6 mSv for a dynamic 99mTc-MAG3 scintigraphy (Fanti 2003). These values are restrained if we compare them with other imaging techniques, such as renal angiography (5–7 mSv) or TC (10 mSv).

In addition, nuclear medicine examinations are easily reproducible. The possibility to safely and reliably repeat an examination, without the risk of main discrepancies, has main relevance in clinical practice,

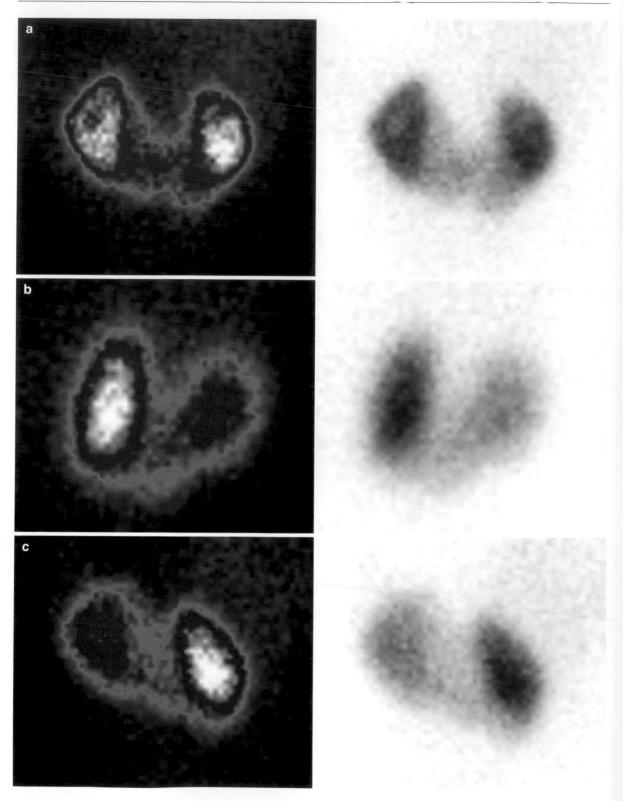

**Fig. 8.2** 99m-Tc DMSA static renal scintigraphy in an infant of 6 months of age with horse shoe kidneys. Images are represented in colour (*warm metal scale*) and in *black* and *white* (*inverted grey scale*). DRF is 49.8% for the right kidney and 50.2% for the left kidney. (**a**) Posterior view; (**b**) posterior left oblique view; (**c**) posterior right oblique view

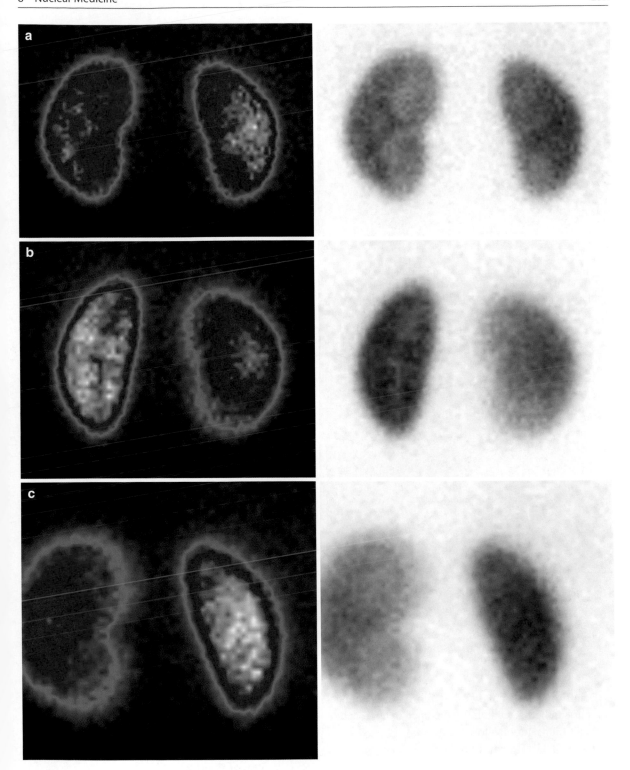

**Fig. 8.3** 99m-Tc DMSA static renal scintigraphy in a 5-year-old child. Images are represented in colour (*warm metal scale*) and in *black* and *white* (*inverted grey scale*). DRF is 53.3% for the right kidney and 46.7% for the left kidney. (**a**) Posterior view; (**b**) posterior left oblique view; (**c**) posterior right oblique view. The study reveals indirect signs of bilateral pielectasia with cortical thinning mainly in the polar regions

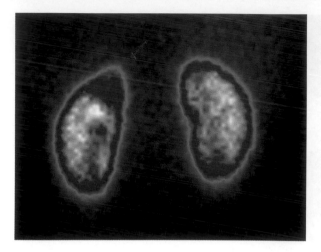
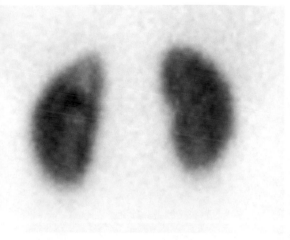

**Fig. 8.4** Posterior view of 99m-Tc DMSA static scintigraphy in a 7-year-old child. DRF is 50.5% for the left kidney and 49.5% for the right kidney. The patient presented a UTI at birth. VCUG showed no VUR and the child was referred for a follow-up static scintigraphy. Both images show a markedly reduced uptake of the tracer in the upper pole of the left kidney (*arrow*) as a result of cortical damage (renal scarring)

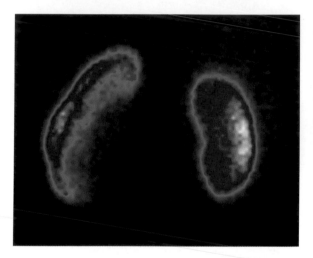
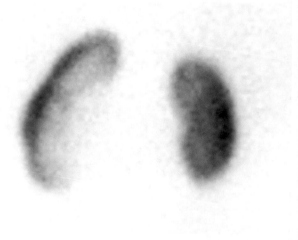

**Fig. 8.5** Posterior view of 99m-Tc DMSA static scintigraphy in an 8-year-old child. DRF is 55.8% for the right kidney and 44.2% for the left kidney. The patient had a prenatally diagnosed left hydronephrosis, resulting in an obstructed PUJ. During the first year of age, the child underwent corrective surgery with Anderson Hynes pyeloplasty. Follow-up static scintigraphy shows a large left kidney with thinned renal parenchyma stretched round the intrarenal collecting system, which is still dilated, but no longer obstructed. The right kidney shows some cortical thinning in the polar regions, more marked on the upper pole, and indirect signs of slightly dilated intrarenal collecting system

especially in those conditions requiring a functional comparison before and after a therapeutic approach or in case of long-term follow-up.

These characteristics render nuclear medicine investigations largely used in renal disorders, with main indications on detection, evaluation, and quantification of renal function, urinary tract dilatation, UTI, renovascular disease, or renal transplantation. However, any potential congenital and acquired condition may benefit from a functional investigation with a renal nuclear medicine examination.

### 8.3.1 Renal Failure

The evaluation of renal function represents an important part of the investigations performed in nuclear medicine. The methods utilized, either based on blood

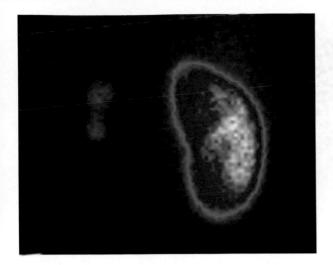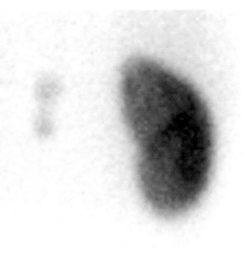

**Fig. 8.6** Posterior view of 99m-Tc DMSA static scintigraphy in an 8-year-old child. DRF is 97% for the right kidney and 3% for the left kidney. The patient presents a prenatally diagnosed hypoplastic left kidney, severely damaged in the intrauterine period. On static scintigraphy, the left kidney presents as a slightly visible area of very small dimensions. The right kidney showed is increased in dimensions, with good functional development and indirect signs of dilated collecting system, especially in the polar regions, secondary to functional compensation

sampling or camera based, are accurate and relatively simple to perform. There exists, however, a proper indication for nuclear medicine examinations in case of deterioration of renal function. Renal failure can be either an acute or a chronic impairment of the excretory function, and in an overwhelming number of cases, can be diagnosed by a specific renal scintigraphy (Fig. 8.7).

When the process develops slowly under a chronic cause, or simply as a consequence of physiologic decline with age, renal failure can be difficult to reveal and its real gravity is easily underestimated. The routine examination is serum creatinine, but it requires an important loss of functioning parenchyma to become abnormal, and can remain within the normal range despite an inulin clearance of 60–80% below normal values (Levey et al. 1991).

In this context renal scintigraphy has a proper indication in the quantification of chronic renal impairment, thanks to the more reliable proportion existing between clearance estimated by nuclear medicine methods and renal function. The strength of nuclear medicine in renal impairment is its ability to assess renal function even in case of very low levels of clearance.

Differently from chronic renal failure, whose reversibility is considered unlikely and therapeutic intervention is mainly limited to the prevention of further progression, in acute renal failure there exists the real possibility of reversibility, and hence, recovery of the function.

Nuclear medicine has no utility in the immediate assessment of acute renal failure, as the priority in the initial phases is the rapid recognition of this life-threatening condition and recovery of the reversible factors.

Acute renal failure is often multifactorial and its causes are usually classified as pre-renal, renal and post-renal. Imaging in acute renal failure has two potential roles, diagnostic and prognostic.

Pre-renal causes of acute failure are usually dehydration or shock, which when prolonged in time may precipitate in acute tubular necrosis (ATN). It is not exactly a necrosis and represents temporary and reversible cessation of renal function. ATN presents an initial phase with oliguria, followed by a progressive improvement of renal function over 7–14 days manifested with a polyuric phase (Hilson 1994). As the perfusion is generally maintained in the initial phase, the typical nuclear medicine appearance in dynamic scintigraphy would be well-vascularized kidneys, but with absent or very poor tracer concentration or excretion. With 99mTc-DTPA, we can see a good vascular pool in the first pass, but no tracer retention and no visualization of the collecting system. With tubular excreted agents (MAG3), the feature changes and dynamic scintigraphy reveals a progressive tracer uptake in the kidneys, with no evidence of excretion.

A prognostic estimation can be done on the basis of the data derived from tubular excreted agents. If tubular

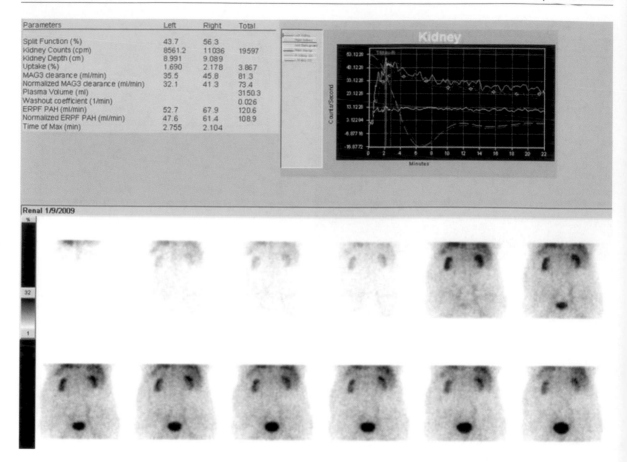

| Parameters | Left | Right | Total |
|---|---|---|---|
| Split Function (%) | 43.7 | 56.3 | |
| Kidney Counts (cpm) | 8561.2 | 11036 | 19597 |
| Kidney Depth (cm) | 8.991 | 9.089 | |
| Uptake (%) | 1.690 | 2.178 | 3.867 |
| MAG3 clearance (ml/min) | 35.5 | 45.8 | 81.3 |
| Normalized MAG3 clearance (ml/min) | 32.1 | 41.3 | 73.4 |
| Plasma Volume (ml) | | | 3150.3 |
| Washout coefficient (1/min) | | | 0.026 |
| ERPF PAH (ml/min) | 52.7 | 67.9 | 120.6 |
| Normalized ERPF PAH (ml/min) | 47.6 | 61.4 | 108.9 |
| Time of Max (min) | 2.755 | 2.104 | |

Renal 1/9/2009

**Fig. 8.7** 99m-TC MAG3 dynamic scintigraphy in an adult patient with chronic renal failure (serum creatinine is 3.8 mg/dL). Renal impairment is symmetric and can be immediately evidenced thanks to the reduced renal dimensions and the high radioactivity seen in the background. The tracer uptake is modest, bilaterally, as confirmed by the reduced amplitude of the renogram curves. The reduced vis a tergo determines, in addition, a slower urinary excretion

function is preserved, typically seen as progressive accumulation of the tracer, the prognosis is generally good. But even if tracer retention is not seen, it does not mean that there will not be any recovery (Hilson 1994).

When the cause of renal failure is a parenchymal disease, nuclear medicine role is somehow limited, as despite giving a value to renal impairment, it has nothing to offer in identifying the specific renal pathology. Size and function criteria are not exclusive for one disease or another. In addition, some parenchymal pathologies, such as glomerulonephritis, diabetes, amyloidosis, or myeloma, may present normal-sized or even enlarged kidneys, with globally reduced function. In these cases and in case of an acute deterioration in chronic failure, nuclear medicine finds a proper indication in a prognostic vision. A reasonably well-perfused kidney suggests potential recovery, although there will be a return to normal function only if before the onset of the acute failure the kidneys were normal.

The less frequent cause of acute renal failure is connected to post-renal problems, almost exclusively due to obstruction, which is one of the reversible causes of renal failure (O'Reilly et al. 2001). The drainage problem must be either bilateral or occurring in a solitary kidney, otherwise it is unlikely to reach renal impairment by a simple obstruction, as the contralateral kidney usually compensates. Although obstruction is generally detected by a dynamic scintigraphy, this is not always the case, as for severe obstruction there can be a potential renal functional exclusion. In these cases diagnosis must be a combination of different imaging techniques for the clinical manifestation.

## 8.3.2 Urinary Tract Dilatation

In clinical practice, one of the principal requests for a nuclear imaging study concerns urinary tract dilatation. The main problem to investigate in urinary tract dilatation is the presence of obstruction, which when left untreated can lead to the loss of renal function. In adults, urinary tract dilatation must always be considered pathologic, as the cause, in an overwhelming number of cases, is an obstruction, or less frequently, a consequence of congenital abnormalities, left undiagnosed. In children, urinary tract dilatation can be related to many different pathological or non-pathological entities, which can not only include exclusively obstruction, but either vesicoureteric reflux (VUR) or other paraphysiological situations, although the most worrisome condition is an obstructive system.

Presentation and diagnosis are different whether the patient is an adult or a child. In adults, obstruction is more frequently referred to a chronic condition, leading to flank pain, renal litiasis, UTI, or a progressive renal deterioration. As an acute event, it is usually a result of urinary stones, or more rarely, a consequence of iatrogenic cause (intervention, compressive masses, etc.). In paediatric population, obstruction is a complex clinical entity, mainly determined by congenital defects concerning potentially any part of the urinary tract (pelvi-ureteric junction, vesicoureteric junction, urethra, etc.). One of the most frequent causes of obstruction in children is related to a unilateral or bilateral hydronephrosis. The pathology can either be diagnosed in the intrauterine period, by means of prenatal ultrasonography, or during childhood. In the later case, clinical presentation may be similar to the adult symptoms, but in some cases the pathology can be completely silent.

Nuclear medicine can make an important contribution in discriminating between obstructed and non-obstructed system, as well as assessing the functional and urodynamic results of a corrective surgery (O'Reilly et al. 1978, 2001). The procedure of choice is diuretic scintigraphy which, compared to other imaging techniques, is essential in distinguishing patients who can benefit from surgery from those who can be treated conservatively (Boubaker et al. 2006; O'Reilly 2003).

In diuretic scintigraphy, the main drainage patterns to take into account can be classified as normal, dilated non-obstructed, equivocal and obstructed pattern.

In adults, referring parameters to assess obstruction are time to activity peak ($T_{max}$) and half time or time to obtain a 50% of the tracer washout (T1/2).

For the interpretation of data, either a visual analysis or a quantitative evaluation can be used. The visual analysis takes into account the aspect of the sequential dynamic images, produced by the summarized frames, but also the trend of the washout curves, rather than the rate of washout by measuring the T1/2 after furosemide. Prompt clearance of the radiopharmaceutical from the renal pelvis with a T1/2 of less than 10 min (up to 15 min) is considered a normal response, while a T1/2 greater than 20 min suggests obstruction (Figs. 8.8 and 8.9). Values between 15 and 20 min are considered indeterminate and should be interpreted with the context of the examination (O'Reilly et al. 1978). Approximately 10–17% of the studies will be difficult to interpret because of an indeterminate response (Taylor and Nally 1995).

Usually, in concordance with the above-described features, the corresponding renograms show indicative shapes. The washout curve for a non-obstructed kidney is more likely of concave shape, whereas the washout curve for an obstructed kidney is usually a rising or convex curve. All the other shapes, not included in obstructed or non-obstructed cases, can be considered equivocal.

Some conditions, however, may lead to stepwise or irregular curves depending on other conditions, such as large fluctuations in blood flow, VUR, double moiety, or intermittent hydronephrosis. Intermittent hydronephrosis may occur as a delayed double peak curve and can be considered as a possible fifth drainage pattern. It occurs usually 10–15 min post-diuretic injection and presents with an initially rapid tracer elimination followed by a sudden cessation of the effect or reversion to a rising curve. This type of response is known as Homsy's sign (Homsy et al. 1988) and is an indicator to an intermittent hydronephrosis. To fully clarify the pattern, a F-15 study is indicated, as in selected cases it will lead to normalization of equivocal studies (Taylor and Nally 1995).

In children, the parameters utilized for adult are not always reliable. In fact, due to the high renal pelvis compliance, even in non-obstructed cases, the response pattern in children may appear equivocal or suggestive for obstruction. In paediatric population, the criteria

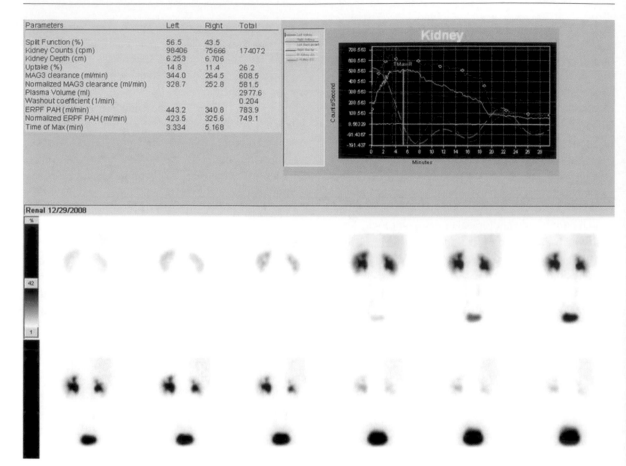

| Parameters | Left | Right | Total |
|---|---|---|---|
| Split Function (%) | 56.5 | 43.5 | |
| Kidney Counts (cpm) | 98406 | 75666 | 174072 |
| Kidney Depth (cm) | 6.253 | 6.706 | |
| Uptake (%) | 14.8 | 11.4 | 26.2 |
| MAG3 clearance (ml/min) | 344.0 | 264.5 | 608.5 |
| Normalized MAG3 clearance (ml/min) | 328.7 | 252.8 | 581.5 |
| Plasma Volume (ml) | | | 2977.6 |
| Washout coefficient (1/min) | | | 0.204 |
| ERPF PAH (ml/min) | 443.2 | 340.8 | 783.9 |
| Normalized ERPF PAH (ml/min) | 423.5 | 325.6 | 749.1 |
| Time of Max (min) | 3.334 | 5.168 | |

Renal 12/29/2008

**Fig. 8.8** 99m-TC MAG3 diuretic scintigraphy in an adult patient with bilateral pelvic dilatation, query obstruction. Images are acquired for 30 min, with the possibility of diuretic administration during the study. Both kidneys show a good tracer uptake, less prominent in the right kidney. The excretory phase is partially delayed, especially on the left kidney. Furosemide was given at 15 min after tracer injection. Sequential summarized frames show a significant washout of the tracer from the collecting system after the diuretic effect. Renogram curves confirm a prompt response to stimulated diuresis, by showing a rapid step-wise decrease in radioactivity. This sort of response is in keeping with dilated non-obstructed collecting systems

for the assessment of obstruction are more complicated and must take into account the factors effecting urinary drainage, such as renal function, hydration status, volume of the collecting, bladder status and gravity effect. However, in the overwhelming majority of the cases, the visual interpretation of the curves can give accurate results.

For a proper diuretic scintigraphy, it is important that a good hydration and paediatric patients can easily undergo dehydration. Therefore, when querying obstruction, a nuclear physician must take into account that a delayed washout can be a result of this condition, even in the absence of renal disorder (Inoue et al. 2004).

In newborns, there exists a physiologic immaturity of the nephrons, which induces to postpone diuretic scintigraphy until the age of 4 weeks. A complete renal maturity is surely present only after the second year of age (Lythgoe et al. 1994). Renal function is another potential cause of altered results in diuretic scintigraphy. Brown et al. (1992) already established that in case of single kidney GFR ≤15 mL/min, the stimulus produced by furosemide is insufficient to give a good diuretic stress on the obstructed site.

In parallel to poor functioning kidneys, huge capacity, as well as bladder distention, can give false positive tests, with poor washout even in the absence of obstruction. In children, this risk is higher, and in any

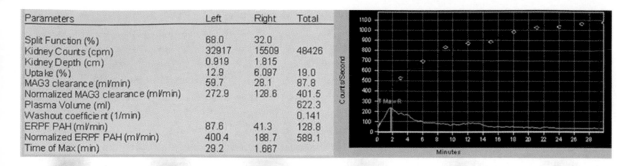

| Parameters | Left | Right | Total |
|---|---|---|---|
| Split Function (%) | 68.0 | 32.0 | |
| Kidney Counts (cpm) | 32917 | 15509 | 48426 |
| Kidney Depth (cm) | 0.919 | 1.815 | |
| Uptake (%) | 12.9 | 6.097 | 19.0 |
| MAG3 clearance (ml/min) | 59.7 | 28.1 | 87.8 |
| Normalized MAG3 clearance (ml/min) | 272.9 | 128.6 | 401.5 |
| Plasma Volume (ml) | | | 622.3 |
| Washout coefficient (1/min) | | | 0.141 |
| ERPF PAH (ml/min) | 87.6 | 41.3 | 128.8 |
| Normalized ERPF PAH (ml/min) | 400.4 | 188.7 | 589.1 |
| Time of Max (min) | 29.2 | 1.667 | |

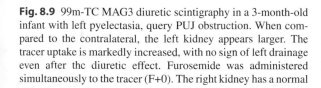

**Fig. 8.9** 99m-TC MAG3 diuretic scintigraphy in a 3-month-old infant with left pyelectasia, query PUJ obstruction. When compared to the contralateral, the left kidney appears larger. The tracer uptake is markedly increased, with no sign of left drainage even after the diuretic effect. Furosemide was administered simultaneously to the tracer (F+0). The right kidney has a normal activity, as demonstrated by the corresponding renogram, with a slightly evident stepwise response to furosemide at the 15th minute. On the *left* there is a gigantic curve, with progressive increase in activity. This feature is a result of a well-compensated PUJ obstruction

case, transient or physiologic hydronephrosis should be excluded, as they occur quite often in newborns (Chertin et al. 2006). In these cases, an F-15 study is preferred, as well as serial examinations to confirm obstruction. The principal advantage of F-15 is the reduction of the rate of equivocal cases from 17 to 3%, with significant importance when comparing results before and after corrective surgery (O'Reilly 2003).

An important parameter to consider, when querying obstruction, is DRF, which represents the contribution of each kidney with a normal range of 45–55% (Gordon et al. 2001). A DRF below 40% or a decrease of more than 5% on serial diuretic studies is generally considered indicative of renal function deterioration, secondary to obstruction, and is therefore, in most cases, used as threshold for surgery.

DRF alone is not always sufficient to assess renal function, as in unilateral impaired kidneys, the contralateral normal one compensates by inducing an apparent fall of DFR, whereas the absolute renal function remains stable (Boubaker et al. 2006).

However, if the kidney retains 20% of its expected function, the result of the diuretic study can be considered diagnostic; otherwise, as renal function deteriorates, an abnormal response cannot be used to distinguish obstruction from poorly functioning kidneys (Taylor and Nally 1995).

False negative results are less common in diuretic scintigraphy, although they can occur in highly compliant renal pelvis, or when there is an intense diuretic response with high pressures through a partially obstructed system (O'Reilly 2003). In these cases renograms may not be clearly obstructive.

### 8.3.3 Urinary Tract Infection

UTI are inflammatory processes affecting the lower and the upper urinary tract (cystitis, cystopyelitis, etc.), as well as the renal parenchyma (pyelonephritis). Principally frequent in children, UTI affects girls twice as often as boys, with 80% of the first infection being diagnosed during the first 2 years of age (Piepsz and Ham 2006). Infection seems to be easily promoted by VUR, especially if of high grade, urinary tract obstruction, renal stones, and incomplete bladder emptying.

The main problem in UTI is the possibility of permanent renal damage (renal scarring) and its long-term consequences, which can lead to hypertension, complications during pregnancy and renal failure (Piepsz and Ham 2006). Especially in case of pyelonephritis, the risk for renal damage is greater and seems to be directly related to the time between diagnosis and treatment, as well as recurrence of UTIs. Thus, a proper prevention and treatment as well as the identification of the underlying predisposing factors become crucial for the prevention of renal scarring, whose gravity is directly related to the probability of long-term complications.

UTI benefits from antibiotic regimens, oral for lower tract infections, and IV for infections affecting the collecting system or renal parenchyma (Taylor and Nally 1995). When a possible predisposing abnormality is diagnosed, an antibiotic prophylaxis can also be indicated.

Renal scarring can be a consequence of different conditions, although the most important association is the one with VUR and bladder dysfunction.

The diagnosis for reflux is usually based on ultrasound, VCUG, or RNC, while for a proper evaluation of renal damage, the best examination is static scintigraphy with cortical agents, such as 99m-Tc DMSA (Piepsz et al. 2001).

The reference method for VUR is VCUG, mandatory as first investigation in boys, where anatomic details of the urethra are necessary. The method has some drawbacks related to radiation burden and the invasiveness of the procedure due to catheterization. The nuclear medicine alternatives for VCUG are represented by RNC, such as DRC and IRC, which give useful information of urinary tract performance, including bladder, with lower radiation burden (Piepsz and Ham 2006) The main limits for RNC, both direct or indirect, are concerned with the rough anatomic information given by the study and with the unreliable definition of VUR grading, especially in low-grade refluxes. Generally for girls, a DRC is sufficient, as urethral anatomy is not usually questioned (De Bruyn and Gordon 2001).

Management of VUR is based on antibiotic prophylaxis and follow-up, especially in neonates with low-grade refluxes, which are expected to resolve spontaneously within the first 2 years of age (Pelido Silva et al. 2006). Despite antibiotic prophylaxis, however, it is not unlikely to have at least an episode of UTI, principally due to an underlying bladder dysfunction (Piepsz and Ham 2006). In case of conservative treatment failure, management includes antireflux surgery. Long-term complications in VUR, such as renal dysfunction or permanent scars, seems to require other underlying abnormalities (i.e. dysplasia) (Hilson 2003). This fact is confirmed by the demonstration that surgical intervention in these cases has no effect on the progression of renal failure (Smellie et al. 2001).

The estimation of renal damage is based principally on cortical scintigraphy (Figs. 8.10 and 8.11). 99mTc-DMSA has a high sensitivity in the detection of parenchymal defects due to infection (80–100%), but cannot differentiate between acute pyelonephritis and permanent renal scars (Piepsz and Ham 2006). In addition, it has a high negative, but a weak positive predictive value. To assess the real significance of DMSA findings in the acute phase, a follow-up evaluation is important, as among the abnormal findings during acute pyelonephritis, the risk for a permanent scar is present in 60% of the cases. There seem to be a strong correlation between the grade of VUR and renal scars, although up to 84% of the refluxing kidneys have a normal DMSA at follow-up (Polito et al. 2006; Moorhty et al. 2005). Thus, some authors propose the use of follow-up DMSA only in children with diagnosed VUR, because they were found to be at high risk of developing renal scars (Polito et al. 2006), while others 3–6 months after the first febrile UTI, to assess patients requiring further investigation (Moorhty et al. 2005).

The timing and frequency of follow-up examinations, however, may vary depending not only on institutional policy, but also on the approved guidelines for UTI assessment.

## 8.3.4 Renovascular Hypertension

Renovascular hypertension (RVH) is a clinical condition manifested by an elevated blood pressure

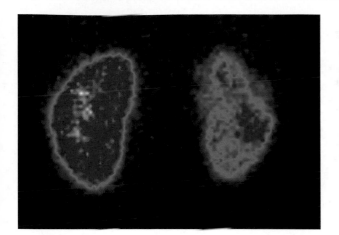
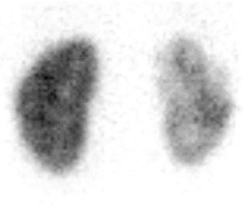

**Fig. 8.10** Posterior view of 99m-Tc DMSA static scintigraphy in a 6-year-old child. DRF is 32.6% for the right kidney and 67.4% for the left kidney. The patient presented with a severe UTI in keeping with an acute pyelonephritis. Static renography, performed during IV antibiotic therapy, documents a severe hypofixation of the tracer on the right kidney, in keeping with diffused parenchymal involvement. The left kidney is slightly involved, presenting with homogeneously reduced tracer uptake

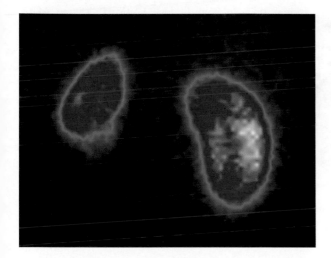
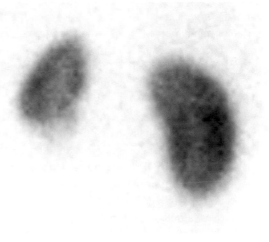

**Fig. 8.11** Posterior view of 99m-Tc DMSA static scintigraphy in a 7-year-old child. DRF is 69% for the right kidney and 31% for the left kidney. The patient presented recurrent UTIs from the first year of age. VCUG documented a double moiety in the left kidney and bilateral VUR. Static scintigraphy in the left kidney shows a severe damage in the lower moiety, which seems functionally excluded, and a severe to moderate parenchymal damage in the upper moiety. On the right kidney there is an initial cortical thinning in the upper pole in the context of dilated intrarenal collecting system

secondary to a stenotic or obstructive lesion within the renal artery. Fifteen to thirty percent of patients with refractory hypertension (Zeller 2005) are reported to have a RVH, which represents overall 3–5% of all hypertensive patients. Not all renal artery stenosis are responsible for RVH, as primary hypertension may coexist, thus diagnosis can be made only retrospectively once the renal artery obstruction has been corrected (Senitko and Fenves 2005). A 50% stenosis of the renal artery is generally considered as threshold for the onset of hemodynamic anomalies, although it is not unlikely to have clinical manifestation even in stenosis narrowing less than 50% of the renal artery lumen (Schreij et al. 1996).

Most frequently (79–90%), renal artery stenosis is due to an atherosclerotic process, affecting commonly older men, while in the remaining 10–30%, it is secondary to fibromuscular dysplasia, predominantly seen in young females (Senitko and Fenves 2005). RVH can also be seen in infants, usually after a renal artery thrombosis post umbilical artery catheterization or coartation of the aorta.

Hemodynamic changes in RVH are a consequence of the activation of the renin-angiotenin system with concomitant release of angiotensin II and aldosterone to maintain physiologic renal perfusion by increasing blood pressure (Radermacher and Haller 2003). The potential recovery of the pathology is mostly feasible in an acute phase, as in a chronic phase, both pharmacologic therapy and relief of the obstruction have been shown as less effective in hypertension recovery (Boubaker et al. 2006). Despite suggestive clinical features, suspicion alone is not sufficient for an invasive procedure such as renal angiography, which remains the gold standard technique for revealing the presence of renal artery stenosis. An accurate, safe and relatively cheap procedure capable of giving remarkable information functional significance of the renal artery lesions is dynamic scintigraphy with ACEi challenging.

ACEi inhibits the effect of compensatory response of the renin-angiotensin system on the renal artery stenosis, by reducing the conversion of angiotensin I to angiotensin II, thereby diminishing the vasoconstriction of the efferent arteriole and decreasing the GFR (Taylor et al. 2003). Standard procedure is well defined and comprises administration of an ACEi, commonly captopril (25–50 mg), 1 h before the scanning (Fommei et al. 1993). In patients with chronic therapy with ACEi, it is recommended to suspend treatment 4–7days prior to the scan.

Main drawbacks are related to reduced accuracy in case of renal impairment, bilateral stenosis, or unilateral stenosis in patients with only one kidney. In order to overcome some of the above-mentioned questions, an association with the baseline test is recommended (Boubaker et al. 2006) (Fig. 8.12).

ACEi scintigraphy can be performed with both glomerular-filtered or tubular excreted agents. Pure glomerular agents, such as DTPA, in affected kidney tend to decrease their uptake after ACEi, which is often manifested as a change in the absolute or relative renal uptake compared to the baseline study (Taylor and Nally 1995). Unless the stenosis is unilateral and severe, the relative uptake of MAG3 does not usually change with respect to baseline study, and RVH can be detected thanks to cortical retention following ACEi. The tracer progressively accumulates in the renal cortex because the reduced glomerular filtration, secondary to the ACEi effect, determines a decreased flow in the renal tubules, and therefore, a delayed washout of the radiotracer.

Both the sequential images and the computer-generated time activity curves provide helpful information about renal size, perfusion, and excretory capacity. There exists a high probability of RVH (>90%) when a marked deterioration of the renogram curve is noted after ACEi when compared to the baseline findings, while the probability is low (<10%) when normal findings are seen during ACEi even in case of abnormal baseline study (Inoue et al. 2004). Other effects diagnosing RVH include a functionally excluded kidney or a delayed $T_{max}$ (>11 min) following ACEi, marked cortical retention of tracer after ACEi, and marked decrease in GFR. A decrease in relative function following ACEi that exceeds 5% is usually considered a significant sign.

The therapeutic option for RVH is not exclusively invasive such as percutaneous transluminal renal angioplasty or surgical intervention, but can also include pharmacological regimens (Senitko and Fenves 2005). Functional testing with ACEi challenging scintigraphy seems to better predict therapeutic outcome of RVH than does renal angiography (Harward et al. 1995), with an overall sensitivity and specificity round 90% (Taylor and Nally 1995).

### 8.3.5 Renal Transplantation

Another clinical indication for a nuclear medicine study is related to the assessment of renal function in case of renal transplantation. It is nowadays a routine procedure, which can dramatically change survival and quality of life of the patients undergoing graft. The general overview of both donor and recipient conceives multidisciplinary investigations, which includes renal nuclear medicine.

At first, a dynamic scintigraphy can be performed in the donor before the intervention, in keeping with the known functional and drainage information the study offers. It is not performed in clinical routine, but

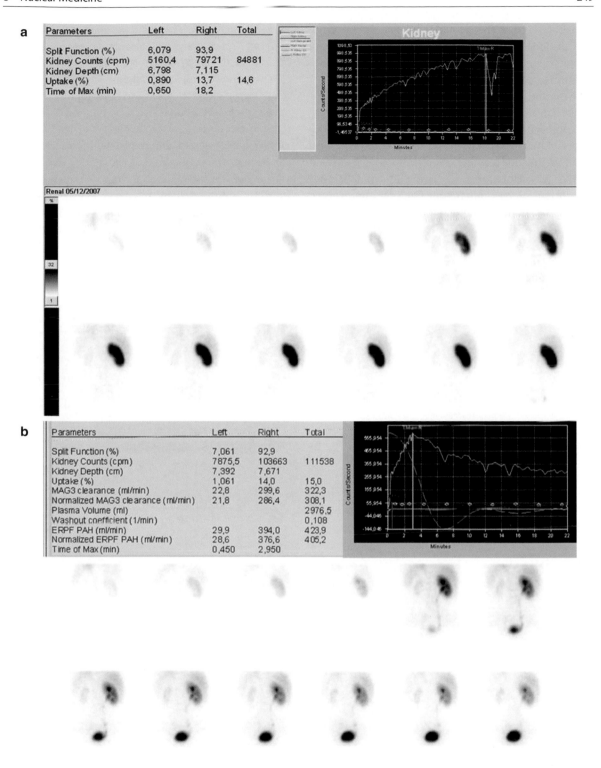

**Fig. 8.12** 99m-TC MAG3 dynamic scintigraphy in an elderly patient with bilateral renovascular disease; severe left renal artery stenosis, query for right kidney function. (**a**) ACEi challenging study 1 h after the administration of 50 mg captopril: the left kidney is almost completely functionally excluded; the right kidney shows a significant delay in tracer uptake, which has a progressive entrapment in the renal parenchyma and almost no urinary tract visualization. Renograms reveal a *left curve* similar to the background activity and a *right curve* in progressive increase. (**b**) Baseline dynamic renography: the left kidney is confirmed as functionally excluded; the right kidney shows a good tracer extraction and an almost normal excretory phase. Slight retardation can be picked out, as the renogram appears less concave in the second part of the curve, when compared to a normal study

in parallel to the other required criteria, the investigation excludes any misdiagnosed pathologic condition related to the excretory renal function and urinary tract performance.

After the transplantation, the main questions to elucidate are related to the possible graft complications, both immediate or delayed ones (Boubaker et al. 2006). Shortly after the operation, there can be a delayed graft, mainly due to acute complications such as rejection, ATN, vascular, or urinary problems. Complications may occur after an initial graft function improvement or longer after the operation. These complications may be a result of the same conditions arisen in the acute phase, but also of late onset conditions, such as chronic allograft nephropathy, renovascular hypertension, UTI, obstructive or refluxing uropathy, etc.

The principal nuclear medicine studies involved in renal transplantation are based on rapidly excreted agents, preferably 99mTc-MAG3 (Fig. 8.13), thanks to its high excretion rate, and more rarely on 99mTc-DTPA. Occasionally, a static scintigraphy, with 99mTc-DMSA, can be performed, query renal damage.

In renal transplantation, an important parameter to assess is represented by renal perfusion; thus when performing a dynamic scintigraphy, the flow phase (blood pool) should be acquired with a rapid frame

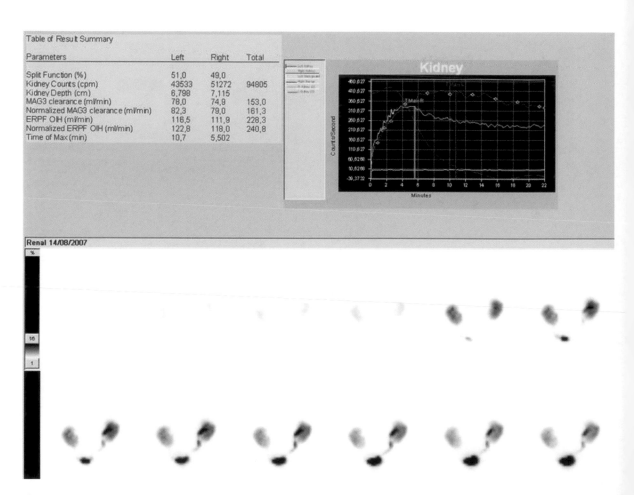

**Fig. 8.13** 99m-TC MAG3 dynamic scintigraphy in an adult patient 1 month after a double renal transplantation. Images are obtained in an anterior view at the level of the lower abdomen. Uptake of the tracer is preserved bilaterally. There is some delay on the parenchymal transit time, especially in the kidney sighted in the left. Non-significant urinary tract obstruction is seen, but there is some urinary stasis in the left collecting system. The study is within a good renal transplantation result, according to the delayed recovery of a complete function after the operation

sequence (1 s per frame). Abnormal findings can range from complete renal exclusion during the perfusion phase, due to a vascular occlusion, to a delayed tracer uptake or cortical retention, in case of arterial stenosis. An acute event may be represented by ATN, which performs similarly to the same condition during an acute renal failure, while acute rejection may appear with a rather reduced perfusion and patchy blood pool image. The later one is the most worrisome condition after renal allograft, although a good selection of recipient and donor reduces the recurrence of this undesirable event.

Renal function post-transplantation may reach almost normal values, represented by a good tracer clearance (mainly ERPF or TER) and reasonably good renogram trend. However, in an overwhelming number of cases, quantitative values are closer to the lower normal limit and renogram curves may show variable drainage patterns. These features must take into account the new anatomic location, which interferes with renal performance both through vascular and drainage phase. In any case, the same clinical indications for nuclear medicine examinations used in native renal disorders can be prescribed for transplanted kidneys too.

### 8.3.6 Renal Cancer

FDG-PET does not seem to be a valid tool for the detection of primary renal malignancy due to a low sensitivity, ranging from 40 to 94%, with no advantage over CT (Fig. 8.14).

Some authors suggested that FDG-PET may be useful for the detection of distant metastasis (Majhail et al. 2003; Kang et al. 2004) from renal carcinoma, a very important issue since the presence of second-arisms is an independent predictor of poor outcome. For retroperitoneal lymph node metastases and/or renal bed recurrence, PET sensitivity and specificity were 75.0% and 100.0% respectively (vs. 92.6% sensitivity and 98.1% specificity for abdominal CT). Also, PET had a sensitivity of 75.0% and a specificity of 97.1% for metastases to the lung parenchyma compared to 91.1 and 73.1%, respectively, for chest CT. PET had a

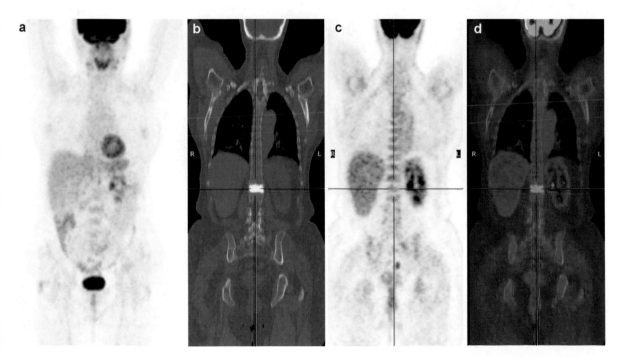

**Fig. 8.14** F-FDG PET–CT scan of a patient studied for re-staging of a clear cell renal cancer. (**a**) No area of pathologic tracer uptake. In the coronal images of CT (**b**), PET (**c**) and fusion (**d**), it is shown a known lesion at the spine which shows no increased uptake

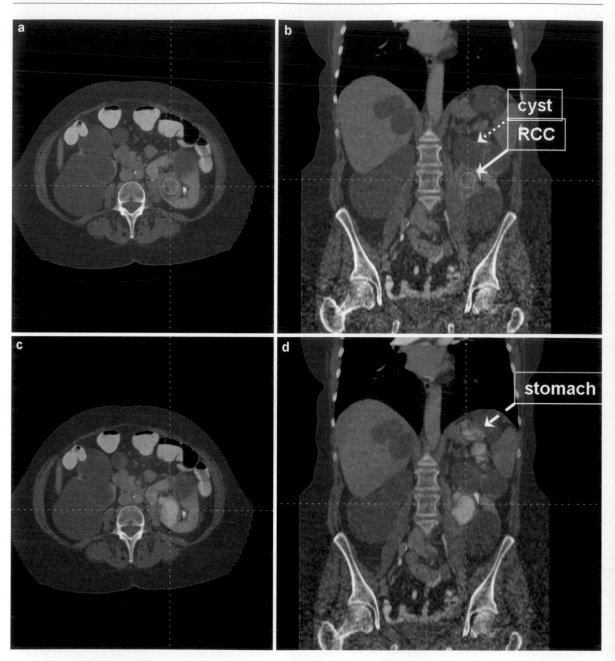

**Fig. 8.15** 124I-cG250 (**a**, **b**) CT, and (**c**, **d**) PET–CT scan of a patient with renal cancer and plycistic renal disease. Neoplastic lesion shows an evident increase of tracer uptake, while cysts are "cold"; tracer uptake in the stomach is related to free iodide (image courtesy of Prof. Divgi, UPenn, PA)

sensitivity of 77.3% and specificity of 100.0% for bone metastases, compared to 93.8 and 87.2% for combined CT and bone scan, respectively. Therefore, FDG-PET may be applied for re-staging renal cancer, especially for the identification of visceral and bone metastasis, while its role in the diagnosis is limited.

124I.cG250 has been shown to accurately identify both primary and metastatic lesions in clear cell renal cancer. Pilot study and preliminary data indicate a very high accuracy of antibody PET (Divgi et al. 2007) and a multicentric trial is currently running to evaluate the role of this approach to study renal cancer (Fig. 8.15).

**Acknowledgments** The authors want to thank the colleagues Cristina Nanni and Roberto Franchi for their precious contribution, constancy and professional support.

# References

Adeyoju AAB, Burke D, Atkinson C et al. (2001) The choice of timing for diuretic renography: the F0 method. BJU Int 88:1–5

Aide N, Cappele O, Bottet P et al. (2003) Efficiency of [(18)F] FDG PET in characterising renal cancer and detecting distant metastases: a comparison with CT. Eur J Nucl Med Mol Imaging 30(9):1236–1245

Anderson PJ, Rangarajan V, Gordon I (1997) Assessment of drainage in PUJ dilatation: pelvic excretion efficiency as an index of renal function. Nucl Med Commun 18(9):823–826

Anger H (1957) A new instrument for mapping gamma-ray emitters. Biol Med Q Rep UCRL 3653:38

Arnold RW, Subramanian G, McAfee JG et al. (1975) Comparison of 99mTc complexes for renal imaging. J Nucl Med 16(5):357–367

Bachor R, Kotzerke J, Gottfried HW et al. (1996) Positron emission tomography in diagnosis of renal cell carcinoma. Urologe A 35:146–150

Bianchi C (1972) Measurement of glomerular filtration rate. Prog Nucl Med 2:21–53

Blaufox MD, Aurell M, Bubeck B et al. (1996) Report of the Radionuclides in Nephrourology Committee on renal clearance. J Nucl Med 37:1883–1890

Boubaker A, Prior JO, Meuwly J et al. (2006) Radionuclide investigation of the urinary tract in the era of multimodality imaging. J Nucl Med 47:1819–1836

Boyd RE, Robson J, Hunt FC (1973) 99-technetium-m gluconate complexes for renal scintigraphy. Br J Radiol 46:604–612

Brown SCW, Upsdell SM, O'Reilly PH (1992) The importance of renal function in the interpretation of diuresis renography. Br J Urol 92:121–125

Brucer M (1990) A chronology of nuclear medicine 1600-1989. Heritage, St Louis, p 141

Bubeck B, Brandau W, Weber E et al. (1990) Pharmacokinetics of technetium-99m-MAG3 in humans. J Nucl Med 31: 1285–1293

Chaiwatanarat T, Pathy AK, Bomanji JB et al. (1993) Validation of renal output efficiency as an objective quantitative parameter in the evaluation of upper urinary ntract obstruction. J Nucl Med 34:845–848

Chantler C, Garnett ES, Parsons V et al. (1969) Glomerular filtration rate measurement in man by single injection method using 51-Cr-EDTA. Clin Sci 37:169–180

Chertin B, Pollack A, Koulikov D et al. (2006) Conservative treatment of ureteropelvic junction obstruction in children with antenatal diagnosis of hydronephrosis: lessons learned after 16 years of follow-up. Eur Urol 49:734–739

Christensen AB, Groth S (1986) Determination of 99m-T-DTPA clearance by a single plasma sample method. Clin Physiol 6:579–588

Christiansen IA, Hevesy G, Lomholt S (1924) Radiochemical method of studying the circulation of bismuth in the body. CR Acad Sci 178:1324

Cosgriff PS, Berry JM (1982) A comparative assessment of deconvolution and diuresis renography in equivocal upper urinary tract obstruction. Nucl Med Comm 3:377–384

De Bruyn R, Gordon I (2001) Postnatal investigation of fetal renal disease. Prenat Diagn 21:984–991

Despopoulus A (1965) A definition of substrate specificity in renal transport of organic anions. J Theor Biol 8:163–192

Divgi C, Pandit Taskar N, Jungbluth AA et al. (2007) Preoperative characterisation of clear-cell renal carcinoma using iodine-124-labelled antibody chimeric G250 (124I-cG250) and PET in patients with renal masses: a phase I trial. Lancet Oncol 8(4):304–310

EANM procedure guidelines: http://www.nucmedinfo.com/Pages/guiedlinebase.html

Eckelman W, Richards P (1970) Instant 99mTc-DTPA. J Nucl Med 11:761

English PJ, Testa HJ, Lawson RS et al. (1987) Modified method of diuretic renography for the assessment of equivocal pelvi-ureteric junction obstruction. Br J Urol 59:10–14

Enlander D, Weber PM, Dos Remedios LV (1974) Renal cortical imaging in 35 patients: superior quality with 99mTc-DMSA. J Nucl Med 15(9):743–749

Eshima D, Taylor A Jr (1992) Technetium-99m ($^{99m}$Tc) mercaptoacetyltriglycine. Uptake on the new 99mTc renal tubular function agent. Semin Nucl Med 22:61–73

Fanti S (2003) Nefrologia. In: Dondi M, Giubboni R (eds) Medicina Nucleare nella pratica clinica. Patron, Bologna, pp 337–365

Fleming JS, Wilkinson J, Oliver RM et al. (1991) Comparison of radionuclide estimation of glomerular filtration rate using technetium-99m diethylene-triaminepentaacetic acid and chromium 51 ethylenediaminetetraacetic acid. Eur J Nucl Med 18:391–395

Fommei E, Ghione S, Hilson AJ et al. (1993) Captopril radionuclide test in renovascular hypertension: a European multicentre study. European Multicentre Study Group. Eur J Nucl Med 20:617–623

Fritzberg AR, Kasina S, Eshma D et al. (1986) Synthesis and biological evaluation of Tc-99m MAG3 as a hippuran replacement. J Nucl Med 27:111–116

Gordon I, Colarihna P, Fettich J et al. (2001) Guidelines for standard and diuresi renography in children. Eur J Nucl Med 28:BP21–BP30

Harward TR, Poindexter B, Huber TS et al. (1995) Selection of patients for renal artery repair using captopril testing. Am J Surg 170:183–187

Hilson AJW (1994) Renal failure. In: Murray IPC, Ell PJ (eds) Nuclear medicine in clinical diagnosis and treatment, vol 1. Churchill Livingstone, New York, pp 319–327

Hilson AJW (2003) Functional renal imaging with nuclear medicine. Abdom Imaging 28:176–179

Hilson AJW, Mistry RD, Maisey MN (1976) Tc-99m-DTPA for the measurement of glomerular filtration rate. Br J Radiol 49:794–796

Homsy YL, Mehta PJ, Huot D et al. (1988) The intermittent hydronephrosis. A diagnostic challnge. J Urol 140:1222–1226

Hosokawa S, Kawamura J, Yoshida O (1978) Basic studies on the intrarenal localization of renal scanning agent Tc-99m DMSA. Acta Urol Jpn 23:61–65

Ikeda S, Fujina A, Ishibash A (1982) Microautoradiography of water soluble Tc99m-labelled compounds with Tc99m-DTPA. Kaku Igaku Jpn Nucl Med 19:1229–1232

Inoue Y, Minami M, Ohtomo K (2004) Isotopic scan for diagnosis of renal disease. Saudi J Kidney Dis Transpl 15:257–264

Inoue Y, Yoshikawa K, Suzuki T et al. (2000) Attenuation correction in evaluating renal function in children and adults by camerabased method. J Nucl Med 41(5):823–829

Kang DE, White RL Jr, Zuger JH, Sasser HC, Teigland CM (2004) Clinical use of fluorodeoxyglucose F 18 positron emission tomography for detection of renal cell carcinoma. J Urol 171(5):1806–1809

Kempi V, Persson RB (1975) Tc99m-DTPA (Sn) dry-kit preparation. Quality control and clearance studies. Nucl Med Stuttg 13:389

Klopper JF, Hauser W, Atkins HL et al. (1972) Evaluation of Tc99m DTPA for the measurement of glomerular iltration rate. J Nucl Med 13:107–110

Levey AS, Manaio MP, Perrone RD (1991) Laboratory assessment of renal disease: clearance, urinaalysisand reanl biopsy. In: Brenner BM, Rector FC (eds). The kidney, 4th edn, vol 1. Saunders, Philadelphia, pp 919–968

Lupton EW, Lawson RS, Shields RA et al. (1984) Diuresis renography and parenchymal transit time studies in the assessment of renal pelvic dilatation. Nucl Med Commun 5: 451–459

Lythgoe MF, Gordon I, Anderson PJ (1994) Effect of renal maturation on the clearance of technetium-99m mercaptoacetyltriglycine. Eur J Nucl Med 21:1333–1337

Majhail NS, Urbain JL, Albani JM et al. (2003) F-18 fluorodeoxyglucose positron emission tomography in the evaluation of distant metastases from renal cell carcinoma. J Clin Oncol 21(21):3995–4000

McAfee JG, Gagne G, Atkins HL et al. (1979) Biological distribution and excretion of DTPA labelled with Tc-99m and In-111. J Nucl Med 20:1273–1278

Montravers F, Grahek D, Kerrou K et al. (2000) Evaluation of FDG uptake by renal malignancies (primary tumor or metastases) using a coincidence detection gamma camera. J Nucl Med 41:78–84

Moorhty I, Easty M, McHugh K, Ridout D (2005) The presence of vesicoureteric reflux does not identify a population at risk fro renal scarring following a first urinary tract infection. Arch Dis Child 90:733–736

Müller-Suur R (1994) Radiopharmaceuticals: thcir intrarenal handling and localization. In: Murray IPC, Ell PJ (eds) Nuclear medicine in clinical diagnosis and treatment, vol 1. Churchill Livingstone, New York, pp 195–212

O'Reilly PH (2003) Consensus Committee of the Society of Radionuclides in Nephrourology. Standardization of the renogram technique for investigating the dilated urinary tract and assessing the results of surgery. BJU Int 91:239–243

O'Reilly PH, Brooman PJC, Mak S et al. (2001) The long term results of Anderson Hynes pyeloplasty. BJU Int 87:1–4

O'Reilly PH, Testa HJ, Lawson RS et al. (1978) Diuresis renography in equivocal urinary tract obstruction. Br J Urol 50: 76–80

Pelido Silva JM, Oliveira EA, Dinz JS et al. (2006) Clinical course of prenatally detected primary vesicoureteral reflux Pediatr Nephrol 21:86–91

Perini R, Pryma D, Divgi C (2008) Molecular imaging of renal cell carcinoma. Urol Clin North Am 35(4):605–611

Peters AM (1994) Graphical analysis of dynamic data: the Patlak-Rutland plot [editorial]. Nucl Med Commun 15:669–672

Piepsz A, Colarihna P, Gordon I et al. (2001) Guidelines for 99mTc-DMSA scintigraphy in children. Eur J Nucl Med 28: BP37–BP41

Piepsz A, Ham HR (2006) Pediatric applications of renal nuclear medicine. Semin Nucl Med 36:16–35

Piepsz A, Ismaili K, Hall M et al. (2005) How to interpret a deterioration of split function? Eur Urol 47:686–690

Piepsz A, Kinthaert J, Tondeur M et al. (1996) The robusteness of the Patlak-Rutland slope fro the determination of split renal function. Nucl Med Commun 17(19):817–821

Piepsz A, Tondeur M, Ham H (2000) NORA: a simple and reliable parameter for estimating renal output with or without furosemide challenge. Nucl Med Commun 21:317–323

Polito C, Rambaldi PF, Signoriello G et al. (2006) Permanent renal parenchymal defects after febrile UTI are closely associated with vesicoureteric reflux. Pediatr Nephrol 21: 521–526

Radermacher J, Haller H (2003) The right diagnostic work-up: investigating renal and renovascular disorders. J Hypertens Suppl 21:S19–S24

Ramdave S, Thomas GW, Berlangieri SU et al. (2001) Clinical role of F-18 fluorodeoxyglucose positron emission tomography for detection and management of renal cell carcinoma. J Urol 166:825–830

Russell CD, Bischoff PG, Rowell KL et al. (1983) Quality control of Tc99m-DTPA for measurement of glomerular filtration. Concise communication. J Nucl Med 24:722–727

Russell CD, Thorstad B, Yester MV et al. (1988) Comparison of technetium-99m MAG3 with iodine-131 hippuran by a simultaneous dual channel technique. J Nucl Med 29: 1189–1193

Schreij G, Ritsema GH, Vreugdenhil G et al. (1996) Steosis and renographic characteristics in renovascular disease. J Nucl Med 37:594–597

Senitko M, Fenves AZ (2005) An update on renovascular hypertension. Curr Cardiol Rep 7:404–411

Smellie JM, Barrat TM, Chantler C et al. (2001) Medical versus surgical treatment in children with severe bilateral vesicoureteric reflux and bilateral nephropathy: randomised trial. Lancet 357:1329–1333

Smith HW (1956) Principles of renal physiology. Oxford University Press, New York

Stacy BD, Thornburn GD (1966) Cr5-ethylene-diaminetetraacetate for the estimation of glomerular filtration rate. Science 1076: 5–38

Stevens E, Rosoff B, Weiner M et al. (1962) Metabolism of the chelating agent diethylene triaminepentaacetic acid C14 DTPA in man. Proc Soc Exp Biol Med 111:235

Taplin GV, Meredith OM, Kade H (1956) The radioisotope renogram. An external test for individual kidney function and upper urinary tract patency. J Lab Clin Med 48:886

Taylor A, Eshima D (1994) renal artery stenosis and ischemia: effect on renal blood flow and extraction fraction. Hypertension 23:96–103

Taylor A, Eshima D, Christin PE et al. (1988) A technetium-99m MAG3 kit formulation: preliminary results in normal volunteers and patients with renal failure. J Nucl Med 29: 616–622

Taylor A, Nally J (1995) Clinical applications of renal scintigraphy. AJR Am J Roentgenol 164(1):31–41

Taylor AT, Blaufox MD, Dubovsky EV et al. (2003) Society of Nuclear Medicine procedure guidelines fro diagnosis of renovascular hypertension, version 3.0, approved June 20, 2003. Available at http://interactice.snm.org/doc/pg_ch16_0403.pdf. Accessed 23 Aug 2006

Treves ST, Harmon WE, Packard AB et al. (2007) Kidneys. In: Treves ST (ed) Pediatric nuclear medicine/PET. Springer Science and Business Media, LLC, New York, pp 239–285

Wang SC, Ting KS, Woo CC (1965) Chelating therapy with Na-DMS in occupational lead and mercury intoxications. Chin Med J 84:437-439

Waxman AD, Tanaceseu D, Siemen JK et al. (1975) Technetium-99m glucoheptonate as a brain scanning agent. A critical comparison with pertechnetate. J Nucl Med 16: 580–581

Zeller T (2005) Renal artery stenosis: epidemiology, clinical manifestation, and percutaneous andovasculaar therapy. J Interv Cardiol 18:497–506

# The Role of Kidney Biopsy in the Diagnosis of Renal Disease and Renal Masses

**9**

Michele Carraro and Fulvio Stacul

## Contents

**Abstract**

> Renal biopsy has become a fundamental diagnostic tool both in nephrology, for the diagnostic assessment of many renal diseases, and in oncology, for the characterization of renal masses.

> A number of different nephrologic diseases can show a similar clinical and laboratory pattern but the histopathological features are different. Biopsy is required as different histological entities are associated with different therapeutic protocols and with different prognoses when considering the renal function. Biopsy of renal masses are becoming more frequent, as this procedure is required in candidates to non surgical treatments, i.e., radiofrequency ablation, and in patients for whom partial nephrectomy may be preferred. The correct patients selection and preparation, the use of modern bioptic devices, the possibility of a real time monitoring of the procedure by means of ultrasound, significantly decreased both patient discomfort and the complication rate of this invasive procedure. Until few years ago renal biopsy was performed in few selected centers, while now it is more widespread but nevertheless it requires a multidisciplinary team where the nephrologist, the radiologist and the pathologist are involved. All these physicians are essential part of the team and are required for the procedure and for the correct diagnostic interpretation.

F. Stacul (✉)
Department of Radiology Ospedale Maggiore,
Piazza Ospitale 1, 34123 Trieste, Italy
e-mail: fulvio.stacul@aots.sanita.fvg.it

M. Carraro
Department of Medicine, Cattinara Hospital,
University of Trieste, Strada di Fiume 447,
34149 Trieste, Italy

E. Quaia (ed.), *Radiological Imaging of the Kidney*,
Medical Radiology, DOI: 10.1007/978-3-540-87597-0_9, © Springer-Verlag Berlin Heidelberg 2011

## 9.1 Introduction

Since its introduction in clinical practice the renal biopsy has become one of the most important diagnostic procedures for the development of the body of knowledge encompassed by modern Nephrology. The renal biopsy leads to the diagnosis of many renal diseases, contributes precise prognostic information on the evolution of the disease, and provides the basis for a successful therapeutic strategy.

This important diagnostic tool has, as an intrinsic characteristic, the requirement for the support of various specialists, each of whom plays a fundamental role in obtaining the maximum quantity of clinical information from the procedure with the minimum of discomfort for the patient at a minimum economic cost. The nephrologist, who is the natural coordinator for the procedure, must define the clinical indications for the biopsy and the degree of risk involved, and in so doing exclude the presence of any absolute contraindication and correct any relative contraindication. The nephrologist is often the material executor of the procedure, must often prepare and preserve the tissue and assure its safe transport to the pathologist, and with the pathologist determines, on the basis of histopathological findings and considering the clinical course of the disease, the clinicopathological diagnosis. Finally, the nephrologist formulates, with the consent of the patient, the therapeutic strategy and follows the clinical course of the disease. The radiologist assists the nephrologist or directly performs the biopsy utilizing the appropriate radiological technique to visualize the kidney. The pathologist uses an array of histological techniques (light microscopy with all the stains considered necessary to make the diagnosis, immunofluorescence microscopy, electron microscopy) to render, on the basis of the histological findings and in concert with the clinical information provided by the nephrologist, the correct diagnosis.

## 9.2 Historical Background

The introduction of renal biopsy in clinical practice is a milestone of modern Nephrology and has provided, together with dialysis and renal transplantation, the decisive push which led to the birth of this specialty that distinguished itself from general internal medicine in the early 1960s.

From the end of the 1800s there were reports of patients with Bright's Disease who did not respond to the therapy of the time and who underwent decapsulation operations with the intent of reducing intrarenal pressure. During these procedures a small surgical biopsy of the renal parenchyma would be performed, and the tissue was analyzed microscopically (Ferguson 1899). Decapsulation procedures were also performed in Europe, and in Campbell 1930 published the histological results of the first series of 23 renal biopsies.

Using a aspiration needle, Alwall in Sweden is credited with performing the first percutaneous renal biopsy in 1944, although the report of the procedure was not published until 1952 (Alwall 1952).

A near forgotten nephrological pioneer, Antonio Pérez Ara (1950), a cuban pathologist who was unaware of the experience of Alwall, began to perform percutaneous renal biopsies in 1948, and the findings of biopsies of eight patients were published in 1950 in a Cuban medical journal. Dr. Perez localized the kidney by pyelography, injecting intravenously 20 mL of iodinated contrast media (Diodrast). The cutaneous site of the biopsy was selected using a radio-opaque grid. The biopsy itself was performed with a trocar which Dr. Perez called a *nephrobiotome*.

The percutaneous renal biopsy became well-known to the general medical public after the Danish physicians Paul Iversen and Claus Brun (1951) described their experience of renal biopsy performed on 60 patients. These investigators used a needle 1 mm in diameter which was attached to a syringe for aspiration. Dr. Iverson together with Dr. Kaj Roholm (1939) had already described in 1939 the use of the needle for liver biopsies. Iverson and Brun obtained renal biopsy specimens which were diagnostic in 53% of the procedures.

In the 1950s the Italian nephrological school notably contributed to the development of the renal biopsy and to the use of various microscope techniques to observe the renal tissue. Among these Italian pioneers, Prof. Fiaschi and his group were the first to introduce renal biopsy as a routine tool in clinical practice. At that time the procedure was relatively complex and required numerous radiological controls which are summarized on Table 9.1.

Electron microscopy for diagnostic purposes was first applied also by Dr. Fiaschi's group between 1955 and 1958, specifically by Naccarato and Andres, in

**Table 9.1** Early percutaneous renal biopsy procedure (Di Gaddo et al. 1954)

| |
|---|
| Patient in prone position |
| Insufflation of a small quantity of oxygen in the retroperitoneal space |
| Radiographic identification of the right kidney |
| Skin tracing on the back and right flank of the kidney position |
| Local anesthesia with novocaine 2% in the tissues surrounding the inferior pole of the right kidney |
| Measurement of perirenal pressure induced by the retroperitoneal air |
| Radiographic control of the anesthesia needle location |
| Insertion of the biopsy needle sleeve |
| Biopsy of the renal tissue |
| Tissue fixation with formaldehyde 3% |
| In case of bleeding injection of small quantities of hemostatic gel |

collaboration with Swedish colleagues from the Karolinska Institute of Stockholm (Fogazzi and Cameron 1999). Finally, the same Italian group, in collaboration with investigators at Columbia University in New York, first applied immunofluorescence microscopy to renal biopsy tissue in 1957, the results of which were published by Seegal et al. (1959), a year before Freedman (1960) and collaborators published what is considered by many the first article on the subject.

## 9.3 Clinical Indications for Renal Biopsy

In the following paragraphs we will analyze the principal points of the decision algorithm that lead to the renal biopsy. The indications for renal biopsy – with the refinements of the histopathological techniques on the one hand and the reduction of biopsy complications, thanks to real-time ultrasound guidance and to needle improvements, on the other – are constantly increasing. For practical purposes we have divided the discussion in two sections – major indications, or those in which the biopsy is considered indispensable for the formulation of the diagnosis and the subsequent therapeutic strategy, and optional uses of the biopsy, the indications for which are still being defined.

### 9.3.1 Major Indications

#### 9.3.1.1 Idiopathic Nephrotic Syndrome

The idiopathic nephrotic syndrome in the adult patient is the clinical situation that classically requires the performance of the renal biopsy, which is justified by the fact that several histological entities can give rise to the syndrome in adults, each of which is associated with its own therapeutic protocols, differing from each other in terms of drugs, dosages, and duration of treatment. Richards et al. (1994) documented that the renal biopsy, performed in adults with the nephrotic syndrome, significantly influenced the choice of therapeutic protocol in 86% of the cases. On the other hand conflicting opinions exist regarding the significance of histological findings for each single glomerular pathology. Regarding the nephrotic syndrome secondary to membranous glomerulopathy, some studies have indicated that the co-presence of focal and segmental glomerulosclerosis is a negative prognostic indicator, both in terms of clinical response to standard therapy and of progression to renal failure (Dumoulin et al. 2003). Other studies, in contrast, have not found that FSGS or other histological variants of membranous nephropathy are as useful as clinical data in predicting the disease outcome (Troyanov et al. 2006). Regarding segmental glomerulosclerosis itself, numerous studies have stressed the importance of the histological characteristics of the biopsy obtained at the first signs of the disease. The presence of the cellular form, and its "collapsing" variant, indicates an inadequate response to conventional therapy and a faster progression towards end-stage renal disease (ESRD), in comparison with the classical histologic variants including perihilar sclerosis and tip lesion (Stokes et al. 2006; Chun et al. 2004). The cellular variant is also highly predictive of segmental glomerulosclerosis recurrence posttransplant (Newstead 2003). Other, less frequent, diagnostic possibilities of the nephrotic syndrome may surprise the nephrologist as he reads the outcome of the biopsy, such as primary amyloidosis, fibrillary glomerulonephritis, membranous nephropathy with characteristics of lupus nephritis without the clinical or serological signs of systemic disease, and finally rare diseases with peculiar histological characteristics such as Fabry's Disease, collagen fibrotic glomerulopathy, L-CAT (lecithin-cholesterol acyltransferase) deficiency nephropathy. In pediatric patients with the nephrotic syndrome renal biopsy is not usually indicated since more than 90% of these patients have minimal change glomerulopathy that usually responds to well-known corticosteroid protocols. Thus the renal biopsy in children is reserved for atypical presentations, such as the persistence of microhematuria, hypertension and low complement levels after 6 weeks of steroid therapy, therapy failure, or for suspected congenital familial nephrotic syndrome.

### 9.3.1.2 Acute Renal Injury

In the absence of data clearly indicating the cause of acute renal failure (thus excluding cases with clear laboratory or radiological evidence of prerenal failure, obstruction, and acute tubular necrosis) renal biopsy becomes a fundamental tool not only for diagnosis but above all for prognosis and for determining the therapeutic protocol. One prospective study has shown that renal biopsy was essential in deciding the treatment and hence the outcome in 71% of acute renal failure patients; the modification of the therapeutic strategy subsequent to the biopsy resulted in clinical benefits which far outweighed the risk of the biopsy (Kobrin and Madaio 1996).

### 9.3.1.3 Renal Allograft Dysfunction

The causes of renal allograft dysfunction correlate with the time from transplantation in which they are found; nevertheless renal biopsy can be essential for determining the diagnosis and the treatment choices.

The failure of the kidney to function immediately following transplantation is termed *delayed graft function*, which is formally defined as the persistence of oliguria or the need for dialysis in the first week post-transplant. Apart from urinary tract obstruction, caused by ureteral necrosis or obstruction, or from thrombosis of the renal artery or vein which can be diagnosed by doppler ultrasonography, the cause of delayed graft function, and in particular the differential diagnosis between postischemic acute tubular necrosis (the most common cause of delayed graft function) and acute rejection, can only be determined by biopsy.

Early posttransplant renal dysfunction is characterized by renal insufficiency 1–12 weeks after transplantation in patients with initial normal functioning of the graft. The major causes of early dysfunction include acute rejection, calcineurin inhibitor (cyclosporin or tacrolimus) nephrotoxicity, urinary tract obstruction or reduced renal perfusion associated with a reduction in effective circulating volume. Other diagnostic possibilities include infections (cytomegalovirus or polyoma virus) and early recurrence of the primary renal disease such as segmental glomerulosclerosis, hemolytic-uremic syndrome and thrombotic thrombocytopenic purpura, Goodpasture's syndrome (antiglomerular basement membrane antibody disease), and interstitial nephritis (Josephson et al. 1999). If one can exclude calcineurin inhibitor toxicity (by briefly reducing the dose and not seeing an improvement in renal function) and urinary tract obstruction, renal biopsy would be highly indicated.

Late acute graft dysfunction is characterized by abrupt worsening of renal function more than 3 months after transplantation. The causes of this situation are essentially the same as those of early posttransplant renal dysfunction, plus the possibility of noncompliance, especially in the case of adolescent recipients. A negative renal ultrasound, particularly the absence of renal artery stenosis, indicates the performance of the allograft biopsy.

Many patients suffer a gradual deterioration of renal function in the years following transplantation, often with persistent proteinuria and hypertension. In this situation, in cases where there is a suspicion of disease recurrence or de novo glomerulonephritis vs. chronic allograft nephropathy or drug nephrotoxicity, renal biopsy can provide valuable information (Briganti et al. 2002), particularly if one is contemplating the conversion of the immunosuppressive regimen.

## 9.3.2 Optional Indications

### 9.3.2.1 Persistent Nonnephrotic Proteinuria

Renal biopsy is not currently indicated, at least in common clinical practice, in patients who present with isolated proteinuria less than 500 mg to 1 g per 24 h, normal renal function, absence of hematuria of glomerular origin (see below), and absence of clinical or laboratory signs suggestive of systemic disease associated with glomerular pathology, such as systemic lupus erythematosus, vasculitis, monoclonal gammopathy, etc. In such cases the prognosis is good in terms of renal function, and there is no indication for therapy with steroids or other immunosuppressants. Current nephrological opinion changes, however, for proteinuria consistently and significantly greater than 1 g per day, particularly when there is a insufficient response to angiotensin converting enzyme inhibitors or angiotensin receptor blockers; in these cases most nephrologists opt for the biopsy. The presence of diabetes mellitus, in particular in the absence of other signs of microangiopathy such as retinopathy, does not always justify the clinical diagnosis of diabetic nephropathy. Studies carried out on patients with diabetes mellitus type 2 and proteinuria have shown that between 10 and 30% of cases result from nephropathy different from classical diabetes (Fioretto et al. 2008), and thus also in the presence of diabetes and proteinuria the renal biopsy should be considered to optimize the therapeutic approach.

### 9.3.2.2 Isolated Glomerular Hematuria

Patients who present with isolated glomerular hematuria (dysmorphic red cells and/or red cell casts in the urinary sediment, dipstick negative for proteinuria, normal renal function, normal blood pressure) usually have a benign prognosis in terms of renal function and do not require drug therapy or particular restrictions in terms of lifestyle. In these cases in which prognostic information is not forthcoming and the nephrologist is not confronted with the necessity of making therapeutic choices, the renal biopsy does not appear to be indicated. One series of patients with these clinical characteristics in which renal biopsy was performed demonstrated thin membrane disease in 43% of cases, IgA nephropathy in 20%, other glomerular pathology (including Alport's syndrome) in 19%, and histologically normal kidneys in 18% (Hall et al. 2004). In another series the renal biopsy modified the therapeutic strategy in only 3% of cases (Richards et al. 1994). An exception could be made for cases of isolated glomerular hematuria associated with a family history of renal disease and particularly of chronic kidney injury. When the patient in question is young, renal biopsy may have a role in genetic counseling. In cases in which the hematuria is associated with nonnephrotic proteinuria the probability of significant glomerular pathology is greater than 70%, and in particular the probability of finding IgA nephropathy is greater than

40% (Hall et al. 2004); in this situation, performance of the renal biopsy should be considered.

### 9.3.2.3 Chronic Kidney Injury

Renal biopsy may have an important diagnostic role also when the patient presents with established chronic renal injury. The leading example is when renal cortical thickness, demonstrated by ultrasound, is greater than 8–10 mm (Barbiano Di Belgiojoso et al. 2002), particularly associated with proteinuria but also in the absence of proteinuria. In patients with proteinuria renal biopsy may identify the glomerular disease responsible for the proteinuria, modify the therapy accordingly, quantify the degree of chronicity of the lesion, as a useful prognostic indicator, and demonstrate pathology which may be destined to recur in a possible future kidney transplant (Pasquali 2008; Lupo et al. 2008). In patients with chronic kidney injury without proteinuria renal biopsy can also play an important diagnostic role with therapeutic implications, as well as defining the chronicity index and the prognosis. An important example is when the biopsy demonstrates an interstitial nephritis which may be susceptible to corticosteroid treatment (Tomson Charles 2003).

## 9.4 Contraindications to the Renal Biopsy

Contraindications to the performance of the renal biopsy can be absolute or relative. In effect the only absolute contraindication, apart from the refusal of the patient to consent to the procedure after having been completely informed regarding the risks and benefits, is the inability of the patient to cooperate with the operator at the moment of the biopsy (as a consequence, for example, of respiratory difficulty or of the impossibility to maintain the correct position during the entire period of the procedure). Relative contraindications include a hemorrhagic diathesis, severe uncontrolled hypertension, the presence of a single kidney (congenital or acquired), a renal neoplastic mass or renal cysts, a renal artery aneurysm, a renal or perirenal abscess, or the presence of hydronephrosis.

A detailed medical history, an accurate physical exam and the timely discontinuation of anticoagulant or antiplatelet drugs, together with a prebiopsy laboratory evaluation of coagulation status would demonstrate, and allow the correction of any bleeding risk before the biopsy procedure. In particular it is necessary to demonstrate before the biopsy that the platelet count is greater than $100,000/mm^3$, that prothrombin time and activated partial thromboplastin times are in the normal range, and that the bleeding time is in the normal range. Significant anemia can also alter bleeding time, and in these cases any additional anemia induced by the biopsy could *per se* worsen the clinical conditions of the patient. A hematocrit value greater than 30% and a hemoglobin concentration greater than 10 g/dL would represent an acceptable safety level. An elevated bleeding time (>8–10 min), together with a carefully obtained history and physical exam, and the hematocrit and hemoglobin values are the major predictors of hemorrhagic risk in patients who undergo renal biopsy (Mattix and Singh 1999). An abnormal bleeding time in the absence of other prohemorrhagic factors does not necessarily prohibit the performance of the biopsy; the procedure can be carried out after premedication with DDAVP (deamino-1-8-d-aggnine vasopressin), which is administered at a mean dose of 0.3 µg/kg 1 or 2 h before the biopsy (Mannucci et al. 1983). For patients in therapy with an anticoagulant, the drug should be discontinued for a period sufficient to reduce the INR to equal or less than 1.5. If the patient is on heparin, the drug should be stopped at least 12–24 h before the procedure, and low molecular weight heparin should be discontinued at least 24 h before the procedure. Aspirin (and perhaps also ticlopidine) should be discontinued 2–3 weeks before the biopsy and nonsteroidal anti-inflammatory drugs at least 2–5 days before the biopsy. Paracetamol can be administered without worry. One should recall that some herbal medicines containing garlic, ginseng and ginko, sold in pharmacies and health food stores as "revitalizers," also have antiaggregant properties.

Uncontrolled hypertension increases bleeding complications following renal biopsy, and since severe and uncontrolled hypertension constitutes a serious disease per se, it also requires a treatment independently of the risk it represents for the renal biopsy. Thus, at the moment of the biopsy the blood pressure should have been corrected to the level as close as possible to the norm.

The presence of a single kidney, whether congenital or acquired, is not a contraindication for renal biopsy in the absence of other risk factors; it is the normal situation for renal transplant patients, who are often the subjects for renal biopsy.

Renal tumors are normally an indication for surgical intervention; renal biopsy may provide useful information regarding the co-presence of parenchymal renal disease by sampling the tissue which are free of tumor in the nephrectomy specimen (partial or total).

Renal cysts do not constitute a contraindication to renal biopsy, provided that a portion of the parenchyma can be found which would allow the percutaneous procedure. Indications for renal biopsy in a patient with polycystic kidney disease would be extremely rare.

The presence of a renal abscess or hydronephrosis requires urgent treatment, regardless of the co-presence of renal parenchymal disease which may be an indication for renal biopsy. Thus, relief of urinary tract obstruction and antibiotic therapy for urinary tract infection, even if asymptomatic, would be considered prerequisites for renal biopsy.

Morbid obesity can cause difficulty in localizing the renal pole to biopsy, and above all, may not allow the renal parenchyma to be reached with the patient in the normal prone position, even with very long biopsy needles. In this situation, the biopsy may be carried out with success with the patient in the supine anterolaterale position or under CT guidance (Gesualdo et al. 2008).

## 9.5 The Preparation of the Patient for Renal Biopsy

### 9.5.1 The Patient Before the Biopsy

Once there is a clinical indication to perform the renal biopsy, absolute contraindications have been excluded, relative contraindications have been remedied, and risks associated with the procedure have been minimized – the biopsy is performed. The patient must be able to cooperate fully, simulating beforehand key moments in the biopsy procedure, such as controlling inspiration and brief moments of apnea. The patient must maintain an immobile posture in the prone position with the upper abdomen resting on a pillow or rigid bedroll, in order to fix the kidney in position.

The day of the procedure the patient must be fasting. In the case of agitation or anxiety mild sedation is useful, but the patient must remain able to cooperate during the procedure. Venous access with an angiocath must be present, connected by an infusion set to a bottle of normal saline, in case of emergency.

## 9.6 The Biopsy Procedure

The biopsy procedure is preceded by selecting the site of the biopsy, which besides anatomic considerations depends on the eventual presence of lesions (for example, cortical scars or cysts) that were seen in the preliminary renal ultrasound (US) examination, and by the choice of biopsy needle. Immediately following the biopsy itself, the tissue is studied under the dissecting microscope to confirm that it is indeed renal parenchyma and is divided according to the various microscopic techniques it must undergo. Thus, a familiarity with the different preservation and fixation methods is required.

### 9.6.1 The Choice of the Biopsy Site

The preferred site of the renal biopsy is the inferior pole of the left kidney because the renal pelvis and large caliber vessels are relatively far from this level. The biopsy procedure is usually carried out under local anesthesia, although in children less than 10 years of age general anesthesia may be preferred. Renal US is the preferred method for localizing the kidney and for monitoring more or less continually the procedure. The renal biopsy and US localization can be performed using more than one protocol, according to how the US is used in the various phases of the biopsy: (a) biopsy after US localization of the kidney (with the actual biopsy performed without visualization); (b) US-assisted biopsy in real time, without a guide on the US probe; (c) US-guided biopsy in real time, with a guide fixed on the probe through which the needle is inserted. The US-guided biopsy in real time is currently considered the safest and most successful option.

### 9.6.2 Biopsy Needle Types

Technological progress has produced biopsy needles which are progressively more efficient and less traumatic. The needles used today can be differentiated on the basis by which the tissue core is obtained. In brief, (a) tweezer-like needles; (b) aspiration needles; and (c) cutting needles are available. Another distinguishing characteristic among needles involves the triggering mechanism of the needle that can be: (a) manual; (b) semiautomatic; or (c) automatic. From the aspiration technique of Iversen and Brun (1951) the renal biopsy needle has evolved to the Vim and Silverman needle modified by Franklin, then to the spring mechanism of the Tru-cut needle and finally to the automatic needles in use today. These needles also have different sizes, and the choice of the various caliber (14-16-18-20 gauge) depends on the necessity to obtain a histologically-sufficient sample, the customs of the biopsy team, and the characteristics of the patient (size, age, native renal biopsy vs. transplant biopsy). Currently the needles most in use in adults have a caliber between 14 and 18 gauge (Fig. 9.1), whereas the biopsy needles for use in children have a caliber between 18 and 20 gauge, or even smaller in renal transplants for cellular aspirates for microhistology. Pathologists tend to prefer the tissue cores from the 14 gauge needle which, because of their greater dimensions, provide sufficient material for all the study preparations (Ferrario and Rastaldi 2003).

Thus, needles differ amongst themselves for several aspects that regard the cutting action and whether this action is partially or totally automatic and also for the needle caliber, the echogenicity of the needle tip, the length of the tissue core, the weight of the handle, etc.

The semiautomatic and automatic models offer some advantages: (a) they can be used single- handedly, and thus a lone operator can both obtain the biopsy and operate the ultrasound probe; (b) the velocity with which the sampling occurs, that is considered the most delicate parameter in terms of hemorrhagic complications, is decidedly superior compared to manual methods (shortening the time that the needle stays in the kidney and thus reducing the possibility of complications associated with movements of the organ or of the needle).

In conclusion, given the wide range of needle types currently available, it is evident that each operator who

**Fig. 9.1** (**a**) A trucut automatic needle with a calliper of 16 gauge, usually employed in diffuse renal diseases; (**b**) A trucut automatic needle with a calliper of 18 gauge, usually employed in focal renal disease; (**c, d**) The mechanism of action of the automatic trucut cutting needle. (**c**) The hollow core needle progress in tissues while the outer cutting edge component (**d**) separates the tissue sample.

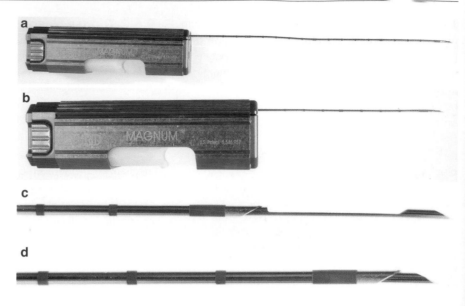

has experience with renal biopsy will use the method and equipment on the basis of his or her personal experience and preferences.

### 9.6.3 Evaluation and Division of the Biopsy Tissue

The tissue obtained by renal biopsy is evaluated immediately following the procedure. In optimal conditions two biopsy core samples of approximately 2 cm each are obtained to provide enough tissue to perform the common microscopic techniques (light microscopy, immunofluorescence, electron microscopy). To confirm that the tissue is kidney and that glomeruli are present, the biopsy core can be quickly viewed under a stereoscopic dissecting microscope, and the division of the material for the various microscopic techniques can be performed immediately following the biopsy procedure. If a dissecting microscope is not available, the biopsy can be divided blindly, sampling pieces from the head and the tail of the tissue cylinder (in the case of a single core) or from the tails of the two cores, two fragments of 1 mm$^2$ for the electron microscope. The remaining part of the tissue core or cores is divided into two equal parts, one of which is placed in fixative for electron microscopy and the other in transport medium (for example, Michel's solution) for immunofluorescence. Alternatively, if the operator is not expert in dividing the tissue, the tissue samples can be placed in a humid transport chamber (for

example, a Petri dish, the base of which is covered which filter paper soaked in saline, and then closed hermetically with parafilm), and divided by the pathologist who receives the samples.

### 9.6.4 Fixatives for Preservation of the Biopsy Tissue

For light microscopy the samples must first be placed in fixative solutions (formalin, paraformaldehyde, or Zenker's or Bouin's alcohol solution. For immunofluorescence the samples are snap frozen in embedding material or are sent in transport medium (for example, Michel's solution) to the pathology laboratory. For electron microscopy the tissue is placed immediately in solution buffered with glutaraldehyde (usually 2.5%) (Fogo 2003).

## 9.7 Percutaneous Biopsy of Renal Masses

### 9.7.1 Indications

Indications for biopsy of focal renal lesions were traditionally limited and well defined. They included: (a) the differential diagnosis of a renal cancer from a metastatic neoplasm or lymphoma; (b) the tissue diagnosis in patients with unresectable tumor and (c) diagnosis of malignancy in candidates to non surgical treatment, i.e., radiofrequency ablation.

In the first clinical setting (patients presenting with renal mass and another malignancy) the indication to biopsy was recently challenged. The most common malignancies metastatic to the kidney are lymphoma and lung carcinoma, but the majority of patients with renal masses diagnosed in the setting of a clinically localized non renal malignancy will not have metastatic disease to the kidney. Sanchez-Ortiz et al. (2004) showed that patients who were found to have metastases to the kidney had evidence of clinical progression or radiographic evidence of other metastases from their non renal malignancy. Therefore a biopsy of the renal mass may not be indicated if the non renal malignancy is clinically localized. The same applies to patients with a renal mass and a history of lymphoma, particularly if the mass is enhancing on CT and there is no other evidence of lymphoma progression.

The second setting includes patients with high stage renal lesions who cannot tolerate resection for medical reasons. In this situation the biopsy can establish the diagnosis of renal cell carcinoma and non surgical therapy can be instituted.

Percutaneous biopsy has an additional important role in patients referred for percutaneous ablation of suspected renal cell carcinoma. Actually, characterization of small renal masses by imaging alone has limitations. Enhancement may be equivocal in small masses. It may be difficult to distinguish renal cell carcinoma from an angiomyolipoma with minimal fat. Moreover approximately 5% of angiomyolipomas do not contain visible fat on CT or MRI and are indistinguishable from small renal cell carcinomas (Wolf 1998; Sant et al. 1984). A number of studies showed that about 30% of small renal masses who underwent surgery were found to be benign (Frank et al. 2003; Gill et al. 2003; Link et al. 2005). In the series reported by Tuncali et al. (2004) 37% of the patients referred for cryotherapy of suspected renal cell carcinoma had a benign renal mass. Therefore they should undergo a biopsy before the treatment session.

Biopsy of focal renal lesions was advocated in evaluating the indeterminate cystic renal mass (Bosniak category 3 and 2F). The availability of multiphasic helical CT has reduced the number of indeterminate renal cyst diagnosis from 5 to 8% in the past to 3% presently (Lang et al. 2002). Imaging-guided biopsy can alter the management of these indeterminate cysts avoiding unnecessary surgery in 39% of patients in the series by Harisinghani et al. (2003) and in 70% of patients in the series by Lang et al. (2002). Israel and Bosniak (2005) challenged this conclusion, claiming that truly indeterminate cystic masses require surgery whether the biopsy specimen is positive or negative.

Furthermore biopsy may be required in patients for whom partial nephrectomy rather than radical nephrectomy may be a preferred alternative treatment. The indications for partial nephrectomy are not completely defined but certainly include (Renshaw et al. 1997) patients at risk for bilateral malignancies (Von Hippel – Lindau disease, tuberous sclerosis), patients who may not tolerate radical nephrectomy for medical reasons, young patients who might benefit from retaining as much renal function as possible, and patients with small renal masses. The difficulty in differentiating a small renal cell carcinoma from a benign lesion, including oncocytoma, angiomyolipoma and metanephric adenoma, was already underscored. Moreover some renal cell carcinomas, i.e., small cromophobe renal cell carcinomas, have a very favorable prognosis, and some patients with this tumor may be ideal candidates for partial nephrectomy (Renshaw et al. 1997). Neuzillet et al. (2004) underline that they select partial nephrectomy for cortical, low grade, clear cell and chromophobic renal cell carcinoma while radical nephrectomy is performed in cases of central, high grade or papillary renal cell carcinoma.

It's worthwhile mentioning that in the future percutaneous biopsy could provide additional information, beyond histology. Actually molecular and genomic features can affect patient prognosis and the biopsy could show genetic profiling able to better differentiate renal tumors with different grades of aggressiveness and metastatic potential (Volpe et al. 2007).

### 9.7.2 Technique

Percutaneous biopsy of a renal mass can benefit either of CT or US guidance with the patient in a prone, semiprone or lateral decubitus position. The majority of the authors prefer a CT guidance (Fig. 9.2) and use a localizing grid placed overlying the region of biopsy. Following initial planning CT, the entrance site is identified, anesthesia with 5–10 mL of 1% lidocaine is performed, a small skin incision is made and a 17-gauge introducer is directed toward the lesion. The tip of the introducer is placed at

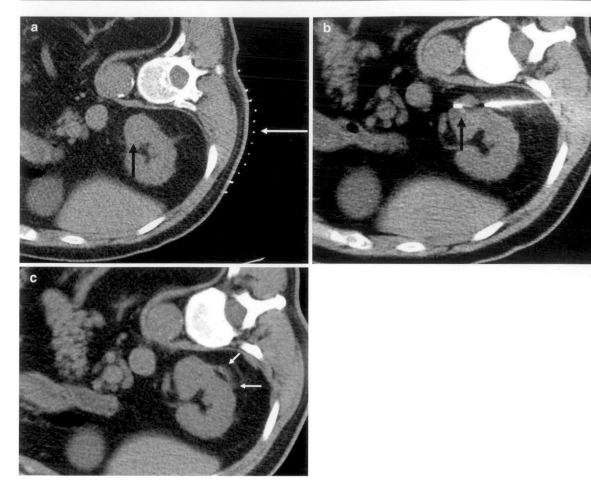

**Fig. 9.2** (**a**) Axial CT of patient in right lateral decubitus position. Preplanning CT performed with grid in position (*white arrow*) allows for planning for the needle entrance site to biopsy medial right renal tumor (*black arrow*). (**b**) Axial CT of patient in right lateral decubitus position. A 17-gauge coaxial needle and 18 gauge core biopsy gun (*black arrow*) are inserted into the right renal mass. (**c**) Axial CT of patient in right lateral decubitus position. Post procedure CT shows very minimal perinephric hemorrhage (*arrows*). A normal finding after renal biopsy (courtesy of Raul N. Uppot, Harvard Medical School)

the periphery of the renal mass to minimize the possibility of seeding along the needle tract. Through the introducer, multiple fine-needle aspirates using a 22-gauge Chiba and multiple (at least two) core biopsy samples using an 18-gauge biopsy gun are obtained. Post procedural CT scanning is performed to evaluate for perirenal hemorrhage or other complications.

After the procedure the patient is observed for a minimum of 4 h during which pulse and blood pressure are monitored at 30 min intervals.

Occasional failures in CT guided biopsies may be related to the needle manipulation outside the CT gantry allowing the needle to accidentally shift away from the intended mass and occasionally the needle would

push away instead of pierce the mass (Lechevallier et al. 2000). Caoili et al. (2002) favored US guidance which allows continuous visualization of the needle as it enters the mass. However, no significant differences in biopsy accuracy arising from mode of imaging guidance (CT or sonography) was reported (Maturen et al. 2007).

Most authors presently prefer performing both fine-needle aspirations and core biopsies. Limitations of performing fine-needle aspiration alone include significant insufficient sample rates (ranging from 5 to 16%) and false negative rates (ranging from 8 to 36%). Moreover the cytologic features of an angiomyolipoma can mimic a malignant tumor. Furthermore oncocytes can be seen in both oncocytomas and renal cell carcinomas. Therefore aspiration can be misleading in these cases.

Larger needles yielded a higher sensitivity and a higher negative predictive value according to Rybicki et al. (2003) and may improve the ability to subclassify and grade renal cell carcinoma (Lechevallier et al. 2000). Moreover the usual core size (1.7×0.1 cm) allows specific histopathological procedures such as immunohistochemical staining or lymphoma immunophenotyping. However these benefits must be weighed against the increased risk of bleeding and pseudoaneurysm formation.

### 9.7.3  Results

Imaging-guided percutaneous biopsy of renal masses is an accurate, useful and safe procedure.

Earlier reports considered fine-needle aspiration procedures and reported poor sensitivity for the detection of malignancy and a high rate of nondiagnostic procedures, while with the use of core needles the sensitivity is as high as 89–100% (Lechevallier et al. 2000; Jaff et al. 2005; Eshed et al. 2004; Maturen et al. 2007). Accuracy superior to 90% in all recent series was reported in the review by Volpe et al. (2007).

It is interesting to realize that percutaneous biopsy has a different accuracy in different clinical settings, as pointed out by Rybicki et al. (2003). They showed that the procedure has a high sensitivity in patients with a known malignancy (90%), in patients with no known malignancy and suspected unresectable tumor (92%) and in nonsurgical patients with a mass suspected to be a resectable renal cell carcinoma (100%).

Furthermore their results are of interest when they are stratified by mass size. The sensitivity was excellent (97%) for masses between 4 and 6 cm, lower for masses 3 cm and less and greater than 6 cm (84% and 87% respectively). Technical difficulties in performing biopsies of small masses and the risk of sampling errors in large masses that are more likely to contain necrosis can explain these results.

Today, core biopsies and fine – needle aspirations appear to be complementary and this is especially true in case of complex cystic masses (Volpe et al. 2007).

The clinical role of the procedure was highlighted by Neuzillet et al. (2004) who considered that biopsy is necessary for management of small (less than 4 cm) renal masses: biopsy actually changed tumor management in 47.8% of their patients who avoided radical nephrectomy. They underscored the high accuracy in identifying histological tumor type. Similar results were reported by Wolf (1998) who avoided surgery in 44% of their patients based on biopsy results. Jaff et al. (2005) reported that the biopsy results significantly improved patient care in 32 out of 46 patients. These data were reinforced by Maturen et al. (2007): biopsy results significantly impacted clinical management in 60.5% of their patients.

It should be mentioned that the accuracy of Fuhrman grade assignment is often suboptimal, as shown by Neuzillet et al. (2004) and by Lechevallier et al. (2000). Interobserver variability and tumor heterogeneity may in part explain this phenomenon (Volpe et al. 2007).

Reported complications of percutaneous biopsy include hemorrhage, pseudoaneurysm and arteriovenous fistula formation, infection, pneumothorax (such complications are discussed in the following section) and needle track seeding. Tumor track seeding is extremely rare: only six cases have been reported (Volpe et al. 2007) and the use of an introducer is designed to prevent this complication. Apparently the risk may increase with the number of needle passes and with noncutting needles.

## 9.8  Renal Biopsy Complications and Follow-Up

The complication rate associated with the performance of percutaneous renal biopsy has significantly decreased in recent years as a result of the technological advances applied to the procedure. The use of automatic biopsy needles and of ultrasound to localize the biopsy site and to visualize the needle course in real time are by now considered routine and virtually indispensable for the execution of a safe procedure. Nevertheless, percutaneous renal biopsy cannot be considered totally exempt from complications, particularly those associated with postbiopsy hemorrhage. Bleeding can occur also when the prebiopsy evaluation, which we discussed in previous paragraphs, has excluded a coagulation defect.

Complications can be divided into major and minor. Major complications (Fig. 9.3) are those which require a clinical intervention, whether transfusions of blood components, the necessity of performing

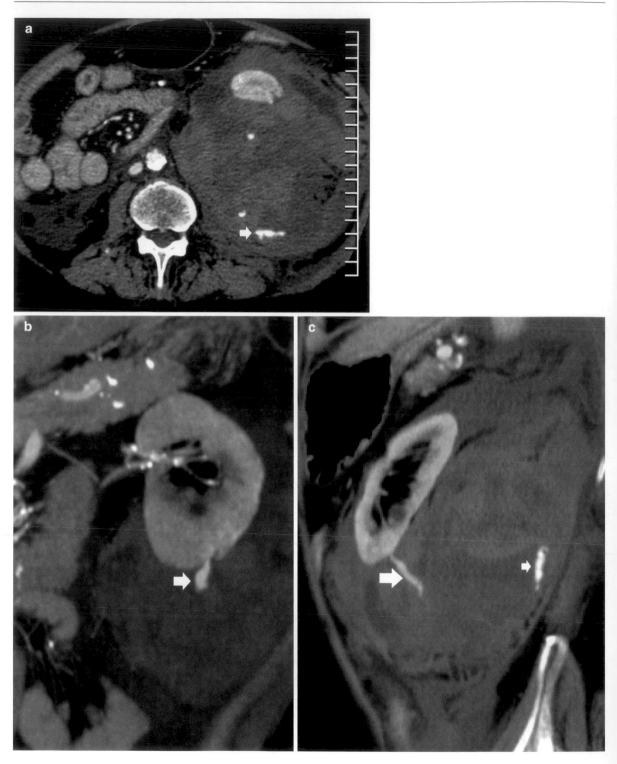

**Fig. 9.3** (**a–c**) Renal bleeding after percutaneous biopsy. (**a**) Contrast-enhanced CT, arterial phase. Transverse plane. A huge perirenal haemirrhagic collection is evident on the perirenal space with anterior dislocation of the left kidney (k). There is evidence of active hemorrhage (*arrow*) after iodinated contrast administration. (**b**) Coronal and (**c**) sagittal reformations. The site of origin of active bleeding (*large arrow*) is visualized after contrast administration. The presence of active blleding is also visualized posteriorly (*small arrow*) as in the transverse plane. Active bleeding was interrupted by selective intra-arterial injection of embolizing material (courtesy of Salvatore Sammartano, Santa Chiara Hospital, Trento, Italy)

an invasive procedure (for example, angiography with embolization of a bleeding vessel, a surgical procedure for draining a large hematoma, a surgical procedure to close a bleeding vessel or fistula tract, or nephrectomy), the formation of an obstruction of the urinary tract with subsequent acute renal insufficiency, postbiopsy sepsis, or the death of the patient. Minor complications are those which do not require a clinical intervention beyond simple observation, such as transient macrohematuria, mild lumbar pain at the biopsy site, or a small perirenal hematoma (less than 5 cm) that will resorb spontaneously without the need for a clinical intervention (Manno et al. 2004).

Complications generally are observed within 24 h from the moment of the biopsy, and this time period corresponds to the period of close monitoring of the patient in the hospital. In a large study composed of both prospective and retrospective cases, 89% of all complications were observed within 24 h, including 91% of the major complications and 87% of the minor complications (Whittier and Korbet 2004). Overall, complications were observed in 13% of the 750 biopsy patients who participated in the study – minor complications were seen in 6.7% (3.1% with macrohematuria which resolved spontaneously and 2.1% with small perirenal hematoma) and major complications were seen in 6.4% (1.6% with macrohematuria, 1.9% hematoma, 0.4% arteriovenous fistula, 0.3% urinary tract obstruction with acute renal insufficiency); one patient (0.13%) died from perirenal hemorrhage following the renal biopsy. A prospective study of 471 biopsies for which ultrasound was obtained 24 h after the procedure regardless of the presence of clinical signs demonstrated a much higher incidence of complications – 34.1% – which was due to the presence of hematoma which were observed in 157 cases (33.3%). The hematoma were clinically silent in 142 cases, and thus clinically relevant cases numbered 15 (3.2%). Major complications occurred in six biopsied patients (1.2%); of these, two presented with arteriovenous fistula and four suffered large hematoma. One patient underwent nephrectomy, and there were no deaths.

In conclusion, recent data have shown that the percutaneous renal biopsy represents an invasive procedure that, if carefully planned and patients with absolute contraindications or intractable relative contraindications are excluded, has a low incidence of complications. In most cases complications are observed within 24 h following the biopsy, and thus, currently, the procedure must be performed after admission to the hospital, the patient without a major complication can be discharged after 24 h of observation, and a follow-up visit is planned 5–7 days following discharge to confirm the absence of complications.

# References

Alwall N (1952) Aspiration biopsy of the kidney, including report of a case of amyloidosis diagnosed in 1944 and investigated at autopsy. Acta Med Scand 143:430–435

Barbiano Di Belgiojoso G, Ferrario F, Genderini A (2002) Borderline indications for renal biopsy. G Ital Nefrol 19(3): 335–349

Briganti EM, Russ GR, McNeil JJ et al. (2002) Risk of renal allograft loss from recurrent glomerulonephritis. N Engl J Med 347(19):1531–1532

Campbell G (1930) The results of decapsulation in nephritis. Arch Dis Child 5:283–290

Caoili EM, Bude RO, Higgins EJ et al. (2002) Evaluation of sonographically guided percutaneous core biopsy of renal masses. AJR Am J Roentgenol 179:373–378

Chun MJ, Korbet SM, Schwartz MM et al. (2004) Focal segmental glomerulosclerosis in nephrotic adults: presentation, prognosis, and response to therapy of the histologic variants. J Am Soc Nephrol 15:2169–2177

Di Gaddo M, Torsoli A, Righini E (1954) Tecnica della biopsia renale transcutanea. Urologia 21:376–380

Dumoulin A, Hill GS, Montseny JJ et al. (2003) Clinical and morphological prognostic factors in membranous nephropathy: significance of focal segmental glomerulosclerosis. Am J Kidney Dis 41(1):38–48

Eshed I, Elias S, Sidi AA (2004) Diagnostic value of CT-guided biopsy of indeterminate renal masses. Clin Radiol 59:262–267

Ferguson (1899) The surgical treatment of nephritis. The Medical Standard, June, 1899. Am J Med Sci 117:223–224

Ferrario F, Rastaldi MP (2003) Caratteristiche ottimali del prelievo bioptico. In: Pasquali S, Roccatello D, Pani A, Manno C, Onetti Muda A, Cagnoli L (eds) Manuale di Terapia delle Nefropatie Glomerulari Milano. Wichtig, Milan, pp 280–285

Fioretto P, Caramori ML, Mauer M (2008) The kidney in diabetes: dynamic pathways of injury and repair. The Camillo Golgi Lecture 2007. Diabetologia 51:1347–1355

Fogazzi GB, Cameron JS (1999) The early introduction of percutaneous renal biopsy in Italy. Kidney Int 56:1951–1961.

Fogo AB (2003) Approach to renal biopsy. Am J Kidney Dis 42(4):826–836

Frank I, Blute ML, Cheville JC et al. (2003) Solid renal tumors: an analysis of pathological features related to tumor size. J Urol 170: 2217–2220

Freedman PH, Peters JH, Kark RM (1960) Localisation of gamma globulin in the diseased kidney. Arch Intern Med 105:524–535

Gesualdo L, Cormio L, Stallone G et al. (2008) Percutaneous ultrasound-guided renal biopsy in supine antero-lateral position: a new approach for obese and non-obese patients. Nephrol Dial Transplant 23(3):971–976

Gill IS, Matin SF, Desai MM et al. (2003) Comparative analysis of laparoscopic versus open partial nephrectomy for renal tumors in 200 patients. J Urol 170:64–68

Hall CL, Bradley R, Kerr A et al. (2004) Clinical value of renal biopsy in patients with asymptomatic microscopic hematuria with and without low-grade proteinuria. Clin Nephrol 62(4):267–272

Harisinghani MG, Maher MM, Gervais DA et al. (2003) Incidence of malignancy in complex cystic renal masses (Bosniak Category III): should imaging-guided biopsy precede surgery? AJR Am J Roentgenol 180:755–758

Israel GM, Bosniak MA (2005) How I do it: evaluating renal masses. Radiology 236:441–450

Iversen P, Brun C (1951) Aspiration biopsy of the kidney. Am J Med 11:324–330

Iversen P, Roholm K (1939) On aspiration biopsy of the liver with remarks on its diagnostic significance. Acta Med Scand 102:1–16

Jaff A, Molinié V, Mellot F et al. (2005) Evaluation of imaging-guided fine-needle percutaneous biopsy of renal masses. Eur Radiol 15:1721–1726

Josephson MA, Chiu MY, Woodle ES et al. (1999) Drug-induced acute interstitial nephritis in renal allografts: histopathologic features and clinical course in six patients Am J Kidney Dis 34(3):540–548

Kobrin S, Madaio MP (1996) Renal biopsy. In: Jacobs HS, Striker GE, Klahr S (eds) The principles and practice in nephrology. Mosby, St. Louis, pp 67–71

Lang EK, Macchia RJ, Gayle B et al. (2002) CT-guided biopsy of indeterminate renal cystic masses (Bosniak 3 and 2F): accuracy and impact on clinical management. Eur Radiol 12:2518–2524

Lechevallier E, Andre M, Barriol D et al. (2000) Fine-needle percutaneous biopsy of renal masses with helical CT guidance. Radiology 216:506–510

Link RE, Bhayani SB, Allaf ME et al. (2005) Exploring the learning curve, pathological outcomes and perioperative morbidity of laparoscopic partial nephrectomy performed for renal mass. J Urol 173:1690–1694

Lupo A, Bernich P, Antonucci F et al. (2008) Kidney diseases with chronic renal failure in the Italian renal biopsy registries. G Ital Nefrol 25 (suppl S44): S20–S26

Manno C, Strippoli GF, Arnesano L et al. (2004) Predictors of bleeding complications in percutaneous ultrasound-guided renal biopsy. Kidney Int 66:1570–1577

Mannucci PM, Remuzzi G, Pusineri F et al. (1983) Deamino-8-D-arginine vasopressin shortens the bleeding time in uremia. N Engl J Med 308(1):8–12

Mattix H, Singh AK (1999) Is the bleeding time predictive of bleeding prior to a percutaneous renal biopsy? Curr Opin Nephrol Hypertens 8:715–718

Maturen KE, Nghiem HV, Caoili EM et al. (2007) Renal mass core biopsy: accuracy and impact on clinical management. AJR Am J Roentgenol 188:563–570

Neuzillet Y, Lechevallier E, Andre M et al. (2004) Accuracy and clinical role of fine needle percutaneous biopsy with computerized tomography guidance of small (less than 4.0 cm) renal masses. J Urol 171:1802–1805

Newstead CG (2003) Recurrent disease in renal transplantation. Nephrol Dial Transplant 18(S 6):vi68–vi74

Pasquali S (2008) Diagnostic strategies in kidney disease with chronic renal failure. G Ital Nefrol 25 (suppl S44):S15–S19

Pérez Ara A (1950) La biopsia puntural del riñón megálico. Consideraciones generales y aportación de un nuevo método. Bol Liga contra Cáncer 25:121–147

Renshaw AA, Granter SR, Cibas ES (1997) Fine-needle aspiration of the adult kidney. Cancer 81:71–88

Richards NT, Darby S, Howie AJ et al. (1994) Knowledge of renal histology alters patient management in over 40% of cases. Nephrol Dial Transplant 9:1255–1259

Rybicki FJ, Shu KM, Cibas ES et al. (2003) Percutaneous biopsy of renal masses: sensitivity and negative predictive value stratified by clinical setting and size of masses. AJR Am J Roentgenol 180:1281–1287

Sanchez-Ortiz RF, Madsen LT, Bermejo CE et al. (2004) A renal mass in the setting of a nonrenal malignancy. When is a renal tumor biopsy appropriate? Cancer 101:2195–2201

Sant GR, Heaney JA, Ucci AAJ et al. (1984) Computed tomographic findings in renal angiomyolipoma: a histologic correlation. Urology 24:293–296

Seegal BC, Hsu JH, Fiaschi E et al. (1959) La tecnica degli anticorpi fluorescenti applicata allo studio della patogenesi della nefrite umana. R Ass Fisiopatol Clin terap 31:1063–1078

Stokes MB, Valeri AM, Markowitz GS et al. (2006) Cellular focal segmental glomerulosclerosis: clinical and pathological features. Kidney Int 70:1783–1792

Tomson Charles RV (2003) Indications for renal biopsy in chronic kidney disease. Clin Med 3:513–517

Troyanov S, Roasio L, Pandes M et al. (2006) Renal pathology in idiopathic membranous nephropathy: a new perspective. Kidney Int 69:1641–1648

Tuncali K, vanSonnenberg E, Shankar S et al. (2004) Evaluation of patients referred for percutaneous ablation of renal tumors: importance of a preprocedural diagnosis. AJR Am J Roentgenol 183:575–582

Volpe A, Kachura JR, Geddie WR et al. (2007) Techniques, safety and accuracy of sampling of renal tumors by fine needle aspiration and core biopsy. J Urol 178:379–386

Whittier WL, Korbet SM (2004) Timing of complications in percutaneous renal biopsy. J Am Soc Nephrol 15:142–147

Wolf JJS (1998) Evaluation and management of solid and cystic renal masses. J Urol 159:1120–1133

# Nonvascular Interventional Radiology Procedures

## 10

Raul N. Uppot

## Contents

R.N. Uppot
Department of Radiology, Division of Abdominal
Imaging & Intervention, Massachusetts General Hospital,
55 Fruit Street, White 270, Boston, MA 02111, USA
e-mail: ruppot@partners.org

E. Quaia (ed.), *Radiological Imaging of the Kidney*,
Medical Radiology, DOI: 10.1007/978-3-540-87597-0_10, © Springer-Verlag Berlin Heidelberg 2011

**Abstract**

> Interventional uroradiology is management of urological diseases using minimally invasive techniques and imaging guidance.

> Using ultrasound, CT, and fluoroscopy and small bore needles, catheters and wires, many urological conditions can be managed and treated including: focal and nonfocal renal biopsies, drainage of renal and perirenal collections, percutaneous nephrostomy and lithotripsy, ureteral stenting and embolization, and suprapubic tube placement.

> Interventional uroradiology can be performed with conscious sedation with minimal risk of complications.

## 10.1 Introduction

Image-guided renal interventions have expanded due to technical advances in imaging capabilities and interventional tools. What was once the realm of operative surgical procedures performed by urologists, is now increasingly becoming minimally invasive, image-guided renal interventions performed by interventional radiologists.

Interventional radiologists can now perform multiple urological interventions including: focal and nonfocal renal biopsies, renal cell cancer ablation (discussed in a different chapter), percutaneous catheter drainage of renal and perirenal fluid collections, percutaneous nephrostomy tube placement, provide access for percutaneous lithotripsy, ureteral balloon dilatation and stenting, ureteral embolization, and suprapubic tube placement.

Urological interventions entail a multidisciplinary approach in close cooperation with urologists and nephrologists. Performing image-guided interventions requires an understanding of the current capabilities of various available imaging modalities and interventional equipment, a mastery of techniques, and a thorough understanding for the indications and contraindications in the management of many urological conditions.

This chapter will review image-guided renal interventions including a review of imaging modalities available, an overview of the tools used for interventional procedures, and techniques for all image-guided nonvascular renal interventions.

## 10.2 Imaging Modalities and Interventional Equipment

Advances in imaging equipment and interventional tools have advanced the field of interventional uroradiology. Imaging modalities used for guiding interventional uroradiology techniques include fluoroscopy, ultrasound, CT, and recently interventional MRI. Each imaging modality has evolved to play a specific role in the management of urological conditions.

In addition, advances in design of percutaneous access needles, wires, and catheters have revolutionized minimally invasive access to the kidneys and renal collecting system.

### 10.2.1 Imaging Modalities

#### 10.2.1.1 Fluoroscopy

Fluoroscopy is real time X-ray visualization of internal organ structures. For many years, fluoroscopy has been used to diagnose many urological conditions. Intravenous pyelograms, retrograde nephrostograms, and cystograms were used to evaluate the kidneys and the urinary collecting system. The natural evolution of fluoroscopy is its use in interventional renal procedures.

Use of fluoroscopy combined with intravenous or retrograde ureteral injection of iodinated contrast allows real-time visualization of the kidneys and renal collecting system. Injected contrast provides excellent contrast between the renal collecting system and the renal parenchyma and can guide many interventional procedures (Fig. 10.1). Image-guided procedures performed using fluoroscopy include percutaneous nephrostomy tube placement, access for percutaneous lithotripsy, ureteral balloon dilatation and stenting, ureteral embolization, and suprapubic tube placement. Limitations of fluoroscopy include: radiation exposure to the patient and the interventional radiologist (Kumar 2008), and only single plane view of the internal organs. Recent advances in fluoroscopy include the ability to tilt the image intensifier (Fig. 10.2) and biplane fluoroscopy to evaluate the internal organs in more than a single plane. Other advances include mechanisms to decrease radiation dose including pulsed fluoroscopy and digital screen image capture.

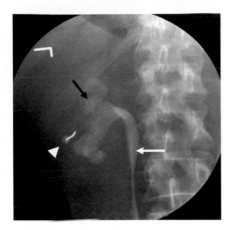

**Fig. 10.1** Spot fluoroscopic image of the left kidney for lithotripsy. Image shows left staghorn calculus (*black arrow*) a ureteral stent had been placed (*white arrow*) and needle (*arrowhead*) is being advanced into midpole calyx after retrograde injection of contrast to opacify the renal collecting system

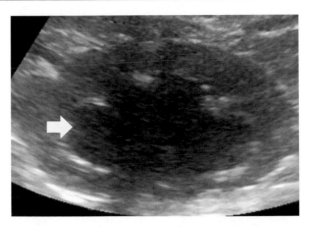

**Fig. 10.3** Sagittal ultrasound of the kidney showing moderate hydronephrosis. The cortex is preserved. The hydronephrosis (*arrow*) can easily be targeted by an access needle for nephrostomy tube placement

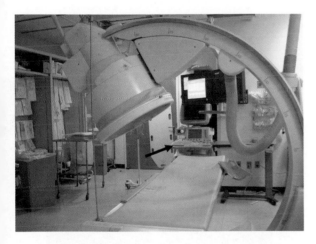

**Fig. 10.2** Photograph of interventional suite showing the ability to tilt image intensifier to aid in interventional procedures involving the urinary system. A nearby ultrasound machine (*arrow*) is also always available for use during interventional procedures

Except for suprapubic tube placement, patients are typically placed in the prone or prone oblique position for most renal interventional procedures.

### 10.2.1.2 Ultrasonography

Ultrasound has also been used for many years diagnostically to evaluate the kidneys. Typically a 2–4 mHz transducer is used to image the kidneys via a flank approach. Sonography can evaluate the size of the kidneys, the appearance of the cortex, the presence of hydronephrosis, and can evaluate for the presence of renal stones or masses (Fig. 10.3).

In the field of interventional uroradiology, ultrasound is used for focal or nonfocal renal biopsies, guiding initial access for nephrostomy tube or nephrolithotomy needle placement, and for suprapubic tube placement. Advantages of ultrasound include real-time visualization, portability, and lack of ionizing radiation. Limitations include need for specialized technical skills to properly scan the renal collecting system and guide the proper placement of needles and/or catheters. Another limitation is the potential for poor visualization of the kidneys due to overlying bowel gas or thickened subcutaneous and retroperitoneal tissues.

### 10.2.1.3 CT

Increasingly, CT scanners are becoming available exclusively for interventional procedures. Modifications to a standard diagnostic CT include addition of CT fluoroscopy, larger diameter gantry, and the availability of multiplanar reformatting (Fig. 10.4), have promoted the use of CT for image-guided procedures. CT is used for renal biopsies, renal tumor ablations, drainage of renal or perirenal collections, and on a few occasions, percutaneous nephrostomy (Egilmez et al. 2007). Advantages of CT include 2D visualization of

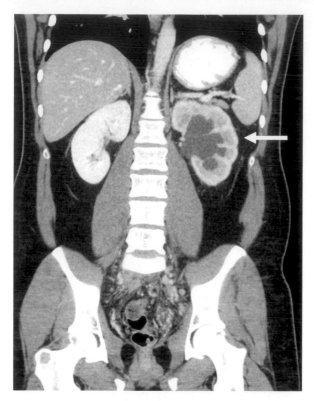

**Fig. 10.4** Coronal reformatted contrast enhanced CT showing left hydronephrosis and delayed left renal nephrogram (*arrow*)

internal organ structures and improved tissue contrast over ultrasound and fluoroscopy. Disadvantages include radiation to the patient and to the radiologist, if CT fluoroscopy feature is used.

### 10.2.1.4 Interventional MRI

Interventional MRI is now being used for image-guided procedures (Fennessy et al. 2008) at a few centers worldwide. It has been used to perform cryoablation of renal tumors (Silverman et al. 2005). The advantages of interventional MRI include superior tissue contrast, multiplanar imaging, and no radiation. Limitations include, limited availability of interventional MRI equipment, and need for MR-safe interventional equipment.

### 10.2.2 Interventional Equipment Tools

In addition to advances in imaging modalities, advances in the design of needles, guidewires and catheters have pushed the field of interventional uroradiology forward.

### 10.2.2.1 Needles

Many interventional uroradiology procedures can be performed due to the availability of small bore 17–22-gauge needles. These needles are available from sizes varying from 6 to 25 cm and allow percutaneous access to the kidney or renal collecting system with minimal damage to the surrounding structures (Lee 2004a). Needles are used for renal biopsies, access to renal or perirenal fluid collections, access to the renal collecting system for nephrostomy tube placement or for lithotripsy.

Coaxial needles may be used to obtain multiple samples through a single puncture (Fig. 10.5), increased patient tolerability for the procedure, and decrease the potential for tumor seeding along the needle tract as reported in a study of breast biopsies using coaxial needles by Helbich et al. (1997).

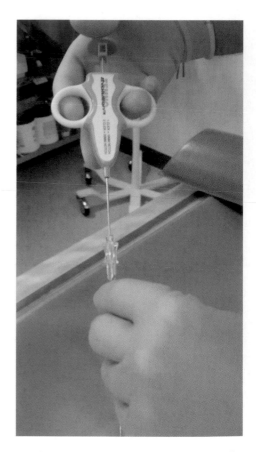

**Fig. 10.5** Photograph of 17 gauge Temno coaxial needle system (Cardinal Health Vaughan, ON) used for our focal renal biopsies

**Fig. 10.10** (**a**) Angiographic image of the left kidney shows 2 cm pseudoaneurysm arising from lower pole branch vessel (*arrow*) after non focal renal biopsy. Patient had persistent hematuria and hematocrit drop prompting angiogram study. (**b**) Angiographic image of the left kidney postcoiling of the pseudoaneurysm shows coils within the left lower pole branch vessel (*arrow*) and the previously visualized pseudoaneurysm is no longer seen

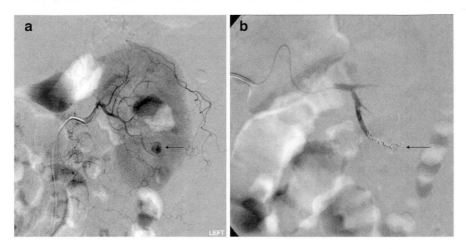

extensive hematuria with blood clots usually requires 24-h admission, serial hematocrits, and possible blood transfusions. On rare occasions, angiography is necessary to evaluate for pseudoaneurysms as a cause for ongoing persistent hemorrhage (Fig. 10.10). Other complications include infection, pneumothorax, hydrothorax, or hemothorax due to a transpleural access, injury to adjacent organs including the liver, spleen, or colon. The risk of needle tract seeding of tumor is low. Overall, needle tract seeding for any abdominal biopsy has been reported to be between 0.003 and 0.009% (Smith 1991). A few cases of needle track seeding from renal mass biopsies have been reported in the literature (Gibbons et al 1977; Kiser et al. 1986; Wehle and Grabstald 1986).

The renal biopsy is covered with greated detail on Chap. 9 which is dedicated to this topic.

## 10.4  US- and CT-Guided Drainage of Renal and Perirenal Collections

### 10.4.1  Indications

Percutaneous aspiration or drainage of renal or pararenal collections is typically performed to address a renal abscess, or decompression of a fluid collection which is causing pain or ureteral obstruction. Although small renal abscesses can initially be managed with antibiotics, larger collections requires percutaneous or surgical intervention for drainage (Lee et al. 2008; Hung et al. 2007).

### 10.4.2  Preparation

Image-guided drainage of renal or perirenal collections can be performed using either ultrasound or CT guidance. Ultrasound guidance can be performed is the collection is a large easy visible fluid collection with no potential to traverse adjacent critical organs (Fig. 10.11). Smaller, more central renal or perirenal collections may require CT-guided drainage. Fluid aspiration is only performed if there is no evidence for an abscess or infection. In most cases, a pigtail catheter is left in position to drain the abscess. In cases of an abscess or infected collection, patients are typically covered with intravenous antibiotics prior to the start of the procedure.

### 10.4.3  Techniques

Two techniques exist for percutaneous drainage of fluid collections including modified Seldinger technique or tandem trocar technique (Lee 2004a–c).

Most institutions perform a CT-guided images using a modified Seldinger technique. In this technique, a needle is inserted under imaging guidance into the targeted fluid collection. Subsequently, the inner stylet is removed and a guidewire is advanced into the fluid collection and its position confirmed with imaging. The needle is then removed and serial dilators are then inserted over the guidewire to achieve dilatation of the tract capable of supporting an 8–12-French catheter. Finally, a pigtail catheter is advanced over the guidewire and its tip curled

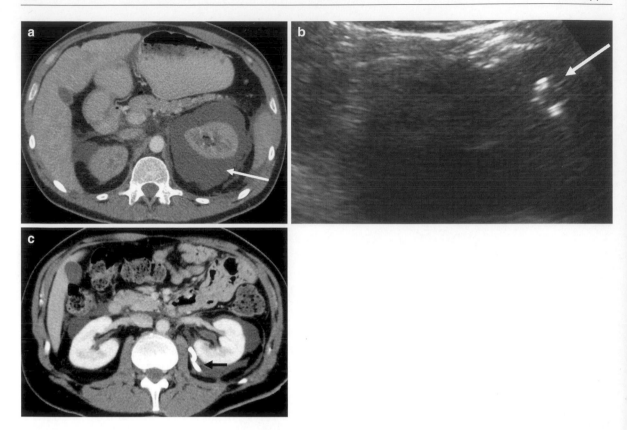

**Fig. 10.11** (**a**) Axial CT showing large left perinephric fluid collection (*arrow*). (**b**) Sagittal ultrasound of the perinephric fluid collection showing ultrasound-guided placement of pigtail catheter (*arrow*) into the collection. (**c**) Axial CT showing decompression of perinephric fluid after placement of pigtail catheter adjacent to the left kidney (*arrow*)

within the collection. The advantages of the modified Seldinger technique include targeting of the organ using a small needle and once the target is reached the guidewire is used as a tract to guide subsequent placement of dilators and catheters. The limitations of a modified Seldinger technique include longer procedure time due to tedious serial dilatation of the tract.

At our institution we perform most of our CT-guided drainages using a tandem trocar technique. In this technique, a needle is inserted under imaging guidance into the targeted fluid collection. Imaging confirms the position and trajectory of the needle. Subsequently, a properly chosen catheter loaded on a sharp-tipped inner stiffener is directly advanced into the collection parallel to the initial needle placement. A final confirmatory CT scan confirms position of the pigtail within the collection. The advantage is of a tandem trocar technique include expedited placement of the catheter directly into the collection and minimizing spread of the infected fluid collection as can occur with use of serial dilators

over a guidewire. The challenge of the tandem trocar technique is that it requires great technical skill to ensure accurate parallel positioning of the catheter relative to the needle to avoid injury to adjacent critical organs.

After placement of pigtail catheter into the collection, all the fluid is aspirated and sent to microbiology and clinical laboratory for evaluation. The cavity is then carefully irrigated with a total of 60 cc of normal saline, in 20 cc aliquotes. Irrigation of the cavity must be performed carefully to avoid over distention of the cavity and pressurized translocation of infected fluid into the renal vasculature, which can precipitate sepsis.

### 10.4.4 Success Rate

The success rate for drainage of renal or perirenal abscesses has been reported to be between 60 and 94% (Lee 2004a–c).

### 10.4.5 Complications

Complications of image-guided drainage include hemorrhage, infection, injury to adjacent organs, and sepsis. Complications of renal or perirenal abscess drainage are low and are reported to be less than 5%.

## 10.5 Percutaneous Nephrostomy

### 10.5.1 Indications

Percutaneous nephrostomy tube placement is used to treat hydronephrosis resulting in renal failure or urosepsis. Image-guided nephrostomy tube placements are typically performed with a combination of both sonography and fluoroscopy (Dyer et al. 2002). Fluoroscopy can occasionally be used exclusively is there is a visible renal collecting system calculus or a retrograde ureteral stent that can be used to opacify the collecting system.

### 10.5.2 Preparation

Review of prior ultrasound or CT imaging is useful to evaluate for the degree of hydronephrosis, potential cause for hydronephrosis, and evaluate for ease of access to the kidney.

### 10.5.3 Technique

Patient's are placed prone oblique on the fluoroscopy table with the ipsilateral side facing the interventional radiologists. Patient's are obliqued 20° to facilitate access to the posterior calix via the avascular plane of Brodel (Papanicolaou 1995; Scatorchia and Berry 2000).

At our institution we use either ultrasound (Fig. 10.12) or retrograde injection of contrast via stent to identify the renal collecting system. The skin is then prepped and draped and anesthetized with 1% lidocaine. After initial needle placement, urine is aspirated from the collecting system and an equivalent amount of diluted contrast is instilled under fluoroscopy (Fig. 10.13a). If the initial needle axis is not adequate, defined as either an anterior

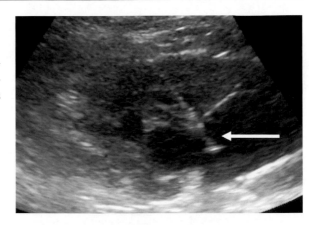

**Fig. 10.12** Sagittal ultrasound of the kidney showing needle (*arrow*) guided into the renal collecting system for placement of a nephrostomy tube

calix, into the renal pelvis, or superiorly via a transpleural access, a second needle may be inserted under fluoroscopic guidance into a lower pole posterior calix (Fig. 10.13b). If the initial needle placement is adequate in a posterior calix below the 12th rib, a guidewire is inserted and subsequent dilatations are performed for eventual placement of a nephrostomy tube (Fig. 10.13c). After placement of a nephrostomy tube, urine is aspirated and sent to microbiology, a final nephrostogram is carefully performed confirming placement of the nephrostomy tube into the collecting system (Fig. 10.13d).

### 10.5.4 Success Rate

If the collecting system is dilated, the success rate approaches 100%. Even for nondilated systems the success rate is as high as 80% (Maher et al. 2000).

### 10.5.5 Complications

The reported overall incidence of major complications is 4% including massive hemorrhage 1–3.6% (Farrell and Hicks 1997; Lee 1994), and pneumothorax 1%. A common complication is sepsis due to overdistention of the renal collecting system or guidewire or catheter manipulations. Other complications include hematuria, subintimal dissection (Fig. 10.14), injury to central renal vasculature (Harris and Walther 1984), adjacent organ injury including spleen, colon, liver, pleura.

**Fig. 10.13** (**a**) Fluoroscopic spot image after initial needle access under ultrasound guidance now used to carefully opacify the left renal collecting system (*arrow*). (**b**) Because initial needle access was above the 12th rib (*black arrow*) a second access was obtained using a sheethed needle directed into lower pole calyx under fluoroscopic guidance (*white arrow*). (**c**) Fluoroscopic spot image showing advancement of a curved wire (*arrow*) into proximal ureter via lower pole access. Access to the proximal ureter allows for a more stable purchase of the guidewire for subsequent dilations and nephrostomy tube placement. (**d**) Fluoroscopic spot image showing final placement of pigtail nephrostomy tube into renal collecting system via lower pole access (*arrow*)

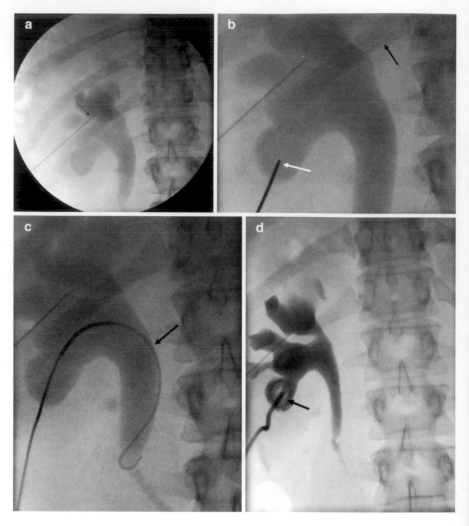

## 10.6 Percutaneous Lithotripsy and Nephrolithotomy

Interventional radiologists, working in close operation with urologists can perform percutaneous lithotripsy. The role of the interventional radiologists is to provide percutaneous access to the renal collecting system, ureter, and bladder so that the urologist can perform lithotripsy in the operating room (Lee 2004a–c).

### 10.6.1 Indications

Indications for lithotripsy include obstructing proximal calcuili or nephrocalculi which cause pain.

### 10.6.2 Preparation

Prior to access for percutaneous lithotripsy, review of prior images is important to confirm the side of percutaneous access, the location of the calculus, the stone burden, and the skin trajectory to access the renal collecting system. At our institution, patient's initially present to the urologist and have a retrograde stent placed that may be used to opacify the renal collecting system during percutaneous access.

### 10.6.3 Technique

Patient's are placed prone on the fluoroscopy table. The skin is prepped draped and anesthetized. Under

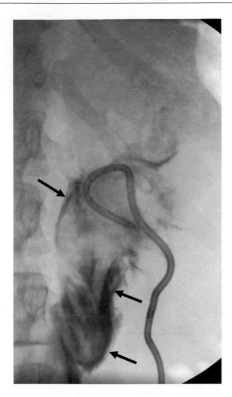

**Fig. 10.14** Fluoroscopic spot image showing attempted right nephrostomy tube placement with catheter incorrectly placed into the subintimal space. The subintimal dissection is identified by outlining of the true renal collecting system by contrast (*arrows*)

fluoroscopic guidance, access to the renal collecting system is obtained via either direct puncture to the calix containing the renal calculi or after opacification of the renal collecting system via the previously placed retrograde stent (Fig. 10.15a). In contradistinction to nephrostomy tube placement via a lower pole calix, the ideal access for percutaneous lithotripsy is via the calix that crosses and allows access to the stones for lithotripsy (Fig. 10.15b). Once access is obtained, a 3 J-wire and an angled guiding catheter are used to manipulate beyond the stone into the proximal ureter and down into the bladder (Fig. 10.15c). Manipulation across the calyceal stones may be difficult and techniques to facilitate crossing the stone include distending the collecting system allowing for the space between the calyceal wall and the stone, or using a combination of the angled guiding catheter and a glidewire. After a guidewire is placed in the bladder the patient may be transferred back to urology for immediate lithotripsy or alternatively, a nephroureteral

stent can be placed and urologist may access the nephroureteral stent at a later date to perform the lithotripsy.

### 10.6.4 Success Rate

For renal stones the success rate is 98.3 and 88.2% for ureteral stones (Segura et al. 1985).

### 10.6.5 Complications

Complications are the same as nephrostomy tube placement including hemorrhage, hematuria, sepsis, adjacent organ injury. The risk of sepsis occurs during the manipulation near potentially infected stones with wires and catheters. Preprocedure antibiotic coverage of the patient is important and close post procedure monitoring is important to look for the risk for sepsis secondary to manipulation next to a potentially infected stone.

## 10.7 Ureteral Stenting

### 10.7.1 Indications

Ureteral stenting is used to treat obstructing stones, obstructing stricture, obstructing bladder mass, or manage a ureteral leak.

### 10.7.2 Preparation

Prior imaging detailing the abnormality within the ureter and associated findings such as hydronephrosis, ureteral or periureteral masses or stones, or urinomas is reviewed.

### 10.7.3 Techniques

Many of the steps for ureteral stenting follow steps for nephrostomy tube placement (detailed above). Patients are placed prone oblique on the fluoroscopy table and

**Fig. 10.15** (**a**) Fluoroscopic spot image showing ureteral stent in position used to opacify the renal collecting system in a retrograde manner (*black arrow*). External clamp (*white arrow*) identified the targeted entry site into midpole calyx. (**b**) Fluoroscopic spot image showing access to left renal collecting system with a small angled catheter (*white arrow*) lateral to the large staghorn stone (*black arrow*). (**c**) Fluoroscopic spot image showing manipulation of angled catheter with the help of a guidewire across the calyceal stone towards the distal ureter (*arrow*)

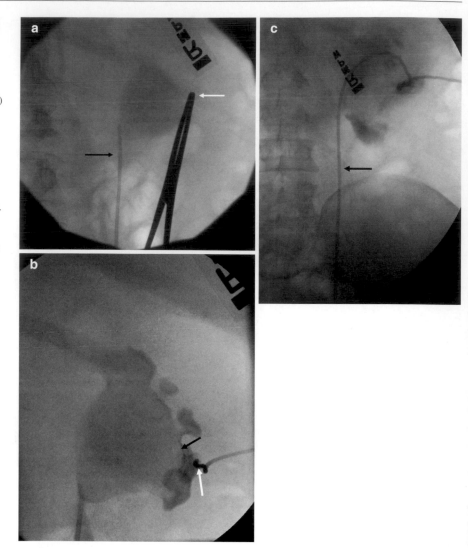

access to the renal collecting system is obtained. After a guidewire is manipulated into the collecting system down the ureter into the bladder, serial dilatations of the tract are performed. We then placed a sheath into the proximal renal collecting system and subsequently advance a double pigtail stent over the guidewire. The distal portion of the stent is deployed into the bladder by retracting the guidewire (Fig. 10.16a). Subsequently, the proximal portion of the pigtail is released into the renal pelvis (Fig. 10.16b). Typically after initial ureteral stent placement we maintain a safety nephrostomy due to the risk of hemorrhage within the collecting system, during guidewire and catheter manipulation, that can subsequently result in obstruction of the stent. After 24–48 h, a nephrostomy

tube injection is performed to confirm patency of the stent and no collecting system hematoma. If the stent is patent and there is no hematoma, nephrostomy tube can be removed.

### 10.7.4 Success Rate

Technical success state for ureteral stent placement approaches 100% (Lee 2004a–c; Lu et al. 1994). These stents have to be changed on a regular basis by the urologist due debris build up and subsequent obstruction. The 3 month patency rate of these stents is reported to be 95 and 54% at 6 months (Lee 2004a–c; Lu et al. 1994).

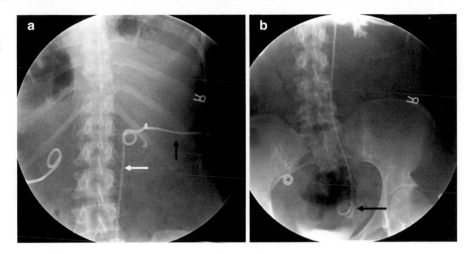

**Fig. 10.16** (**a**) Fluoroscopic spot image showing proximal pigtail deployment of ureteral stent (*white arrow*). A safety nephrostomy is seen (*black arrow*). (**b**) Fluoroscopic spot image showing distal pigtail deployment of ureteral stent (*arrow*)

### 10.7.5 Complications

Complications include hemorrhage, hematuria, sepsis, ureteral injury including perforation or subintimal dissection.

## 10.8 Ureteral Ballooning of Strictures

### 10.8.1 Indications

Balloon dilatation of the ureter may be used to treat benign ureteral strictures. Ureteral strictures can be the result of prior trauma/postoperative, instrumentation, radiation, or pelvic mass (Fig. 10.17a).

### 10.8.2 Preparation

Prior imaging including fluoroscopic studies, CT, ultrasound, or MR urograms are reviewed to identify the location, length, and potential cause for stricture. Patients typically already have either nephrostomy, nephroureteral stent, or internalized stent.

### 10.8.3 Techniques

Under fluoroscopic guidance with the patient placed prone, the ureter is accessed via the previously placed nephrostomy or nephroureteral stent. These site of the stricture is crossed with a stiff guidewire.

A balloon sized to the normal ureter is then advanced over the stiff guidewire to the point of narrowing (Fig. 10.17b). The balloon is then insufflated carefully to 20 atm. until the visualized balloon waist is opened (Fig. 10.17c). Overdistention of the balloon risks the potential for ureteral injury. After balloon dilatation, typically a nephroureteral or internalized ureteral stent is left in place for several weeks. Removal of the stents is achieved after inserting a guidewire, removing the stent over the guidewire, and performing an antegrade injection of the ureter adjacent to the guidewire, detailing the resolution of the stricture and showing no evidence of extravasation from the ureter.

### 10.8.4 Success Rate

In cases of ureteral injuries diagnosed late after cesarean section, approximately 75% of strictures were successfully managed with ureteral dilation and stents alone. Only 25% needed to undergo surgery for operative repair (Ustunsoz et al. 2008).

### 10.8.5 Complications

In addition to bleeding, and infection, ureteral balloon dilatation carries the added risk of ureteral laceration.

**Fig. 10.17** (**a**) Fluoroscopic
spot image showing proximal
right renal hydronephrosis
due to distal stricture at
ureteral-ileal loop (*arrow*).
(**b**) Fluoroscopic spot image
showing guidewire and
partially inflated balloon
across the distal right ureteral
anastomotic stricture. See
small waist of stricture
(*arrow*). (**c**) Fluoroscopic
spot image showing full
inflated balloon opening up
the ureteral stricture (*arrow*)

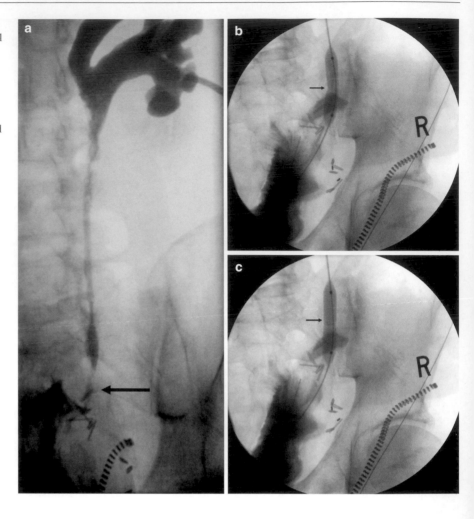

## 10.9  Ureteral Embolization

### 10.9.1  Indications

Ureteral embolization is a rare procedure and is only
performed in patients who have an inoperable pelvic
tumor or leak (Fig. 10.18a) and who require permanent
urinary diversion via nephrostomy tubes.

### 10.9.2  Preparation

Prior nephrostogram and cross sectional imaging is
reviewed before planning for coil placement.

### 10.9.3  Techniques

Under fluoroscopic guidance with the patient placed
prone, the ureter is accessed via the previously
placed nephrostomy or nephroureteral stent. An initial
nephrogram is performed identifying the entire course
of the ureter. Subsequently a guidewire is inserted into
the nephrostomy tube and the nephrostomy tube is
removed and replaced with a 5 French angled guiding
catheter. The angled guiding catheter is then advance
to the distal ureter overling the pelvic brim and multiple 10/5 and 8/4 tornado coils are stacked within a
short segment of the ureter (Fig. 10.18b). In addition to
the coils a gelfoam/contrast slurry is injected into the
clump of coils. Repeat injections of the ureter with the
angled guiding catheter should show slowing of flow

**Fig. 10.18** (**a**) Fluoroscopic spot image of the distal left ureter showing extravasation from the distal left ureteral leceration (*arrow*). (**b**) Fluoroscopic spot image post ureteral coil embolization showing contrast extending proximal to the level of the coiled ureter (*arrow*) with no evidence of extravasation

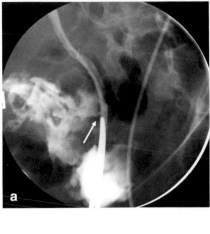
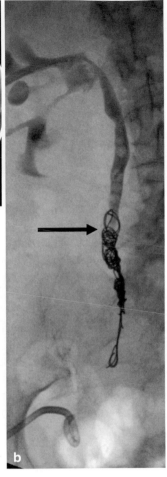

past the area of embolization. Complete ureteral embolization is typically not possible at the first attempt. Typically it takes several weeks for a reactive process of the ureter to scar and may require a second or third.

### 10.9.4  Success Rate

Farrell et al. (1997) reported a success rate of 100% in 34 patients who underwent ureteral embolization for urinary incontinence and fistulas.

### 10.9.5  Complications

Reported complications include coil migration into the renal pelvis in 2 patients and nephrostomy

tube occlusion requiring replacement in 3 patients (Farrell et al. 1997).

## 10.10  Sovrapubic Tube Placement

### 10.10.1  Indications

Sovrapubic tubes allow decompression of the bladder via small bore tube placed through the anterior pelvic wall and allow for long term drainage of the kidney while avoiding the complications of infection and urethral irritation and trauma from a chronic urethral foley. Indications include treatment for bladder outlet obstruction, neurogenic bladder, keeping a perforated bladder decompressed, and diverting urine from a urethral injury.

### 10.10.2 Preparation

Review of prior cross sectional imaging through the pelvis can identify the location of the sigmoid colon, small bowel loops and possible hernias that may lie anterior to the bladder. Typically a urethral foley is placed prior to sovrapubic tube insertion to allow for retrograde distension of the bladder. Patients are given preprocedure antibiotics.

### 10.10.3 Techniques

Patients are placed prone on the procedure table and are sedated. The skin is prepped and draped and anesthetized. A location just superior to the palpated pubic symphysis just lateral to the midline is chosen as the entry site. A sovrapubic tube can be directly placed using a trocar device under ultrasound guidance (Fig. 10.19). Alternatively the bladder can be accessed via fluoroscopy (Fig. 10.20) using a sheathed needle and the tract serially dilated to the appropriate size catheter. Once the catheter is advanced into the bladder, its position is confirmed under ultrasound or fluoroscopy.

### 10.10.4 Success Rate

Success rate has been reported to approach 100% (Lee et al. 1994).

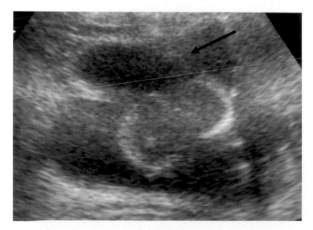

**Fig. 10.19** Transverse ultrasound image of a distended bladder showing ultrasound-guided placement of foley catheter loaded onto a trocar (*arrow*) into the bladder

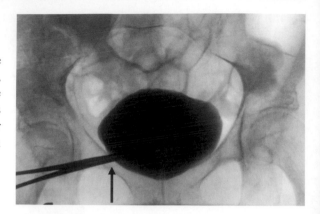

**Fig. 10.20** Fluoroscopic spot image showing opacification of the bladder with contrast injected via urethral foley catheter. The external clamp is used to identify entrance site of the sheathed needle (*arrow*) for eventual placement of a suprapubic catheter

### 10.10.5 Complications

Specific complications include bladder or bowel perforation, infection or bleeding.

### 10.10.6 Conclusion

Interventional uroradiology has evolved the management of many urological conditions. Advances in imaging equipment and interventional tools have promoted the acceptance of this field as a viable option for management of many urological conditions. Interventional radiologists performing these procedures must have an understanding for the indications and risks for managing many of these urological conditions and acquire the technical skills. Widespread use of interventional MRI and use of navigational tools for image-guided procedures will increase the accuracy and speed by which these procedures will be performed.

### References

Caoili EM, Bude RO, Higgins EJ et al. (2002) Evaluation of sonographically guided percutaneous core biopsy of renal masses. AJR 179(2):373–378

Dechet CB, Zincke H, Sebo TJ et al. (2003) Prospective analysis of computerized tomography and needle biopsy with permanent sectioning to determine the nature of solid renal masses in adults. J Urol 169(1):71–74

Dyer RB, Regan JD, Kavanagh PV et al. (2002) Percutaneous nephrostomy with extensions of the technique: step by step. Radiographics 22:503–525

Egilmez H, Oztoprak I, Atalar M et al. (2007) The place of computed tomography as a guidance modality in percutaneous nephrostomy: analysis of a 10-year single-center experience. Acta Radiol 48(7):806–813

Eshed I, Elias S, Sidi AA (2004) Diagnostic value of CT-guided biopsy of indeterminate renal masses. Clin Radiol 59: 262–267

Farrell TA, Hicks ME (1997) A review of radiologically guided percutaneous nephrostomies in 303 patients. J. Vasc Interv Radiol 8:769–774

Farrell TA, Wallace M, Hicks ME (1997) Long-term results of transrenal ureteral occlusion with use of Gianturco coils and gelatin sponge pledgets. J Vasc Interv Radiol 8:449–452

Fennessy FM, Tuncali K, Morrison PR et al. (2008) MR imaging-guided interventions in the genitourinary tract: an evolving concept. Radiol Clin N Am 46:149–166

Gibbons RP, Bush WH Jr, Burnett LL (1977) Needle tract seeding following aspiration of renal cell carcinoma. J Urol 118(5):865–867

Hara I, Miyake H, Hara S et al. (2001) Role of percutaneous image-guided biopsy in the evaluation of renal masses. Urol Int 67(3):199–202

Harris RD, Walther PC (1984) Renal arterial injury associated with percutaneous nephrostomy. Urology 23:215–217

Helbich TH, Mayr W, Schick S et al. (1997) Coaxial technique: approach to breast core biopsies. Radiology 203(3):684–690

Herts BR, Baker ME (1995) The current role of percutaneous biopsy in the evaluation of renal masses. Semin Urol Oncol 13:254–261

Hung CH, Liou JD, Yan MY et al. (2007) Immediate percutaneous drainage compared with surgical drainage of renal abscess. Int Urol Nephrol 39(1):51–55

Jemal A, Siegel R, Ward E et al. (2006) Cancer statistics, 2006. CA Cancer J Clin 56(2):106–130

Kiser GC, Totonchy M, Barry JM (1986) Needle tract seeding after percutaneous renal adenocarcinoma aspiration. J Urol 136(6)1292–1293

Kumar P (2008) Radiation safety issues in fluoroscopy during percutaneous nephrolithotomy. Urol J 5(1):15–23

Lechevallier E, Andre M, Barriol D et al. (2000) Fine-needle percutaneous biopsy of renal masses with helical CT guidance. Radiology 216(2):506–510

Lee BE, Seol HY, Kim TK et al. (2008) Recent clinical overview of renal and perirenal abscesses in 56 consecutive cases. Korean J Intern Med 23(3):140–148

Lee MJ (2004a) Image-guided percutaneous biopsy. In: Kaufman JA, Lee MJ (eds) The requisites: vascular & interventional radiology, 1st edn. Mosby, St. Louis, pp 469–488

Lee MJ (2004b) Percutaneous abscess and fluid drainage. In: Kaufman JA, Lee MJ (eds) The requisites: vascular & interventional radiology, 1st edn. Mosby, St. Louis, pp 489–520

Lee MJ (2004c) Percutaneous genitourinary interventions. In: Kaufman JA, Lee MJ (eds) The requisites: vascular & interventional radiology, 1st edn. Mosby, St. Louis, pp 602–635

Lee WJ, Patel U, Patel S et al. (1994) Emergency percutaneous nephrostomy: results and complications. J Vasc Interv Radiol 5(1):135–139

Lu DS, Papanicolaou N, Girard M et al. (1994) Percutaneous internal ureteral stent placement: review of technical issues and solutions in 50 consecutive cases. Clin Radiol 49(4): 256–261

Maher MM, Fotheringham T, Lee MJ (2000) Percutaneous nephrostomy. Semin Interv Radiol 17:329–339

Neuzillet Y, Lechevallier E, Andre M et al. (2004) Accuracy and clinical role of fine needle percutaneous biopsy with computerized tomography guidance of small (less than 4.0 cm) renal masses. J Urol 171(5):1802–1805

Papanicolaou N (1995) Renal anatomy relevant to percutaneous interventions. Semin Intervent Radiol 12:163–172

Richter F, Kasabian NG, Irwin RJ Jr et al. (2000) Accuracy of diagnosis by guided biopsy of renal mass lesions classified indeterminate by imaging studies. Urology 55(3):348–352

Rybicki FJ, Shu KM, Cibas ES et al. (2003) Percutaneous biopsy of renal masses: sensitivity and negative predictive value stratified by clinical setting and size of masses. AJR 180(5): 1281–1287

Scatorchia GM, Berry RF (2000) A review of renal anatomy. Semin Interv Radiol 17:323–328

Segura JW, Patterson DE, LeRoy AJ et al. (1985) Percutaneous removal of kidney stones: review of 1000 cases. J Urol 134(6)1077–1081

Shah RB, Bakshi N, Hafez KS et al. (2005) Image-guided biopsy in the evaluation of renal mass lesions in contemporary urological practice: indications, adequacy, clinical impact, and limitations of the pathological diagnosis. Hum Pathol 36(12): 1309–1315

Silverman SG, Tuncali K, van Sonnenberg E et al. (2005) Renal tumors: MR imaging-guided percutaneous cryotherapy – initial experience in 23 patients. Radiology 236:716–724

Smith ED (1991) Complications of percutaneous abdominal fine-needle biopsy. Radiology 178:253–258

Tuncali K, van Sonnenberg E, Shankar S et al. (2004) Evaluation of patients referred for percutaneous ablation of renal tumors: importance of a preprocedure diagnosis. AJR 183: 575–582

Ustunsoz B, Ugurel S, Duru NK et al. (2008) Percutaneous management of ureteral injuries that are diagnosed late after cesarean section. Korean J Radiol 9(4):348–353

Wehle MJ, Grabstald H (1986) Contraindications to needle aspiration of a solid renal mass: tumor dissemination by renal needle aspiration. J Urol 136:446–448

Wood BJ, Khan MA, McGovern F et al. (1999) Imaging guided biopsy of renal masses: indications, accuracy and impact on clinical management. J Urol 161(5):1470–1474

Wunderlich H, Hindermann W, Al Mustafa AM et al. (2005) The accuracy of 250 fine needle biopsies of renal tumors. J Urol 174(1):44–46

# Congenital and Development Disorders of the Kidney

# 11

Veronica Donoghue

## Contents

**Abstract**

> This chapter gives a brief outline of the embryology of the renal tract and discusses anomalies of position and fusion of the kidneys, renal agenesis and anomalies in renal size. It also discusses in detail the various types of congenital renal cystic disease and the causes of congenital renal collecting system dilatation.

## 11.1 Embryology of the Kidneys, Ureters and Bladder

The kidney development begins at the fifth week of gestation from an outpouching of the mesonephric duct which becomes the ureteric bud. This later forms the ureter and collecting system of the kidney. At approximately the seventh week of gestation age the glomeruli and tubules arise from mesenchymal tissue called the metanephric blastema. If the ureteric bud and the metanephric blastema fail to communicate the kidney does not develop. All nephrons and the ureteric bud branches have developed by 32–36 weeks of gestation. The bladder arises from the superior urogenital sinus which in turn arises from the cloaca. The bladder trigone arises from the mesonephric ducts into which the ureters fuse. As the foetus develops the kidneys rotate and migrate cranially and reach their final level by the eighth to the eleventh week of gestation. As they migrate they also undergo 90° medial rotation. Each kidney receives its blood supply from its neighbouring vessels (Benz-Bohm 2008). For a more detailed description of the kidney embryology, please see Chap. 1.

V. Donoghue
Radiology Departments, Children's University Hospital,
Temple Street, Dublin 1, Ireland
e-mail: veronica.donoghue@cuh.ie

E. Quaia (ed.), *Radiological Imaging of the Kidney*,
Medical Radiology, DOI: 10.1007/978-3-540-87597-0_11, © Springer-Verlag Berlin Heidelberg 2011

## 11.2 Positional and Fusion Anomalies

### 11.2.1 Ectopic Kidney

Failure of a kidney to migrate from its position of embryonal development to its retroperitoneal adult location results in simple renal ectopia. The condition is frequently referred to by the final position in which the kidney lies i.e. the pelvis, lumbar, abdominal or thoracic locations. It may be accompanied by malrotation of the affected kidney and it is frequently smaller than normal (Daneman and Alton 1991). The diagnosis may be made during routine antenatal ultrasonography and is also frequently made incidentally during ultrasonography for other clinical indications. Ultrasonography is sufficient to make the diagnosis in most cases. The adrenal gland may have an elongated appearance in an empty renal fossa (Fig. 11.1). A Tc99m DMSA scan may be helpful if the kidney is difficult to visualize because of overlying bowel loops and is particularly helpful to assess the degree of functioning renal tissue. If there is evidence of a dilated pelvis and calyces a Tc99m Mag 3 renogram is useful to determine if there is obstruction to drainage. The size of the kidney and amount of renal cortex can also be assessed using MRI (Kavanagh et al. 2005). In recent years there have been developments in the technique of MR

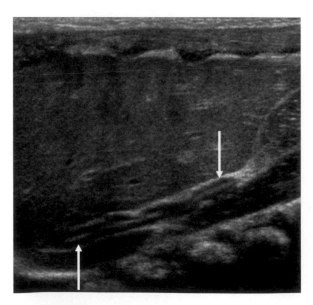

**Fig. 11.1** Elongated right adrenal gland in a child with absent right kidney (*arrows*)

urography but it is not yet widely available. As vesicoureteric reflux is present in up to 70% of these kidneys a voiding cystourethrogram may be required. The contralateral kidney may be abnormal in approximately 50% of patients. Other associated anomalies include genital anomalies (Downs et al. 1973), skeletal, cardiovascular (Malek et al. 1971), and gastrointestinal anomalies (Ritchey 1992).

### 11.2.2 Horseshoe Kidneys

The horseshoe kidney is the most common fusion anomaly and its incidence is approximately 1:400 (Glenn 1959). The mechanism of fusion is unknown but it is thought to occur early in development after the ureteral bud enters the metanephric blastema. The kidneys lie on either side of the midline and their lower poles are connected by either a band of renal parenchymal or fibrous tissue (Fig. 11.2). This isthmus usually lies anterior to the great vessels. In a very small number of cases the isthmus connects the upper poles and rarer still is the "doughnut" kidney where both the upper and lower poles are fused.

The diagnosis can be made using renal ultrasonography. The lower poles of the kidneys are medially located and the renal pelvis may be anterior. Transverse images demonstrating the isthmus is essential to make the diagnosis and to distinguish from malrotation without fusion. Tc99m DMSA scan is excellent at identifying the orientations of the kidneys and the functioning renal tissue of the isthmus. It is especially useful when the amount of functioning renal parenchyma is small. If necessary the diagnosis can be confirmed using MRI, IVU or post-intravenous CT.

Thirty-three percent of patients with horseshoe kidneys have at least one other abnormality (Boatman et al. 1972). Associated anomalies include those of the central nervous system, gastrointestinal tract, cardiovascular and skeletal systems. Horseshoe kidneys have been reported in 20% of patients with Trisomy 18 (Boatman et al. 1972) and 7% of patients with Turner's syndrome (Lippe et al. 1988).

Hydronephrosis occurs in approximately 30% of patients due to pelviureteric junction obstruction due to a high ureteral insertion or an anomalous renal vessel. Dilatation may also be due to reflux which has been noted in approximately 50% of children with

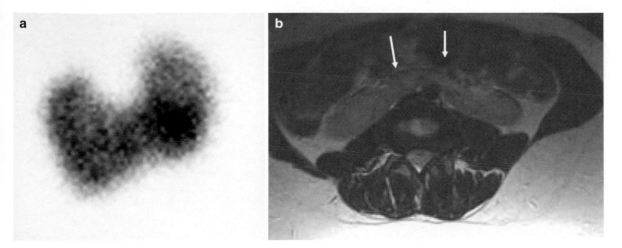

**Fig. 11.2** (**a**) DMSA renogram demonstrating horseshoe kidneys with a connecting inferior band of renal tissue. (**b**) Connecting band in horseshoe kidneys identified incidentally in a patient who had an MRI of the spine (*arrows*)

horseshoe kidneys. There is an increased incidence of Wilms' tumour (Mesrobian et al. 1985).

### 11.2.3 Crossed Fused Ectopia

This is the second most common fusion anomaly after horseshoe kidney. The crossed ectopic kidney lies on the contralateral side to the insertion of its draining ureter into the bladder. Crossed ectopia with fusion occurs in 85% of cases and without fusion in less than 10% (McDonald and McClellan 1957; Abeshouse and Bhisitkul 1959).

Solitary and bilateral crossed renal ectopia are very rare. There are six types of crossed renal ectopia with fusion. The most common type is when the upper pole of the crossed kidney lies inferior to and is fused with the normally located kidney (Fig. 11.3). Its renal pelvis is anterior representing incomplete rotation. The next most common type is inferior ectopia where both pelves have opposite orientation indicating complete rotation.

The diagnosis is suspected on sonography but it may be impossible to distinguish between fused and unfused kidneys. This may also be difficult to determine on intravenous urography because the poles often overlap. Tc99m DMSA scintigraphy with SPECT (Applegate et al. 1995), CT or MRI may be necessary to establish the diagnosis. MRI and CT angiography will also help to outline the vascular

supply which may be quite variable. Vesicoureteric reflux is the most common associated anomaly and therefore a voiding cystourethrogram is indicated in these patients.

### 11.3 Renal Agenesis and Anomalies in Size

### 11.3.1 Renal Agenesis

Renal agenesis is the result of failure of the ureteric bud to connect with the metanephric blastema during the appropriate stage of development. A blind ending ipsilateral ureter of varying length may be present.

Bilateral renal agenesis is rare and estimated by Potter to occur in 1:48,000 cases (Potter 1972). The bladder is absent in approximately 50% of cases and when present the trigone is usually underdeveloped. The association of pulmonary hypoplasia, bowel anomalies, clubbed lower extremities and a typical facial appearance led Potter to describe the syndrome. There may also be associated genital anomalies.

Prenatally the diagnosis is usually made by sonography. There is severe oligohydramnios and failure to visualize foetal kidneys and a urinary bladder. The condition is incompatible with life.

Unilateral renal agenesis is often clinically silent. Ultrasonographic screening of 132,686 school children

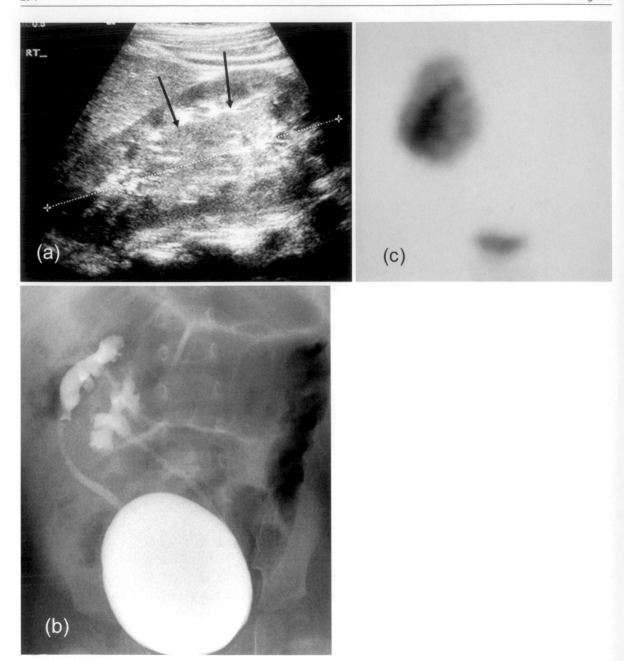

**Fig. 11.3** Patient with crossed fused ectopia. (**a**) US at location of renal fusion (*arrows*). (**b**) VCUG demonstrating reflux into both collecting systems. (**c**) DMSA scan mimics a single right kidney

revealed an incidence of 1:12,800 children (Sheih et al. 1989).

The left kidney is absent more frequently than the right. There is aplasia of the ipsilateral adrenal gland in less than 10% of cases. The contralateral kidney may be ectopic, malrotated or have vesicoureteric reflux.

It may also be associated with genital abnormalities and is associated with syndromes such as Turners, Klippel–Feil, Polands and Mayer–Rokitansky.

When the diagnosis is made antenatally, postnatal sonography is required for confirmation and to evaluate the kidney on the opposite side. If the ipsilateral adrenal gland is present it is often elongated (Fig. 11.1). There may be compensatory hypertrophy of the opposite kidney but at birth the kidney may be normal in size and undergo compensatory hypertrophy later. Tc 99m DMSA scan is extremely useful in confirming the diagnosis and in assessing the size of the contralateral kidney. However, this study must be correlated with the ultrasound findings as a multicystic dysplastic kidney (MCDK) is also non-functioning and will mimic renal agenesis on scintigraphy.

As there is a strong association with vesicoureteric reflux a voiding cystourethrogram is recommended in these infants. An MRI scan is useful in assessing associated genital anomalies (Lang et al. 1999).

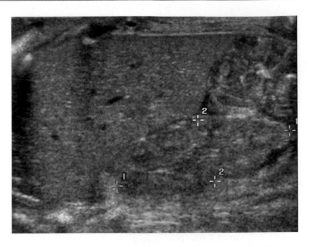

**Fig. 11.4** Hypoplastic right kidney (*between cursors*). The kidney is small with a smooth outline

### 11.3.2 Renal Hypoplasia

True renal hypoplasia, which is a small kidney with essentially normal renal parenchyma with fewer renal lobules and calyces and a normal ureter is a rare congenital abnormality. It originates as a result of disturbed differentiation of metanephrogenic tissue or problems with the induction of tissue differentiation (Riccabona and Ring 2008). It may be combined with dysplastic elements. The kidney may be ectopic or malrotated and is prone to recurrent infections. Hypoplastic kidneys must be distinguished from acquired small kidneys such as those due to renal artery stenosis, renal vein thrombosis or infection.

Segmental renal hypoplasia or Ash-Upmark kidney is when one or more renal lobes fail to develop. Patients suffer from hypertension.

Renal hypoplasia may be diagnosed incidentally. Ultrasonography demonstrates small kidneys with a smooth outline (Fig. 11.4). In segmental hypoplasia the appearance may be similar to that of reflux nephropathy with indentation and thinning of the cortex together with calyceal dilatation and distortion. Some authors (Arant et al. 1979) believe that segmental hypoplasia is an acquired lesion as it is commonly associated with vesicoureteric reflux even in the absence of demonstrable infection.

Voiding cystourethrography is recommended in patients with renal hypoplasia to outrule reflux. Tc 99m DMSA scintigraphy confirms the smooth outline of the kidney without focal defects. Intravenous urography is not indicated.

## 11.4 Renal Cystic Disease

Renal cystic disease can be divided into conditions of developmental origin such as MCDK and cystic renal dysplasia and conditions of genetic origin such as autosomal recessive polycystic kidney disease (ARPKD), autosomal dominant polycystic kidney disease (ADPKD), juvenile nephronophthisis (NPHP), medullary cystic kidney disease complex and glomerulocystic kidney disease (GCKD).

### 11.4.1 Renal Cystic Disease of Developmental Origin

#### 11.4.1.1 Multicystic Dysplastic Kidney

MCDK is the most common cystic renal lesion in children. A variety of proposed aetiologies have been associated with the underlying pathogenesis of MCDK. These include genetic disturbances, teratogens, in utero infections and urinary tract outflow obstruction (Hains et al. 2009; Lazebnik et al. 1999).

The incidence is 1:4,000 live births and is twice as common in males. The condition is usually unilateral and usually involves the entire kidney. It may be segmental (Jeon et al. 1999) or may involve one pole of a duplex system or one kidney in crossed ectopia (Kiddoo et al. 2005).

Abnormalities of the contralateral kidney are present in approximately one third of patients (Lazebnik et al. 1999). These include vesicoureteric reflux (18%) and pelviureteric junction obstruction (12%) (Atiyeh et al. 1992). Other associated conditions may include ipsilateral genital anomalies and cardiac anomalies.

Nowadays most patients are detected antenatally by ultrasound screening. Foetal MRI may be helpful in difficult cases (Kiddoo et al. 2005) (Fig. 11.5).

Postnatal imaging is usually by ultrasonography, to confirm the diagnosis and to assess the contralateral kidney. It shows a multicystic kidney with cysts of varying sizes which do not communicate and the intervening renal tissue is echogenic (Fig. 11.6). Scintigraphy using Tc 99m DMSA shows a non-functioning kidney (Fig. 11.6). There is no general consensus on the routine use of voiding cystourethrography to determine if there is reflux into the contralateral kidney.

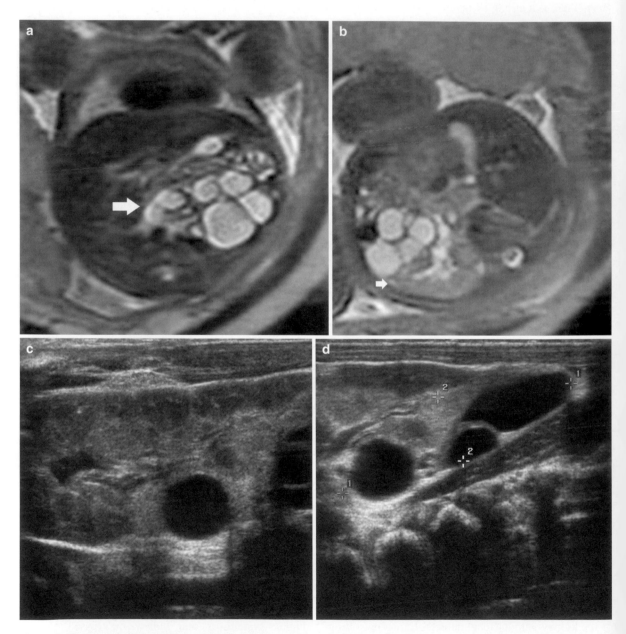

**Fig. 11.5** T2 MRI in a fetus with crossed fused ectopia. (**a**) The anterior lower kidney demonstrates multiple cysts in keeping with a multicystic dysplastic kidney (MCDK) (*arrow*). (**b**) Normal posterior kidney (*arrow*). Postnatal US outlining the normal kidney (**c**) which is fused to the posterior MCDK (**d**)

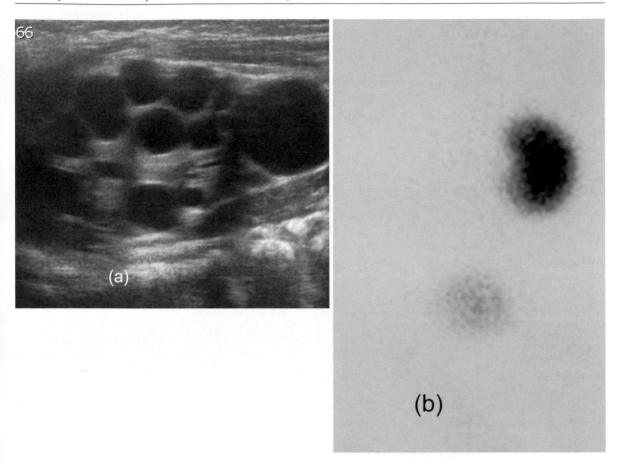

**Fig. 11.6** Infant with MCDK. (**a**) US showing multiple cysts of varying size with intervening abnormally echogenic tissue. (**b**) DMSA scan confirms a non-functioning kidney on the same side

The management of MCDK is usually conservative as its natural history is that of spontaneous atrophy. Follow-up imaging is usually with ultrasonography. Wilms' tumour has been reported in a patient with MCDK (Oddone et al. 1994) and hypertension has been reported in 23% patients (Kiyah et al. 2009).

### 11.4.1.2 Cystic Renal Dysplasia

Renal dysplasia is the result of a developmental anomaly characterized by abnormal structural organization and development of metanephric elements. The kidneys may have multiple cysts. It is frequently associated with urinary tract obstruction and is seen in association with posterior urethral valves, Prune belly syndrome and pelviureteric junction obstruction. This suggests that obstruction and urinary retention may cause abnormal renal development (Shibata and Nagata 2003).

Antenatal MRI may compliment antenatal ultrasonography in establishing the diagnosis (Fig. 11.7).

Postnatally on ultrasonography the kidneys are usually normal to small in size with increased cortical echogenicity, loss of corticomedullary differentiation and scattered small cysts (Fig. 11.8). Voiding cystourethrography may be indicated. Tc 99m Mag 3 renography is helpful to confirm if there is associated obstruction to drainage and Tc 99m DMSA may be required to assess functioning renal tissue.

## 11.4.2 Renal Cystic Disease of Genetic Origin

### 11.4.2.1 Autosomal Recessive Polycystic Kidney Disease

ARPKD is an inherited disease characterized by nonobstructive fusiform dilatation of the renal collecting ducts resulting in enlarged kidneys. Liver disease is present in all patients with the manifestations varying

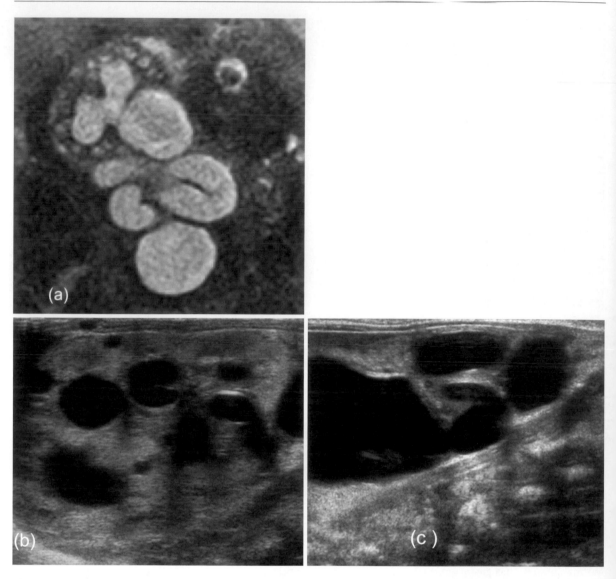

**Fig. 11.7** (**a**) Foetal T2 MR showing a single kidney with significant hydronephrosis and hydroureter. There are multiple small cysts in keeping with cystic dysplasia (**b**). Postnatal US confirm the diagnosis (**c**)

according to the patients age at presentation. The principal pathologic features are periportal fibrosis and biliary duct ectasia. When there is significant liver involvement it is referred to as congenital hepatic fibrosis (Turkbey et al. 2009). The condition is often referred to as infantile polycystic disease as over 90% of patients suffer from renal insufficiency during childhood. It occurs in approximately 1:40,000 live births with a gene defect on chromosome 6 (Zerres et al. 1994).

Antenatally there may be oligohydramnios, very large kidneys and absence of bladder filling. MRI may compliment the ultrasound findings (Cassart et al. 2004).

Infants who are severely affected may have pulmonary hypoplasia and Potter's phenotype and may die from respiratory failure. In selected cases removal of one or both kidneys may improve the respiratory status but the child will usually require dialysis.

Postnatal ultrasonography usually shows enlarged echogenic kidneys with no corticomedullary differentiation. Small cysts up to 3 mm in diameter may be seen and these are usually located peripherally (Boal and Teele 1980). The cysts may be too small to be seen and the echogenic pattern may have a speckled appearance (Fig. 11.9). As the child gets older the kidneys may

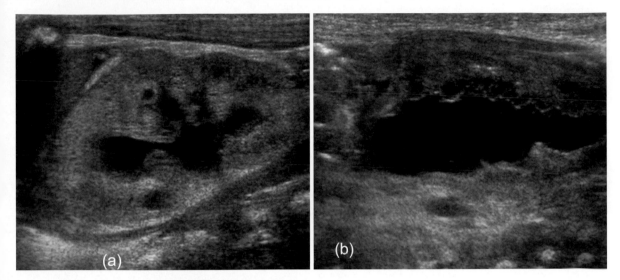

**Fig. 11.8** Newborn with cystic renal dysplasia secondary to posterior urethral valves. (**a**) Left kidney: showing increased cortical echogenicity with loss of the corticomedullary differentiation and multiple cysts. There is renal collecting system dilatation. (**b**) Very irregular thick-walled urinary bladder due to posterior urethral valves

increase further in size and the cysts may enlarge. A family history helps to confirm the diagnosis. Further imaging is only required to follow the condition and this is best performed with sonography. Monitoring of hepatic involvement is necessary to detect complications of portal hypertension. The combined use of conventional and high resolution ultrasonography with MR cholangiography allows detailed definition of the extent of the kidney and hepatobiliary manifestations without requiring ionizing radiation and contrast agents (Turkbey et al. 2009) (Fig. 11.9).

### 11.4.2.2 Autosomal Dominant Polycystic Kidney Disease

ADPKD occurs in approximately 1:1,000 live births. The specific form which develops depends on which of the three genes, PKD1, PKD2 or PKD3 become mutated. In 90% of patients the affected gene is located on the short arm of chromosome 16.

The condition may be detected during infancy and childhood either by selective screening where there is a family history or incidentally. It usually presents during adulthood and is often referred to as adult polycystic kidney disease.

The cysts arise from the nephrons and collecting tubules with which they communicate directly and islands of normal parenchyma are interspersed between the cysts.

Ultrasonography is the imaging modality of choice to investigate these patients. In infants and children the kidneys may be normal but cysts can be seen in the neonatal period (Fig. 11.10). The cysts increase in number over time, may become very large and irregularly distributed throughout the kidney and these may compress normally functioning renal tissue. This will be seen as hyperechoic parenchyma on sonography. The cysts may be complicated by secondary haemorrhage, infection or rupture. Complimentary CT or MRI is rarely necessary.

Intracranial aneurysms associated with the condition have been described in neonates and young children (Proesmans et al. 1982). These may be diagnosed using MR angiography.

### 11.4.2.3 Medullary Cystic Disease and Nephronophthisis

Medullary cystic disease (MCDC) and NPHP are grouped together as they share many features. NPHP is an autosomal recessive disorder with early onset symptoms and medullary cystic kidney disease is inherited as an autosomal dominant disorder which usually affects patients in their thirties.

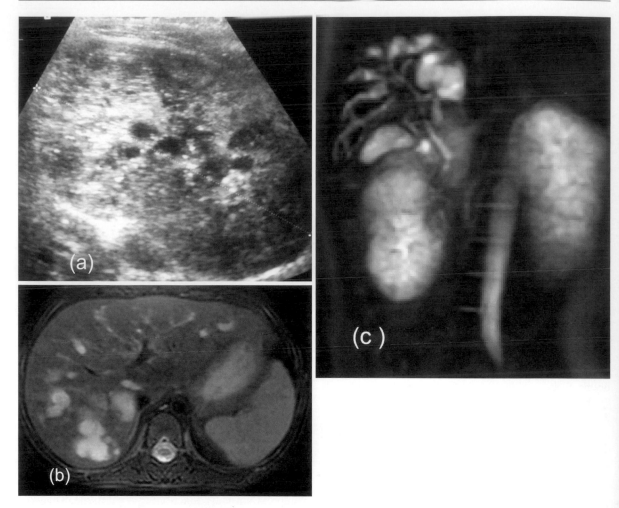

**Fig. 11.9** Newborn with ARPKD. (**a**) The kidney is large, echogenic and contains multiple cysts, some of which are tiny giving rise to a speckled appearance. (**b**) Axial T2 MRI and (**c**) Volume acquisition in the same patient at 2 years showing significant biliary ductal ectasia

Pathologically they cause cysts restricted to the renal medulla or corticomedullary junction in addition to tubular atrophy, tubular basement membrane disintegration and interstitial fibrosis.

Extrarenal manifestations of NPHP include occulomotor apraxia (Cogan syndrome), retinitis pigmentosa (Senior–Loken syndrome), cone-shaped epiphyses and liver fibrosis (Mainzer–Saldino syndrome), optic nerve coloboma with cerebellar vermis hypoplasia (Joubert's syndrome type B), and cranioectodermal dysplasia and electroretinal abnormalities (Sensenbrenner syndrome).

Initially in both conditions the kidneys may be normal. Later they may become slightly hyperechoic and decrease in size. There may be loss of corticomedullary differentiation and cysts may be seen at the corticomedullary junction. Eventually the kidneys become small and scarred. The condition is confirmed by a family history and molecular genetics (Hildebrandt and Otto 2005).

### 11.4.2.4 Glomerulocystic Kidney Disease

Glomeulocystic kidneys can be classified into three main groups (Bernstein 1993).

(a) GCKD comprising non-syndromal autosomal dominant hereditary and sporadic forms.
(b) Glomerulocystic kidneys in hereditary malformation syndromes such as tuberous sclerosis, orofaciodigital

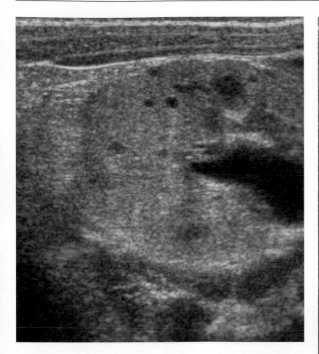

**Fig. 11.10** Transverse US view of kidney in an infant with strong family history of ADPKD. There is some loss of the corticomedullary differentiation and multiple small cysts

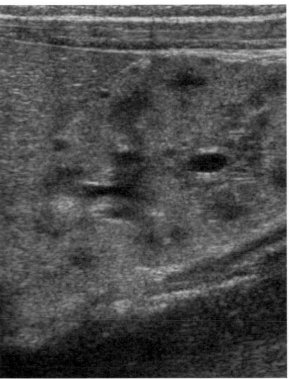

**Fig. 11.11** Renal US in a newborn infant with Zellweger's syndrome. There are a number of small peripheral cysts

syndrome, Trisomy 13, short rib polydactyly syndrome and Jeune's syndrome.

(c) Glomerulocystic kidneys occurring as a minor component in other syndromes such as Zellweger's syndrome where the cysts present are usually inconsequential.

On ultrasonography small cysts are identified and are predominantly in the renal cortex particularly in the sub-capsular region (Fig. 11.11). The kidneys may become enlarged with diffuse increased echogenicity and loss of corticomedullary differentiation (Mercado-Deane et al. 2002). Punctate calcification, medullary fibrosis and reduction in renal size may also occur.

Differentiation from ARPKD may be very difficult (Fredericks et al. 1989; Fitch and Stapleton 1986).

## 11.5 Renal Tract Dilatation

Renal tract dilatation can be associated with obstruction or may be present without obstruction such as with vesicoureteric reflux (Hiorns and Gordon 2008).

### 11.5.1 *Renal Pelvis Dilatation*

Renal pelvis dilatation is frequently detected by routine antenatal ultrasonography. The condition is usually unilateral but may be bilateral. However, it is still discovered in children who present with a urinary tract infection, loin pain or haematuria, occasionally with a history of preceding trauma. In this latter group investigation and immediate treatment is required. There is no uniform consensus regarding when and how to investigate infants with an antenatal diagnosis of renal pelvis dilatation as there are reports that in many patients there is significant improvement or normalization of the dilatation over time. Guidelines for investigation have been published and adopted by the European Society of Paediatric Radiology (Riccabona et al. 2008).

The initial investigation of antenatally diagnosed renal pelvis dilatation is with ultrasonography. Postnatally, the ideal time is 5 days of age or older when the infant is satisfactorily hydrated. This will also help to confirm that the ureter is not dilated and also will help exclude a bladder abnormality. A diagnosis of dilatation is confirmed when the anteroposterior diameter of the renal pelvis is 10 mm or more (Hiorns and Gordon 2008) (Fig. 11.12).

When the diagnosis is confirmed diuretic renography using Tc 99m Mag 3 is the next investigation to confirm whether there is obstruction or not (Fig. 11.13). An intravenous diuretic is given either at the time of injection of the radiopharmaceutical or approximately 15 min after the injection. The study results must be correlated with the ultrasound and clinical findings as the results may be difficult to interpret because of the poor renal function in the neonatal age group (Koff et al. 1988; Gordon et al. 1991).

As vesicoureteric reflux may be associated with pelviureteric junction obstruction some institutions perform a voiding cystourethrogram on all infants with renal pelvis dilatation but there is no documented role for its routine use. Recently MR urography has been used to assess pelviureteric junction obstruction but as software to assess renal function is not universally available this exam is not widely performed.

There is also no consensus on which patients with dilatation require surgery. Many authors have concluded that there is no indication for immediate pyeloplasty in infants with prenatally diagnosed hydronephrosis who demonstrate good renal function postnatally (Ransley et al. 1990; Koff 1998; Gordon et al. 1991; Riccabona 2004).

However, progressive dilatation on sonography or a reduction in renal function of 5–10% on Tc 99m Mag 3 renography requires surgical intervention.

### 11.5.2  Renal Pelvis and Ureter Dilatation

Congenital ureter dilatation can be divided into non-refluxing obstructive megaureter and refluxing non-obstructive megaureter.

Primary obstructive megaureter is due to structural alteration of the muscular layers of the distal ureter. This results in abnormal peristalsis and progressive dilatation of the ureter.

The condition may be diagnosed antenatally or may present in children with a urinary tract infection, abdominal pain or haematuria.

As with dilatation of the renal pelvis, ultrasonography is the initial investigation of choice, followed by Tc 99m Mag 3 renography to assess drainage and function. Voiding cystourethrography is also indicated in these children to outrule reflux as a cause for the dilatation. Intravenous urography or antegrade pyelography may be required occasionally if there is difficulty in assessing drainage on the radionuclide studies (Fig. 11.14). MR urography has replaced intravenous urography and Tc 99m Mag 3 renography in some

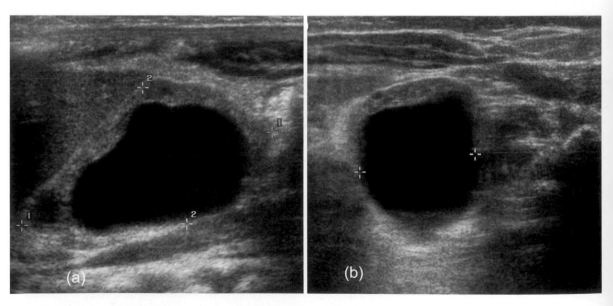

**Fig. 11.12** Newborn with pelviureteric junction obstruction. There is marked dilatation of the renal pelvis (**a**) and with an AP renal pelvis diameter greater than 2 cm (**b**)

**Fig. 11.13** Mag 3 renogram on the same patient as Fig. 11.12 showing poorer uptake of the radiopharmaceutical and no excretion in the obstructed right kidney (**a**). A delayed image at 1 h post-injection shows significant residual radiopharmaceutical in the dilated renal pelvis (**b**)

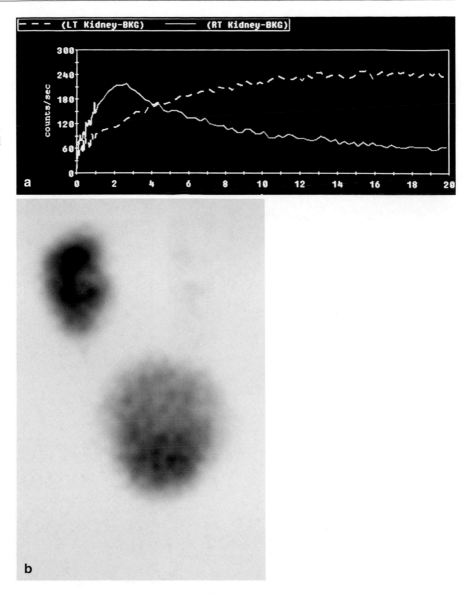

centres (Grattan Smith 2008; Grattan Smith et al. 2008) but MR software to assess renal function is not yet universally available.

Patients with refluxing non-obstructive dilatation may be diagnosed prenatally but they most commonly present with a urinary tract infection. Reflux may be of primary origin or may result from bladder outlet obstruction secondary to posterior urethral valves or a neuropathic urinary bladder for example in infants with a myelomeningocoele.

Isolated primary reflux may be suspected on ultrasonography particularly when ureteral dilatation is intermittent (Fig. 11.15), is associated with thickening or

increased echogenicity of the wall of the renal pelvis or ureter or when there is focal or diffuse cortical loss. The diagnosis is made definitively by voiding cystourethrography, contrast enhanced voiding cystosonography or radionuclide cystography. If significant reflux is confirmed a Tc 99m DMSA scan should be performed to exclude focal renal defects and to assess differential renal function. The importance of reflux in the clinical context of an asymptomatic infant or in a child with a urinary tract infection is not clear. A review of the world literature (Hiorns and Gordon 2008) suggested that in children with a urinary tract infection, vesicoureteric reflux on its own was not sufficient or necessary for renal damage.

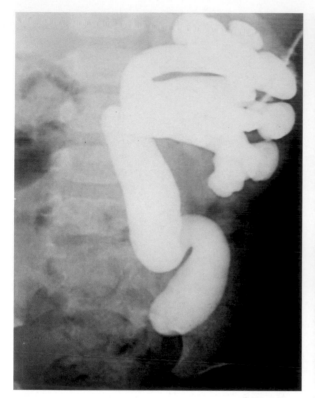

**Fig. 11.14** Antegrade pyelogram outlining a very dilated left collecting system and ureter. There is complete obstruction at the distal ureter

### 11.5.3 Duplex Kidney with Ureter Dilatation

Renal duplication is the most common malformation of the urinary tract and is frequently seen in children who present with urinary tract infection (Stokland et al. 2007). It results from two ureteral buds leading to two separate renal pelves and ureters within a single kidney.

If there is no dilatation, the abnormality may not be clinically significant. Duplex kidneys with dilatation of the upper or lower moiety collecting systems in children usually follow the Weigert–Meyer rule whereby the ureter draining the upper moiety inserts ectopically, medial and inferior to the normal opening. The opening may be associated with a ureterocoele and its ureter may be obstructed. This ureterocoele may also obstruct the lower pole ureter. There may be reflux into the ureter draining the lower pole moiety

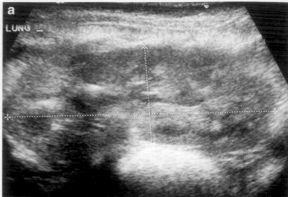

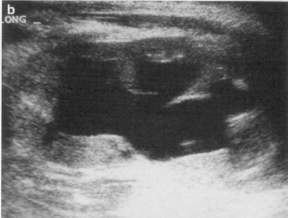

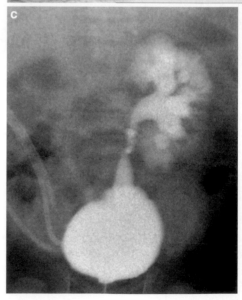

**Fig. 11.15** Infant with antenatal history of renal pelvis dilatation. Postnatal US demonstrates intermittent dilatation of the left renal collecting system (**a**, **b**). VCUG shows left Grade V reflux (**c**)

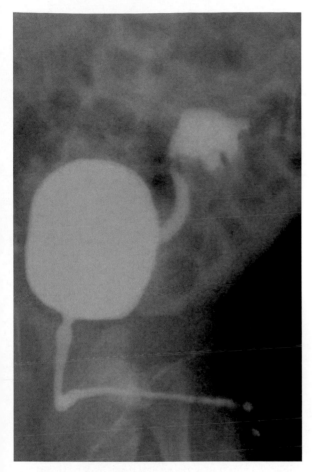

**Fig. 11.16** VCUG in an infant with a left duplex system. There is significant reflux into the lower moiety of a left duplex system

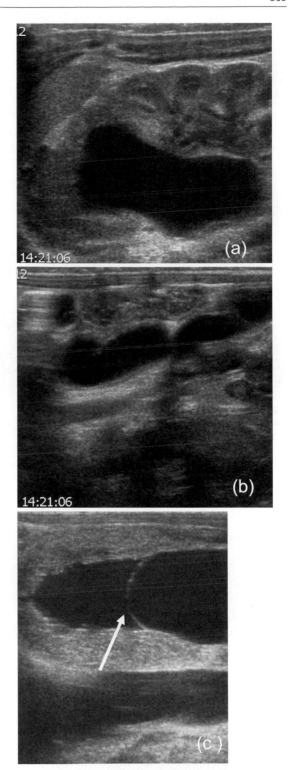

**Fig. 11.17** Newborn with right duplex system. Renal US shows dilated upper moiety collecting system (**a**) and ureter (**b**). There is a large ureterocoele in the bladder (*arrow*) which is thick-walled (**c**)

and it may be dilated (Fig. 11.16). If there is dilatation the diagnosis is often made antenatally.

Postnatally the diagnosis is confirmed using ultrasonography which also allows confirmation of a ureterocoele if this is present (Fig. 11.17). Occasionally the degree of cortical loss in the upper pole is so marked that the only abnormality may be a dilated collecting system which may mimic a cystic suprarenal mass. A voiding cystourethrogram may also help in identifying a ureterocoele (Fig. 11.18) and will identify reflux into the ureters.

If there is a large ureterocoele present it is usually incised cystoscopically to relieve the obstruction. Following this procedure it is necessary to assess the function in the upper pole moiety and this is best done by either a Tc 99m DMSA or a Tc 99m Mag 3

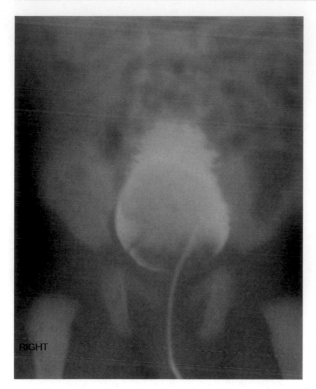

**Fig. 11.18** VCUG in newborn demonstrating contrast outlining a large ureterocoele

renogram. If there is very poor residual function a secondary heminephrectomy is performed.

## 11.5.4 Posterior Urethral Valves

Posterior urethral valves were first described by Young in the early 1900s. He classified the abnormality into three types:

Type 1 is described as a bicuspid membrane which extends from the posterior verumontanum to the proximal membranous urethra. This accounts for the vast majority of valves.

Type 2 is described as mucoal folds extending from the verumontanum to the bladder neck. It is now thought that these are not obstructing valves.

Type 3 valves are thought to represent incomplete dissolution of the urogenital membrane distal to the verumontanum. Young's classification does not have any clinical significance and it has been challenged (Dewan et al. 1992). It is now proposed that most congenital posterior urethral obstructions are anatomically similar.

The vast majority of newborns with obstructive posterior urethral valves are detected antenatally. Less severe forms may not present until later in childhood. Foetal intervention for posterior urethral valves has been undertaken in some centres and carries a considerable risk to the foetus with a foetal mortality of 43%. There is no conclusive evidence that it improves renal function in these infants (Holmes et al. 2001).

After birth ultrasound examination is usually performed early. Classically there is a variable degree of hydronephrosis and hydroureter. There may be thinning of the renal parenchyma. The renal cortex may show increased echogenicity and contain small cysts due to associated renal dysplasia (Fig. 11.8). The bladder wall is usually thickened and may be very distended with urine and it may be possible to identify a dilated posterior urethra. A perinephric urinoma may be present due to calyceal rupture as a result of increased pressure (Fig. 11.19). The diagnosis is confirmed by voiding cystourethrogram and the bladder is usually catheterized retrogradely. There is dilatation of the posterior urethra (Fig. 11.20) and occasionally bands are seen representing the valves. The diagnosis can be made when the infants voids with the catheter in position but if there is any doubt about the diagnosis it is best to also obtain images during voiding when the catheter has been removed. The bladder wall is often thickened and trabeculated and there may be diverticulae. Vesicoureteric reflux of varying severity is commonly identified (Fig. 11.20) and there may also be reflux of contrast into the seminal vesicles.

Tc 99m DMSA scintigraphy is useful in assessing the amount of functioning renal tissue.

Following valve ablation the management of children with posterior urethral valves depends on the degree of renal impairment.

## 11.5.5 Prune Belly Syndrome

Prune belly syndrome, also known as Eagle–Barrett Syndrome is characterized by a deficiency of the abdominal musculature, urinary tract dilatation and undescended testes. The vast majority of patients are boys with approximately 3–4% occurring in females. The pathogenesis is uncertain. It affects 1: 30,000–40,000 live births. It is associated with Trisomy 18 and 21 and cardiac defects such as Tetralogy of Fallot and

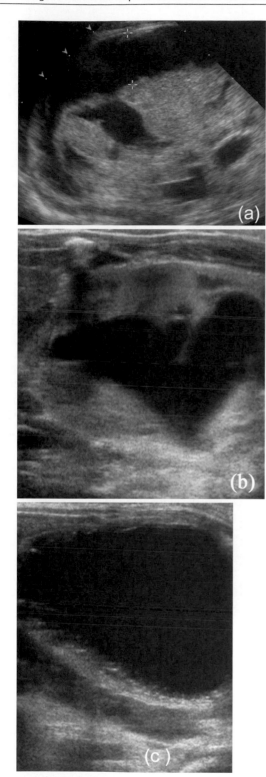

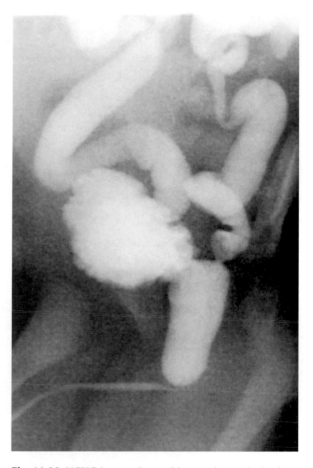

**Fig. 11.20** VCUG in a newborn with posterior urethral valves. There is marked dilatation of the posterior urethra. The urinary bladder is very thick-walled and there is marked reflux into dilated and tortuous ureters

**Fig. 11.19** US in a newborn with posterior urethral valves. There is bilateral hydronephrosis (**a**, **b**) with a right perinephric urinoma between cursors (**a**). The urinary bladder is very distended and thick-walled

ventricular septal defects are reported in 10% of patients. There may be associated pulmonary hypoplasia.

If there is upper tract dilatation the diagnosis may be suspected on prenatal ultrasonographic screening but the condition may be very difficult to distinguish from other causes of dilatation such as bladder outlet obstruction due to posterior urethral valves.

Postnatally, ultrasonography will show dilatation of the collecting systems and ureters of varying degrees. The bladder may be large but in contrast to bladder outlet obstruction due to posterior urethral valves the bladder wall is not thickened (Fig. 11.21). On voiding cystourethrography the large bladder, if present, will be confirmed and emptying of the bladder may be incomplete. There may be a persistent urachus. Bilateral vesicoureteric reflux is common with very dilated and tortuous ureters. The bladder neck may be open with

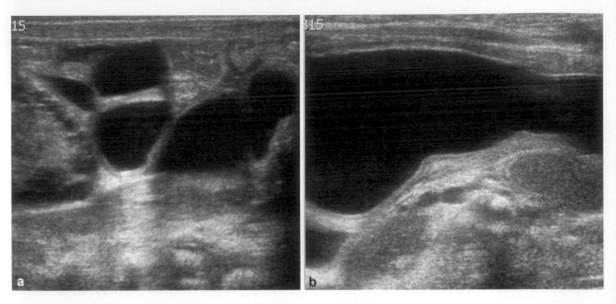

**Fig. 11.21** Infant with Prune belly syndrome US shows marked dilatation of the ureters (**a**). The urinary bladder is very distended with a normal thickness of the bladder wall (**b**)

some elongation and dilatation of the posterior urethra (Fig. 11.22). A prostatic utricle remnant is seen occasionally.

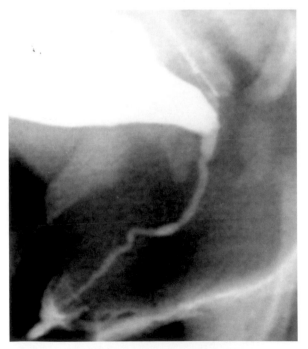

**Fig. 11.22** VCUG in a boy with Prune belly syndrome via a suprapubic catheter. There was persistent opening of the posterior urethra during the study with elongation of the posterior urethra

Further imaging with Tc 99m DMSA scintigraphy is often required later to assess the differential renal function and overall functional impairment. It also demonstrates focal areas of abnormal function. MR urography is very rarely required in these infants but if anatomic information is required it may be useful.

Treatment in infants with Prune belly syndrome is usually conservative and the overall prognosis depends on the degree of pulmonary hypoplasia and renal dysplasia.

## 11.6 Congenital Renal Tumours

Perinatal renal tumours are extremely rare. The commonest solid renal mass in this age group is the mesoblastic nephroma. It is also referred to as foetal renal hamartoma. Most cases are clinically benign. The tumour is usually large and involves a large area of the kidney (Woodward et al. 2005). Characteristically the mass is hyperechoic on ultrasonography with increased vascularity on Doppler examination. Contrast enhanced CT and MRI shows a rim of normal kidney surrounding the tumour. The imaging appearances mimic Wilms' tumour which is extremely rare prior to 2 years of age. A few cases of congenital renal rhabdoid tumours have been reported.

# References

Abeshouse BS, Bhisitkul I (1959) Crossed renal ectopia with and without fusion. Urol Int 9:63–91

Applegate K, Connolly L, Treves T (1995) Tc-99m DMSA imaging of crossed fused renal ectopia. Clin Nucl Med 20: 947–948

Arant BS Jr, Soteol-Avila C, Bernstein J (1979) Segmental "hypoplasia" of the kidney (Ash-Upmark). J Pediatr 95: 931–939

Atiyeh B, Husmann D, Baum M (1992) Contralateral renal abnormalities in multicystic dysplastic kidney disease. J Pediatr 121:65–67

Benz-Bohm G (2008) Urinary tract embryology, anatomy and anatomical variants. In Fotter R (ed) Pediatric uroradiology, 2nd edn. Springer, Berlin, pp 55–66

Bernstein J (1993) Glomerulocystic kidney disease: nosological considerations. Pediatr Nephrol 7:464–470

Boal Dk, Teele R (1980) Sonography of infantile polycystic kidney disease. AJR Am J Roentgenol 135:575–580

Boatman DL, Kolln CP, Flocks RH (1972) Congenital anomalies associated with horseshoe kidney. J Urol 107:205–207

Cassart M, Massez A, Metens T et al. (2004) Complementary role of MRI after sonography in assessing bilateral urinary tract anomalies in the fetus. AJR Am J Roentgenol 182: 689–695

Daneman A, Alton DJ (1991) Radiographic manifestations of renal anomalies. Radiol Clin North Am 29:351–363

Dewan PA, Zappala SM, Ransley PG et al (1992) Endoscopic reappraisal of the morphology of congenital obstruction of the posterior urethra. Br J Urol 70:439–444

Downs RA, Lane JW, Burns E (1973) Solitary pelvic kidney: its clinical implications. Urology 1:51–56

Fitch SJ, Stapleton FB (1986) Ultrasonographic features of glomerulocystic disease in infancy: similarity to infantile polycystic kidney disease. Pediatr Radiol 16:400–402

Fredericks BJ, de Campo M, Chow CW et al. (1989) Glomerulocystic renal disease: ultrasound appearances. Pediatr Radiol 19:184–186

Glenn JF (1959) Analysis of 51 patients with horseshoe kidney. N Engl J Med 261:684–687

Gordon I, Dhillon HK, Gatanash H et al. (1991) Antenatal diagnosis of pelvic hydronephrosis: assessment of renal function and drainage as a guide to management. J Nucl Med 32: 1649–1654

Grattan Smith JD (2008) MR urography: anatomy and physiology. Pediatr Radiol 38(suppl 2):S275–S285

Grattan Smith JD, Little SB, Jones RA (2008) MR urography evaluation of obstructive uropathy. Pediatr Radiol 38 (suppl 1):S49–S46

Hains DS, Bates CM, Ingraham S et al. (2009) Management and etiology of the unilateral multicystic dysplastic kidney: a review. Pediatr Nephrol 24:233–241

Hildebrandt F, Otto F (2005) Cilia and centrosomes: a unifying pathogenic concept for cystic kidney disease? Nat Rev Genet 6:928–940

Hiorns M, Gordon I (2008) Upper urinary tract dilatation in newborns and infants. In Fotter R (ed) Pediatric uroradiology, 2nd edn. Springer, Berlin, pp 237–250

Holmes N, Harrison MR, Baskin LS (2001) Fetal surgery for posterior urethral valves: long-term postnatal outcomes. Pediatrics 108:1–7

Jeon A, Cramer BC, Walsh E et al. (1999) A spectrum of segmental multicystic renal dysplasia. Pediatr Radiol 29:309–315

Kavanagh EC, Ryan S, Awan A et al. (2005) Can MRI replace DMSA in the detection of renal parenchymal defects in children with urinary tract infections? Pediatr Radiol 35: 275–281

Kiddoo DA, Bellah RD, Carr MC (2005) Cross fused ectopic multicystic dysplastic kidney with associated ureterocoele. Urology 66:432

Kiyah A, Yilmaz A, Turhan P et al. (2009) Unilateral multicystic dysplastic kidney: a single center experience. Pediatr Nephrol 24:99–104

Koff SA (1998) Neonatal management of unilateral hydronephrosis: role for delayed intervention. Urol Clin North Am 25:181–186

Koff SA, McDowell GC, Byard M (1988) Diuretic radionuclide assessment of obstruction in the infant: guidelines for successful interpretation. J Urol 140:1167–1168

Lang IM, Babyn P, Oliver GD (1999) MR imaging of paediatric uterovaginal anomalies. Pediatr Radiol 29:163–170

Lazebnik N, Bellinger MF, Ferguson JE et al. (1999) Insights into the pathogenesis and natural history of fetuses with multicystic dysplastic kidney disease. Prenat Diagn 19:418–423

Lippe B, Geffner ME, Dietrich RB et al. (1988) Renal malformations in patients with Turner's syndrome: imaging in 141 patients. Pediatrics 82:852–856

Malek RS, Kelalis PP, Burke EC (1971) Ectopic kidney in children and frequency of association with other malformations. Mayo Clin Proc 46:461–467

McDonald JH, McClellan DS (1957) Crossed renal ectopia. Am J Surg 93:995–1002

Mercado-Deane MG, Beeson JE, John SD (2002) US of renal insufficiency in neonates. Radiographics 22:1429–1438

Mesrobian HJ, Kelalis PP, Hrabovsky E et al. (1985) Wilms' tumour in horseshoe kidneys: a report from the National Wilms' Tumour Study. J Urol 133:1002–1003

Oddone M, Marino C, Sergi C et al. (1994) Wilms' tumour arising in a multicystic kidney. Pediatr Radiol 24:236–238

Potter EL (1972) Normal and abnormal development of the kidney. Year Book, Chicago

Proesmans W, Van Damme B, Casaer P et al. (1982) Autosomal dominant polycystic kidney disease in the neonatal period: association with a cerebral arteriovenous malformation. Pediatrics 70:971–975

Ransley PG, Dhillon HK, Gordon I et al. (1990) The postnatal management of hydronephrosis diagnosed by prenatal ultrasound. J Urol 144:584–587

Riccabona M (2004) Assessment and management of newborn hydronephrosis. World J Urol 22:73–78

Riccabona M, Avni FE, Blickman JG et al. (2008) Imaging recommendations in paediatric uroradiology: minutes of the ESPR workgroup session on urinary tract infection, fetal hydronephrosis, urinary tract ultrasonography and voiding cystourethrography, Barcelona, Spain, June 2007. Pediatr Radiol 38:138–145

Riccabona M, Ring E (2008) Renal agenesis, dysplasia, hypoplasia and cystic disease of the kidney. In Fotter R (ed) Pediatric uroradiology, 2nd edn. Springer, Berlin, pp 187–210

Ritchey M (1992) Anomalies of the kidney. In Kelalis PP, King LR, Belman AB (eds) Clinical pediatric urology, vol 1, 3rd edn. Saunders, Philadelphia, pp 500–528

Sheih CP, Liu MB, Hung CS et al. (1989) Renal abnormalities in schoolchildren. Pediatrics 84:1086–1090

Shibata S, Nagata M (2003) Pathogenesis of human renal dysplasia: an alternative scenario to the major theories. Pediatr Int 45:605–609

Stokland E, Jodal U, Sixt R et al. (2007) Uncomplicated duplex kidney and DMSA scintigraphy in children with urinary tract infection. Pediatr Radiol 38:826–828

Turkbey B, Ocak I, Daryanini K et al. (2009) Autosomal recessive polycystic kidney disease and congenital hepatic fibrosis (ARPKD/CHF) Pediatr Radiol 39:100–111

Woodward PJ, Sohaey R, Kennedy A et al. (2005) A comprehensive review of fetal tumors with pathological correlation. Radiographics 25:215–242

Zerres K, Mucher G, Bachner L et al. (1994) Mapping of the gene for autosomal recessive polycystic kidney disease (APPKD) to chromosome 6p21;cen. Nat Genet 7: 429–432

# Renal Cystic Disease

**12**

Kyongtae T. Bae, Alessandro Furlan, and Fadi M. El-Merhi

## Contents

## Abstract

> *Renal cystic disease* is a heterogeneous entity including developmental (*simple* and *complex cysts, localized cystic diseases, extraparenchymal sinus cysts, medullary sponge kidney* and *multicystic dysplastic kidney*), acquired (*acquired cystic kidney disease*) and heritable (*autosomal dominant polycsystic kidney disease, autosomal recessive polycystic kidney disease, tuberous sclerosis complex, von Hippel–Lindau disease*) disorders. Various imaging modalities are used for the diagnosis and clinical evaluation of renal cystic diseases. While ultrasound is more commonly used as a screening modality, CT and MR imaging are more widely used in clinical settings for characterizing renal cystic lesions, assessing cysts complications and differentiating benign from malignant cystic lesions. The diagnosis of a specific renal cystic disease can be made by a review of the patient's clinical history in conjunction with radiographic findings. Key imaging features useful for the diagnosis of renal cystic disease include the location, distribution, size, and composition of renal cysts as well as other coexisting noncystic renal lesions and characteristic extrarenal findings.

K.T. Bae (✉) and A. Furlan
Department of Radiology, University of Pittsburgh,
3362 Fifth Avenue, Pittsburgh, PA 15213, USA
e-mail: baek@upmc.edu

F.M. El-Merhi
Department of Radiology, University of Texas,
San Antonio, TX, USA

## 12.1 Introduction

A *renal cyst* represents a dilated fluid-filled segment of a nephron or a collecting tubule (Gardner 1988). According to the classic definition, a *cystic kidney* is a kidney containing three or more cysts, and *renal cystic disease* is the illness resulting from a cystic kidney (Gardner 1988). Renal cystic disease is a heterogeneous entity that comprises heritable, developmental, and acquired disorders. Throughout the past decade, considerable progress has been made in reaching a consensus for standardized terminology and classification of renal cystic disease among radiologists, pathologists, nephrologists, and urologists, as shown in Table 12.1 (Churg and World Health Organization. Collaborating Centre for the Histological Classification of Renal Diseases 1987). Some of these entities are exceedingly rare and beyond the scope of this article.

**Table 12.1** Classification of renal cysts

| |
|---|
| I. Simple renal cysts, solitary and multiple |
| II. Complex renal cysts |
| III. Extraparenchymal renal cysts |
|    A. Parapelvic cysts |
|    B. Peripelvic cysts |
| IV. Localized, segmental and unilateral renal cysts |
| V. Acquired renal cystic disease |
| VI. Polycystic kidney disease |
|    A. Autosomal dominant polycystic kidney disease |
|      1. Glomerulocystic disease of newborn |
|      2. Classic polycystic disease of older children and adults |
|        (a) PKD1 gene (chromosome 16, encoding for polycystin-1) |
|        (b) PKD2 gene (chromosome 4, encoding for polycystin-2) |
|    B. Autosomal recessive polycystic kidney disease |
|      1. Polycystic disease of newborns and infants |
|      2. Polycystic disease of older children and adults |
|        (a) Medullary ductal ectasia |
|        (b) Congenital hepatic fibrosis |
|        (c) Caroli's disease |
| VII. Renal cysts in hereditary malformation syndromes |
|    A. Tuberous sclerosis complex |
|    B. von Hippel–Lindau syndrome |
|    C. Zellweger cerebrohepatorenal syndrome |
|    D. Jeune asphyxiating thoracic dystrophy |

**Table 12.1** (continued)

| |
|---|
|    E. Oral-facial-digital syndrome I |
|    F. Brachyesomelia-renal syndrome |
| VIII. Renal medullary cysts |
|    A. Medullary sponge kidney |
|    B. Hereditary tubulointerstitial nephritis (medullary cystic kidney) |
|      1. Familial juvenile nephronophthisis |
|      2. Medullary cystic disease |
|      3. Renal-retinal dysplasia complex |
| VII. Renal cystic dysplasia |
|    A. Multicystic kidney |
|    B. Cystic dysplasia associated with lower urinary tract obstruction |
|    C. Diffuse cystic dysplasia, syndromal and nonsyndromal |
| VIII. Drug or toxin-induced renal cysts |
| IX. Glomerulocystic kidney disease |
|    A. Infantile-onset dominant polycystic kidney disease |
|    B. Syndromal glomerular cystic disease |
|    C. Nonsyndromal glomerular cysts |

Renal cysts are common radiographic and clinical abnormalities. While renal cysts are frequently discovered as incidental findings in clinical diagnostic imaging studies, dedicated imaging studies can be performed to confirm a suspected diagnosis. The diagnosis of a specific renal cystic disease can be made by a review of the patient's clinical history in conjunction with radiographic findings. Key imaging features useful for the diagnosis of renal cystic disease include: renal cyst location (i.e., uni- or bilateral kidney involvement renal cortex, medulla, pelvis or exophytic); cyst distribution (i.e., sparse, dense); cyst size; cyst composition (simple, complex, hemorrhagic, proteinacious, calcium); dimension (aspect) and functional state of the affected kidney; other coexisting noncystic lesions in the kidney, and cystic and noncystic lesions in other organs (e.g., liver, pancreas or spleen). Other clinical features, such as age at presentation, familiar history of disease and degree of renal functional impairment, may also help establish the diagnosis (Tables 12.2 and 12.3).

**Table 12.2** Imaging features of cystic kidney disorders

| Entity | Age at detection | Number of cysts | Renal cyst distribution | Cyst size | Kidney size | Renal complications and associated tumors | Extrarenal findings |
|---|---|---|---|---|---|---|---|
| Simple, complex cysts | Adult | Few (increases with age) | Uni- or bilateral; mainly cortical | Variable | Normal | Nonspecific | None |
| Extraparenchymal cysts | Adults | Few | Uni- or bilateral; juxtapelvis | Medium to large | Normal | Nonspecific | None |
| Localized cystic disease | Adult | Few | Unilateral, clustered; whole or regional | Medium to large | Normal | Nonspecific | None |
| Acquired cystic disease | Adult | Few to many (increases with dialysis) | Bilateral mainly cortical | Variable | Atrophic | Increased renal cell carcinoma | None |
| Autosomal dominant polycystic kidney disease | All ages | Few to numerous (progressively increase) | Bilateral; diffuse | Variable | Normal to large | Hypertension and renal failure | Hepatic cysts; cerebral aneurysms |
| Autosomal recessive polycystic kidney disease | Neonate, Juvenile | Few to numerous | Bilateral; diffuse | Small | Normal to large | Hypertension and renal failure | Congenital hepatic fibrosis; Caroli disease |
| Tuberous sclerosis | All ages | Few to many | Bilateral; mainly cortical | Small | Normal | Angiomyolipomas | Dermatologic findings; retinal hamartomas |
| von Hippel–Lindau | All ages | Few to many | Bilateral; mainly cortical | Variable | Normal | Renal cell carcinoma (multicentric, bilateral) | Pancreatic cysts; retinal hemangioblastoma; pheochromocytoma |
| Medullary sponge kidney | Adult | Few | Bilateral medullary | Small | Normal | Medullary nephrocalcinosis | None |
| Multilocular cystic nephroma | Juvenile and adult form | Few | Unilateral; corticomedullary | Medium to large | Normal | Likely benign; potential malignancy controversial | None |
| Multicystic dysplastic kidney | Infant and adult form | Few to many (progressively involute) | Unilateral; diffuse | Variable | Enlarged; involuted | Vesicoureteral reflux; controlateral UPJ obstruction | None |
| Lithium nephropathy | Adult | Numerous | Bilateral; diffuse | Small | Normal | Nonspecific | None |

**Table 12.3** Renal cystic diseases assorted by the renal laterality and key differential diagnostic features

| Unilateral | Bilateral | | Uni- or bilateral |
|---|---|---|---|
| Localized cystic disease: clustered | Genetic | ADPKD: hepatic cysts, often big kidneys | Simple, complex cysts |
| | | ARPKD: small cysts, hepatic fibrosis | Parapelvic cysts: mimicking hydronephrosis |
| MLCN: thick capsule, herniates to pelvis | | TS: AMLs | |
| | | VHL: RCCs, pancreatic cysts | |
| MCDK: no normal parenchyma, involutes | Nongenetic | Acquired: atrophic kidneys, dialysis history | |
| | | MSK: medullary calculi, few tiny cysts | |
| | | Lithium: tiny cysts, lithium history | |

*MLCN* multilocular cystic nephroma; *MCDK* multicystic dysplastic kidney; *ADPKD* autosomal dominant polycystic kidney disease; *ARPKD* autosomal recessive polycystic kidney disease; *TS* tuberous sclerosis complex; *AML* angiomyolipoma; *VHL* von Hippel–Lindau disease; *RCC* renal cell carcinoma; *MSK* medullary sponge kidney

Various imaging modalities are used for the diagnosis and clinical evaluation of renal cystic diseases. Renal ultrasound is readily available and can be safely performed in a wide range of patients. It does not emit radiation or require normal renal function for the procedure and can be used as a screening tool for polycystic kidney disease (Parfrey et al. 1990; Ravine et al. 1994). Ultrasound also has the advantage of being cost-effective and easily tolerated by patients for repetitive studies. The down-side to ultrasound imaging is that it is operator-dependent and may be less accurate and reproducible than CT or MR imaging, particularly for detecting small cysts.

While ultrasound is more commonly used as a screening modality, CT and MR imaging are more widely used in clinical settings for characterizing renal cystic lesions, assessing cysts complications and differentiating benign from malignant cystic lesions. CT with iodinated contrast is an efficient, accurate imaging technique for renal structures. However, it involves the emission of ionizing radiation and the use of an iodinated contrast medium which may harm patients with existing impaired renal function. MR imaging has been demonstrated to be superior to ultrasound and CT for the visualization of small renal cysts (Nascimento et al. 2001). T2-weighted MR imaging sequences are best for detecting the presence of fluid-filled cavities. In particular, short-breath-hold strongly T2-weighted sequences such as, half-Fourier single-shot turbo spin-echo and RARE, have been proven very useful in depicting structures containing static fluids. MR imaging is also the imaging modality of choice for the evaluation of morphological and physiological changes associated with renal cystic disease (EL-Merhi and Bae 2004). Contrast-enhanced CT and gadolinium-enhanced MRI are used to determine enhancement within a renal lesion and can differentiate a cyst (no enhancement) from a cystic neoplasm (enhancement). In addition, with the availability of 3D urography studies by CT and MR, the conventional excretory urography (i.e., IVP) has limited roles in evaluating patients with renal cystic diseases.

## 12.2 Simple Cysts

*Simple cysts* are the most common renal lesions in adults. The incidence, number, and size of renal cysts increase with age, reported in up to 27% of patients greater than 50 years of age (Laucks and McLachlan 1981; Tada et al. 1983). Renal cysts can be solitary, multiple, or bilateral, and they commonly arise in the renal cortex. They are benign asymptomatic lesions, most of which are incidentally discovered on ultrasound or CT examinations.

On ultrasound, simple cysts classically present as round, anechoic lesion with acoustic enhancement and no appreciable wall thickness. On CT imaging, simple cysts are round with no perceptible walls and are well-demarcated from the adjacent renal parenchyma (Fig. 12.1). The CT attenuation values of renal cysts are typically less than 20 HU (water attenuation). On MR imaging, simple renal cysts present with the same morphologic features as demonstrated on CT. They appear very bright on T2-weighted images and maintain homogeneous signal void on T1-weighted images (Fig. 12.2) (Hartman et al. 2004).

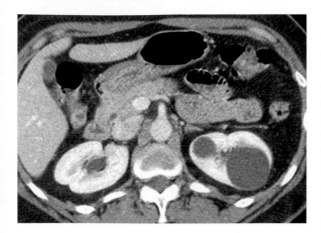

**Fig. 12.1** Simple cyst. Contrast-enhanced CT image of the left kidney shows two simple cysts of water attenuation with no complexity or perceptible wall

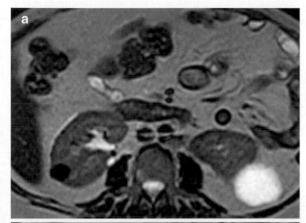

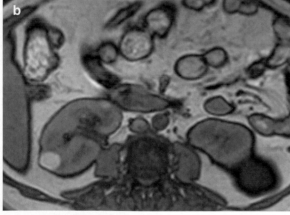

**Fig. 12.2** Simple and complex cysts. (**a**) Axial T2-weighted and (**b**) T1-weighted MR images show an exophytic simple cyst on the left and a complex cyst on the right kidney. While the simple cyst shows bright T2 and dark T1 signal intensities, the complex cyst demonstrates the opposite signal intensity characteristics

The absence of contrast enhancement is critical to differentiate renal cysts from renal tumors with a cystic component. Although renal cysts should not enhance after administration of intravenous contrast material (Thomsen et al. 1997), some cysts may appear to enhance (*pseudo-enhancement*). This is because of multiple technical and image-related factors that are directly associated with the presence of iodinated contrast material within adjacent renal parenchyma (Fig. 12.3) (Bae et al. 2000; Coulam et al. 2000; Maki et al. 1999). The degree of *pseudo-enhancement* in CT is typically less than 10–20 HU but varies with multiple factors (size, location of cysts, CT scanners, reconstruction algorithm) (Bae et al. 2000; Birnbaum et al. 2007; Coulam et al. 2000; Wang et al. 2008). In addition to pseudo-enhancement, small cysts deep in the renal parenchyma may be subjected to a partial volume averaging with adjacent contrast-enhanced renal parenchyma and may appear to enhance (Silverman et al. 2008). To minimize the partial volume averaging effect on the enhancement assessment, it is critical to use appropriate image slice thickness; typically the thickness should be less than the diameter of the lesion.

Pseudo-enhancement may be also observed in contrast-enhanced MR imaging. Various features found in MR imaging, including motion artifacts, inherent noise, and partial volume averaging, can cause the appearance of enhancement (Ho et al. 2002). The optimal percentage of enhancement thresholds for distinguishing cysts from malignancies is reported to be 15%, with the optimal timing for measurement at 2–4 min after the administration of contrast material (Ho et al. 2002). Some researchers advocate the review of the subtracted images (enhanced minus unenhanced MR images) for the detection of subtle contrast enhancement within renal lesions (Hecht et al. 2004) (Fig. 12.4).

## 12.3 Complex Cysts

Simple renal cysts may be complicated by internal hemorrhage, infection, or other processes that may appear on imaging with complex radiologic features suggestive of cystic renal neoplasm. On US imaging, complex cysts may present with internal echo, septum, wall thickening, calcification, and acoustic shadowing. Similarly, heterogeneous morphologic features of complex cysts are delineated and characterized on CT and MR imaging. Some of the findings of complex

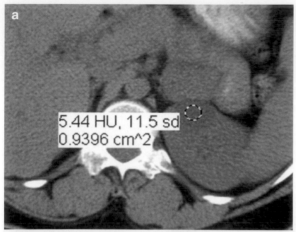

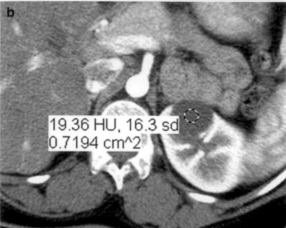

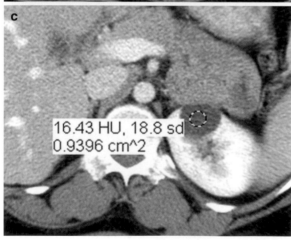

**Fig. 12.3** Pseudo-enhancement in simple cyst. The attenuation of simple cyst is measured by placing a region-of-interest (ROI) on CT images obtained (**a**) before the administration of contrast medium, (**b**) after the administration of contrast medium at the corticomedullary phase, and (**c**) at the nephrographic phase. Pseudo-enhancement is measured approximately 14 HU (=19−5) at the corticomedullary and 11 HU (=16−5) at the nephrographic phase

cysts, such as irregular wall thickening, dense calcification, and multiple septa, can also be seen in cystic renal neoplasm (Hartman et al. 2004). A classification system of renal cystic lesions on CT, the Bosniak Classification of Renal Cystic Disease, grouped renal cysts into four categories based on imaging appearance in an attempt to predict the risk of malignancy and determine the risk and management of complex cysts and cystic neoplasm (Bosniak 1986). This will be discussed further in Chap. 26.

Complex cysts may present as hyperdense cysts (attenuation greater than water) in CT due to internal hemorrhage or proteinaceous content (Sagel et al. 1977). Since hyperdense cysts show no significant contrast enhancement, they can be differentiated from renal neoplasms based on the assessment of enhancement. However, hyperdense cysts discovered incidentally at CT with only a single phase of contrast enhancement may not be easily distinguishable from solid renal masses solely based on CT attenuation. A recent study reported that on portal venous phase contrast-enhanced CT scans, attenuation greater than 70 HU or moderate or marked internal heterogeneity favor a diagnosis of renal cell carcinoma (RCC) over a diagnosis of hyperdense renal cyst (Suh et al. 2003).

MR imaging is useful to evaluate complex cystic renal masses. Hemorrhage or protein within complex cysts may cause T1 shortening and present with higher signal intensity than water on T1-weighted image (Brown and Semelka 1995; Marotti et al. 1987) (Fig. 12.2). Hemorrhagic cysts may show variable signal intensities on T2-weighted images, depending on the stage of blood products (Brown and Semelka 1995; Hilpert et al. 1986; Marotti et al. 1987). Although the presence of calcification within renal lesions is difficult to identify with MR imaging, the same morphologic features can be used to characterize complex cystic lesions, as with CT. Lack of gadolinium contrast enhancement is an important MR feature to differentiate complex cysts from renal cystic neoplasms. Since complex cysts are typically hyperintense on T1-weighted images, a careful comparison between the pre- and postcontrast MR images and the use of subtraction technique are often required to accurately assess the enhancement within complex cysts (Fig. 12.4) (Brown and Semelka 1995; Hilpert et al. 1986; Marotti et al. 1987).

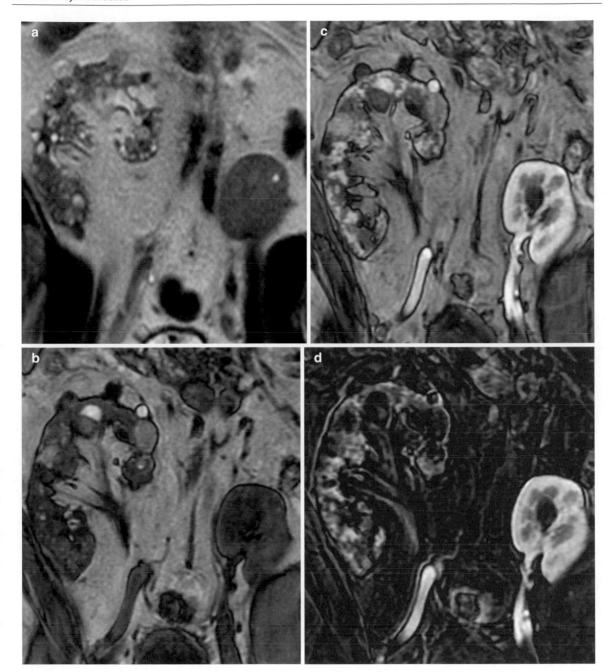

**Fig. 12.4** Subtraction MR imaging useful for assessing contrast enhancement. (**a**) Coronal T2-weighted, (**b**) T1-weighted pregadolinium, (**c**) T1-weighted postgadolinium enhanced, and (**d**) subtraction of post minus pregadolinium T1-weighted images show the native right kidney with multiple simple and complex cysts and the transplanted left pelvic kidney

## 12.4 Extraparenchymal Renal Sinus Cysts

*Extraparenchymal cysts* commonly occur in the renal sinus. These cysts are usually called *parapelvic* or *peripelvic cysts* because of their locations adjacent to the renal pelvis (Amis and Cronan 1988; Rha et al. 2004). Although parapelvic cysts (originating in the renal parenchyma and extending into the renal sinus) and peripelvic cysts (originating in the sinus presumably from lymphatic obstruction) differ in their origins, they are radiographically indistinguishable and are described interchangeably. These cysts are often discovered incidentally and frequently multiple in nature. They replace the renal sinus fat and may displace or compress adjacent structures, including the renal pelvis and calyces, parenchyma, and vessels (Schwarz et al. 1993).

Renal sinus (parapelvic or peripelvic) cysts are benign and do not require treatment or imaging follow-up. Although these cysts do not communicate with collecting system, they may simulate hydronephrosis because of their proximity to the collecting system. One useful sign for the differentiation of renal sinus cysts from hydronenphrosis is that, whereas renal sinus cysts are centered predominantly in the renal hilum with relatively sparing of the upper and lower apexes of the renal sinus (Fig. 12.5), hydronephrosis is usually evident throughout the entire renal sinus (Fig. 12.6). When the diagnosis is still uncertain, postcontrast delayed CT and

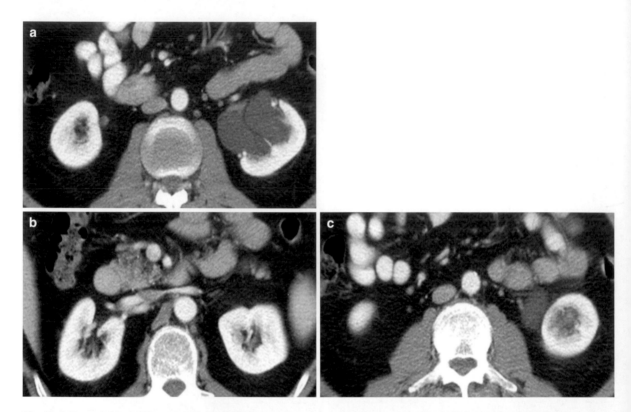

**Fig. 12.5** Parapelvic cyst. Contrast-enhanced CT images show (**a**) parapelvic cyst at the level of hilum and no visualization of cysts in the renal sinus at (**b**) the upper and (**c**) lower pole of the left kidney

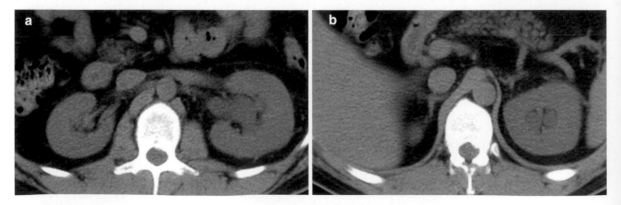

**Fig. 12.6** Hydronephrosis. Unenhanced CT images show diffusely dilated collection system at the levels of (**a**) hilum, (**b**) upper pole, (**c**) lower pole, and (**d**) an obstructing calculus in the left mid ureter. The left kidney is also enlarged and edematous

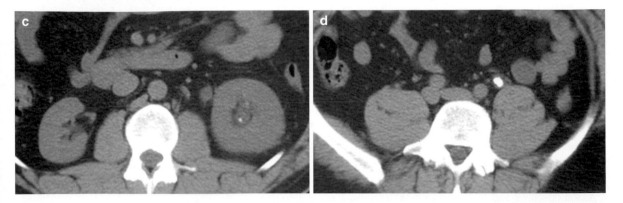

**Fig. 12.6** (continued)

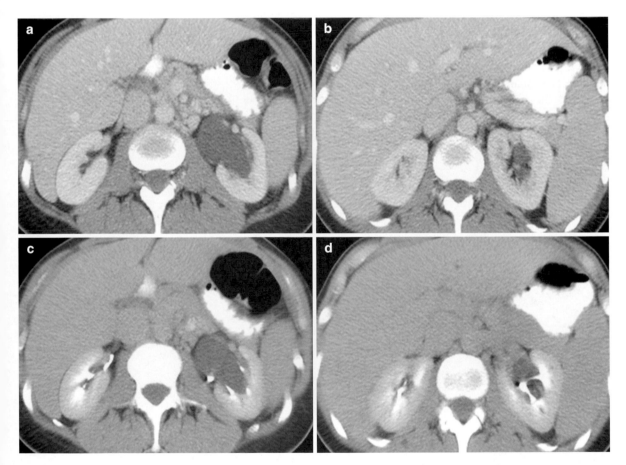

**Fig. 12.7** Parapelvic cyst in contrast-enhanced and delayed CT. (**a**, **b**) Contrast-enhanced and (**c**, **d**) delayed CT images show a large left renal parapelvic cyst which does not enhance but is surrounded by delayed excretion of contrast medium within the collecting system

MR images can help differentiate unenhanced renal sinus cysts (which compress or displace enhanced collecting system) from a contrast-enhanced dilated pyelocalyceal system (Fig. 12.7) (Morag et al. 1983; Nahm and Ritz 2000). It should be noted that the signal intensity of the contrast-enhanced collecting system in MR imaging varies depending on the delayed phases and on the concentration of gadolinium contrast excreted into the collecting system (EL-Merhi and Bae 2004).

## 12.5 Localized Cystic Disease

*Localized cystic disease* is a benign condition of unknown pathogenesis characterized by a cluster of simple cysts localized in only one kidney (Slywotzky and Bosniak 2001) (Fig. 12.8). It is also known as *segmental cystic disease of the kidney* (affecting only part of the kidney) or *unilateral cystic disease of the kidney* (affecting the entire kidney). Cysts are limited to one kidney and the contralateral kidney is normal. No association with renal tumor or renal insufficiency has been reported (Brenner and Rector 2008). Differential diagnoses for localized cystic disease include multiloculated cystic neoplasm, such as multilocular cystic nephroma and multiloculated RCC (Hartman et al. 1987, 2004). The multilocular cystic neoplasm usually has thick capsule that may demonstrate contrast enhancement. The absence of a capsule surrounding the cluster of cysts, the presence of normal parenchyma between the individual cysts and the presence of cysts outside the cluster confirm the diagnosis of localized cystic disease (Slywotzky and Bosniak 2001). Finally, when presenting in children, autosomal dominant polycystic kidney disease (ADPKD) may be a differential diagnostic consideration and can be further evaluated by phenotype screening of family members or by a long-term follow-up imaging (Slywotzky and Bosniak 2001).

## 12.6 Acquired Cystic Kidney Disease

*Acquired cystic kidney disease (ACKD)* is a progressive disorder, characterized by the occurrence of bilateral renal cysts in patients with end stage renal disease; most commonly in patients on chronic hemodialysis or peritoneal dialysis. Although the pathogenesis of cyst development is not fully understood, the prevalence and severity of ACKD depends on the duration of dialysis; reaching 40–60% of patients by 5 years and over 90% by 10 years of dialysis (Grantham and Levine 1985;

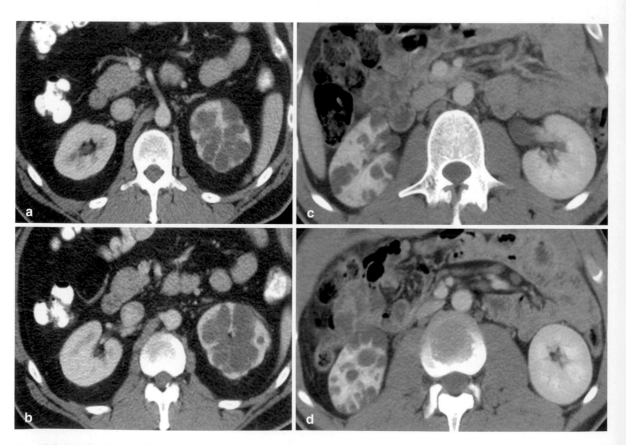

**Fig. 12.8** Localized cystic disease in two patients. Contrast-enhanced CT images show localized cystic disease involving (**a**, **b**) the left kidney of a 45-years-old male and (**c**, **d**) the right kidney of a 19-years-old male. The patients were asymptomatic and had normal renal function. The contralateral kidney was normal

Ishikawa 1985; Levine 1996; Levine et al. 1984). Cysts in ACKD vary in size from microscopic to several centimeters in diameter, and hemorrhagic cysts occur in approximately 50% of patients (Levine et al. 1991) (Fig. 12.9). The affected kidneys are usually atrophic at the time of cyst development. However, in some cases following many years of dialysis, the kidneys may have an enlarged appearance due to development of extensive renal cysts and resemble ADPKD (Bakir et al. 1999) (Fig. 12.10). Patients are usually asymptomatic, but may present with flank pain, hematuria or more serious complications, such as retroperitoneal hemorrhage or renal malignancy. ACKD is associated with increased incidence of RCC (approximately 7% of cases), which is estimated to as much as 40 times

greater than in the general population (Takebayashi et al. 2000). Compared to the sporadic form, RCC associated with ACKD is usually of a papillary type, bilateral and multiple (Schwarz et al. 2007).

Ultrasound imaging of ACKD typically demonstrates multiple cysts of varying size in small echogenic kidneys. However, fibrotic shrunken end-stage kidneys are difficult to image with sonography (Taylor et al. 1989). Contrast-enhanced CT or MR imaging is more sensitive to determine the extent of the disease, cyst complications, and renal carcinomas (Choyke 2000; Levine et al. 1984; Takebayashi et al. 1999; Taylor et al. 1989). Because of limited or absent renal function of these individuals and the presence of numerous simple and complex cysts, MRI is the preferred modality

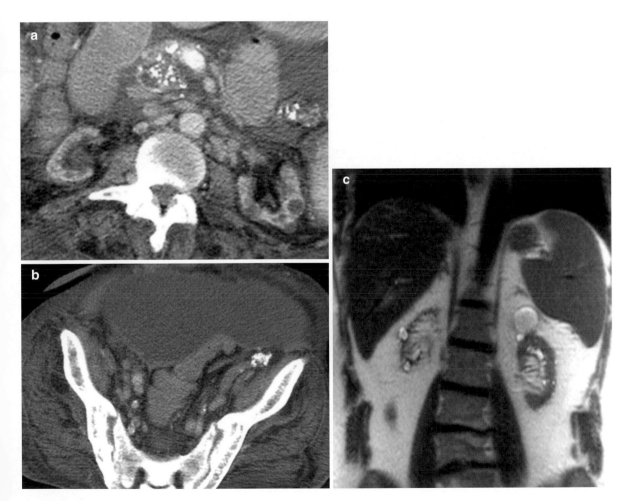

**Fig. 12.9** Acquired renal cystic disease. (**a**) Contrast-enhanced CT image shows multiple small cysts in bilateral atrophic kidneys in patient with end-stage renal disease undergoing peritoneal dialysis. (**b**) CT image of the pelvis demonstrates an involuted renal allograft in the left pelvis and dense bony changes associated with renal osteodystrophy. (**c**) Coronal T2-weighted MR image shows numerous acquired cysts and atrophic kidneys in another patient on hemodialysis

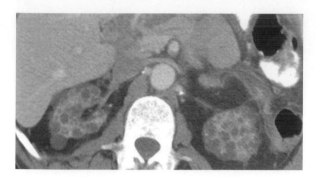

**Fig. 12.10** Acquired renal cystic disease mimicking polycystic kidney disease (PCKD). Contrast-enhanced CT image shows diffuse cystic enlargement of the kidneys simulating PCKD in a patient on hemodialysis. However, in contrast to autosomal dominant polycystic kidney disease (ADPKD) or autosomal recessive polycystic kidney disease (ARPKD), extrarenal findings such as hepatic cysts or fibrosis are absent. The kidney is also not enlarged despite severe renal cystic involvement

for evaluation of potential renal malignancies, however, contrast-enhanced CT may also be used if patients are receiving dialysis (Takebayashi et al. 1999).

Screening for RCC has been recommended after 3 years of dialysis, followed by annual or semiannual studies, preferably with CT (Levine et al. 1991). However, this approach has been questioned since RCC is actually a relatively rare cause of death among dialysis patients making the screening not cost-effective (Mindell 1989). Therefore, for a patient on dialysis the decision on surveillance for RCC should be based on patient's characteristics, such as age, general medical condition, and risk factors such as prolonged dialysis, large kidneys and male sex. After successful transplantation, the cysts regress and the kidneys return to their baseline atrophic size. Transplant recipients with ACKD seem to present a higher prevalence of RCC (19–54%), therefore, annual ultrasound surveillance of the native kidneys is useful in this high risk-population (Schwarz et al. 2007).

## 12.7 Polycystic Kidney Diseases

### 12.7.1 Autosomal Dominant Polycystic Kidney Disease

*ADPKD* is the most common inherited renal disorder that is characterized by the progressive development of multiple cysts and marked renal enlargement leading

to renal insufficiency (Churchill et al. 1984; Gabow et al. 1990; Grantham et al. 2006a; Harris et al. 2006; Parfrey et al. 1990). It occurs in 1:700–1:1,000 individuals, affecting approximately 600,000 Americans, and is the fourth leading cause of end-stage renal disease in the world (Davis et al. 1991). ADPKD is caused by mutations within either of two genes, PKD1 and PKD2. Approximately 85% of affected individuals have the PKD1 gene (located on chromosome 16 and encoding for polycystin-1) and the remaining 15% have the PKD2 gene (located on chromosome 4 and encoding for polycystin-2) (Parfrey et al. 1990). Both genotypes are characterized by the progressive enlargement of innumerable cysts derived from tubules and associated renal volumes growth (Fig. 12.11). However, compared to individuals with PKD2, those with PKD1 tend to have more cysts at the baseline, larger mean cyst and kidney volumes, and are associated with an earlier onset of renal insufficiency and higher morbidity and mortality (Grantham et al. 2006b; Harris et al. 2006; Kimberling et al. 1993). In the process of cystogenesis, the genetic defect seems to only affect at the

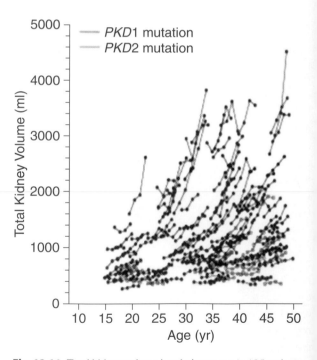

**Fig. 12.11** Total kidney volume in relation to age in 185 patients with identified PKD1 (*red*) or PKD2 (*blue*) mutations. The kidneys of patients with PKD1 mutations were generally larger at baseline and expanded at faster rates than those of patients with PK2 mutations. From (Grantham et al. 2006b); Copyright 2006 Massachusetts Medical Society. All rights reserved

level of cyst initiation, since the rate of cystic enlargement does not depend on the gene mutation (Harris et al. 2006). Interestingly, male gender may be important to the rate of cystic expansion, suggesting a hormonal influence on the process (Harris et al. 2006).

In individuals with a positive family history, the diagnosis of ADPKD can be established by radiologic imaging and demonstration of renal cysts. The kidneys are affected bilaterally in almost all instances, but may be quite asymmetric. Early in the disease, the kidney is close to normal in size with a sizable amount of normal renal parenchyma. With disease progression however, the kidney gradually enlarges as the cysts increase in number and size, and replace normal parenchyma (Fig. 12.12). The increase in cystic volume may be accompanied with an increase in noncystic renal parenchyma volume that mostly corresponds to indiscernible microcysts and inflammatory fibrotic tissue replacing normal parenchyma. Renal ultrasonography is commonly used for initial screening of the children of an affected individual. According to Ravine et al. (1994), sonographic diagnostic criteria for ADPKD for individuals with a family history of PKD1 include: at least two unilateral or bilateral cysts in individuals aged <30 years; two cysts in each kidney aged 30–59 years; and four cysts in each kidney aged ≥60 years or older. Of note, this sonographic diagnostic criterion is not applicable for individuals without a family history of ADPKD. The diagnostic sensitivity is also reduced in detecting individuals with PKD2 because renal cysts may present later in life than those with PKD1 (Nicolau et al. 1999; Pei et al. 2009). Furthermore, the sonographic criteria cannot be used with CT or MR imaging because these imaging modalities have higher sensitivity than ultrasound for the detection of renal cysts, particularly small cysts (Harris et al. 2006; Nascimento et al. 2001).

ADPKD may be clinically discovered because of symptoms related to the growth or complications of the cysts including palpable abdominal mass, flank pain, hematuria, or urinary tract infection (Fig. 12.13). This diagnosis can be confirmed by radiologic imaging demonstrating bilateral multiple cysts and renal enlargement and by the exclusion of features specific to other renal cystic diseases. Most ADPKD renal cysts are simple cysts (Fig. 12.12) and have low signal intensity on T1-weighted images and prominently high signal intensity on T2-weighted images, but the signal intensity of complex cysts affected by hemorrhage or infection may vary (Fig. 12.13). Hemorrhagic cysts are often multiple

and subcapsular in location and common in kidneys with a heavy cyst burden (Levine et al. 1985). On unenhanced CT images intracyst hemorrhage causes cyst hyperdensity (Levine and Grantham 1985). On MR imaging, the signal intensity of hemorrhagic cysts is high on T1-weighted images and often low on T2-weighted images, but the T2 signal intensity may vary depending on the chronicity of the blood products (Huch Boni et al. 1996). Subcapsular and perinephric hematomas may occur as a consequence of rupture of hemorrhagic cysts (Fig. 12.14). Calcification of the cyst wall resulting from old hemorrhage is common while renal calculi and infection occur more frequently than in the normal population. Although the risk of RCC is not increased with ADPKD (Grantham 2008; Levine and Grantham 1992; Torres et al. 2007), differentiation of hemorrhagic cysts from renal neoplasm on CT or MR imaging is determined by contrast enhancement.

ADPKD is associated with many extra-renal, cystic and noncystic manifestations (Torres et al. 2007). Hepatic cysts are the most common extrarenal manifestation and their prevalence and aggregate total hepatic cyst volume increase with age. One study (Bae et al. 2006) reported that hepatic cysts were evident in 94% of patients ≥35 years and were more prevalent and larger in total cyst volume in females. Other organs that may contain cysts include pancreas, spleen, epididymis, seminal vesicle, uterus, ovary, and thyroid. ADPKD is also associated with saccular berry aneurysm of the Circle of Willis (particularly in individuals with family history), aortic dissection, cardiac valvular disease, and colonic diverticular disease.

ADPKD is a slow progressive disease, complicated by hypertension and renal failure. Renal replacement therapy is required in 45% of patients by the age of 60 (Churchill et al. 1984; Parfrey et al. 1990). Once renal insufficiency develops in ADPKD, a rapid decline in renal function leading to end-stage renal disease ensues. To maximize the benefits of the treatment, it is crucial to identify patients who are at a high risk for end-stage renal disease early in the course of their disease while they still maintain good renal function. For this purpose, radiologic imaging is an important biomarker for the ADPKD progression. While there is high inter- and intra-individual variability in progression to end-stage renal disease, increased renal size or renal volume is associated with a poorer renal outcome (Dalgaard 1957). An on-going clinical cohort study of ADPKD subjects

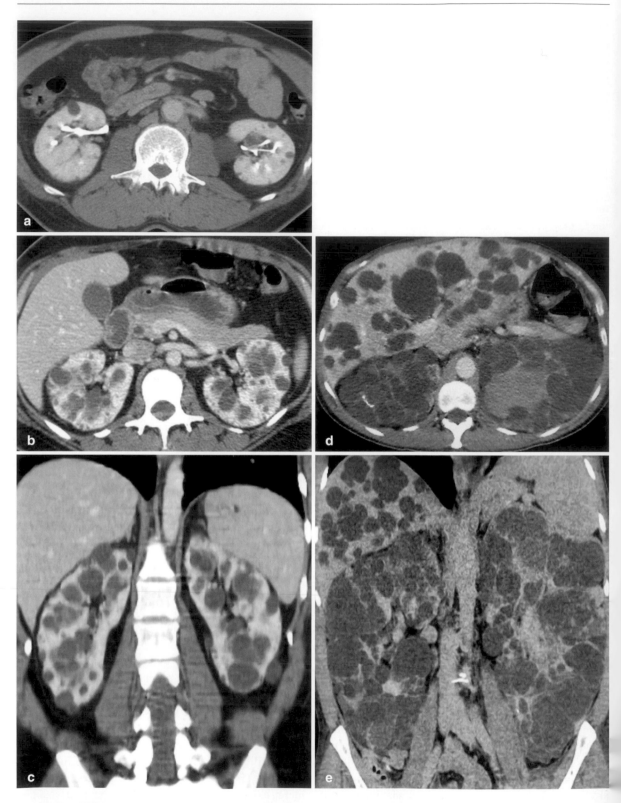

**Fig. 12.12** ADPKD in three different disease severity. Contrast-enhanced CT images of the kidneys shows numerous renal cysts of varying size and attenuation from (**a**) 46-years-old male with normal renal function, (**b**, **c**) 27-years-old female with GFR of 63 mL/min/1.73 m², and (**d**, **e**) 47-years-old male on dialysis. The patient with the most advanced ADPKD shows extensive hepatic cysts and little remaining enhancing renal parenchyma

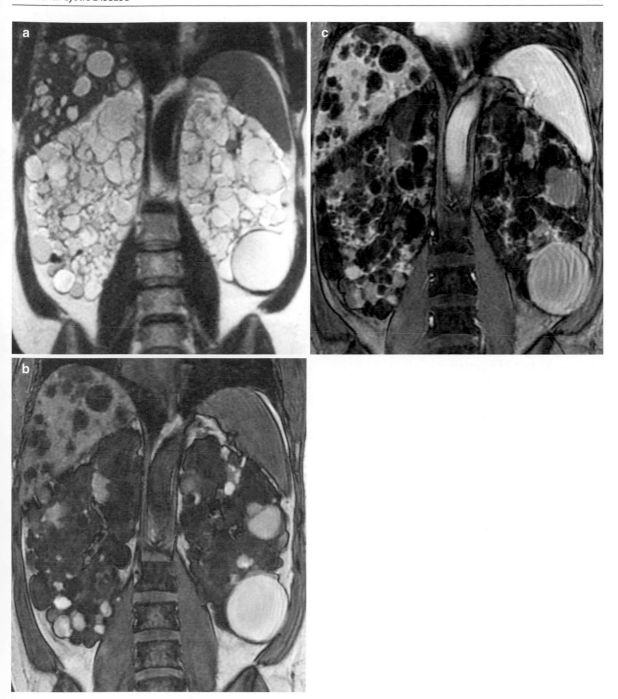

**Fig. 12.13** ADPKD on MR images. (**a**) T2-weighted coronal image shows innumerable cysts of bright signal intensity occupying markedly enlarged bilateral kidneys. (**b**) On unenhanced T1-weighted image, simple cysts are of dark signal intensity, whereas complex cysts present with intermediate to bright signal intensities. (**c**) Contrast-enhanced T1-weighted image shows scant amount of enhancing renal parenchyma remains surrounding the renal cysts. Extensive hepatic cysts are also present

receiving annual MR imaging has reported that kidney enlargement resulting from the expansion of cysts is continuous and quantifiable and is associated with the decline of renal function (Chapman et al. 2003; Grantham et al. 2006a) (Fig. 12.11). In this ADPKD cohort, the kidney volume growth occurred with a mean rate of increase of 5.3%/year (Chapman 2008), and higher rates of kidney enlargement were associated with a more rapid decrease in renal function (Grantham et al. 2006a).

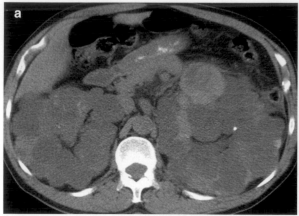
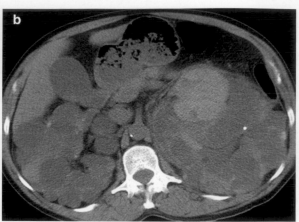
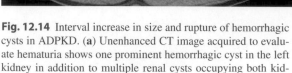

**Fig. 12.14** Interval increase in size and rupture of hemorrhagic cysts in ADPKD. (**a**) Unenhanced CT image acquired to evaluate hematuria shows one prominent hemorrhagic cyst in the left kidney in addition to multiple renal cysts occupying both kidneys. (**b**) Repeated CT scan obtained 5 days later to assess a drop in hematocrit reveals interval increase in size and rupture of the left renal hemorrhagic cyst

### 12.7.2 Autosomal Recessive Polycystic Kidney Disease

*Autosomal recessive polycystic kidney disease (ARPKD)* is a genetic disease transmitted by autosomal recessive inheritance (the mutated gene PKHD1 is located in chromosome 6p12) with an estimated frequency of 1:20,000 live births (Zerres et al. 1998). It is characterized by renal tubular ectasia (manifesting as multiple bilateral renal cysts) and hepatic ductal plate malformation (leading to hepatic fibrosis and Caroli's disease) (Chilton and Cremin 1981). ARPKD is divided into four groups depending on the age of onset: antenatal; neonatal; infantile; and juvenile subtypes. In general, the earlier the onset of disease, the more severe the renal findings and the less pronounced the hepatic involvement (Lonergan et al. 2000). The neonatal subtype is the most common, and the neonates with this type succumb to pulmonary insufficiency in the first few days of life (Habif et al. 1982). Children with ARPKD present at a later age may survive into their teens or early adulthood.

Sonographic findings of ARPKD include bilateral, enlarged and hyperechoic kidneys. The echogenicity is attributed to the unresolved 1–2 mm cystic dilatation of the collecting tubules that increases the number of acoustic interfaces (Boal and Teele 1980). Recently, there has been an increase in the role of MR imaging in pregnant women for the evaluation of fetuses; especially those fetuses with equivocal second trimester ultrasound. On MR imaging, fetuses with ARPKD have enlarged bilateral kidneys with high signal intensity on T2-weighted images attributed to the innumerable, irresolvable small cysts. At unenhanced CT, the kidneys are smooth, enlarged and low in attenuation. After contrast material injection, the kidneys show a striated appearance as they excrete contrast material slowly through the dilated collecting ducts (Lonergan et al. 2000). In older children with ARPKD, the liver may show bile-duct dilatation and evidence of portal hypertension and varices (Fig. 12.15). Hepato-biliary abnormalities in these patients are assessed by means of ultrasonography and MR cholangiography (Turkbey et al. 2009).

## 12.8 Renals Cysts in Hereditary Malformation Syndromes

### 12.8.1 Tuberous Sclerosis Complex

*Tuberous sclerosis (TS)* is a multiorgan hereditary disorder, transmitted by autosomal dominant trait. Classical clinical features of TS, as seen in Bourneville–Pringle syndrome, are mental retardation, seizures, and cutaneous lesions. Angiomyolipomas (AMLs) and cysts are common renal lesions associated with TS. AMLs are hamartomatous lesions consisting

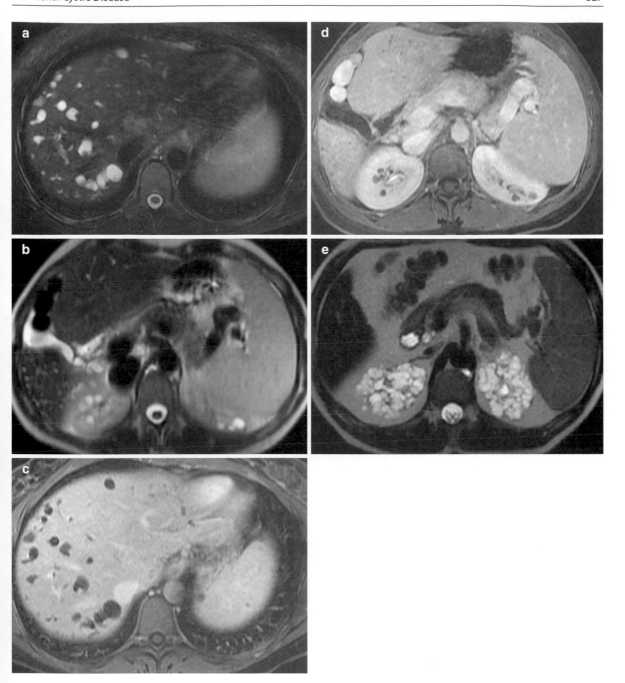

**Fig. 12.15** Autosomal recessive polycystic kidney disease. (**a, b**) T2-weighted axial and (**c, d**) contrast-enhanced T1-weighted axial MR images show few small bilateral renal cysts and saccular dilatation of intrahepatic bile ducts consistent with Caroli's disease. Some dilated bile ducts demonstrate the *central dot sign* (corresponding to intraluminal portal veins). The patient has normal renal function but stigmata of portal hypertension including splenomegaly and mesenteric varices. (**e**) T2-weighted axial image from another patient shows numerous small cysts replacing most of bilateral kidneys which are not enlarged. This patient is status post liver and kidney transplant, and the spleen is persistently enlarged

of abnormal blood vessels, smooth muscle, and adipose tissue occurring in 70–80% of adults and children with TS (Casper et al. 2002; Ewalt et al. 1998).

These lesions are often bilateral and multiple; have the tendency to increase in size over time or to bleed into the subcapsular and perinephric regions (Lemaitre et al. 1995; Reichard et al. 1998). Renal cysts have been reported to occur from 17 to 47% of patients with TS (Casper et al. 2002; Ewalt et al. 1998). These are usually bilateral and multiple with varying sizes and tend to involve both the cortex and medulla (Stapleton et al. 1980).

On ultrasound the diagnosis may be suspected in case of multiple bilateral anechoic renal cysts and hyperechoic lesions suggesting AMLs. However, lesion hyperechogenicity is not specific for AMLs since small RCCs may have the same appearance (Forman et al. 1993). CT and MR imaging are required for the confirmation of fat within the lesion (Pereira et al. 2005). Specifically, fat suppressed MR imaging techniques, such as spectral fat-saturation and chemical-shift imaging may be used to detect minimal amounts of fat and resolve indeterminate cases at CT (Fig. 12.16). Nevertheless, fat-deficient AML may be difficult to differentiate from renal-cell carcinoma. Renal cysts may be the earliest and only manifestation of this disorder in infancy and sometimes can be confused with the diagnosis of ADPKD (Mitnick et al. 1983). However, the combination of small cysts and AMLs is virtually pathognomonic of TS (Levine et al. 1997; Thomsen et al. 1997).

### 12.8.2 von Hippel–Lindau Disease

*von Hippel–Lindau* (VHL) disease is an autosomal dominant hereditary phakomatosis characterized by the development of a variety of benign and malignant tumors in different organs. VHL has a prevalence of 1:39,000–53,000 and is associated with inactivation of a tumor suppressor gene located in the short arm of chromosome 3. Several phenotypes exist. Common manifestations include hemangioblastomas of the central nervous system and retina, renal cysts and RCCs, pancreatic cysts and islet cell tumors, pheochromocytomas, and epididymal cystadenoma (Levine et al. 1982).

Renal cyst is a very common visceral manifestation of VHL occurring in 76% of patients (Levine et al. 1982). The cysts mainly occur in the renal cortex, are typically multiple, bilateral, and small; ranging in size from 0.5 to 3.0 cm in diameter (Figs. 12.17 and 12.18). They may mimic ADPKD but are not associated with renal failure (Choyke et al. 1995). RCCs are common, developing in 20–45% of patients

with VHL, and account for one third of the deaths in patients with VHL. Compared to sporadic forms, RCCs in VHL tend to occur in an earlier age (mean age, 37 years), bilaterally, and either as solid hypovascular masses or as complex cystic masses (Choyke et al. 1990; Taouli et al. 2003) (Fig. 12.18). Close tumor surveillance and detection with appropriate management such as renal nephron-sparing surgeries are important because if left untreated, RCC carries a poor prognosis and widely metastasize (Choyke et al. 1995). Ultrasound is highly sensitive for the detection of renal cysts; however, its value in screening RCCs for patients with VHL is limited because of its low accuracy in detecting small renal tumors. Accurate detection of solid renal cell tumors requires contrast-enhanced CT or MR imaging (Leung et al. 2008).

### 12.9 Medullary Sponge Kidney

*Medullary sponge kidney (MSK)* or precalyceal canalicular ectasia is a nonhereditary disorder, characterized by cystic dilatation of the collecting ducts (ducts of Bellini) of the medullary pyramids (Harrison and Rose 1979). The cysts are variable in size from 1 to 8 mm and are confined to the papillary portion of the pyramids. The cysts distribution is usually bilateral and rarely unilateral or segmental (Bernstein 1976). MSK presents predominantly in adults and rarely in children. Although MSK is usually a benign disorder that may remain asymptomatic and undetected for life, it is associated with an increased frequency of calculi and infection. The dilated ducts contain calcified deposits and approximately 50% contain nephrolithiasis (medullary nephrocalcinosis).

On gray-scale ultrasound the renal medulla appears typically hyperechoic due to the calcified deposits (Fig. 12.19). The diagnosis of MSK was traditionally made on excretory urography, where the appearance varies from linear striations ("paint brush") to small round contrast collections ("papillary blush") (Fig. 12.19) that may contain some filling defects reflecting calculi deposits (Davidson Alan 1985). This appearance is the direct result of pooling of contrast material within the dilated collecting tubules located within the tips of the renal papilla. Today, 3D volume-rendered imaging acquired during the urographic phase of a MDCT

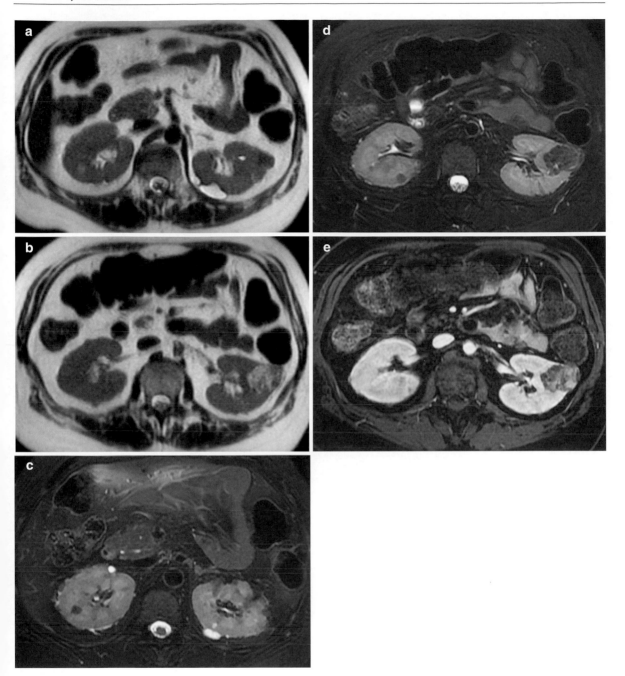

**Fig. 12.16** Tuberous sclerosis. T2-weighted axial MR images (**a**, **b**) without and (**c**, **d**) with fat saturation show several small cortical or exophytic renal cysts and fat signal lesions consistent with angiomyolipomas (AMLs) in both kidneys. AMLs are bright to intermediate signal intensities on the images without fat saturation but dark on the images acquired with fat saturation. (**e**) Contrast-enhanced T1-weighted image with fat saturation shows a heterogeneous contrast enhancement within a large AML in the left kidney

(Fig. 12.20) or MR urogram can establish the diagnosis of MSK demonstrating the characteristic findings seen on excretory urography (Maw et al. 2007; Semelka Richard 2002). The sonographic findings of MSK include dilated, anechoic spaces and intensively echogenic shadow produced by the deposits of calcium (Thomsen et al. 1997).

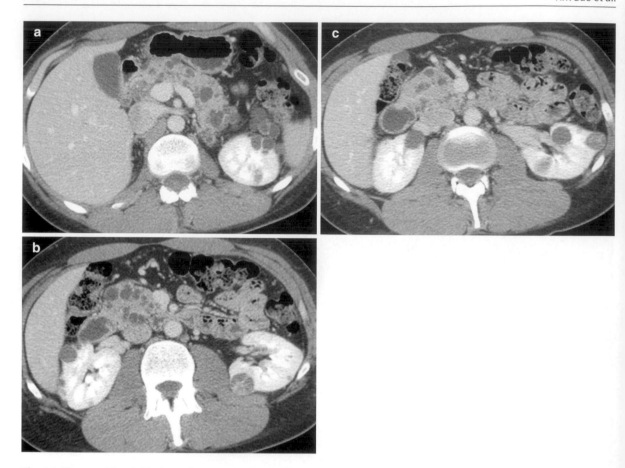

**Fig. 12.17** von Hippel–Lindau disease. (**a–c**) Contrast-enhanced CT images show multiple cysts in pancreas and both kidneys. The renal cysts are predominantly cortical. Two enhancing, partially exophytic cystic masses in the left kidney are consistent with renal cell carcinomas (RCC). A small enhancing exophytic cystic lesion in the left kidney is also concerning for a RCC

## 12.10 Multicystic Dysplastic Kidney

*Muticystic dysplastic kidney (MCDK)* is a nonhered-ited, developmental disorder characterized by multiple renal cysts replacing functional renal parenchyma in the affected whole or segmented kidney. It is the most common cystic malformation of the kidney among infants and it is found in approximately 1:4,000 live births (Winyard and Chitty 2001). The development of dysplasia seems to be associated to complete obstruction of the ureters during nephrogenesis (Nagata et al. 2002). These cysts are of variable sizes and numbers, usually unilateral (80–90%) with little or no normal renal parenchyma. It is often associated with ipsilateral renal anomalies such as vesicoureteral reflux (25%) and with contralateral renal anomalies (40%) of which ureteropelvic junction obstruction is the most common (Karmazyn and Zerin 1997).

MCDK is usually diagnosed in utero or at birth, representing one of the most common abdominal masses in the newborn (Hashimoto et al. 1986). Characteristic sonographic findings include multiple, small, noncommunicating cysts, and absence of normal parenchyma among the cysts (Sanders and Hartman 1984). On fetal MR imaging, large multiple or septated renal cysts without detectable renal parenchyma may be seen in the affected kidney. In addition, MRI has the potential to differentiate between obstructed kidney and MCDK and to predict progression of disease (Greenbaum et al. 2008). On CT and MR imaging, MDCK characteristically presents as a small cystic mass with peripheral calcification in the expected location of a kidney

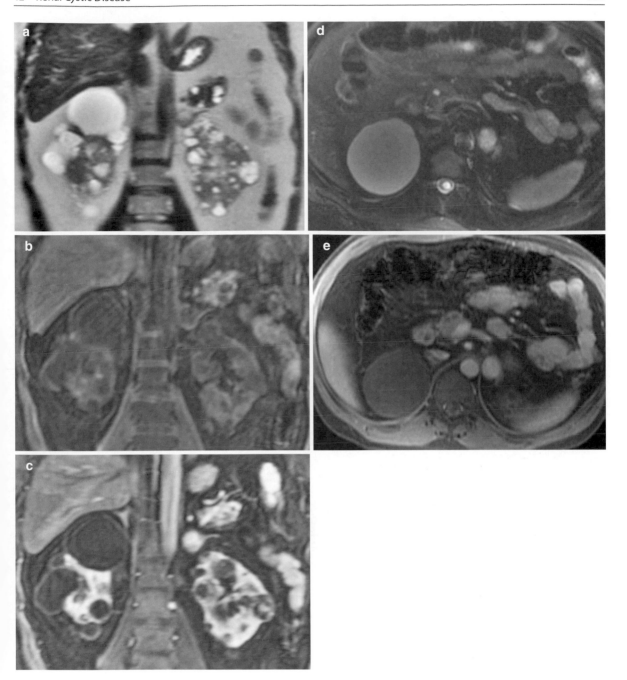

**Fig. 12.18** von Hippel–Lindau disease. (**a**) T2-weighted coronal, (**b**) T1-weighted coronal unenhanced, and (**c**) T1-weighted coronal enhanced MR images show numerous cysts in both kidneys. An exophytic renal cyst in the lateral interpole of the left kidney shows an enhancing soft-tissue nodule strongly suggestive of RCC. Several pancreatic cysts are shown in the pancreatic tail. In addition, a T2 bright, enhancing mass consistent with a pheochromocytoma is present in the left adrenal gland, as confirmed in the axial (**d**) T2-weighted and (**e**) T1-weighted enhanced MR images

(Fig. 12.21). As involution of MDCK is frequently observed, which can be followed sonographically, routine nephrectomy is not recommended and is reserved for some cases with hypertension or malignant transformation, or cases with an exceptionally large cystic kidney (Vester et al. 2008).

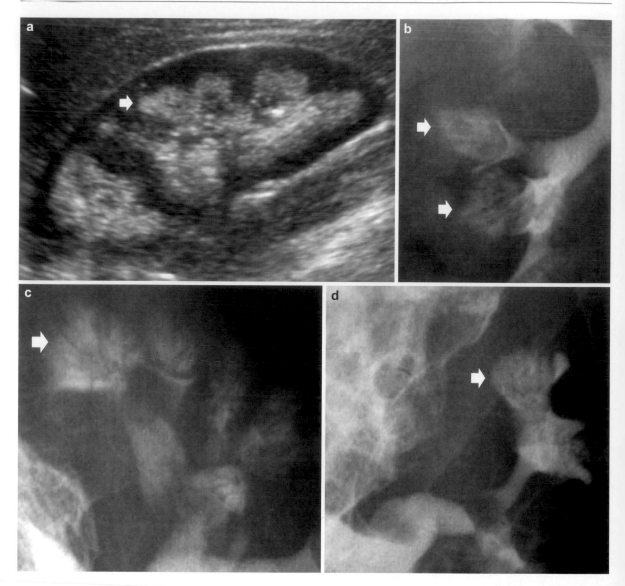

**Fig. 12.19** (**a–d**) Medullary sponge kidney (MSK). (**a**) Gray-scale ultrasound. Longitudinal scan. On gray-scale ultrasound the renal medulla appears typically hyperechoic (*arrow*) due to the calcified deposits. (**b–d**) On excretory urography, the appear-ance of the MSK varies from linear striations ("paint brush," *arrows* in (**b**) and (**c**)) to small round contrast collections ("papillary blush" *arrow* in (**d**)) (courtesy of Prof. Emilio Quaia)

## 12.11  Chronic Lithium Nephropathy

Long-term treatment with lithium salts may dam-age the renal tubuli and result in chronic tubuloint-erstitial nephropathy, clinically manifesting as nephrogenic diabetes insipidus and chronic renal disease (Boton et al. 1987). Up to 62% of patients with chronic lithium nephropathy present with mul-tiple small cysts, usually less than 2 mm in diameter and localized in both the cortex and the medulla (Markowitz et al. 2000) (Fig. 12.22). Due to the small size of the cysts, ultrasonography imaging may not show discrete cysts. MR imaging demon-strates the characteristic pattern of renal cysts asso-ciated with lithium nephropathy as multiple, uniformly and symmetrically distributed micro-cysts in normal-sized kidneys (Farres et al. 2003; Meier et al. 2007).

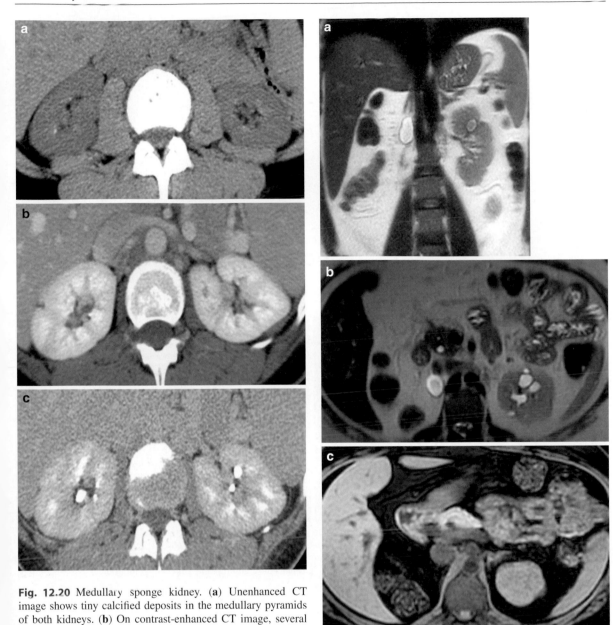

**Fig. 12.20** Medullary sponge kidney. (**a**) Unenhanced CT image shows tiny calcified deposits in the medullary pyramids of both kidneys. (**b**) On contrast-enhanced CT image, several small cysts are shown in the medulla of the left kidney. Right renal cysts imaged in different sections are not visualized. (**c**) Excretory CT image shows pooling of contrast material within the dilated collecting tubules (papillary blush) of both kidneys

**Fig. 12.21** Muticystic dysplastic kidney. (**a**) T2-weighted coronal, (**b**) T2-weighted axial, and (**c**) T1-weighted axial MR images show a round simple cystic mass with no discernible renal parenchyma in the expected location of the right kidney. A few cysts are present in relatively normal appearing left kidney

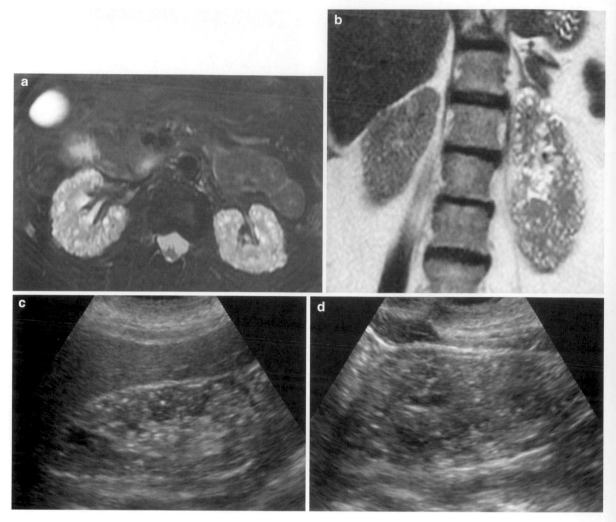

**Fig. 12.22** Lithium nephropathy. (**a**) T2-weighted axial with fat saturation and (**b**) T2-weighted oblique coronal without fat saturation MR images demonstrate innumerable tiny cysts occupying, uniformly and near symmetrically, the cortex and medulla in both kidneys. (**c**) Right and (**d**) left renal ultrasound images show that both kidneys are normal in size but almost entirely replaced by innumerable tiny echogenic foci

# References

Amis ES Jr, Cronan JJ (1988). The renal sinus: an imaging review and proposed nomenclature for sinus cysts. J Urol 139(6):1151–1159

Bae KT, Heiken JP, Siegel CL et al. (2000) Renal cysts: is attenuation artifactually increased on contrast-enhanced CT images? Radiology 216(3):792–796

Bae KT, Zhu F, Chapman AB et al. (2006) Magnetic resonance imaging evaluation of hepatic cysts in early autosomal-dominant polycystic kidney disease: the Consortium for Radiologic Imaging Studies of Polycystic Kidney Disease cohort. Clin J Am Soc Nephrol 1(1):64–69

Bakir AA, Hasnain M, Young S et al. (1999) Dialysis-associated renal cystic disease resembling autosomal dominant polycystic kidney disease: a report of two cases. Am J Nephrol 19(4):519–522

Bernstein J (1976) A classification of renal cysts. Perspect Nephrol Hypertens 4:7–30

Birnbaum BA, Hindman N, Lee J et al. (2007) Renal cyst pseudoenhancement: influence of multidetector CT reconstruction algorithm and scanner type in phantom model. Radiology 244(3):767–775

Boal DK, Teele RL (1980) Sonography of infantile polycystic kidney disease. AJR Am J Roentgenol 135(3):575–580

Bosniak MA (1986) The current radiological approach to renal cysts. Radiology 158(1):1–10

Boton R, Gaviria M, Batlle DC (1987) Prevalence, pathogenesis, and treatment of renal dysfunction associated with chronic lithium therapy. Am J Kidney Dis 10(5):329–345

Brenner BM, Rector FC (2008) Brenner & Rector's the kidney, 8th edn. Saunders Elsevier, Philadelphia

Brown ED, Semelka RC (1995) Magnetic resonance imaging of the adrenal gland and kidney. Top Magn Reson Imaging 7(2):90–101

Casper KA, Donnelly LF, Chen B et al. (2002) Tuberous sclerosis complex: renal imaging findings. Radiology 225(2):451–456

Chapman AB (2008) Approaches to testing new treatments in autosomal dominant polycystic kidney disease: insights from the CRISP and HALT-PKD studies. Clin J Am Soc Nephrol 3(4):1197–1204 (CJN.00060108)

Chapman AB, Guay-Woodford LM, Grantham JJ et al. (2003) Renal structure in early autosomal-dominant polycystic kidney disease (ADPKD): The Consortium for Radiologic Imaging Studies of Polycystic Kidney Disease (CRISP) cohort. Kidney Int 64(3):1035–1045

Chilton SJ, Cremin BJ (1981) The spectrum of polycystic disease in children. Pediatr Radiol 11(1):9–15

Choyke PL (2000) Acquired cystic kidney disease. Eur Radiol 10(11):1716–1721

Choyke PL, Filling-Katz MR, Shawker TH et al. (1990) von Hippel-Lindau disease: radiologic screening for visceral manifestations. Radiology 174(3 pt 1):815–820

Choyke PL, Glenn GM, Walther MM et al. (1995) von Hippel-Lindau disease: genetic, clinical, and imaging features. Radiology 194(3):629–642

Churchill DN, Bear JC, Morgan J et al. (1984) Prognosis of adult onset polycystic kidney disease re-evaluated. Kidney Int 26(2):190–193

Churg J, World Health Organization. Collaborating Centre for the Histological Classification of Renal Diseases (1987) Renal disease: classification and atlas, 1st edn. Igaku-Shoin, New York

Coulam CH, Sheafor DH, Leder RA et al. (2000) Evaluation of pseudoenhancement of renal cysts during contrast-enhanced CT. AJR Am J Roentgenol 174(2):493–498

Dalgaard OZ (1957) Bilateral polycystic disease of the kidneys: a follow-up of two hundred eighty-four patients and their families. Acta Med Scand 328(suppl):1–233

Davidson Alan J (1985) Radiology of the kidney. Saunders, Philadelphia

Davis F, Coles GA, Harper PS et al. (1991) Polycystic kidney disease re-evaluated: a population-based study. Q J Med 79:477

EL-Merhi FM, Bae KT (2004) Cystic renal disease. Magn Reson Imaging Clin N Am 12(3):449–467; vi

Ewalt DH, Sheffield E, Sparagana SP et al. (1998) Renal lesion growth in children with tuberous sclerosis complex. J Urol 160(1):141–145

Farres MT, Ronco P, Saadoun D et al. (2003) Chronic lithium nephropathy: MR imaging for diagnosis. Radiology 229(2):570–574

Forman HP, Middleton WD, Melson GL et al. (1993) Hyperechoic renal cell carcinomas: increase in detection at US. Radiology 188(2):431–434

Gabow PA, Chapman AB, Johnson AM et al. (1990) Renal structure and hypertension in autosomal dominant polycystic kidney disease. Kidney Int 38(6):1177–1180

Gardner KD Jr (1988) Cystic kidneys. Kidney Int 33(2):610–621

Grantham JJ (2008) Clinical practice. Autosomal dominant polycystic kidney disease. N Engl J Med 359(14):1477–1485

Grantham JJ, Chapman AB, Torres VE (2006a) Volume progression in autosomal dominant polycystic kidney disease: the major factor determining clinical outcomes. Clin J Am Soc Nephrol 1(1):148–157

Grantham JJ, Levine E (1985) Acquired cystic disease: replacing one kidney disease with another. Kidney Int 28(2):99–105

Grantham JJ, Torres VE, Chapman AB et al. (2006b) Volume progression in polycystic kidney disease. N Engl J Med 354(20):2122–2130

Greenbaum LA, Hidalgo G, Chand D et al. (2008) Obstacles to the prescribing of growth hormone in children with chronic kidney disease. Pediatr Nephrol 23(9):1531–1535

Habif DV Jr, Berdon WE, Yeh MN (1982) Infantile polycystic kidney disease: in utero sonographic diagnosis. Radiology 142(2):475–477

Harris PC, Bae KT, Rossetti S et al. (2006) Cyst number but not the rate of cystic growth is associated with the mutated gene in autosomal dominant polycystic kidney disease. J Am Soc Nephrol 17(11):3013–3019

Harrison AR, Rose GA (1979) Medullary sponge kidney. Urol Res 7(3):197–207

Hartman DS, Choyke PL, Hartman MS (2004) From the RSNA refresher courses: a practical approach to the cystic renal mass. Radiographics 24(suppl 1):S101–S115

Hartman DS, Davis CJ, Sanders RC et al. (1987) The multiloculated renal mass: considerations and differential features. Radiographics 7(1):29–52

Hashimoto BE, Filly RA, Callen PW (1986) Multicystic dysplastic kidney in utero: changing appearance on US. Radiology 159(1):107–109

Hecht EM, Israel GM, Krinsky GA et al. (2004) Renal masses: quantitative analysis of enhancement with signal intensity measurements versus qualitative analysis of enhancement with image subtraction for diagnosing malignancy at MR imaging. Radiology 232(2):373–378

Hilpert PL, Friedman AC, Radecki PD et al. (1986) MRI of hemorrhagic renal cysts in polycystic kidney disease. AJR Am J Roentgenol 146(6):1167–1172

Ho VB, Allen SF, Hood MN et al. (2002) Renal masses: quantitative assessment of enhancement with dynamic MR imaging. Radiology 224(3):695–700

Huch Boni RA, Debatin JF, Krestin GP (1996) Contrast-enhanced MR imaging of the kidneys and adrenal glands. Magn Reson Imaging Clin North Am 4(1):101–131

Ishikawa I (1985) Uremic acquired cystic disease of kidney. Urology 26(2):101–108

Karmazyn B, Zerin JM (1997) Lower urinary tract abnormalities in children with multicystic dysplastic kidney. Radiology 203(1):223–226

Kimberling WJ, Kumar S, Gabow PA et al. (1993) Autosomal dominant polycystic kidney disease: localization of the second gene to chromosome 4q13-123. Genomics 18:467–472

Laucks SP Jr, McLachlan MS (1981) Aging and simple cysts of the kidney. Br J Radiol 54(637):12–14

Lemaitre L, Robert Y, Dubrulle F et al. (1995) Renal angiomyolipoma: growth followed up with CT and/or US [comment]. Radiology 197(3):598–602

Leung RS, Biswas SV, Duncan M et al. (2008) Imaging features of von Hippel-Lindau disease. Radiographics 28(1):65–79; quiz 323

Levine E (1996) Acquired cystic kidney disease. Radiol Clin North Am 34(5):947–964

Levine E, Collins DL, Horton WA et al. (1982) CT screening of the abdomen in von Hippel-Lindau disease. AJR Am J Roentgenol 139(3):505–510

Levine E, Cook LT, Grantham JJ (1985) Liver cysts in autosomal-dominant polycystic kidney disease: clinical and computed tomographic study. AJR Am J Roentgenol 145(2):229–233

Levine E, Grantham JJ (1985) High-density renal cysts in autosomal dominant polycystic kidney disease demonstrated by CT. Radiology 154(2):477–482

Levine E, Grantham JJ (1992). Calcified renal stones and cyst calcifications in autosomal dominant polycystic kidney disease: clinical and CT study in 84 patients. AJR Am J Roentgenol 159(1):77–81

Levine E, Grantham JJ, Slusher SL et al. (1984) CT of acquired cystic kidney disease and renal tumors in long-term dialysis patients. AJR Am J Roentgenol 142(1):125–131

Levine E, Hartman DS, Meilstrup JW et al. (1997) Current concepts and controversies in imaging of renal cystic diseases. Urol Clin North Am 24(3):523–543

Levine E, Slusher SL, Grantham JJ et al. (1991) Natural history of acquired renal cystic disease in dialysis patients: a prospective longitudinal CT study. AJR Am J Roentgenol 156(3):501–506

Lonergan GJ, Rice RR, Suarez ES (2000) Autosomal recessive polycystic kidney disease: radiologic-pathologic correlation. Radiographics 20(3):837–855

Maki DD, Birnbaum BA, Chakraborty DP et al. (1999) Renal cyst pseudoenhancement: beam-hardening effects on CT numbers. Radiology 213(2):468–472

Markowitz GS, Radhakrishnan J, Kambham N et al. (2000) Lithium nephrotoxicity: a progressive combined glomerular and tubulointerstitial nephropathy. J Am Soc Nephrol 11(8):1439–1448

Marotti M, Hricak H, Fritzsche P et al. (1987) Complex and simple renal cysts: comparative evaluation with MR imaging. Radiology 162(3):679–684

Maw AM, Megibow AJ, Grasso M et al. (2007) Diagnosis of medullary sponge kidney by computed tomographic urography. Am J Kidney Dis 50(1):146–150

Meier M, Beigel A, Schiffer L et al. (2007) Magnetic resonance imaging in a patient with chronic lithium nephropathy. Nephrol Dial Transplant 22(1):278–279

Mindell HJ (1989). Imaging studies for screening native kidneys in long-term dialysis patients. AJR Am J Roentgenol 153(4):768–769

Mitnick JS, Bosniak MA, Hilton S et al. (1983) Cystic renal disease in tuberous sclerosis. Radiology 147(1):85–87

Morag B, Rubinstein ZJ, Hertz M et al. (1983) Computed tomography in the diagnosis of renal parapelvic cysts. J Comput Assist Tomogr 7(5):833–836

Nagata M, Shibata S, Shu Y (2002) Pathogenesis of dysplastic kidney associated with urinary tract obstruction in utero. Nephrol Dial Transplant 17(suppl 9):37–38

Nahm AM, Ritz E (2000) The renal sinus cyst-the great imitator. Nephrol Dial Transplant 15(6):913–914

Nascimento AB, Mitchell DG, Zhang XM et al. (2001) Rapid MR imaging detection of renal cysts: age-based standards. Radiology 221(3):628–632

Nicolau C, Torra R, Badenas C et al. (1999) Autosomal dominant polycystic kidney disease types 1 and 2: assessment of US sensitivity for diagnosis. Radiology 213(1):273–276

Parfrey PS, Bear JC, Morgan J et al. (1990) The diagnosis and prognosis of autosomal dominant polycystic kidney disease. N Engl J Med 323(16):1085–1090

Pei Y, Obaji J, Dupuis A et al. (2009) Unified criteria for ultrasonographic diagnosis of ADPKD. J Am Soc Nephrol 20(1):205–212

Pereira JM, Sirlin CB, Pinto PS et al. (2005) CT and MR imaging of extrahepatic fatty masses of the abdomen and pelvis: techniques, diagnosis, differential diagnosis, and pitfalls. Radiographics 25(1):69–85

Ravine D, Gibson RN, Walker RG et al. (1994) Evaluation of ultrasonographic diagnostic criteria for autosomal dominant polycystic kidney disease 1. Lancet 343(8901):824–827

Reichard EA, Roubidoux MA, Dunnick NR (1998) Renal neoplasms in patients with renal cystic diseases. Abdominal Imaging 23(3):237–248

Rha SE, Byun JY, Jung SE et al. (2004) The renal sinus: pathologic spectrum and multimodality imaging approach. Radiographics 24(suppl 1):S117–S131

Sagel SS, Stanley RJ, Levitt RG et al. (1977) Computed tomography of the kidney. Radiology 124(2):359–370

Sanders RC, Hartman DS (1984) The sonographic distinction between neonatal multicystic kidney and hydronephrosis. Radiology 151(3):621–625

Schwarz A, Lenz T, Klaen R et al. (1993) Hygroma renale: pararenal lymphatic cysts associated with renin-dependent hypertension (Page kidney). Case report on bilateral cysts and successful therapy by marsupialization. J Urol 150(3):953–957

Schwarz A, Vatandaslar S, Merkel S et al. (2007) Renal cell carcinoma in transplant recipients with acquired cystic kidney disease. Clin J Am Soc Nephrol 2(4):750–756

Semelka Richard C (2002) Abdominal-pelvic MRI. Wiley-Liss, New York, UK

Silverman SG, Israel GM, Herts BR et al. (2008) Management of the incidental renal mass. Radiology 249(1):16–31

Slywotzky CM, Bosniak MA (2001) Localized cystic disease of the kidney. AJR Am J Roentgenol 176(4):843–849

Stapleton FB, Johnson D, Kaplan GW et al. (1980) The cystic renal lesion in tuberous sclerosis. J Pediatr 97(4):574–579

Suh M, Coakley FV, Qayyum A et al. (2003) Distinction of renal cell carcinomas from high-attenuation renal cysts at portal venous phase contrast-enhanced CT. Radiology 228(2):330–334

Tada S, Yamagishi J, Kobayashi H et al. (1983) The incidence of simple renal cyst by computed tomography. Clin Radiol 34(4):437–439

Takebayashi S, Hidai H, Chiba T et al. (1999) Using helical CT to evaluate renal cell carcinoma in patients undergoing hemodialysis: value of early enhanced images. AJR Am J Roentgenol 172(2):429–433

Takebayashi S, Hidai H, Chiba T et al. (2000) Renal cell carcinoma in acquired cystic kidney disease: volume growth rate determined by helical computed tomography. Am J Kidney Dis 36(4):759–766

Taouli B, Ghouadni M, Correas JM et al. (2003) Spectrum of abdominal imaging findings in von Hippel-Lindau disease. AJR Am J Roentgenol 181(4):1049–1054

Taylor AJ, Cohen EP, Erickson SJ et al. (1989) Renal imaging in long-term dialysis patients: a comparison of CT and sonography. AJR Am J Roentgenol 153(4):765–767

Thomsen HS, Levine E, Meilstrup JW et al. (1997) Renal cystic diseases. Eur Radiol 7(8):1267–1275

Torres VE, Harris PC, Pirson Y (2007) Autosomal dominant polycystic kidney disease. Lancet 369(9569):1287–1301

Turkbey B, Ocak I, Daryanani K et al. (2009) Autosomal recessive polycystic kidney disease and congenital hepatic fibrosis (ARPKD/CHF). Pediatr Radiol 39(2):100–111

Vester U, Kranz B, Hoyer PF (2010) The diagnostic value of ultrasound in cystic kidney diseases. Pediatr Nephrol 25(2):231–240

Wang ZJ, Coakley FV, Fu Y et al. (2008) Renal cyst pseudoenhancement at multidetector CT: what are the effects of number of detectors and peak tube voltage? Radiology 248(3): 910–916

Winyard P, Chitty L (2001) Dysplastic and polycystic kidneys: diagnosis, associations and management. Prenat Diagn 21(11):924–935

Zerres K, Rudnik-Schoneborn S, Steinkamm C et al. (1998) Autosomal recessive polycystic kidney disease. J Mol Med 76(5):303–309

# Renal Parenchymal and Inflammatory Diseases

## Emilio Quaia

**13**

## Contents

### Abstract

> Renal parenchymal diseases may be characterized by gray-scale and color and power Doppler ultrasound (US). The most typical appearance of renal parenchymal diseases on gray-scale US is a diffuse increase in echogenicity of parenchyma of both kidneys with an increased or a reduced visibility of renal pyramids. Color and power Doppler analysis of intrarenal flows may reveal an increase in the resistive index value (>0.7). Even though gray-scale and Doppler US provide morphological and functional evaluations of renal parenchymal diseases, they do not present high specificity and sensitivity in the characterization of the different renal parenchyma disease.

Renal parenchyma diseases may be intrinsic or may occur as manifestations of systemic disease (Andreoli 1992). Intrinsic renal parenchyma disease include glomerular and tubulointerstitial disorders, while glomerular involvement in systemic diseases occurs in various form of vasculitis, diabetes, and metabolic and hemathological diseases. Renal parenchyma diseases are often nonspecific in their clinical manifestations – as hematuria, proteinuria (>150 mg/day in adults, or 140 mg/m$^2$/day in children), azotemia, hypertension, or metabolic acidosis.

Ultrasound (US) is usually the first imaging procedure used to evaluate the kidneys in a patient presenting with proteinuria, hematuria or renal failure details (Huntington et al. 1991; Martinoli et al. 1999). A sensitivity of 62–77%, a specificity of 58–73% and a positive predictive value of 92% for detecting microscopically

E. Quaia
Department of Radiology, Cattinara Hospital, University of Trieste, Strada di Fiume 447, 34149 Trieste, Italy
e-mail: quaia@univ.trieste.it

E. Quaia (ed.), *Radiological Imaging of the Kidney*,
Medical Radiology, DOI: 10.1007/978-3-540-87597-0_13, © Springer-Verlag Berlin Heidelberg 2011

proved renal parenchymal changes have been reported for US (Platt et al. 1988; Page et al. 1994). In early clinical stages of renal parenchymal diseases, kidneys may appear normal on US, whereas as parenchymal diseases progress, changes in echogenicity and echotexture of renal parenchyma usually manifest.

Different renal parenchymal diseases present the same US appearance and US-guided biopsy may be necessary to determine the exact histological cause of renal failure (Platt et al. 1988; Di Nardo et al. 1989; Tikkakoski et al. 1994). Increased renal echogenicity is suggestive of renal parenchymal diseases including glomerulonephritis, pyelonephritis, nephrotic syndrome, obstructive nephropathy, hemoglobinuria, myoglobinuria, renal vein thrombosis, acute tubular necrosis, interstitial nephritis, and renal involvement of malignancies in childhood (Kasap et al. 2006). Even though gray-scale and Doppler US provide morphological and functional evaluations of renal parenchymal diseases, they do not present high specificity and sensitivity in the characterization of the different renal parenchyma disease, since different renal parenchymal diseases may reveal the same appearance on US, whereas the same renal parenchymal disease may present different appearances on US according to the stage of renal disease and to clinical situation. Anyway, renal parenchymal diseases may reveal some characteristic patterns on US, even though renal parenchymal disease characterization cannot be considered feasible by US in the majority of cases. Doppler US is a useful tool in renal parenchymal diseases and ARF follow-up, during and after medical treatment.

The role of nonenhanced functional MR imaging in the assessment of renal function and renal parenchyma diseases is described on Chap. 34.

Nuclear medicine has an important role in the diagnostic work-up of patients with renal parenchyma diseases. The diagnostic capabilities of nuclear medicine, and particularly, of single photon emission tomography (SPECT) are described on Chap. 8.

## 13.1 Glomerulonephritis, Tubulo-Interstitial Nephritis, and Vasculitides

Two major types of disorders affect the glomerulus: the acute nephritic syndrome characterized mainly by inflammatory and/or necrotizing lesions within glomeruli, and the nephrotic syndrome, a predominantly noninflammatory derangement of the glomeruli characterized by an abnormally permeable glomerular filtration barriers to macromolecules so that massive proteinuria occurs (>3.5 g/day in adults or 40 mg/m$^2$/h in children) even though the glomerular filtration rate (GFR) may be normal (Andreoli 1992). Glomerular diseases may be classified into three groups: (1) primary renal diseases which manifest as acute nephritic syndrome (glomerulonephritis) with abrupt onset of hematuria and proteinuria, red cell casts, and decreased GFR (acute renal failure); (2) primary renal diseases which manifests with nephrotic syndrome; (3) secondary involvement of the glomerulus by a variety of systemic diseases, with either a nephritic or nephrotic syndrome (Couser 1992).

Two immunologic mechanisms of glomerular disease are accepted: (1) Deposition of antibody to glomerular basement membrane antigens (Goodpasture's syndrome), or (2) Discontinuous or granular deposition of immunoglobulin and complement within (a) the glomerular mesangium (IgA nephropathy, Henoch-Schönlein purpura, and early lupus nephritis), (b) along the subendothelial surface of the capillary wall between endothelial cells and the glomerular basement membrane (severe lupus nephritis, type I membranoproliferative glomerulonephritis), (c) on the outer subepithelial surface of the capillary wall (membranous nephropathy, and poststreptococcal glomerulonephritis). Most glomerular antibody deposits contain predominantly immunoglobulin G (IgG), which activates complement via the classic complement pathway (Couser 1992). The histologic lesions include diffuse (e.g. poststreptococcal glomerulonephritis) or focal (e.g. IgA nephropathy) glomerular involvement, hypercellularity involving glomerular endothelial and/or mesangial cells or epithelial cells in Bowman's space (this resulting in glomerular crescents in severe diseases), and neutrophils and mononuclear cell infiltrates with narrowing or occlusion of the capillary loops. In some other glomerulopathies other histologic lesions can be found. In minimal change nephrotic syndrome there is absence of abnormalities on light microscopy, and of immune deposits on immunofluorescence while the typical lesions is represented by diffuse epithelial cell foot fusion often associated with moderate focal or diffuse proliferation of mesangial cells. Focal glomerulosclerosis is an histologic lesion found in some patients with otherwise typical minimal change nephrotic syndrome, consisting in focal mesangial proliferation affecting some glomeruli and some capillary loops within an affected glomerulus (Couser 1992).

In the acute interstitial nephritis, the primary abnormality is damage to the tubulointerstitial system of the kidney, with secondary glomerular damage. Thus renal tubular function tends to be deranged disproportionately to reductions in the GFR. Characteristically, in acute interstitial nephritis mononuclear cells infiltrate the interstitium, particularly in the renal cortex (McKinney 1992). Inflammatory cells may invade the tubular wall and may be associated with areas of tubular necrosis. The infiltrate may be diffuse or patchy, and the extent of the infiltrate corresponds in general to the degree of renal function impairment (McKinney 1992). Tubulointerstitial renal disorders often damage the juxtaglomerular apparatus and tend to impair renin production with consequent hyporeninemia and hypoaldosteronism, impaired urinary concentration in response to water deprivation, modest degree of salt wasting, hyperkalemia, and hyperchloremic metabolic acidosis (Andreoli 1992). Isolated tubular defects, as renal glicosuria, aminoaciduria, and tubular acidosis, are frequently observed. With prolonged acute interstial nephritis, interstitial fibrosis may develop, and the pathologic picture may merge into that of chronic interstitial nephritis.

The most common systemic diseases resulting in glomerular involvement, beside diabetic nephropathy, are the various form of vasculitis. Renal vasculitides affecting the kidney comprise polyarteritis nodosa, Wegener granulomatosis, rheumatoid vasculitis, cryoglobulinemia related vasculitis, hypersensitivity vasculitis (leukocytoclastic vasculitis angiitis), Henoch-Schönlein purpura, and antineutrophil cytoplasmic antibodies (ANCA) positive vasculitides.

### 13.1.1 Glomerulonephritis and Tubulo-Interstitial Nephritis

On US the most typical appearance of renal parenchymal diseases is a diffuse increase in echogenicity of parenchyma of both kidneys with an increased or a reduced visibility of renal pyramids. The number of hyaline casts per glomerulus is related to loss of

visualization of cortico-medullary junction and of pyramids (Hricak 1982). Renal sinus may appear inhomogeneous on US for septal thickness, fibrosis, atrophy and loss of adipose tissue with a progressive lower renal sinus–renal parenchyma differentiation. Patients with renal diseases involving primarily the tubulointerstitial compartment most frequently present abnormal RI values, while patients with glomerular disease often have normal RI values.

Renal enlargement is related to the extent of glomerular hyper-cellularity and crescent formation, whereas cortical echogenicity is related to severity of glomerular sclerosis, crescent formation, interstitial inflammatory cell infiltration, tubular atrophy and interstitial fibrosis. In glomerulonephritis with a prevalent mesangial matrix and basement membrane involvement, such as IgA nephropaty (Fig. 13.1), membranous GN (Fig. 13.2), minimal change glomerulonephritis, and focal glomerulosclerosis cortical echogenicity is usually normal or slightly increased since glomerular component accounts only for 8% of renal parenchyma. As renal disease progresses, histological changes spread among the three primary parenchymal components, nephron, vessels and interstitium, and hyperechoic renal parenchyma results. In crescentic and proliferative glomerulonephritis which present glomerular, interstitial and vascular involvement and in tubulo-interstitial nephritis, renal parenchyma is often hyperechoic. The RIs values are usually elevated in diseases of the tubulo-interstitial compartment (Mostbeck et al. 1991; Sugiura et al. 2004; Ikee et al. 2005), whereas they are often normal in kidneys with glomerular pathologies (Figs. 13.1 and 13.2), except in crescentic and proliferative glomerulonephritis where they are frequently increased. The RIs values are significantly correlated to the amount of arteriolosclerosis, glomerular sclerosis, oedema and interstitial fibrosis. These findings are nonspecific, and RIs analysis does not distinguish different forms of renal medical disorders. Waveform Doppler US analysis is useful in the follow-up of renal parenchymal diseases to predict noninvasively the improvement or worsening of renal function according to RIs values. In renal acute crescentic and proliferative glomerulonephritis and tubulo-interstitial diseases color and power Doppler usually reveal a decreased renal parenchymal perfusion, which correlates with increased RIs values measured on interlobar–arcuate arteries.

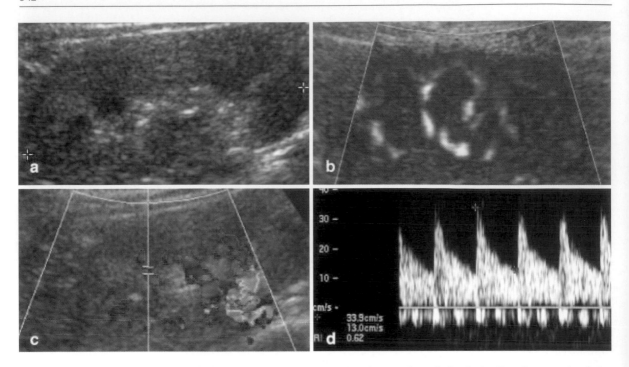

**Fig. 13.1** (**a–d**) IgA nephropathy. (**a**) Kidneys present normal morphological appearance on gray-scale ultrasound, and (**b**) normal renal parenchymal vascularization is revealed by power Doppler ultrasound. (**c, d**) On duplex Doppler normal resistive index values (0.62) are revealed

## 13.1.2 Renal Vasculitides

Since vascular and interstitial components are the most represented in renal parenchyma, and since they are both involved in renal vasculitides, US may reveal early involvement. Renal vasculitides, such as Wegener granulomatosis (Fig. 13.3) and polyarteritis nodosa (Fig. 13.4) manifest as an increased cortical echogenicity with reduced cortico-medullary differentiation. US may also reveal multiple cortical hypoechoic areas of variable size and shapes with cortical distortion, expressing regions of parenchymal oedema. The RIs values are significantly correlated with creatinine level and presence of interstitial disease.

Polyarteritis nodosa is a systemin necrotizing vasculitis of medium and small arteries which consists of foci of fibrinoid necrosis that begin in the media. Renal involvement occurs in 90% of patients with polyarteritis nodosa. Inflammation then spreads to involve the intima and adventitia, and results in small aneurysms and vascular thrombosis. These small aneurysms occur at the bifurcation of interlobular or arcuate arteries and are best seen at digital subtraction angiography (Fig. 13.5) even though they can be effectively identified by contrast-enhanced

CT during the corticomedullary phase (Fig. 13.6). Subsequent renal ischemia occurs and renin-mediated hypertension is common. The small aneurysms seen in polyarteritis nodosa may occasionally rupture with resultant intraparenchymal or perinephric hematoma. Bilateral multiple small wedge-shaped hypovascular area (Figs. 13.6 and 13.7) are identified in the renal parenchyma on contrast-enhanced CT (Pope et al. 1981; Ozaki et al. 2009) corresponding to multiple renal cortical infarctions from vasculitis of the interlobar and arcuate arteries. Perirenal hematoma by aneurismal rupture represents another typical imaging findings (Wilms et al. 1986; Ozaki et al. 2009).

## 13.2 Systemic Diseases Involving the Kidney

## 13.2.1 Diabetic Nephropathy

Renal disease is an important cause of morbidity in patients with diabetes mellitus and kidney is involved in 30–50% of patients with longstanding type-I

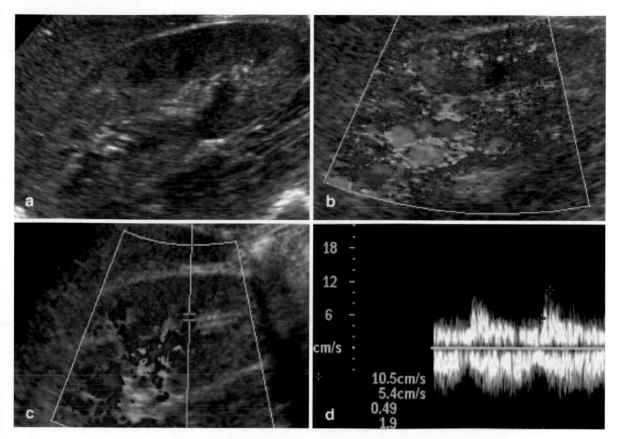

**Fig. 13.2** (**a–d**) Membranous glomerulonephritis. (**a**) Kidneys reveal a slight increase in cortical echogenicity with an increased cortico-medullary differentiation on gray-scale ultrasound. (**b**) Normal renal parenchymal vascularization is revealed by color Doppler ultrasound, whereas on (**c**, **d**) Duplex Doppler normal resistive index values (0.49) are revealed

insulin-dependent diabetes mellitus (juvenile onset diabetes mellitus) and in 1–2.5% of patients with noninsulin-dependent diabetes mellitus (Soldo et al. 1997). Diabetes mellitus determines the development of end-stage renal disease in approximately 25–40% of patients entering chronic dialysis (Myers 1992). Although dialysis and transplantation prevent death from uremia, the 5 year survival in diabetic patients with end-stage renal disease is much worse than that of nondiabetic patients. Therefore, it is important to recognize the very early stage of diabetic nephropathy and to institute appropriate therapy, especially when urinary albumin excretion is >300 mg/day.

Diabetic glomerulopathy, a complex disorder associated with a diffuse expansion of collagenous component of the glomerulus with accumulation of extracellular matrix resulting in an expansion of mesangium and thickening of glomerular basement membrane (diffuse intercapillary glomerulosclerosis), is the predominant

cause of renal failure (Myers 1992). The diabetic patient is also prone to other renal disease, including pyelonephritis, papillary necrosis, and obstructive nephropathy which lead to renal failure, and diabetic patients with glomerulopathy are more susceptible to these associated renal diseases (Myers 1992). Several factors have been implicated in the development of diabetic nephropathy including poor glycemic control (fasting plasma glucose >140–160 mg/dL), genetic factors, hemodynamic abnormalities (increased GFR), systemic hypertension, altered vascular permeability, metabolic disturbance, and hyperlipidemia. According to Diabetes Control and Complications Trial Research Group (DCCT) (1993) and United Kingdom Prospective diabetes study (UKPDS) (2005) the tight glycemic control has been shown to be the primary prevention from all microvascular complications in the diabetic patient including nephropathy, retinopathy, and neuropathy

Early abnormalities of glomerular function appear almost in all patients with type-I insulin-dependent

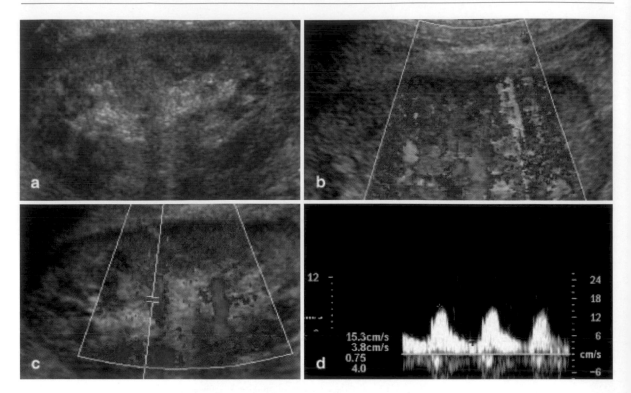

**Fig. 13.3** (**a–d**) Wegener granulomatosis. (**a**) On gray-scale ultrasound, kidneys reveal a clear increase in renal parenchymal echogenicity with a low cortico-medullary diffferentiation, whereas on color Doppler ultrasound (**b**) a clear reduction of renal parenchymal perfusion is documented. (**c, d**) Duplex Doppler reveals diffusely increased resistive index values (0.75)

diabetes mellitus, but only part of them will develop a progressive proteinuric form of diabetic glomerulopathy. The stage 1 of diabetic glomerulopathy is devoid of clinical symptoms and signs of glomerulopathy, and it manifests with a 20–40% elevation of the GFR above that found in age-matched normal control subjects due to a generalized hypertrophy of the glomeruli (Myers 1992). Stage 2 of diabetic glomerulopathy is characterized by increasing proteinuria (with a microalbuminuria >250 µg/min), declined GFR, and development of hypertension and edema. Diffuse thickening of the glomerular basement membrane is noted along with increased mesangial volume. The stage 3 of diabetic glomerulopathy represents the last 2–3 years advanced stage of what is a 20–25 years process, and it is characterized by the development of azotemia and progressive worsening of hypertension and edema. At this stage, the mesangium further expands and occupies a greater portion of the glomerular volume while the thickness of the glomerular basement membrane is not necessarily increased. Frequently, characteristic nodular hyaline-like deposits situated at the periphery of the glomerulus, named nodular glomerulosclerosis or intercapillary glomerulosclerosis or Kimmelstiel-Wilson lesions, are evident in the center of the peripheral glomeruli (Olefsky 1992).

Diabetic patients, with initial renal involvement, present enlarged kidneys, increased parenchymal thickness, and increase of the renal parenchyma echogenicity with increased visibility of renal pyramids and cortico-medullary differentiation on gray-scale US (Fig. 13.8). This appearance is related to the increased GFR in the initial stages of renal disease, whereas in diabetic patients with mild renal involvement, renal length and parenchymal thickness are usually normal. In diabetic patients undergoing hemodialysis renal length is reduced. In advanced diabetic nephropathy, renal parenchyma echogenicity may appear increased or normal according to vascular and interstitial compartment involvement, whereas renal margins are usually diffusely irregular. Multiple irregularities of the renal cortex profiles with indentation between renal calyces may simulate fetal lobations even though in diabetic nephropathy the overall parenchyma thickness

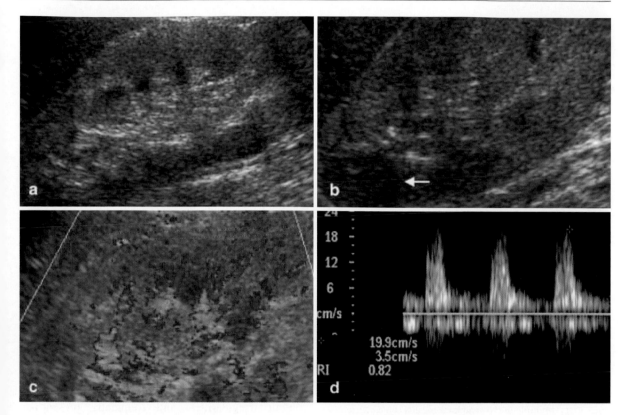

**Fig. 13.4** (**a–d**) Polyarteritis nodosa. (**a**) On gray-scale ultrasound, kidneys reveal a clear increase in renal parenchymal echogenicity, with a poor cortico-medullary differentiation, and (**b**) some hypoechoic cortical areas (*arrow*) which can be expression of localized cortical oedema. (**c**) Reduced renal parenchymal vascularization is documented on color Doppler ultrasound, whereas (**d**) a clear increase in resistive index values (0.82) is revealed by pulsed Doppler

is reduced by atrophy (<12 mm). The RIs are typically elevated in advanced diabetic nephropathy, whereas RIs are often normal in the early stage of disease (Platt et al. 1994). The RIs are highly correlated with serum creatinine concentration and creatinine clearance rate, whereas an elevated RI (≥0.70) is associated with impaired renal function, increased proteinuria and poor prognosis (Platt et al. 1994).

### 13.2.2 Hypertension

Coexistence of hypertension and decreased renal function may be due to nephrosclerosis secondary to hypertension, or primary renal disease with secondary hypertension. Nephrosclerosis represents the second most common diseases that result in referral of patients for transplantation (Curtis 1992). Even though hypertension is better treated than in the past, yet the incidence of end-stage renal failure due to hypertension has not decreased. Kidney transplantation in this group of patients often restores normal renal function and normal blood pressure control.

Benign nephrosclerosis is the term used for the renal pathology associated with sclerosis of renal arterioles and small arteries due to medial and intimal thickening as a response to hemodynamic changes, aging, genetic defects, or some combination of these and to hyaline deposition in arterioles (Alpers 2005). The resultant effect is focal ischemia of the renal parenchyma supplied by vessels with thickened walls and consequent narrowed lumen (Alpers 2005). Some degree of nephrosclerosis is present at autopsy with increasing age preceding or in the absence of hypertension. Hypertension and diabetes mellitus increase the incidence and severity of the lesions. Malignant nephrosclerosis is the form of renal disease associated with the malignant or accelerated phase of hypertension (Alpers 2005). This pattern of hypertension may occasionally develop in previously

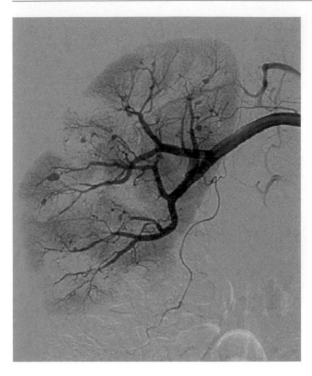

**Fig. 13.5** Polyarteritis nodosa. 51-year-old man with fever of unknown origin. Digital subtraction angiography of the right renal artery. Multiple microaneurysms located at the interlobular and arcuate arteries. Irregularities, narrowing, ectasia, and occlusion in small arteries are also identified. Multiple wedge-shaped hypoperfusion areas are demonstrated (courtesy of Dr. Kumi Ozaki, Kanazawa, Japan)

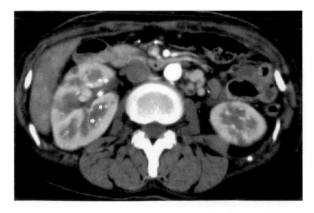

**Fig. 13.6** Polyarteritis nodosa. A 48-year-old women. Contrast-enhanced CT during corticomedullary phase shows multiple multiple microaneurysms (*arrows*) located at the interlobular and arcuate arteries and multiple wedge-shaped hypoperfusion areas in both kidneys (courtesy of Dr. Kumi Ozaki, Kanazawa, Japan)

normotensive individuals but often is superimposed on pre-existing essential benign hypertension, secondary forms of hypertension (renal, endocrine, vascular, or neurogenic), or an underlying chronic renal disease, particularly glomerulonephritis or reflux nephropathy (Alpers 2005). Kidneys present a size which is related to the duration and severity of the hypertensive disease. Small petechial hemorrhages may appear on the renal cortical surface from rupture of arterioles or glomerular capillaries. The two histologic landmarks of malignant nephrosclerosis are the fibrinoid necrosis of arterioles, and the hyperplastic arteriolitis with the typical onion-skinning appearance.

The renal vascular alterations of hypertension depend on the severity of the blood pressure elevation and whether the process accelerates to malignant hypertension. Arteriolosclerosis of small cortical renal arteries, interlobar, arcuate and interlobular, is a common features of kidney in patients with systemic arterial hypertension (Quaia and Bertolotto 2002). In nephroangiosclerosis both kidneys are usually symmetrically reduced in their diameters with reduction of the renal parenchyma thickness, cortical scars or renal contour irregularities, and frequently present an increased cortical echogenicity with increased corticomedullary differentiation (Fig. 13.9a). Color and power Doppler US reveal nonspecific reduction of vascularization. If compared to normal patient population, renal RIs are typically increased (>0.7 and frequently around 0.8) (Fig. 13.9b). Renal perforating arteries and veins (Bertolotto et al. 2000) are much more visible in kidneys of nephroangiosclerotic patients in comparison with normal subjects, since they enlarge in nephroangiosclerosis and present normally directed flows from the kidney towards renal capsule. Renal RIs are increased with values ranging from 0.8 and 0.98.

### 13.2.3 Lupus Systemic Erythematosus

Systemic lupus erythematosus is an autoimmune disease involving multiple organs. The kidneys are the most commonly affected organs, with significant associated morbidity and mortality and renal involvement in 15–85% of cases (Kim and Kim 1990). Renal lesions in systemic lupus erythematosus are classified into five types: type 1, normal or minimal-change disease; type 2, mensangial glomerulonephritis; type 3, focal

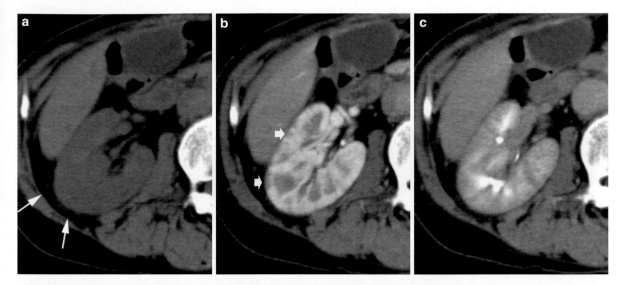

**Fig. 13.7** (**a–c**) Polyarteritis nodosa. Seventy-one-year-old man with fever of unknown origin (**a**) Unenhanced CT shows diffuse enlargement and slight thickening of Gerota's fascia (*arrows*). (**b**) Contrast-enhanced CT during corticomedullary phase shows multiple small wedge-shaped less-enhanced areas (*arrows*). The margin between the cortex and medulla is indistinct during the excretory phase (**c**) (courtesy of Dr. Kumi Ozaki, Kanazawa, Japan)

proliferative glomerulonephritis; type 4, diffuse proliferative glomerulonephritis; type 5, membranous glomerulonephritis (Kim and Kim 1990).

Gray-scale US has been reported to have a sensitivity of 95% in lupus nephritis detection (Longmaid et al. 1987). In lupus nephritis kidneys may present reduced or increased dimensions and an increased cortical echogenicity with reduced cortico-medullary differentiation. US may also reveal multiple cortical hypoechoic areas of variable size and shapes with cortical distortion, expressing regions of parenchymal oedema. The RIs values are significantly correlated with creatinine level and presence of interstitial disease, whereas normal RIs values are considered as a good prognostic factor (Platt et al. 1997).

### 13.2.4 *Metabolic and Hematological Disease-Related Nephropathies*

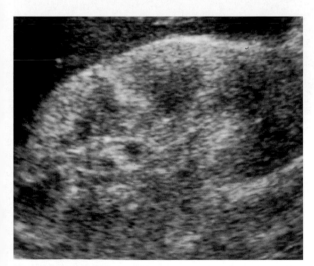

**Fig. 13.8** Diabetic nephropathy. Gray-scale US. Longitudinal scan. Enlarged kidneys and increased parenchymal thickness with diffuse increase of the renal parenchyma echogenicity with increased visibility of renal pyramids and cortico-medullary differentiation

In hyperoxaluria, and particularly in enteric hyperoxaluria due to enhanced absorption of dietary oxalate in patients with ileal disease, kidneys present normal or reduced dimensions with smooth margins, and a hyperechoic renal cortex and medulla. In gout nephropathy hyperechoic papillary spots or a diffuse hyperechoic medulla may be observed. Renal stones are usually present while kidneys present normal or reduced dimensions with smooth margins. In nephrocalcinosis hyperechoic calcium depositions are observed mainly in renal cortex but also in renal pyramids.

The kidneys are frequently involved in all forms of systemic amyloidosis, and represent a major complications of the disease (Amendola 1990) both in the

**Fig. 13.9** (**a**, **b**) Seventy-years-old patient with slightly increased creatinine levels (1.5 mg/dL) and hypertension (170/110 mmHg). (**a**) Longitudinal US scan of the left kidney. Reduction of the renal parenchyma thickness, renal contour irregularities, and increased cortico-medullary differentiation. (**b**) Increased value of the resistive index (0.9) measured on a segmental artery

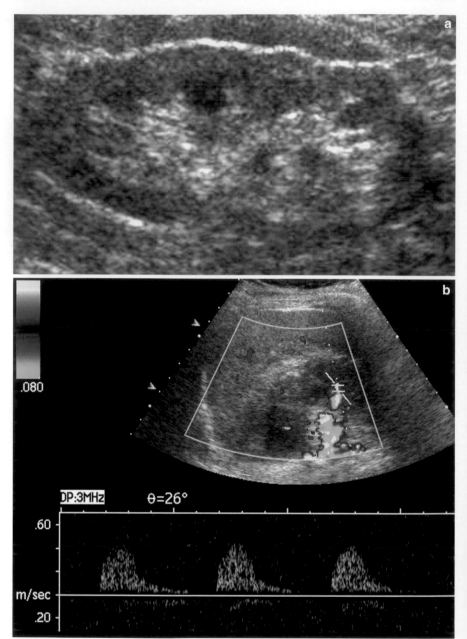

AL (amyloid light chain) and AA (amyloid-associated) types (Kim and Kim 1990). Amyloidosis can occur without any associated disease (primary amyloidosis) or in association with chronic destructive disease such as chronic osteomyelitis, rheumatoid arthritis, tuberculosis, or malignancies (secondary amyloidosis) (Kim and Kim 1990). Microscopically, amyloid is first deposited in the mesangium of the glomerulus and later extends along the basement membrane of the glomerula capillaries, producing a thickened appearance (Amendola 1990).

In amyloidosis (Fig. 13.10), as in leukemia and multiple myeloma, both kidneys appear enlarged and hyperechoic with reduced or normal or increased cortico-medullary and cortical-sinus differentiation on gray-scale US. The RIs values are usually increased. Glycogenosis results in liver and kidney involvement (Fig. 13.11), with hepatomegaly, hypoglycemia, and hyperuricemia.

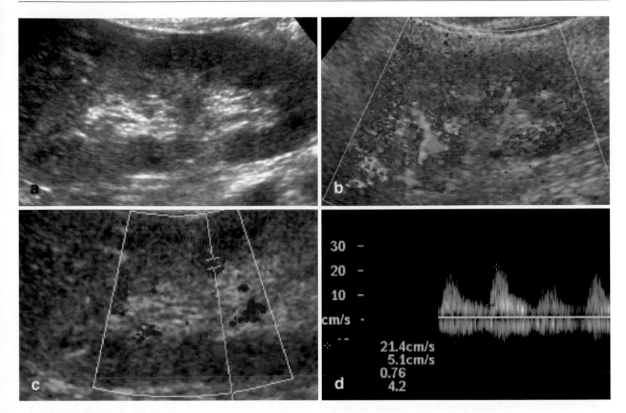

**Fig. 13.10** (**a–d**) Renal amyloidosis. (**a**) On gray-scale ultrasound, kidneys reveal increased renal parenchymal echogenicity, with low corticomedullary differentiation, whereas (**b**) reduction of renal parenchymal perfusion is documented by color Doppler ultrasound. (**c, d**) Duplex Doppler reveals diffusely increased RIs values (0.76)

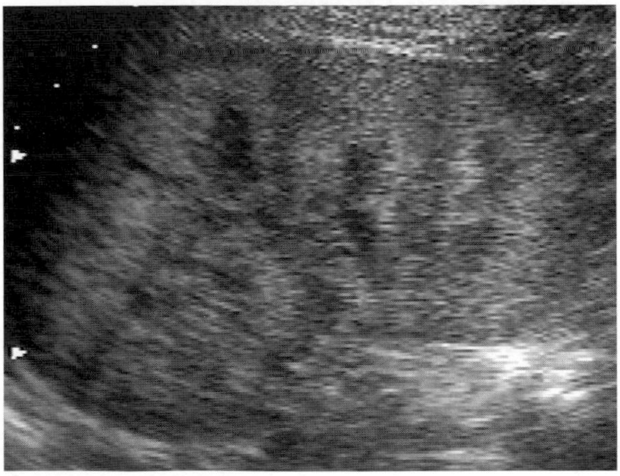

**Fig. 13.11** Type-I glycogenosis. Gray-scale US. Longitudinal scan. Enlarged kidneys and increased parenchymal thickness with diffuse increase of the renal parenchyma echogenicity with reduced visibility of renal pyramids and cortico-medullary differentiation

### 13.2.5 HIV-Associated Nephropathy

HIV-associated nephropathy (originally called AIDS-associated nephropathy) consists in a focal and segmental glomerulosclerosis (Saag 1992). Histologically the glomerulus shows a global collapse of the glomerular capillaries, increased mesangial sclerosis, and a proliferative cap of visceral epithelial cells with dilatation of the Bowam space and universal tubular damage (Saag 1992). This type of medical nephropathy may occur at any stage of HIV infection. Clinically, HIV-associated nephropathy should be suspected in the HIV patient with deteriorating renal function, nephrotic range proteinuria, and azotemia in the absence of hypertension. AIDS-associated nephropathy is an immunological phenomenon and is characterized by marked proteinuria and rapid-onset renal failure (Symeonidou et al. 2009). US reveals normal-sized or enlarged kidneys, with increased cortical echogenicity related to focal and segmental glomerulosclerosis and

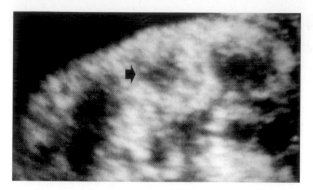

**Fig. 13.12** HIV-associated nephropathy. Gray-scale US. Longitudinal scan. Diffuse increase of the renal parenchyma echogenicity with reduced visibility of renal pyramids (*arrow*)

to dilated renal tubules filled by proteinaceous material (Miller et al. 1993). Both kidneys appear enlarged and echogenic with obliteration of the renal sinus fat appearance and reduced or loss cortico-medullary differentiation on gray-scale US (Fig. 13.12) with a reduced visibility of renal pyramids. Hyperechoic nephromegaly is a nonspecific finding but when associated with pelvocalyceal thickening the diagnosis of HIV-associated nephropaty should be considered (Hamper et al. 1988; Wachsberg et al. 1995).

Beside HIV-associated nephropathy, patients with HIV infection may present renal opportunistic infections, neoplasia, and highly-active antiretroviral therapy. The lack of T helpe lymphocytes (CD4 cells) leads these patient category towards opportunistic infections including *Pneumocystis jirovecii* and mycobacterial and fungal infections (see Chap. 17). Patients infected with HIV are more susceptible to neoplasia including renal non-Hodgkin's lymphoma (see Chap. 25) and Kaposi sarcoma. Highly-active antiretroviral therapy may determine direct toxic effects on the kidneys from certain drugs such as tenofovir or didanosine, or nephrolithiasis which is a recognized side effect of indinavir and nelfinavir (Symeonidou et al. 2009), and other side effects including dyslipidemia, insulin resistance, and hypertension which may lead to renal artery stenosis.

## 13.3 Drug Nephropathies

Most drug nephropathies involve mainly the tubular–interstitial compartment. Even though acute interstitial nephritis is a rare complication of drug therapy, the

high frequency with which these drugs are used it account for a substantial portion of all cases of acute renal failure. Penicillins, sulfonamides, antituberculous drugs, nonsteroidal anti-inflammatory drugs, and allopurinol are among the most important drugs involved in acute interstitial nephritis. Beside, mononuclear cell infiltrate, eosinophils are typically present in the renal interstitium (McKinney 1992). In analgesic nephropathy kidneys may reveal hyperchoic spots on renal pyramids due to papillary calcifications, which can be observed also in sarcoidosis, primary hyperparathyroidism, diabetes mellitus, medullary sponge kidney and in long dialysis treatment. Renal papillary necrosis occurs in 70–80% of patients with analgesic nephropathy but may be observed also in diabetes mellitus, obstructive uropathy, sickle cell disease, acute or chronic pyelonephritis, acute tubular necrosis and renal vein thrombosis. In those cases with a clear renal collecting system dilatation, US may detect papillary necrosis as an hyperechoic filling defect without acoustic shadowing (Hoffman et al. 1982). In heavy metals and other drugs nephropathy US does not reveal any pathological modifications also when acute renal failure occur. Diffuse incrementation of renal RIs may be observed. Iodinated contrast media may be responsible for acute renal failure. US reveals normal kidneys with increased RIs which reduce progressively after medical treatment.

## 13.4 Pediatric Renal Parenchymal Diseases

The most common vascular renal diseases in neonates and infants are renal vein thrombosis, renal corticomedullary necrosis and renal artery thrombosis secondary to dehydration, sepsis, blood loss and severe hypoxia. Even though hyperechogenicity of renal parenchyma is a nonspecific parameter in pediatric patients, a relationship between degree of cortical echogenicity and histopathological changes on renal biopsy has been shown (Erwin et al. 1985). The more frequent renal parenchymal disease in children is acute glomerulonephritis, where kidneys may appear normal or enlarged, with or without hyperechoic renal cortex, with normal or increased RIs and with a normal or reduced renal parenchymal perfusion on color and power Doppler. Other pediatric renal parenchymal diseases associated

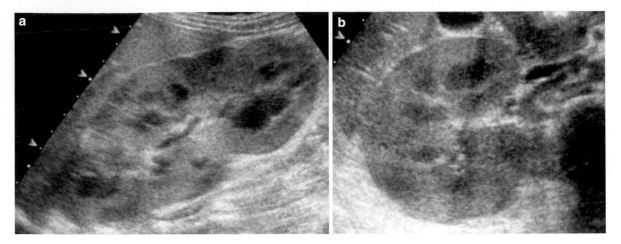

**Fig. 13.13** (**a**, **b**) Renal involvement in acute lymphatic leukemia in a pediatric patients. Gray-scale US. Longitudinal (**a**) and transverse scan (**b**). Enlarged kidneys and increased parenchymal thickness with diffuse increase of the renal parenchyma echogenicity with increased visibility of renal pyramids and cortico-medullary differentiation

with increased renal echogenicity are type-I glycogenosis, glomerulosclerosis, oculocerebral syndrome, renal dysplasia, oxalosis, renal amyloidosis, acute multifocal pyelonephritis, sickle cell anemia, primary polycythaemia, and acute lymphatic leukemia (Fig. 13.13). In children with systemic hypertension, US reveals dotted echogenic spots at the cortico-medullary junction caused by a diffuse calcifying process involving the lamina elastica of the interlobar and arcuate arteries.

Nephrotic syndrome is uncommon in pediatric patients and may be related to progressive glomerulonephritis, infections, collagen vascular diseases, amyloidosis or neoplasms. In nephrotic syndrome kidneys may appear normal on US or may be enlarged with increased parenchymal echogenicity.

Haemolytic uraemic syndrome is a microangiopathic haemolytic anemia that causes thrombocytopaenia, renal failure and hypertension, and occurs principally in children about 3–10 days following episodes of gastroenteritis or viral upper respiratory tract infections. A similar syndrome occurs less frequently in adults, often associated with complications of pregnancy or during the postpartum period (postpartum acute renal failure) or associated with the use of oral contraceptives or also following treatment with a variety of antineoplastic agents. Renal cortex appears typically hyperechoic with sharp delineation of hypoechoic pyramids and increased cortico-medullary differentiation, probably related to swelling of glomerular endothelial and mesangial cells, and to the presence of platelet aggregates and fibrin thrombi in the lumen of glomerular capillaries. Markedly elevated RIs are found. Nephrocalcinosis is rare in children and associated mainly with hypercalcaemic status, renal tubular diseases, enzymatic disorders, prolonged furosemide therapy and Tamm-Horsfall proteinuria.

## 13.5 Renal Medullary and Papillary Necrosis

Renal papillary necrosis is the necrosis of renal papilla within renal medulla secondary to interstitial nephritis or ischemia. At intravenous excretory urography renal papillary necrosis manifests as a triangular or bulbous cavitation adjacent to calyx. It may be bilateral if related to a systemic or disseminated cause and often results from analgesic nephropathy, diabetes, and sickle cell trait. or diabetes or unilateral if it is due to obstruction, infection, or venous thrombosis. Unilateral disease is associated with severe unilateral acute pyelonephritis, obstruction, and renal vein thrombosis. Sloughing of the papilla often results in gross hematuria, renal colic, and obstruction. Papillary necrosis can be bilateral or unilateral.

Papillary necrosis is a condition which may result from any of several disease processes. The common etiology of papillary necrosis is diabetes, nonsteroidal anti-inflammatory medication abuse or overuse or analgesic nephropathy (specifically aspirin and phenacetin), sickle cell disease, pyelonephritis and tuberculosis, renal vein thrombosis, and obstructive uropathy (Chul Jung et al. 2006). The papillary necrosis seen in tuberculosis and severe pyelonephritis is a direct result of the infection. All or some of the necrotic papilla may be resorbed or sloughed into the collecting system. The pathophysiology of papillary necrosis seen in the other diverse group of diseases appears to be ischemia to the papillae. The medullary papillae are especially susceptible to ischemic insult because of the low oxygen tension, high blood osmolality, and relatively poor perfusion in the papillary tips. If the ischemic process in the medullary region is caused by a temporary spasm and normal circulation is restored within a reasonable period, or if predisposing conditions are corrected within a reasonable period, the involved tissues may recover. However, if ischemia continues and perfusion is not restored, irreversible coagulation necrosis, tubular fibrosis, and lobar infarcts result (Chul Jung et al. 2006).

Traditionally, renal papillary necrosis has been diagnosed primarily with the use of intravenous excretory urography. Nowadays computed tomography (CT) urography is not used to detect renal papillary necrosis, even though there are relatively few published reports about the CT features of the condition. Multi–detector row CT can demonstrate these findings even more clearly and directly than single–detector row CT, because of the advantages of thinner sections and multiplanar reformations (Chul Jung et al. 2006) and can depict necrosis as clearly as does excretory urography and thus allow accurate diagnosis of the condition. The radiologic appearance of papillary necrosis depends on the severity and chronicity of the

necrosis. Different morphologic patterns have been described according to the extension of necrosis. In the advanced stage of necrosis, clefts originate from the fornices and extend into and dissect the medullary pyramids and papillae, ultimately causing the papillae to slough. Renal papillary necrosis is visible when contrast material (e.g., at IV urography) in the urinary collecting system fills a necrotic cavity located centrally or peripherally in the papillae.

Calyceal deformities in renal papillary necrosis occur in three forms: early, medullary and papillary. The earliest and most subtle changes result in papillary swelling (necrosis in situ) that is often impossible to observe radiologically without serial urograms. The medullary form (Figs. 13.14 and 13.15), corresponding to a central medullary necrosis, takes place at the tip of the papilla and it appears as microcavities surrounded by the papilla fornices (Figs. 13.16 and 13.17).

The papillary form, a necrosis of a larger portion of the papilla, may represent the evolution of the medullary form or it may represents an ab-initio necrotic process beginning at the base of the papilla. Detachment of necrotic papillae starts in the central part of the calyx, and a round or oval cavity opens (Figs. 13.18 and 13.19). The detachment of necrotic papillae usually begins in the region of the caliceal fornices, and the resulting defect is triangular in shape (Figs. 13.20 and 13.21). Clefts that originate from the fornices and that undermine and ultimately sever the papillary tip are classic manifestations of renal papillary necrosis. The entire necrotic papilla or portions of it may be retained within the excavated calyx, in which case contrast material will surround the unextruded papillary tip producing a signet ring sign when the calix is filled with contrast material. This results in circular or irregular filling defects. The devitalized papilla also may act as a nidus for calcification.

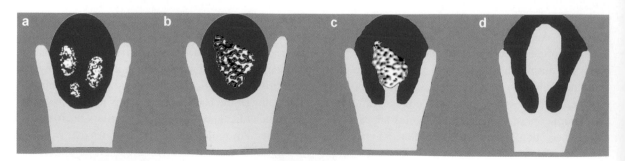

**Fig. 13.14** (**a–d**) Scheme. Different stages of the renal medullary necrosis. The renal papilla is represented in red while the renal calyces are represented in *yellow*. The process begins as papillary swelling or necrosis in situ (**a**, **b**), and progressively becomes central medullary necrosis taking place at the tip of the papilla appearing as microcavities (**c**, **d**) surrounded by the papilla fornices

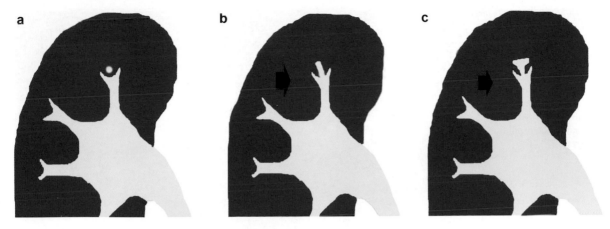

**Fig. 13.15** (**a–c**) Scheme. Different stages of the renal medullary necrosis as it appears on intravenous excretory urography or CT urography. The renal parenchyma, including the renal papilla, is represented in *red* while the renal calyces are represented in *yellow*. The central medullary necrosis progressively extends up to a central cavity (*arrow*) surrounded by renal calyces

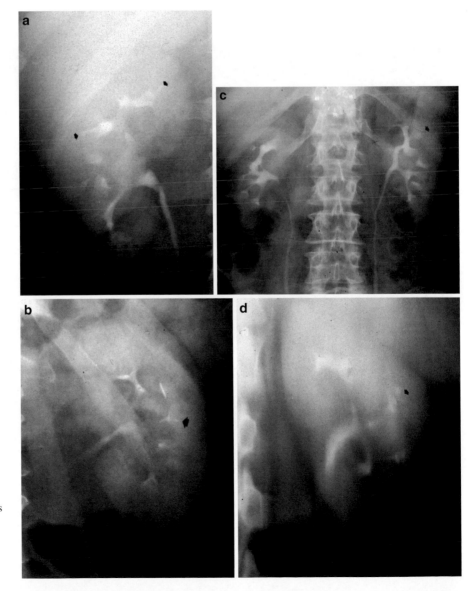

**Fig. 13.16** (**a–d**) Renal medullary necrosis. Intravenous excretory urography. Different patterns of renal medullary necrosis (*arrows*) appearing in the center of renal papilla surrounded by the papilla fornices

**Fig. 13.17** (**a**, **b**) Renal medullary necrosis. CT urography. (**a**) Transverse image; (**b**) coronal reformation. Renal medullary necrosis takes place at the tip of the papilla, and appears as plus image (*arrow*) in the medullary necrosis surrounded by the papilla fornices

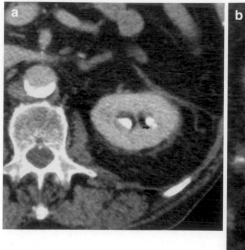
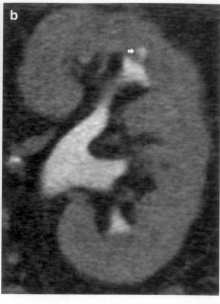

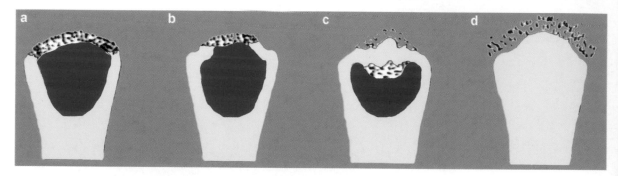

**Fig. 13.18** (**a–d**) Scheme. Different stages of the renal papillary necrosis. The renal papilla is represented in *red* while the renal calyces are represented in *yellow*. (**a**) The detachment of necrotic papillae begins in the region of the caliceal fornices. (**b**) Clefts originating from the fornices progressively surrounds the papillary tip. (**c**) The entire necrotic papilla or portions of it may be retained within the excavated calyx, in which case contrast material will surround the unextruded papillary tip producing a signet ring sign when the calix is filled with contrast material. (**d**) Sloughing of the necrotic papilla causes the calyx to be blunted

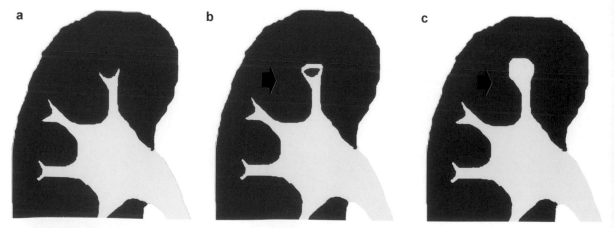

**Fig. 13.19** (**a–c**) Scheme. Different stages of the renal papillary necrosis as it appears on intravenous excretory urography or CT urography. The renal parenchyma, including the renal papilla, is represented in *red* while the renal calyces are represented in *yellow*. The renal papilla is progressively surrounded by clefts (*arrow*) originating from the adjacent fornices and a cavity results after expulsion of the renal papilla

**Fig. 13.20** (**a–d**) Renal papillary necrosis. Intravenous excretory urography. Different patterns of renal papillary necrosis (*arrows*)

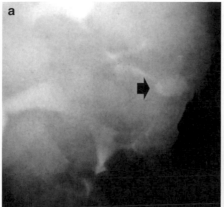

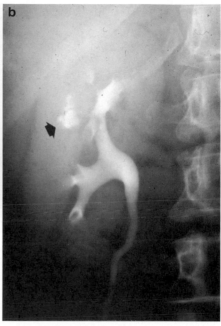

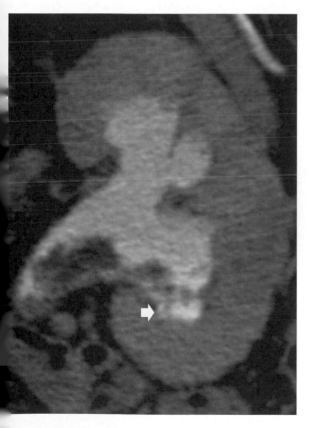

**Fig. 13.21** Renal papillary necrosis. CT-urography. Renal papillary necrosis (*arrow*) with sloughing of the necrotic papilla. Hypodense blood coagula are also evident at the level of the pyelo-ureteral junction

Sloughing of the necrotic papilla causes the calyx to be blunted. This blunted calyx (Fig. 13.21) may be distinguished from that seen in reflux nephropathy (i.e., one that is associated with a deep cortical scar), whereas the renal contour of papillary necrosis is normal or gently undulating. Blunted calyces may also be seen in congenital megacalyces. Megacalycosis is an asymptomatic congenital disorder with imaging features that are characterized by enlarged calyces and normal renal pelvis and ureter. Typically, megacalycosis involves all of the calyces uniformly and there is a greater number of calyces than normal (i.e., >15). Papillary necrosis tends to be dissimilar from calyx to calyx, and the number of calyces is not increased.

The differential diagnosis for extracalyceal cavities also involves pyelocalyceal diverticulum, as differentiation between these entities can be difficult. Calyceal diverticula are uroepithelium-lined outpouchings of the collecting system into the renal parenchyma. Typically, calyceal diverticula connect to the calyceal fornix and project into the renal cortex (including a column of interlobar cortex) and not into the medulla.

# References

Alpers CE (2005) The kidney. In: Kumar V, Abbas AK, Fausto N (eds) Robbins and Cotran pathologic basis of disease. Elsevier Saunders, Philadelphia, pp 955–1021

Amendola MA (1990) Amyloidosis of the urinary tract. In: Pollack HM, McClennan BL, Dyer R, Kenney PJ (eds) Clinical urography. Saunders, Philadelphia, pp 2909–2920

American Diabetes Association (2005) Implications of the United Kingdom Prospective Diabetic Study. Diabetes Care 26 (suppl):S28–S32

Andreoli TE (1992) Approach to the patient with renal disease. In: Wyngaarden JB, Smith LH, Bennett JC (eds) Cecil textbook of medicine. Saunders, Philadelphia, pp 477–482

Bertolotto M, Quaia E, Galli G et al.(2000) Color Doppler sonographic appearance of renal perforating vessels in subjects with normal and impaired renal function. J Clin Ultrasound 28:267–276

Chul Jung D, Kim SH, Jung SI et al. (2006) Renal papillary necrosis: review and comparison of findings at multidetector row CT and intravenous urography. Radiographics 26:1827–1836

Couser WG (1992) Glomerular disorders. In: Wyngaarden JB, Smith LH, Bennett JC (eds) Cecil textbook of medicine. Saunders, Philadelphia, pp 551–568

Curtis JJ (1992) Renal transplantation. In: Wyngaarden JB, Smith LH, Bennett JC (eds) Cecil textbook of medicine. Saunders, Philadelphia, pp 546–551

Di Nardo R, Iannicelli E, Leonardi D et al. (1989) Echographic aspects of kidney diseases and comparison with needle biopsy. Ann Ital Med Int 4:207–212

Erwin B, Carroll B, Muller H (1985) A sonographic assessment of neonatal renal parameters. J Ultrasound Med 4:217–220

Hamper UM, Goldblum LE, Hutchins GM et al. (1988) Renal involvement in AIDS: sonographic-pathologic correlation. AJR Am J Roentgenol 150:1321–1325

Hoffman J, Schnur M, Koenigsberg M (1982) Demonstration of renal papillary necrosis by sonography. Radiology 145:785–787

Hricak H (1982) Renal medical disorders: the role of sonography. In: Sanders RC (ed) Ultrasound annual 1982. Raven, New York, p 43

Huntington DK, Hill SC, Hill MC (1991) Sonographic manifestations of medical renal disease. Semin Ultrasound CT MR 12:290–307

Ikee R, Kobayashi S, Hemmi N et al. (2005) Correlation between the resistive index by Doppler ultrasound and kidney function and histology. Am J Kidney Dis 46:603–609

Kasap B, Soylu A, Türkmen M et al. (2006) Relationship of increased renal cortical echogenicity with clinical and laboratory findings in pediatric renal disease. J Clin Ultrasound 34:339–342

Kim SH, Kim B (1990) Renal parenchyma disease. In: Pollack HM, McClennan BL, Dyer R, Kenney PJ (eds) Clinical urography. Saunders, Philadelphia, pp 2652–2687

Longmaid HE, Rider E, Tymkiw J (1987) Lupus nephritis: new sonographic findings. J Ultrasound Med 6:75–79

Martinoli C, Bertolotto M, Pretolesi F et al. (1999) Kidney: normal anatomy. Eur Radiol 9 (suppl 3):389–393

McKinney TD (1992) Tubulointerstitial diseases and toxic nephropathies. In: Wyngaarden JB, Smith LH, Bennett JC (eds) Cecil textbook of medicine. Saunders, Philadelphia, pp 568–579

Miller FH, Parikh S, Gore RM (1993) Renal manifestations of AIDS. Radiographics 13:587–596

Mostbeck GH, Kain R, Mallek R et al. (1991) Duplex Doppler sonography in renal parenchymal disease. Histopathologic correlation. J Ultrasound Med 10:189–194

Myers BD (1992) Diabetes and the kidney. In: Wyngaarden JB, Smith LH, Bennett JC (eds) Cecil textbook of medicine. Saunders, Philadelphia, pp 590–593

Olefsky JM (1992) Diabetes mellitus. In: Wyngaarden JB, Smith LH, Bennett JC (eds) Cecil textbook of medicine. Saunders, Philadelphia, pp 1291–1310

Ozaki K, Miyayama S, Uschiogi Y et al. (2009) Renal involvement of polyarteritis nodosa: CT and MR findings. Abdom Imaging 34:265–270

Page JE, Morgan SH, Eastwood JB et al. (1994) Ultrasound findings in renal parenchymal disease: comparison with histological appearances. Clin Radiol 49:867–870

Platt JF, Rubin J, Bowerman R et al. (1988) The inability to detect kidney disease on the basis of echogenicity. AJR Am J Roentgenol 151:317–319

Platt JF, Rubin JM, Ellis JH (1994) Diabetic nephropathy: evaluation with renal duplex Doppler US. Radiology 190:343–346

Platt JF, Rubin JM, Ellis JH (1997) Lupus nephritis: predictive value of conventional and Doppler US and comparison with serologic and biopsy parameters. Radiology 203:82–86

Pope TL, Buschi AJ, Moore TS et al. (1981) CT features of renal polyarteritis nodosa. AJR Am J Roentgenol 136:986–987

Quaia E, Bertolotto M (2002) Renal parenchymal diseases: is characterization feasible with ultrasound? Eur Radiol 12:2006–2020

Saag MS (1992) Renal, cardiac, endocrine, and rheumatologic manifestations of HIV infection. In: Wyngaarden JB, Smith LH, Bennett JC (eds) Cecil textbook of medicine. Saunders, Philadelphia, pp 1952–1957

Soldo D, Brkljacic B, Bozikov V et al. (1997) Diabetic nephropathy. Comparison of conventional and duplex Doppler ultrasonographic findings. Acta Radiol 38:296–302

SugiuraT, Nakamori A, Wada A et al. (2004) Evaluation of tubulointerstitial injury by Doppler ultrasonography in glomerular diseases. Clin Nephrol 61:119–126

Symeonidou C, Hameeduddin A, Hons B et al. (2009) Imaging features of renal pathology in the huma immunodeficiency virus-infected patients. Semin Ultrasound CT MRI 30:289–297

The Diabetes Control and Complications Trial Research Group–DCCT (1993) The effect of intensive treatment of diabetes on the development and progression of long-term complications in insulin-dependent diabetes mellitus. N Engl J Med 329(14):977–986

Tikkakoski T, Waahtera K, Makarainen H et al. (1994) Diffuse renal disease. Diagnosis by ultrasound guided cutting needle biopsy. Acta Radiol 35:15–18

Wachsberg RH, Obolevich AT, Lasker N (1995) Pelvocalyceal thickening in HIV-associated nephropaty. Abdom Imaging 20:371–375

Wilms G, Oyen R, Waer M et al. (1986) CT demonstration of aneurysms in polyarteritis nodosa. J Comput Assist Tomogr 10:513–515

# Obstructive Uropathy, Pyonephrosis, and Reflux Nephropathy in Adults

**14**

Emilio Quaia, Paola Martingano, and Marco Cavallaro

## Contents

**Abstract**

> Urinary tract obstruction is a clinical situation which may clearly defined by imaging. The different causes of renal obstruction may be easily detected by ultrasound (US) and characterized thanks to the panoramicity of the new imaging modality such as computed tomography urography (CTU) and magnetic resonance urography (MRU). Pyonephrosis represents the chronic suppurative infection in an obstructed kidney. Gray-scale US with tissue harmonic imaging represents the most sensitive imaging technique to detect pyonephrosis. The vesico-ureteral reflux is the retrograde flow of urine from the bladder toward the kidney.

Urinary tract obstruction is a common cause of renal dysfunction and one of the most frequent causes of reversible renal failure. Obstructive uropathy refers to the structural or functional changes in the urinary tract that impede the normal flow of urine (Klahr 1992) and it is observed in all age groups. It occurs in a variety of clinical settings and is a relatively common cause of impaired renal function (obstructive nephropathy).

Urinary tract obstruction can occur anywhere in the urinary tract from the renal papilla to the urethral meatus and may be determined by a plenty of causes including congenital and acquired disorders. Obstruction may be completely asymptomatic even though, most frequently, it manifest with clear clinical symptoms. The clinical manifestations of urinary tract obstruction depend on the level, degree, and duration of obstruction, the rate

E. Quaia (✉), P. Martingano and M. Cavallaro
Department of Radiology, Cattinara Hospital, University
of Trieste, Strada di Fiume 447, 34149 Trieste, Italy
e-mail: quaia@univ.trieste.it

E. Quaia (ed.), *Radiological Imaging of the Kidney*,
Medical Radiology, DOI: 10.1007/978-3-540-87597-0_14, © Springer-Verlag Berlin Heidelberg 2011

of distension of the renal collecting system, whether the obstruction is unilateral or bilateral, and whether the renal obstruction is accompanied by complications, particularly infections. Pain, due to stretching of the renal collecting system or the renal capsule, is a common presenting symptom in obstructive uropathy and particularly in patients with ureteral calculi. Bilateral ureteral obstruction (e.g., benign prostatic hypertrophy) or unilateral urinary tract obstruction in patients with solitary kidney or with preexisting impaired renal function lead to anuria and acute postrenal failure (see Chap. 29) with hypertension and uremia. Gross hematuria may be seen in obstruction, particularly when it is due to renal stone or neoplasia. In the presence of gross hematuria, clots may cause ureteral obstruction. Other clinical manifestations include tubular disorders followed by nephrogenic diabetes insipidus with water and sodium depletion, and metabolic acidosis, and pain. Obstructive uropathy also carries with it the possible complication of urinary tract infection and pyonephrosis (Andreoli 1992).

Clinically, partial obstruction is more common than complete obstruction (Talner et al. 2000a). Chronic partial obstruction may cause intermittent flank pain which can be elicited by administration of diuretics and/or excessive fluid intake (Klahr 1992). In patients with partial or incomplete obstruction of the urinary tract, the urinary output may be normal or increased (polyuria). Some partial obstructions may exist for several time, even years, with no or mild impairment of renal function. Severe long-standing partial obstruction

usually results in medullary and cortical atrophy, similar to that seen with chronic total obstruction. Partial obstruction often leads to greated pyelectasis than does complete obstruction for a similar temporal range, even though no relationship has been noted between the degree of pyelocaliciectasis and renal function.

The usual morphologic manifestation of obstructive uropathy is hydronephrosis which corresponds to the dilatation of the renal pelvis and calyces (pyelocaliectasis) associated or not with obstruction or parenchymal thinning (Talner et al 2000a). Hydrocalyx (hydrocalycosis) is a localized hydronephrosis due to obstruction of the infundibulum to a calyx or a groups of calyces. Most clinically significant obstructions cause at least minimal hydronephrosis, but not all hydronephrosis is caused by obstruction (e.g., vesicoureteral reflux commonly causes nonobstructive hydronephrosis). Hydronephrosis presents four grades (Fig. 14.1). The first grade indicates a mild pyelocaliectasis with renal calyces maintaining the normal morphology; the second grade indicates pyelocaliectasis with the renal calyces with a balloon shape; the third grade indicate the presence of a progressive thinning of renal parenchyma with renal calyces which are eventually assimilated in one single sac in the fourth grade. Hydronephrosis does not develop in every patient with obstructive uropathy. In 3–5% of patients with obstructive uropathy hydronephrosis is not present (Curry et al. 1982; Rascoff et al. 1983; Naidich et al. 1986), especially in early obstruction, hypovolemia and dehydratation, nephrosclerosis, and retroperitoneal disease (retroperitoneal fibrosis or carcinomatosis).

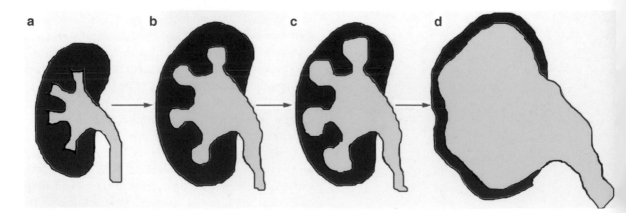

**Fig. 14.1** (**a–d**) Scheme. Hydronephrosis grading. (**a**) First grade of hydronephrosis. Mild dilatation of the intra-renal urinary tract; (**b**) second grade of hydronephrosis with mild pyelocaliectasis with renal calyces maintaining the normal mor- phology; (**c**) third grade with pyelocaliectasis and renal calyces with a balloon shape; (**d**) fourth grade with a progressive thinning of renal parenchyma and renal calyces which are eventually assimilated in one single sac

During obstruction, the kidneys undergo functional and biochemical alterations. Acute ureteral obstruction leads to a decrease in the renal blood flow and glomerular filtration rate, ultimately resulting in interstitial fibrosis and irreversible renal damage if untreated (Vaughan et al. 2004). Renal damage is initiated by high intratubular pressure, with initial renal vasodilatation followed by progressive vasoconstriction and decrease in renal blood flow, cellular atrophy, and necrosis. In addition, parenchymal infiltration by macrophages and T lymphocytes may cause scarring of the kidney (Klahr 1992). The rise in the intratubular pressure decreases the net hydrostatic filtration pressure across glomerular capillaries, resulting in a progressive decrease of GFR.

Since the consequences of obstructive uropathy are potentially reversible, prompt diagnosis and appropriate treatment are essential to prevent the permanent loss of renal function, which is directly related to the degree and duration of the obstruction. The site of obstruction determines the approach in these patients. If the obstruction is distal to the bladder, the placement of urethral catheter may be sufficient. Sometimes a suprapubic cystostomy is required. If the obstruction is located in the upper urinary tract, placement of percutaneous nephrostomy or passage of a retrograde ureteral catheter may be necessary. Anyway, relief of obstruction at any stage is frequently followed by renal shrinkage with a variable pattern of postobstructive atrophy of renal parenchyma. In patients with sepsis appropriate antibiotic therapy is also indicated, while in some patients with acute renal failure dialysis may be required (Klahr 1992). Surgical intervention can be delayed in low-grade or partial chronic urinary tract obstruction. Prompt relief of obstruction is indicated when there are repeated episodes of urinary tract infections, the patient has significant symptoms, there is urinary retention, or there is evidence of recurrent or progressive renal damage (Klahr 1992).

# 14.1  Obstructive Uropathy

## 14.1.1  Imaging Findings

The first imaging examination to be employed in obstructive uropathy is ultrasound (US). Multidetector computed tomography (CT) urography is currently thought to be the most sensitive and comprehensive imaging examination for the evaluation of the entire urinary tract and also in the assessment of obstructive uropathy (Caoili et al. 2002). Magnetic resonance (MR) urography is employed in the assessment of the morphology of the dilated urinary tract (Nolte-Ernsting et al. 2003), while MR excretory urography includes a dynamic functional study and it is useful in the functional assessment of the obstructed kidney (Teh et al. 2003). Even though several authors (Rohrschneider et al. 2002; Teh et al. 2003; Lefort et al. 2006) have shown substantial agreement between dynamic MR renography and isotopic renography in the renal function and excretion, technetium-99m diethylenetriamine pentaacetic acid or MAG3-technetium-99m diuretic renography remain the reference standards in the assessment of the renal function in the renal tract obstruction.

### 14.1.1.1  Ultrasound

US is the most sensitive imaging technique in detecting renal hydronephrosis. US is accurate in detecting and assessing the grade of hydronephrosis (Fig. 14.2), even though it may reveal false-negative results, such as renal obstruction without dilatation (early obstruction, hypovolemia and dehydratation, retroperitoneal disease), or false-positive results such as dilation of the urinary tract in nonobstructed patients (extrarenal pelvis, parapelvic cysts, prominent renal vasculature, postobstructive dilatation, ureterovescical reflux, and congenital megacalices). There is no correlation between the grade of hydronephrosis and the grade of obstruction. Nowadays, the employment of microbubble-based contrast agents allow an accurate assessment of renal parenchyma perfusion (Quaia et al. 2009) which can be reduced in the acute or chronic urinary tract obstruction.

Renal vasoconstriction is the key factor in the pathophysiological course of acute and chronic obstruction and increased RIs values result. Resistive Index (RI) assessment is a separate and distinct parameter from collecting system dilatation to assess urinary obstruction (Platt 1996). Duplex Doppler sonography has been reported to be an useful noninvasive imaging method for the diagnosis of renal obstruction. RIs elevation (Fig. 14.3) occurs by 6 h of clinical acute renal

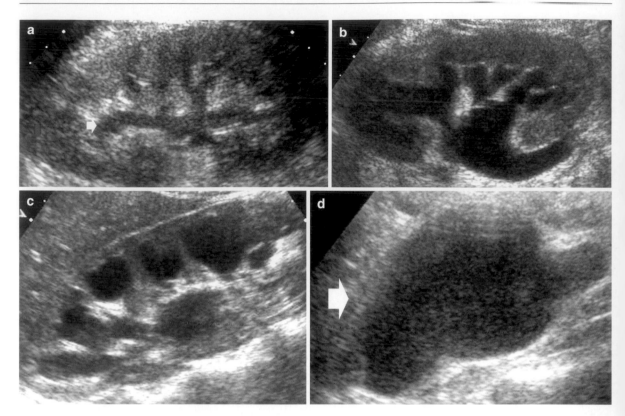

**Fig. 14.2** (**a–d**) Ultrasound, longitudinal scan. Hydronephrosis grading. Progressive dilatation of the intrarenal collecting system and pyelocaliectasis with a progression reduction of the renal cortical thickness. (**a**) First grade of hydronephrosis with mild dilatation of the intra-renal urinary tract (*arrow*). (**b**) Second grade of hydronephrosis with pyelocaliectasis and normal morphology of renal calyx. (**c**) Third grade of hydronephrosis with pyelocaliectasis and renal calyces with a balloon shape. (**d**) Fourth grade of hydronephrosis with a progressive thinning of renal parenchyma

obstruction and may precede pyelocaliectasis. A mean RI >0.7, a difference >0.06–0.08 between the mean RI of the two kidneys, and a progressive increase in RI following fluid administration and diuretics have been considered diagnostic of obstruction (Platt 1992; Quaia and Bertolotto 2002). A significant fall in RIs values is reported after nephrostomy. In general, there should be a rapid return to normal RIs if obstruction is relieved within 5 h, whereas RIs may take days or even weeks to return to baseline levels if obstruction is present for at least 18–24 h.

The evaluation of renal parenchyma RIs presents a controversial role in the acute renal colic with a sensitivity from 19 to 92% and a specifity from 88 and 98% according to the different series (Platt et al. 1989; Tublin et al. 1994; Lee et al. 1996). This is determined by the absence of a true reference standard to diagnose renal obstruction and by the possible presence of

partial and intermittent obstruction. Normal RI likely reflects the lack of obstruction of sufficient degree to produce vasoconstriction (Platt 1996).

### 14.1.1.2 Unenhanced Spiral CT

Unenhanced spiral or multidetector-row CT is now considered the reference imaging techniques for one specific form of urinary obstruction, namely urolithiasis (see Chap. 15). The direct finding is the visualization of the calculus itself. Indirect signs include renal pelvis and ureteral dilatation (frequency, 65–90%), perinephric and periureteral stranding (36–82%), rim sign around the ureter (frequency 50–77%), renal enlargement (frequency 36–71%), renal sinus fat blurring, and decreased attenuation of the renal parenchyma (Smith et al. 1995; Niall et al. 1999). It has to

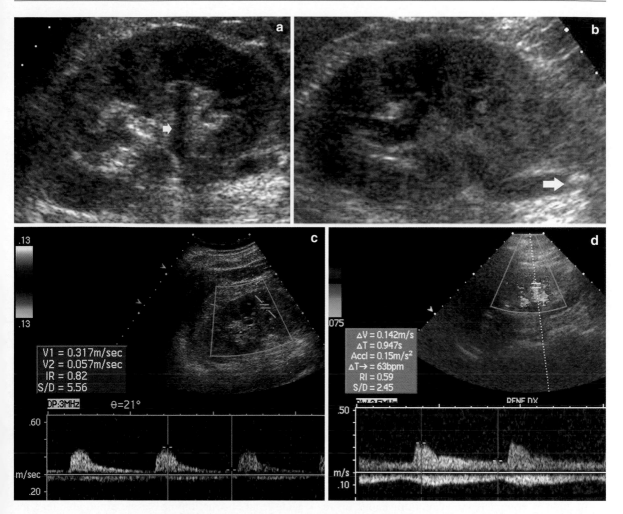

**Fig. 14.3** (**a–d**) Urinary tract obstruction due to ureteral stone. (**a**) US longitudinal scan of the right kidney revealing a mild pyelocaliectasis (*arrow*) with a normal morphology of renal calyces and normal thickness and dimension of renal paren-chyma; (**b**) renal obstruction is caused by a stone (*arrow*) in the proximal part of the ureter; (**c**) resistive index are increased (0.82) in the segmental arteries of the obstructed kidney, while it is normal (0.59) in the controlateral kidney (**d**)

be underlines that the reduced attenuation of the renal parenchyma is not specific for the renal colic since it may be caused also by interstitial edema in acute pyelonephritis, and by venous congestion in renal vein thrombosis.

### 14.1.1.3  Intravenous Excretory Urography and CT Urography

Before the advent of helical CT and CT urography, intravenous excretory urography was indicated in the diagnosis of renal hydronephrosis, in the identification of the stone, in the differentiation from other calcific densities, and to provide functional informations about the kidney. Even until the late 1990s, intravenous excretory urography because of its superior spatial resolution, was still considered the examination of choice for evaluating the urothelium (Silverman et al. 2009). Intravenous excretory urography presents a detection rate of urinary stones ranging from 70 to 90% (Miller et al. 1998). Intravenous excretory urography reveals the grade and extent of dilation of the urinary collecting system proximal to obstruction with the evidence of the site of obstruction. In acute renal obstruction the classic urographic features are

**Fig. 14.4** (**a**, **b**) Acute urinary tract obstruction due to an urinary stone located in the intramural tract of the left ureter. Intravenous excretory urography. (**a**) Increasing nephrographic density on the left kidney (*arrow*) with delayed contrast excretion (**b**). Renal calyces appeared 1 h after iodinated contrast injection also with evidence also of dilatation of the collecting system and ureter

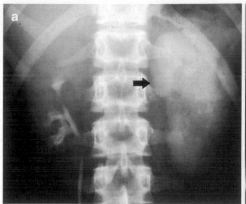
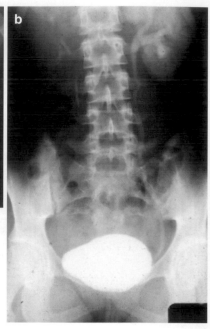

dimensional increase of the kidney, an increasing nephrographic density defined as obstructive nephrogram and delayed contrast excretion with delayed calyceal appearance on excretory urography (Fig. 14.4) also with variable dilatation of the collecting system and ureter (Talner et al. 2000a). Dilatation is often mild or lacking in the acute obstructive uropathy, even when obstruction is complete. Anwyay, intravenous excretory urography is a time consuming imaging technique especially in obstructed patients, and it implied high radiation dose and iodinated contrast agents administration. Moreover, intravenous excretory urography is not advocated in acute ureteral obstruction due to iodinated contrast – induced diuresis.

On CT urography it is difficult to obtain a single image of all urinary collecting system segments in an opacified and distended state. Furosemide improves the urinary tract and ureteral opacification and distension (Silverman et al. 2006) with a greater effect than saline by increasing the urinary flow rate and the delivery of contrast medium to the middle and distal ureter. Postprocessing techniques are similar in most centers. A combination of rendering techniques has been used, including multiplanar reformat (MPR), curved planar reformat (CPR), and thin-slab or thick-slab average intensity projection (AIP), volume rendering (VR), or maximum intensity projection (MIP) 3D images.

The urographic signs of acute and chronic obstruction have their counterparts on CT-urography. CT-urography reveal the grade and extent of dilation of the urinary collecting system proximal to obstruction with the evidence of the site of obstruction (Fig. 14.5). The obstructed kidney swells slightly because of enlargement of the tubules and interstitial edema. In acute renal obstruction the classic urographic features are an increasing nephrographic density defined as obstructive nephrogram and delayed contrast excretion with delayed calyceal appearance on excretory urography also with variable dilatation of the collecting system and ureter (Talner et al. 2000a). Dilatation is often mild or lacking in the acute obstructive uropathy, even when obstruction is complete.

Chronically obstructed kidneys may be small, normal, or large. The volume is determined by many factors, the most important being the duration and degree of obstruction and the distensibility of the collecting system (Talner et al. 2000a). The obstruction of the urinary tract, if not treated, usually determines a progressive atrophy of the renal parenchyma. In postobstructive renal atrophy renal medulla and cortex are both reduced in their thickness (Fig. 14.5). Chronic obstructive uropathy may also present a nondilated renal collecting system in 4–6% of cases (Naidich et al. 1986). This may be determined by the tumoral infiltration of the ureteral wall, or to chronic incomplete obstruction of the ureter which may be suddenly complicated by an acute event such as infection.

Most of the false positive findings of US, including extrarenal pelvis and parapelvic cysts simulating urinary tract obstrucion, are easily differentiated from true obstruction by CT urography (Fig. 14.6).

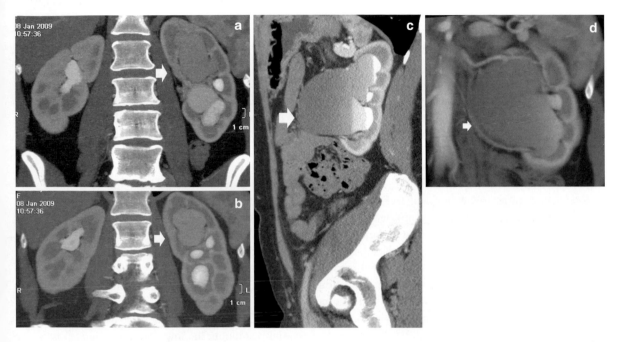

**Fig. 14.5** (**a–d**) Ureteropelvic junction obstruction in a 21-years-old woman due to an arterial crossing vessel (accessory renal artery). (**a, b**) Multidetector CT urography; (**c**) curved multiplanar reformation; dilatation of the left intra-renal collecting system (*arrow*) with reduction of renal cortex thickness due to chronic obstruction. (**d**) 3D maximum intensity projection. Evidence of the crossing vessel (*arrow*) determining the ureteropelvic junction obstruction

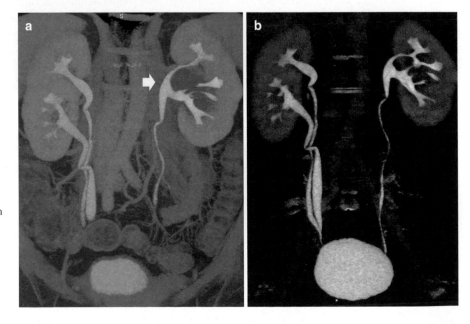

**Fig. 14.6** (**a, b**) Parapyelic cysts simulating urinary tract obstruction. (**a**) 3D maximum intensity projection depicts the spatial morphology and the relationship between the cysts and the renal calyces. (**b**) Color-coded volume rendering (VR) confirms calyceal distorsion

## 14.1.1.4 MR Urography

MR urography has received a relatively lower attention than multidetector CT urography, being hampered by the low spatial resolution, which is crucial for calyceal evalution and by the requirement of updated MR units. The use of a phased array body coil is preferable because of the improved signal-to-noise ratio (SNR). The imaging protocol for evaluation of the kidney at our institution on a 1.5-Tesla (T). Currently 1–1.5-T systems are generally used for abdominal imaging, but the advent of 3-T MRI systems brings a twofold increase in the SNR. The increase in SNR can be spent on higher resolution or on even faster imaging. When combined with parallel imaging techniques such as sensitivity encoding (SENSE), the speed of any sequence can be increased by up to a factor of four or higher.

Excellent contrast resolution and lack of ionizing radiation make MR urography a useful technique for non invasively evaluating the entire urinary tract, especially when ionizing radiation is to be avoided, such as in pediatric or pregnant patients. A number of studies have shown that MR urography is a useful examination for investigating the causes of urinary tract dilatation and diagnosing urinary tract obstruction in adult and pediatric populations (Roy et al. 1998; Shokeir et al. 2004; Kocaoglu et al. 2005). Fast imaging techniques are essential because of respiratory motion of the kidneys, and MR scan should be performed within one breath-hold according to patient compliance. The patient should get clear instructions on breath-hold technique. If the patient has difficulty with breath-holding, a short period of hyperventilation before breath-holding may be helpful. If the sequence is too long to perform in one breath-hold, respiratory triggering can be used. Another technique of respiratory motion control is respiratory gating by use of a navigator pulse. Breathold imaging at the end of expiration should be performed in compliant patients, while nonbreathold imaging should be performed in noncompliant patients. Nonbreathold imaging should include single-shot sequences, magnetization-prepared gradient echo, half-Fourier single-shot technique (HASTE) – providing a shorter echo time, poorer signal-to-noise-ratio and reduced contrast-to-noise-ratio if compared to TSE T2-weighted sequence, respiratory gating or respiratory triggering, or MR imaging navigators.

The static-fluid MR urography utilizes unenhanced, heavily T2-weighted pulse sequences to image the urinary tract (Nikken and Krestin 2007) including half-Fourier single-shot echo-train spin-echo sequences (such as HASTE), thick-slab RARE, or respiratory-triggered three-dimensional echo-train spin-echo sequences. On the heavily T2 weighted images, the urinary tract is hyperintense because of its long relaxation time, independent of the excretory renal function (Fig. 14.7). Additional spectral fat suppression can help to further improve the contrast between urinary tract fluid and retroperitoneum. Static-fluid MR urography sequences are typically used in the coronal plane, although other imaging planes can be used. Two fundamental techniques may be employed: (1) single-slice projection images in which a single 6–8 cm slice is employed, and (2) multislice technique employing sequential static-fluid acquisitions by a 3D multiple slice technique with longer acquisition time to ensure visualization of the entire ureters and assess for a fixed narrowing or obstruction. This technique is ideally suited for patients with dilated or obstructed collecting system.

The advantages of single-slice projection are the short acquisition time (6–8 s), absence of motion artifacts, no necessity of postprocessing, and the possibility to identify the location of obstruction. The main drawbacks of the single-slice technique are the low spatial resolution, the low SNR, and the impossibility to define the cause of obstruction. The advantages of multislice technique are reduced partial volume averaging artifact, and the increased spatial and contrast resolution. The drawbacks of multislice technique are the longer acquisition time compared to the single slice technique and the superimposing extraurinary fluid. When MR urography is combined with assessment of the renal parenchyma and soft tissues of the abdomen and pelvis, precontrast T1- and T2-weighted images on the axial or coronal plane are obtained of the abdomen and pelvis.

In excretory MR urography, intravenous gadolinium is combined with a T1-weighted 3D gradient echo (GRE) sequence. Excretory MR urography provides high-quality images of both nondilated and obstructed collecting systems. When information about vascular structures is critical, such as the evaluation of congenital uretropelvic junction obstruction in which a crossing vessel is suspected, an MR angiography-type sequence is performed in the coronal plane. Alternatively, a dynamic, axial, fat-suppressed sequence can be performed through the kidneys to capture the precontrast, corticomedullary, nephrographic, and excretory phases.

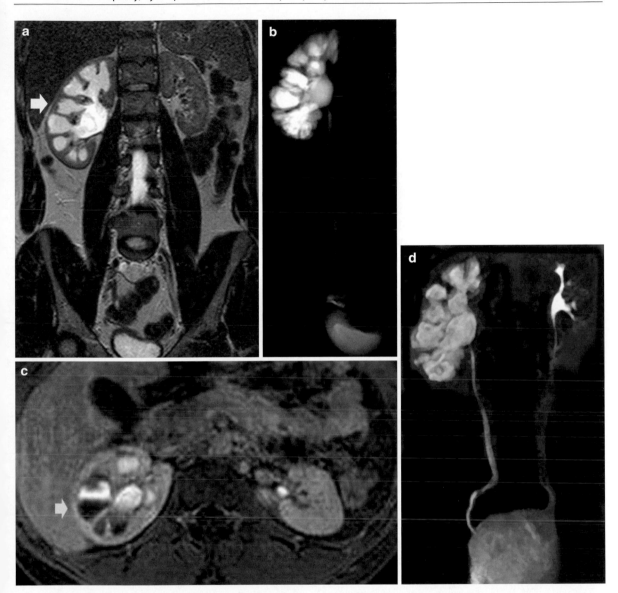

**Fig. 14.7** (**a–d**) Urinary tract obstruction due to ureteropelvic junction obstruction. (**a**) T2-weighted turbo spin-echo sequence. Coronal plane. (**b**) Static-fluid MR urography. Dilatation of the right intra-renal collecting system (*arrow in* **a**) with reduction of renal cortex thickness due to chronic obstruction. (**c**) T1-weighted 3D Gradient Echo MR sequence. Excretory phase after gadolinium injection. Dilatation of the right intra-renal collecting system (*arrow*) with contrast excretion and evidence of the T2* effect gadolinium with descreas of urine signal intensity. (**d**) Excretory MR urography, 5 min after iodinated contrast injection. Maximum Intensity projection 3D image. Dilatation of the right intra-renal collecting system with clear visualization of the intra-renal and extrarenal urinary tract.

Excretory phase images are then typically obtained approximately 5 min after intravenous gadolinium chelate is administered at a dose of 0.05–0.1 mmol/kg and are usually accomplished with some type of fat-suppressed three-dimensional gradient-echo sequence. Having patients raise their arms over their heads during coronal acquisitions reduces wrap-around artifact.

Excretory MR urography performed after intravenous gadolinium chelate administration without pharmacologic intervention is often lacking due to suboptimal ureteral distention, uneven distribution of the contrast material in the collecting systems, and the hypointense T2* effect of concentrated gadolinium (Hagspiel et al. 2005). Therefore, some combination of intravenous hydration and diuretic administration is typically used adjunctively (Karabacakoglu et al. 2004). Furosemide (0.05–0.1 mg/kg) is the diuretic typically used for excretory MR urography and can be used successfully in adults at doses as low as 5 mg. Oral hydration is discouraged, as the high T2 signal intensity of fluid within the bowel can interfere with the visualization of the urinary tract during static-fluid MR urography, particularly when maximum intensity projections are rendered.

For excretory MR urography, the thinnest partitions that maintain acceptable SNR and anatomic coverage should be prescribed. Breath-holding is essential for excretory phase imaging, as acquisition times of 20–30 s are typical with most widely available three-dimensional gradient-echo sequences. A through-plane resolution of 2–3 mm is usually achievable with currently available MR systems operating at 1.5–3.0 T. The use of parallel imaging techniques reduces acquisition times with a modest penalty in SNR. For patients with limited breath-holding capacity, the urinary tract can be imaged in segments. Static-fluid MR urography sequences should be performed prior to excretory MR urography sequences, as excreted gadolinium chelate can reduce the signal intensity of urine on T2-weighted images. Also, the bladder is best evaluated on T1-weighted images within the first few minutes after intravenous contrast material administration, but before excreted gadolinium chelate reaches the bladder via the ureters.

By combining sequences designed to evaluate the collecting systems, ureters, and bladder with sequences designed to evaluate the kidneys (particularly for masses), a comprehensive assessment of the urinary tract became possible. The all in one technique includes SE T1-weighted, dual-echo GRE T1-weighted, TSE T2 –weighted with fat suppression, diffusion sequences, static-fluid MR urography, and excretory MR urography. The general MR protocol consists of the following sequences: (1) Coronal T2-weighted HASTE (TR infinite, TE 120 ms, flip angle 90°, breath-hold), serving as a localizer, but also supplying valuable T2-weighted information. The limitation of this sequence is a relatively low SNR; (2) Transverse T2-weighted turbo spin-echo sequence with fat suppression (TR 2,000 ms, TE 100 ms, flip angle 90°, respiratory triggering). This sequence provides for more detailed T2-weighted information; (3) Transverse T1-weighted gradient echo sequence, in-phase and opposed-phase (TR 180 ms, TE 2.3 ms/4.6 ms, flip angle 90°, breath-hold), preferably as a dual-echo sequencet; (4) Static-fluid MR urography; (5) Transverse

or coronal 3D T1-weighted fast spoiled gradient echo sequence for dynamic imaging (TR 130 ms, TE 1.0 ms, flip angle 90°), using 30 mL intravenous gadolinium contrast, immediately followed by three breath-hold periods with four scan series per breath-hold. In this way precontrast and postcontrast images in arterial, nephrographic, and excretory phase are obtained. (6) Coronal 3D fast gradient echo with fat suppression, obtained immediately after the dynamic series for delayed contrast-enhanced images (TR 3 ms, TE 2 ms, flip angle 15°) corresponding to the MR excretory urography.

## 14.1.2 Causes of Obstruction

### 14.1.2.1 Congenital Anomalies

Congenital anomalies of the renal collecting system are one of the principal causes of renal tract obstruction (Table 14.1). The most common obstruction of normally placed ureters in children occurs in the

**Table 14.1** The different congenital and acquired causes of renal tract obstruction

| Causes |
| --- |
| *Congenital* |
| Hydrocalyx[a] |
| Calyceal diverticulum[b] |
| Ureteropelvic junction obstruction |
| Ureteral obstruction (namely primary obstructive megaureter) |
| Urethral valves |
| *Acquired* |
| Scarring (inflammation, surgery, trauma) |
| Intraluminal ureteral obstruction (stone, blood clot, sloughed papilla, tumors) |
| Extraluminal ureteral obstruction |
| Postsurgical ureteral obstruction |
| Radiation ureteral stricture |
| Retroperitoneal fibrosis |
| Pelvic lipomatosis |
| Pregnancy |
| Gynecological causes (endometriosis, pelvic inflammatory disease) |
| Gastrointestinal disease (Crohn's disease, diverticulitis, acute pancreatitis, tumors) |
| Benign prostatic hypertrophy and prostatic carcinoma |

*Note:* Specific causes of obstruction
[a]Obstruction of the infundibulum to a calyx(ices) due to intrinsic or extrinsic causes
[b]A urine-containing cavity lined with transitional epithelium and connected to the fornix of a minor calyx by a narrow isthmus

juxtavesical segment and is called primary obstructive megaureter.

Megapolycalicosis (Fig. 14.8) is defined as a congenital dilatation of the renal calices without evidence of obstruction. In absence of complications such as infection and stones, megapolycalicosis would not have a particular clinical relevance if not for the possible misinterpretation as hydronephrosis. Megaureter is frequently associated to megapolycalicosis. Postobstructive renal atrophy must be differentiated from megapolycalicosis and reflux nephropathy based on the ratio between

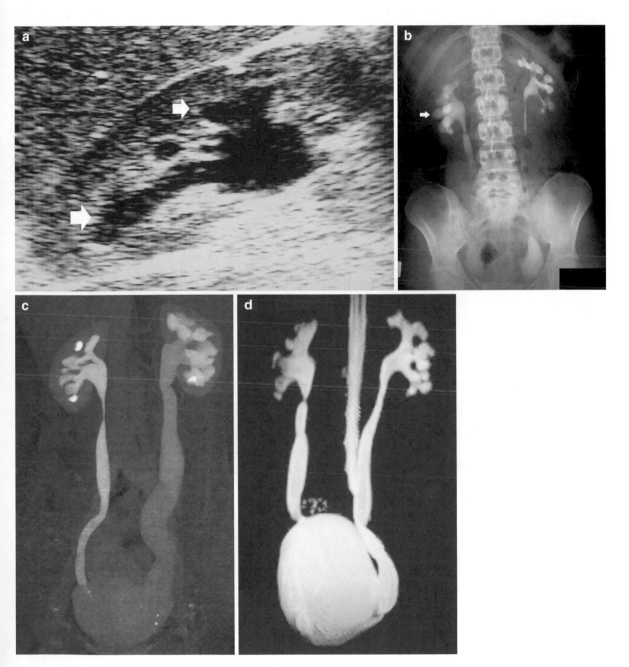

**Fig. 14.8** (**a–d**) Congenital megaureter in 22-years-old woman. (**a**) Ultrasound. Dilatation of the intra-renal collecting system (*arrow*). (**b**) Intravenous excretory urography; (**c**) CT urography; (**d**) Static-fluid MR urography. Evident dilatation of the calices (*arrow*) in both kidneys without evidence of obstruction. Bilateral megaureter (*arrows*) is associated to megapolycalicosis

renal medulla and cortex. In normal cases the ratio between the renal medulla and cortex is 1.5–2 to 1. In megapolycalicosis the renal medulla presents a reduced thickness while the cortex is normal and the ratio medulla/cortex is near to 1.

Other cause of ureteral obstruction are ureteral valve, ureteral atresia, circumcaval (retrocaval, post-caval) ureter. An ectopically inserting ureter draining the upper moiety of a kidney with duplication of the urinary tract is frequently involved in obstruction.

### 14.1.2.2 Ureteropelvic Junction Obstruction

Ureteropelvic junction obstruction, also named pelvi-ureteric junction obstruction or idiopathic, pelvic, or congenital hydronephrosis, is defined as an obstruction of the flow of urine from the renal pelvis to the proximal ureter. It represents a major cause of obstructive uropathy at all ages and is the most common cause of neonatal hydronephrosis (Talner et al. 2000b). This pathologic entity may have congenital or acquired causes, and requires frequently a surgical treatment consisting in open or laparoscopic pyeloplasty, or endopyelotomy. The idiopatic ureteropelvic junction obstruction is a major cause of obstructive uropathy at all ages and is the most common cause of neonatal hydronephrosis. Pelvic kidneys are associated with an increased incidence of ureteropelvic junction obstruction, and of stone formation. Other causes are reported in Table 14.2. It has been suggested that accessory renal arteries in the lower pole of either kidney that cross the ureteropelvic junction contribute to ureteropelvic junction obstruction in up to 11% of children (Hoffer and Lebowitz 1985) and 52% of adults (Lowe and Marshall 1984).

It is twice more frequent in the left than in the right kidney, occurs more frequently (about 90% of cases) in kidneys with an extrarenal pelvis, and it is the most common form of urinary tract obstruction in pediatric patients. Unilateral obstruction is more frequent than bilateral obstruction (10–30% of cases). It manifests with acute flank pain.

On US, the renal pelvis appears disproportionately large compared to dilated calyces. CT urography with multiplanar reformations (MPRs) is the most accurate imaging technique to identify the cause of ureteropelvic junction obstruction including crossing vessels. Pyelocaliectasis with ureteropelvic junction narrowing with normal caliber ureter downstream is evident on imaging (Fig. 14.9). Ureteropelvic junction

**Table 14.2** The different congenital and acquired causes of ureteropelvic junction obstruction

| Causes |
| --- |
| *Congenital* |
| Anomalies of rotation |
| Intrinsic stenosis |
| Segment disfunction (adynamic segment) |
| Kinkings or angulations |
| Adhesions or bands |
| Crossing vessel (lower-pole renal artery) |
| Horseshoe kidney |
| High insertion of the ureter |
| Urethral valves |
| |
| *Acquired* |
| Scarring (inflammation, surgery, trauma) |
| Reflux |
| Malignant tumors (transitional cell carcinoma, squamous cell carcinoma, metastasis) |
| Benign tumors (polyps, mesodermal tumor) |
| Intraluminal lesions (stone, clots, papilla, fungus ball, cholesteatoma) |

Note: Specific causes of ureteropelvic junction obstruction

obstruction may be segmental involving the superior or inferior moiety in patients with duplication of the renal collecting system or with a bifid renal plevis (Fig. 14.10). Longstanding uteropelvic junction obstruction may manifest with severe hydronephrosis and marked parenchymal atrophy and minimal contrast excretion (Fig. 14.11).

### 14.1.2.3 Urolithiasis and Acute Renal Colic

Renal colic refers to the passage of a renal calculus from the renal pelvis into the ureter characterized by acute pain, generally beginning in the flank and radiating into the groin (Andreoli 1992). Renal colic pain constitutes the most common cause of patients with an acute abdomen seen in emergency department. Renal colic due to calculi obstructing the uretero-pelvic junction, the pelvic brim where the ureter crosses the iliac vessels, or the ureterovescical junction represents the most common cause for acute renal obstruction, and 40–60% of patients referred for CT for a suspicion of colic pain have an obstructing renal stone (Taourel et al. 2008).

Renal stones form by an initial crystallization of a nidus (nucleation) from a supersaturated urine with subsequent crystal growth and aggregation of the nidus into macroscopic stone (Pak 1992). The most frequent type of stones are calcium stones (75–80%) – calcium oxalate and/or calcium phosphate –, struvite stones

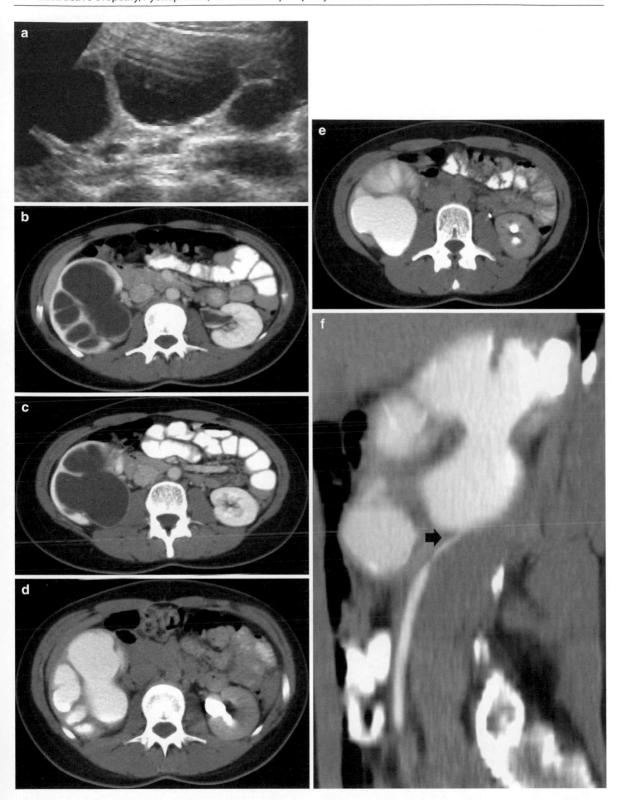

**Fig. 14.9** (**a–f**) Ureteropelvic junction obstruction in a 21-years-old woman presenting with acute flank pain. (**a**) Ultrasound. Four-grade hydronephrosis of the right kidney. (**b, c**) Contrast-enhanced CT. Excretory phase. The right kidney presents a fourth-grade hydronephrosis with no evidence of contrast excretion due to urinary tract obstruction. (**d, e**) Delayed CT scan 20 min after iodinated contrast administration. (**f**) Coronal reformation of the scan obtained 20 min after contrast administration. Ureteropelvic junction obstruction with pyelocaliectasis and ureteropelvic junction narrowing (*arrow*) with normal caliber ureter downstream

**Fig. 14.10** (**a**, **b**) Segmental ureteropelvic junction obstruction in a 42-years-old female patient with bifid renal pelvis who had surgery for vesico-ureteral reflux during childhood and presenting with acute flank pain. Contrast-enhanced CT, nephrographic phase. (**a**) Transverse plane. (**b**) Coronal reformation. Segmental dilatation of the intrarenal urinary tract due to surgical scarring of the ureteropelvic junction at the lower pole of the right kidney (*arrow*)

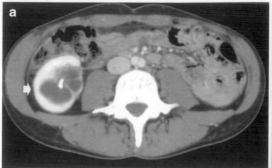
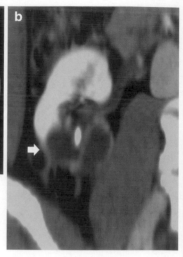

**Fig. 14.11** (**a**–**c**) Longstanding uteropelvic junction obstruction with chronic urinary tract obstruction. CT scans (**a**, **b**) and multiplanar reformat (**c**) showing the typical findings of longstanding ureteropelvic obstruction. There is severe hydronephrosis with marked parenchymal atrophy (*arrow* in **a**). Minimal contrast excretion is noted (*arrow* in **b**). Lower scan showed absence of ureteral dilatation

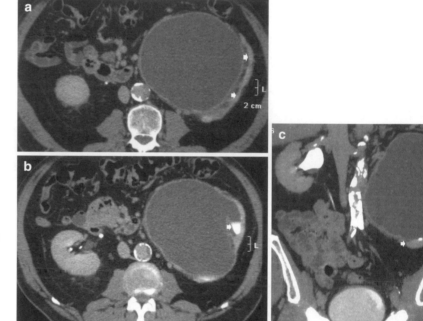

(15–20%) – magnesium ammonium phosphate (struvite) or magnesium ammonium phosphate plus calcium phosphate (triple phosphate), uric acid stones (5–10%), and cystine stones (1–3%). Rare type of stones are matrix stones (mucoproteins), xanthine stones, and protease inhibitor stones (Indinavir-induced in patients with AIDS). Some metabolic conditions, including hypercalciuria, hyperoxaluria, gout, and cystinuria, and urinary tract infections with urea-splitting organisms, present an increased incidence of renal stone in comparison to the normal population.

Most ureteral stones originate in a calyx, but stones occasionally form de novo in a dilated ureter or ureteral segment. The principal locations of renal stones are calyceal, renal pelvis, or ureteropelvic junction. Ureteral calculi are located distally in the ureter or ureterovesical junction. Milk of calcium consists in calcium carbonate and calcium phosphate. Stones less than 5 mm in diameter do not usually require surgical intervention or instrumentation, and about 90% of these stones pass spontaneously. If the stones are 5–7 mm in diameter only about half pass, while stones larger than 7 mm in diameter usually are not passed spontaneously (Klahr 1992). If the stone completely occlude the ureter and does not move, surgical intervention or instrumentation is necessary. The probability of renal calculi causing ureteral obstruction with acute postrenal failure is small unless one kidney is already nonfunctional and a stone obstructs the outflow of urine from the other kidney (Andreoli 1992).

US is considered as the first-line imaging modality in a patient with acute renal colic to identify indirect signs of urinary obstruction as hydronephrosis, hydroureter, and urinomas. The detection of urinary stones and clarity of posterior shadowing are significantly improved by US harmonic imaging (Ozdemir et al. 2008). Twinkling artifact – also named color comet-tail artifact (Tchelepi and Ralls 2009) – facilitates the detection of stones and provide informations on their chemical composition.

It is determined by the random Doppler shift in the shadow of the stone, it depends from the roughness of the surface of the stone, and it is not visible in the stones of calcium oxalate. The detection of ureteral jets by color Doppler does not imply the absence of obstruction since ureteral jets may be identified also in partial ureteral obstruction (Burge et al. 1991; Cox et al. 1992). The visibility of the ureteral jets depends on the flow velocity and density gradient between the urine in the bladder and ureter. This represents a time consuming assessment and it is not routinely employed.

The best imaging modality to confirm the diagnosis of a urinary stone in a patient with acute flank pain is unenhanced helical CT of the abdomen (see Chap. 15). The best diagnostic clues are the visualization of the calculus itself (Fig. 14.12) with proximal hydronephrosis and perinephric stranding. Regardless of composition, almost all renal stones are

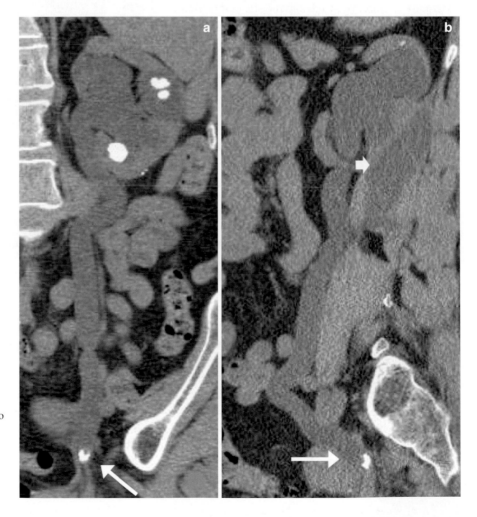

**Fig. 14.12** (**a**, **b**) Ureteral obstruction due to renal stone. Unenhanced CT, curved planar reformations. Dilatation of the intra-renal urinary tract and ureter due to a single stone (*large arrow*) obstructing the distal ureter. Intra-renal stones are also evident. Evidence of posterior renal urinoma (*small arrow*)

detected at unenhanced CT because the attenuation of stones is higher than that of surrounding tissue, even though the attenuation of uric stones is lower than the attenuation of calcium stones (Taourel et al. 2008). Imaging is important also to rule our other important cause of acute renal colic including renal and urinary tract infections, renal infarction, and hemorrhagic conditions of the perinephric and sub-capsular spaces, renal parenchyma, or the collecting system.

In acute renal colic the classic urographic features are those of acute ureteral obstruction including dimensional increase of the kidney, obstructive nephrogram, delayed contrast excretion and delayed calyceal appearance and variable dilatation of the collecting system and ureter. CT-urography reveal the grade and extent of dilation of the urinary collecting system proximal to obstruction with the evidence of the site of obstruction (Figs. 14.13 and 14.14). Static-fluid MR urography is employed to define the site and cause of ureteral obstruction in a functionally excluded kidney or in delayed contrast excretion on excretory intravenous urography (Fig. 14.15), or in patients with urinary tract duplication and urinary tract obstruction (Figs. 14.16–14.19).

### 14.1.2.4 Other Benign Causes of Obstructive Uropathy

• *Retroperitoneal fibrosis.* Retroperitoneal fibrosis is a chonic inflammatory process localized in the lumbar retroperitoneum. The development of inflammation and fibrosis in the retroperitoneum most often results in a periaortic mass that causes pain and constitutional symptoms. The fibrous layer extends along the aorta through a plaquelike infiltrative soft-tissue process (Surabhi et al. 2008). Retroperitoneal fibrosis typically is localized to the distal abdominal (infrarenal) aorta and the common iliac arteries; involvement of the pelvis is uncommon. Its organ involvement results in urinary tract obstruction, bowel dysfunction, and venous compression with leg swelling, or thrombosis (Swartz 2009). The syndrome appears autoimmune in nature, but has no specific immunologic markers. There is a primary or idiopatic form which is the

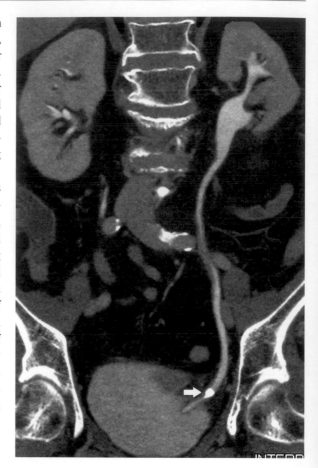

**Fig. 14.13** Acute ureteral obstruction due to stone on the distal premural left ureter. CT urography. Mild dilatation of the renal pelvis and ureters. The renal stone is visualized in the distal tract of the left ureter (*arrow*)

most common including about two third of the cases. The secondary form include one third of cases and it is principally related to drugs (methysergide, β-blocker, hydralazine, ergotamide, LSD) and diseases stimulating desmoplastic reaction (malignant tumors, metastases, Hodgkin lymphoma, carcinoid tumor, hematoma, radiation, retroperitoneal injury, surgery, infection, urinary extravasation, or abdominal aortic aneurysm). There is a 3:1 male-to-female preponderance among those affected by the disease. Perirenal involvement may be secondary to extension from retroperitoneal fibrosis, may occur without associated retroperitoneal fibrosis, or may be one of various manifestations of multifocal fibrosclerosis.

**Fig. 14.14** (**a–d**) Uteropelvic junction obstruction in an horseshoe kidney due to renal stone. (**a**) Gray-scale ultrasound. Fourth-grade hydronephrosis of the left kidney due to a renal stone (calipers) located at the ureteropelvic junction. (**b**) CT urography. Dilatation of the urinary tract of the left kidney (*large arrow*) with evidence of the obstructing renal stone (*small arrow*). (**c**, **d**) Curved multiplanar reformats. Evident dilatation of the intra-renal urinary tract (*arrow*) due to the urinary stone at the ureteropelvic junction

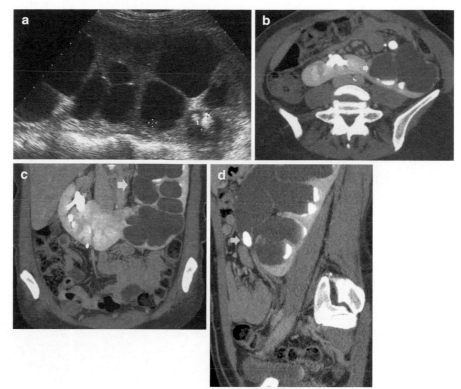

**Fig. 14.15** (**a–d**) Acute ureteral obstruction due to stone on the distal premural left ureter. Excretory urography. (**a**) Plain radiograph of the abdomen. A dense opacity (*arrow*) is evident on the left pelvic region. (**b**) Excretory urography, 15 min after contrast administration. Increased nephrographic density and delayed contrast excretion with delayed calyceal appearance (*arrows*) and variable dilatation of the collecting system and ureter. (**c**, **d**) Static-fluid MR urography. Evident dilatation of the renal pelvis and ureters (*white arrows*). The renal stone is visualized in the distal tract of the left ureter (*black arrow*)

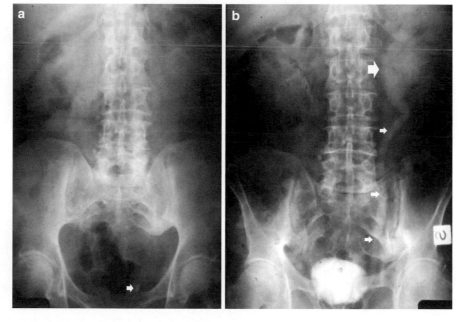

**Fig. 14.15** (continued)

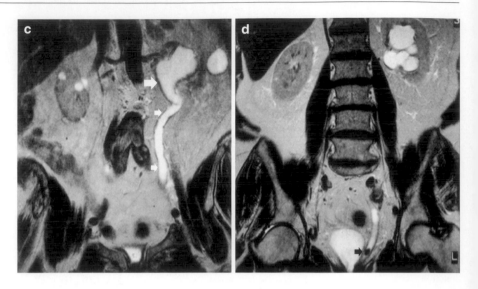

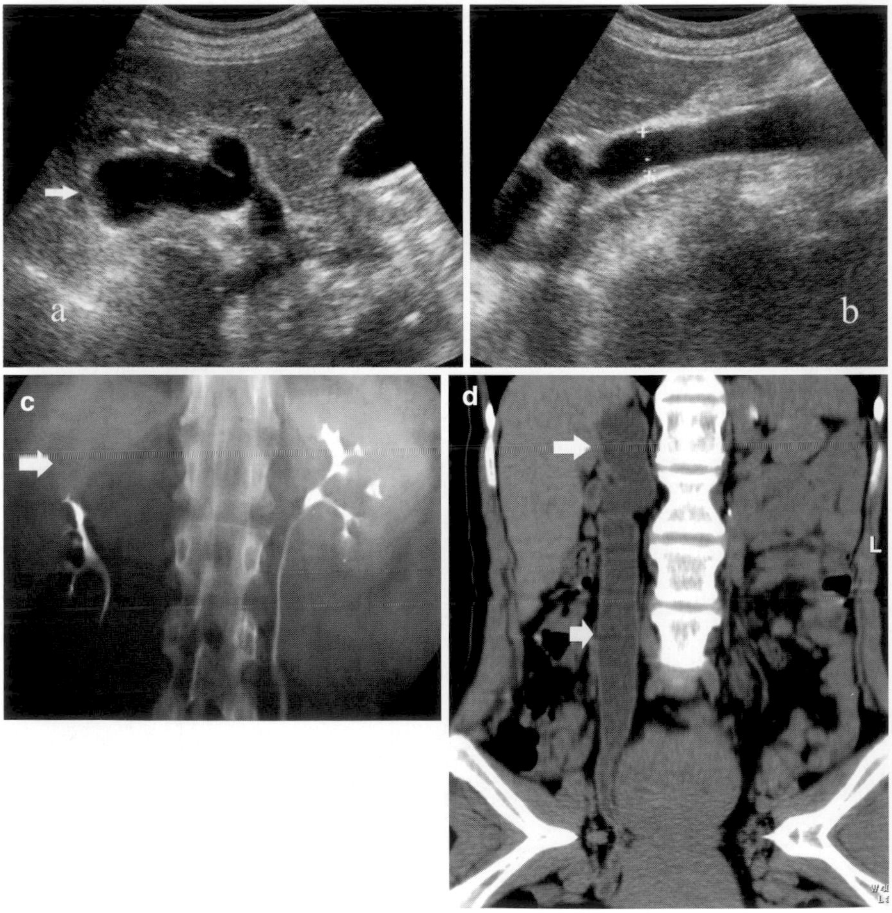

**Fig. 14.16** (**a–d**) Distal ureteral obstruction due to a renal stone in a 21-years-old woman in a duplicated collecting system. Patients presents with an abdominal pain with irradiation to the right flank and groin. Ultrasound, transverse (**a**) and longitudinal (**b**) scan. The upper pole mojety (*arrow*) appears dilated with no evidence of ureteral filling defects as the ureter (calipers). (**c**) Excretory urography. Absent opacification of the upper pole moiety (*arrow*) due to obstruction. (**d**) Unenhanced CT, coronal reformation. Dilation of the upper moiety and of the whole ureter (*arrows*)

**Fig. 14.17** (**a, b**) Distal ureteral obstruction in a duplicated collecting system in the right kidney. (**a**) Static-fluid MR urography. Evident dilatation of the upper pole moiety (*arrow*) and ureter in the right kidney. (**b**) TSE T2-weighted MR sequence, transverse plane. A renal stone (*arrow*) is evident on the distal right ureter inside the intramural tract

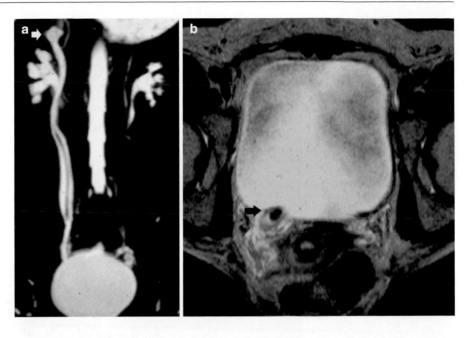

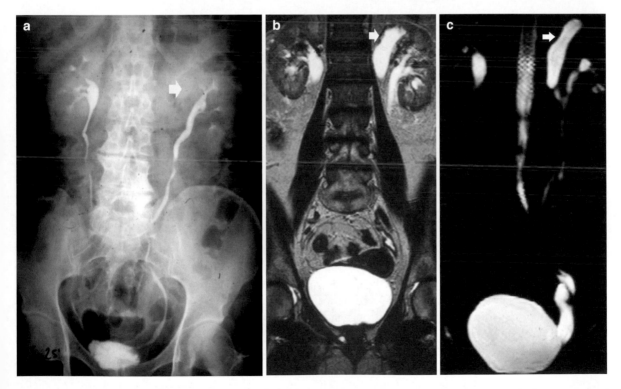

**Fig. 14.18** (**a–c**) Segmental obstruction due to a renal stone in a left duplicated intra-renal collecting system. (**a**) Excretory urography. Absent opacification of the upper moiety in a dupli-cated left urinary tract. (**b**) TSE T2-weighted MR sequence, and (**c**) static-fluid MR urography. Evident dilatation of the upper pole moiety (*arrow*) and ureter in the left kidney

**Fig. 14.19** (**a–c**) Obstruction of the middle ureter due to a renal stone in a 41-years-old woman with a duplicated collecting system. Patients presents with an abdominal pain with irradiation to the right flank and groin. (**a**) Ultrasound, longitudinal scan. The lower pole mojety of the right kidney appears dilated (*arrow*) with no evidence of ureteral filling defects. (**b**) Excretory urography. Absent opacification of the lower pole moiety (*arrow*) of the right kidney. (**c**) Static-fluid MR urography. Evident dilatation of the lower pole moiety (*arrow*) and ureter in the right kidney and identification of the level of obstruction

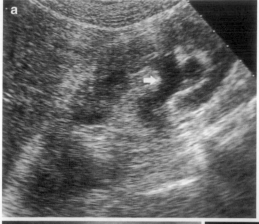

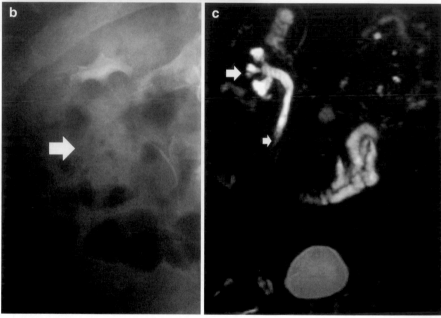

Three stages of the disease have been described, ranging from chronic active inflammation to fibrous scarring. The principal feature at cross-sectional imaging is a mantle of soft-tissue encasing the aorta, inferior vena cava, and ureters (Fig. 14.20). In most patients, the fibrous plaque forms a centrally located soft-tissue mantle of variable thickness extending from the renal hilum to the common iliac vessels (Witten 2000). The mass usually surrounds the aorta and vena cava, and caudal extension involves the bifurcation of these vessels and the common iliac vessels sometimes with the involvement of the kidneys, pancreas, spleen or mediastinum. The ureters lie on the anterolateral aspect of the fibrotic mass and may be encased by the mass for a varying distance with dilatation of the ureters above the level of involvement. The T2-weighted MR signal intensity and dynamic enhancement characteristics depend on the stage of the disease. Whereas areas affected by active inflammation demonstrate high T2 signal intensity and early contrast enhancement, areas of fibrosis show low T2 signal intensity and delayed contrast enhancement. Perirenal fibrosis that occurs in association with retroperitoneal fibrosis or as part of multifocal fibrosclerosis is not difficult to detect at imaging. However, the imaging features of isolated perirenal fibrosis are nonspecific, and a biopsy may be required to achieve a definitive diagnosis. Differential diagnoses include aortitis (perianeurysmal inflammation or fibrosis due to hypersensitivity to atheromatous plaques), ruptured abdominal aortic aneurysm, retroperitoneal metastases and lymphoma, and retroperitoneal hemorrhage.

**Fig. 14.20** (**a–c**) Urinary tract obstruction due to retroperitoneal fibrosis. Contrast-enhanced CT, excretory phase. (**a**) Dilatation of the intra-renal urinary tract of the right kidney. (**b**, **c**) Encasement of both ureters and infrarenal aorta by a soft-tissue mass (*arrow*) corresponding to a granulomatous tissue in retroperitoneal fibrosis

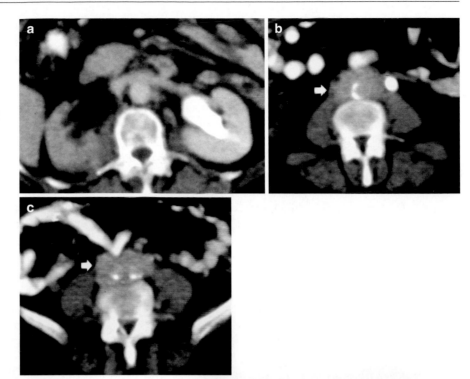

- *Renal pelvis blood clot.* Acute obstruction in a patient with macroscopic hematuria is often caused by blood clot. Clots in the renal pelvis may be identified in patients with bleeding diathesis and, particularly, in patients undergoing anticoagulative pharmacologic treatment, or in trauma. The clot assumes the configuration of the ureter and eventually lyses or passes into the bladder after several minutes to hours. As important elements for the differential diagnosis, clots move or disappear on follow-up scans, and do not show contrast enhancement. CT urography identifies multiple filling defects in the renal pelvis and ureter (Fig. 14.21). Sloughed papilla, fungus balls, or cholesteatoma may also cause obstruction of the urinary tract and should be considered in the differential diagnosis.

- *Pregnancy.* Physiologic hydronephrosis of pregnancy is the most commonly encountered cause of ureteral dilatation in pregnancy and may be present in over one-half of women by the third trimestre (Leyendecker et al. 2004). It results from compression of the ureter between the gravid uterus and iliopsoas muscle. Static MR urography techniques are virtually identical to the heavily T2-weighted sequences employed for MR cholangiopancreatography and accurately depict the level and, in many cases, the cause of ureteral obstruction without requiring intravenous injection of gadolinium-based

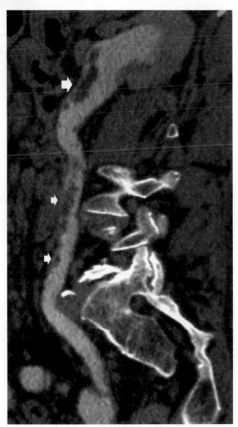

**Fig. 14.21** Multidetector CT urography. Curved planar reformation. Multiple coagula manifesting as multiple filling defects (*arrows*) in the renal and extrarenal urinary tract simulating a diffuse transitional cell carcinoma

contrast material which should be avoided in pregnancy (Leyendecker et al. 2004). Urolithiasis is the most common cause of urological-related abdominal pain in pregnant women, and it may be observed in 1/200–1/2,000 women during pregnancy depending on the population. It is important to distinguish between physiologic hydronephrosis and stone disease. Hydronephrosis of pregnancy is characterized by smooth tapering of the ureter at the level of the sacral promontory (Roy et al. 1995). Left-sided colic is more likely to represent the presence of a stone. The presence of a filling defect within the ureter or an unusual site of obstruction (e.g., ureteropelvic junction or ureterovesical junction) suggests that the obstruction is not physiologic. Perinephric or periureteral edema or fluid may be present in the setting of obstructive calculi.

• *Postsurgical obstruction.* Transient obstruction or permanent stricture may develop after any procedure on the ureter including retrograde and aterograde catheterization. Postsurgical (Fig. 14.22) and radiation (Fig. 14.23) ureteral strictures represent an important part of iatrogenic cause of urinary tract obstruction.

• *Benign neoplasms.* Uterine fibromas may rarely determine ureteral compression with urinary tract dilatation (Fig. 14.24). Prostatic enlargement is a common cause of partial or complete obstruction to urine outflow. Benign prostatic hypertrophy causing urethral obstruction with bilateral or unilateral urinary tract obstruction in patients with solitary kidney (Fig. 14.25) or with preexisting impaired renal function may determines acute postrenal failure. In contrast to the case in ureteral obstruction, the urinary bladder distends and often results in overflow urinary incontinence (paradoxical iscuria). The patient may therefore present with azotemia secondary to a profound reduction in glomerular filtra-

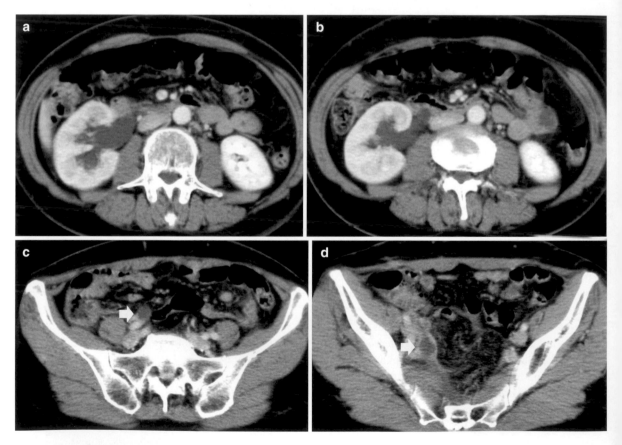

**Fig. 14.22** (**a–d**) Urinary tract obstruction due to surgical stricture of the right ureter in a 64-years-old female patient who had right ovariectmy 15 days before. Contrast-enhanced CT, nephrographic phase. Persistent corticomedullary phase with nephrographic phase delay on the right obstructed kidney. Second grade hydronephrosis with dilatation of the whole right ureter (*arrows*) and evidence of peri-ureteric fibrosis in the premural tract of the right ureter

**Fig. 14.23** (**a**, **b**) Urinary tract obstruction due to radiation stricture of the right ureter due radiation therapy in a 65-years-old female patient who had radical nephro-ureterectomy of the left kidney. Contrast-enhanced CT, coronal (**a**) and sagittal (**b**) reformations. Third-grade hydronephrosis with dilatation of the whole right ureter due to peri-ureteric fibrosis (*arrow*) in the premural tract of the right ureter

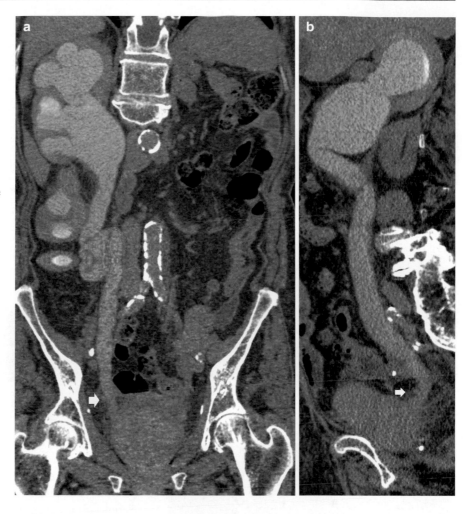

tion and yet have significant volumes of urine flow (Andreoli 1992).

### 14.1.2.5  Malignancies Causing Obstructive Uropathy

- *Ureteral tumors.* Transitional cell papilloma and carcinoma account for almost 90% of primary urteral tumors. On intravenous urography and, nowadays, on multidetector CT urography, it is difficult to obtain a single image of all urinary collecting system segments in an opacified and distended state and intravenous saline (250 mL) or furosemide injection improve the urinary tract and ureteral opacification and distension. It is not just about depicting anatomy, since opacification and distenstion helps in detection of small urothelial neoplasms of the ureter.

Ureteral tumors clinically manifest as gross hematuria. CT urography shows an intraluminal filling defect, a localized ureteral dilatation surrounding and below the tumor (*goblet sign*), cupping of the contrast material over the convex margin of the lesion, and/or hydronephrosis (Fig. 14.26). The kidney may appear functionally excluded at intravenous urography and renal hydronephrosis with ureteral obstruction is identified by static-fluid MR urography (Fig. 14.27). It is important to note that dilatation and obstruction of the urinary tract may be present or not when ureteral tumor is identified. Small transition cell carcinomas of the ureter may determine little or no obstruction of the upper urinary tract (Fig. 14.28) due to the remaining space for urine to flow around the papillary tumor.

- *Nonureteral tumors.* Bladder carcinoma (Fig. 14.29), pelvic carcinomas (cervical carcinoma, and

**Fig. 14.24** (**a**, **b**) Urinary tract obstruction due to extrinsic ureteral compression from large uterine fibroma. TSE T2-weighted MR sequence. Dilatation of the right urinary tract (*arrows*) due to extrinsic compression from an uterine fibroma (u). (**b**) Static-fluid MR urography. Dilatation of the right urinary tract

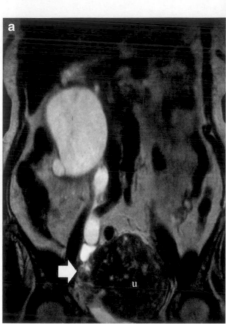
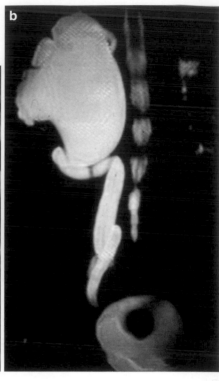

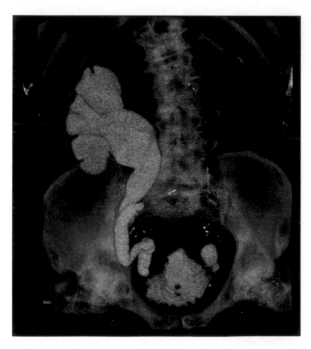

**Fig. 14.25** Urinary tract obstruction due to benign prostatic hypertrophy in a patient with previous left nephrectomy. CT urography. VR 3D color-coded image. Third-grade hydronephrosis and hydroureter due to benign prostatic hypertrophy with bladder wall hypertrophy and diverticula

infiltrating ovary carcinomas) or uterine fibromas, prostatic adenocarcinomas, metastatic pelvic lymph nodes, and retroperitoneal malignancies may obstruct the ureters and cause renal failure. Neoplasms are the primary cause of obstruction of the pelvic brim and ureterovescical junction. Extraureteral malignancies, such as disseminated retroperitoneal lymphoma or retroperitoneal lymph node metastases (Fig. 14.30), may determine urinary tract obstruction by direct extension to the ureter, diffuse metastasis with encasement of the periureteral tissues and/or ureteric wall, or mucosal metastasis.

### 14.1.3 Obstructive Nephropathy and Postrenal Acute Renal Failure

Azotemia and oliguria occur in urinary tract obstruction only when the urinary tract is obstructed bilaterally or when obstruction occur in a sole functioning kidney as in individual with renal agenesis or with renal transplantation. Postrenal acute renal failure

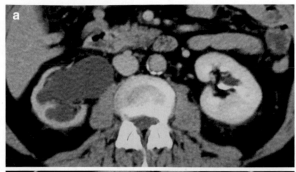

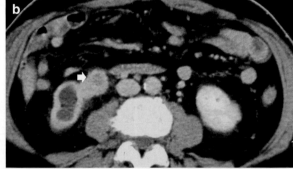

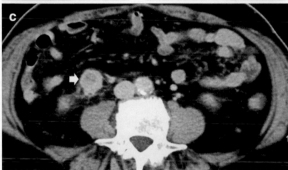

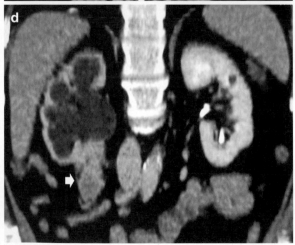

**Fig. 14.26** (**a–d**) Urinary tract obstruction due to ureteral tumor with dilatation of the urinary tract and late contract excretion. (**a–c**) CT, excretory phase, and (**d**) coronal reformation. Hydronephrosis in the right kidney due to an ureteral tumor (*arrow*) localized in the upper ureter

account for 5–25% of cases of acute renal failure. The degree of azotemia depends upon the extent of obstruction; partial obstruction may produce only moderate degrees of azotemia, while complete obstruction of the urinary tract obviously produces anuria (Andreoli 1992). Obstruction of the urinary flow can irreversibly damage the kidney. If the obstruction is partial or nearly complete, renal function may be preserved for as long as 4–5 weeks following the onset of obstruction (Andreoli 1992).

The clinically important distinction of renal obstruction from nonobstructive dilatation cannot be resolved by gray-scale US, even though the accuracy of US to rule out obstruction increases in patients with an high pretest probability of urinary tract obstruction.

Doppler US may provide unique data not available from conventional US in postrenal acute renal failure. Demonstration of high RI in patients with acute renal failure and hydronephrosis increases the diagnostic confidence for a diagnosis of obstruction.

(For postrenal acute renal failure see also Chap. 29).

## 14.2 Pyonephrosis

The chronic suppurative infection in an obstructed kidney is defined pyonephrosis. Although acute infections often occur in an obstructed system, true pyonephrosis is observed when chronic obstructive changes of the urinary tract are evident. Any cause of chronic ureteral obstruction predisposes to pyonephrosis. Urinary calculus disease is a common cause (about 50% of cases), while the other possible causes are malignant disease of retroperitoneum and pelvis, retroperitoneal fibrosis, postoperative fibrosis, and congenital obstruction (especially ureteropelvic junction obstruction). Purulent debris consisting of sloughed urothelium and a mixture of inflammatory cells collects in the obstructed upper urinary tract, namely the calyces and renal pelvis. The associated pyelonephritis causes eventual destruction of the renal parenchyma (Kenney 1990). The infecting organism is almost always a common urinary pathogen, namely a gram-negative bacterium, including *Escherichia coli*, *Proteus mirabilis*, *Klebsiella pneumoniae*, and *Pseudomonas aeruginosa*.

The clinical presentation is often acute, with acute flank pain, fever, chills, and leukocytosis. Subacute presentation with a low-grade fever,

**Fig. 14.27** (**a–b**) Urinary
tract obstruction due to left
ureteral tumor with dilatation
of the urinary tract and
functionally excluded kidney.
(**a**) Intravenous excretory
urography. Functionally
excluded left kidney with
absent excretion of the
iodinated contrast agent. (**b**)
Static-fluid MR urograpgy.
Hydronephrosis in the left
kidney due to an ureteral
tumor (*arrow*) localized in
the distal ureter

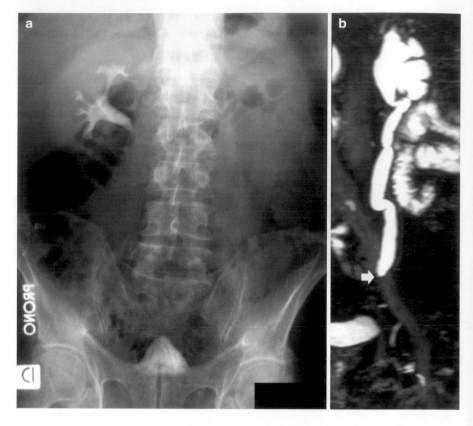

**Fig. 14.28** (**a–b**) Urinary
tract obstruction due to
ureteral tumor with mild
dilatation of the urinary tract.
(**a**) CT urography. Curved
planar reformat. An irregular
thickening of the distal
ureteral wall (*arrow*) is
evident during the excretory
phase. (**b**) Volume rendering
3D image confirms the
presence of urothelial tumor
of the distal ureter (*arrow*)

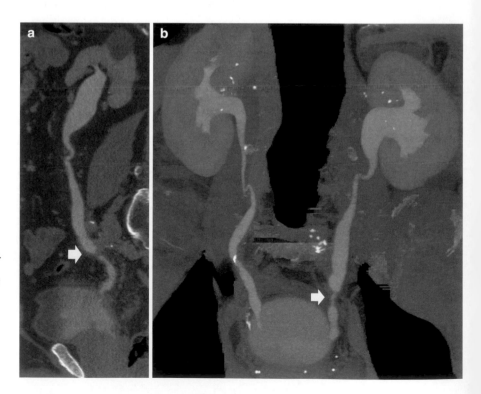

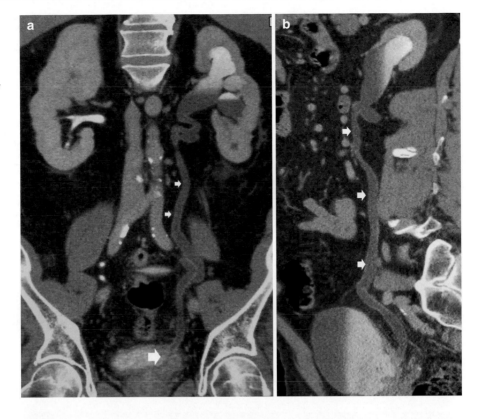

**Fig. 14.29** (**a**, **b**) Left urinary tract chronic obstruction due to bladder carcinoma of the trigonus. Coronal (**a**) and curved planar (**b**) reformations show hydronephrosis and mild ureteral dilatation (*small arrows*) on the left kidney due to bladder carcinoma in the trigonal zone (*large arrow*)

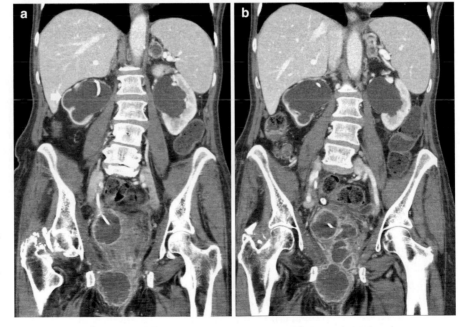

**Fig. 14.30** (**a**, **b**) Urinary tract obstruction due to extrinsic compression from diffuse pelvic lymph node metastases from ovary cancer. Contrast-enhanced CT, coronal reformat. Bilateral dilatation of the upper urinary tract with fourth-grade hydronephrosis on the right kidney

weight loss, anorexia, and dull pain is not uncommon (Kenney et al. 1990). Patients with urinary tract infection and elevated serum creatinine levels should undergo US examination to exclude obstruction, because pyonephrosis may quickly result in irreversible renal damage or sepsis. US examination with tissue harmonic imaging technology is extremely sensitive in detecting pyonephrosis (Fig. 14.30). The infected urine or pus within the obstructed collecting system determine the evidence

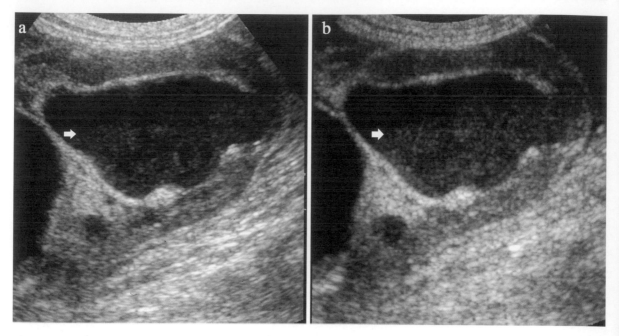

**Fig. 14.31** (**a**, **b**) Renal pyonephrosis. (**a**) Conventional gray-scale ultrasound. Dilatation of the upper urinary tract with an echoic content (*arrow*) laying in the dependent portion of the dilated urinary system. (**b**) Tissue harmonic imaging allows a better depiction of the laying echoic content (*arrow*) with a more clear separation of the urine from the debris

of diffusely dispersed fine echoes in the dilated renal collecting system, or echoes laying in the dependent portions of the dilated pelvis (Figs. 14.31 and 14.32). Usually, CT is not needed because diagnosis and treatment can be managed by US followed by percutaneous aspiration and drainage. CT may be performed to differentiate pyonephrosis from other causes with a similar clinical presentation, to evaluate the site and the cause of renal obstruction, and to assess the perinephric extension of the infection. The typical presentation is hydronephrosis with high density (>20 Hounsfield units) of the contents of the renal collecting system. After contrast injection, a decreased enhancement of renal parenchyma compared to the other kidney is shown reflecting the loss of renal function, with absent or very low opacification of the renal calyces (Figs. 14.32 and 14.33). A typical finding is the contrast laying over the debris in the dilated obstructed renal collecting system due to the high density of the pus in the collecting system, which is the contrary of the usual situation in the contrast layers in the dependent portion of the dilated system. The perinephric extension of the infection is indicated by alteration in the perinephric and retroperitoneal fat planes. The nuclear medicine shows a nonfunctioning kidney (Fig. 14.34).

Adequate drainage with the percutaneous aspiration of purulent urine from the collecting system remains the most accurate modality to confirm the diagnosis, besides to represent the best therapy for pyonephrosis in conjunction with appropriate antibiotics. After the initial percutaneous aspiration, a percutaneous nephrostomy tube should be inserted.

## 14.3 Reflux Nephropathy in Adults

The vesico-ureteral reflux is the retrograde flow of urine from the bladder toward the kidney. Reflux nephropathy is a condition in which the kidneys are damaged by the backward flow of urine into the kidney, and is the most common urinary tract abnormality in children, with 1–2% incidence in the general population (Ascenti et al. 2004; Valentini et al. 2004) and is an important cause of renal failure. Together with congenital megacalyces, vesicoureteral reflux represents the most common cause of nonobstructive dilatation of the renal collecting system. Sterile vesico-ureteral reflux in

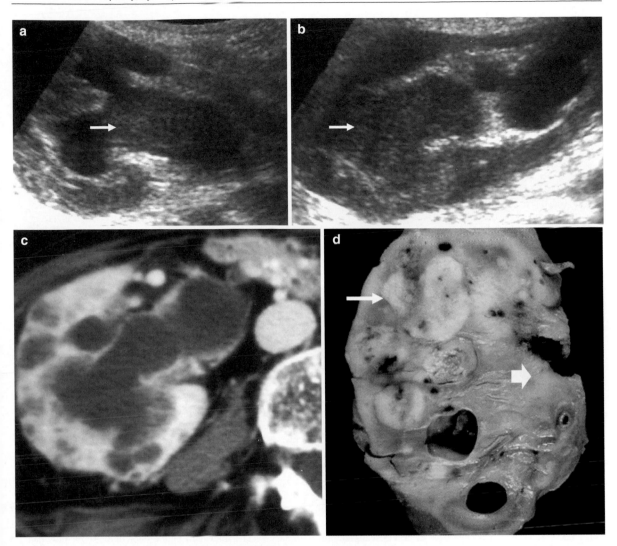

**Fig. 14.32** (**a–d**) Renal pyonephrosis in a 75-years-old woman presenting with acute flank pain, hematuria, fever, and leukocytosis. Ultrasound (**a**: transverse scan; **b**: longitudinal scan) shows a mild dilatation of the upper urinary tract with an echoic content (*arrow*) laying in the dependent portion of the dilated urinary system. Contrast-enhanced CT (**c**) shows renal hydronephrosis with absent opacification of the renal calyces, and multiple round hypodense parenchymal lesions which were interpreted as renal abscesses. No perinephric extension of the infection is evident. The percutaneous drainage was attempted without success and nephrectomy was performed. The surgical specimen (**d**) shows a whitish tumor infiltrating the renal parenchyma (*long arrow*), the renal sinus, and the ureteropelvic junction (*large arrow*). Microscopic analysis showed a infiltrative sarcomatoid-cell type renal cell carcinoma

adults with normal urinary tracts and no evidence of urinary tract obstruction is of uncertain significance (Spataro 1990). Vesico-ureteral reflux is occasionally evident in the presence of benign prostatic hypertrophy, neuropathic bladder, bladder carcinoma, drug-induced cystitis, granulomatous cystitis, or iatrogenic-induced ureteral office injury. Anyway, also in adults the vesico-ureteral reflux may predispose to pyelonephritis in the presence of lower urinary tract infection.

Previously known as chronic atrophic pyelonephritis, reflux nephropathy is usually due to urinary reflux and episodic urinary infection beginning in infancy and childhood. It is often present in young adult with hypertension and renal insufficiency. It can be unilateral or bilateral and leads to focal or global decrease in renal size with notch or valley in the surface of the kidney immediately opposite a dilated calyx with a calviform shape (Fig. 14.35). Symptoms include blood in the urine,

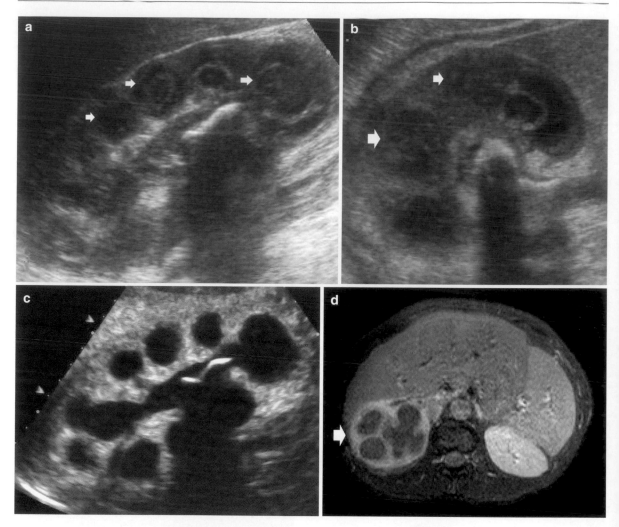

**Fig. 14.33** (**a–d**) Renal pyonephrosis. (**a, b**) US scan, longitudinal and axial planes. Multiple renal stones are evident on the right renal pelvis with the typical posterior acoustic shadowing with evident intra-renal urinary tract dilatation with hyperechoic content (*arrows*). (**c**) Contrast-enhanced US, 35 s after sulfurhexafluoride microbubble injection, shows the normal perfusion of renal parenchyma with evidence of the dilatation of the urinary tract (*arrows*) with suppression of the signal provided by the hyperechoic content and consequent higher signal-to-noise ratio. (**d**) Axial 3D fast gradient-echo with fat suppression, obtained immediately after the dynamic series after gadolinium-based contrast agent injection during the nephrographic phase, confirms the intra-renal urinary tract dilatation on the right kidney with absent contrast excretion within the renal calyces

burning or stinging with urination, dark or foamy urine, flank or back pain, nicturia, and urinary frequency and hypertension and proteinuria due to glomerulosclerosis. The best diagnostic clue is the contrast instilled into the bladder which opacifies the ureter and may reach the intrarenal collecting system, often only transiently.

The International Reflux Study Committee grading system classifies the vesico-ureteral reflux in 5 grades: I: reflux into the ureter not reaching the renal pelvis; II: reflux reaching the renal pelvis but without evidence of calyx blunting; III: mild caliceal blunting; IV: progressive caliceal and ureteral dilatation; V: very dilated and tortuous collecting system, intrarenal reflux. In adults, findings of parenchymal scarring, ureteral dilatation, or calyceal clubbing should suggest to perform voiding cystourethrography.

The typical deformities of renal papillae due to calyceal distortions with a typical claviform morphology which can be identified on intravenous excretory urography (Fig. 14.36) or CT urography (Fig. 14.37). Parenchymal alterations, including decrease in renal size and notch of the renal parenchyma surface, may be identified on contrast-enhanced CT or MR imaging (Fig. 14.38). In 10% of adults requiring

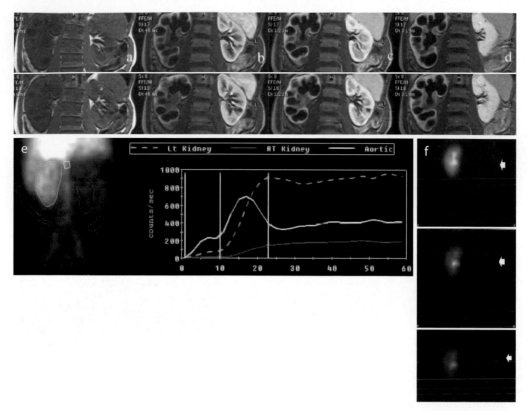

**Fig. 14.34** (**a–f**) Renal pyonephrosis. Coronal 3D T1-weighted breath-hold fast spoiled gradient echo sequence before (**a**) and after intravenous gadolinium-based contrast agent injection reveal dilatation of the intra-renal urinary tract of the right kidney with alteration of the corticomedullary (**b**, **c**), nephrographic and nephrographic phase (**d**) in comparison with the other kidney with absent contrast excretion. (**e**) SPECT imaging with absent concentration of the radiotracer on the right kidney. (**f**) Dynamic functional SPECT examination. Perfusion study. The different vascular profile of the left kidney (*blue*), right kidney (*pink*), and aorta (*white*) shows the reduced functionality of the right kidney

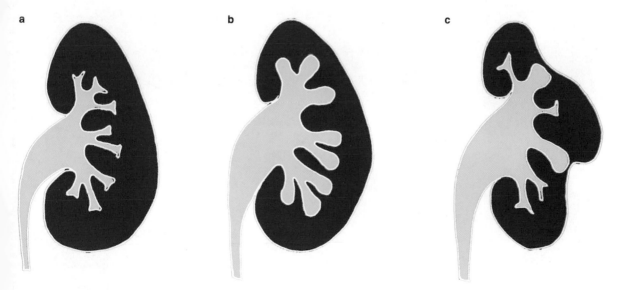

**Fig. 14.35** (**a–c**) Renal morphology changes due to different causes. (**a**) Normal kidney; (**b**) Postobstructive renal atrophy; (**c**) Reflux nephropathy. In reflux nephropathy a notch or valley in the surface of the kidney appears immediately opposite a dilated calyx with a calviform shape

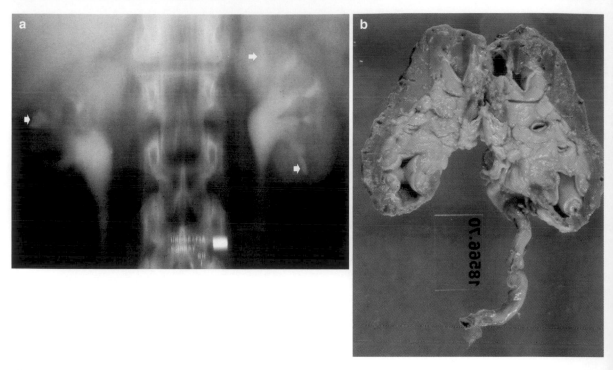

**Fig. 14.36** (**a**, **b**) Chronic reflux nephropathy in a 60-years old woman. (**a**) Intravenous excretory urography, nephropyeloto-mography. Calyceal distortions (*arrows*) with a typical claviform morphology due to chronic vesicoureteral reflux. (**b**) Surgical specimen. Dilatation of the intra-renal urinary tract

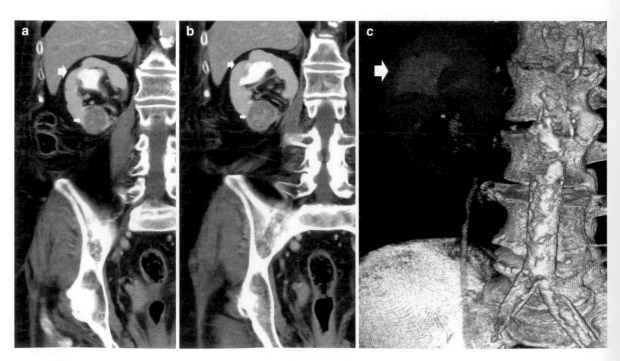

**Fig. 14.37** (**a–c**) Reflux nephropathy in a 65-years old man. (**a**, **b**) CT urography, calcyceal distortion. Calyceal distortion with a typical claviform morphology (*large arrow*) due to chronic vesicoureteral reflux with adjacent renal parenchyma scar. A synchronus renal parenchyma solid tumor (*small arrow*) is identified. (**c**) VR, color-coded image. Calyceal dilatation and distortion of the calyces of the upper renal pole (*large arrow*)

**Fig. 14.38** (**a–f**) Reflux nephropathy in the left kidney of a 55-years old man. (**a, b**) T2-weighted spectral fat saturation inversion recovery (SPIR); (**c, d**) T2-weighted turbo spin-echo (TSE); (**e, f**) T1-weighted spoiled gradient echo with fat suppression after gadolinium-based agent injection. (**a, c, e**) Normal kidney; (**b, d, f**) Typical parenchymal alterations (*arrows*) in a kidney with vesico-ureteral reflux

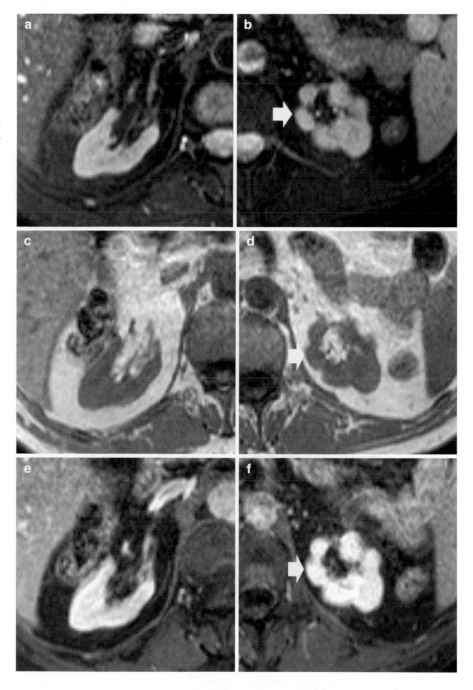

renal replacement therapy for end-stage renal disease the cause is reflux nephropathy. Acute inflammatory responses to the infection result in renal parenchymal damage and subsequent renal scarring. Loss of functioning renal mass prompt compensatory changes in renal hemodynamics that, over time, are maladaptive and result in glomerular injury and sclerosis. Vesico-ureteral reflux presents with acute urinary infection, with a frequency ranging from 20 to 50%.

Traditionally, retrograde voiding cystourethrography (Fig. 14.39) or radionuclide cystography still remain the reference standard techniques for the diagnosis of vesico-ureteral reflux. Vesicoureteral reflux is effectively shown by either voiding cystourethrography or by radionuclide cystography. Nuclear cystography is more sensitive to detect transient episodes of reflux and provides a lower dose of radiation, is favored for screening and follow-up in children. Contrast-enhanced voiding sonocystography

**Fig. 14.39** (**a–d**) Reflux nephropathy. Voiding cystourethrography in a 10-years-old male patient. Initial left vesico-ureteral reflux evident during the progressive retrograde opacification of the bladder (**a**). Complete vesicoureteral reflux (**b**) after completion of bladder retrograde opacification. (**c**, **d**) Controlateral vesico-ureteral reflux during minction

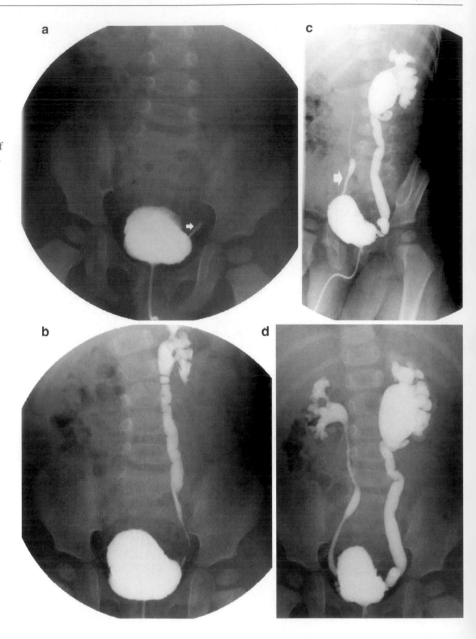

(Fig. 14.40) now appears as a valuable alternative method, due to absence of radiation dose and properties of microbubble-based contrast agents (Mentzel et al. 1999; Darge et al. 2001; Valentini et al. 2004). Recently, contrast-enhanced voiding sonocystography (Fig. 14.40) has been proposed both for the diagnosis and follow-up of vesico-ureteral reflux in children (Berrocal et al. 2001; Ascenti et al. 2004). Several studies have showed the high diagnostic accuracy of contrast-enhanced voiding sonocystography compared to voiding cystourethrography (Valentini et al. 2001) and direct radionuclide cystography (Ascenti et al. 2003) to detect and grading (Darge and Troeger 2002) the vesico-ureteral reflux in children. Because of its accuracy, contrast-enhanced voiding sonocystography could replace radiological voiding cystourethrography in the detection of vesico-ureteral reflux in girls, the follow-up in boys, and in the management of recurrent infection in children presenting with normal radiological voiding cystourethrography (Galloy et al. 2003). Anyway, further studies have proved the efficacy of voiding sonocystography to detect and grading the vesico-ureteral reflux in adult patients who

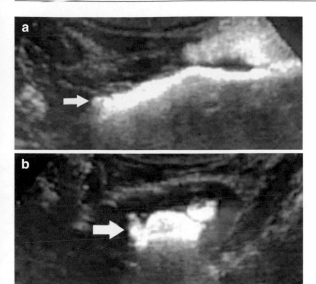

**Fig. 14.40** (**a**, **b**) Reflux nephropathy. Voiding cistoureterosonography in a 12-years-old female patient. Reflux of microbubbles (**a**) in a moderately dilated left ureter (*arrows*). Evidence of microbubbles in the pelvicalyceal system with almost complete cancellation of background tissues (**b**) (courtesy of Prof. Ascenti, University of Messina, Italy)

the bladder to the ureter, renal pelvis, and renal calyces or when color signals are seen in the urinary tract. The associated morphologic signs (dilated or nondilated ureter, renal pelvis and calyces) contribute to vesico-ureteral reflux assessment with the use of five grades assigned on the basis of contrast-enhanced voiding sonocystography, which makes this system comparable to the most frequently used radiographic system of vesico-ureteral reflux grading: Grade I, echoes or color signals in the ureter above the ureteral orifice; grade II, echoes or color signals extending up to the renal pelvis and calyces, with no ureteral dilatation; grade III, ureter, renal pelvis, and calyces containing echoes or color signals, with mildly dilated ureter; grade IV, echoes or color signals in dilated ureter, renal pelvis and calyces; grade V, echoes or color signals in markedly dilated ureter, renal pelvis and calyces. Sensitivity and specificity of contrast-enhanced voiding sonocystography in revealing vesico-ureteral reflux in children range from 69 to 100% and from 87 to 97%, respectively (Berrocal et al. 2001; Ascenti et al. 2003, 2004).

had undergone renal transplantation with previous evidence of urinary tract infection (Valentini et al. 2004).

From the technical point of view the voiding sonocystography is easy to perform. The bladder is emptied after aseptic introduction of a 5–8 French infant feeding tube. The bladder is then filled with 200–250 mL of room-temperature saline solution. Microbubble contrast agent is administered in a volume of 10% of the bladder volume. After microbubbles administration a suspension of a small volume of saline solution was injected in order to push the residual contrast agent through the catheter. In this way, echogenic microbubbles are easily identified in the bladder, which is filled by anechoic saline solution. The microbubbles first reach the ventral region of the bladder creating a posterior strong acoustic shadowing and obscuring the dorsal region of the bladder. By increasing slowly the acoustic power of insonation, microbubbles are distributed into the vesical lumen. Then, acoustic power is switched at the lowest level (mechanical index: 0.04–0.2) to get a satisfactory visualization of microbubbles. During microbubbles administration, the bladder, ureter, renal pelvis and calyces were evaluated by color or contrast-specific harmonic US modes. The same evaluation is repeated during the voiding phase. Diagnosis of vesico-ureteral reflux is assigned on the basis of echoes refluxing from

# References

Andreoli TE (1992) Approach to the patient with renal disease. In: Wyngaarden JB, Smith LH, Bennett JC (eds) Cecil textbook of medicine. Saunders, Philadelphia, pp 477–482

Ascenti G, Zimbaro G, Mazziotti S et al. (2003) Vesicoureteral reflux: comparison between urosonography and radionuclide cystography. Pediatr Nephrol 18:768–771

Ascenti G, Zimbaro G, Mazziotti S et al. (2004) Harmonic US imaging of vesicoureteric reflux in children: usefulness of a second generation US contrast agent. Pediatr Radiol 34:481–487

Berrocal T, Gaya F, Arjonilla A et al. (2001) Vesicoureteral reflux: diagnosis and grading with echo-enhanced cystosonography versus voiding cystourethrography. Radiology 221:359–365

Burge HJ, Middleton WD, McClennan BL et al. (1991) Ureteral jets in healthy subjects and in patients with unilateral ureteral calculi: comparison with color Doppler US. Radiology 180(2):437–442

Caoili EM, Cohan RH, Korobkin M et al. (2002) Urinary tract abnormalities: initial experience with multi-detector row CT urography. Radiology 222:353–360

Cox IH, Erickson SJ, Foley WD et al. (1992) Ureteric jets: evaluation of normal flow dynamics with color Doppler sonography. AJR Am J Roentgenol 158:1051–1055

Curry NS, Gobien RP, Schabel SI (1982) Minimal dilatation obstructive nephropathy. Radiology 143:531–534

Darge K, Troeger J (2002) Vesicoureteral reflux grading in contrast-enhanced voiding urosonography. Eur J Radiol 43:122–128

Darge K, Zieger B, Rohrschneider W et al. (2001) Contrast-enhanced harmonic imaging for the diagnosis of vesicoureterorenal reflux in pediatric patients. AJR Am J Roentgenol 177:1411–1415

Galloy MA, Mandry D, Pecastaings M et al (2003) Sonocystography: a new method for the diagnosis and follow-up of vesico-ureteric reflux in children. J Radiol 84:2055–2061

Hagspiel KD, Butty S, Nandalur KR et al. (2005) Magnetic resonance urography for the assessment of potential renal donors: comparison of the RARE technique with a low-dose gadolinium-enhanced magnetic resonance urography technique in the absence of pharmacological and mechanical intervention. Eur Radiol 15:2230–2237

Hoffer FA, Lebowitz RL (1985) Intermittent hydronephrosis: a unique feature of ureteropelvic junction obstruction caused by a crossing renal vessel. Radiology 156:655–658

Karabacakoglu A, Karakose S, Ince O et al. (2004) Diagnostic value of diuretic-enhanced excretory MR urography in patients with obstructive uropathy. Eur J Radiol 52:320–327

Kenney PJ (1990) Imaging of chronic renal infections. Am J Roentgenol 155(3):485–494

Kenney PJ, Breatnach ES, Stanley RJ (1990) Pyonephrosis. In: Pollack HM (ed) Clinical urography. Saunders, Philadelphia, pp 843–849

Klahr S (1992) Obstructive uropathy. In: Wyngaarden JB, Smith LH, Bennett JC (eds) Cecil textbook of medicine. Saunders, Philadelphia, pp 579–584

Kocaoglu M, Ilica AT, Bulakbasi N et al. (2005) MR urography in pediatric uropathies with dilated urinary tracts. Diagn Interv Radiol 11:225–232

Lee HJ, Kim SH, Jeong YK et al. (1996) Doppler sonographic resistive index in obstructed kidneys. J Ultrasound Med 15(9):613–618

Lefort C, Marouteau-Pasquier N, Pesquet AS et al. (2006) Dynamic MR urography in urinary tract obstruction: implementation and prelimininary results. Abdom Imaging 31:232–240

Leyendecker JR, Gorengaut V, Brown JJ (2004) MR imaging of maternal diseases of the abdomen and pelvis during pregnancy and the immediate postpartum period. Radiographics 24:1301–1316

Lowe FC, Marshall FF (1984) Ureteropelvic junction obstruction in adults. Urology 23:331–335

Mentzel HJ, Vogt S, Patzer L et al (1999) Contrast-enhanced sonography of vesicoureterorenal reflux in children: prelminary results. AJR Am J Roentgenol 173:737–740

Miller OF, Rineer SK, Reichard SR et al. (1998) Prospective comparison of unenhanced spiral computed tomography and intravenous urogram in the evaluation of acute flank pain. Urology 52(6):982–987

Naidich JB, Rackson ME, Mossey RT et al. (1986) Nondilated obstructive uropathy: percutaneous nephrostomy performed to reverse renal failure. Radiology 160:653–657

Niall O, Russell J, MacGregor R et al. (1999) A comparison of noncontrast computerized tomography with excretory urography in the assessment of acute flank pain. J Urol 161(2):534–537

Nikken JJ, Krestin GP (2007) MRI of the kidney – state of the art. Eur Radiol 17:2780–2793

Nolte-Ernsting CC, Staatz G, Tacke J et al. (2003) Mr urography today. Abdom Imaging 28:191–209

Ozdemir H, Demir MK, Temizöz O et al. (2008) Phase inversion harmonic imaging improves assessment of renal calculi: a comparison with fundamental gray-scale sonography. J Clin Ultrasound 36(1):16–19

Pak CYC (1992) Renal calculi. In: Wyngaarden JB, Smith LH, Bennett JC (eds) Cecil textbook of medicine. Saunders, Philadelphia, pp 603–608

Platt JF (1992) Duplex Doppler evaluation of native kidney dysfunction. Obstructive and nonobstructive disease. AJR Am J Roentgenol 158:1035–1042

Platt JF (1996) Urinary obstruction. Radiol Clin North Am 34(6):1113–1129

Platt JF, Rubin JM, Ellis JH (1993) Acute renal obstruction: evaluation with intrarenal duplex Doppler and conventional US. Radiology 186:685–688

Platt JF, Rubin JM, Ellis JH et al. (1989) Duplex Doppler US of the kidney: differentiation of obstructive and nonobstructive dilatation. Radiology 171:515–517

Quaia E, Bertolotto M (2002) Renal parenchymal diseases: is characterization feasible with ultrasound?. Eur Radiol 12:2006–2020

Quaia E, Nocentini A, Torelli L (2009) Assessment of a new mathematical model for the computation of numerical parameters related to renal cortical blood flow and fractional blood volume by contrast-enhanced ultrasound. Ultras Med Biol 35(4):616–627

Rascoff JH, Golden RA, Spinowitz BS et al.(1983) Nondilated obstructive uropathy. Arch Intern Med 143:696–698

Rohrschneider WK, Haufc S, Wiesel M et al. (2002) Functional and morphologic evaluation of congenital urinary tract dilatation by using combined static-dynamic MR urography: findings in kidneys with a single collecting system. Radiology 224:683–694

Roy C, Saussine C, Guth S et al. (1998) MR urography in the evaluation of urinary tract obstruction. Abdom Imaging 23:27–34

Roy C, Saussine C, Jahn C et al. (1995) Fast imaging MR assessment of ureterohydronephrosis during pregnancy. Magn Reson Imaging 13:767–772

Shokeir AA, El Diasty T, Eassa W et al. (2004) Diagnosis of noncalcareous hydronephrosis: role of magnetic resonance urography and noncontrast computed tomography. Urology 63:225–229

Silverman SG, Akbar SA, Mortele KJ et al. (2006) Multidetector row CT urography of normal urinary collecting system: furosemide versus saline as adjunct to contrast medium. Radiology 240:749–755

Silverman SG, Leyendecker JR, Amis SE (2009) What is the current role of CT urography and MR urography in the evaluation of the urinary tract. Radiology 250:309–323

Smith RC, Rosenfield AT, Choe KA et al. (1995) Acute flank pain: comparison of non-contrast-enhanced CT and intravenous urography. Radiology 194(3):789–794

Spataro RF (1990) Inflammatory conditions of the renal pelvis and ureter. In: Pollack HM (ed) Clinical urography. Saunders, Philadelphia, pp 884–901

Surabhi VR, Menias C, Prasad SR et al. (2008) Neoplastic and non-neoplastic proliferative disorders of the perirenal space: cross-sectional imaging findings. Radiographics 28:1005–1017

Swartz RD (2009) Idiopathic retroperitoneal fibrosis: a review of the pathogenesis and approaches to treatment. Am J Kidney Dis: doi:10.1053/j.ajkd.2009.04.019

Talner LB, O'Reilly PH, Roy C (2000a) Urinary obstruction. In: Pollack HM, McClennan BL (eds) Clinical urography. Saunders, Philadelphia, pp 1846–1966

Talner LB, O'Reilly P, Wasserman NF (2000b) Specific causes of urinary obstruction. In: Pollack HM, McClennan BL (eds) Clinical urography. Saunders, Philadelphia, pp 1967–2136

Taourel P, Thuret R, Hoquet MD et al. (2008) Computed tomography in the nontraumatic renal causes of acute flank pain. Semin Ultrasound CT MRI 29:341–352

Tchelepi H, Ralls PW (2009) Color comet-tail artefact: clinical applications. AJR Am J Roentgenol 192:11–18

Teh HS, Ang ES, Wong WC et al. (2003) MR renography using a dynamic gradient-echo sequence and low-dose gadopentetate dimeglumine as an alternative to radionuclide renography. AJR Am J Roentgenol 181:441–450

Tublin ME, Dodd GD, Verdile VP (1994) Acute renal colic: diagnosis with duplex Doppler US. Radiology 193(3):697–701

Valentini AL, De Gaetano AM, Minordi LM et al. (2004) Contrast-enhanced voiding US for grading of reflux in adult patients prior to antireflux ureteral implantation. Radiology 233:35–39

Valentini AL, Salvaggio E, Manzoni C et al (2001) Contrast-enhanced gray-scale and color Doppler voiding urosonography versus voiding cystourethrography in the diagnosis and grading of vesicoureteral reflux. J Clin Ultrasound 29:65–71

Vaughan ED Jr, Marion D, Poppas DP et al. (2004) Pathophysiology of unilateral ureteral obstruction: studies from Charlottesville to New York. J Urol 172(6 pt 2):2563–2569

Witten DM (2000) Retroperitoneal fibrosis. In: Pollack HM, McClennan BL (eds) Clinical urography. Saunders, Philadelphia, pp 2878–2894

# Nephrocalcinosis and Nephrolithiasis

Siân Phillips and Gareth R. Tudor

## Contents

### Abstract

> The presence of renal calculi in humans has been identified in mummies discovered as long ago as 4,000 BC, affecting humans for millennia. The underlying aetiology of both nephrocalcinosis and nephrolithiasis is complex. An appreciation of the processes involved in calculus formation aids in the understanding of the diagnosis and management of the disease. The progression of imaging technology has promoted increasingly sensitive and specific techniques in the diagnosis of nephrocalcinosis and nephrolithiasis. Currently, non-contrasted computed tomography has superceded the excretory intravenous urogram in the investigation of acute renal colic because of diagnostic accuracy and ease of application. An understanding of current imaging technology and techniques is necessary to allow its appropriate application in the diagnosis and ongoing management of nephrocalcinosis and nephrolithiasis.

## 15.1 Introduction

Nephrolithiasis has been a recognised human disease for millennia. They were found in entombed Egyptian mummies dating back as far as 4,000 BC. The earliest recognised discovery in El Amara in a teenage boy. Nephrolithiasis is defined as calcification that lies in the collecting system, bladder, ureter and calyceal system. The majority of calculi are found in the

S. Phillips (✉) and G.R. Tudor
Abertawe Bro Morgannwg University Health Board,
Department of Radiology, Princess of Wales Hospital,
Coity Road, Bridgend, Wales CF31 1RQ, UK
e-mail: sian.phillips@abm-tr.wales.nhs.uk

E. Quaia (ed.), *Radiological Imaging of the Kidney*,
Medical Radiology, DOI: 10.1007/978-3-540-87597-0_15, © Springer-Verlag Berlin Heidelberg 2011

pelvicalyceal system and can be passed into the ureter. Nephrocalcinosis is renal calcification that occurs in the renal parenchyma.

With the discovery of modern X-ray by Roentgen, the value of imaging was recognised in the diagnosis and management of nephrolithiasis and nephrocalcinosis. Calcification is easily identified by standard X-rays and computed tomography (CT). The latter bearing the advantage of identification of calculi which are radiolucent on conventional radiographs. This has lead to the increased utilisation of CT in the imaging of nephrolithiasis and nephrocalcinosis. The first paper on intravenous urography was published in 1932, which described the features of a delayed nephrogram and dilated collecting system in a patient with renal colic. This technique was considered to be the most reliable method in the assessment of renal calculi until the advent of helical CT in the early 1990s.

In the UK, acute nephrolithiasis accounts for 1.8/10,000 hospital admissions with an incidence of 7/1,000, with similar figures reported the USA (Sandhu et al. 2003). In the era of increased abdominal cross-sectional imaging, renal calculi are increasingly diagnosed as an incidental finding. The aim of imaging is to identify the presence of nephrocalcinosis and nephrolithiasis and its physiological impact and to plan further management.

## 15.2 Nephrocalcinosis

The term nephrocalcinosis describes the deposition of calcium salts in the renal parenchyma. Nephrocalcinosis is a condition, which is a manifestation of different diseases caused by hypercalcemia and hypercalciuria, and can be subdivided into *medullary nephrocalcinosis* or *cortical nephrocalcinosis*. Macroscopic nephrocalcinosis can be classified into two groups, calcification in normal and abnormal tissue. Chemical nephrocalcinosis, relating to the increase of intracellular calcium and microscopic nephrocalcinosis, is not visualised with standard imaging. Metastatic calcification is calcium in normal tissues which is usually due to abnormal biochemistry, i.e., elevated serum calcium. The resultant metabolic imbalance leads to metastatic calcification when the solubility of calcium and phosphate or oxalates in extra cellular fluid is exceeded.

Dystrophic calcification is calcium seen in abnormal tissues such as vessels, haematoma, tumours and inflammatory masses and occurs when the solubility of the product of calcium and phosphate is exceeded due to pH changes or a reparative process. This is not considered to be true nephrocalcinosis.

### 15.2.1 Causes and Incidence of Nephrocalcinosis

The true incidence of nephrocalcinosis is difficult to establish. Mortensen and Emmett (1954) described the causes of nephrocalcinosis in 91 cases. More recently, Wrong and Feest (1976) described the causes in 375 patients. Cortical nephrocalcinosis accounts for 2.4% of causes, and medullary nephrocalcinosis accounts for the remaining 97.6%. The three most common causes of medullary nephrocalcinosis being quoted as primary hyperparathyroidism, renal tubular acidosis type 1 and medullary sponge kidney (Figs. 15.1 and 15.2).

### 15.2.2 Cortical Nephrocalcinosis

Cortical nephrocalcinosis is generally due severe destructive cortical disease, often seen in patients with end-stage renal failure (Fig. 15.3). It is seen outlining the periphery of the kidney and along the columns of Bertin.

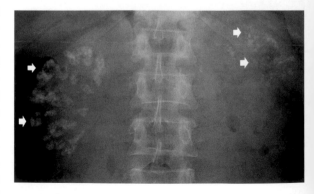

**Fig. 15.1** Plain abdomen radiography demonstrating parenchymal calcifications (*arrows*) in a patient with medullary sponge kidney

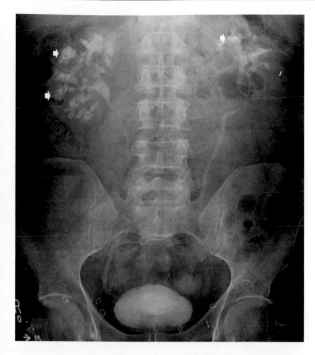

**Fig. 15.2** Intravenous excretory urography demonstrating parenchymal calcifications (*arrows*) in a patient with medullary sponge kidney

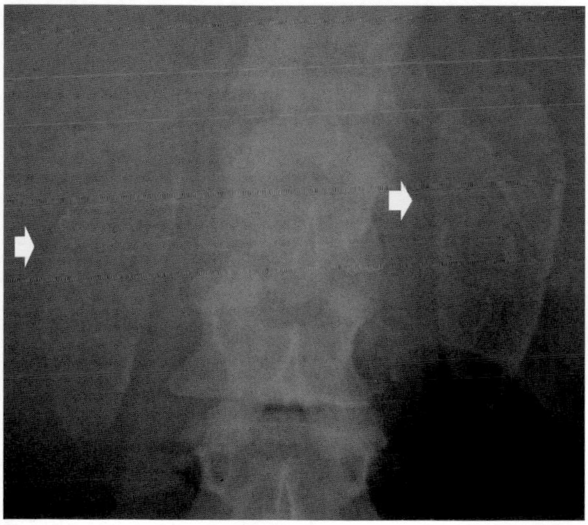

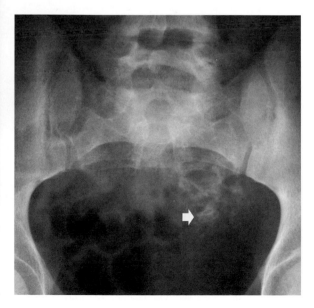

**Fig. 15.3** Plain abdomen radiography demonstrating bilateral uniform cortical nephrocalcinosis (*arrows*)

hypercalcemia and/or hypercalciuria involving many conditions which lead more frequently to nephrolithiasis (hyperparathyroidism, vitamin D intoxication, beryllium poisoning, systemic sarcoidosis, milk-alkali syndrome, hyperthyroidism, Addison disease, idiopathic hypercalcaemia of infancy, increased bone catabolism associated with myeloma, disseminated metastatic bone disease, leukaemia, and immobilisation hyperparathyroidism), and chronic renal infections (tuberculosis, AIDS organisms, chronic pyelonephritis) and rejected renal transplants. Ethylene glycol (antifreeze) poisoning can cause marked ballooning and hydropic or vacuolar degeneration of the proximal convoluted tubules and actually corresponds to a form of acute tubular necrosis. Calcium oxalate crystals are usually found in the tubular lumen in such poisonings since ethylene glycol can lead to secondary hyperoxaluria.

Any form of chronic glomerulonephritis can give rise to nephrocalcinosis. The calcification in these cases is seen as fine, granular densities on standard X-rays. Acute cortical necrosis gives rise to patchy calcification, often related to episodes of hypovolaemic shock and eclampsia. Other described causes of cortical nephrocalcinosis include chronic pyelonephritis, Alport's syndrome, renal transplants (Fig. 15.4), oxalosis, polycystic kidney disease and trauma.

Cortical nephrocalcinosis may be identified in many pathologic conditions such as acute tubular necrosis, chronic glomerulonephritis, Alport syndrome, prolonged

**Fig. 15.4** Plain radiograph of the pelvis demonstrating cortical calcification (*arrow*) in a transplant kidney

### 15.2.3 Medullary Nephrocalcinosis

This form of nephrocalcinosis constitutes the most frequently identified type. Medullary nephrocalcinosis is characterised by diffuse calcium deposition within the renal medulla. Underlying causes include medullary sponge kidney, distal renal tubular acidosis, hyperparathyroidism, milk-alkali syndrome, hypervitaminosis D, chronic pyelonephritis, chronic glomerulonephritis, sarcoidosis, glycogen storage disease, Wilson's disease, sickle cell anaemia, infections of the renal medulla, renal papillary necrosis and hyperuricemic (gout, Lesch–Nyhan syndrome) or hypokalemic conditions (primary hyperaldosteronism, long-term furosemide therapy, and Bartter's syndrome). This appears radiologically as small clusters of calcification in the pyramids (Fig. 15.5). In some causes the pathophysiology is well understood, such as oxalosis and analgesic nephropathy (Figs. 15.6 and 15.7). In other cases, the pathophysiology is less well understood, with characteristic association with hypercalcaemia or hypercalciuria. Hyperparathyroidism and renal tubular acidosis are the most commonly recognised causes of medullary nephrocalcinosis along with medullary sponge kidney.

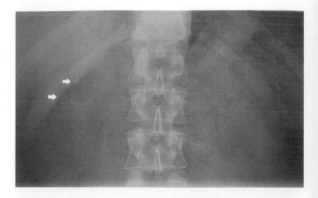

**Fig. 15.5** Plain abdomen radiography demonstrating pyramidal calcification in the right upper pole (*arrows*)

#### 15.2.3.1 Abnormal Calcium Metabolism

All hypercalcaemic or hypercalciuric states can give rise to medullary nephrocalcinosis. The most common is primary hyperparathyroidism secondary to an adenoma, which causes increased mobilisation of calcium from bone. Hypervitaminosis D, which causes increased absorption of calcium, is a well recognised cause of hypercalcaemia and nephrocalcinosis. This may be accidental, self induced or iatrogenic. The latter occurs despite normocalcaemia. Other causes include milk-alkali syndrome, sarcoidosis, immobilisation and hyperthyroidism.

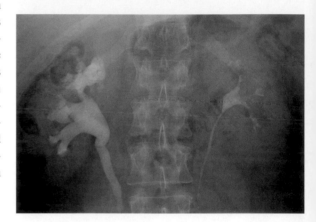

**Fig. 15.6** Intravenous excretory urography in a patient with analgesic nephropathy and a sloughed papilla causing hydronephrosis on the right kidney

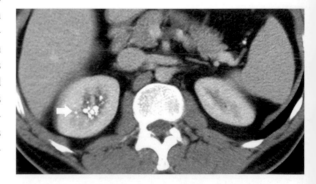

**Fig. 15.7** Contrast-enhanced computed tomography (CT) demonstrating pyramidal calcifications (*arrow*) in a patient with analgesic nephropathy

#### 15.2.3.2 Renal Tubular Diseases

Distal renal tubular acidosis is the second most common cause of medullary nephrocalcinosis. Most forms of distal renal tubular acidosis have a high incidence of nephrocalcinosis. The degree of nephrocalcinosis is more severe in these conditions than other causes. Calcium phosphate is believed to be deposited in the collecting ducts after precipitating from the urine.

Fanconi's syndrome, Wilson's disease and Amphotericin B toxicity are recognised common causes of secondary renal tubular acidosis. Proximal renal tubular acidosis does not manifest itself radiologically.

### 15.2.3.3 Medullary Sponge Kidney

The underlying aetiology in medullary sponge kidney is an anatomical defect of cystic dilatation of the distal collecting ducts. There is no underlying metabolic defect. Radiologically, this presents with dense papillary calcification, which has a characteristic appearance (Figs. 15.8–15.10). The disease may manifest itself unilaterally or segmentally.

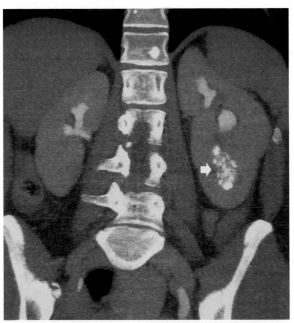

**Fig. 15.10** CT urography. Coronal reformats. Renal sponge kidney with regional medullary nephrocalcinosis (*arrow*) (from the editor E. Quaia)

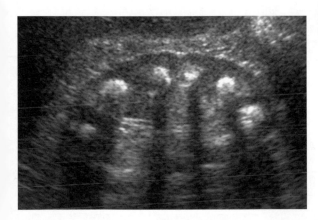

**Fig. 15.8** Ultrasound (US) demonstrating extensive medullary calcifications, manifesting with focal hyperechogenicity with posterior acoustic shadowing, in a patient with medullary sponge kidney

## 15.3 Nephrolithiasis

Nephrolithiasis is the description of the formation and passing of urinary tract calculi. The terms nephrolithiasis (refers to the kidney) and urolithiasis (refers to the ureter) indicate the presence of calcification(s) within the lumen of the collecting system, ureter and bladder. The commonest clinical manifestation is presentation with acute renal colic. Overall, world prevalence of nephrolithiasis is quoted at 2–3% (Menon and Resnick 2002); however this does vary around the world with different incidences quoted, depending on genetic background, race and climate. Calculus formation is related to an affluent lifestyle in developed countries. Peak incidence occurs in the fourth and fifth decade (Freeman and Sells 2008). Clinically, patients present with acute, severe loin pain when a renal calculus becomes impacted in the ureter causing obstruction, dysuria, stangury, haematuria and recurrent urinary tract infections. They can also present incidentally and chemically with dipstick haematuria, pyuria, sterile pyuria and proteinuria. However, calculi are often asymptomatic, identified as incidental findings on cross-sectional imaging. These incidental findings

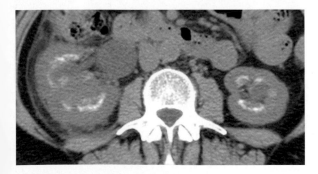

**Fig. 15.9** Unenhanced CT demonstrating extensive parenchymal calcification in a patient with medullary sponge kidney with perinephric stranding and an enlarged kidney

are, however, important as it can have important lifestyle implications including exclusion from certain occupations such as an airline pilot.

The clinical and metabolic presentation of stone disease can also change over time within various geographical regions. With careful clinical investigation and follow-up, it has been recognised that a cause for calculus formation can be elucidated in 97% of cases (Rivers et al. 2000). Seventy percent of renal calculi contain calcium, and it is recognised in patients with this form of calculus disease will form further calculi within 7 years (Asplin et al. 1996) (Fig. 15.11).

The principal locations of renal calculi are calyceal, renal pelvis, or ureteropelvic junction. If extracorporeal shock wave lithotripsy (ESWL) is considered, the size, location, and chemical composition of the urinary stones and the assessment of anatomic and functional anomalies in the upper urinary tract are of great importance in-order to assess and ensure the smooth passage of the fragmented calculi (Saw et al. 2000; Boll et al. 2009). ESWL is an out-patient procedure, usually administered without anaesthesia. ESWL represents the most common mode of therapy for renal stones, and it is indicated for any type of stones, even though it works better for softer stones such as uric acid stones. A variety of stone characteristics, such as stone size, location and composition, may affect the success of ESWL. ESWL is indicated in the treatment of renal stones <2 cm in diameter.

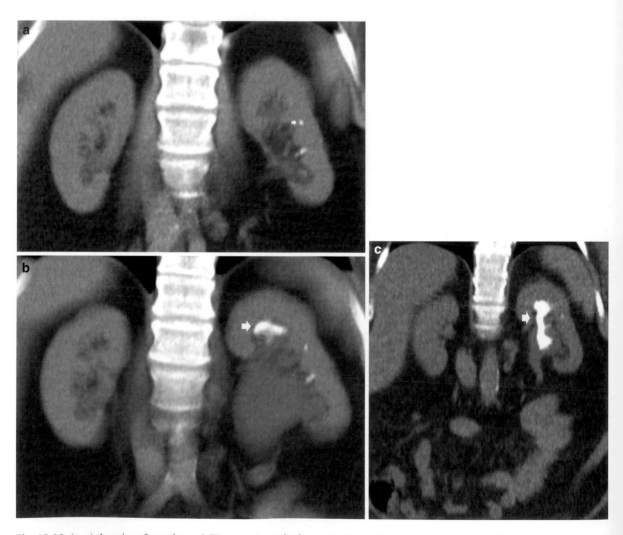

**Fig. 15.11** (**a–c**) A series of unenhanced CT coronal acquired over an 18 month period demonstrating initially a calculus (arrow) in the ureter causing hydronephrosis (**a**), then the progressive development of a staghorn calculus (*arrows*) (**b–c**)

Ureteric calculi are located distally in the ureter or ureterovesical junction. The American Urological Association published management guidelines for ureteric calculi (Segura et al. 1997). These guidelines recommend that patients whose calculi have a low probability of spontaneous passage (on the basis of their size and location) should be offered intervention. Newer semirigid, fibreoptic ureteroscopes can now be passed with minimal trauma, and in many cases, without dilatation. ESWL remains the first-line treatment for ureteric calculi, regardless of their site with better results for radiopaque stones less than 1 cm in diameter. For proximal ureteral stones of 1 cm or larger, ESWL, ureteroscopy, and percutaneous nephrolithotomy (PCNL) are all acceptable treatments (Teichman 2004). An endoscopic procedure (double J stent) can be inserted prior to ESWL in some cases, such as solitary kidney or large calculi. This decreases the number of complications. ESWL is contraindicated in pregnant patients, bleeding diathesis, uncontrolled hypertension, active urinary tract infections, and obstruction distal to the stone. Complications include vascular injury, perirenal haematoma, or subcapsular haematoma.

## 15.3.1 Incidence and Epidemiology

Risk of developing nephrolithiasis in the adult population varies in different parts of the world. The highest quoted incidence of nephrolithiasis is in Saudi Arabia at 20.1%, with incidences of 1–5% in Asia, 5–9% in Europe and 12–13% in Canada and North America (Ramello et al. 2000). Nephrolithiasis presents a peak incidence between 20 and 50 years of age, and overall male-to-female ratio of 4:1. Epidemiological factors for stone forming disease include race, sex, age, inherited and individual predisposing factors such as obesity. Environmental factors that influence formation include climate, socio-economic, diet and fluid intake.

### 15.3.1.1 Race and Sex

A higher incidence is quoted in males in the Caucasian population, which has been attributed to genetic make up. However, it is noted that the incidence difference in

Black Americans disappears when they adopt a Caucasian diet (Ramello et al. 2000). Conversely, the ratio is quoted as 0.5–0.7, respectively, male-to-female ratios in Black American and Hispanics (Michaels et al. 1994). The higher prevalence of nephrolithiasis in males has been attributed to the effect of androgens (Fan et al. 1999). Recent studies from the USA suggest that there is a changing gender prevalence of stone disease with a change from a 1.7:1 to −1.3:1 male-to-female ratio (Scales et al. 2007). This is speculated to be due to lifestyle factors and obesity.

### 15.3.1.2 Age

In idiopathic disease in males, a normal distribution of age is described with a peak incidence at 35 years. Females have a biphasic distribution peak, one at 30 years and the second at 55 years. This is thought to be secondary to calcium reabsorption secondary to the menopause.

### 15.3.1.3 Inherited Diseases

The incidence quoted for disease such as cystinuria (autosomal recessive) and hyperoxaluria is scant. Multiple predisposing factors have been identified including general factors (male gender), inherited conditions (polycystic kidney disease, renal tubular acidosis, hyperparathyroidism, cystinuria, and hypercalciuria), medications (triamterene, sulphonamides, carbonic anhydrase inhibitors, indinavir, acatazol amide, corticosteroids), low urine volume, hypercalciuria (hyperparathyroidism, sarcoidosis), hyperoxaluria, and hypocitraturia (distal renal tubular acidosis). The prevalence of cystinuria is estimated at 2% in the general population.

### 15.3.1.4 Individual Predisposing Factors

Obesity is associated with an increased risk of renal calculi, especially in females with a BMI over 40. Hypertensive patients are more likely to suffer from renal calculus disease. Factors influencing this are complex and may be due to the antihypertensive therapy and other dietary factors.

### 15.3.1.5 Environmental Factors

Calculus disease is more prevalent in a temperate climate. This has been described secondary to decreased fluid intake combined with high plasma vitamin D serum levels secondary to sun exposure.

### 15.3.1.6 Socio-Economic Factors

Calculus disease is seen as a disease of more affluent nations.

### 15.3.1.7 Diet

A high-protein diet has influence on calculus formation risk and calculus composition. Uric acid and calcium oxalate calculi are more prevalent in those with a diet high in animal proteins. The role of dairy products in the pathogenesis of renal calculus disease remains in debate.

## 15.3.2 Pathophysiology

Despite significant progress in the treatment of renal calculi, the degree of understanding of the pathogenesis of renal calculus disease has not paralleled this. It has been described that urinary supersaturation is necessary for clinical stone formation. This precipitates crystals to form in the urine. The crystals are believed to be retained in the tubules of the kidney. Several substances found in urine have been demonstrated to precipitate crystal formation, e.g., pyrophosphate, Tamm-Horsfall proteins and magnesium. Noncrystalline organic material, matrix, is then combined with crystal to form calculi. The mode that this occurs remains a source of ongoing research. Several theories have been proposed for pathogenesis. One such theory is crystal-induced renal injury secondary to hyperoxaluria, free particle hypothesis. This proposes that there is a rapid crystal growth in the tubular lumen resulting in crystals being trapped in the papillary collecting duct, resulting in stone formation. An intravascular phenomenon has been proposed with calculi forming as a result of this phenomenon in the vasa recta.

Insufficient or abnormal urinary inhibitor, which depends on the balance of supra-saturation and urinary inhibitors. Nano bacteria have been proposed as cytotoxic gram-negative bacteria are also implicated in other diseases such as atherosclerosis and periodontal disease. Urinary stasis secondary to anatomic abnormalities is also an identified cause, e.g., hydronephrosis, pelvoureteric junction obstruction and horseshoe kidney. Randall's plaques were described over 60 years ago, this suggested that calculi formed around calcium salt deposits in the tip of the renal papilla.

## 15.3.3 Types of Calculi

### 15.3.3.1 Calcium Calculi

Calcium oxalate stones account for 60% of all renal stones. This is followed by calcium phosphate types (hydroxy-apatite 20% and brushite 2%). Hypercalcaemia is the most important pathophysiological risk factor. This can be divided into three categories:

1. Absorptive hypercalciuria due to increased stone absorption of calcium.
2. Renal hypercalcaemia due to renal tubular resorption of calcium, which precipitates increasing PTH secretion due to low serum calcium.
3. Resorptive hypercalcaemia associated with primary hyperparathyroidism.

Other causes of hypercalcuria include malignancy, sarcoidosis, hyperparathyroidism and vitamin D toxicity. Hyperoxaluria, hyperuricosuria and gout can also give rise to calcium oxalate calculi.

Calcium oxalate calculi are dense and therefore relatively well identified on abdominal radiographs.

### 15.3.3.2 Cystine Stones

Cystinuria is an autosomal recessive disease that results in a defect in the renal tubular absorption of amino acids, which in turn results in cystinuria. These calculi are only identified on abdominal radiographs if they contain calcium.

### 15.3.3.3 Struvite or Infective Calculi

Struvite calculi are composed of magnesium and ammonium phosphate and account for between 7 and 13% of all renal calculi in the western world (Gleeson and Griffith 1993). They are formed secondary to infection by urease-producing bacteria, most commonly Proteus mirabilis. Struvite does not crystallise in the urine if the pH is less than 7.19. As urinary tract infections are more frequent in women, struvite calculi are seen in females more frequently than males (2:1). Pure struvite calculi are relatively rare; the most common manifestation of struvite calculi is triple stones, calcium-magnesium-ammonium phosphate stones. This is the most common composition of staghorn calculi (Figs. 15.11–15.13) and are clearly seen on abdominal radiographs. Pure struvite stones are radiolucent.

### 15.3.3.4 Uric Acid Calculi

The incidence of a uric acid stones varies from 40% in Israel to 10% in the USA. They are associated with obesity and type II diabetes. Three factors contributing to uric acid stones are hyperuricosuria, acidic urine and low urinary volume. Low urine pH is often related to medication and also associated with chronic diarrhoea and an ileostomy. A low urinary volume, less than 2 L/day, is considered to predispose to calculus formation. Hyperuricosuria is related to several inherited metabolic disorders such as Lesch Nynan syndrome and

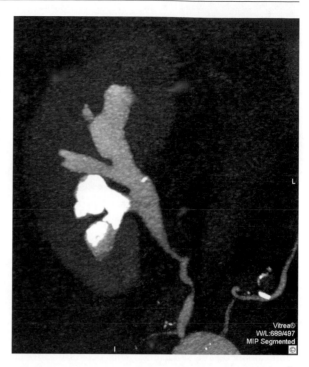

**Fig. 15.13** CT urography. Coronal reformat.

glycogen storage disease types I, III, Va and VII. Uric acid stones are radiolucent on abdominal radiographs. They, however have sufficient density to be demonstrated in CT and cast an acoustic shadow on ultrasound (US).

### 15.3.3.5 Xanthine Calculi

Xanthine calculi are seen in patients with hereditary xanthuria and those undergoing treatment with allopurinol. They are rare calculi with a density similar to that of uric acid calculi and have similar imaging characteristics.

### 15.3.3.6 Matrix Calculi

Like struvite calculi, matrix calculi are typically seen in patients with underlying proteus infections, as well as other infections such as *Escherichia coli* and *Candida albicans*. Their composition is mainly of coagulated mucoids with very little calcium component. They are radiolucent on abdominal X-rays.

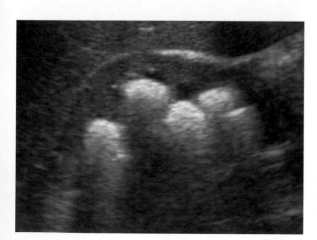

**Fig. 15.12** Grey-scale ultrasound. Longitudinal scan. Staghorn renal stone with multiple hyperechogenicities with posterior acoustic shadowing in the renal pelvis

### 15.3.3.7 Indinavir Calculi

Indinavir sulphate is a drug used widely to treat HIV infections. It is a protease inhibitor, and during clinical trials, 4% of patients receiving the therapy developed calculi. Indinavir crystals are precipitated in the urine forming calculi. These are radiolucent on both plain radiographs and CT (Schwartz et al. 1999). Calcium oxalate and phosphate precipitate within the indinavir crystals, and with time, the density all of the calculi will increase enough to become visible on CT and abdominal radiographs. Contrast-enhanced CT in the delayed phase is valuable in the diagnosis of non calcified indinavir calculi (Blake et al. 1998).

### 15.3.3.8 Oxalate Calculi

Oxaluria may be primary or secondary relating to underlying disorders such as inflammatory bowel disease and short, small bowel syndrome. This occurs due to fat malabsorption leading to saponification of calcium, leaving oxalate unbound, which is then absorbed in the mucosa of the colon.

Patients with coeliac disease as well as Crohn's disease have increased absorption of oxalate from the colon. Patients with inflammatory bowel disease are at increased risk of urolithiasis of all types, with a reported prevalence of 2–12% (Mcleod and Churchill 1992). Increased consumption of leafy green vegetables that are high in oxalate can also give rise to hyperoxaluria. This results in nephrocalcinosis and progressive formation of calcium oxalate stones. The majority of patients with calcium oxalate stones may not have any detectable abnormality of oxalate metabolite or hyperoxaluria. Oxalate calculi are usually radio-opaque on abdominal radiographs.

## 15.4  Imaging

### 15.4.1  Background and Principles

The main aims of imaging in patients with acute flank pain that can be related to renal colic are the detection of calculi or the non-stone disease; detection of nonurinary disease related to flank pain; assessment of size, number and location of the stone(s); detection of complications and evaluation of the contralateral kidney.

Four imaging techniques are employed to diagnose renal colic are: (1) plain abdominal radiography (kidney-ureter-bladder radiograph; KUB); (2) US; (3) intravenous urography; (4) helical CT.

Identifying the position of calculi anatomically will influence clinical management and intervention. Imaging should establish the physiological impact of the calculus, again influencing the ongoing management of renal disease. Abdominal radiography and intravenous urography were the main stay of imaging strategies until the end of the last century, along with US assessment. The advent of helical CT has seen these modalities largely superseded by a non-contrasted helical CT and excretory CT urography.

### 15.4.2  Abdominal Radiographs

The majority (90%) of renal tract calculi are dense enough to be identified on standard KUB abdominal radiographs (Spirnak et al. 1990) (Figs. 15.14 and 15.15). Renal calculi are usually single, polymorphic and with homogeneous opacity. Phleboliths typically appear as multiple round or oval opacities with a

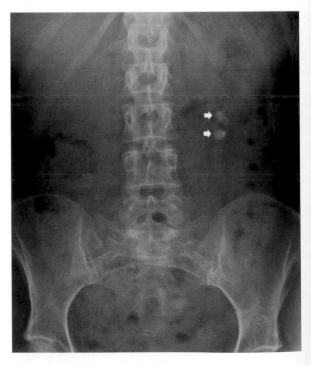

**Fig. 15.14** Plain abdomen radiography demonstrating calculi (*arrows*) within calyces of the left kidney

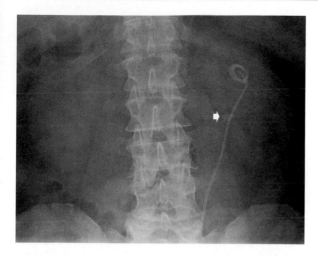

**Fig. 15.15** Plain abdomen radiography with ureteric stent in situ demonstrating a calculus (*arrow*) within the renal pelvis

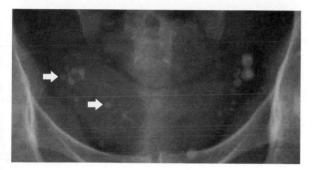

**Fig. 15.16** Plain abdomen radiography. Pelvic pleboliths appearing as multiple round or oval opacities with a central lucency (*arrows*), and lateral to the inferior portion of the sacrum

central lucency, and lateral to the inferior portion of the sacrum (Fig. 15.16). The sensitivity of the plain abdominal radiography in the detection of urinary calculi ranges from 44 to 77%, while the specificity ranges from 80 to 87% (Svedström et al. 1990; Haddad et al. 1992; Dalla Palma et al. 2001).

One of the main limitations of this technique is the presence of bowel gas and faecal material within the large bowel, which can obscure small calculi. The principal reasons for the limited visibility of renal stones on the plain radiography are bone overlapping and extra-urinary calcifications including vascular calcifications, calcified lymph nodes, focal zones of compact bone, and phleboliths. Patient body habitus can also give rise to interpretation difficulties. In patients presenting with loin pain, the KUB radiograph is often the initial investigation; however, it has been argued that this investigation is not necessary in the investigation of acute renal colic if unenhanced CT is utilised (Kennish et al. 2008).

The KUB is an extremely valuable tool in the follow-up of known renal calculi, especially those undergoing treatment and intervention for calculus disease (Fig. 15.15).

### 15.4.3 Intravenous Excretory Urography

In the USA, this examination has largely been superseded by unenhanced helical CT. However, in Europe and other parts of the world, this technique continues to be utilised where access to CT scanning may be limited. Intravenous excretory urography is a time- consuming technique, especially in obstructed patients; adds the risks of iodinated contrast administration; and is not suggested in acute ureteral obstruction due to contrast-induced diuresis.

The technique involves the intravenous administration of low osmolality non-ionic contrast medium and examination of the renal tract with targeted abdominal X-rays at selected time intervals. This will identify the position and anatomical location of calculi, along with a degree of obstruction if the calculus has passed into the ureter (Fig. 15.17).

The reported sensitivity of this technique for identifying calculi is 84–95%, but this falls when small calculi are considered (Miller and Kane 2000). The main disadvantage of this technique is the possible patient adverse reaction to intravenous contrast media, although this is small with non-ionic contrast media. Also, precise anatomical delineation is suboptimal if interventional techniques are considered. In this case, a CT should be performed for superior anatomical reference. The examination is contraindicated in patients with renal impairment and a serum creatinine over 150 μmol/L. It is recognised that some calculi are not identified with this technique with a detection rate of 69% (Dalla Palma et al. 2001). The utilisation of linear tomography has largely disappeared.

Digital tomography is a new technique that demonstrates promise, but this has yet to be fully evaluated in the context of other imaging modalities in the evaluation of the renal tract (Fig. 15.18). The findings of renal tract obstruction on intravenous urography include absent nephrogram, delayed nephrogram, renal enlargement, delayed pyelogram, extravasation of contrast, hydronephrosis, asymmetry in contrast density and delayed emptying of the collecting system.

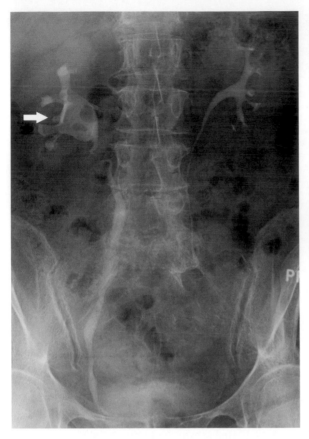

**Fig. 15.17** Intravenous excretory urography demonstrating a right staghorn calculus (*arrow*) appearing as a complex filling defect in the dilated renal pelvis

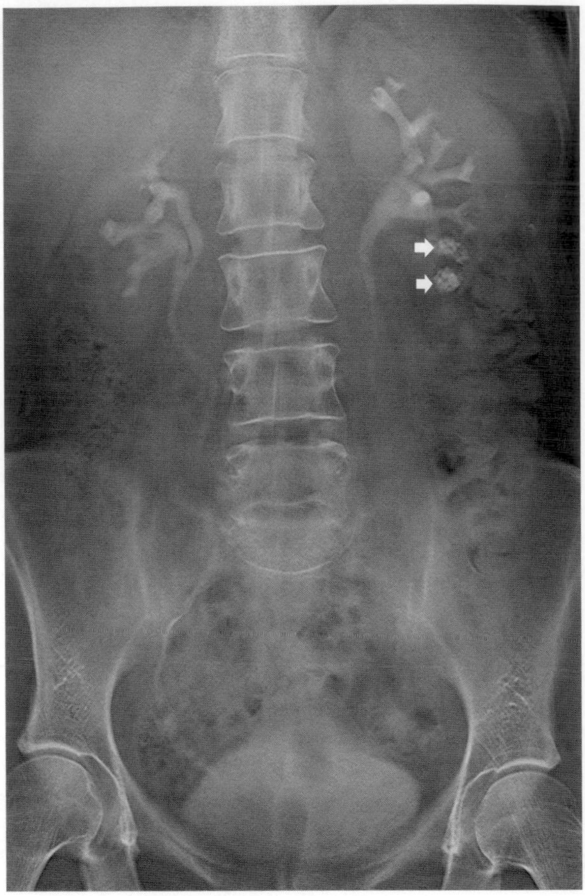

**Fig. 15.18** Digital tomosynthesis IVU demonstrating renal calculi (*arrows*) within the lower pole calyces of the left kidney

### 15.4.4 *Ultrasound*

US can be employed to detect hydronephrosis, to identify calculi, to assess the renal size and renal parenchyma thickness and detect complications. In non-hydrated patients, US presents a sensitivity of 24–73% (Fowler et al. 2002) and a specificity of 74%, while the sensitivity becomes 85–100% and the specificity 83–100% in hydrated patients (Middleton et al. 1988; Svedström et al. 1990; Haddad et al. 1992; Dalla Palma et al. 1993). US has a low sensitivity (20–30%) and high specificity (90%) in the detection of renal calculi ureteral stones, US presents a moderate sensitivity (60–70%) and high specificity (90–95%) (Fowler et al. 2002) in the detection of ureteral calculi. The main variables affecting the US sensitivity in detecting urinary stone are the calculus size and position, and patient body habitus, while calculus composition does not affect the diagnostic sensitivity and specificity of US. US allows the evaluation of the kidney and pelvis provided that the bladder is distended.

Renal and ureteral calculi are characteristically identified on US as echogenic foci with an acoustic shadow (Fig. 15.19). Renal calculi need to be 5 mm to be identified consistently on US, and US can identify calculi that are radiolucent on KUB X-ray. The detection of urinary stones and clarity of posterior shadowing are significantly improved by harmonic imaging (Ozdemir et al. 2008). The other US findings in a patient with renal colic, besides the direct identification of the calculus, consist of increased echogenicity of renal parenchyma, pelvicalyceal and ureteric dilatation, and subcapsular collections (urinomas) (Fig. 15.20).

Doppler US techniques are utilised to demonstrate haemodynamic changes that occur with obstruction,

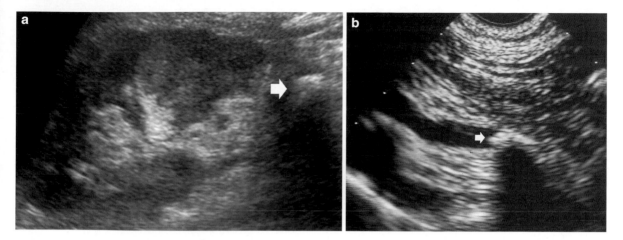

**Fig. 15.19** (**a**) Grey-scale ultrasound. Longitudinal scan. A calculus (*arrow*) with posterior acoustic shadowing is visualised in the lower pole of the left kidney. (**b**) Grey-scale ultrasound Longitudinal scan. A calculus (*arrow*) with posterior acoustic shadowing is visualised in the distal ureter

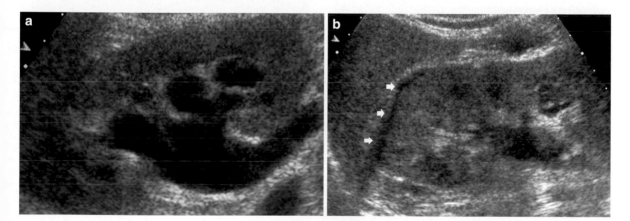

**Fig. 15.20** (**a–b**) Gray-scale ultrasound. Indirect signs of renal colic. (**a**)Dilatation of the intrarenal urinary tract; (**b**) subcapsular collections corresponding to urinoma (*arrows*) (courtesy of Prof. E. Quaia)

which results in intrarenal vascular resistance with associated rise in the resistance resistive index (RI). Duplex Doppler sonography has been reported to be a useful non-invasive imaging method for the diagnosis of renal obstruction. A mean RI >0.7, a difference >0.08–0.1 between the mean RI of the two kidneys, and a progressive increase in RI following fluid administration and diuretics have been considered diagnostic of obstruction (Platt 1992; Platt et al. 1992, 1993). The evaluation of renal parenchyma RIs presents a controversial role in the acute renal colic with a sensitivity from 19 to 92% and a specificity from 88 to 98% according to the different series (Platt et al. 1989a, b; Tublin et al. 1994; Lee et al. 1996; Platt 1996). This is determined by the absence of a true

reference standard to diagnose renal obstruction and by the possible presence of partial and intermittent obstruction.

It has been suggested that colour Doppler US along with KUB X-ray could be adopted the initial investigation of renal colic; however this has not been adopted in general clinical practice (Haddad et al. 1994). Twinkle artefact – also named colour comet-tail artefact (Campbell et al. 2004; Tchelepi and Ralls 2009) or sparkle sign – facilitates the detection of calculi, providing information on their chemical composition. It is determined by the random Doppler shift in the shadow of the stone and depends on the roughness of the surface of the stone. It is not visible in calcium oxalate calculi. Twinkle artefact may also be helpful in identifying calculi that are poorly echoic and lacking discrete shadowing (Fig. 15.21).

The detection of ureteral jets by colour Doppler does not imply the absence of obstruction since ureteral jets may be identified also in partial ureteral obstruction (Burge et al. 1991; Cox et al. 1992). The visibility of the ureteral jets depends on the flow velocity and density gradient between the urine in the bladder and ureter. This represents a time-consuming assessment and is not routinely employed.

The role of US in the follow-up of renal calculi is limited, with KUB and CT being more informative (Fowler et al. 2002). US is the preferred imaging modality in pregnancy over excretory urography, with incidence of renal stones equal to that in the non-pregnant female. This technique enables visualisation of the kidney and identification of calculi and obstruction without utilisation of ionising radiation. Filling defects on intravenous urography can be identified as being either soft tissue (e.g., clot or tumour) or renal calculi, on the basis of US. The role of US in the follow-up of renal calculi, which are being conservatively managed or undergoing treatment with extracorporeal shockwave lithotripsy (ESWL), is limited. It is difficult to reproduce measurements consistently with poorer spatial resolution and the associated issues surrounding a user-dependent technique.

## 15.4.5 Computed Tomography

The advent of multidetector row helical CT has revolutionised the imaging of renal calculi and nephrocalcinosis. Multidetector row CT allows image acquisition in a single breath-hold with thin-collimation (Figs. 15.22 and 15.23). With ever-improving technology, this has allowed improvement in spatial, temporal and contrast resolution the images obtained are of ever-increasing quality. The ability to perform multiplanar reformats (MPR) in orthogonal, oblique and curved planes, along with volume rendering and reconstruction techniques, optimises the anatomical delineation of the study. Accurate determination of the stone burden is a

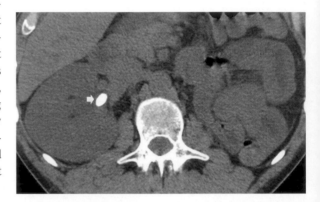

**Fig. 15.22** Unenhanced CT scan demonstrating a right renal pelvis calculus (*arrow*) in a patient with solitary kidney

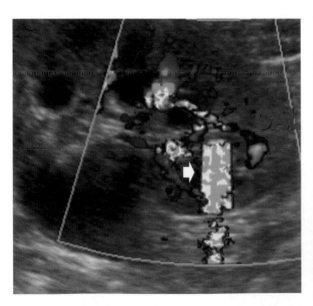

**Fig. 15.21** Ultrasound image demonstrating the sparkle sign or twinkle artefact sign (*arrow*) due to a calculus in a lower pole calyx (Courtesy of Dr F Bowyer)

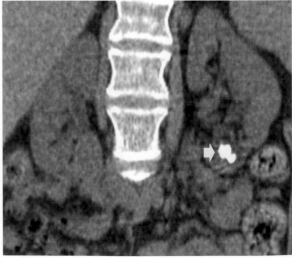

**Fig. 15.23** Coronal CT reformations showing lower pole calculi (*arrow*) in the left kidney

major advantage of this technique over IVU and linear tomography. The ability of CT to diagnose nonopaque calculi was recognised as far back as the 1970s (Segal et al. 1978). Ninety nine percent of calculi can be identified on CT, even though they are radiolucent on standard radiographs. Indinavir and pure matrix calculi are sometimes not identified on CT. There are two main techniques described for imaging of the renal tract by CT, non-contrasted helical CT and excretory CT urography.

### 15.4.5.1 Unenhanced CT

This technique was developed in the mid 1990s (Smith et al. 1995). It is currently the mainstay in the evaluation of renal calculi, especially in the USA and large parts of Europe, where some departments have completely abandoned intravenous urography in favour of

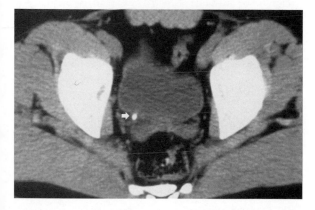

**Fig. 15.24** Unenhanced CT image demonstrating a ureteral stone (*arrow*) in the distal right ureter

CT techniques (Amis 1999; Silverman et al. 2009). This simple technique does not involve any patient preparation, oral or intravenous contrast with minimal imaging time. There is an increased radiation dose compared with intravenous urography, hence low-dose techniques are advocated (Tack et al. 2003; Hamm et al. 2002; Nawfel et al. 2004) (Figs. 15.24 and 15.25).

An optimally protocoled CT examination with low exposure factors does maintain its diagnostic accuracy (Meagher et al. 2001; Memarsadeghi et al. 2005). Unenhanced CT is more effective than intravenous urography in precisely identifying ureteric stones and is equally effective as IVU in the determination of the presence or absence of ureteric obstruction (Smith et al. 1995). Nowadays, thin-section 1-mm-collimation with a low pitch is possible in multidetector CT imaging of the urinary tract. Examinations are usually performed by using 120 kVp tube voltage, and 16 (detector rows) × 0.75-mm (section thickness), 64×0.5-mm, or 32×1-mm collimation, and 2-mm interval reconstruction. The tube current (100–330 mA, with a mean of 150 mA) is adjusted for each examination, according to patient body habitus, by using automated dose modulation algorithm.

The technique has a high sensitivity (94–100%) and specificity (93–98%) (Dalla Palma et al. 2001) with the added benefit of being able to identify alternative pathologies, which can mimic renal colic, such as pyelonephritis, hepatobiliary disease and vascular conditions (Rucker et al. 2004). Although this technique is more expensive than US and IVUs, it is considered to be more cost effective (Pfister et al. 2003). Patients are scanned in the supine position in a single breath hold. Prone scanning is advocated to demonstrate renal calculi

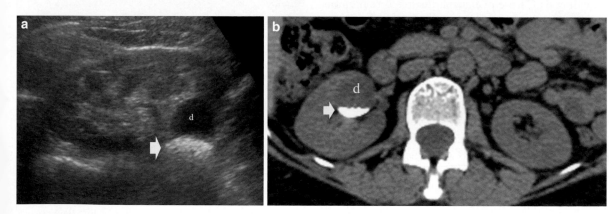

**Fig. 15.25** (**a**) Ultrasound of the right kidney demonstrating echogenic stone (*arrow*) within a calyceal diverticulum indicated by the letter *d*. (**b**) Unenhanced CT demonstrating the renal stone (*arrow*) within a calyceal diverticulum indicated by the letter *d*

that have passed to the vesicoureteric junction VUJ (Levine et al. 1999). The ability to reconstruct images in coronal and sagittal planes is beneficial. Reformatted images can then be performed in the coronal plane. Clinicians often prefer coronal reformatted images to review the data as it replicates the visual presentation of an intravenous urogram.

Unenhanced CT shows direct and indirect findings of colic pain due to stone. The direct finding is the visualisation of the calculus itself (Figs. 15.22–15.25). Regardless of composition, almost all renal stones are detected at unenhanced CT because the attenuation of stones is higher than that of surrounding tissue, even though the attenuation of uric stones is lower than the attenuation of calcium stones (Taourel et al. 2008). Indirect signs include ureteral dilatation (frequency: 65–90%) (Fig. 15.26a) with or without perirenal urinoma (Fig. 15.26b), perinephric (Fig. 15.27) and periureteral (Fig. 15.28) stranding (36–82%), renal enlargement (frequency 36–71%) and reduced attenuation (>5 HU) of the renal parenchyma (pale kidney sign) (Georgiades et al. 2001; Goldman et al. 2004), renal sinus fat blurring (Fig. 15.29) (Smith et al. 1996; Niall et al. 1999; Sourtzis et al. 1999), and the rim sign around the ureter (frequency 50–77%) (Fig. 15.30).

An early sign of acute ureteric obstruction is the effacement of pelvicalyceal fat, perinephric oedema or stranding in the perinephric space and may evolve into a frank perinephric fluid collection. Boridy et al. (1999) described this as being due to urine in infiltrating into the perinephric space along the bridging septa of Kuhn, possibly a result of pyelolymphatic backflow (Fig. 15.27). Differential diagnoses that should always be considered in patients presenting with perinephric stranding on CT are pyelonephritis, renal vein thrombosis and renal infarction.

The most important challenge in the interpretation of unenhanced CT in the evaluation of patients with suspected urolithiasis is the frequent inability to identify the ureter among periureteral vessels and to differentiate urinary calculi from extra-urinary calcifications, in particular from phleboliths. The rim sign is specific for the urinary stone, while the comet-tail sign is specific for phleboliths (Fig. 15.31). The comet-tail sign consists in the eccentric tapering of soft tissue extending from one surface of the calcification. Moreover, most phleboliths are round or oval, while most renal or ureteral calculi are slightly angular in shape. Phleboliths may contain a central lucent area, even though this is rarely observed on CT (Traubici et al. 1999).

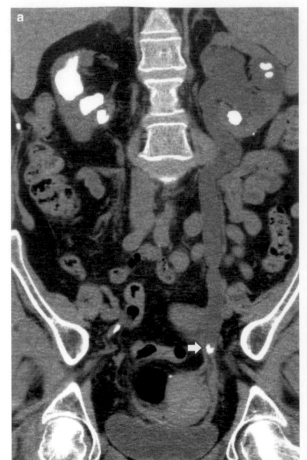

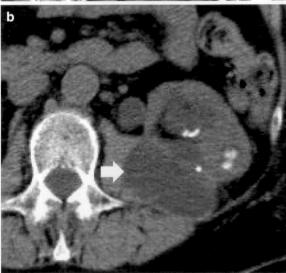

**Fig. 15.26** (**a**, **b**) Indirect signs of renal calculi. (**a**) Unenhanced CT. Coronal reformation. Left urinary tract dilatation due to an obstructing ureteral stone (*arrow*). Multiple renal calculi are evident on the left kidney, while staghorn calculosis is depicted on the right kidney. (**b**) Unenhanced CT. Transverse plane. Peri-renal urinoma (*arrow*) (courtesy of Prof. E. Quaia)

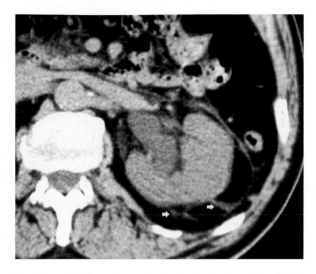

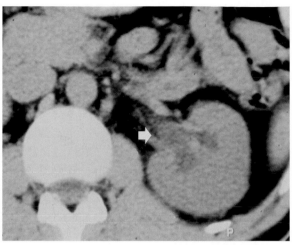

**Fig. 15.27** Indirect signs of renal calculi. Unenhanced CT. Transverse plane. Perinephric strandings (*arrows*) surrounding the enlarged left kidney with dilatation of the intrarenal urinary tract (courtesy of Prof. E. Quaia)

**Fig. 15.29** Indirect signs of renal calculi. Unenhanced CT. Transverse plane. Renal sinus fat blurring (*arrow*) with increased density of the sinus fat (courtesy of Prof. E. Quaia)

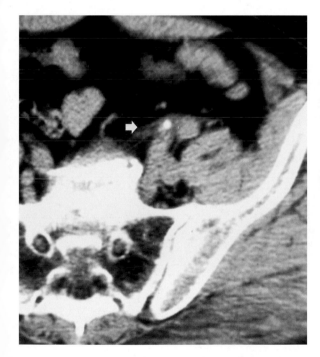

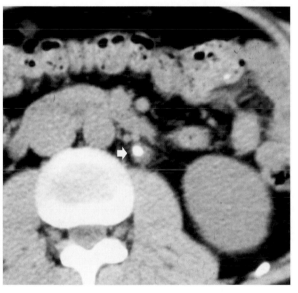

**Fig. 15.30** Indirect signs of renal calculi. Unenhanced CT. Transverse plane. Rim sign (*arrows*) around the dilated ureter with a renal calculi (courtesy of Prof. E. Quaia)

**Fig. 15.28** Indirect signs of renal calculi. Unenhanced CT. Transverse plane. Periureteral strandings (*arrow*) with dilatation of the distal ureter presenting a stone (courtesy of Prof. E. Quaia)

Another important task of unenhanced CT is the differentiation of renal colic from other causes of acute flank pain including diverticulitis or appendicitis, pelvic masses, large renal tumours, bowel obstruction, and aortic aneurysm. Most of these pathologic entities are identified on unenhanced CT. The advantage of unenhanced CT to evaluate for renal calculi in the acute setting is the identification of extra renal diagnoses such as appendicitis, gynaecological disease, and most notably, ruptured abdominal aortic aneurysms whose clinical presentation can frequently mimic renal colic.

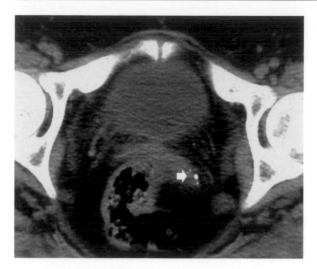

**Fig. 15.31** Indirect signs of renal calculi. Unenhanced CT. Transverse plane. Comet-tail (*arrows*) adjacent to pelvic phleboliths consisting of eccentric tapering of soft tissue extending from one surface of the calcification (courtesy of Prof. E. Quaia)

Site, size and density of renal calculi can be determined by CT, a density of greater than 1,000 HU being considered to be less responsive to ESWL (Joseph et al. 2002). Theoretically, CT also has the ability to identify the chemical composition of renal calculi; this, however, has not been adopted into clinical practice (Hillman et al. 1984; Deveci et al. 2004). The dual energy CT attenuation value can be used to predict the chemical composition of the stones in vitro (Grosjean et al. 2008; Thomas et al. 2009; Boll et al. 2009). This ability indicates the strength of CT as an imaging tool over that of intravenous urography or US. The identification of cystine and calcium oxalate would be beneficial as they are relatively resistant to ESWL. Nakada et al. (2000) described the ability to differentiate between uric acid and calcium oxalate stones in the clinical setting. Three-dimensional (3D) reconstructions can add greater anatomical information. Which is beneficial when intervention is considered, it may influence the choice of ESWL and PCNL.

Since the radiation exposure from KUB is 0.5–0.9 mSv, from intravenous urography is 1.33–3.5 mSv, while from regular dose CT is 4.3–16.1 mSv, the employment of low-dose unenhanced CT is advocated. In single slice CT, the higher the pitch, the lower the corresponding dose, however, in multidetector CT, the lower the current tube (mA) the lower the corresponding dose (Mahesh et al. 2001). With the most recent low-dose CT protocols,

it is possible to achieve a dose of 0.97–1.35 mSv (Knöpfle et al. 2003), while with ultra-low-dose CT (20 mA), a dose of 0.5–0.7 mSv (Kluner et al. 2006).

### 15.4.5.2 CT Urography

This technique is the CT examination of renal imaging tract after the administration of intravenous contrast, with delayed imaging to visualise the collecting systems and lower tracts during the excretory phase.

CT urography is being introduced for 3D evaluation of those patients with complex renal calculus disease in whom PCNL is considered (Patel et al. 2009). This technique allows optimal anatomical delineation both for renal (Fig. 15.32) and urinary stones (Figs. 15.33 and 15.34). The most common indication for this procedure is the investigation of microscopic haematuria in the examination of the urothelium for upper and lower tract

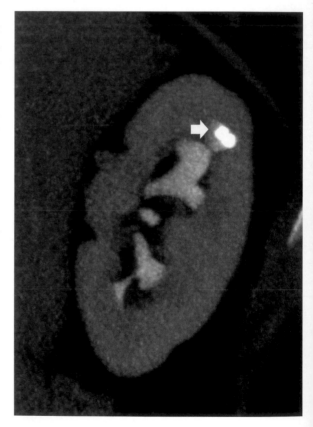

**Fig. 15.32** CT urography. Coronal reformation. Renal calculus within a calyceal diverticulum (*arrow*) on the upper calyces of the left kidney (courtesy of Prof. E. Quaia)

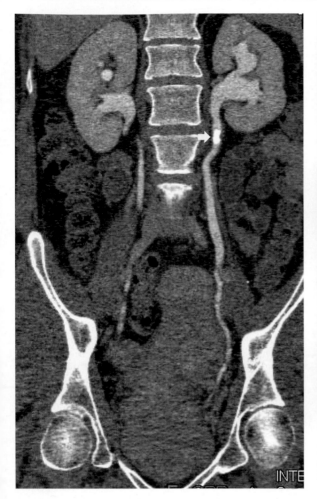

**Fig. 15.33** CT urography. Coronal reformation. Mild hydronephrosis on the left kidney with an obstructing calculus in the proximal ureter (*arrow*). Right pelvicalyceal drainage is normal with IV contrast seen in the right ureter (courtesy of Prof. E. Quaia)

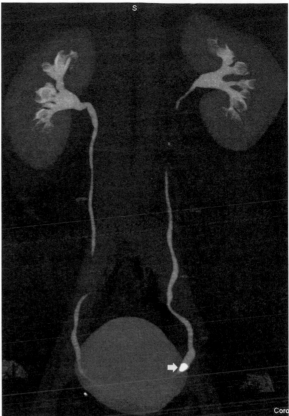

**Fig. 15.34** CT urography. Maximum intensity projection. A calculus is visualised in the distal ureter (*arrow*) (courtesy of Prof. E. Quaia)

neoplastic lesions (Silverman et al. 2009). The technique utilised varies widely from department to department; optimal protocols have yet to be decided (Townsend et al. 2009). There are reports of dual-energy contrast enhanced CT, relating to the ability of this technique to subtract the contrast-enhanced data set, creating virtual unenhanced CT images (Scheffel et al. 2007).

## 15.4.6 Other Techniques

Magnetic resonance urography (MRU) has been universally adopted as a non-ionising radiation investigation of the renal tract. The technique has a limited role in the evaluation of renal calculi, although has demonstrated benefit on examination of the renal tract in specific groups such as those of pregnant patients presenting with symptoms of ureteric colic. It can be useful to differentiate between physiological hydronephrosis and ureteric calculi. This technique enables reconstruction of the images from the raw data set to present images that mimic a conventional IVU. Spatial resolution is, however, poor. There may also be difficulty in differentiating filling defects seen on MRU, the appearances of early urothelial tumours and small calculi being very similar (Girish et al. 2004).

# References

Amis ES Jr (1999) Epitaph for the urogram. Radiology 213: 639–640

Asplin JR, Favus MJ, Coe FL (1996) Nephrolithiasis. In: Brenner BM (ed) The kidney. WB Saunders, Philadelphia, PA, pp 1893–1935

Blake SP, McNicholas MM, Raptopoulos V (1998) Non opaque crystal deposition causing ureteric obstruction in patients with HIV undergoing indinavir therapy. AJR 171:717–720

Boll DT, Patil NA, Paulson EK et al. (2009) Renal stone assessment with dual-energy multidetector CT and advanced post-processing techniques: improved characterization of renal stone composition – pilot study. Radiology 250:813–820

Boridy IC, Kawashima A, Goldman SM et al. (1999) Acute ureteolithiasis: nonenhanced helical CT findings of perinephric oedema for prediction of degree of ureteral obstruction. Radiology 213:663–667

Burge HJ, Middleton WD, McClennan BL et al. (1991) Ureteral jets in healthy subjects and in patients with unilateral ureteral calculi: comparison with color Doppler US. Radiology 180(2):437–442

Campbell SC, Cullinnan JA, Rubens DJ (2004) Slow flow or no flow? Color and power Doppler US pitfalls in the abdomen and pelvis. Radiographics 28:497–506

Cox IH, Erickson SJ, Foley WD et al. (1992) Ureteric jets: evaluation of normal flow dynamics with color Doppler sonography. AJR 158:1051–1055

Dalla Palma L, Pozzi-Mucelli R, Stacul F (2001) Present-day imaging of patients with renal colic. Eur Radiol 11:4–17

Dalla Palma L, Stacul F, Bazzocchi M et al. (1993) Ultrasonography and plain film versus intravenous urography in ureteric colic. Clin Radiol 47(5):333–336

Deveci S, Co kun M, Tekin M et al. (2004) Spiral computed tomography: role in determination of chemical compositions of pure and mixed urinary stones-an in vitro study. Urology 64:237–240

Fan J, Chandhoke PS, Grampas SA (1999) Role of sex hormones in experimental calcium oxalate nephrolithiasis. J Am Soc Nephrol 10:S376–S380

Fowler KA, Locken JA, Duchesne JH et al. (2002) US for detecting renal calculi with nonenhanced CT as a reference standard. Radiology 222:109–113

Freeman SJ, Sells S (2008) Investigation of loin pain. Imaging 20:38–56

Georgiades CS, Moore CJ, Smith DP (2001) Differences of renal parenchymal attenuation for acutely obstructed and unobstructed kidneys on unenhanced helical CT: a useful secondary sign? AJR 175:325–330

Girish G, Chooi WK, Morocos SK (2004) Filling defect artefacts in magnetic resonance urography. Eur Rad 14:145–150

Gleeson MJ, Griffith DP (1993) Struvite calculi. Br J Urol 71:503–511

Goldman SM, Faintuch S, Ajzen SA et al. (2004) Diagnostic value of attenuation measurements of the kidney on unenhanced helical CT of obstructive ureteolithiasis. AJR 182:1251–1254

Grosjean R, Sauer B, Guerra RM et al. (2008) Characterization of human renal stones with MDCT: advantage of dual energy and limitations due to respiratory motion. AJR 190:720–728

Haddad MC, Sharif HS, Abomelha MA et al. (1994) Colour Doppler sonography and plain abdominal radiography in the management of patients with renal colic. Eur Radiol 4: 529–532

Haddad MC, Sharif HS, Shahed MS et al. (1992) Renal colic: diagnosis and outcome. Radiology 184:83–88

Hamm M, Knopfle E, Wartenberg S et al. (2002) Low dose unenhanced helical computerized tomography for the evaluation of acute flank pain. J Urol 167:1687–1691

Hillman BJ, Drach GW, Tracey P et al. (1984) Computed tomographic analysis of renal calculi. AJR 142:549–552

Joseph P, Mandal AK, Singh KL et al. (2002) Computerized tomography attenuation value of renal calculus: can it predict successful fragmentation of the calculus by extracorporeal shock wave lithotripsy? A preliminary study. J Urol 167:1968–1971

Kennish SJ, Bhatnagar P, Wah TM et al. (2008) Is the KUB radiograph redundant for investigating acute ureteric colic in the non-contrast enhanced computed tomography era? Clin Radiol 63:1131–1135

Kluner C, Hein PA, Gralla O et al. (2006) Does ultra-low-dose CT with a radiation dose equivalent to that of KUB suffice to detect renal and ureteral calculi? J Comput Assist Tomogr 30(1):44–50

Knöpfle E, Hamm M, Wartenberg S et al. (2003) CT in ureterolithiasis with a radiation dose equal to intravenous urography: results in 209 patients. Rofo 175(12): 1667–1672

Levine J, Neitlich J, Smith RC (1999) The value of prone scanning to distinguish ureterovesical junction stones from ureteral stones that have passed into the bladder: leave no stone unturned. AJR 172:977–981

Mahesh M, Scatarige JC, Cooper J et al. (2001) Dose and pitch relationship for a particular multislice CT scanner. AJR 177(6):1273–1275

McLeod RD, Churchill DN (1992) Urolithiasis complicating inflammatory bowel disease. J Urol 148:974–978

Meagher T, Sukmar VP, Collingwodd J et al. (2001) Low dose computed tomography in suspected acute colic. Clin Radiol 56:873–876

Memarsadeghi M, Heinz-Peer G, Schaefer-Prokop et al. (2005) Unenhanced multi-detector row CT in patients suspected of having urinary stone disease: effect of section width on diagnosis. Radiology 235:530–536

Menon M, Resnick MI (2002) Urinary lithiasis: etiology, diagnosis, and medical management. In: Walsh PC, Retik AB, Darracott VE Jr (eds) Campbell's urology. WB Saunders, Philadelphia, PA, pp 3229–3305

Michaels EK, Nakagawa Y, Miura N et al. (1994) Racial gender variation in gender frequency of calcium urolithiasis. J Urol 152:2228–2231

Middleton WD, Dodds WJ, Lawson TL et al. (1988) Renal calculi: sensitivity for detection with US. Radiology 167:239–244

Miller OF, Kane CJ (2000) Unenhanced helical computed tomography in the evaluation of acute flank pain. Curr Opin Urol 10:123–129

Mortensen JD, Emmett JL (1954) Nephrocalcinosis: a collective and clinicopathological study. J Urol 71:398–406

Nakada SY, Douglas GH, Attai S et al. (2000) Determination of stone composition by noncontrast spiral computed tomography in the clinical setting. Urology 55:816–819

Nawfel RD, Judy PF, Schleipman AR et al. (2004) Patient radiation dose at CT urography and conventional urography. Radiology 232:126–132

Niall O, Russell J, MacGregor R et al. (1999) A comparison of noncontrast computerized tomography with excretory urography in the assessment of acute flank pain. J Urol 161(2): 534–537

Ozdemir H, Demir MK, Temizöz O et al. (2008) Phase inversion harmonic imaging improves assessment of renal calculi: a comparison with fundamental gray-scale sonography. J Clin Ultrasound 36(1):16–19

Patel U, Walkden RM, Ghani KR et al. (2009) Three-dimensional CT pyelography for planning of percutaneous nephrostolithotomy: accuracy of stone measurement, stone depiction and pelvicalyceal reconstruction. Eur Radiol 19:1280–1288

Pfister SA, Deckaret A, Laschke S et al. (2003) Unenhanced helical computed tomography vs intravenous urography in patients with acute flank pain:accuracy and economic impact in a randomized prospective trial. Eur Radiol 13:2513–2520

Platt JF (1992) Duplex Doppler evaluation of native kidney dysfunction. Obstructive and nonobstructive disease. AJR 158: 1035–1042

Platt JF (1996) Urinary obstruction. Radiol Clin North Am 34:1113–1129

Platt JF, Rubin JM, Ellis JH (1989a) Distinction between obstructive and non obstructive pyelocaliectasis with Duplex Doppler sonography. AJR 153:997–1000

Platt JF, Rubin JM, Ellis JH et al. (1989b) Duplex Doppler US of the kidney: differentiation of obstructive and nonobstructive dilatation. Radiology 171:515–517

Platt JF, Rubin JM, Ellis JH (1993) Acute renal obstruction: evaluation with intrarenal duplex Doppler and conventional US. Radiology 186:685–688

Ramello A, Vitale C, Marangella M (2000) Epidemiology of nephrolithiasis. J Nephrol 13(suppl 3):S65–S70

Rivers K, Shetty S, Menon M (2000) When and how to evaluate a patient with nephrolithiasis. Urol Clin North Am 27:203–213

Rucker CR, Menias CO, Bhalla S (2004) Mimics of renal colic: alternative diagnoses at unenhanced helical CT. Radiographics 27:S11–S28

Sandhu C, Anson KM, Patel U (2003) Urinary tract stones – part I: role of radiological imaging in diagnosis and treatment planning. Clin Radiol 58:415–421

Saw KC, McAteer JA, Monga AG et al. (2000) Helical CT of urinary calculi: effect of stone composition, stone size, and scan collimation. AJR 175:329–332

Scales CD, Curtis LH, Norris R et al. (2007) Changing gender prevalence of stone disease. J Urol 177:979–982

Scheffel H, Stolzman P, Frauenfelder T et al. (2007) Dual-energy contrast-enhanced computed tomography for the detection of urinary stone disease. Invest Radiol 42:823–829

Schwartz B, Schenkman N, Armenakas N et al. (1999) Imaging characteristics of indinavir calculi. J Urol 161:1085–1087

Segal AJ, Spataro RF, Linke CA et al. (1978) Diagnosis of non-opaque calculi by computed tomography. Radiology 129: 447–450

Segura JW, Preminger GM, Assimos DG et al. (1997) Ureteral Stones Clinical Guidelines Panel summary report on the management of ureteral calculi. J Urol 158:1915–1921

Silverman SG, Leyendecker JR, Amis ES Jr (2009) What is the current role of CT urography and MR urography in the evaluation of the urinary tract? Radiology 250:309–323

Smith RC, Rosenfield AT, Choe KA et al. (1995) Acute flank pain: comparison of non-contrasted CT and intravenous urography. Radiology 194:789–794

Smith RC, Verga M, Dalrymple N et al. (1996) Acute ureteral obstruction: value of secondary signs of helical unenhanced CT. AJR 167(5):1109–1113

Sourtzis S, Thibeau JF, Damry N et al. (1999) Radiologic investigation of renal colic: unenhanced helical CT compared with excretory urography. AJR 172(6):1491–1494

Spirnak JP, Resnick MI, Banner MP (1990) Calculus disease of the urinary tract. In Davidson AJ, Hartman D (eds) Radiology of the kidney and urinary tract. WB Saunders, Philadelphia, PA, pp 53–96

Svedström E, Alanen A, Nurmi M (1990) Radiologic diagnosis of renal colic: the role of plain film, excretory urography and sonography. Eur J Radiol 11(3):180–183

Tack D, Sourtzis S, Dellpierre I et al. (2003) Low dose multidetector CT of patients with suspected renal colic. AJR 180:305–311

Taourel P, Thuret R, Hoquet MD et al. (2008) Computed tomography in the nontraumatic renal causes of acute flank pain. Semin Ultrasound CT MRI 29:341–352

Tchclepi H, Ralls PW (2009) Color comet-tail artifact: clinical applications. AJR 192:11–18

Teichman JMH (2004) Acute renal colic from ureteral calculus. N Engl J Med 350:684–693

Thomas C, Patschan O, Ketelsen D et al. (2009) Dual-energy CT for the characterization of urinary calculi: in vitro and in vivo evaluation of a low-dose scanning protocol. Eur Radiol 19:1553–1559

Townsend BA, Silverman SG, Mortele KJ et al. (2009) Current use of computed tomographic urography: survey of the Society of Uroradiology. J Comput Assist Tomogr 33: 96–100

Traubici J, Neitlich JD, Smith RC (1999) Distinguishing pelvic phleboliths from distal ureteral stones on routine unenhanced helical CT: is there a radiolucent center? AJR 172:13–17

Wrong OM, Feest TG (1976) Nephrocalcinosis. In: Peters DK (ed) Advanced medicine no 12. Pitman Medical, London, pp 394–206

# Acute Renal Infections

**16**

Alfredo Blandino, Silvio Mazziotti, Fabio Minutoli,
Giorgio Ascenti, and Michele Gaeta

## Contents

## Abstract

> Urinary tract infections (UTI) are a very common urologic disease and one of the most common infectious disorders among human beings. Women are more prone to develop urinary tract infections than men, in the vast majority of the cases due to *Escherichia coli*.

> In adults, diagnosis of UTI is characteristically based on typical clinical symptoms and laboratory findings. Imaging is usually requested for patients who do not respond to antimicrobial therapy, especially when there is a strong suspicion of involvement of the upper urinary tracts and kidney, i.e. acute pyelonephritis.

> Computed tomography (CT) is the modality of choice in evaluating acute bacterial pyelonephritis. In fact, CT performed immediately after contrast material injection and at delayed intervals provides highly specific features and an accurate assessment of intra- and extrarenal complications, represented mainly by renal and extrarenal abscesses and gas forming infections.

> Conversely, ultrasound (US), contrast-enhanced ultrasound, and magnetic resonance imaging (MRI) can also be useful in some limited circumstances.

> Nuclear medicine plays an important role in evaluating acute pyelonephritis in children.

A. Blandino (✉), S. Mazziotti, F. Minutoli, G. Ascenti,
and M. Gaeta
Department of Radiological Science, University of Messina,
Policlinico "G. Martino", Gazzi, Messina, Italy
e-mail: ablandino@unime.it

E. Quaia (ed.), *Radiological Imaging of the Kidney*,
Medical Radiology, DOI: 10.1007/978-3-540-87597-0_16, © Springer-Verlag Berlin Heidelberg 2011

# 16.1 Acute Bacterial Pyelonephritis

## 16.1.1 Clinical Features and Pathophysiology

Two definitions can be proposed for acute bacterial pyelonephritis:

- A clinical definition, based on clinical and laboratory findings.
- A pathologic definition, related to the anatomopathological macro and microscopic abnormalities.

Although pyelonephritis is defined as inflammation of the renal pelvis and kidney, the diagnosis is clinical (Schaeffer and Schaeffer 2007).

Acute pyelonephritis is a typical clinical syndrome characterized by an abrupt onset of chills, high-grade fever (>38.5°C), and unilateral or bilateral flank pain with costovertebral tenderness. These so-called *"upper tract signs"* are frequently accompanied by urinary frequency and urgency, dysuria, and soprapubic pain; finally, in rare circumstances, gastrointestinal symptoms such as abdominal pain, vomiting, and diarrhea can be present. Asymptomatic progression of acute to chronic pyelonephritis may result in the absence of overt symptoms, especially in compromised host (Schaeffer and Schaeffer 2007).

Laboratory findings comprise pyuria and bacteriuria, leukocitosis within the blood with a predominance of neutrophils, elevated C-reactive protein level, and increased erythrocyte sedimentation rate. Additionally, creatinine clearance can be decreased and generally, blood cultures may be positive.

Urinalysis reveals numerous white blood cells (WBCs), chains of cocci, and large numbers of leukocyte casts in the urinary sediment; the latter being very specific for acute pyelonephritis.

Besides, two types of infections can be found, complicated and uncomplicated, generally related to the interaction between the uropathogens and the host (Talner et al. 1994). The virulence factors of the bacteria, the inoculum size as well as the inadequacy of host protection mechanisms are responsible for the favorable infection of the urinary tract (Schaeffer and Schaeffer 2007).

The term *uncomplicated* refers to infections in a healthy patient, generally women in the premenopausal state, with a structurally and functionally normal urinary tract (Schaeffer and Schaeffer 2007). The vast majority of these patients respond successfully to treatment and the infecting organisms are eradicated by a short course of oral antimicrobial therapy.

In these circumstances, the onset of infection is in the lower urinary tract, the bladder, with an isolated or recurrent bacterial cystitis or acute pyelonephritis; prompt response to antibiotic therapy do not require any imaging studies.

Conversely, *complicated infections* occur in patients that, for clinical, functional, or morphological conditions, have a major risk of infections, a decrease in the efficacy of therapy, and the possibility of resistance to the antimicrobial therapy.

The vast majority of these patients are men, and the most important factors responsible for complicated infections are the following: (a) functional or congenital or acquired anatomic abnormalities of the urinary tract (e.g., vesico-ureteral reflux (VUR), calculi, or urinary tract obstruction, altered bladder function, prostatic hypertrophy, carrier of an indwelling catheter or intermittent catheterization, etc.). (b) Pregnancy, (c) altered host resistance or increased virulence and/or antimicrobial resistance of pathogens (e.g., elderly, diabetes, immunosuppression, hospital-acquired infections, renal transplantation, neutropenia, HIV-positive patients, chronic renal insufficiency, recent antimicrobial agent use, or recent hospitalization in the previous month).

Diabetic patients are of particular concern because they are prone to develop acute complicated pyelonephritis; moreover, it is sometimes very difficult to get the correct diagnosis on clinical grounds in patients with diabetes, because as many as 50% of these patients will not suffer from the so called "upper tract signs" like flank pain or costovertebral tenderness that are very helpful in differentiating pyelonephritis from simple cystitis or lower urinary tract infections (UTIs). As such, an early or more aggressive approach to imaging in patients with diabetes may be beneficial (Dunnick et al. 2001).

*Escherichia coli* is by far the most common cause of infections, accounting for 80% of community-acquired and 50% of hospital-acquired infections. Two other common gram-negative Enterobacteriaceae, *Proteus* and *Klebsiella*, and gram-positive *Escherichia faecalis*, *Staphylococcus aureus*, and *saprophyticus* are responsible for the rest of most community-acquired infections. The other most common pathogens that cause nosocomial infections are *Enterobacter*, *Klebsiella*, *Pseudomonas aeruginosa*, *Citrobacter*, and *E. faecalis* (Dunnick et al. 2001).

Sometimes, the age of the patients or the predisposing condition can influence the predominance of the infecting organism. For example, Latham et al. (1983) state that *Staphylococcus saprophyticus* is now recognized as causing approximately 10% of symptomatic lower UTIs in young sexually active females, whereas, less common pathogens like Gardenella vaginalis and Ureaplasma urealyticum may infect patients with an indwelling catheter (Fairley and Birch 1989).

The infection can start via two/three routes:

*Ascending route.* This is the most frequent due to ascending urethral infection with usual urinary bacteria, and the pathophysiology of acute ascending pyelonephritis is best discussed as a continuum of the disease (Craig et al. 2008).

Uropathogenic strains resident in bowel flora, such as *E. coli*, are able to adhere to and colonize the perineum and urethra, and successively migrate to the bladder where they establish an inflammatory response in the urothelial cells. Adherence of bacteria to the introital and urothelial mucosa plays an essential step in ascending UTIs. Moreover, gram-negative *E. coli* produces a number of adhesins that permit it to attach to the urinary mucosa.

Sometimes, some specific conditions can further favor this route of infections. For example, women who use spermicidal agents are more prone to develop UTI. The flora normally present in the vaginal introitus, the urethra, and the perineal region contains microorganisms that form an obstacle against uropathogenic colonization. The use of antimicrobial or spermicidal agents alters the normal protective flora, thus increasing the receptivity of the epithelial cells to the pathogens.

Once reaching the bladder, the pathogens can migrate up the ureter to the central collecting system. Clinical and experimental evidence strongly indicate that most episodes of pyelonephritis are due to the upward retrograde ascent of bacteria from the bladder to the renal pelvis and to the parenchyma (Dunnick et al. 2001).

In children, this commonly occurs as a result of VUR; conversely, in adults, in whom a frank reflux is very uncommon, bacteria are thought to ascend to the kidney via the ureter against the antegrade flow of urine. In the latter evenience, edema associated with bladder infections may alter the ureterovesical junction to permit reflux; once the pathogens reach the ureter, they may ascend to the upper urinary tract and renal parenchyma. However, any condition that interfere with the normal ureteral peristaltic function can greatly increase this process.

It is well known from the literature that certain virulence strains of bacteria, for example *E. coli*, are capable of producing surface adhesin proteins termed P fimbriae and endotoxins that facilitate upward migration along the ureter. The P fimbriae, in fact, facilitates bacterial adhesion to the cells of the urothelium (Schaeffer and Schaeffer 2007).

The endotoxins are believed to inhibit ureteral peristalsis by blocking the alpha-adrenergic nerves within the smooth muscle, thus having a significant antiperistaltic effect and creating a functional obstruction. This functional obstruction endangered the forward flow of urine, which is a normal protective mechanism against upper UTIs (Schaeffer and Schaeffer 2007).

Whatever may be the cause of ureteral obstruction, as well as the dilation of the ureters and pelvis secondary to pregnancy-related hormonal alterations, it has a significant antiperistaltic effect thus explaining the frequency of acute pyelonephritis in these kinds of patients.

Owing to the ascension of bacterial pathogens, an infected-inflamed ureter and renal pelvis, i.e., ureteropyelitis, supervenes; continuing their retrograde ascent, the bacteria enter the renal parenchyma via the collecting duct at the papillary tips, causing an infectious-inflammatory response within the collecting tubule and into the renal interstitium (Kawashima et al. 2000).

The intensity of the inflammatory reaction depends on several factors like the bacterial virulence and host defense; moreover, an increase of the intrapelvic pressure from ureteral obstruction or VUR, particularly in case of high degree intrarenal reflux, can exacerbate the inflammatory pyelo-tubulo-interstitial process.

Inflammation of the pyelocaliceal lining, even though not very prominent, is usually depicted histologically in acute parenchymal infections, thus explaining the correct definition of this pathologic process, pyelonephritis.

Once the bacteria reaches the collecting tubules, leukocytes migrate from the interstitium into the tubule lumina; leukocytes then liberate enzymes that destroy the tubule cells and so the bacterium invades the interstitium by 48–72 h (Talner et al. 1994). A true tubulo-interstitial nephritis arise with inflammatory cells, mononuclear cells, and neutrophils, present both in the tubule and in the interstitial tissue. The inflammation radiates centrifugally from the papilla to the cortex along the medullary rays (Talner et al. 1994).

At the peak of inflammation, tubules are filled with leukocytes and other materials thus creating a focal intrarenal obstruction. Simultaneously, an intense vasoconstriction of the arteries and arterioles arise in the affected renal parenchyma, which generally shows a patchy distribution, sometimes lobar.

Normally, both macro and microscopically, there is a clear-cut demarcation between the involved and bordering spared portions of the renal parenchyma.

Macroscopically, the involved parenchyma presents as radiating yellow-white stripes or a wedge radiating through the full thickness of the parenchyma, from the papillae to the kidney surface, following the medullary beams.

Severe tubulo-interstitial inflammation causes parenchyma swelling with an increase in the size of the affected kidney. Renal inflammation can spread to the bridging septa of the perinephric fat space, to the Gerota fascia, and, very rarely, to the extrarenal space.

*Hematogenous route.* This route of infection is less common in human than the ascending route and it occurs especially in patients addicted to drug taken via a parenteral route, in immunocompromised or pediatric patients, or in patients having an extrarenal source of infection such as teeth, skin, or heart valve.    ·

Hematogenous infection is invariably due to *S. aureus* or Streptococcus species (Papanicolaou and Pfister 1996).

In contrast to the ascending route, the lesions begin in the cortex and involve the medullary region 24–48h after bacterial inoculation. Initially, the lesions are round, small, multiple, and peripheral, without any lobar distribution; after 48 h, it is not possible to make a distinction between the ascending and hematogenous route based on the distribution, due to the spreading of the inflammation.

Experimental data support that the infection is enhanced when the kidney is obstructed (Smellie and Normand 1975).

*Lymphatic route.* There is scanty evidence that lymphatic route play a significant role in acute pyelonephritis.

The anatomical disposition of the lymphatic vessels permits the pathogens to travel from the low urinary tract toward the kidney; moreover, in severe bowel infections or retroperitoneal abscesses, direct extension of the bacteria via the lymphatics may result.

Finally, it should be highlighted that in the past, a variety of terms were coined to describe these severe acute renal infections. Such terms include acute bacterial nephritis, focal or lobar bacterial nephritis, lobar nephronia, etc. (Talner et al. 1994).

The Society of Uroradiology recommends a simplified nomenclature based on the conventional and widely accepted term of acute pyelonephritis, which reunites most of the clinical, pathologic, and radiologic features of acute bacterial infections of the kidney. In order to delineate the severity and the distribution of the infection, they suggest to use focal, diffuse, and with or without renal enlargement.

### 16.1.2 Imaging

The role of imaging in the evaluation of patients with suspected UTI has been much debated.

In general, routine radiologic imaging in not required and not performed in the majority of uncomplicated cases of acute pyelonephritis in adults (Craig et al. 2008; Stunel et al. 2007). In fact, there is good evidence that imaging does not alter the clinical care in 90% of patients with pyelonephritis, because these patients respond successfully to antibiotics in 48–72 h. The validity of the 72-h period was confirmed by Soulen et al., who demonstrate that 95% of uncomplicated pyelonephritis became afebrile within 48 h of congruous antimicrobial therapy and nearly 100% did so within 72 h.

In selected clinical scenario early imaging is required, and specifically:

- In patients who are not responding to the appropriate intravenous antibiotic therapy within the first 72 h (occurring in approximately 5% of cases).
- In patients with unusually severe symptom or with atypical signs and symptoms in whom other disease entity are suspected.
- In patients having a high risk to develop severe life-threatening complications (e.g., diabetic and elderly patients, immunocompromised patients, such as those with HIV, transplantated on immunosuppressant therapy, and patients receiving cytotoxic chemotherapy).
- In patients with signs and symptoms of urinary tract obstruction.
- In patients with recurrent infections suggesting bacterial persistence within the urinary tract.

Finally, as stated by Craig et al., diagnostic imaging has an important role "to look for previously occult structural or functional abnormalities that may require intervention and to evaluate the extent of organ damage subsequent to a resolved acute infection."

Once the decision has been made to proceed with diagnostic imaging of an acute renal pyelonephritis, it is very important to choose the correct modality.

Available imaging modality include intravenous or escretory urography (IVU or EU), ultrasound (US), computerized tomography (CT), magnetic resonance (MR), and nuclear medicine (NM), each of them with their own benefit, indication, and limitation (Demertzis and Menias 2007; Craig et al. 2008; Stunel et al. 2007; Browne et al. 2004).

### 16.1.2.1 IVU

In the past, IVU was commonly performed in the evaluation of acute pyelonephritis.

Several studies have demonstrated that IVU is normal in 75% of uncomplicated acute pyelonephritis cases (Webb 1997; Baumgarten and Baumgarten 1997; Browne et al. 2004). In the remaining 25%, the IVU findings normally seen in cases of acute renal infections include (a) diffuse renal enlargement, related to the accompanying edema, (b) delayed and attenuated renal nephrogram, sometimes with a striated appearance of the involved portion of renal parenchyma, (c) delayed contrast medium filling of the renal collecting system with decreased opacity, (d) dilation or efface-ment of the collecting system.

In general, more severe and diffuse the interstitial inflammatory disease more evident is the degree of radiographic abnormality and the degree of impairment of contrast excretion (Dunnick et al. 2001).

Calicectasis may occur as the result of acute pyelo-nephritis; this feature has been attributed to the decreased or inhibited peristaltic activity induced by the endotox-ins elaborated by gram-negative pathogens, but in the vast majority of cases, this finding implies past or pres-ent urinary tract obstruction (Dunnick et al. 2001).

Nevertheless, IVU in not sensitive enough to dem-onstrate parenchymal abnormalities, micro and macro renal abscesses and perirenal involvement (Browne et al. 2004).

One of the main remaining information of IVU could be the detection of urinary tract obstruction, although this can now be better obtained be other modalities. According to recent literature, IVU should not be used for the evaluation of acute pyelonephritis (Craig et al. 2008; Stunel et al. 2007).

### 16.1.2.2 US

US is relatively insensitive in the evaluation of acute pyelonephritis, when compared with contrast-enhanced CT. In some prospective studies, US fails to demon-strate abnormalities in 75–80% of patients with uncom-plicated infections and often underestimates the severity of the attack, even in cases of multifocal dis-ease or perinephric extension (Craig et al. 2008; Stunel et al. 2007; Browne et al. 2004; Majd et al. 2001).

Despite this lack of sensitivity and specificity, US is frequently used as a first-line imaging technique to evaluate the urinary tract in patients with symptoms of pyelonephritis, especially in young people. Moreover, US can still be considered the technique of choice in the evaluation of pregnant women with acute bacterial pyelonephritis due to the lack of ionizing radiation (Stunel et al. 2007).

In about 20% of cases, generalized renal edema, due to inflammation and congestion, can be detected by ultrasound examination demonstrating an overall kidney length in excess of 15 cm or, alternatively, an increased length higher than 1.5 cm with respect to the unaffected kidney (Vourganti et al. 2006).

Differences in the renal parenchymal echogenicity due to edema (hypoechoic) or hemorrhage (hyper-echoic), together with the loss of corticomedullary dif-ferentiation, are indicative, even if not specific findings, of acute pyelonephritis at US (Fig. 16.1a).

Dilatation of the collecting cavities in the absence of demonstrable obstructive cause can be appreciated by US and correlate with the inhibition of normal ureteral peristalsis, due to the action of bacterial endotoxins.

In cases of fungal infection, US may demonstrate the presence of fungal debris with the formation of fungus balls in the pelvi-caliceal system with conse-quent urinary obstruction. In addition, collection of air, due to gas-forming infections, may be seen in the blad-der or collecting system (Vourganti et al. 2006).

Improvements in ultrasound techniques with power Doppler ultrasonography, demonstrating areas of parenchymal hypoperfusion, have resulted in better accuracy of US. Although experimental studies in

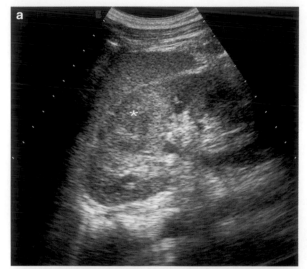

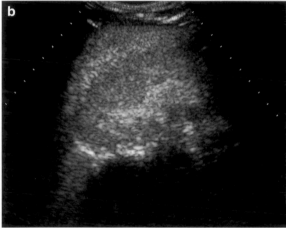

**Fig. 16.1** (**a**, **b**) Young woman with acute focal pyelonephritis studied with ultrasound (US). (**a**) Ultrasound of the left kidney in a patient with fever and leukocytosis shows mild enlargement of the renal parenchyma with loss of cortico-medullary differentiation in the middle part of the kidney (*asterisk*). (**b**) Contrast-enhanced ultrasound (CEUS) does not show any difference in the enhancement of the whole left kidney

animal models show a poor diagnostic accuracy in comparison with CT and scintigraphy, a positive power Doppler US can obviate the need for further examinations (Majd et al. 2001).

Contrast-enhanced ultrasonography (CEUS) has been recently reported as a useful tool to better demonstrate areas of poor perfusion related to pyelonephritis as a result of compression and vasoconstriction of arterial and arteriolar vessels, caused by inflammatory infiltration (Mitterberger et al. 2007). Comparative studies realized on animal models showed a significant increase of accuracy of the CEUS with respect to the

Power Doppler in the diagnosis of acute pyelonephritis, with values of sensibility comparable to those of MRI or CT imaging (Farhat et al. 2002).

However, this technique has not yet found a general use in the evaluation of the infected kidney and, in our experience, does not considerably improve the accuracy of US (Fig. 16.1b).

In our opinion, the main advantage of CEUS in acute pyelonephritis lies in excluding the growth of an abscess which requires a drainage in patients who does not respond to medical therapy (Fig. 16.2).

CEUS is, conversely, a fundamental diagnostic tool to image pediatric patients suspected of having VUR, using first generation, or preferably second generation contrast agents with urosonography (Ascenti et al. 2004; Zimbaro et al. 2007).

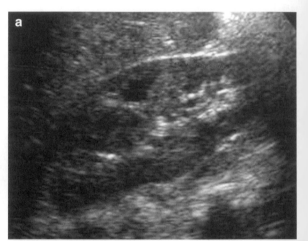

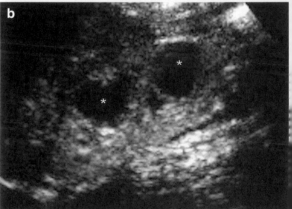

**Fig. 16.2** (**a**, **b**) Diabetic patient with right kidney abscesses. (**a**) Conventional ultrasound of the right kidney does not show any focal or diffuse lesion inside the renal parenchyma. (**b**) CEUS shows two round hypoechoic foci in the renal parenchyma (*asterisks*) suggestive of renal abscesses

## 16.1.2.3 CT

CT is considered the most appropriate imaging technique for the diagnosis and follow-up of patients with acute bacterial pyelonephritis. Its main roles are to delineate the extent of the disease and to identify significant complications or urinary obstruction.

Unenhanced CT is extremely useful for the detection of renal enlargement, hemorrhage, inflammatory masses, obstruction, calculi, parenchymal calcifications, and urinary tract gas and therefore, it should be always performed first in the imaging protocol (Kawashima et al. 1997; Kawashima et al. 2000). Involved areas occasionally present with lower attenuation due to edema or necrosis; in rare hemorrhagic bacterial nephritis, unenhanced CT demonstrates wedge-shaped or rounded areas of increased attenuation determined by parenchymal bleeding (Rigsby et al. 1986; Craig et al. 2008) (Fig. 16.3).

However, the above-described findings are frequently absent; therefore, contrast-enhanced scans often have to be performed following the unenhanced study.

Helical and multidetector CT allows studying the different phases of excretion after intravenous contrast medium administration. A rational CT protocol for investigating patients with suspected acute pyelonephritis requires performing precontrast imaging followed by postcontrast acquisition at approximately 50–100 s after injection, and to continue with delayed imaging especially if urinary tract obstruction is

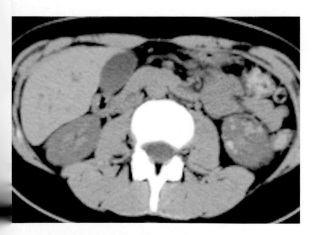

**Fig. 16.3** Hemorrhagic acute bacterial pyelonephritis. Unenhanced computerized tomography (CT) examination shows multiple round or oval high density foci within the left kidney (reprinted, with permission from Craig et al. (2008)

suspected (Stunel et al. 2007). These parameters are designed to take advantage of the nephrographic phase considered to be superior in depicting the full extent of lesions and to better define the characteristic abnormalities of acute pyelonephritis (Wyatt et al. 1995). Further, delayed CT scans at 3 h or more can help to differentiate acute pyelonephritis from hypoattenuating areas caused by other pathologies like infarcts and tumors.

After the injection of contrast material, acute pyelonephritis usually appears as one or more wedge-shaped zones of lesser enhancement extending from the papilla in the medulla to the kidney capsule with a lobar distribution and poor corticomedullary differentiation. Enhancement of the involved region may be either homogeneous or irregular, but attenuation is always minor than normal parenchyma (Figs. 16.4a, b and 16.5).

Vasospasm, tubular obstruction, and/or interstitial edema originate areas of poor or nonfunctioning parenchyma which may determine this pattern of differential enhancement (Kawashima et al. 1997; Gold et al. 1983; Hoddick et al. 1983). The tendency of these three disorders to decrease the contrast agent flow through the tubule helps to explain the pattern of delayed and persistent enhancement seen in delayed scans obtained 3–6 h after contrast medium administration (Dalla Palma et al. 1995) (Fig. 16.4c).

In acute pyelonephritis, the alternating bands of increased and decreased attenuation, which correspond to the differential enhancement of infected and not infected parenchyma, are sharply defined at the edge. During the healing process, the differential enhancement becomes more and more faint until it will either completely normalize or evolve to a scar, as demonstrated by parenchymal volume reduction (Fig. 16.6).

The alternating bands of hyper and hypoattenuation parallel to the axes of the tubules and collecting ducts, which characterize the so-called "striated nephrogram" typical of acute pyelonephritis, can be correlated to the obstructed tubules alternated to normal tubules; stasis of the contrast material secondary to the obstruction of the collecting system is the reason for these striations, which have a lobar distribution, may be uni- or multifocal, and can be uni or bilateral (Fig. 16.7). However, it is noteworthy that this CT finding is not pathognomonic of acute pyelonephritis and can also be seen in poorly hydrated patients and in normal kidneys when contrast agents with low osmolarity are used.

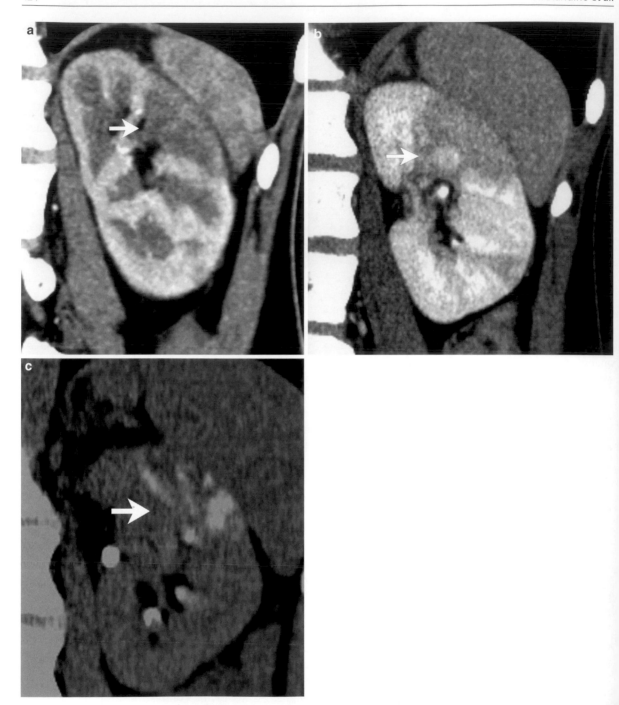

**Fig. 16.4** (**a–c**) Postcontrast coronal multiplanar reconstruction CT images in a patient with acute focal bacterial pyelonephritis of the left kidney. A wedge-shaped area of low attenuation radiating from the medulla to the cortical surface with loss of corticomed-ullary differentiation (*arrow*) is well demonstrated both in the arterial (**a**) as well as in the nephrographic phase (**b**) of the study. Delayed CT acquisition during the excretory phase (**c**) shows par-tial, persistent enhancement of the low attenuation area (*arrow*)

The finding of round, not wedge-shaped peripheral hypoattenuating renal lesions in the clinical setting of pyelonephritis should raise the suspect of hematogenous seeding (Fig. 16.8); nonetheless, when these lesions coalesce or involve the entire kidney, it may not be possible to distinguish between the ascending and hematogenous infection (Talner et al. 1994; Lee et al. 1980) (Fig. 16.9).

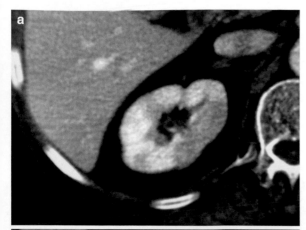

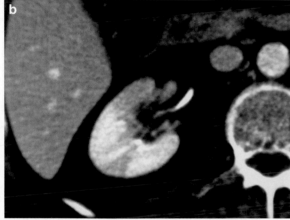

**Fig. 16.5** (**a**, **b**) Male patient with multifocal acute bacterial pyelonephritis of the right kidney. Contrast-enhanced CT scans obtained at different levels show multifocal regions of diminished enhancement both in the upper (**a**) as well as in the middle part (**b**) of the right kidney

Differential diagnosis for focal hypoattenuating areas includes a mass, areas of renal infarction, tumors, or scarring, in particular, when these CT findings are identified in the absence of clinically suspected pyelonephritis. The hypoattenuating areas caused by infarcts and tumors persist even after antibiotic treatment, whereas changes resolve following treatment when they are caused by pyelonephritis; moreover, scarring rarely occurs in adult patients. Furthermore, delayed CT scans can help differentiate tumor from inflammatory mass by showing persistent enhancement in areas of previously diminished enhancement (Fig. 16.4c).

CT commonly demonstrates secondary signs of renal infection and its complications. These signs include focal or global enlargement of the kidney, obliteration of the renal sinus and perinephritic fat planes, calyceal effacement caused by the swelling of the adjacent affected renal parenchyma, pelvicalyceal wall thickening and enhancement secondary to ascending infections, soft tissue perinephritic stranding, and thickening of the Gerota fascia (Goldman and Fishman 1991; Pickhardt et al. 2000; Soulen et al. 1989).

In particular, pelvicalyceal wall thickening and enhancement secondary to ascending infection may be the only imaging feature of acute pyelonephritis when CT is performed early, before renal damage is macroscopically evident with this imaging technique (Figs. 16.10 and 16.11).

It is important to observe that perinephric stranding alone should be interpreted with caution, because even in the presence of acute symptoms, it may relate to previous infections, trauma, or vascular disease (Urban and Fishman 2000).

Soft tissue filling defect in the collecting system may represent sloughed tissue from papillary necrosis, inflammatory debris, or blood clots.

Diffuse pyelonephritis is characterized by renal enlargement, poor enhancement, and poor excretion of contrast medium in proportion to the severity of infection (Fig. 16.12).

Finally, it also has to be noted that acute pyelonephritis is often a dynamic process in which the areas of the kidney characterized by improvement can be adjacent to the areas of progression.

### 16.1.2.4 Nuclear Medicine

As far as NM examinations are concerned, the use of $^{99m}$Tc-glucoheptonate or dimercaptosuccinic acid (DMSA) should be considered for the detection of acute pyelonephritis and renal scarring (Eggli and Tulchinsky 1993). Cortical scintigraphy, indeed, has shown superior sensitivity in detecting pyelonephritis and renal scars compared with IVU or renal ultrasonography (Eggli and Tulchinsky 1993; Bjorgvinsson et al. 1991; Hatch and Ouwenga 2006).

Since $^{99m}$Tc-DMSA is less affected than glucoheptonate by the interference of urinary radiotracer excretion, it appears to be the most appropriate radiotracer. Its uptake is related to the relative amount of functioning renal tissue and does not measure a specific localization process. The exact mechanism by which it localizes in the kidney is unclear although glomerular filtration, tubular secretion, and tubular resorption have been suggested to play a role; it seems that the tracer is taken up by the peritubular vessels. Approximately,

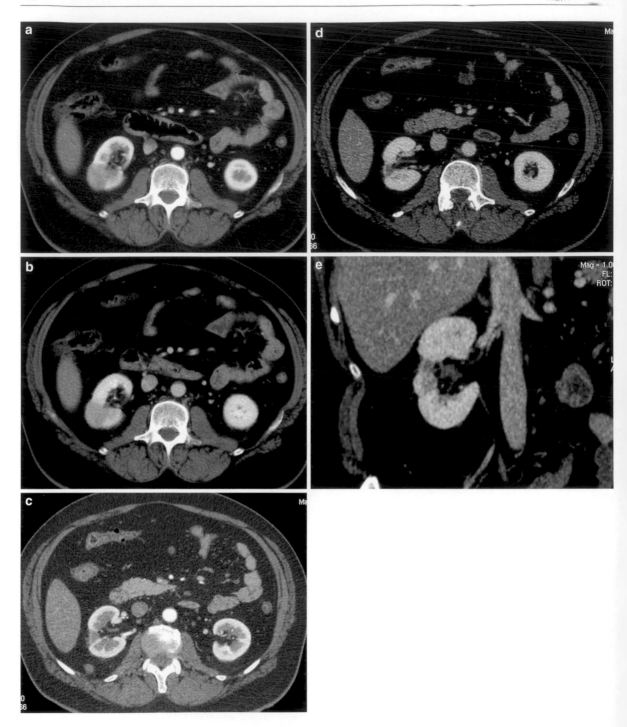

**Fig. 16.6** (**a–e**) Favorable evolution in a case of not-complicated acute focal pyelonephritis of the right kidney. Contrast enhanced-CT scans obtained during arterial (**a**) and nephrographic (**b**) phase show focal swelling with a round-shaped area of decreased attenuation radiating from the papilla to the posterior surface in the middle part of the right kidney. The 2-month follow-up shows the positive evolution of renal infection residuating with parenchymal volume reduction and renal scar, well demonstrated both in the arterial phase (**c**) as well as in the axial (**d**) and the coronal reconstructed (**e**) images of the nephrographic phase (case courtesy of G. Regine, MD, S. Camillo Hospital, Rome, Italy)

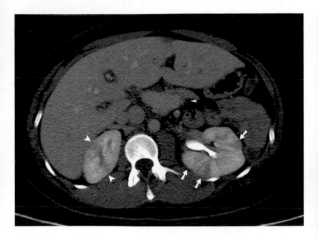

**Fig. 16.7** Bilateral and multifocal acute bacterial pyelonephritis. The nephrographic phase of contrast-enhanced CT scan shows the typical striated pyelogram pattern in the left kidney (*arrows*) of an adult woman with bilateral acute bacterial pyelonephritis. Note also some focal wedge-shaped areas of the disease in the right kidney (*arrowheads*)

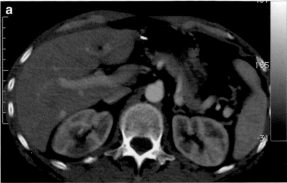

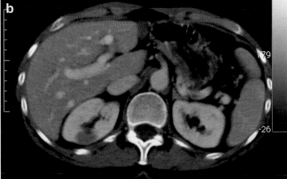

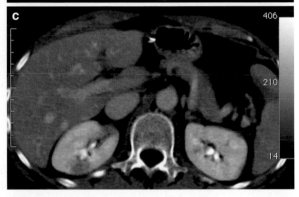

**Fig. 16.8** (**a–c**) Drug abusing patient with clinical signs of acute pyelonephritis. Contrast-enhanced CT scans during arterial (**a**), nephrographic (**b**), and excretory (**c**) phases demonstrate the presence of a round, peripheral hypoattenuating lesion in the posterior upper half of the right kidney, suspected for hematogenous pyelonephritis

40–50% of $^{99m}$Tc-DMSA accumulate in the cortical tubules within 1 h and remain for 24 h. Images (posterior and anterior views) are obtained about 3 h after injection, preferably with high resolution collimators. The examination delivers a significant radiation dose to the patient (3.15R to the kidneys and 4.25R to the renal cortices for a 185-MBq injected dose) (Hatch and Ouwenga 2006; Piepsz et al. 1999).

The normal DMSA scan demonstrates nearly equal distribution of radiopharmaceutical throughout the cortex (the outer part corresponding to the cortex is more active than the inner part, the medulla and the collecting system); the contours of the kidney are generally round although a contour can be flat without suggesting a lesion. Moreover, kidney may appear triangular or "pear shaped." Kidney rotation and/or the normal contrast of the hypoactive poles with the hyperactive columns of Bertin may cause false interpretation of the images (Piepsz et al. 1999).

There is no consensus on cortical scintigraphy in acute renal infection (Hatch and Ouwenga 2006; Piepsz et al. 1999).

Several authors suggest that acute renal scintigraphy is not necessary because half of the acute lesions are transitory and disappear (Stokland et al. 1996); others consider that clinical and biological arguments constitute a weak evidence for acute pyelonephritis and that patients with lack of clinical and biological signs or with negative or equivocal urine cultures may still have UTI with obvious acute renal lesions (Conway and Cohn 1994). Only 58% of experts in one consensus study (Piepsz et al. 1999) were using a cortical imaging study during the acute phase of an infection;

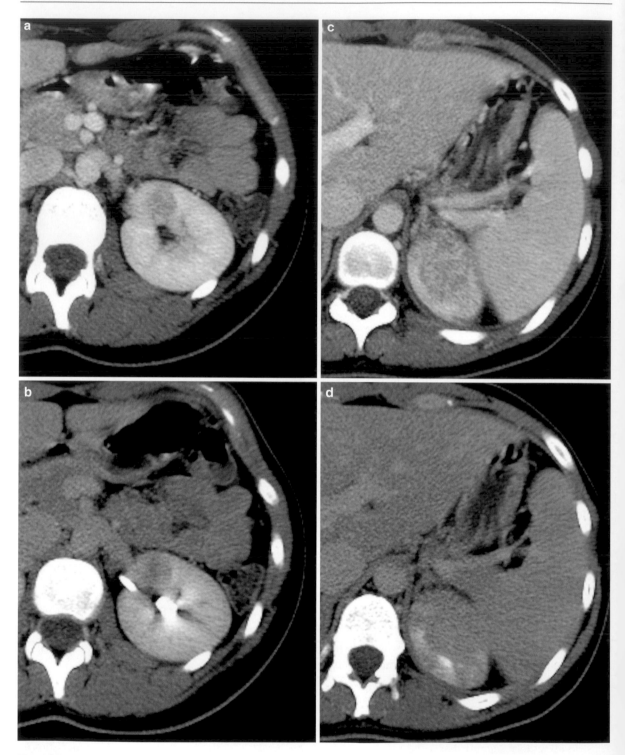

**Fig. 16.9** (**a–d**) Multifocal hematogenous pyelonephritis in 50-year-old patient with bacterial endocarditis. Enhanced CT scans obtained during parenchymal nephrographic phase (**a**) and excretory phase (**b**) show the presence of a round peripheral hypoattenuating lesion in the anterior lip of the left kidney compatible with the diagnosis of hematogenous pyelonephritis. Contrast-enhanced CT scans obtained during nephrographic (**c**) and excretory (**d**) phases at the level of the upper pole of the kidney show a huge coalescent hypodense lesion not allowing differentiation between ascending and hematogenous infection (case courtesy of M. Mandalà, MD, Hospital Cannizzaro, Catania, Italy)

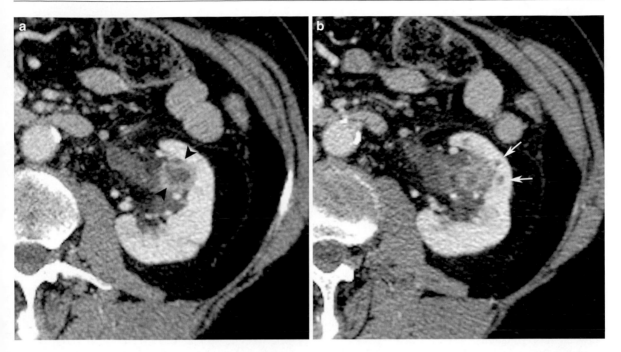

**Fig. 16.10** (**a**, **b**) Young male patient with left pyelitis. Contrast-enhanced CT scan (**a**) shows thickening and enhancement of the calyceal wall (*arrowheads*). A CT scan obtained at a lower level (**b**) demonstrates the presence of round, small areas of low density at the apex of the papillae (*thin arrows*) representative of early pyelonephritis with renal parenchyma involvement (case courtesy of G. Regine, MD, S. Camillo Hospital, Rome, Italy)

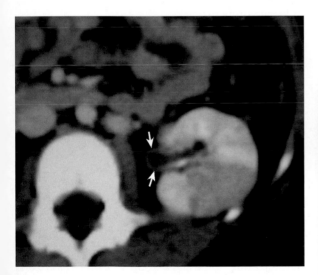

**Fig. 16.11** Diabetic patient with left kidney pyelitis and focal acute pyelonephritis. Mild thickness with faint enhancement of the pelvic wall suggesting acute pyelitis is well appreciable on the axial contrast-enhanced CT scan (*arrows*). Note also the huge wedge-shaped area of parenchymal involvement suggesting focal pyelonephritis (case courtesy of V. Magnano San Lio, MD, Garibaldi Hospital, Catania, Italy)

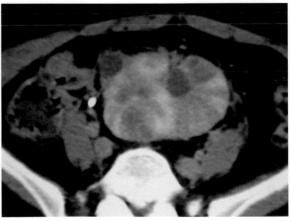

**Fig. 16.12** Acute diffuse pyelonephritis in pelvic kidney. Contrast-enhanced CT scan reveals enlargement of the pelvic kidney, loss of contrast enhancement with multifocal regions of diminished enhancement radiating from the papillae to the cortical surface. Note also a small exophytic simple renal cyst

among those who perform acute DMSA, 22% did it for any first UTI, 22% for any UTI, and 56% only in case of high suspicion of acute pyelonephritis. There is consensus that acute DMSA should be performed without delay (3–7 days).

Pyelonephritic lesions appear as focal, multiple, or diffuse reduction in the accumulation of the radiopharmaceutical, probably because of local ischemic changes in the infected segments of renal parenchyma (Fig. 16.13).

It has been demonstrated on animal models that the presence of a scintigraphic abnormality strongly correlates with the extension of the anatomic lesion. In the clinical practice, however, scintigraphic abnormalities in case of acute UTI are not specific unless any other underlying disease such as renal abscess, hydronephrosis, cysts, or complicated duplex kidney has been excluded. It is mandatory, therefore, to combine scintigraphy with ultrasound which allows differentiation between these situations.

Many reports suggest that SPECT shows more lesions than planar images (Piepsz et al. 1999).

Determination of the relative left and right DMSA uptake is generally performed (on the posterior view with or without lateral view for the correction of kidney depth; one can also determine the geometric mean using both the anterior and posterior views; no consensus is reached whether or not the background should be subtracted). The normal lowest value for relative uptake is approximately 45%. The normal side to side distribution can completely miss bilateral small kidney; inversely, the normal unilateral duplex

situation can be associated with abnormally high relative function. For some authors, a percentage below 45% during acute UTI predicts permanent damage (Piepsz et al. 1999; De Sadeleer et al. 1993). Hydronephrosis is not a contraindication for a DMSA scintigraphy, but constitutes a pitfall giving rise to the overestimation of the relative function on the side of obstruction because of the accumulation of the excreted radiotracer.

There is a wide consensus among NM physicians for a systematic use of cortical scintigraphy in the detection of sequelae, namely renal scarring after an episode of pyelonephritis, whatever the number of previous infections; there is no consensus concerning the adequate moment for the detection of sequelae (3–6–12 months); however, most of the authors suggest that DMSA examination should not be performed until at least 6 months after acute infection (Hatch and Ouwenga 2006; Piepsz et al. 1999; Stokland et al. 1999; Sixt and Stokland 1998).

Renal parenchymal scintigraphy has demonstrated that the scars occur at the same site as the region in which pyelonephritis is detected. The best predictor of renal sequelae is probably the presence of a renal abnormality during the acute phase of infection. Therefore, the risk of developing persistent scars is low when early scintigraphy is normal and this may influence further strategy.

Many argue that if the DMSA study is normal at the time of acute UTI, no further investigation is required, because the kidneys have not been involved and thus there will be no late sequelae. Others use the acute DMSA study to determine the intensity of antibiotic therapy (Rossleigh 2007).

### 16.1.2.5 MRI

MRI is not normally employed in patients suffering from acute renal infections.

Nevertheless, MRI is an emerging, strong modality for the evaluation of kidney and urinary tract pathology, including acute and chronic renal infections, and it may eventually prove of high value when utilized appropriately and in selected cases.

Renal MRI potentially offers a cost-effective and radiation-free alternative in the radiological diagnosis of acute pyelonephritis. Due to the lack of ionizing radiation, it is especially useful in patients for whom exposure to X-rays should be avoided (e.g., pregnant

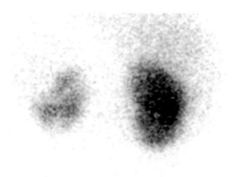

**Fig. 16.13** $^{99m}$Tc-DMSA scintigraphy (posterior view) in a patient with suspected acute pyelonephritis shows reduced accumulation of the radiopharmaceutical in the left kidney mainly involving the upper pole. The relative left and right dimercaptosuccinic acid (DMSA) uptake was 32 and 68%, respectively. Ultrasonography (not shown) was negative

women). Moreover, it should be used in patients with allergy to iodinated contrast agents.

Conventional MRI findings reproduce the pathologic change that characterizes acute pyelonephritis, with signal changes reflecting the distribution of edema within the renal parenchyma.

Kidney can show focal or diffuse enlargement with the affected inflammatory areas following the expected signal intensity of edematous lesions, i.e., low signal intensity on T1-weighted images and high intensity on T2-weighted images, with loss of normal corticomedullary differentiation (Craig et al. 2008; Stunel et al. 2007). The edematous inflammatory areas are better depicted using T2-weighted images with fat suppression (FS) technique (Fig. 16.14).

Perirenal stranding or small amount of perinephric fluid can be seen, but these are aspecific signs found in several other renal and perirenal pathological conditions.

MRI with gadolinium is very helpful in exactly depicting areas of renal parenchyma involvement. The MRI features are quite similar to those of CT scan, with focal or diffuse, round or wedge-shaped area of decreased enhancement compared with the normal enhancement of the not-involved neighboring renal parenchyma (Fig. 16.15).

In order to increase the conspicuity of intrarenal lesion, Lonergan et al. (1998) proposed an alternative MRI protocol in a series of children aged 2–16 years suffering from acute pyelonephritis.

In fact, using a gadolinium-enhanced inversion-recovery MR imaging it is possible to use the negative enhancement effect of the paramagnetic contrast agent. The normally well-perfused renal parenchyma become hypointense or dark, because gadolinium decreases the signal intensity on inversion recovery images ("contrast negative effect"); conversely the less well-perfused areas of acute inflammation remain high in signal intensity, due to the concomitant effects of edema and poor delivery and concentration of gadolinium (Figs. 16.16 and 16.17).

According to Lonergan et al., "gadolinium-enhanced inversion recovery MR imaging allows the detection of a greater number of pyelonephritic lesions than does renal cortical scintigraphy, making MR imaging a viable diagnostic modality for the evaluation of suspected pyelonephritis in children."

The results of the present study are in agreement with the clinical application of the same authors' previous work on the use of MR imaging with the gadolinium-enhanced fast inversion-recovery sequence in

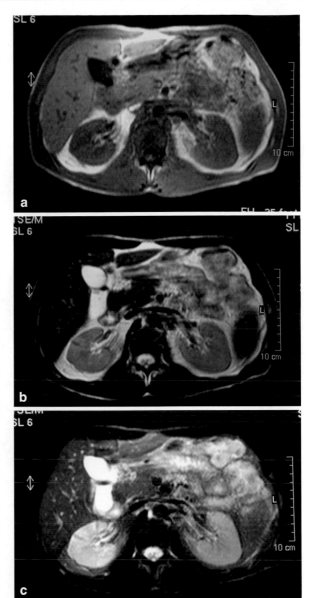

**Fig. 16.14** (**a–c**) Conventional MRI in a young woman with right acute bacterial pyelonephritis. (**a**) Gradient-echo T1-weighted axial magnetic resonance (MR) image passing through the middle part of both the kidneys does not show any difference in size and signal intensity between the right and left kidney. (**b**) Axial T2-weighted fast spin-echo image show a faint and diffuse high signal intensity of right renal parenchyma. (**c**) Axial T2-weighted fast spin-echo image with fat suppression (FS). The high intensity of the affected renal parenchyma, due to diffuse edema, is highlighted and well recognizable (case courtesy of G. Cardone, MD, S. Raffaele Hospital, Milan, Italy)

experimental pyelonephritis in piglets, where the authors reported a high sensitivity (91%) and specificity (93%) for the detection of pyelonephritic lesions (Pennington et al. 1996).

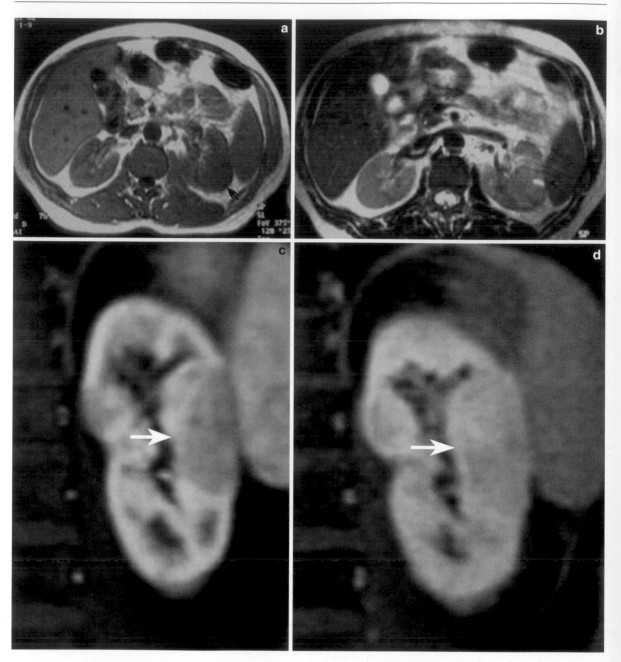

**Fig. 16.15** (**a–d**) Patient with acute focal bacterial pyelonephritis of the left kidney. (**a**) Gradient-echo axial T1-weighted MR image passing through the middle part of the kidney. Mild enlargement of left kidney with focal swelling of the posterior middle portion (*arrow*). (**b**) Axial T2-weighted fast spin-echo shows round mild hyperintense area in the posterior part of the left kidney; a small preexisting hyperintense cyst compressed from the involved parenchyma is shown (*arrowhead*). (**c, d**) Contrast-enhanced T1-weighted gradient-echo coronal images. The involved renal parenchyma by the acute bacterial inflammation is well appreciable both in the arterial (**c**) as well as in the nephrographic phase (**d**) of the study as a peripheral hypointense wedge-shaped area (*arrow*) (case courtesy of M. Scialpi, MD, University of Perugia, Italy)

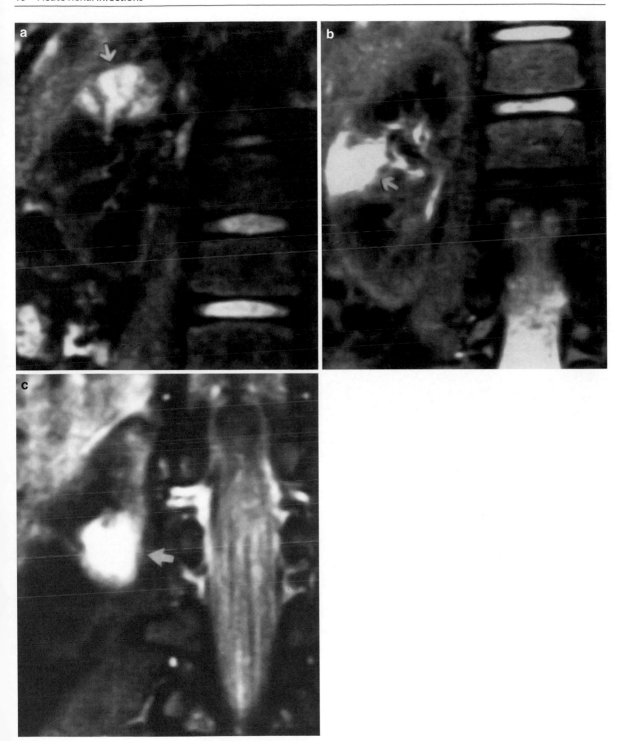

**Fig. 16.16** (**a–c**) Young patient with multifocal acute bacterial phyelonephritis. Coronal gadolinium-enhanced inversion-recovery MR images (2,000/16/160, 90° flip angle) at three different levels show foci of high signal intensity (*arrows*) consistent with multifocal pyelonephritis in the right kidney. In this sequence, normal well-perfused renal parenchyma become dark ("negative contrast agent"), whereas, the affected area of pyelonephritis remain high in signal intensity, due to a combination of edema and poor delivery and concentration of Gd (reprinted, with permission from Lonergan et al. (1998)

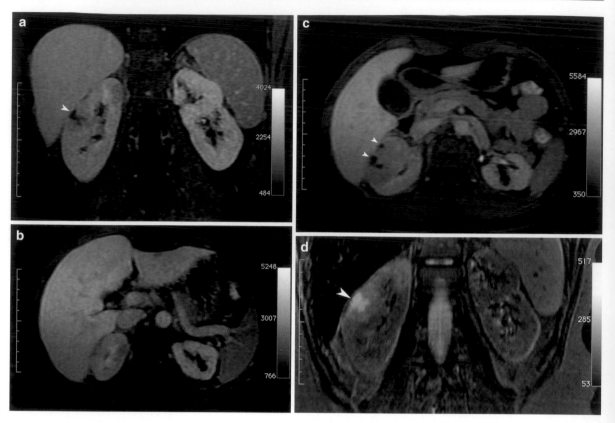

**Fig. 16.17** (**a–d**) Young woman with unilateral multifocal acute right kidney phyelonephritis. (**a**) Postcontrast coronal T1-weighted gradient-echo image with FS shows two focal area of decreased enhancement located respectively in the upper pole and in the middle part of the right kidney. (**b–c**) Axial contrast-enhanced T1-weighted images with FS well demonstrate the wedge-shaped hypointense area in the upper (**b**) and in the middle part of the

kidney (**c**), a feature consistent with acute pyelonephritis. In the larger inflammatory lesion, tiny areas of early colliquation are well appreciable (*arrowheads* in **a** and **c**). (**d**) Coronal gadolinium-enhanced inversion-recovery MR images shows with good accuracy both the involved part of renal parenchyma as well as the early peripheral colliquation in the larger lesion (*arrowhead*) (case courtesy of S. Pappalardo, MD, Sirina Hospital, Taormina, Italy)

Moreover, the value of this kind of approach in children and young patients was also successively confirmed by Weiser et al. (2003).

Conventional MR study may be added with MR-urography in order to delineate the urinary tract in cases where infection is related to a dilated system.

It is a well-known fact that "static-fluid MR urography" or "MR pyelography" is a well-suited technique for the assessment of dilated system (Blandino et al. 2003), with the presence of fluid-fluid level within a dilated urinary system on MR pyelography suggesting a complicated hydronephrosis, generally a hydro-pyo-nephrosis (Magno et al. 2004; Geoghegan et al. 2005).

The combination of conventional MR imaging and MR-urography allows the comprehensive assessment of renal infection and its complications, with the so called "all in one" or "one stop shopping" approach.

It should be mentioned that there are potential pitfalls related to MRI.

Stone disease and gas-forming infections can cause signal voids which are difficult to depict and consequently limits the accuracy of MRI. While these are rare in children, they are common in adult patients, especially in high-risk patients like diabetics, thus limiting the value of MRI in these clinical grounds.

Finally, recent reports in literature have highlighted the possible role of diffusion-weighted (DW) imaging in acute renal infection.

Verswijvel et al. (2002) have shown that areas of acute pyelonephritis have restricted proton diffusion with a lower ADC value; so, it can be easily demonstrated and differentiated from the normal parenchyma on the DW images (Fig. 16.18).

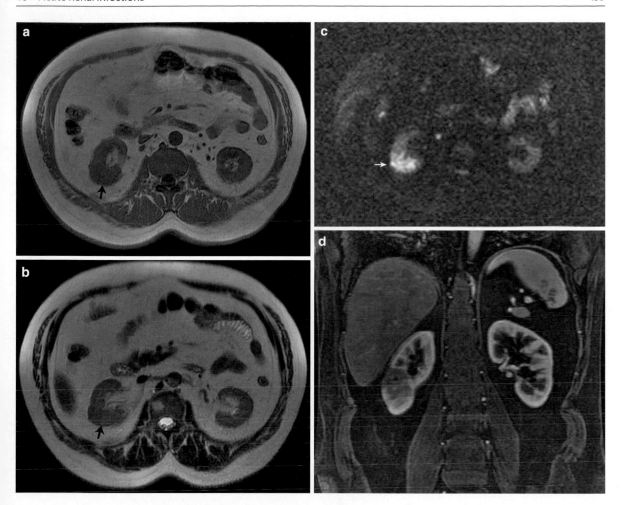

**Fig. 16.18** (**a–d**) patient with acute focal bacterial pyelonephritis. On conventional axial T1-weighted (**a**) and T2-weighted (**b**) images, there is only a focal swelling of the posterior part of the lower pole of the right kidney (*arrows*), with subtle focal hyperintensity on T2-weighted image. (**c**) On axial diffusion-weighted (DW) image, the acute focal pyelonephritic lesion is well depicted as a hyperintense focal area (*arrow*) due to the restriction of proton diffusion. (**d**) The peripheral hypointense wedge-shaped infected region in the middle part of right kidney is well shown in this postcontrast coronal T1-weighted image with FS (case courtesy of G. Regine, MD, S. Camillo Hospital, Rome, Italy)

Cova et al. (2004) and Chan et al. (2001) in a small series of patients with hydronephrosis and hydropyonephrosis have demonstrated on MR diffusion imaging, a very clear cut-off between the ADC value of the renal pelvis in infected and noninfected cases.

The explanation rely on the very high viscosity and cellularity of the thick, adhesive fluid in the urinary tracts of the pyonephrotic kidney, thus providing a very low ADC which explain its hyperintensity on DW images and hypointensity on ADC maps, indicating restricted diffusion.

Both of the studies prove the efficacy of the technique in acute renal infections, but according to Verswijvel et al., "refinement of the technique, in-depth investigation of the pathological background of the MR findings, and evaluation of its clinical value needed further investigation."

## 16.2 Renal and Perinephric Abscess

### 16.2.1 Clinical Features and Pathophysiology

Renal abscess is a collection of purulent material confined to the renal parenchyma.

Before the antimicrobial era, 75–80% of renal abscesses formed as a result of hematogenous dissemination of staphylococci organisms, generally *S. aureus*, usually from a site in the skin or in the bone. Since about 1970, gram-negative organisms have been implicated in the majority of renal abscesses in the adult population. Consequently, the hematogenous renal seeding is not likely to be the primary pathway for gram-negative abscess formation, which is generally due to the ascending infection associated with tubular obstruction (Schaeffer and Schaeffer 2007).

Generally, in the vast majority of patients suffering from acute pyelonephritis, the inflammatory process is reversible, but severe vasospasm and inflammation can occasionally result in liquefactive necrosis and abscess formation. In these circumstances, there is a coalescence of multiple small micro-abscesses that are present as a part of acute pyelonephritis.

Diabetic patients who are predisposed to develop an abscess has a complication of acute pyelonephritis, with almost 75% of all renal parenchymal abscesses occurring in this patient population. Moreover, gram-negative enteric species occur in the setting of VUR, renal stone disease, neurogenic bladder, and immunocompromised states; septic emboli in drug abusers are increasingly becoming a common cause of renal abscess formation.

Renal abscess may be solitary or may form in multiple sites simultaneously in the kidney, the latter generally suggesting a hematogenous dissemination.

Gas-forming renal abscesses are exceedingly rare, especially in the absence of the usual common risk factors (diabetes, obstruction, calculi) (Joseph et al. 1996).

Perinephric abscess normally results from the rupture of an acute renal cortical abscess into the perinephric space, but not infrequently develops directly from acute pyelonephritis. Perinephric abscesses may also form as a result of pyelosinus extravasation of the infected urine or from hematogenous seeding from an external source of infection. Another infrequent but not rare mechanism is the direct extension into the perinephric space from an infection in an adjacent organ (i.e., a ruptured appendix or diverticulitis) (Dunnick et al. 2001).

A paranephric abscess originates from a perinephric infection that ruptures through Gerota's fascia into the pararenal space.

Signs and symptoms of intra- or extrarenal abscess are not specific, and not infrequently, clinical differenti-

ation of these conditions from less virulent forms of bacterial infection of the kidney is very difficult.

A renal abscess should be always suspected when appropriate antimicrobial therapy does not lead to clinical response in a few days. In most cases, symptoms of urinary infections are present for periods longer than 2 weeks. Interestingly, up to 20–25% of patients with an abscess have negative urine culture, especially if the process is walled off (Thornbury 1991).

In some patients, the referred pain to the groin, the thigh, and the hip may be the clue that the infection has spread outside the kidney (Dunnick et al. 2001).

## 16.2.2 Imaging

IVU is no longer used in the diagnosis of renal abscess due to its poor value. It can however demonstrate the features of acute pyelonephritis, like kidney enlargement, decreased focal or diffuse opacity of the renal parenchyma, and the obstruction or urinary tract malformation; the latter is responsible for acute renal infection.

Ultrasonography is particularly useful in the diagnosis of a renal abscess that may be either intra- or extraparenchymal. The kidney is usually enlarged with the distortion of the normal outer contour.

Acute abscesses will appear as a hypoechoic mass with posterior through transmission and indistinct margins, indistinguishable from less severe focal nephritis. A mature abscess usually appear as a fluid-filled mass with a thickened distinct wall. Occasionally, mobile debris may be seen within the collection (Fig. 16.19a). In about 50% of mature abscesses, contrast enhancement of the wall can be demonstrated with CEUS (Fig. 16.19b), and differential diagnosis with neoplastic complex cysts as the multiloculated cystic carcinoma must be considered; in these circumstances, diagnosis is based on clinical and laboratoristic data.

CT is the procedure of choice for the detection and follow-up of renal abscess.

The appearance of CT images may significantly change within 24-h. Early liquefaction within a region of tubulo-interstitial inflammation produces small peripheral cortical areas of hypoattenuation (near water attenuation), often irregular and poorly marginated; these areas do not enhance after contrast medium administration (Soulen et al. 1989) (Fig. 16.20).

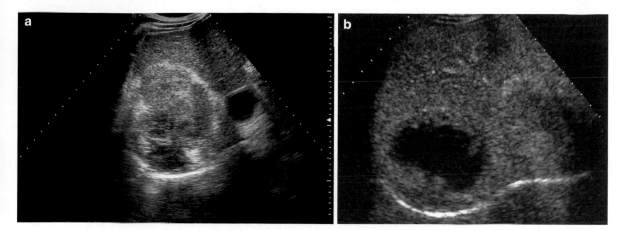

**Fig. 16.19** (**a**, **b**) Huge right kidney abscess in an elderly diabetic man. Conventional ultrasound (**a**) shows a large hypoisoechoic mass in the upper pole of the right kidney. After the introduction of contrast medium (CEUS) (**b**), both the central unenhanced area of the abscess as well as the thickened walls are well demonstrated

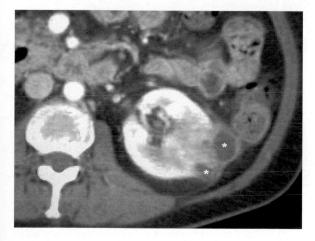

**Fig. 16.20** Patient with typical clinical features of complicated acute pyelonephritis evolving toward abscess formation. Within the low-attenuation areas of acute pyelonephritis, contrast-enhanced CT of the left renal parenchyma shows two early abscesses (*asterisks*) with secondary involvement of the adjacent perinephric space

The early abscess can be surrounded by a zone of decreased enhancement, probably representing infected but nonnecrotic parenchyma (Fig. 16.21), and may appear hyperdense on delayed scans. Conversely, the typical mature abscess is sharply demarcated from the surrounding parenchyma and shows a peripheral rim of enhancement in up to half of the cases (Fig. 16.22). These characteristic rims are pseudocapsules with variable wall thickness in which nodularity is frequently observed; they are best visualized after contrast administration during the excretory phase. Septations can be observed within the abscess. Renal parenchyma surrounding the abscess can be normal, or it may show the alterations typical of pyelonephritis. Areas of gas within an inflammatory mass, though uncommon, are pathognomonic of an abscess (Joseph et al. 1996).

Patients with CT abscess often show fascial and septal thickening and perinephritic fat obliteration (Figs. 16.20 and 16.21b, c).

Perinephric abscesses appear on CT scans as areas of soft tissue or fluid attenuation within the perirenal space that, in some cases, may involve the psoas muscle and may extend to the pelvis and groin (Fig. 16.22).

MR plays no role in the diagnosis and evaluation of intrarenal abscess. It is a useful substitute in cases in which CT exams cannot be performed, like in pregnancy (Puvaneswary et al. 2003) or in iodinated allergic patients.

On MRI, intrarenal abscess generally appears as on ovoid or rounded thick-walled lesion with an inhomogeneous low-signal intensity on T1-weighted images and with increased signal intensity on T2-weighted images consistent with the fluid (Fig. 16.23).

Cellular debris forming a fluid-fluid level can be found inside the mass as well as irregular septations. Edema or thin stripes of fluid can be seen in the perinephric space on T2-weighted images, especially in lesions located near the renal cortex.

Extrarenal extension of an abscess with the involvement of perinephric or paranephric spaces is well depicted by means of CT or MRI (Figs. 16.21b, c and 16.24).

Percutaneous drainage of intra- or extrarenal abscess under radiologic guidance is the preferred method of therapy. Ultrasonic or CT guidance may be

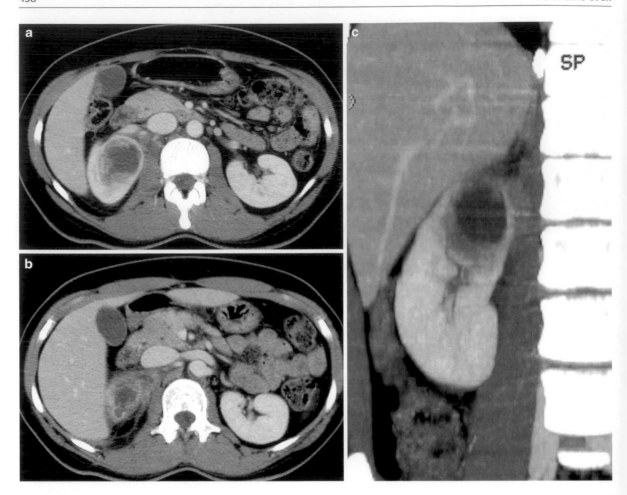

**Fig. 16.21** (**a–c**) Contrast-enhanced CT in a patient with early renal abscess. The lesion in the nephrographic phase (**a**) appears as a not-enhancing fluid-filled rounded area with an irregular thick halo of diminished enhancement representing infected but not necrotic parenchyma. CT scan at the level of the upper pole of the kidney (**b**) shows the involvement of the perinephric space. Coronal multiplanar reconstruction (**c**) well demonstrates both parenchymal and perinephric involvement

used, depending upon the size and location of the purulent fluid collections.

## 16.3 Gas-Forming Renal Infections

The presence of gas within the renal parenchyma or inside the excretory system may be due to a variety of benign or pathological entities.

The most frequent sources include the iatrogenic introduction of air during a surgical or radiological procedure, enteric fistula formation, external penetrating trauma, and bland tissue infarction with necrosis.

Surely, the most severe, life-threatening cause is urinary infection with gas-forming bacteria, with gram-negative microorganisms like *E. coli* in 70% of cases, followed by Klebsiella, Proteous, Entcrobacter, Pseudomonas, and Aerobacter, considered the most frequent bacteria responsible.

Gas-forming infections are usually associated with diabetes in the majority of cases, but they also occur in patients with altered host resistance with a depressed cell-mediated immune response, or in patients with urinary tract obstruction and infections.

Poor glycolysis at the tissue level in diabetic patients results in an increase of glucose concentration, followed by fermentation of this excess of glucose by bacteria with carbon dioxide and nitrogen production (Grayson et al. 2002).

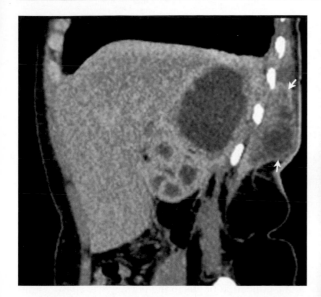

**Fig. 16.22** Patient with mature abscess in the right kidney with the involvement of the posterior muscular wall. Contrast-enhanced CT of the upper pole of the right kidney shows a round unenhanced collection with near-water attenuation and only a subtle rim of enhancement. The multiloculated fluid-filled collections inside the muscle of the posterior abdominal wall are well appreciable (*arrows*)

Gas-forming infections include two distinct clinical entity, emphysematous pyelonephritis and emphysematous pyelitis.

### 16.3.1  Emphysematous Pyelonephritis

Emphysematous pyelonephritis refers to a severe life-threatening gas forming infection with acute necrotizing parenchymal and perirenal infection (Craig et al. 2008; Kawashima et al. 1997).

In the vast majority of cases (85–90%), it is associated with diabetes, but it also occurs in nondiabetic patients with altered immunity, UTI, papillary necrosis, and significant renal functional impairment. Urinary tract obstruction due to renal stone disease, transitional cell carcinoma, or sloughed papillae was once considered to be an essential part of emphysematous pyelonephritis, together with diabetes and gram-negative organisms (Joseph et al. 1996); however, it was found in only 40% of 55 patients studied by Michaeli et al. (1984). Conversely, urinary tract obstruction is a frequent coexisting condition found in emphysematous pyelonephritis of nondiabetic patients.

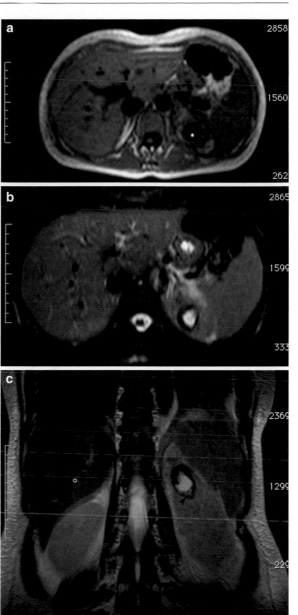

**Fig. 16.23** Young woman with focal abscess in the left kidney. (**a**) Axial Gradient-echo T1-weighted image shows a round hypointense lesion with hazy border in the upper pole of the left kidney (*asterisk*). The round fluid-filled abscess with irregular thick low-signal intensity wall in the upper pole of the kidney is well demonstrated both in the axial (**b**) and in the coronal (**c**) turbo spin-echo T2-weighted images. Note also some debris in the lower part of the abscess (*arrowhead* in **c**)

It seems reasonable to suppose that impaired host response, caused by local or systemic conditions, allows pathogens having the capability of producing carbon dioxide to use necrotic tissue as a substrate to generate gas in vivo (Dunnick et al. 2001).

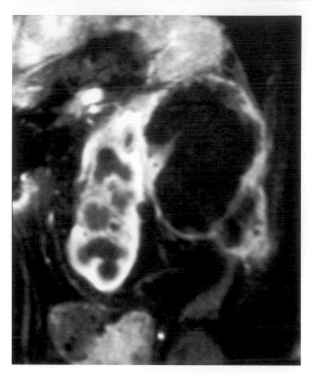

**Fig. 16.24** Huge peri- and pararenal left kidney abscess. Postcontrast sagittal T1-weighted gradient-echo image with FS shows a large loculated fluid-filled lesion with thick, irregular enhancing wall located in the perirenal and pararenal space (case courtesy of M. Scialpi, MD, University of Perugia, Italy)

It occurs exclusively in adult patients, with women affected twice as often as men and it is usually unilateral, although some case reports of bilateral forms are described in the literature.

Usual clinical presentation is very severe with rapid onset of chills, fever, flank pain, and vomiting; not infrequently, patients are lethargic and confused, with several associated medical problems such as hyperglycemia, acid-base irregularity, dehydration, and electrolyte imbalance (Grayson et al. 2002). Without early therapeutic intervention, the condition becomes rapidly progressive with fulminant septic shock, carrying an overall mortality rate of approximately 50% (Stunel et al. 2007).

Emphysematous pyelonephritis is a surgical emergency with nephrectomy recommended for patients with a fulminant clinical course, unsuccessful drainage, and for patients who do not improve after a few days of therapy.

Early medical management includes aggressive fluid support, hyperglycemic control in diabetic patients, intravenous broad-spectrum antimicrobial therapy,

correction of electrolyte, and acid-base irregularities. If a kidney is obstructed, surgical or preferentially percutaneous drainage is requested.

Especially in nondiabetic patients, improvement in antibiotics with combined interventional procedure has decreased the mortality (Papanicolaou and Pfister 1996).

X-ray of the abdomen may demonstrate gas bubble overlying the renal fossa in approximately 85% of cases (Evanoff et al. 1987).

In "early" cases, there are few bubbles of gas within the renal parenchyma, a feature often mistaken for bowel gas. With the rapid progression of the disease, it is possible to detect mottled or crescent-shaped gas collection in the renal parenchyma, sometimes radially oriented, corresponding to the renal pyramids. A crescentic collection of gas in the perinephric space within the Gerota's fascia indicates a more advanced stage of renal necrosis.

On imaging, US demonstrates an enlarged kidney with high-amplitude, nondependent echoes within the renal parenchyma or collecting system.

Definitive US differentiation of hyperechoic foci due to intraparenchymal and collecting system gas from those due to calcifications or stones can be difficult.

Usually, the gas reverberations produce characteristic low-level posterior reverberation artifacts known as "dirty shadowing," different from "clean" posterior shadowing produced by calcium (Vourganti et al. 2006).

The presence of adjacent bowel gas may also cause interpretive errors in the US evaluation of emphysematous pyelonephritis.

Furthermore, US is poor in differentiating between emphysematous pyelonephritis type 1 or 2, underestimates the depth of parenchymal involvement and perinephric extension of infection, and cannot detect small microabscesses that are common in early acute infections.

Although in the past, diagnosis of emphysematous pyelonephritis may have been made using IVU (mottled gas in nonfunctioning kidney), it is generally agreed that currently, the most reliable diagnostic imaging modality is CT.

CT allows to demonstrate the presence and extent of gas in the renal parenchyma and in subcapsular, perinephric or pararenal space, and also the presence of perinephric fluid collections or renal or perirenal abscesses, as well as the source of obstruction when present.

Administration of intravenous contrast material often reveals asymmetric renal enhancement or delayed excretion and, during the nephrogram phase, will help to recognize areas of focal tissue necrosis or abscess formation.

Two types of emphysematous pyelonephritis with different prognostic significance have been differentiated by Wan et al. on the basis of CT findings (Wan et al. 1996).

Type 1 represents the typical emphysematous pyelonephritis and is characterized by parenchymal destruction with streaky, mottled, bubbly, or loculated gas collections, but no perinephric fluid or focal abscess. In classic emphysematous pyelonephritis, gas may extend to the subcapsular, perinephric, and pararenal spaces and may cross to the controlateral retroperitoneal spaces, even when the other kidney is not infected.

Type 2 emphysematous pyelonephritis is characterized by the presence of bubbly or loculated gas in the renal parenchyma or by gas in collecting system with associated renal or perirenal fluid collections that are thought to be a sign of favorable immune response. The so-called "emphysematous pyelitis" should be considered as distinct, although the definition of type 2 emphysematous pyelonephritis can include this subset of gas-forming renal infections.

Type 1 has a more aggressive course and a significantly higher mortality rate (69% vs. 18% of type 2) (Wan et al. 1996).

CT is the modality of choice for evaluating patients with emphysematous pyelonephritis (Fig. 16.25). Conversely, MRI has no role in the detection of gas in the urinary system.

### 16.3.2 Emphysematous Pyelitis

Emphysematous pyelitis is a less aggressive and severe form of gas-forming renal infection, with gas localized to the renal collecting system (calyces or pelvis) (Craig et al. 2008; Grayson et al. 2002).

Emphysematous pyelitis is more common in women; it is often associated with obstructing conditions and 50% of the patients are diabetic. *E. coli* is the most common infecting pathogens, and pyuria is almost always evident on urinalysis (Joseph et al. 1996).

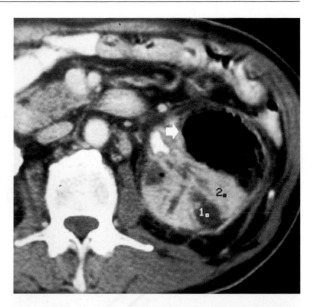

**Fig. 16.25** Diabetic patient with emphysematous pyelonephritis. Contrast-enhanced CT, nephrographic phase. Evidence of intrarenal air component (*arrow*). (**1**) Simple cyst. (**2**) Normal parenchyma

The overall mortality rate is significantly less than that for emphysematous pyelonephritis, in the range of 15–20% of cases. In the absence of obstruction, surgical or interventional drainage are seldom performed and the infectious process will likely respond to intravenous antimicrobial therapy. Nephrectomy should be reserved to the more aggressive form, with the persistence of gas despite the conservative medical therapy.

Plain film demonstrates gas inside the ureteral or pelvicaliceal system, but the tiny bubbles of gas, the so called "air pyelogram," can be obscured by the overlying gas inside the bowel; moreover, noninfectious source of air (e.g., trauma, reflux of air or gas from the bladder following a surgical or interventional radiologic procedure, gastro-intestinal or colonic fistula) should be excluded.

US findings are typically nondependent high-amplitude echoes within the renal pelvic or calices representing the foci of air, associated with posterior "dirty acoustic shadowing." This type of "dirty shadowing" can be differentiated from the more distinct acoustic "clean shadowing" that occurs posterior to renal calculi (Sommer and Taylor 1980).

CT represents the technique of choice, allowing an accurate differentiation of the less severe form of emphysematous pyelitis from the more aggressive emphysematous pyelonephritis.

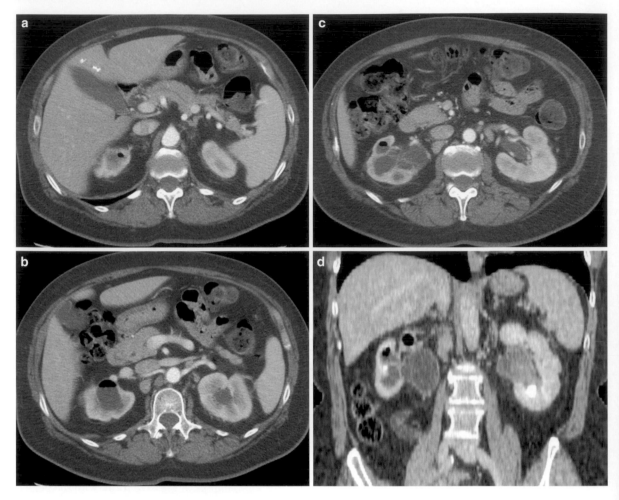

**Fig. 16.26** (**a–d**) Patient with emphysematous pyelitis. Contrast-enhanced CT scans obtained at different levels of the kidneys (**a–c**) and coronal multiplanar reconstruction (**d**) well show the dilated collecting system with gas bubbles and air-fluid levels within the right calyces

Typical CT features are a dilated collecting system, gas bubbles, or gas-fluid levels within the renal caliceal system or renal sinus, and the lack of parenchymal gas (Fig. 16.26).

## References

Ascenti G, Zimbaro G, Mazziotti S et al. (2004) Harmonic us imaging of vesicoureteric reflux in children: usefulness of a second generation us contrast agent. Paediatr Radiol 34: 481–487

Baumgarten DA, Baumgarten BR (1997) Imaging and radiologic management of upper urinary tract infections. Urol Clin North Am 24:545–569

Bjorgvinsson E, Majd M, Eggli KD (1991) Diagnosis of acute pyelonephritis in children: comparison of sonography and 99mTc-DMSA. AJR Am J Roentgenol 157:539–543

Blandino A, Minutoli F, Gacta M et al. (2003) MR pyelography in the assessment of hydroureteronephrosis: single-shot thick-slab rare versus multislice Haste sequences. Abdom Imaging 28:433–443

Browne RFJ, Zwirewich C, Torreggiani WC (2004) Imaging of urinary tract infection in the adult. Eur Radiol 14:168–183

Chan JHM, Tsui EYK, Luk SH et al. (2001) MR diffusion-weighted imaging of kidney: differentiation between hydronephrosis and pyonephrosis. J Clin Imaging 25:110–113

Conway JJ, Cohn RA (1994) Evolving role of nuclear medicine for the diagnosis and management of urinary tract infection. Editor's column. J Pediatr 124:87–90

Cova M, Squillace E, Stacul F et al. (2004) Diffusion-weighted MRI in the evaluation of renal lesions: preliminary results. Br J Radiol 77:851–857

Craig WD, Wagner BF, Travis MD (2008) Pyelonephritis: radio-logic-pathologic review. Radiographics 28:255–276

Dalla Palma L, Pozzi-Mucelli F, Pozzi-Mucelli RS (1995) Delayed CT findings in acute renal infection. Clin Radiol 50:364–370

De Sadeleer C, De Boe V, Keuppens F et al. (1993) Can the outcome of renal abnormalities be predicted on the basis of the initial Tc-99m DMSA scintigraphy? Eur J Nucl Med 20:867

Demertzis J, Menias CO (2007) State of the art: imaging of renal infections. Emerg Radiol 14:13–22

Dunnick NR, Sandler CM, Newhouse JH et al. (2001) Textbook of uroradiology, 3rd edn. Lippincott William & Wilkins, Philadelphia, PA, pp 150–177

Eggli DF, Tulchinsky M (1993) Scintigraphic evaluation of paediatric urinary tract infection. Semin Nucl Med 23:199–218

Evanoff GV, Thompson CS, Foley R et al. (1987) Spectrum of gas within the kidney: emphysematous phyelonephritis and emphysematous phyelitis. Am J Med 83:149–154

Fairley KF, Birch DF (1989) Detection of bladder bacteriuria in patients with acute urinary symptoms. J Infect Dis 159:226–231

Farhat W, Traubici J, Sherman C et al. (2002) Reliability of con-trast enhanced sonography with harmonic imaging for detect-ing early renal scarring in experimental pyelonephritis in a porcine model: preliminary results. J Urol 168:1114–1117

Geoghegan T, Govender P, Torreggiani WC (2005) MR-urography depiction of fluid-debris levels: a sign of phyonephrosis. AJR Am J Roentgenol 185:560

Gold RP, McClennan BL, Rottenberg RR (1983) CT appearance of acute inflammatory disease of the renal interstitium. AJR Am J Roentgenol 141:343–349

Goldman SM, Fishman EK (1991) Upper urinary tract infection: the current role of CT, ultrasound, and MRI. Semin Ultrasound CT MR 12:335–360

Grayson DE, Abbott RM, Levy AD et al. (2002) Emphysematous infections of the abdomen and pelvis: a pictorial review. Radiographics 22:543–561

Hatch DA, Ouwenga MK (2006) Pediatric urology. In: Henkin RE (ed) Nuclear medicine. Mosby, Philadelphia, PA, pp 1089–1107

Hoddick W, Jeffrey RB, Goldberg HI et al. (1983) CT and sonography of renal and perirenal infections. AJR Am J Roentgenol 140:517–520

Joseph RC, Amendola MA, Artze ME et al. (1996) Genitourinary tract gas: imaging evaluation. Radiographics 16:295–308

Kawashima A, Sandler CM, Goldman SM (2000) Imaging in acute renal infection. BJU Int 86:70–79

Kawashima A, Sandler CM, Goldman SM et al. (1997) CT of renal inflammatory disease. Radiographics 17:851–866

Latham RH, Running K, Stamm WE (1983) Urinary tract infec-tions in young adult women caused by staphylococcus sap-rophyticus. JAMA 250:3063–3066

Lee JK, McClennan BL, Melson GL et al. (1980) Acute focal bacterial nephritis: emphasis on gray scale sonography and computed tomography. AJR Am J Roentgenol 135:87–92

Lonergan GJ, Pennington DJ, Morrison JC et al. (1998) Childhood pyelonephritis: comparison of gadolinium-enhanced MR imaging and renal cortical scintigraphy for diagnosis. Radiology 207:377–384

Magno C, Blandino A, Anastasi G et al. (2004) Lithiasic obstruc-tive uropathy. Hydronephrosis characterization by magnetic resonance pyelography. Urol Int 72:40–42

Majd M, Nussbaum Blask AM, Markle BM et al. (2001) Acute pyelonephritis: comparison of diagnosis with 99mTc-DMSA SPECT, spiral CT, MR imaging, and power Doppler US in an experimental pig model. Radiology 218:101–108

Michaeli J, Mogle P, Perlberg S et al. (1984) Emphysematous pyelonephritis. J Urol 131:203–208

Mitterberger M, Pinggera GM, Colleselli D et al. (2007) Acute pyelonephritis: comparison of diagnosis with computed tomography and contrast-enhanced ultrasonography. BJU Int 101:341–344

Papanicolaou N, Pfister RC (1996) Acute renal infections. Radiol Clin North Am 34:965–995

Pennington DJ, Lonergan GJ, Flack CE et al. (1996) Experimental phyelonephritis in piglets: diagnosis with MR imaging. Radiology 201:199–205

Pickhardt PJ, Lonergan GJ, Davis CJ et al. (2000) Infiltrative renal lesions: radiologic-pathologic correlation. Radiographics 20:215–243

Piepsz A, Blaufox D, Gordon I et al. (1999) Consensus on renal cortical scintigraphy in children with urinary tract infection. Semin Nucl Med 29:160–174

Puvaneswary M, Bisits A, Kosken B (2003) Renal abscess with paranephric extension in a gravid woman: ultrasound and magnetic resonance findings. Australas Radiol 49:230–232

Rigsby CM, Rosenfield AT, Glickman MG et al. (1986) Hemorrhagic focal bacterial nephritis: findings on gray-scale sonography and CT. AJR Am J Roentgenol 146:1173–1177

Roberts JA (1991) Etiology and pathophysiology of pyelone-phritis. Am J Kidney Dis 17:1–9

Rossleigh MA (2007) Renal infection and vesico-ureteric reflux. Semin Nucl Med 37:261–268

Schaeffer AJ, Schaeffer MD (2007) Infections of the urinary tract. In: Vein AJ, Kavoussi LR, Novick AC et al. (eds) Campbell-Walsh urology, 9th edn. Saunders, Philadelphia, PA, pp 135–198

Sixt R, Stokland E (1998) Assessment of infective urinary tract disorders. Q J Nucl Med 42:119–125

Smellie JM, Normand IC (1975) Bacteria, reflux, and renal scar-ring. Arch Dis Child 50:581–585

Sommer FG, Taylor KJW (1980) Differentiation of acoustic shadowing due to calculi and gas collections. Radiology 135:399–403

Soulen MC, Fishman EK, Goldman SM et al. (1989) Bacterial renal infections: role of CT. Radiology 171:703–707

Stokland E, Hellstrom M, Jacobsson B et al. (1996) Early Tc-99m DMSA scintigraphy in symptomatic first-time uri-nary tract infection. Acta Paediatr 85:430–436

Stokland E, Hellstrom M, Jacobsson B et al. (1999) Imaging of renal scarring. Acta Paediatr Suppl 88:13–21

Stunel H, Bucley O, Feeney J et al. (2007) Imaging of acute pyelonephritis in adult. Eur Radiol 17:1820–1828

Talner LB, Davidson AJ, Lebowitz RL et al. (1994) Acute pyelo-nephritis: can we agree on terminology? Radiology 192:297–305

Thornbury JR (1991) Acute renal infections. Urol Radiol 12:209–213

Urban BA, Fishman EK (2000) Tailored helical CT evaluation of the acute abdomen. Radiographics 20:725–749

Verswijvel G, Vandecaveye V, Gelin G et al. (2002) Diffusion-weighted MR imaging in the evaluation of renal infection: preliminary results. JBR-BRT 85:100–103

Vourganti S, Agarwal PK, Bodner DR et al. (2006) Ultrasonographic evaluation of renal infections. Radiol Clin North Am 44:763–775

Wan YL, Lee TY, Bullard MJ et al. (1996) Acute gas-producing bacterial renal infection: correlation between imaging findings and clinical outcome. Radiology 198:433–438

Webb JAW (1997) The role of imaging in adult acute urinary tract infection. Eur Radiol 7:837–843

Weiser AC, Amukele SA, Leonidas JC et al. (2003) The role of gadolinium enhanced magnetic resonance imaging for children with suspected cute pyelonephritis. J Urol 169: 2308–2311

Wyatt SH, Urban BA, Fishman EK (1995) Spiral CT of the kidneys: role in characterization of renal disease I. Nonneoplastic disease. Crit Rev Diagn Imaging 36:1–37

Zimbaro G, Ascenti G, Visalli C et al. (2007) Contrast-enhanced ultrasonography (voiding urosonography) of vesico-ureteral reflux: state of the art. Radiol Med 112:1211–1224

# Chronic Renal Infections and Renal Fungal Infections

**17**

Emilio Quaia, Leonardo Giarraputo, Paola Martingano, and Marco Cavallaro

## Contents

### Abstract

> Chronic renal infections are becoming increasingly rare because of the availability of effective antibiotics, and early detection and treatment of both acute renal and urinary tract infections and conditions predisposing a patient to chronic infections. The aim of the present chapter is to illustrate the fundamental imaging features of the different forms of chronic renal infections, and the modern imaging of renal tuberculosis with multidetector CT urography. From pathological point of view the chronic renal infections include two types, interstitial chronic pyelonephritis and granulomatous pyelonephritis, namely xanthogranulomatous, malacoplakia and renal tuberculosis. In this chapter the findings and the role of ultrasonography (US), computed tomography (CT), intravenous excretory urography, and CT urograhy in the different chronic renal infections are reviewed.

From the pathological point of view the chronic renal infections include two types, interstitial chronic pyelonephritis and granulomatous pyelonephritis, namely xantogranulomatous pyelonephritis, renal tuberculosis, and malacoplakia (Dalla Palma and Pozzi Mucelli 2000). Imaging allows to depict both factors causing obstruction and infection such as stones and the renal and extrarenal extension of the disease. We shall focus on the following pathological entities: chronic pyelonephritis, renal tuberculosis, xanthogranulomatous pyelonephritis, renal replacement lipomatosis, malacoplakia, and cholesteatoma, and chronic renal infections in AIDS and renal fungal infections. We

E. Quaia (✉), L. Giarraputo, P. Martingano, and M. Cavallaro
Department of Radiology, Cattinara Hospital, University
of Trieste, Strada di Fiume 447, 34149 Trieste, Italy
e-mail: quaia@univ.trieste.it

E. Quaia (ed.), *Radiological Imaging of the Kidney*,
Medical Radiology, DOI: 10.1007/978-3-540-87597-0_17, © Springer-Verlag Berlin Heidelberg 2011

shall not deal with chronic pyonephrosis and of chronic abscess, because the features are common to the correspective acute disease.

## 17.1 Chronic Pyelonephritis

Chronic pyelonephritis is a somewhat controversial disease from a pathogenetic standpoint. Despite the ongoing debate on whether the condition is an active chronic infection, arises from multiple recurrent infections, or represents stable changes from a remote single infection, its radiologic appearance is the same (Craig et al. 2008). Chronic pyelonephritis is a chronic tubulo-interstitial

fibrosing nephritis with long-standing recurrent infection and ongoing renal destruction, that may be unilateral or bilateral and involves renal parenchyma, renal calices and renal pelvis. On the other hand, the term chronic pyelonephritis does not fit with the residuum of old disease not presently active (e.g., reflux nephropathy). Chronic pyelonephritis is more frequent in diabetic population, with 20–40% of incidence compared to 2–6% in normal population according to autopsy series. Kidneys are dimensionally reduced with atrophy, parenchymal scars, irregular margins and cortical thinning and hypertrophy of residual normal tissue, and dilation of corresponding renal calices – calyceal clubbing secondary to retraction of the papilla from overlying scar – (Figs. 17.1 and 17.2), dilatation of the calyceal system (Craig et al.

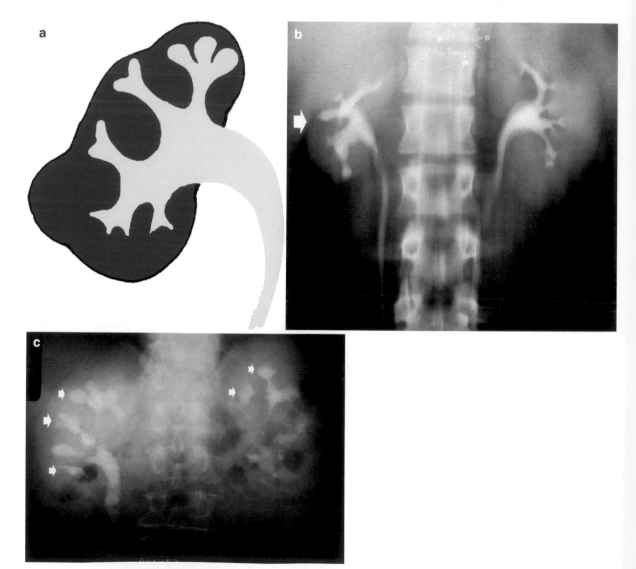

**Fig. 17.1** (a–c) Chronic pyelonephritis. (a) Typical calyceal deformations. (b, c) Intravenous excretory urography. Progressive caliceal distortion (*arrows*) due to the underlying renal parenchyma damage and scarring

**Fig. 17.2** (**a–d**) Chronic pyelonephritis. Multidetector CT urography. Coronal reformations. (**a, b**) Right kidney. Calyceal distortion and clubbing (*arrows*) due to the underlying renal parenchyma damage with renal parenchyma scarring and focal reduction of renal parenchyma thickness. (**c, d**) Left kidney. Diffure reduction of the renal parenchyma thickness with caliceal distortion (*arrows*)

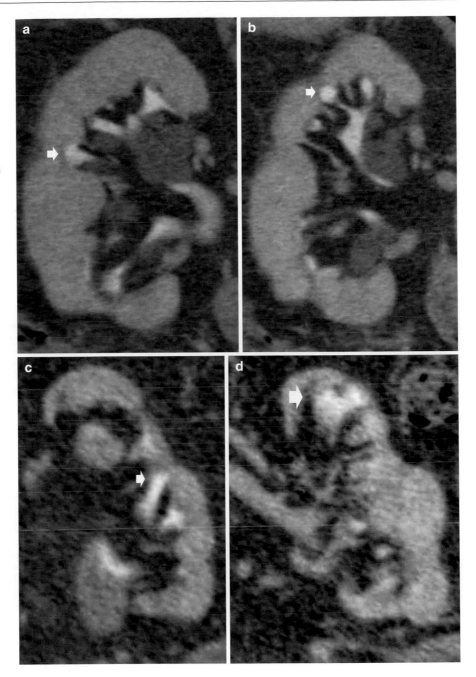

2008, and increased parenchymal echogenicity with poor corticomedullary differentiation. Hypertension is frequently a long-term sequela.

The goals of imaging in chronic recurrent pyelonephritis are the detection of chronic renal damage, and the detection of abnormalities that are often the cause of recurrence. However it should be stressed that there are no radiologic features that at a single point in time reliably indicate activity of the process. Therefore the goals of radiological investigations become the detection of abnormalities that are often the cause of the recurrence (i.e., infectious stones) and the detection of the chronic renal damage. In the past, intravenous excretory urography and nephrotomography, and nowadays CT urography are often capable to achieve these two goals. Findings related to the chronic renal damage (decrease of the kidney size, parenchymal scars, caliceal distortion – Fig. 17.1) are easily depicted at intravenous excretory urography.

Multidetector computed tomography (CT) urography and magnetic resonance (MR) imaging readily identify the chronic renal parenchyma damage and calyceal distortion and clubbing (Fig. 17.2).

## 17.2 Renal Tuberculosis

Genitourinary tuberculosis is the most common manifestation of extrapulmonary tuberculosis (Engin et al. 2000; Harisinghani et al. 2000) accounting for 15–20% of infections outside the lungs (Gibson et al. 2004). Approximately 4–8% of patients with pulmonary tuberculosis will develop clinically significant genitourinary infection (Gibson et al. 2004). *Mycobacterium tuberculosis* reaches the genitourinary organs, particularly the kidneys, by the hematogenous seeding from disease in the lungs. The seeding occurs at the time of the initial lung infection with seeding of *Mycobacterium tuberculosis* in the periglomerular and peritubular capillary bed. Small granulomas form in the renal cortex bilaterally, adjacent to the glomeruli, and remain stable for many years (Kenney 1990). A high rate of perfusion and favorable oxygen tension increase the likelihood of bacilli proliferating in this location (Gibson et al. 2004). In patients with intact cellular immunity, the disease remains confined to the renal cortex, while in some patients, breakdown of host defense mechanisms leads to reactivation of the cortical granulomas with enlargement and coalescenze and organisms spread into the real medulla causing a papillitis which may extend into the collecting system (Kenney 1990). In fact, after capillary rupture the organisms migrate to the proximal tubule and loop of Henle with eventual development of enlarging, caseating granulomas and papillary necrosis. Granuloma formation, caseous necrosis, and cavitation are stages of progressive infection, which can eventually determine the loss of renal function and calcification of the entire kidney (autonephrectomy).

The renal disease remains quiescent until there is an insult to the host's immunity at which time reactivation occurs. Patients with genitourinary tuberculosis typically have local symptoms including frequent voiding and dysuria. Hematuria can be either microscopic or macroscopic. Symptoms may also include back, flank, or abdominal pain (Simon et al. 1977; Gibson et al. 2004). Constitutional symptoms such as fever, weight loss, fatigue, and anorexia are less common (Simon et al. 1977; Gibson et al. 2004). Laboratory abnormalities include pyuria, proteinuria, and hematuria. Standard urine cultures can be normal. Furthermore, the presence of routine urinary tract pathogens can delay the diagnosis of coexistent tuberculosis (Gibson et al. 2004). *Mycobacterium tuberculosis* is isolated from the urine in 80–95% of patients with genitourinary tuberculosis. In adults renal tuberculosis is the most known etiology of infundibolar strictures with consequent hydrocalyx. Obstruction may develop early or during the healing phase, even while the patient is receiving antituberculous therapy.

It must be underlined that each finding of renal tuberculosis can be caused by other diseases, but multiple abnormalities are usually present and allow a correct diagnosis. That's why renal tuberculosis is called the "great imitator." On the plain film and unenhanced CT the kidney may appear large, normal sized or small. Despite hematogenous seeding of both kidneys, clinically significant disease is usually limited to one side and approximately 75% of renal tuberculous involvement is unilateral.

The gray-scale US appearance of renal tuberculosis is not specific. US is advisable to evaluate the nonfunctioning kidney after iodinated contrast agent injection and for the follow-up antitubercular therapy. Kidney may appear large, normal sized or small, and calcifications are common. Hydronephrosis or hypoechoic parenchymal lesions, which correspond to parenchymal abscesses resulting from caseating necrosis, may be observed.

CT urography, as in the past intravenous excretory urography, is now considered the correct imaging technique to assess the upper urinary tract, including the involvement in renal tuberculosis. The most common CT finding arc renal calcifications (37–71%) (Gibson et al. 2004) which follow different patterns. Calcifications may be amorphous, granular, lobar, or curvilinear and frequently extend beyond the kidney (e.g., psoas muscle).

CT urography allows a more accurate evaluation of the amount of residual functioning parenchyma and of the extrarenal spread (Kenney 1990). Nowadays CT urography represents the most accurate imaging techniques to reveal early manifestations of renal tuberculosis (Fig. 17.3). The earliest morphologic alterations of

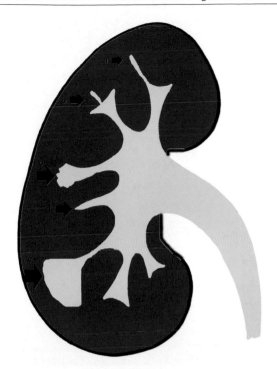

**Fig. 17.3** The early morphologic alterations of renal parenchyma determined by tuberculosis. The fundamental calyceal alterations in renal tuberculosis: calyceal erosion (**a**), medullary necrosis (**b**), papillary necrosis (**c**), and infundibular stricture without (**d**) or with hydrocalyx (**e**)

renal parenchyma corresponding to calyceal alterations determined by tuberculosis include calyceal erosion ("moth-eaten calyx") (Fig. 17.4a) with progression towards medullary (Fig. 17.4b) or papillary necrosis (Fig. 17.4c, d). The pathologic features of renal TB are extremely different and frequently different features coexist (Fig. 17.4b). Common sites of tuberculous strictures are the calyceal neck with hydrocalyx (Figs. 17.5a and 17.6) or phantom calyx (Figs. 17.5b–d and 17.7), infundibulum of a calyx with hydrocalyx or regional or focal hydrocalycosis (Fig. 17.8), the uretero-pelvic junction with dilatation of the entire renal pelvis, calyces and infundibola (Fig. 17.9), or the lower ureteral segment. Tubercular strictures often cohexist with adjacent renal parenchyma scarring. The development of infundibular, pelvic, or ureteral strictures is nearly pathognomonic of renal tuberculosis (Kenney 1990). An infundibular stricture may result in a "phantom calyx" when that segment of the kidney becomes nonfunctional (Fig. 17.5b–d) (Kenney 1990). CT is very accurate in demonstrating parenchymal gross calcifications (Fig. 17.8).

Renal tuberculosis may manifest as extensive cavitation (open or extensive forms) or fibrosclerosis (closed forms) (Becker 1988; Wang et al. 1997). The open or extensive form (Fig. 17.10) corresponds to the extension of the caseified tissue necrosis to the intrarenal excretory tract (Fig. 17.11). Parenchymal masses can develop which may be calcified (Kenney 1990). Communication of the granulomas with the collecting system (Fig. 17.12) can lead to regional spread of the bacilli into the renal pelvis, ureters, urinary bladder, and accessory genital organs. Extensive cavitation may determine renal caseation, whereas fibrosing reaction of the urinary tract results in obstructive hydronephrosis. When the process spreads into the collecting system, the three ways of evolution of the disease: (1) extensive cavitation (Figs. 17.13 and 17.14); (2) fibrosclerosis with resulting noncommunicating cavities (Figs. 17.14–17.17); (3) recurrent "poussées."

The closed or fibrosclerotic form (Fig. 17.18) presents a better outcome to therapy and consists in the extension of the caseified necrosis toward the renal parenchyma. The host's healing response induces fibrosis with calcium deposition, focal fibrosis with progressive parenchymal scarring, stricture formation and dilatation of the intrarenal urinary tract and autonephrectomy (no functional contrast excretion). The fibrosclerotic forms of renal TB may appear as: (1) pure fibrosclerosis with parenchymal scar (Fig. 17.19) often with evidence of noncommunicating cavities (Fig. 17.20); (2) reactivation of the granulomatous process over a permanent status of fibrosclerosis with caseous necrosis and cavitation, or mixed fibrosclerotic and cavitating form, and resulting communicating or noncommunicating cavities with the intrarenal urinary tract (Fig. 17.21). Both forms determine parenchymal calcifications, deformation of the adjacent renal calices from the simple narrowing of the calyx to medullary and papillary necrosis to obstructive hydronephrosis or hydrocalyx.

The end stage of renal tuberculosis corresponds to extensive renal parenchyma caseation and cavitation (Fig. 17.22) resulting in the putty kidney (Fig. 17.23) with the entire kidney becoming small, scarred, and densely calcified (Goldman et al. 1985) with autonephrectomy. In the putty kidney a calcified and thick materials fills a dilated collecting system (Fig. 17.24).

**Fig. 17.4** (**a–d**) Renal tuberculosis. (**a**) Intravenous excretory urography. Calyceal distortion due to initial erosion (*small arrows*); (**b**) Intravenous excretory urography. Renal medullary necrosis (*arrow*) with evidence also of infundibular stricture (*arrowhead*) and adjacent hydrocalyx; (**c**) Intravenous excretory urography. Papillary necrosis (*arrows*). (**d**) CT urography. Maximum intensity projection. Renal medullary necrosis (*arrow*) in one of the renal calices of the lower group

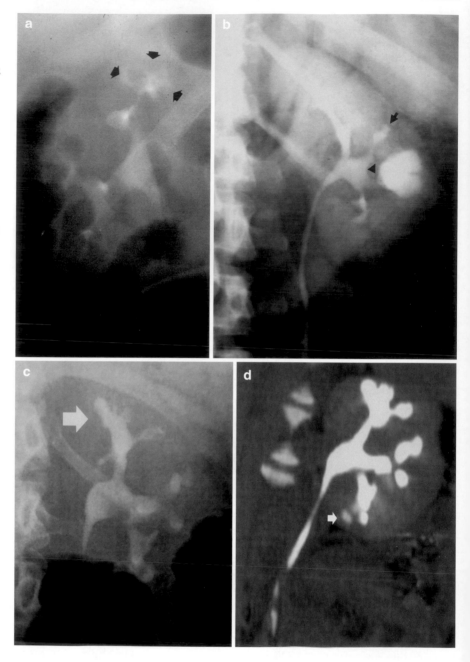

## 17.3 Xanthogranulomatous Pyelonephritis

Xanthogranulomatous pyelonephritis (XGP) is a granulomatous infection characterized by destruction and replacement of renal parenchyma and surrounding tissues with lipid-laden macrophages (xanthoma cells). Females and diabetic patients are more frequently affected. The peak incidence age is the sixth decade of life. This chronic infection is attributed to chronic obstruction or to *Proteus* or *E. coli* infection in 60% of cases. Clinically, XGP manifests with back pain, malaise, weight loss, and urinary tract symptoms such as frequency and dysuria which may be absent in up to 60% of the cases. XGP is almost always unilateral (Parker and Clark 1989). Diffuse XGP form

**Fig. 17.5** (**a–d**) Renal tuberculosis. (**a**) Intravenous excretory urography. Tubercular stricture (*small arrow*) with evidence of hydrocalyx (*large arrow*) and adjacent calyceal erosion (*long arrow*). (**b**) Intravenous excretory urography, and (**c, d**) nephrotomography. Tubercular infundibular stricture (*arrows*) with phantom calyx. (**d**) Renal infundibular stricture (*arrowheads*) often cohexists with adjacent renal parenchyma scar

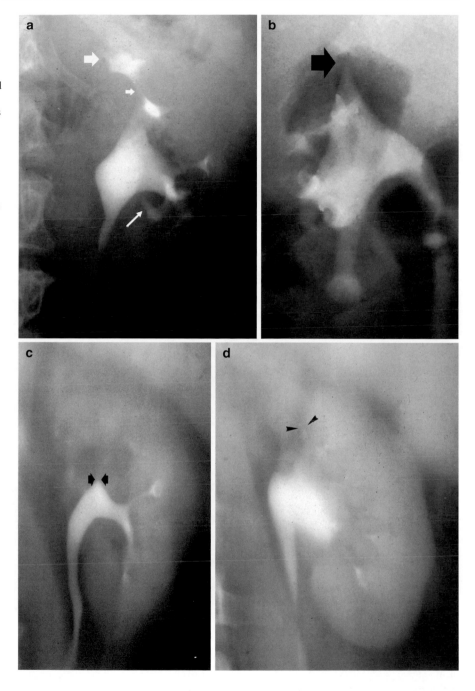

(Subramanyam et al. 1982) is much more frequent (85–90%) than focal (tumefactive) form (Kawashima et al. 1997). Three XGP stages are described: (1) Confined to the kidney; (2) Extension to the Gerota's fascia; (3) Involvement of the paranephric spaces and other retroperitoneal structures.

US reveals a multifocal enlargement of the kidney or a pseudotumoral unifocal pattern (Hartman et al. 1984;

Brown et al. 1996). Furthermore multiple anechoic or hypoechoic areas with echoic content (dylated calyces and/or cavitary collections filled by inflammatory products) surrounded by a thin hyperechoic zone that represents the surrounding inflammatory reaction, and apparent parenchymal thickening (xanthomatous tissue) can be recognized. Stones and renal enlargement may also be identified. The focal (tumefactive form) of

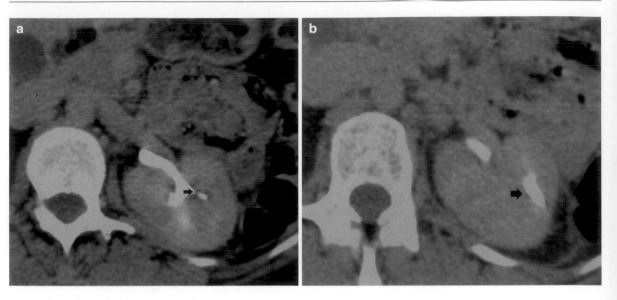

**Fig. 17.6** (**a–b**) Renal tuberculosis. (**a, b**) CT urography. Transverse scan. (**a**) Infundibular stricture (*arrow*) due to fibrosclerosing tuberculosis with narrowing of the infundibulum. (**b**) Dilatation of an upper renal calyx (hydrocalyx)

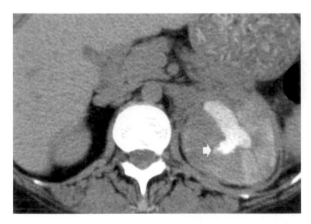

**Fig. 17.7** Renal tuberculosis. CT urography. Transverse scan. Infundibular stricture (*arrow*) due to fibrosclerosing tuberculosis with narrowing of the infundibulum and phantom calyx

XGP may be considered a pseudotumoral lesion (Soler et al. 1997) – see also Chap. 22. The principal differential diagnoses include renal cell carcinoma, transitional cell carcinoma of the kidney, renal lymphoma, and hypertrophic chronic pyelonephritis.

Intravenous excretory urography (IVU) can detect three main different features in the diffuse form: calcifications and stones (79% of cases); renal enlargement and absent excretion of contrast agent in the affected kidney (76%) (Grainger et al. 1982). Stones are usually large and centrally located, often staghorn in type.

CT shows the same three findings detectable by IVU, namely calcifications – stone – and renal enlargement (Fig. 17.25), and additional important features as well, i.e., spherical low-density non enhancing areas (from −15 to +30 HU) surrounded by enhancing rims corresponding to intrarenal collections (Fig. 17.26), possible finer calcifications within the xanthomatous mass, frequent involvement of perinephric region (Fig. 17.27) and adjacent structures with thickening of the Gerota's fascia (Goldman et al. 1984; Claes et al. 1987), and sometimes gas component (Fig. 17.28). The focal form appears as a large hypodense nonenhancing mass possibly with rim enhancement and associated calculus, or as a focal area of renal enlargement with one or more hypo- or anechoic masses. In the focal form all modalities may fail in characterizing lesion. The newer investigative modalities and an increased awareness of XGP should make preoperative diagnosis possible in at least 2/3 of the cases. CT in particular appears to offers a reliable means of diagnosis and spread evaluation. MRI does not seem to give better information than CT.

On cross-sectional imaging the focal form of XGP appears as a non specific renal mass (Fig. 17.29). On examination of the macroscopic specimen, the focal (tumefactive) form manifests as a focal renal mass of yellow tissue with regional necrosis and hemorrhage mimicking renal cell carcinoma. Calculi are better

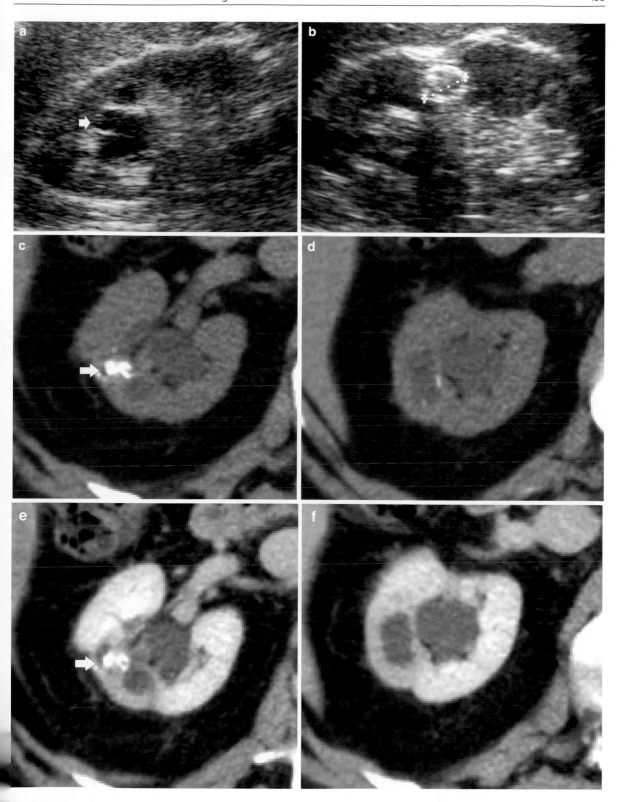

**Fig. 17.8** (**a–g**) Renal tuberculosis. (**a, b**) Ultrasound scan, longitudinal view. Segmental dilatation of the upper urinary tract (*arrow*) with focal calcification within the renal parenchyma (*calipers*) and retraction of the renal profile. Unenhanced (**c, d**) and contrast-enhanced CT (**e, f**) show the renal parenchyma calcifications (*arrow*) with segmental dilatation of the intrarenal urinary tract. (**g**) CT urography, maximum intensity projection. Segmental dilatation of the upper urinary tract (*arrow*) due to fibrosclerosing tuberculosis with tuberculous stricture at the superior infundibulum with regional hydrocalycosis (*arrow*)

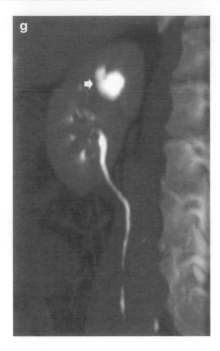

**Fig. 17.8** (continued)

depicted with CT but may be seen at MR imaging as areas of signal void within the collecting system. At MR imaging, the renal parenchyma is compressed by dilated calices and replaced by abscess cavities with intermediate signal intensity on T1-weighted images and high signal intensity on T2-weighted images. Cavity walls may show marked enhancement after contrast material administration. Although the focal form of the disease may be misinterpreted as a renal neoplasm, the presence of a staghorn calculus, appropriate clinical presentation (e.g., chronic pyelonephritis in diabetic patients), and the characteristic imaging findings strongly suggest the diagnosis.

The perirenal space is commonly involved in a wide variety of neoplastic and nonneoplastic conditions including chronic fibrosis, often with xanthogranulomatous features (Fig. 17.30). The most frequent nontumoral pathology of the perirenal space is the secondary perirenal involvement from retroperitoneal fibrosis (Surabhi et al. 2008). Perirenal fibrosis that occurs in association with retroperitoneal fibrosis or as

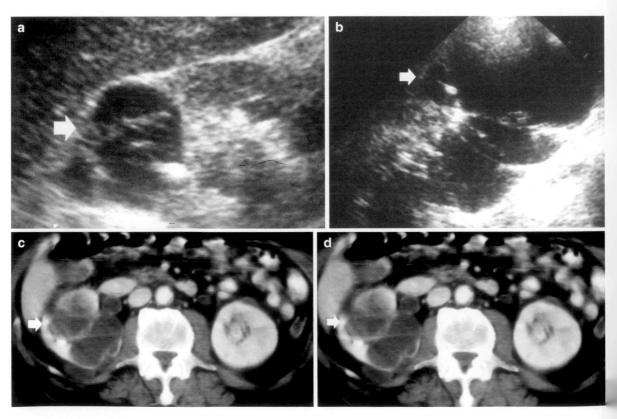

**Fig. 17.9** (**a**–**d**) Sixty-three-year-old patients with renal tuberculosis. Contrast-enhanced nephrographic phase CT. US (**a**: transverse scan; **b**: longitudinal scan). Dilatation of the renal pelvis (*arrow*), which is confirmed by contrast-enhanced CT (**c**, **d**). Renal tuberculosis determines a fibrosclerosis of the uretero-pelvic junction with consequent markedly dilated calices and renal parenchyma thinning

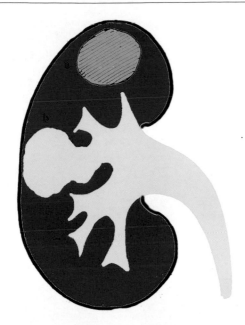

**Fig. 17.10** Renal tuberculosis with caseified tissue necrosis. Open forms. The extensive cavitation of renal parenchyma results in noncommunicating (**a**) or communicating cavities (**b**) with the intrarenal excretory tract with deformation of the adjacent renal calices from the simple narrowing of the calyx, medullary and papillary necrosis, up to obstructive hydronephrosis

part of multifocal fibrosclerosis is not difficult to detect at imaging. However, the imaging features of isolated perirenal fibrosis are nonspecific, and a biopsy may be required to achieve a definitive diagnosis.

## 17.4 Renal Replacement Lipomatosis

Renal replacement lipomatosis (RRL) is a rare reactive pathological entity that is characterized by focal or extensive fat tissue proliferation and renal parenchymal atrophy. It is usually associated with chronic inflammation and calculi. Large hyperplastic fat cells in the renal sinus are diagnostic of RRL. Fat tissue proliferation may be localized in renal sinus, renal hilus and in perirenal and periureteral spaces with severe atrophy of renal parenchyma and enlargement of the kidney. It is usually associated with chronic inflammation, calculi (75%) or XGP (Acunas et al. 1990). Association with renal tuberculosis was also reported (Casas et al. 2002). Plain radiograph characteristically demonstrates a staghorn calculus and, sometimes, a lucent mass.

US reveals an enlarged kidney outlined by a thin hypoechoic rim corresponding to the residual renal parenchyma, stones with posterior acoustic shadowing and sometimes the extension of the echogenicity of the renal sinus to renal parenchyma (Subramanyam et al. 1983). Both XGP and RRL generally coexist and a complete distinction between these two entities is possible only by histological features.

Replacement lipomatosis of the kidney is characterized by extensive renal sinus lipomatosis with parenchymal atrophy. It is usually associated with chronic inflammation and with calculi. In addition to

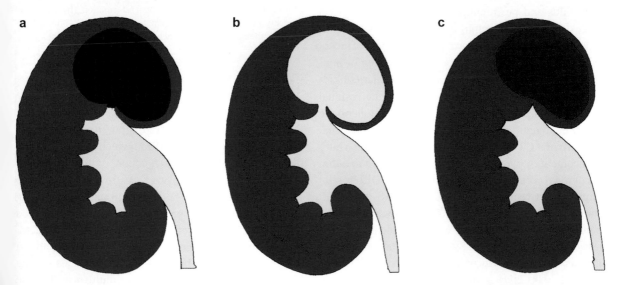

**Fig. 17.11** (**a–c**) Evolution of the open forms of renal tuberculosis. The caseified tissue necrosis (**a**) progressively spreads to the renal urinary tract (**b**). The progressive fibrosclerosis results in a noncommunicating cavity (**c**)

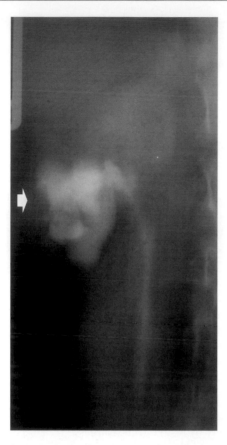

**Fig. 17.12** Open or extensive form. Intravenous excretory urography–nephrotomography with cavitation and extension of the caseified tissue necrosis to the intrarenal excretory tract

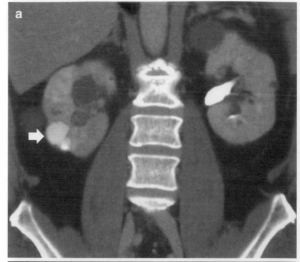

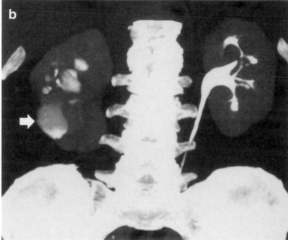

**Fig. 17.13** (**a**) CT urography, coronal reformation. (**b**) Maximum intensity projection. A parenchymal cavity (*arrow*) communicating with the renal excretory tract is visualized on the right kidney

renal sinus, replacement lipomatosis may involve renal hilus and perirenal and sometimes periureteral spaces. Plain radiograph characteristically demonstrates a staghorn calculus and, sometimes, a lucent mass. IVU demonstrates a poorly functioning or nonfunctioning kidney, while US shows an enlarged kidney, outlined by a thin hypoechoic rim (the residual renal parenchyma), stones and the extension of the highly echogenic appearance of the sinus to the renal parenchyma. CT demonstrates stones and diffuse fatty replacement of parenchyma which is reduced to a thin rim of renal cortex (Figs. 17.31 and 17.32). Differential diagnosis between replacement lipomatosis and XGP can be difficult. However in XGP the low attenuation material filling the dilated calyces typically ranges between −15 and +30 HU, while in replacement lipomatosis an attenuation of pure fatty tissue (between −60 and −100 HU) is observed. Sometimes the two diseases coexist.

## 17.5 Renal Malacoplakia

Renal malacoplakia is a rare granulomatous infection (Stanton and Maxted 1981) which occurs because of abnormal monocyte function with accumulation of bacteria incompletely destroyed forming the Michaelis – Guttman bodies (Hartman et al. 1980; Kenney 1990). This pathologic entity is attributed to chronic renal infection by Gram negative bacteria, and most frequently *E. coli*. Most frequently it involves the bladder, but it can be observed also in the kidney. There are two forms, the multifocal and the unifocal. The multifocal form consists in the diffuse enlargement of the kidney with evidence of intrarenal well-delimited yellowish masses with hemorrhagic and necrotic components. The unifocal form appears as a single mass with the same features of the multifocal form. Renal malacoplakia is also a rare cause of acute renal failure (Tam et al. 2003) and obstructive nephropathy due to ureteral and bladder involvement (Sanchez et al. 2009).

IVU usually shows a large smooth kidney without hydronephrosis and often non visualization of

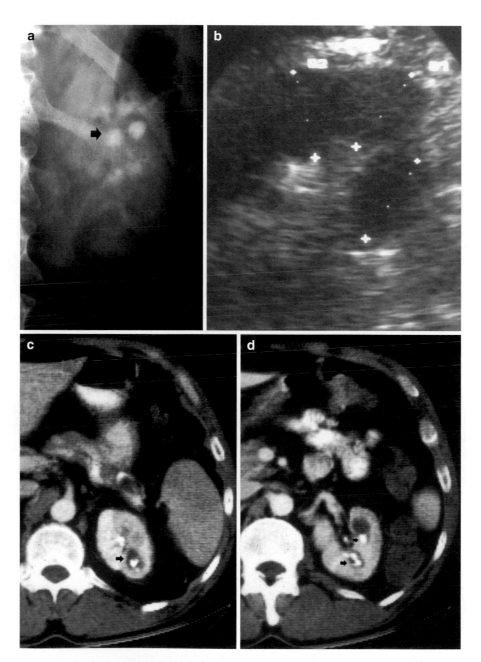

**Fig. 17.14** (**a–f**) Diffuse cavitating open form of renal tuberculosis. (**a**) Intravenous urography, and (**b**) gray-scale ultrasound. Evidence of multiple cavities (*arrow*) on the upper pole of the left kidney communicating with the intrarenal collecting system. (**c–f**) Contrast-enhanced CT during the excretory phase. The left kidney shows diffuse parenchymal cavitation with resulting communicating (*arrows* in **c** and **d**) and noncommunicating cavities (*arrow* and caliper in **e** and **f**)

**Fig. 17.14** (continued)

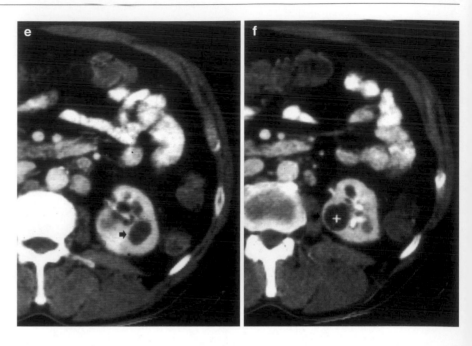

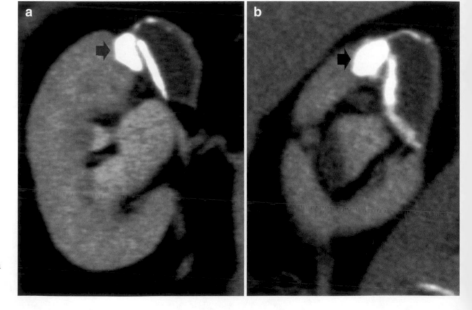

**Fig. 17.15** (**a**, **b**) Renal tuberculosis. CT urography, Coronal (**a**) and sagittal (**b**) reformations of the right kidney. Fibrosclerosing tuberculosis with gross calcification (*arrow*) at the level of the renal parenchyma and adjacent noncommunicating cavity

collecting system. Sometimes small filling defects in the pelvis, ureters and bladder are detected. US shows a large kidney with poorly defined masses of variable echogenicity. The central echo complex in the sinus is distorted and compressed. CT also shows a renal enlargement with hypodense solid masses (Fig. 17.33) with do not enhance, often with involvement of the renal excretory tract which appears compressed or infiltrated. Perinephric extension can be detected. Because of its rarity, renal malacoplakia is usually not considered preoperatively, but the diagnosis could be suggested when above patterns are shown in a patient with urinary tract infection by *E. coli*, especially with a known focus of non renal malacoplakia.

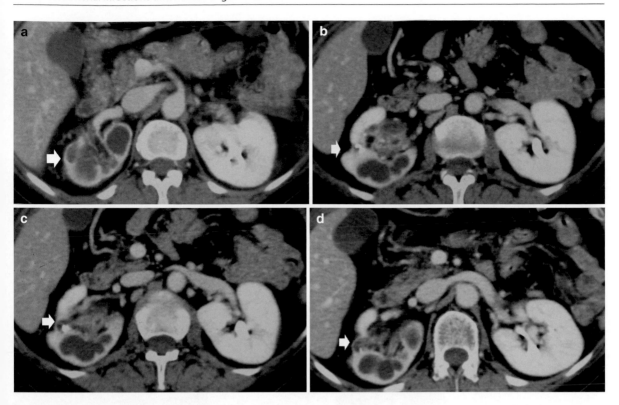

**Fig. 17.16** (**a–d**) Open form of renal tuberculosis with diffusion into the intrarenal collecting system extensive cavitation and fibrosclerosis with resulting noncommunicating cavities. Contrast-enhanced CT during the excretory phase. Extension of the caseified tissue necrosis to the intrarenal excretory tract with parenchymal fibrosclerosis with calcifications and irregularities of the renal margins (*arrow*) and resulting noncommunicating cavities

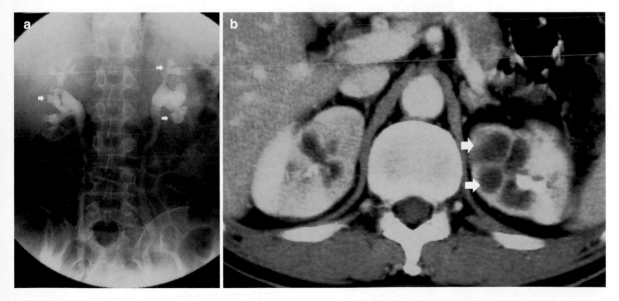

**Fig. 17.17** (**a–d**) Open form with diffusion into the intrarenal collecting system extensive cavitation and fibrosclerosis with resulting noncommunicating cavities. (**a**) Intravenous excretory urography. Irregularities in the morphology and deformations of the renal calcyces (*arrows*). (**b–d**) Contrast-enhanced CT during the excretory phase. Renal parenchyma extensive necrosis with noncommunicating cavities (*arrows*) in both kidneys, and parenchymal fibrosclerosis with calcifications and irregularities of the renal margins

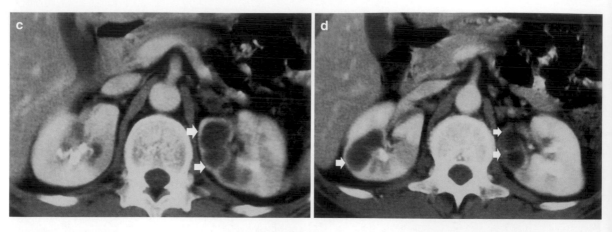

**Fig. 17.17** (continued)

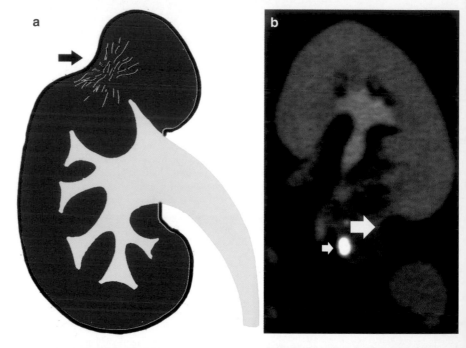

**Fig. 17.18** (**a**) Scheme. Closed form of renal tuberculosis. The pathologic process extends towards the renal parenchyma with progressive fibrosclerosis (*arrow*) and distortion of the adjacent renal calices. (**b**) CT-urography. Typical parenchyma fibrosclerosis (*large arrow*) with adjacent gross parenchymal calcification (*small arrow*)

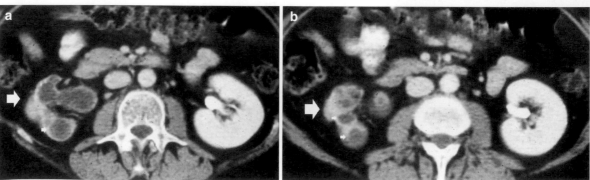

**Fig. 17.19** (**a, b**) Closed form of renal tuberculosis. Contrast-enhanced CT during the excretory phase. The right kidney shows extensive parenchymal fibrosclerosis (*large arrows*) with scar, dilatation of the intrarenal excretory tract (*small arrows*), and loss of excretory function with autonephrectomy (no contrast excretion is evident)

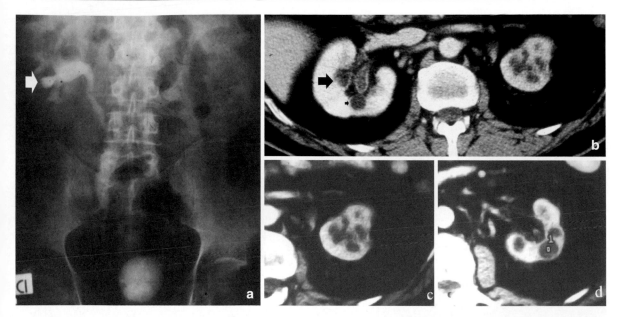

**Fig. 17.20** (**a–d**) Closed form of renal tuberculosis. (**a**) Intravenous urography. Dilatation of the upper (*arrow*) and lower urinary tract with no evidence of contrast excretion in the left kidney. (**b–d**) Contrast-enhanced CT during the excretory phase. (**b**) The right kidney shows parenchymal fibrosclerosis with clear irregularities of the renal parenchyma margins, calyceal deformation and dilatation (*large arrow*) due to the renal parenchyma sclerosis and one noncommunicating cavity (*small arrow*). (**c, d**) The left kidney shows extensive fibrosclerosis with parenchymal scar, necrosis with cavitation and multiple noncommunicating cavities due to reactivation of the caseating process over fibrosclerosis

## 17.6 Cholesteatoma

Long-standing urinary tract infection (particularly with TB) can cause squamous metaplasia of the collecting system (Molina et al. 1988). Desquamation of these epithelial cells forms an intraluminal collection of keratin, which is called a cholesteatoma. The nonspecific symptoms include dysuria, hematuria, and colic. On urography or retrograde pyelography a filling defect is seen with a characteristic laminated appearance caused by contrast material entering interstices in the mass. Calcification can occur, which may in part account for the fact that on CT the attenuation is higher than the usual soft-tissue filling defect (Figs. 17.34 and 17.35). This is not a premalignant condition. Nevertheless, there may be progressived estruction and rapid reaccumulation of debris if the lesion is merely extracted.

## 17.7 Renal Infections in AIDS Patients

The urinary tract is relatively spared from the effects of AIDS (urological symptoms occur in 16% of all patients) and chronic infections are definitely unusual. In *Pneumocystis carinii, Citomegalovirus* and *Mycobacterium avium intracellulare* acquired immuno-deficiency syndrome (AIDS)-correlated disseminated infections, US may reveal diffuse echogenic spots on renal cortex which correspond to punctate calcifications (Miller et al. 1993). *Mycobacterium tuberculosis* may also involve the kidney in AIDS patients manifesting as renal abscesses on US, CT, and MR imaging and pyonephrosis in the acute setting. *Mycobacterium avium intracellulare* asymmetrically involved the renal cortex and medulla (Falkoff et al. 1987).

Disseminated infection by *Candida albicans* determine focal microabscesses in the liver, spleen, pancreas and kidneys, which appear as multiple small hypoechoic lesions on US. *Pneumocystis jirovecii* is a fungus that is most commonly associated with the AIDS-defining illness *Pneumocystis carinii* pneumonia (Symeonidou et al. 2009). The renal infection from *Pneumocystis jirovecii* include atypical cortical nephrocalcinosis (Bergman et al. 1991).

In AIDS patients, *Mucormycosis* usually manifests as disseminated or focal invasion of renal parenchymal vessels, with cortical infarcts and medullary necrosis (Fig. 17.36) (Keogh et al. 2003; Sharma et al.

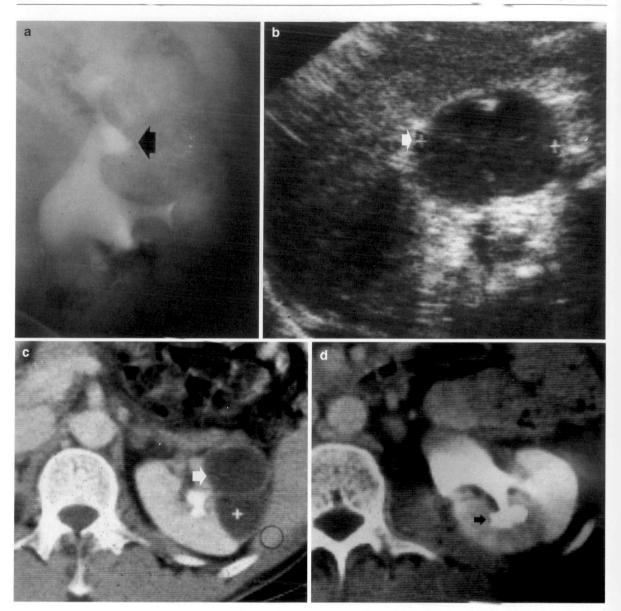

**Fig. 17.21** (**a**–**d**) Closed fibrosclerotic form of renal tuberculosis. (**a**) Intravenous excretory urography. Tubercular infundibular stricture with phantom calyx (*arrow*). (**b**) Ultrasound, longitudinal scan. Evidence of an hypoechoic lesion (*arrow*) in the upper pole of the kidney within the renal parenchyma corresponding to a cavitation. (**c**, **d**) Contrast-enhanced CT during the excretory phase. (**c**) The same cavitation (*arrow*) appears noncommunicating with parenchymal thinning. (**d**) Coexisting communicating cavitation (*arrow*) is also visualized

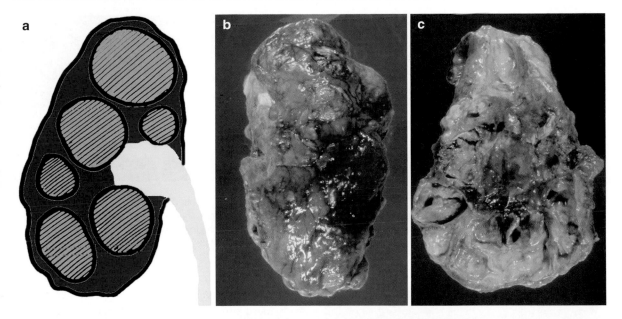

**Fig. 17.22** (**a–c**) Putty kidney. Extensive cavitation determines diffuse renal parenchyma caseation and calcification. (**a**) Scheme; (**b**, **c**) anatomical macroscopic specimen

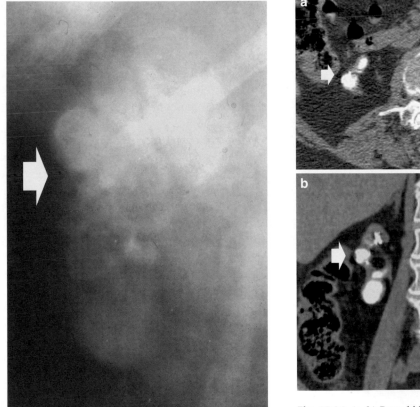

**Fig. 17.23** Plain radiograph. Putty kidney with diffuse calcification (*arrow*) of the renal parenchyma

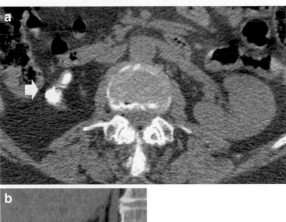

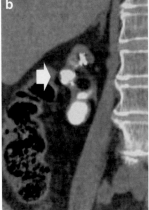

**Fig. 17.24** (**a**, **b**) Putty kidney. (**a**) Unenhanced CT, transverse plane; (**b**) coronal reformation. The entire right kidney (*arrow*) appears small, scarred, and densely calcified. A calcified and thick materials fills a dilated collecting system

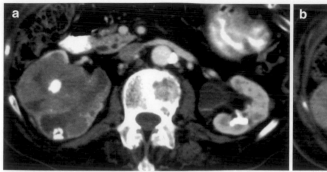
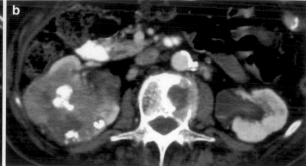

**Fig. 17.25** (**a**, **b**) Diffuse xanthogranulomatous pyelonephritis diffused to both kidneys, mainly to the right kidney. Contrast-enhanced CT, nephrographic phase. CT shows multiple low-density nonenhancing areas surrounded by enhancing rims corresponding to intrarenal collections, and staghorn renal stones without involvement of perinephric region and Gerota's fascia

2006). Diffuse calcifications are also visualized by CT and don't necessarily mean healed, inactive disease.

## 17.8 Renal Fungal Infections

Urinary infections through the hematogenous route (fungemia) can occur with any of the fungi known to produce clinically important disease in humans. Fungal infections, namely from *C. albicans* and *Aspergillus,* usually affect diabetic or immunocompromised patients. Fungal infections of the kidney may manifest as swollen pyelonephritis with swollen kidneys and patchy areas of low attenuation on CT (Symeonidou et al. 2009). Complicating microabscesses may be identified on US and CT, often as unilateral heterogeneous renal or perinephric mass that may be associated with varying degree of hydronephrosis (Symeonidou et al. 2009).

Renal infection from *C. albicans* is probably the most common and is usually an acute infection following systemic candidemia. However sometimes chronic infections occurs. In such cases intravenous excretory urography can identify renal scars, blunted calyces, papillary necrosis, infundibolar stenoses and irregularly marginated or shaggy-contoured filling defects (fungus balls). Fungi are filtered by the glomerulus and then become lodged in the distal tubules where they proliferate and produce multiple medullary and cortical abscesses. A pyelic fungus ball is seen more often in patients with renal candidiasis, and it is usually associated with diabetes, immunosuppression, and urinary obstruction. Such balls appears as echogenic masses in the collecting system without posterior acoustic shadowing at US, and as filling defects on intravenous excretory urography (Fig. 17.37) and as soft-tissue filling defect by CT. Multiple low attenuation lesions on the renal parenchyma, corresponding to microabscesses, may be identified at contrast-enhanced CT. Fungus ball can be treated with percutaneous nephrostomy, and antifungal medication.

Fungal pyelonephritis is much less frequent than bacterial pyelonephritis and present an high mortality rate. *C. albicans* is the most common fungal pathogen involved in genitourinary infections, followed by other species of *Candida* and *Aspergillus*. The kidney is the most frequently involved organ in systemic candidiasis and diabetics, and immunocompromised patients are particularly susceptible to this form of pyelonephritis (Stunell et al. 2007). *C. albicans* determines acute infection of the renal parenchyma and collecting system in the form of acute pyelonephritis (Fig. 17.38). Other renal fungal infections, including actinomycosis (Fig. 17.39), manifest with diffuse renal parenchyma involvement on contrast-enhanced CT, often with diffusion to the ipsilateral perirenal space.

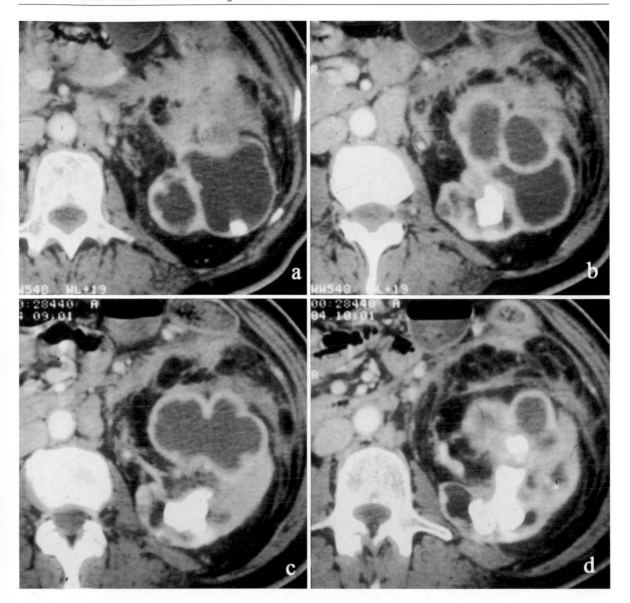

**Fig. 17.26** (**a–d**) Diffuse xanthogranulomatous pyelonephritis confined to the kidney. CT shows multiple low-density nonenhancing areas surrounded by enhancing rims corresponding to intrarenal collections, and renal stone without involvement of perinephric region and Gerota's fascia

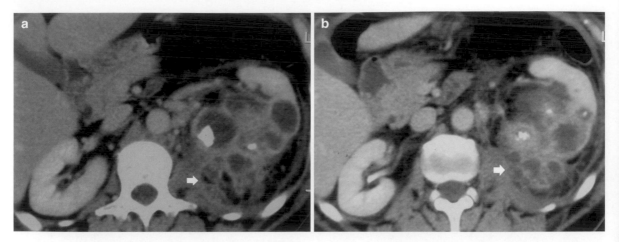

**Fig. 17.27** (**a–b**) Diffuse xanthogranulomatous pyelonephritis with extrarenal diffusion. CT shows multiple low-density non-enhancing areas surrounded by enhancing rims corresponding to intrarenal collections, and renal stone with involvement of the perinephric region, Gerota's fascia, and pararenal posterior space (*arrow*) of the retroperitoneum

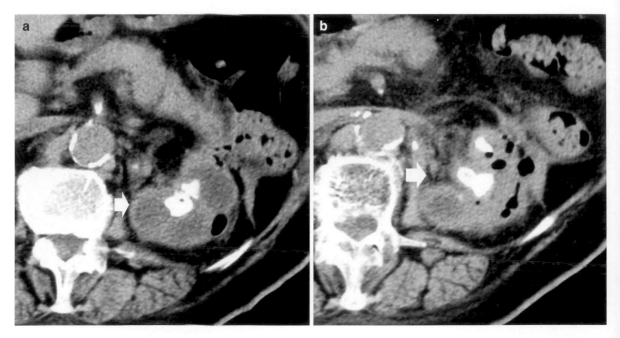

**Fig. 17.28** (**a, b**) Diffuse xanthogranulomatous pyelonephritis with extrarenal diffusion and gas component. CT shows multiple low-density nonenhancing areas surrounded by enhancing rims corresponding to intrarenal collections, and renal stone with involvement of perinephric region, Gerota's fascia, and pararenal posterior space of the retroperitoneum. A gas component is evident within the renal collection

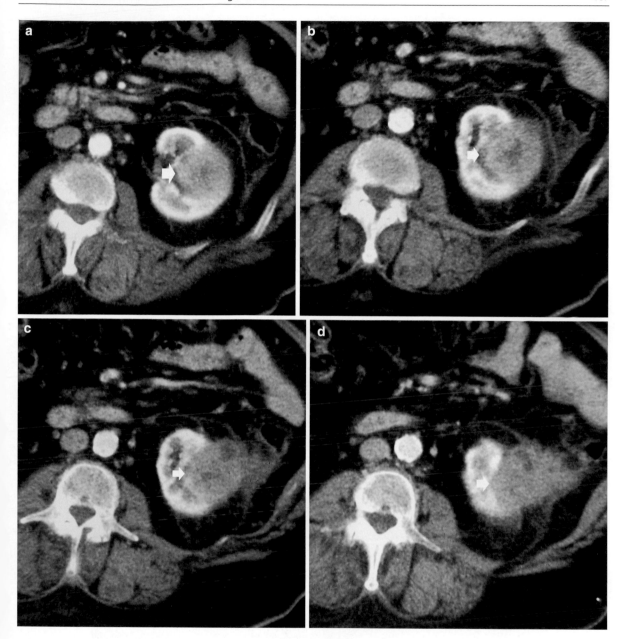

**Fig. 17.29** (**a–d**) Focal xanthogranulomatous pyelonephritis. Axial contrast-enhanced CT during the excretory phase. The focal form of xanthogranulomatous pyelonephritis on the left kidney. The focal (tumefactive) form manifests as a focal renal mass (*arrow*) with extension to the perinephric space

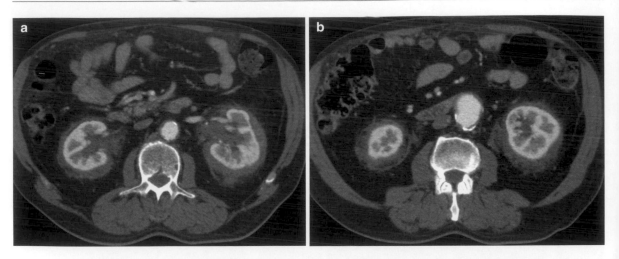

**Fig. 17.30** (**a**, **b**) Xanthogranulomatous fibrotic process of the perirenal space. Axial contrast-enhanced CT obtained during the corticomedullary phase depicts a rindlike soft-tissue layer surrounding both kidneys

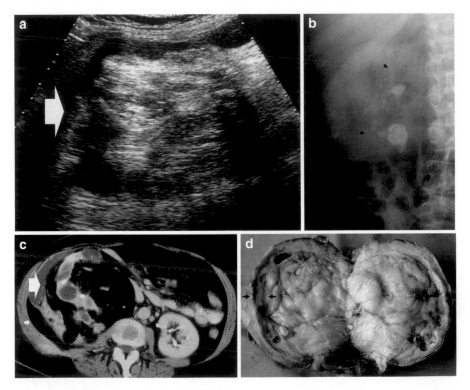

**Fig. 17.31** Renal replacement lipomatosis (RRL) of the right kidney with xanthogranulomatous pyelonephritis. (**a**) Gray-scale ultrasound, longitudinal scan. Renal enlargement (*arrow*) with heterogeneous appearance. (**b**) Plain radiograph. Extensive radiolucency in the right renal pelvis (*arrows*) with staghorn calculosis. (**c**) Contrast-enhanced CT, excretory phase. Extensive renal sinus lipomatosis with parenchymal atrophy and renal staghorn stones with renal hilus involvement. The renal parenchyma which is reduced to a thin rim of renal cortex. The replacement lipomatosis (*arrow*) invades the perirenal space, the anterior pararenal space, and the posterior pararenal space (*small arrow*). (**d**) Gross specimen. Diffuse fatty infiltration of the perirenal space and renal sinus with compression of the renal parenchyma (*arrows*)

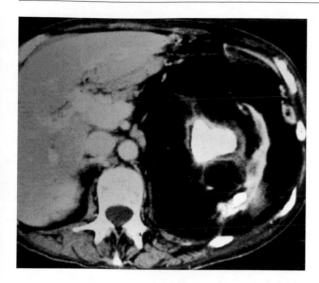

**Fig. 17.32** Renal replacement lipomatosis of the left kidney with xanthogranulomatous pyelonephritis. Replacement lipomatosis of the kidney is characterized by extensive renal sinus lipomatosis with parenchymal atrophy and renal staghorn stones with renal hilus and perirenal involvement. CT demonstrates stones and diffuse fatty replacement of parenchyma which is reduced to a thin rim of renal cortex

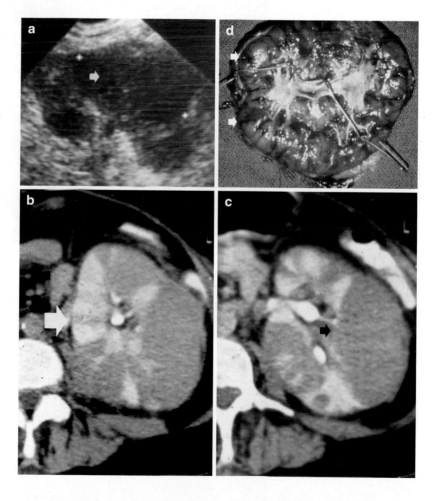

**Fig. 17.33** (**a–d**) Malacoplachia of the left kidney. US (**a**) shows a renal enlargement with evidence of hypodense solid masses on CT (**b**, **c**) compressing the excretory tract. (**d**) Gross pathologic specimen

**Fig. 17.34** (**a**, **b**)
Cholesteatoma (*arrow*).
Unenhanced (**a**) and
contrast-enhanced CT (**b**).
CT the attenuation is higher
than the usual soft-tissue
filling defect

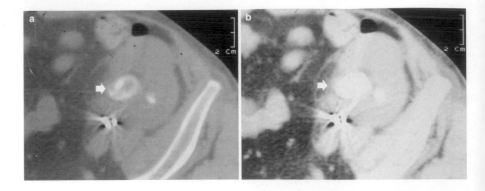

**Fig. 17.35** (**a**, **b**)
Cholesteatoma. CT urogra-
phy, coronal reformations.
(**a**) Diffuse thickening of the
renal pelvis wall (*arrow*) is
visualized in a patient with
long-standing urinary tract
infection due to reflux
nephropathy depicted by
renal parenchyma scar and
calyceal distortion with a
claviform shape; (**b**) a filling
defect with a laminated shape
(*arrow*) is evident within the
renal pelvis corresponding to
renal cholesteatoma

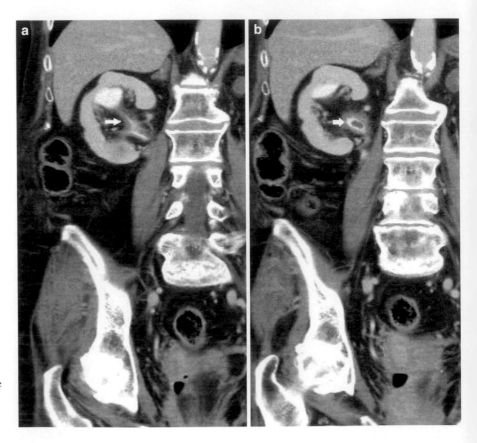

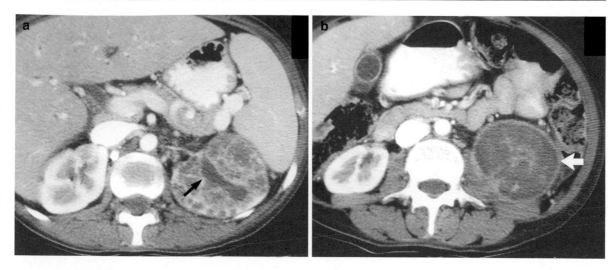

**Fig. 17.36** (**a**, **b**) Renal mucormycosis. (**a**) Thirty-five-year-old woman with left flank pain who was HIV-positive and had history of IV drug abuse. Contrast-enhanced axial CT scan acquired through upper pole of left kidney shows upper caliceal hydronephrosis (*arrow*) and heterogeneous enhancement with numerous small hypodensities throughout renal parenchyma.

(**b**) Thirty-five-year-old woman with left flank pain who was HIV-positive and had history of IV drug abuse. Contrast-enhanced axial CT scan acquired through lower pole of the left kidney shows large hypodense area (*arrow*) corresponding to abscess (*Reprinted with permission from the American Journal of Roentgenology*)

**Fig. 17.37** (**a**, **b**) Renal fungal infection in a immunocompromised patient with a pelvic kidney and renal candidiasis.
(**a**) Gray-scale US. Fungus balls appears as solid lesions (*arrow*) within the upper collecting system.
(**b**) Intravenous excretory urography. Fungus balls appears as filling defects (*arrow*) within the upper collecting system

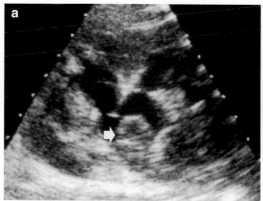

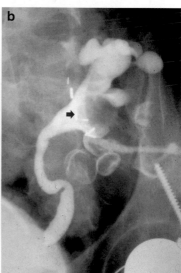

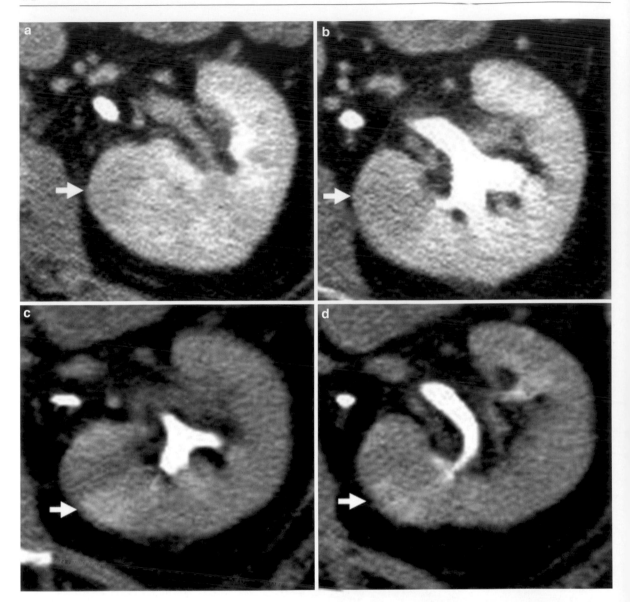

**Fig. 17.38** (**a–d**) Acute pyelonephritis from *C. albicans* in a 72-year-old patients. Contrast-enhanced CT. Transverse plane. (**a**, **b**) Nephrographic-excretory phase. Involvement of the right kidney which presents increased dimensions and heterogeneous density (*arrows*) in the posterior region. (**c**, **d**) Delayed phase obtained 3 h after iodinated contrast injection. Those areas (*arrow*) which appeared heterogeneous during the excretory-nephrographic phase revealed delayed enhancement due to pyelonephritis

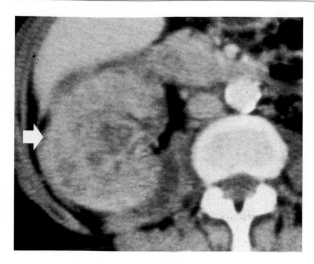

**Fig. 17.39** Renal cryptococcosis. Contrast-enhanced CT. Transverse plane. Involvement of the right kidney (*arrow*) which appears dimensionally increased and with heterogeneous density due to patchy areas also with diffusion to the perirenal space

# References

Acunas B, Acunas G, Rozanes I et al. (1990) Coexistent xanthogranulomatous pyelonephritis and massive replacement lipomatosis of the kidney: CT diagnosis. Urol Radiol 12:88–90

Becker JA (1988) Renal tuberculosis. Urol Radiol 10:25–30

Bergman JM, Wagner C, Cameron R (1991) Renal cortical nephrocalcinosis: a manifestation of extrapulmonary *Pneumocystis carinii* infection in the acquired immunodeficiency syndrome. Am J Kidney Dis 17:712–715

Brown PS, Dodson M, Weintrub PS (1996) Xanthogranulomatous pyelonephritis: report of nonsurgical management of a case and review of the literature. Clin Infect Dis 22:308–314

Casas JD, Cuadras P, Mariscal A et al. (2002) Replacement lipomatosis related to renal tuberculosis: imaging findings in one case. Eur Radiol 12:810–813

Claes H, Vereecken R, Oyen R et al. (1987) Xanthogranulomatous pyelonephritis with emphasis on computerized tomography scan. Urology 9:389–393

Craig WD, Wagner BJ, Travis MD (2008) Pyelonephritis: radiologic-pathologic review. Radiographics 28:255–276

Dalla Palma L, Pozzi Mucelli F (2000) Imaging of chronic renal infections. Radiologe 40:537–546

Engin G, Acunas B, Acunas G et al. (2000) Imaging of extrapulmonary tuberculosis. RadioGraphics 20:471–488

Falkoff GE, Rigsby CM, Rosenfield AT (1987) Partial, combined cortical and medullary nephrocalcinosis: US and CT pattern in AIDS-associated MAI infection. Radiology 162:343–344

Gibson MS, Puckett ML, Shelly ME (2004) Renal tuberculosis. Radiographics 24:251–256

Goldman SM, Fishman EK, Hartman DS et al. (1985) Computed tomography of renal tuberculosis and its pathological correlates. J Comput Assist Tomogr 9:771–776

Goldman SM, Hartman DS, Fishman EK et al. (1984) CT of Xanthogranulomatous pyelonephritis: radiologic-pathologic correlation. AJR Am J Roentgenol 141:963–969

Grainger RG, Longstaff AJ, Parsons MA (1982) Xanthogranulomatous pyelonephritis: a reappraisal. Lancet 19(1): 1398–1401

Harisinghani MG, McLoud TC, Shepard JO et al. (2000) Tuberculosis from Head to Toe. Radiographics 20:449–470

Hartman DS, Davis CJ Jr, Goldman SM et al. (1984) Xanthogranulomatous pyelonephritis: sonographic-pathologic correlation of 16 cases. J Ultrasound Med 3:481–488

Hartman DS, Davis C Jr, Lichtenstein JE, Goldman SM (1980) Renal parenchymal malacoplakia. Radiology 136:33–42

Kawashima A, Sandler CM, Goldman SM et al. (1997) CT of renal inflammatory disease. Radiographics 17:851–866

Keogh CF, Brown JA, Phillips P et al. (2003) Renal mucormycosis in an AIDS patient: imaging features and pathologic correlation. AJR Am J Roentgenol 180:1278–1280

Kenney P (1990) Imaging of chronic renal infections. AJR Am J Roentgenol 155:485–494

Molina RP, Dulabon DA, Roth RB (1988) Renal cholesteatoma. Urology 31 (2):152–154

Miller FH, Parikh S, Gore RM, Nemcek AA Jr, Fitzgerald SW, Vogelzang RL (1993) Renal manifestations of AIDS. Radiographics 13:587–596

Parker MD, Clark RL (1989) Evolving concepts in the diagnosis of xanthogranulomatous pyelonephritis. Urol Radiol 11:7–15

Sanchez LM, Sanchez SI, Bailey JL (2009) Malacoplakia presenting with obstructive nephropathy and bilateral ureteral involvement. Nat Rev Nephrol 5(7):418–422

Sharma R, Shivanand G, Kumar R et al. (2006) Isolated renal mucormycosis: an unusual case of acute renal infarction in a boy with aplastic anemia. Br J Radiol 79:e19–e21

Simon HB, Weinstein AJ, Pasternak MS et al. (1977) Genitourinary tuberculosis: clinical features in a general hospital population. Am J Med 63:410–420

Soler R, Pombo F, Gayol A et al. (1997) Focal xanthogranulomatous pyelonephritis in a teenager: MR and CT findings. Eur J Rad 24:77–79

Stanton MJ, Maxted W (1981) Malakoplakia: a study of the literature and current concepts of pathogenesis, diagnosis and treatment. J Urol 125:139–146

Stunell H, Buckley O, Feeney J et al. (2007) Imaging of acute pyelonephritis in the adult. Eur Radiol 17:1820–1828

Subramanyam BR, Bosniak MA, Horii SC et al. (1983) Replacement lipomatosis of the kidney: diagnosis by computed tomography and sonography. Radiology 148:791–792

Subramanyam BR, Megibow AJ, Raghavendra BN et al. (1982) Diffuse xanthogranulomatous pyelonephritis: analysis by computed tomography and sonography. Urol Radiol 4:5–9

Surabhi VR, Menias C, Prasad SR et al. (2008) Neoplastic and non-neoplastic proliferative disorders of the perirenal space: cross-sectional imaging findings. Radiographics 28:1005–1017

Symeonidou C, Hameeduddin A, Hons B et al. (2009) Imaging features of renal pathology in the huma immunodeficiency virus-infected patients. Semin Ultrasound CT MRI 30:289–297

Tam VK, Kung WH, Li R et al. (2003) Renal parenchymal malacoplakia: a rare cause of ARF with a review of recent literature. Am J Kidney Dis 41(6):E13–E17

Wang LJ, Wong YC, Chen CJ (1997) CT features of genitourinary tuberculosis. J Comput Assist Tomogr 21:254–258

# Renal Vascular Abnormalities

# 18

Therese M. Weber and Mark E. Lockhart

## Contents

T.M. Weber (✉) and M.E. Lockhart
Department of Radiology, University of Alabama at
Birmingham, 619 19th Street, South, JT N312, Birmingham,
AL 35249-6830, USA
e-mail: tweber@uabmc.edu

## 18.1 Renal Vascular Abnormalities

Traditionally the evaluation of renal vascular abnormalities was performed with conventional angiography. Cross-sectional imaging now plays an important and increasing role in evaluating renal vascular abnormalities in both the native and transplant kidneys. Normal anatomy and disease processes will be reviewed, emphasizing the various strengths and weaknesses of ultrasound, computed tomographic angiography (CTA) and magnetic resonance angiography (MRA).

Ultrasound plays a primary imaging role in surveillance of the transplant kidney in an effort to avoid complications and extend the life and function of the transplant kidney. Ultrasound also plays an extremely important role in screening for renal artery stenosis (RAS) in the native kidneys. The quality and accuracy of ultrasound evaluation for RAS is extremely dependent on the volume of cases, as well as the skill and experience of the sonographers and sonologists interpreting the examinations. In the future, there will be greater utilization of renal Doppler ultrasound due to the continued increase in incidence of renal insufficiency, concerns for use of iodinated contrast material and radiation exposure, and increased concern for the association of renal insufficiency and nephrogenic systemic fibrosis (NSF). However, CTA and MRA with multiplanar reformatted images provide exquisite anatomic detail, and they will continue to play a significant role in genitourinary imaging.

E. Quaia (ed.), *Radiological Imaging of the Kidney*,
Medical Radiology, DOI: 10.1007/978-3-540-87597-0_18, © Springer-Verlag Berlin Heidelberg 2011

## 18.2 Arterial Disease

### 18.2.1 *Renovascular Hypertension*

The vast majority of hypertensive patients have essential hypertension, with only a small minority having a renovascular etiology. Renovascular hypertension is more common in patients younger than 20 years of age or older than 50 years of age. In contrast, the onset of essential hypertension is usually between 30 and 50 years of age, and there is usually a family history of hypertension. Rapid acceleration or severe hypertension and severe hypertensive retinopathy also suggests a renovascular etiology.

Renovascular hypertension is renin-mediated and occurs as a physiologic response to renal ischemia. Renin, an enzyme produced in the juxtaglomerular apparatus of the kidney, acts on the circulating serum protein angiotensinogen to produce the inactive hormone angiotensin I, which, is converted to the active hormone angiotensin II. Angiotenesin II increases blood pressure by stimulating aldosterone secretion from the adrenal cortex which causes arteriolar vasoconstriction. This process exerts antidiuretic and antinatriuretic effects on the proximal renal tubule by promoting sodium reabsorption.

The afferent arteriole, which acts as a baroreceptor is the most important factor governing renin release. The transmural pressure across this arteriole may decrease as a result of reduced perfusion pressure or decreased compliance of the arteriole. The hypertension in patients with renovascular hypertension is dependent on the high circulating levels of angiotensin II. Therefore, an angiotensin II antagonist or the converting enzyme inhibitor, captopril, may be used to control the hypertension.

Even though many different processes may cause stenosis of the main renal artery, the most common etiologies are atherosclerosis and fibromuscular dysplasia (FMD). Less common etiologies include congenital, Takayasu's aortitis, middle aortic syndrome, irradiation, or an association with neurofibromatosis. Hypertension may rarely be related to parenchymal abnormalities such as pyelonephritis, glomerulopathies, ureteral obstruction, trauma, and renal mass lesions. Reninoma is a renin-secreting tumor of the juxtaglomerular cells which more frequently occurs in patients under 20 years of age, and is more common in females (Dunnick et al. 1983).

#### 18.2.1.1 Atherosclerosis

Approximately two-thirds of cases of significant stenosis of the main renal artery are related to atherosclerosis. Blood pressure does not rise until the stenosis is 60% or greater. The stenotic lesion usually occurs at the origin of the renal artery or within the first 2 cm, and is usually circumferential, but may be eccentric. Bilateral renal arteries are frequently affected. Atherosclerosis is more common in men than women and is accelerated by smoking. Additional risks for atherosclerotic renovascular disease include longstanding hypertension, diabetes, and dyslipidemia. The onset of hypertension related to atherosclerosis is at a considerably later age than in patients with FMD.

### 18.2.2 *Renal Artery Stenosis (RAS)*

Potential clinical criteria used to select patients who should be imaged to evaluate for RAS include the following:

1. Age extremes, usually younger than 20 or older than 50 years.
2. Recent onset of hypertension (less than 1 year).
3. Rapid acceleration of hypertension.
4. Malignant hypertension.
5. A flank bruit.

Renal Doppler ultrasound offers distinct advantages as the initial screening tool for RAS. These advantages include lack of ionizing radiation, lack of potentially nephrotoxic intravenous contrast, and lack of potential risk of NSF in patients with renal insufficiency. NSF is a rare debilitating and occasionally fatal skin disorder which has recently been associated with intravenous gadolinium contrast administration. In patients with significant renal insufficiency, ultrasound now has become the safest imaging modality for detection of RAS (Thomsen 2006; Broome et al. 2007).

Ultrasound imaging of the renal vasculature can be challenging due to the deep location of the renal vessels, overlying bowel gas, and the large body habitus of many patients. Proper training in the performance and interpretation of the ultrasound examination, as well as a strong quality control program, are critical to improving study quality and diagnostic accuracy. Recent studies have shown that in trained hands the sensitivity and specificity of renal Doppler ultrasound for RAS is up to 95% and 90%, respectively (Bokhari and Faxon 2004). Renal Doppler ultrasound technique, however, is an operator-dependent imaging modality. The two main methods for RAS detection are direct visualization of the narrowing and evaluation of the downstream effects of the stenosis on the segmental renal arteries, which is the indirect method. It is important to visualize the entire main renal artery at ultrasound. Turbulent flow may suggest RAS. Increased velocities at the point of stenosis may appear as color aliasing, which should be further evaluated with spectral Doppler. A peak systolic velocity (PSV) of greater than 2 m/s has been suggested as the threshold for Doppler diagnosis of 60% diameter reduction of the renal artery (Fig. 18.1) (Olin et al. 1995; Pellerito 2002). Another common criterion is a PSV ratio of the renal artery relative to the aorta greater than 3.5. In a recent meta-analysis, PSV was the best predictor of RAS, with sensitivity and specificity of 85% and 92%, respectively (Williams et al. 2007). In many cases, it may not be technically possible to demonstrate the entire length of the main renal artery. Another tool that can be used in this setting is evaluation of the intrarenal arterial waveform morphology (Stavros et al. 1992). Spectral Doppler may show a dampened waveform with spectral broadening and blunting of the systolic upstroke – the tardus-parvus waveform morphology (Fig. 18.2) (Kliewer et al. 1993; Downey 1998). However, it is important to remember that absence of the tardus-parvus waveform does not exclude RAS. Vessel compliance may be reduced in patients with atherosclerotic disease, making the tardus-parvus waveform morphology less obvious (Demirpolat et al. 2003).

An additional advantage that renal Doppler ultrasound has over other imaging modalities is its ability to predict which patients may benefit from therapeutic intervention of RAS. Radermacher et al., in a large prospective study, showed that patients with elevated RI of greater than 0.80 will not improve after renal artery stenting (2001). A subsequent study, however, showed that 29% of patients with renal insufficiency and RI of greater than 0.80 showed improved renal function after revascularization, and perhaps more important, 50% showed improvement in hypertension (Garcia-Criado et al. 2005).

Continued improvement in multidetector CT technology has had a profound impact on reconstructed three-dimensional (3D) images that aid in the diagnosis of RAS. Accessory renal arteries are well-detected with CTA which is an important advantage of CTA, as many of the false-positive and false-negative results are related to accessory arteries. RAS in either the main or an accessory renal artery are now accurately detected with CTA. The sensitivity and specificity of CTA in detecting RAS of 50% or more are approximately 90% and 97%, respectively. The sensitivity is even greater when only stenoses of 75% or greater are considered (Johnson et al. 1999; Urban et al. 2001). MRA techniques used to detect RAS, such as time-of-flight and phase-contrast sequences, may be limited by turbulent blood flow and respiratory motion. 3D gadolinium enhanced MRA avoids these problems by acquiring a complete data set within a single breath-hold. CTA and MRA both have the additional advantage of increasing diagnostic accuracy by providing multiple different ways to view the data. These options include multiplanar reconstruction, shaded surface display, and maximum intensity projection techniques.

### 18.2.2.1 Fibromuscular Dysplasia

FMD, the second most common cause of renovascular hypertension, represents almost one-third of cases of renovascular hypertension. It typically affects women between 30 and 55 years of age. FMD is classified as intimal, medial, or adventitial, as the process may involve any layer of the renal artery.

Intimal fibroplasia is a process of concentric accumulation of collagen beneath the internal elastic membrane. This creates a smooth stenosis, usually located in the midportion of the renal artery. This process is more common among children and is progressive.

Medial fibroplasia is the most common type of FMD and represents about 90% of cases. In this process smooth muscle is replaced by collagen that forms thick ridges. These ridges alternate with areas of small aneurysm formation and result in the classic "string of beads" appearance (Luscher et al. 1987; Harrison and McCormack 1971), which can be seen with conventional arteriography, CTA, or MRA (Fig. 18.3). This type of FMD is most commonly seen in women 15–50 years of age, and usually responds well to percutaneous transluminal angioplasty. FMD can also be seen in cephalic, visceral, and peripheral arteries. FMD may be seen in the carotid and vertebral arteries, but tends to spare the intracranial arteries.

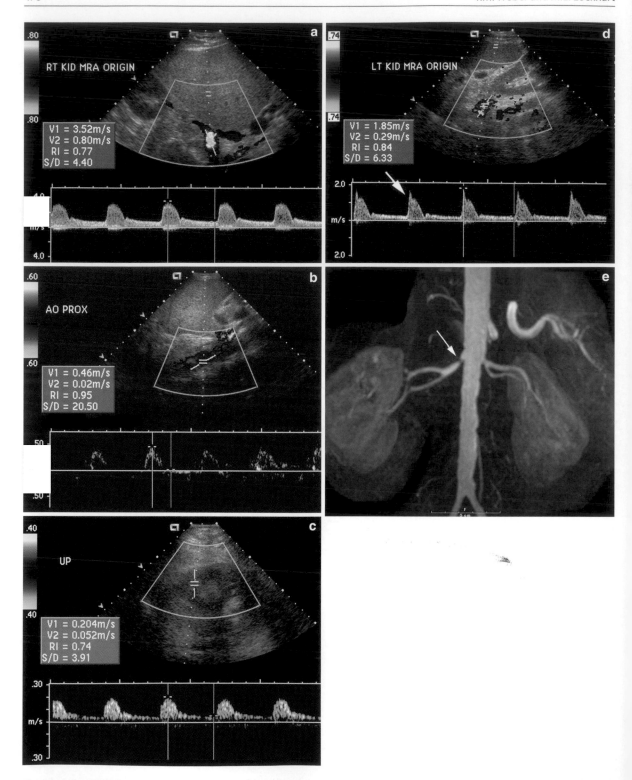

**Fig. 18.1** (a–e) Renal artery stenosis. (a) Duplex Doppler shows turbulent flow within the right main renal artery with elevated peak velocity 352 cm/s, far above the 2 m/s threshold. (b) Peak aortic velocity is 46 cm/s, yielding a ratio of 7.7. (c) Loss of early systolic peak in the segmental artery waveforms help support the diagnosis. (d) For comparison, the left renal artery has normal systolic acceleration and early systolic peak (*arrow*). (e) Coronal MRA confirms high-grade stenosis of the right renal artery (*arrow*)

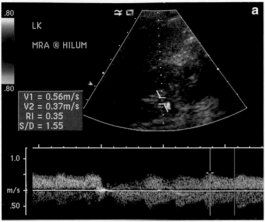
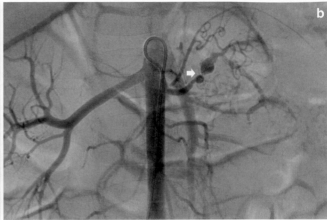

**Fig. 18.2** (**a**, **b**) Renal artery stenosis. (**a**) On duplex Doppler in a 3-year-old with hypertension, there is delayed systolic acceleration with tardus-parvus waveform morphology. (**b**) On conventional angiography, renal artery stenosis (*arrow*) at the bifurcation of the left main renal artery is clearly visible with associated poststenotic dilatation, likely related to fibromuscular dysplasia (FMD)

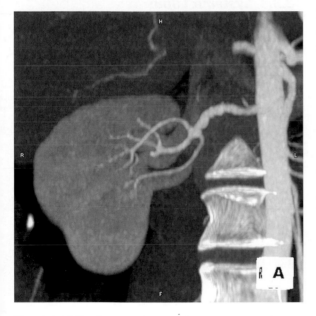

**Fig. 18.3** FMD. Contrasted CTA with maximum intensity projection reconstruction in a 41-year-old female shows beaded irregular appearance of the distal main renal artery with classic appearance of medial fibroplasia

## 18.2.2.2 Takayasu's Aortitis

Takayasu's disease is a granulomatous arteritis that tends to involve the aorta and its major branches. This disease is seen in patients younger than 35 years of age, with a marked female and Asian predominance.

Hypertension is a common complication of this disease and may be caused by coarctation of the aorta or main RAS.

### 18.2.2.3 Neurofibromatosis

In neurofibromatosis, the renal artery is encased by ganglioneuromatous or neurofibromatous tissue. RAS develops from intimal proliferation, thinning of the media, and fragmentation of the elastic tissue. Neurofibromatosis is a rare cause of RAS.

### 18.2.2.4 Middle Aortic Syndrome

This rare syndrome, which occurs in young patients, most commonly in the second decade of life, consists of diffuse narrowing of the abdominal aorta, often involving the visceral and renal arteries. Hypertension is typically severe. An abdominal bruit and diminished femoral pulses in a young patient should suggest the diagnosis. The prognosis is poor, with death most frequently from cerebral hemorrhage, hypertensive encephalopathy, stroke, and congestive heart failure. This disease process does not respond well to transluminal angioplasty and primary treatment is surgical revascularization. Arteriography, CTA or MRA can show the smooth tapering of the distal thoracic or abdominal aorta. Narrowing frequently is severe and most marked in the infrarenal aorta. The renal arteries are commonly affected with long stenoses. In contrast, Takayasu's disease usually affects slightly older patients than middle aortic syndrome and the patients have other manifestations of arteritis, such as fever and elevated sedimentation rate. The great vessels of the chest are often involved in Takayasu's disease, but not in patients with middle aortic syndrome.

## 18.3 Diseases of the Intrarenal Arteries

Disease processes that tend to involve the intrarenal arteries include collagen vascular diseases such as polyarteritis nodosa, Wegener's granulomatosis, and systemic lupus erythematosus (SLE); as well as, intravenous drug abuse, scleroderma, radiation nephritis, and arteriolar nephrosclerosis. These disease processes tend to be associated with multiple microaneurysms.

### 18.3.1 Polyarteritis Nodosa (PAN)

Renal involvement occurs in 90% of patients with PAN. This disease process consists of foci of fibrinoid necrosis that begin in the media. Inflammation then spreads to involve the intima and adventitia, and results in small aneurysms and vascular thrombosis. Subsequent renal ischemia occurs and renin-mediated hypertension is common. The small aneurysms seen in PAN may occasionally rupture with resultant intraparenchymal or perinephric hematoma. These small aneurysms occur at the bifurcation of interlobular or arcuate arteries and are best seen at arteriography. These small aneurysms, although typical of PAN, are not pathognomonic. Similar aneurysms may be seen in SLE, Wegener's granulomatosis, intravenous drug abuse, and renal metastases. Please, see also Chap. 13.

### 18.3.2 Wegener's Granulomatosis

Renal disease may be absent in the limited form of Wegener's granulomatosis. In the full syndrome,

however, a rapidly progressive glomerulonephritis is life threatening. Hematuria and proteinuria are the most common manifestations of the renal involvement. The radiographic findings in the kidneys are nonspecific and may include microaneuryms, renal infarction, parenchymal scarring, and areas of hemorrhage. Wegener's granulomatosis occurs most commonly in the fourth and fifth decades and is slightly more common in males. In addition to renal involvement, the disease process primarily consists of necrotizing granulomas of the respiratory tract and focal necrotizing angiitis of the small arteries and veins. Upper airway involvement may present with sinusitis, otitis media, pharyngitis, mucosal ulcerations and epistaxis.

### 18.3.3 Systemic Lupus Erythematosus (SLE)

Most patients with SLE have renal involvement and renal failure is a frequent cause of death. The larger renal vessels tend to be unaffected; however, interlobular arteries may undergo inflammatory changes and become narrowed resulting in focal glomerulonephritis with thickening of the basement membrane on histologic preparations which results in a "wire loop" appearance. Before the onset of renal failure, the kidneys will usually appear normal radiographically. Although common, renal infarcts are usually too small to be seen. Ultrasound examination is often normal; however, an elevated resistive index may predict worsening renal function.

### 18.3.4 Intravenous Drug Abuse

Intravenous drug abuse vasculitis is similar in clinical and pathologic manifestations to PAN. The radiographic findings, indistinguishable from other vasculitides, may consist of multiple aneurysms 1–5 mm in diameter occurring at bifurcations, vascular stenoses, and complete vascular occlusion with infarction. Methamphetamine is a common drug used in patients who develop a vasculitis; however, these patients are frequently exposed to multiple drugs.

### 18.3.5 Scleroderma

Scleroderma consists of vascular and connective tissue fibrosis with narrowing of the interlobular arteries and possible fibrinoid necrosis of the afferent arterioles. Scleroderma most frequently occurs in the fourth and fifth decades and is significantly more common in women. The kidneys may be affected in up to 80% of patients and renal failure is often the cause of death. Radiographic renal manifestations are nonspecific. Hypertension is common. The microaneurysms seen with the vasculitides are not seen with scleroderma.

### 18.3.6 Radiation Nephritis

Radiation nephritis is a degenerative process that affects the tubules and glomeruli of the kidney. The vascular changes of fibrinoid necrosis occur late in the course of the process and involve primarily arcuate and interlobar arteries.

### 18.3.7 Embolism and Infarction

The source of renal artery emboli is most commonly cardiac disease such as atrial enlargement secondary to valvular disease or dyskinetic left ventricle after myocardial infarction. Other sources for smaller emboli include an ectatic or aneurysmal aorta or cholesterol plaques. The appearance of renal embolism is best demonstrated on CT with absence of contrast enhancement in the affected renal tissue. Typically infarcts are seen as wedge-shaped, low attenuation areas within an otherwise normal-appearing kidney. If the entire kidney is infarcted, it will appear large with a more rounded configuration. In cases where the renal artery is occluded, capsular branches remain patent and may enhance the outer rim of the kidney (Fig. 18.4) a sign named "cortical rim sign." Contrasted CT or MRI best demonstrates this preservation of the outer 2–4 mm of cortex. In some cases of high-grade stenosis of an intrarenal artery there may be decreased opacification of the ischemic area, depending on the timing relative to contrast administration. If delayed images are obtained after contrast has washed out of the normal renal parenchyma, there may be persistent enhancement of this hypoperfused area. Atrophy will begin after the acute phase of renal

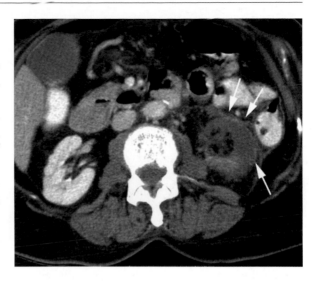

**Fig. 18.4** Renal infarction. Contrasted axial CT shows global hypoenhancement of the left kidney. Subtle rim enhancement (*arrows*) is related to collateral flow from capsular arteries

infarction, yielding a residual cortical scar. If the entire kidney is affected by occlusion of the main renal artery, global renal atrophy will result. Although there may be no appreciable renal function, renin may still be produced and may cause hypertension.

### 18.3.8 Arterial Thrombosis

Atherosclerosis is the most common cause for renal artery thrombosis. Acute thrombosis of the renal artery may occur after trauma, most commonly with blunt abdominal trauma. The acceleration–deceleration forces may produce intimal tears with subsequent dissection of the renal artery and thrombosis. Renal artery thrombosis may also occur as an angiographic interventional complication in cases of subintimal dissection, and is more likely to occur during attempted transluminal angioplasty than during diagnostic renal arteriograms. Color Doppler ultrasound is the best diagnostic imaging study for confirmation, with absence of intrarenal arterial signal.

### 18.3.9 Renal Artery Aneurysm

Aneurysms of the renal arteries are uncommon. There is an association between renal artery aneurysms and hypertension, as many patients with renal artery aneurysm are hypertensive. Renin-mediated hypertension may be the result of extrinsic compression of the main renal artery or an intrarenal branch artery by the aneurysm, or by thrombus formation and occlusion of a branch artery. Renal artery aneurysms may contain clot which may result in renal emboli with or without infarction. The risk of rupture is small but more likely in hypertensive or pregnant patients (Tham et al. 1983). Calcified aneurysms rarely rupture. On abdominal radiograph a calcified aneurysm and a tortuous splenic artery may look similar. On ultrasound, an aneurysm may appear as a hypoechoic mass along the course of the renal artery. The Doppler signal depends on the amount of thrombus, the size of the neck of the aneurysm, and presence of any calcification. On CT, calcification along the wall of the aneurysm is seen on unenhanced CT images. They may be saccular and commonly occur at branch points (Fig. 18.5). After contrast administration, variable enhancement is seen depending on the amount of thrombus within the aneurysm. Likewise, renal artery aneurysms can be demonstrated on MRI. In the setting of trauma, there is disruption of at least part of the wall, termed pseudoaneurysm (Fig. 18.6). A pseudoaneurysm is an acute finding and less likely to have associated calcifications. It may be associated with active extravasation of blood.

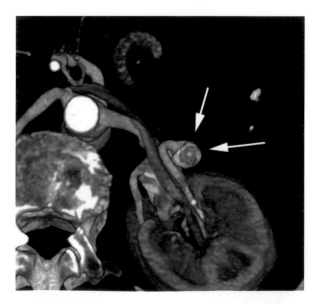

**Fig. 18.5** Renal artery aneurysm. Volume reconstruction of CTA shows small saccular aneurysm (*arrows*) at the bifurcation of the main renal artery

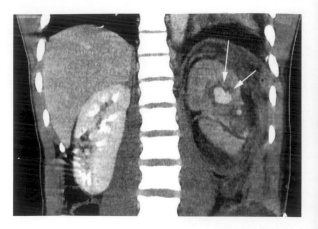

**Fig. 18.6** Renal pseudoaneurysm. Coronal reconstructions of a contrasted CT in a trauma patient shows an irregular intraparenchymal collection of contrast (*arrows*) within the left kidney. There is associated laceration of the renal cortex

## 18.3.10 Arteriovenous Fistula and Malformations (AVF and AVM)

An abnormal communication between the arterial and venous circulations that bypasses the capillary bed can be congenital, acquired or idiopathic. Congenital AVMs are more often found in women than men, and hematuria is the most common presenting complaint. AVF in native kidneys is most often associated with a history of biopsy. Color Doppler ultrasound is now the best noninvasive imaging modality to evaluate AVMs and AVFs, and may show a large tortuous cluster of vessels with increased, abnormal flow (Fig. 18.7). Spectral Doppler waveforms of the renal arteries feeding the AVF will show high velocity, low resistance flow because the abnormal communication bypasses the renal capillary bed. The main renal vein is often dilated, and Doppler may show arterialized waveforms near the AVF.

On CT or MR, the appearance of an AVF will be similar with a cluster of dilated vessels and a dilated renal vein. Early filling of the ipsilateral renal vein is to be expected and may be seen depending upon the timing of the contrast bolus. Multiplanar reconstruction of CT or MR data improves visualization of the anatomy beyond the limits of ultrasound and may aid in surgical planning.

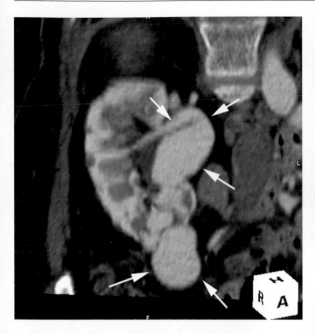

**Fig. 18.7** Arteriovenous malformation. Contrasted CTA of a 72-year-old female demonstrates severe saccular dilatation of venous structures in the renal hilum (*arrows*) and dilatation of the early-filling renal vein extending into the IVC

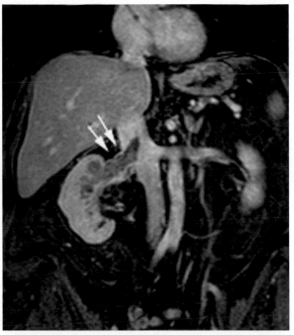

**Fig. 18.8** Renal vein thrombosis. Magnetic resonance angiogram in a 69-year-old female with renal cell carcinoma demonstrates extension of low-signal clot through the renal vein (*arrows*) into the IVC

## 18.4 Venous Disease

### 18.4.1 Renal Vein Thrombosis (RVT)

RVT is more common in the pediatric population, as compared to adults. RVT is most often caused by an underlying abnormality in hydration, the clotting system, or the kidney itself (Llach et al. 1980). Other etiologies include trauma, tumor extension, retroperitoneal fibrosis, acute pancreatitis, and retroperitoneal surgery. RVT associated with tumor extension of renal cell carcinoma is different from bland thrombus and may show arterialized flow on spectral Doppler, CTA or MRA (Sheth et al. 2001). Renal Doppler is the first-line noninvasive imaging modality for diagnosing RVT. Characteristic findings include an enlarged renal vein containing low level echoes and absence of flow. Additionally the kidney may be enlarged with increased echogenicity of the renal parenchyma. When acute RVT is suspected, it is critical to visualize the entire renal vein with color flow Doppler because collateral flow may develop quickly in the native kidney. Another possible

sonographic finding is monophasic waveforms in the renal venous system which is abnormal but not specific for RVT (Mulligan et al. 1992). Imaging of the IVC should be included when evaluating for RVT to determine cephalad extend of thrombus, which can affect surgical management in cases of renal cell carcinoma.

CT and MR can also be used to identify renal vein thrombus, detect a renal mass, and evaluate cephalad extent of IVC thrombus. The coronal images are especially helpful to show the cephalad extent of IVC thrombus (Fig. 18.8). Rapidly acquired gradient-recalled echo MR images can be obtained without intravascular contrast in cases of renal insufficiency or in patients with a contraindication to iodinated contrast material.

### 18.4.2 Varicocele Formation

Varicocele, defined as dilatation of the pampiniform venous plexus, is more common on the left because of anatomical factors including angle of insertion of the

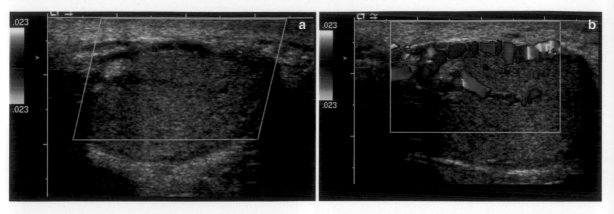

**Fig. 18.9** Intratesticular varicocele. (**a**) Color Doppler shows small amount of parenchymal flow within the testicle at rest. (**b**) On repeat color Doppler during valsalva, there is significantly increased flow in a dilated tortuous vessel within the testicular parenchyma, consistent with varicocele

gonadal vein into the left renal vein and the potential for compression of the left renal vein by the SMA. Isolated right varicocele is uncommon and should raise the question of right renal hilar mass or adenopathy compressing venous outflow. Diagnosis of varicocele is most commonly made with scrotal ultrasound with demonstration of dilated veins greater than 2–3 mm in diameter within the spermatic cord and extratesticular region. Valsalva or standing position will improve varicocele detection by increasing venous distension. Rarely, the varix may be intratesticular (Fig. 18.9). In a recent study by Karazincir et al., the incidence of retroaortic left renal vein was found to be significantly higher in patients with varicocele compared with control patients. The detection of retroaortic renal vein is possible by ultrasound and may be a useful finding in patients with unexplained varicocele (Karazincir et al. 2007).

### 18.4.4 Renal Lymphangiomatosis

Renal lymphangiomatosis, a rare disorder, may be seen as cystic masses in the perinephric space immediately adjacent to the kidney. In this disorder the lymphatic tissue fails to develop a normal communication with the rest of the lymphatic system, with resultant obstruction of larger lymphatics that drain through the renal pelvis. This entity is usually bilateral, may be hereditary, and may be exacerbated by pregnancy. Multiple cystic perinephric masses may be seen with ultrasound, CT, or MRI. This entity should not be confused with autosomal dominant polycystic kidney disease which will have innumerable cysts scattered throughout the renal parenchyma (Leder 1995).

For vascular abnormalities of the transplanted kidney see Chap. 30

### 18.4.3 Gonadal Vein Thrombosis

Thrombosis of the gonadal veins unrelated to tumor thrombus is most often seen in women during the postpartum period. Postpartum ovarian vein thrombosis has a predilection for the right side. Other etiologies of ovarian vein thrombosis include gynecologic surgery or pelvic inflammatory disease. MR and CT are the preferred imaging modalities for diagnosing ovarian vein thrombosis, as ultrasound is frequently limited by bowel gas.

### References

Bokhari SW, Faxon DP (2004) Current advances in the diagnosis and treatment of renal artery stenosis. Rev Cardiovasc Med 5:204–215

Broome DR, Girguis MS, Baron PW et al. (2007) Gadodiamide-associated nephrogenic systemic fibrosis: why radiologists should be concerned. AJR Am J Roentgenol 188:586–592

Demirpolat G, Ozbek SS, Parildar M et al. (2003) Reliability of intrarenal Doppler sonographic parameters of renal artery stenosis. J Clin Ultrasound 31:346–351

Downey D (1998) The retroperitoneum and great vessels, 2nd ed. Mosby, St. Louis, pp 453–486

Dunnick NR, Hartman DS, Ford KK et al. (1983) The radiology of juxtaglomerular tumors. Radiology 147:321–326

Garcia-Criado A, Gilabert R, Nicolau C et al. (2005) Value of Doppler sonography for predicting clinical outcome after renal artery revascularization in atherosclerotic renal artery stenosis. J Ultrasound Med 24:1641–1647

Harrison EG Jr, McCormack LJ (1971) Pathologic classification of renal arterial disease in renovascular hypertension. Mayo Clin Proc 46:161–167

Johnson PT, Halpern EJ, Kuszyk BS et al. (1999) Renal artery stenosis: CT angiography–comparison of real-time volume-rendering and maximum intensity projection algorithms. Radiology 211:337–343

Karazincir S, Balci A, Gorur S et al. (2007) Incidence of the retroaortic left renal vein in patients with varicocele. J Ultrasound Med 26:601–604

Kliewer MA, Tupler RH, Carroll BA et al. (1993) Renal artery stenosis: analysis of Doppler waveform parameters and tardus-parvus pattern. Radiology 189:779–787

Leder RA. Genitourinary case of the day. Renal lymphangiomatosis. AJR Am J Roentgenol 165:197–198

Llach F, Papper S, Massry SG. The clinical spectrum of renal vein thrombosis: acute and chronic. Am J Med 69:819–827

Luscher TF, Lie JT, Stanson AW et al. (1987) Arterial fibromuscular dysplasia. Mayo Clin Proc 62:931–952

Mulligan SA, Koslin DB, Berland LL (1992) Duplex evaluation of native renal vessels and renal allografts. Semin Ultrasound CT MR 13:40–52

Olin JW, Piedmonte MR, Young JR et al. (1995) The utility of duplex ultrasound scanning of the renal arteries for diagnosing significant renal artery stenosis. Ann Intern Med 122:833–838

Pellerito, JS. Renal artery stenosis. Paper presented at: Advances in Sonography; October 26, 2002; San Francisco, CA pp 140–142

Radermacher J, Chavan A, Bleck J et al. (2001) Use of Doppler ultrasonography to predict the outcome of therapy for renal-artery stenosis. N Engl J Med 344:410–417

Sheth S, Scatarige JC, Horton KM et al. (2001) Current concepts in the diagnosis and management of renal cell carcinoma: role of multidetector ct and three-dimensional CT. Radiographics 21 Spec No:S237–S254

Stavros AT, Parker SH, Yakes WF et al. (1992) Segmental stenosis of the renal artery: pattern recognition of tardus and parvus abnormalities with duplex sonography. Radiology 184:487–492

Tham G, Ekelund L, Herrlin K et al. (1983) Renal artery aneurysms. Natural history and prognosis. Ann Surg 197:348–352

Thomsen HS (2006) Nephrogenic systemic fibrosis: a serious late adverse reaction to gadodiamide. Eur Radiol 16:2619–2621

Urban BA, Ratner LE, Fishman EK (2001) Three-dimensional volume-rendered CT angiography of the renal arteries and veins: normal anatomy, variants, and clinical applications. Radiographics 21:373–386; questionnaire 549–355

Williams GJ, Macaskill P, Chan SF et al. (2007) Comparative accuracy of renal duplex sonographic parameters in the diagnosis of renal artery stenosis: paired and unpaired analysis. AJR Am J Roentgenol 188:798–811

# Imaging of Renal Trauma

**19**

Stuart E. Mirvis

## Contents

S.E. Mirvis
Department of Radiology and Maryland Shock-Trauma Center,
University of Maryland School of Medicine, 22 South Greene
Street, Baltimore, MD, 21201, USA
e-mail: smirvis@umm.edu

**Abstract**

> This chapter reviews the imaging diagnosis, classification, and role of radiology in selection of treatment of acute injury and complications of renal trauma. In the era of rapid MDCT (multidetector computed tomography) screening of blunt polytrauma patients scanning involves either selected body segments or, increasingly common, continuous scanning from the cranium through the pelvis, to quickly assess the scope and severity of traumatic pathology throughout the body. MDCT offers the most complete assessment of the parenchyma, collecting system, and renal function of any diagnostic modality. The kidneys are naturally included in every abdominal-pelvic CT performed for blunt trauma and in most cases of penetrating trauma in any case where retroperitoneal injury is possible based on site and trajectory of the penetrating object. As in all patients sustaining major trauma it is the entire clinical scenario especially the hemodynamic status of the patient that determines whether or not CT can or should be obtained. The essential information acquired by CT permits identification of all injuries allowing injury severity to be determined. The injury score has utility for deciding if, when, and what treatment is mandated to achieve an optimal outcome, including preservation of maximal renal function, minimizing early and delayed complications, and determining if further diagnostic studies by CT or other modalities, as nuclear scintigraphy or retrograde pyelography are warranted.

E. Quaia (ed.), *Radiological Imaging of the Kidney*,
Medical Radiology, DOI: 10.1007/978-3-540-87597-0_19, © Springer-Verlag Berlin Heidelberg 2011

## 19.1 Renal Injury Overview

Renal injury occurs in 8–10% of patients sustaining blunt and penetrating trauma (Bower et al. 1978; Lee et al. 2007). The majority of blunt trauma patients have relatively minor injury, which can be observed. Blunt impact injury is far more common in most settings than penetrating injury accounting for 66–90% of cases of renal injury (Baverstock et al. 2001; Dunfee et al. 2008; Gourgiotis et al. 2006; Lee et al. 2007; Miller and McAninch 1995; Shariat et al. 2007) Blunt injuries are most often caused by motor vehicle collisions, falls, and direct impact from assault or sports competition.

Patients who are hemodynamically unstable on admission from any injury mechanism and cannot be resuscitated and stabilized quickly are most likely going to surgery immediately. In some cases where injury to the kidneys is suspected based on the presence of hematuria, location of impact, or wounds and intraoperative findings, an intravenous pyelogram (IVU) may be obtained in the operating room to assess the gross integrity of the renal parenchyma and collecting system with possible postoperative CT performed. A single-film 3-min post contrast injection radiograph verifies visualization of both kidneys, detects most major renal parenchymal injuries (Roberts et al. 1987) and is accurate for staging penetrating trauma in 68% of penetrating injury (Armenakas et al. 1999). The intraoperative IVU is not likely to detect minor injuries, but these are seldom of clinical consequence.

Computed tomography is the diagnostic study of choice for assessing renal injury, is typically readily available and assesses all areas of possible concurrent injury at one time. CT is particularly sensitive for minor parenchymal injuries, subcapsular, peri- and pararenal hematomas without gross displacement or distortion of the kidney, detection of renal bleeding, vascular and collecting system injury. Details of CT methodology are considered below.

## 19.2 Hematuria and Hemodynamic Stability

Suspicion for the presence of renal injury at admission depends mainly on two factors including evidence of direct flank impact and the extent of hematuria. Flank ecchymoses or hematoma, pain on flank palpation, and the presence of lower rib fractures indicate direct impact over the kidney and increase the likelihood of renal injury. The presence of hematuria and, perhaps more significantly, its quantity can be an indicator of renal injury, but this remains the subject of some debate. A study by Hardeman et al. found that 84% of patients with gross hematuria after blunt trauma had renal injury (1987). In a study of 1,588 blunt trauma patients without shock or hematuria by Miller and McAnich, they found only three with significant renal injuries (1995). A study of 2,873 blunt trauma patients from four separate studies with microscopic hematuria found only ten with significant renal injuries (Miller and McAninch 1995). When patients had gross hematuria or microscopic hematuria in the presence of shock 78 of 422 had Grade II-V renal injury (see below ) (Stein et al. 1994). In a study by Shariat et al. of 429 patients, the presence of gross hematuria, hypotension, and flank pain are associated with higher injury grades in the setting of blunt trauma (2007). In the author's practice at the University of Maryland Shock-Trauma Center microscopic hematuria in a hemodynamically stable patient is not an indication for an imaging assessment of the kidneys. Table 19.1 provides a summary of indications for renal imaging in blunt trauma (Mirvis et al. 2001). Lack of hematuria or shock does not exclude a major renal injury. Also, hematuria may be absent in 10–20% of renal injuries (Roberts et al. 1987) and in 25–50% of ureteropelvic junction and vascular pedicle injuries (Kawashima et al. 1997).

## 19.3 Penetrating Renal Trauma

Penetrating trauma accounts for about 10% of cases encountered in acute traumatic injuries of flank and back. Between 15 and 42% of these injuries are accompanied by microscopic hematuria, but the absence of hematuria does not exclude major injury to the renal parenchyma, pedicle, and proximal collecting system. Federle et al. (1987) reported 13 patients with renal pedicle injuries among 41 sustaining penetrating renal injury. Rather than surgical exploration, currently most hemodynamically stable patients with these injuries undergo contrast-enhanced MDCT to determine the location and extent of injury. In most cases the injury can be managed nonoperatively as was true for 20 of 27 patients reported by Federle et al. (1987).

**Table 19.1** Imaging management of potential renal injury

| Clinical presentation | Imaging study |
|---|---|
| Stable with penetrating flank /back injury | Chest, abdomen and pelvic CT using intravenous, oral, and rectal contrast Consider angiography to exclude pseudoaneurysm |
| Gross hematuria – hemodynamically stable and or adequately resuscitated | Abdominal and pelvic CT with oral and IV contrast |
| Persistent hemodynamic instability – requires emergency intervention (surgery or angiography) | Intraoperative IVP when stable or delayed abdomen and pelvic CT |
| Hemodynamically stable with microscopic hematuria without other indication for abdominal-pelvic CT | Observation until hematuria resolved |
| Hemodynamically stable with microscopic hematuria and with other clinical indication for abdominal-pelvic CT | Abdomen and pelvic CT with oral and IV contrast |
| Hemodynamically stable with or without microscopic hematuria, but findings of direct flank impact (lower rib fracture(s), lumbar transverse process fracture(s), flank ecchymosis or pain on palpation | Abdomen-pelvic CT with oral and IV contrast |

In a study of 143 patients with penetrating renal injuries Armenakas et al. found the majority were minor parenchymal wounds with 54% of all injury grades using the AAST classification managed conservatively with only three failures for delayed hemorrhage (1999). In this study 61% of patients had injuries involving adjacent structures including liver, spleen, and diaphragm.

In the author's practice penetrating flank and back injuries are investigated as part of an Abdominal -pelvic MDCT study. Arterial phase, portal venous phase and 3–5 min delayed phase images are acquired. All patients with penetrating torso injury receive oral, rectal, and intravenous contrast. The arterial phase images are vital to demonstrate early contrast blushes that indicate bleeding or pseudoaneurysms in order to distinguish these from urine extravasation that may be seen on delayed images after opacification of the collecting system.

Penetrating flank and back injuries can be divided in three broad categories: (1) Injury limited to retroperitoneum with no direct involvement of visceral structure, (2) Injury involving visceral structure(s), but limited to retroperitoneum, and (3) Injuries extending into the intraperitoneal compartment. It is not necessary to perform peritoneal lavage, laparoscopy, and laparotomy to assess the peritoneal compartment as this is reliably accomplished by high quality MDCT. The presence of oral/colonic contrast is vital to utilize to maintain high accuracy. Patients with no visceral injury are managed conservatively, while those with intraperitoneal extension require laparotomy and potential retroperitoneal exploration. Patients with direct renal injury may or may not require surgery depending on the precise injury. To diagnose the full extent of penetrating injury the course of the penetrating object needs to be followed. Ballistic objects may follow irregular paths due to deflection (as by bone) and also have create a volume of destruction due to their cavitation wave that extends potentially well beyond their direct tract. Renal injury can certainly arise from nonflank and back penetrating torso injuries and are assessed as part of the total abdomen-pelvic study.

## 19.4 Renal Injury Grading

The AAST grading system in based on surgical findings some of which can be diagnosed by MDCT (Table 19.2) (Moore et al. 1989). However, several

**Table 19.2** American Association for the Surgery of Trauma renal injury grading scale (modified from Moore et al. 1989)

| AAST injury grade | Description |
|---|---|
| I | Renal contusion or subcapsular hematoma with intact capsule |
| II | Superficial cortex laceration that does not extend to deep medulla or collecting system or nonexpanding hematoma |
| III | Deep laceration(s) with or without urine extravasastion |
| IV | Laceration(s) extending into collecting system with contained urine leak |
| V | Shattered renal parenchyma, renal vascular pedicle injury or devitalized kidney |

**Table 19.3** MDCT grading of renal trauma (Maryland shock-trauma center)

| Grade | Injury type |
|---|---|
| I | Laceration(s) restricted to cortex<br>Renal contusion<br>Less than 1 cm diameter subcapsular hematoma<br>Perinephric hematoma not filling Gerota's space<br>No on-going bleeding<br>Segmental renal infarction |
| II | Laceration (s) extend to medulla with intact collecting system<br>Greater than 1 cm diameter subcapsular hematoma with intact renal function<br>Perinephric hematoma filling, but not distending Gerota's fascia<br>No on-going bleeding |
| III | Injury extends into renal collecting system with urine extravasation limited to retroperitoneum<br>Perinephric hematoma that distends Gerota's fascia, but is confined to retroperitoneum<br>No on-going bleeding |
| IV | Fragmented parenchyma (3 + fragments) – typically devitalized tissue and large perirenal hematoma<br>On-going bleeding<br>Urine extravasation into peritoneal cavity or continually expanding collection<br>Subcapsular hematoma that compromises renal perfusion<br>Renal pelvic or complete uretero-pelvic junction tear<br>Vascular pedicle injury<br>Intrarenal pseudoaneurysm or arterio-venous fistula |

types of renal injury are not included in the AAST that are also commonly encountered by MDCT. The following grading system was developed at the author's trauma center to address these additional pathologic findings and how they potentially impact treatment (Table 19.3) (Mirvis et al. 2001).

## 19.5 Injury Grading and Intervention

The majority of renal injuries are minor constituting 74–98% (Thomason et al. 1989). Most patients with Grades I and II injury are managed successfully nonoperatively, while grades IV and V often require intervention (Cannon et al. 2008; Shariat et al. 2007; Shefler et al. 2007; Wright et al. 2006). In a study by Shariat et al. of 77 patients with grade IV injury (66% blunt injury and 34% penetrating 32 had renal exploration with 63% managed by renorrhaphy and 37% with nephrectomy (2008). In a retrospective review of a data base with 2,467 patients, Santucci et al. correlated need for renal surgery with injury grade as follows: grade I=0%, grade II=0%, grade III=3%, grade IV=9%, and grade V equals 86% (2001). Nephrectomy is more commonly required for high grade penetrating injury (Wright et al. 2006). Some predictive factors for nonconservative management of renal injury includes separation of the renal poles, nonvisualization of the ipsilateral ureter, multiple points of urinary extravasation, high transfusion requirements, and surgery for concurrent nonrenal injuries (Cannon et al. 2008; Shariat et al. 2008).

Renal injuries typically requiring intervention include vascular injuries (active bleeding or pseudoaneurysm), collecting system disruption, major hematoma and persistent or enlarging urinoma (Figs. 19.1–19.4). Often percutaneous interventions as angiographic embolization , catheter or ureteric stent placement, and intrarterial stenting for main renal artery injury (Dowling et al. 2007) are successful (Figs. 19.5 and 19.6). Though less common than blunt renal injuries, penetrating trauma has a higher likelihood to produce vascular injury and such injuries may manifest in the subacute, or late period after injury. Delayed, focused renal CT-angiography may be prudent to perform in cases of deep or widespread parenchymal or hilar involvement.

## 19.6 CT Findings of Renal Injury

### 19.6.1 Minor: Contusion – Laceration

Contusions (Fig. 19.7) are seen as ill-defined low attenuation regions with irregular margins. They may appear with "striated nephrograms" on contrast-enhanced CT patterns due to areas of edema that create differentiate flow through the parenchyma. On delayed noncontrast enhanced CT contusions may appear as areas of punctate contrast extravasation on the background of nonenhanced parenchyma (Lang et al. 2009; Mirvis 1996). Superficial laceration(s) are linear to

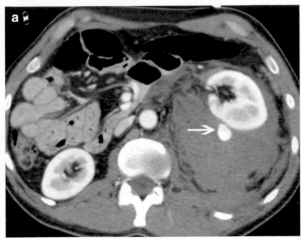

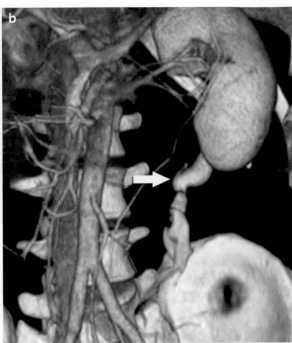

**Fig. 19.1** High grade renal injury. (**a**) CT image with intravenous contrast obtained in a 35-year-old man after 25-foot fall shows a large left perinephric hematoma displacing the kidney anteriorly. Active bleeding arises from the posterior aspect (*arrow*).

(**b**) Volume 3-D image demonstrates bleeding tracking inferior to the kidney (*arrows*). Note the collecting system has not yet opacified helping to distinguish bleeding from urine leak

irregular low attenuation areas limited to the renal cortex and superficial medullary region and typically have a small amount of associated perinephric blood. It should be noted that both lacerations and contusions are best seen on the arterial phase scan when there is peak renal cortical enhancement and are typically less conspicuous on delayed portal and pyelogram phases.

### 19.6.2 *Minor: Focal Renal Infarct*

Segmental renal infarcts are relatively common from blunt renal trauma and usually involve the poles. These injuries result from stretching of renal branch vessels, an accessory renal artery, or capsular arteries and subsequent thrombosis (Lewis et al. 1996) (Fig. 19.8). These infarcts appear as sharply-marginated wedge-shaped regions. Often there are no concurrent renal injuries. Renal angiography is usually not indicated as these injuries, in the author's experience, do not lead to subsequent hemorrhage and do not required embolization as isolated injuries.

### 19.6.3 *Minor: Subcapsular Hematoma*

Subcapsular hematomas are relatively rare, particularly in older adults as it is difficult to strip the capsule from the cortex to allow bleeding into the potential space. Usually the capsule tears resulting in a perinephric hematoma. These hematomas are limited in expansion by the renal capsule creating a convex bulge into the renal parenchyma (Fig. 19.9). Large subcapsular hematomas may produce enough pressure against the parenchyma to delay renal perfusion. In most cases these injuries will resolve without intervention and will be self-limited by increasing subcapsular pressure.

### 19.7 CT Finding of Major Renal Injury

Grade III injuries are more significant and may require intervention. Among them are renal fractures extending to the collecting system with contained urine leak, large perinephric hematomas, without on-going bleeding, and renal parenchymal splits (Fig. 19.10).

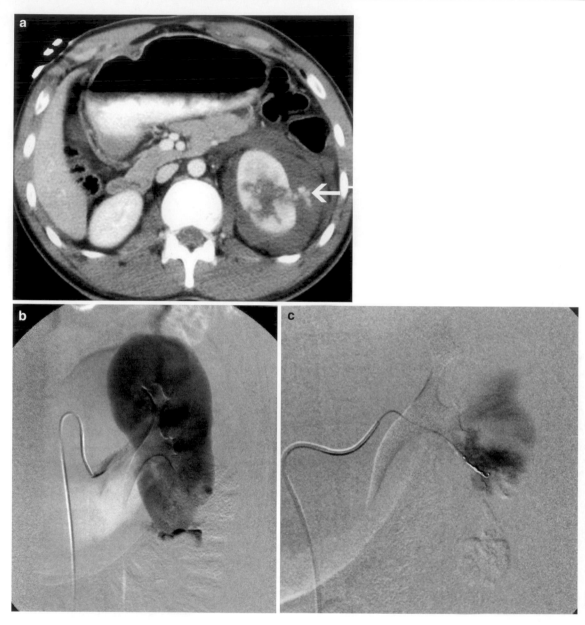

**Fig. 19.2** Active renal bleeding treated by coil embolization. (**a**) Twenty-one-year-old man sustaining injured in fall sustaining deep lacerations through the mid-left kidney. There is on-going bleeding into the peri-nephric hematoma (*arrow*). (**b**) Selective renal arteriogram verifies bleeding from lower pole branch. (**c**) The bleeding is occluded after superselective segmental branch coil embolization

### 19.7.1  Urine Leaks

Urine leaks are visualized as low density fluid collections on arterial phase CT scanning with progressive contrast filling seen on portal venous, or more likely 3–5 min delayed scans (Figs. 19.3 and 19.11). Usually the collections are limited to the perinephric space, remain stable in size, and resolve without intervention. Patency of the pelvocalyceal and ureter is required to allow decompression of a urinoma through a

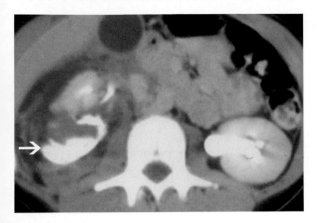

**Fig. 19.3** Urinoma. Urinoma (*arrow*) collects dependent to the right kidney with urine draining from the central collecting system. Antegrade flow through the ureter is intact

low-pressure route and may require double-J catheter stenting. Rarely, urinomas may become infected and require percutaneous drainage. Progressive urinoma enlargement indicates no or poor antegrade collecting system flow.

### 19.7.2 Hematoma

Large perinephric hematomas typically arise from small arterial branch bleeding, although renal venous injuries can also produce a large quantity of perinephric bleeding as well (Fig. 19.12). The hemorrhage may be limited to Gerota's space or extend through adjacent torn fascia into the pararenal spaces, with the potential to spread widely in the larger potential volume. The kidney is typically displaced by the hematoma. Large amounts of peri or pararenal blood can lead to hemodynamic compromise or instability. Treatment of a large peri/pararenal hematoma depends on the clinical course and associated injuries. If there is no active renal bleeding at the time of the CT study, bleeding may recur and lead to rapid hypotension.

### 19.7.3 Parenchymal Disruption

Major parenchymal injuries are represented by deep lacerations that extend into the medulla and collecting system. They include renal splits with isolated portions of renal parenchyma (Fig. 19.4). Usually there is some

degree of nonviable areas of parenchyma, but the majority of the parenchyma remains functional. There is usually a large amount of perinephric hematoma filling or distending Gerota's space. There should be no evidence of ongoing bleeding for this injury to be considered major.

These injuries will often show a significant degree of resolution, even with a complete split, with restoration of normal renal function assuming the majority of the parenchymal is intact (Fig. 19.10). However, these parenchymal injuries should be followed by repeat CT at 24–48 h after initial CT to verify stability as delayed hemorrhage can be difficult to detect clinically and may require urgent interventional embolization or surgical treatment. Progression of symptoms as increasing pain or evidence of delayed bleeding, infection, or delayed urine leak certainly mandate follow-up CT.

## 19.8 CT of Catastrophic Renal Injury

Injuries of grade IV severity account for approximately 5% of all renal injuries and usually require surgical or image guided intervention [36]. These injuries include major vascular injury, renal parenchymal fragmentation usually associated with partial devascularization, renal pelvis disruption, expanding perirenal hematoma, active bleeding, and persistent/uncontrolled urine leakage, including renal vascular pedicle avulsions or complete traumatic occlusions, and renal pelvic avulsions (Figs. 19.1, 19.2, 19.5, and 19.13).

### 19.8.1 Vascular Injury

In blunt trauma with anteroposterior deceleration the kidneys are displaced laterally. This motion stretches the intima beyond its elastic limits leading to intimal disruption. Later clot forms within the lumen around the intimal tear. Initial clot-formation may lead to complete renal artery thrombosis. The artery typically becomes occluded in the proximal one-third of the vessel (Fig. 19.14). The nonperfused kidney often appears uninjured (Fig. 19.15). During contrast-enhanced CT the involved kidney will show no or only

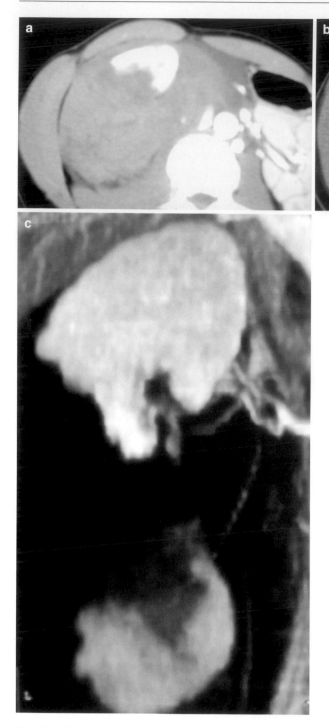

**Fig. 19.4** Catastrophic renal injury – split. (**a**, **b**) There is a huge hematoma surrounding fragments of transected right kidney. (**c**) Coronal reformation shows renal split along the transverse plane (Part **c** was revised)

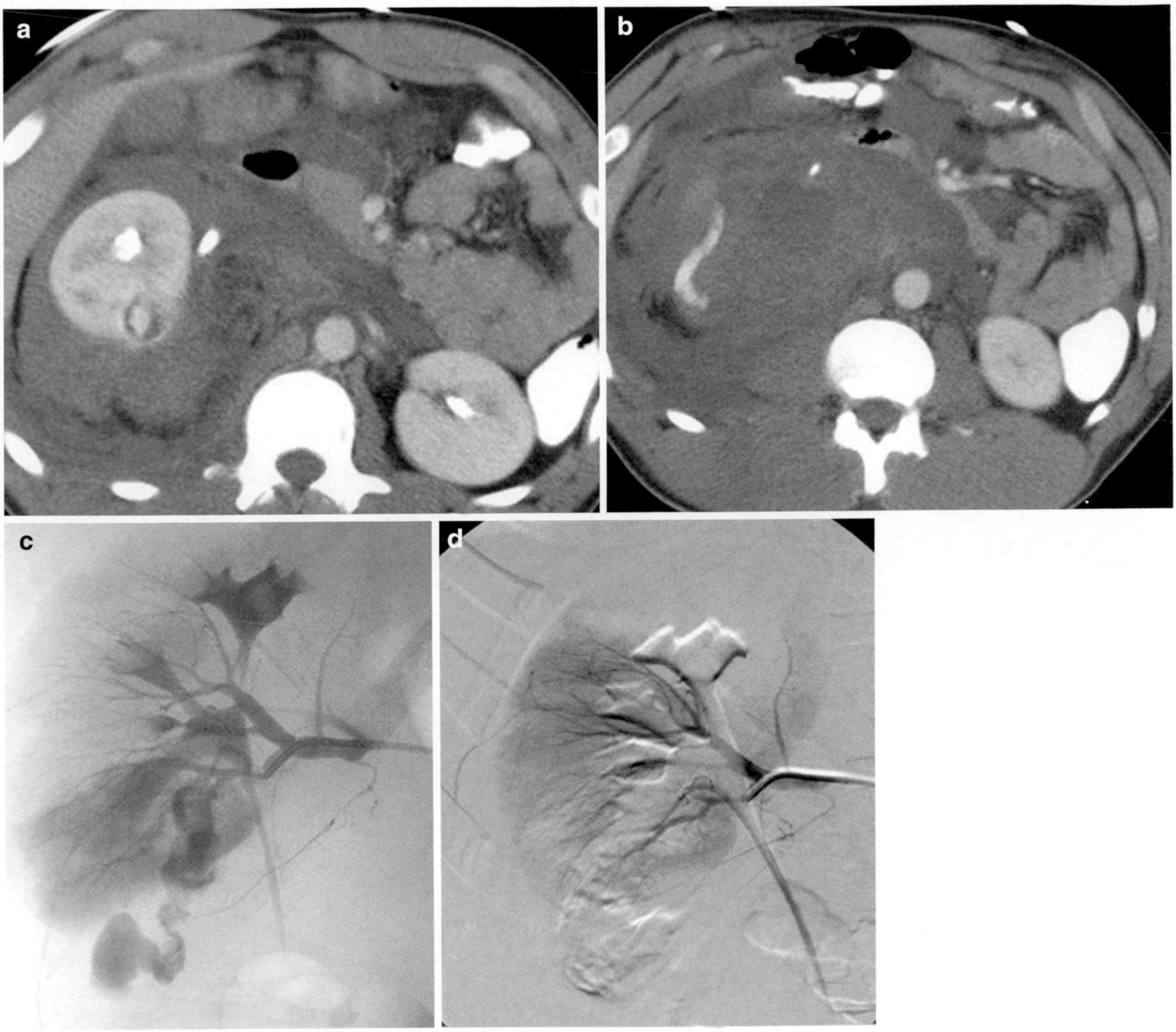

**Fig. 19.5** Embolization for active renal bleeding in 28-year-old male stabbing victim. (**a**) CT image with intravenous contrast shows large right perirenal hematoma with focus of active bleeding in posterior aspect (*arrow*). (**b**) Large hematoma and some iodinated recent bleeding lies caudal to kidney. (**c**) Image from renal arteriogram displays site of bleeding from lower pole segment branch tracking inferior to kidney. (**d**) After proximal coil placement bleeding has been arrested

superficial parenchymal enhancement (from intact capsular vessels (Fig. 19.16). The size of the kidney may appear uniformally diminished from lack of circulating blood. There may be residual areas of perfusion from accessory renal arteries or branches arising proximal to the occlusion. There may be retrograde opacification of the main renal vein and intrarenal veins due to retrograde flow for the inferior vena cava due to decreased renal venous pressure (Cain et al. 1995) (Fig. 19.17). This is especially likely if the contrast is administered via the femoral vein. The opacified intrarenal veins may resemble a normal collecting system suggesting normal function, although there will be no renal parenchymal enhancement seen. Standard MCDT with arterial phase enhancement is quite adequate to establish the diagnosis of renal artery occlusion and angiography is not required unless performed as part of attempted revascularization.

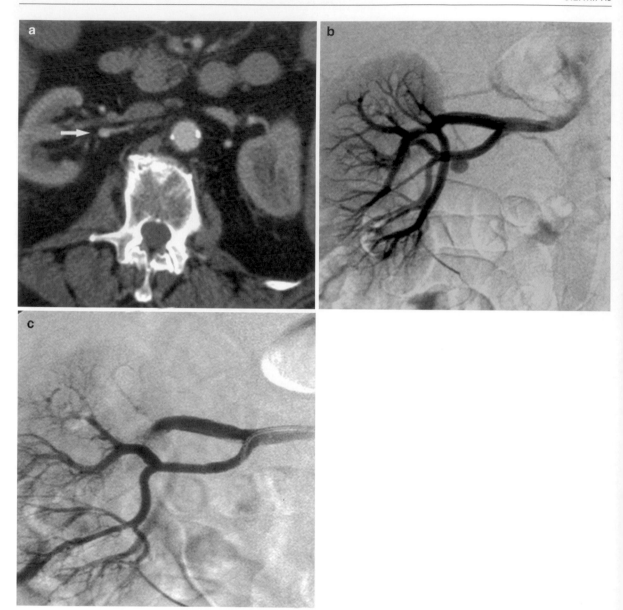

**Fig. 19.6** Renal artery stenting. (**a**) CT image of blunt trauma patient shows a small pseudoaneurysm of the renal artery (*arrow*). (**b**) Selective right renal angiogram verifies aneurysm. (**c**) Pseudoaneurysm successfully covered with stent graft

The amount of time the kidney remains viable in the warm body is debated. Usually flow must be restored with 2 h of injury (Hoffman et al. 1974; Mirvis 1989). Revascularization may be successful after longer periods due to collateral blood supply maintaining viability. Another reason that long warm ischemic times have been described is that the time from injury to actual complete renal artery occlusion may vary considerably. An incomplete renal artery occlusion from the initial injury can maintain partial perfusion of the kidney sustaining viability until flow has been completed disrupted. Once high grade renal artery occlusion is recognized immediate surgical or intervention stent repair of the renal artery is needed to optimize tissue viability. Traumatic occlusion of both renal arteries occurs rarely, with but can be difficult to

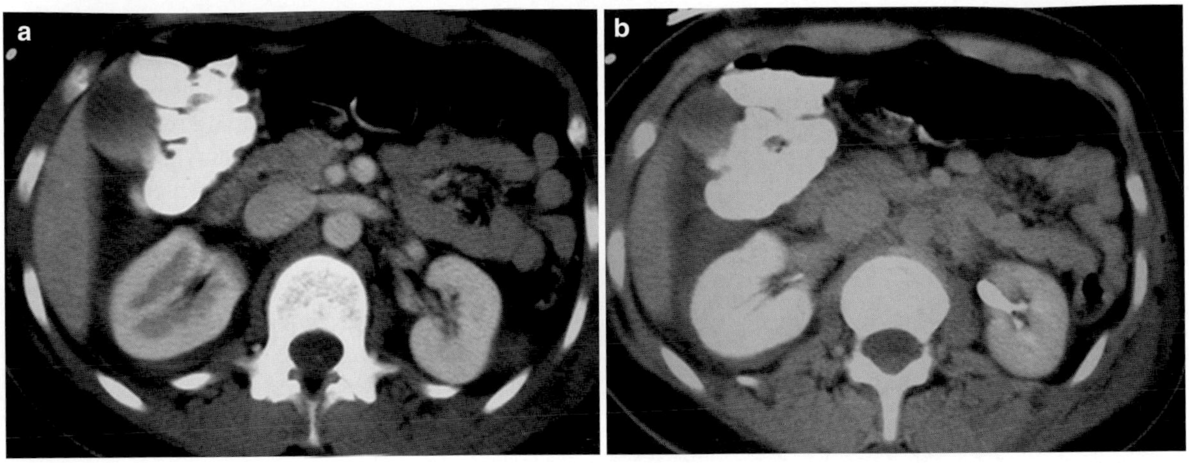

**Fig. 19.7** Renal contusion. (**a**, **b**) CT images acquired post blunt trauma in arterial and portal venous phases shows enlarged right kidney with delayed nephrogram and pyelogram compared to the left kidney. Finding is most consistent with diffuse renal contusion. Free fluid is seen in hepatorenal recess

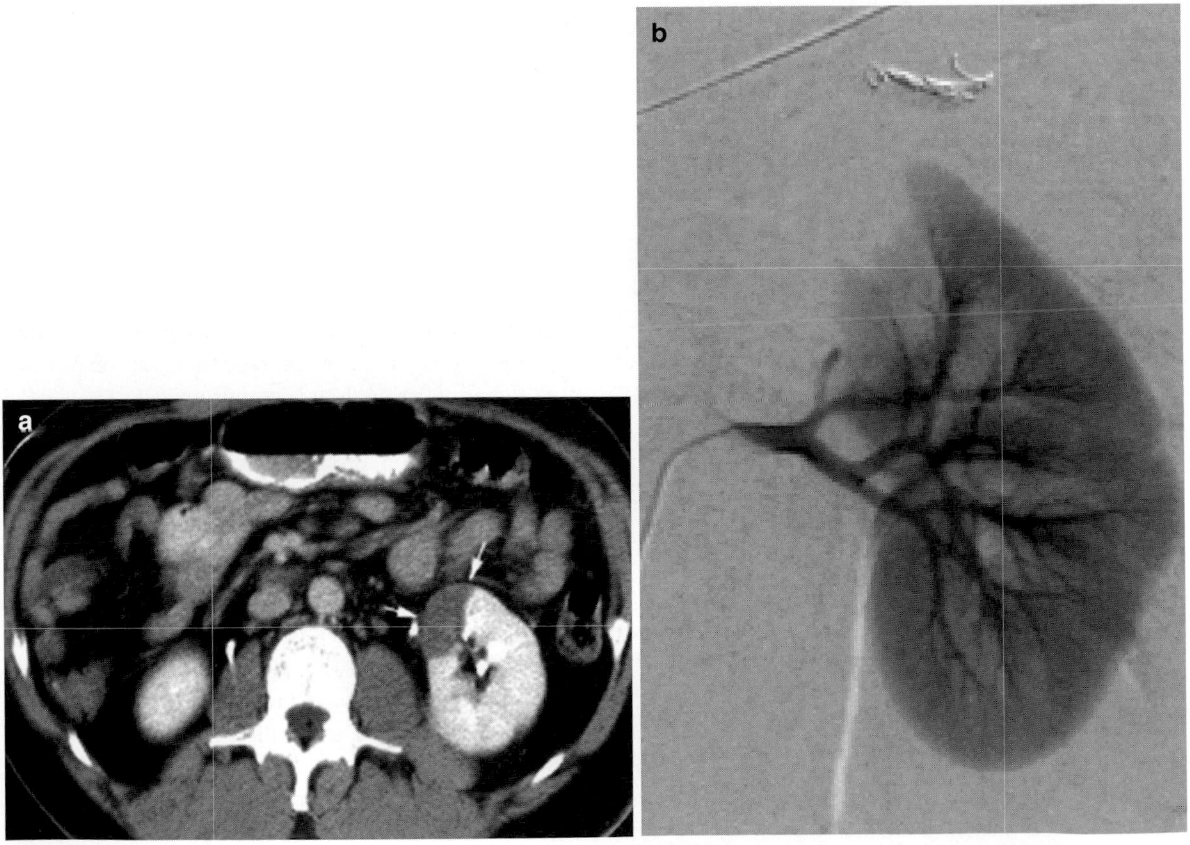

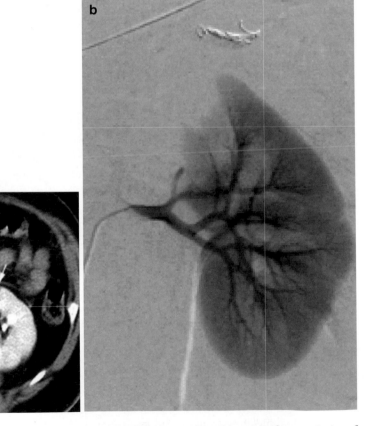

**Fig. 19.8** Segmental renal infarct after trauma. (**a**) CT image acquired in the portal venous phase shows wedge-shaped area of nonenhancement in the anterior upper segment of left kidney (*arrows*). (**b**) Selective renal arteriogram confirms occlusion of segmental vessels supplying superior pole of the kidney. No specific treatment was undertaken

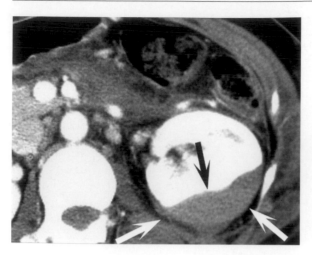

**Fig. 19.9** Subcapsular renal hematoma. Arterial phase CT image shows compression of the enhanced renal parenchyma (*black arrow*) from overlying hematoma confined by renal capsule (*white arrows*)

by angiographic embolization to provide selective vascular interruption and preserve maximal parenchyma. Patients who become hemodynamically unstable with active bleeding require surgical intervention for this injury. In general, while the nephrectomy rate is higher for treatment of bleeding of renal origin by surgery than embolization, patients treated by surgery usually have more severe injuries or required exploration for concurrent surgical injury. High-resolution intravenous contrast-enhanced CT can also directly diagnose renal arterial and venous injuries, including intimal tears and pseudoaneurysms, allowing early interventional repair.

### 19.8.3 Collecting System Injury

Deep renal lacerations extending to the collecting system can result in urine leaks from ruptures in the calyces or renal pelvis. Such injuries are usually detected on delayed contrast-enhanced CT images where the collecting systems have had ample time to opacify (Figs. 19.10 and 19.13). Urinomas may result from urine leaks particularly if there is increased pressure in the collecting system from limited antegrade urine flow (Figs. 19.3 and 19.10). If urine is leaking into a low-pressure system such as the peritoneal or pleural cavity aggressive urinary diversion by catheter drainage or surgical intervention is likely to be required. Most urinomas are self-limited injuries resolving without intervention, but may require drainage for infection or when free antegrade urine flow is compromised.

Injuries to the renal pelvis and particularly the uretero-pelvic junction probably result from overstretching of the collecting system at the time of blunt impact. On arterial phase CT images, before iodinated urine has reached the collecting system, only serous attenuation fluid will be noted in proximity to the collecting system. The collecting system may remain unopacified in the portal phase scan as well, but in some patients early opacification may appear providing evidence of high density urine around the collecting system. Contrast typically accumulates around the medial and inferior aspect of the kidney in proximity to the tear with an uretero-pelvic injury site. In any patient showing fluid around the collecting system in the arterial or portal

discern since the renal parenchyma maintains equivalent CT density bilaterally in the angiography and portal venous CT studies (Klink et al. 1992). A delayed CT study at least 3 min post contrast injection will verify lack of collecting system opacification.

### 19.8.2 Bleeding

On-going hemorrhage arising from the injured kidney is typically visualized on the arterial phase as a linear hyperdensity. Since the collecting system is unopacified on the arterial scan there is no possibility of confusing extravasated vascular contrast from leaking urine. The leaking contrast has a density typically within 15 HU of an adjacent enhanced renal artery (Cerva et al. 1996) (Figs. 19.1, 19.2, and 19.5). On portal phase or delayed imaging the contrast material appears to extend further away from its site of origin and to decrease in density from dilution of nonopacified blood. The extravasated vascular contrast is surrounded by a lower density hematoma, which is not the case with leaking opacified urine (Figs. 19.1, 19.2, 19.5, and 19.18). In the author's practice active bleeding from the kidney is managed

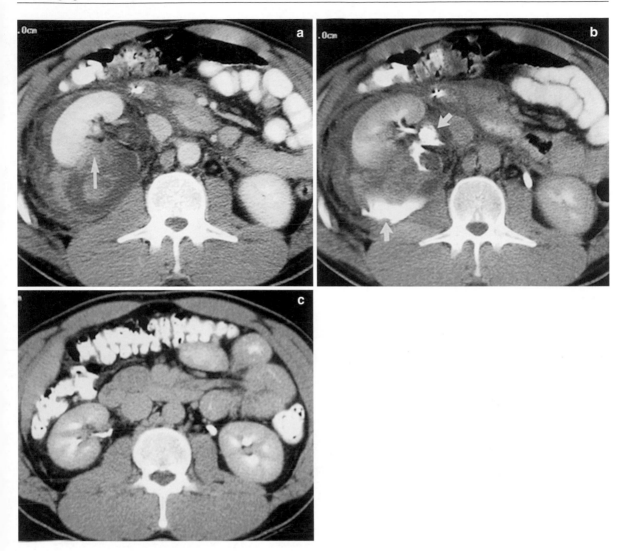

**Fig. 19.10** Major renal injury. (**a**) CT image shows deep laceration through posterior right kidney with ischemic parenchyma (*arrow*) and free fluid principally in the posterior perirenal space. (**b**) Delayed image at 3 min post injection shows extravasated urine pooling dependently and around pelvocalyceal junction (*arrows*). (**c**) Despite severity in injury non operative management follow-up CT 6 months after injury shows essentially normal right renal anatomy

phase scans, 3–5 min pyelogram images are required to assess the collecting system. At this time, collecting system tears should be apparent (Fig. 19.19). If there is opacification of the distal ureter the tear is partial, but if there is no distal ureteral contrast visualized more likely complete. If there is fluid around the collecting system but the patient is off the scanner delayed follow-up by radiography or CT can verify or exclude collecting system disruption as the cause of the perirenal fluid. Avulsion or major tears of the renal pelvis are likely to demonstrate more diffuse contrast extravasation around the pelvis with no or partial visualization of the collecting system. Differentiation of pelvic from proximal ureteral tears is important to determine whether stenting can potentially manage the ureteral injury or surgical repair of the pelvis is required.

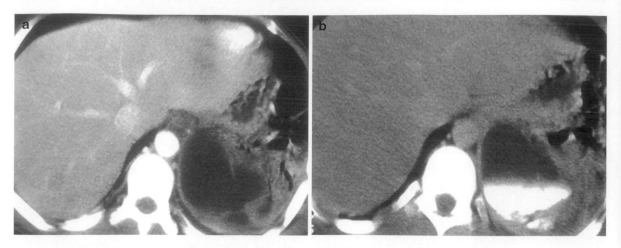

**Fig. 19.11** Urinoma, delayed opacification. (**a**) Arterial phase CT image shows low attenuation fluid collection in left posterior subphrenic space. (**b**) Delayed scan at 5 min after injection shows delayed filling of collection with iodinated urine, verifying urinoma

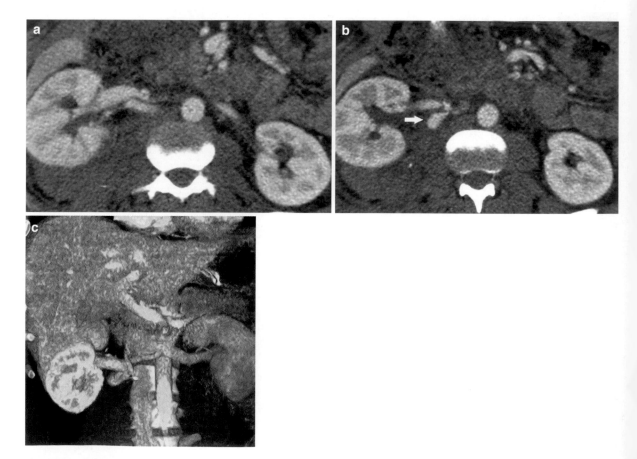

**Fig. 19.12** Renal vein injury. (**a**) CT image in arterial phase shows large right perirenal and anterior pararenal hematoma. (**b**) Adjacent image demonstrates pseudoaneurysm arising from proximal renal vein (*arrow*). (**c**) Volumetric 3D image better shows size and orientation of pseudoaneurysm

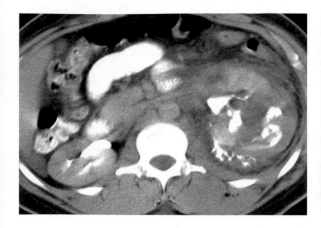

**Fig. 19.13** Catastrophic renal parenchymal injury. Delayed CT image shows extensive injury to left kidney with large perirenal and anterior pararenal hematoma and multiple foci of urine extravasation

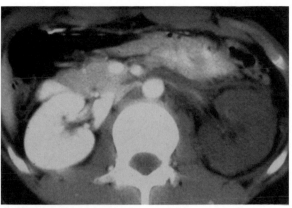

**Fig. 19.15** CT of renal artery occlusion. Arterial phase CT image after blunt injury demonstrates no enhancement of intact left kidney. There is some hemorrhage around the narrowed irregular renal artery

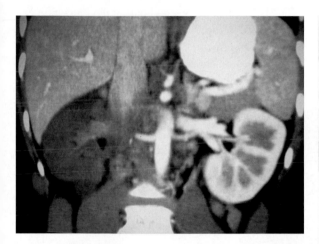

**Fig. 19.14** Renal artery occlusion. Coronal reformatted CT reveals occlusion of the right renal artery after blunt trauma in typical location at junction of proximal third and distal two-thirds of artery

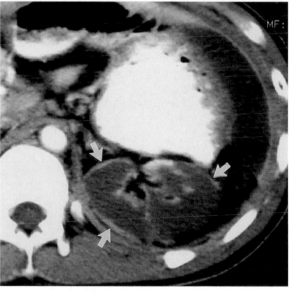

**Fig. 19.16** CT of renal ischemia. Arterial phase CT image indicates residual perfusion of the renal capsule (*arrows*) and possible medullary collateral branches. Otherwise the kidney is nonperfused

## 19.9 Injury of the Abnormal Kidney

Patients with underlying renal abnormalities are at increased risk of injury from a given impact or the impact or the injury are at an increased risk of sustaining injuries from a given impact or the injury may be more severe than to a normal kidney. Schmidlin et al. found that, 19% of patients who sustained a renal injury had a preexisting renal abnormality (1998).

Congenital abnormalities as horseshoe ectopic, polycystic kidneys, and congenital ureteropelvic junction obstruction are at an increased risk of sustaining injuries after abdominal trauma (Li et al. 2007). Patients with chronic hydronephrosis, renal infection, simple renal cysts, and renal cell cancers are also at increased risk of sustaining renal after even minimal impact (Figs. 19.20 and 19.21). Hematuria in patients with renal injury should be followed to resolution. Persistent hematuria could indicate the presence of an underlying renal tumor or vascular lesion.

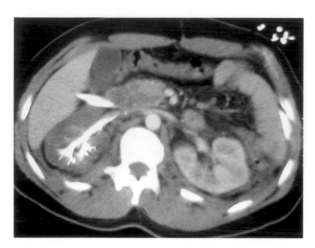

**Fig. 19.17** CT of renal arterial occlusion. CT study was obtained in the arterial phase with contrast injection into the inferior vena cava. Contrast refluxes into the right renal veins due to reversed pressure gradient. It is important not to mistake this appearance as due to pyelogram

## 19.10 Imaging Findings and Management

Most renal injuries, 90–95%, can be treated conservatively without surgery (Matthews and Spirnak 1995). In the author's center minor injuries to the kidneys are not usually followed up by further CT studies unless dictated by the development of new symptoms potentially of renal origin.

Management of patients with major renal injuries will depend on the precise extent of injury, the stability of the injury, and the patient's overall clinical status. Many major injuries including collecting system leaks, large peri -and pararenal hematomas, and major parenchymal lacerations and partial devitalization can be managed without surgery or may require only percutaneous treatment. One or more follow-up CT studies are recommended in patients with major renal injury who are treated conservatively to verify lack of injury progression, beginning resolution and lack of

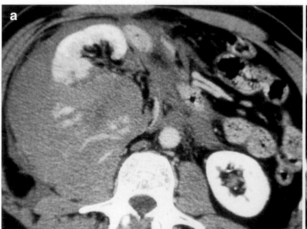
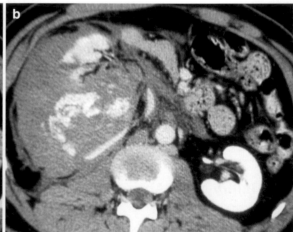

**Fig. 19.18** Active renal hemorrhage. (**a**, **b**) Two images from arterial phase CT shows multifocal areas of bright extravasasted arterial contrast surrounded by large perirenal hematoma. The image is acquired before opacification of the renal collecting system. (**c**) 3D volume image shows extensive bleeding above the right kidney. A small artery connects main renal body from superiorly displaced fragment

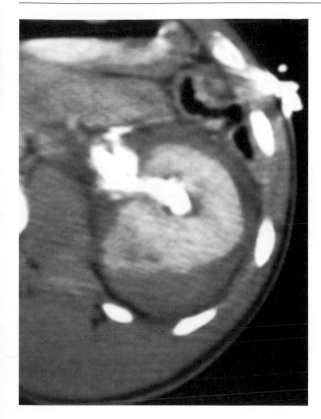

**Fig. 19.19** Uretero-pelvic junction injury. A coned down delayed phase CT image obtained on a 28-year-old man ejected 50-feet in motor vehicle collision shows extravasated opacified urine around lower renal pelvis and proximal ureter. There is a focal posterior renal contusion and perirenal fluid

complications as on-going bleeding, urinioma or infection.

Indications for renal surgical exploration include major renal artery injury (avulsion or occlusion) resulting in either nonperfusion of the kidney on CT or hemodynamic instability after resuscitation due to rapidly expanding hemorrhage that may lead to exsanguination (Sagalowsky et al. 1983). Over the past several years, the role of emergent nephrectomy has diminished for some types of severe renal injuries, with a resultant increase in the rate of renal salvage (Titton et al. 2002). Increasingly, patients with active bleeding and vascular injury are being managed by interventional radiology with stenting for vascular injuries, such as pseudoaneurysm or traumatic arterio-venous malformation and selective embolization of arterial bleeding (Figs. 19.3,

19.5, and 19.6). Percutaneous transcatheter embolization with either gelatin sponge (Gelfoam; Upjohn, Kalamazoo, MI) or stainless steel coils is the preferred method of treatment of bleeding traumatic lesions of the kidney to maximize renal function and viable renal parenchyma (Titton et al. 2002).

## 19.11  Complications of Renal Injury

Complications of renal trauma are most common in patients with higher grades of renal injury. In a retrospective review over 4 years, Blankenship et al. found urologic complications in no patient with grade I injury, 15% in grade II, 38% in grade III, 43% in grade IV, and 100% of grade V (2001). For this reason the article recommends repeat CT scanning in 2–4 days after trauma in all patients with injury grades III-V to identify complications that may require intervention (Blankenship et al. 2001). Complications of renal injury include urinoma, infection, delayed appearance of vascular injury, and hypertension (Fig. 19.22).

### 19.11.1  Persistent Urinoma

A urinoma that has enlarged or is unchanged in size at follow-up CT after 3 or more days or when output from an adequately placed percutaneous drainage catheter does not decrease during the first few days after insertion indicates a persistent leak most likely due to inadequate reduction of pressure on the collecting system injury (Kantor et al. 1989; Matthews and Spirnak 1995). In cases of persistent leakage an antegrade nephrostomy in combination with antegrade ureteral stent placement or placement of a nephroureterostomy catheter is usually warranted to decrease pressure on the collecting system injury and promote healing.

### 19.11.2  Hypertension

Hypertension is a rare complication of renal trauma, typically renin dependent and usually related to renal artery lesions or parenchymal injury (Chedid et al. 2006). In a

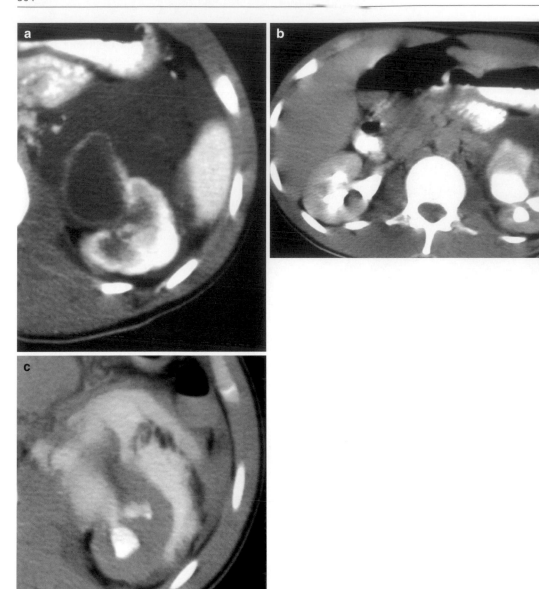

**Fig. 19.20** Rupture of renal pelvis – uretero-pelvic junction obstruction. (**a**) CT in arterial phase in 19-year-old male assault victim shows distended urine filled collecting system with large quantity of perirenal low attenuation fluid anterior to the kidney. (**b**) Delayed image shows filling of pelvis with iodinated urine and leak into peripelvic region. (**c**) Further delayed CT image demonstrates more extensive extravasation from collecting system

**Fig. 19.21** Ruptured collecting system: UPJ obstruction. (**a**) Arterial phase CT image shows right kidney is markedly distended by hydronephrosis with small diameter proximal ureter. There is surrounding low attenuation urine. (**b**) Adjacent CT image shows ruptured markedly thinned renal pelvis with surrounding urine

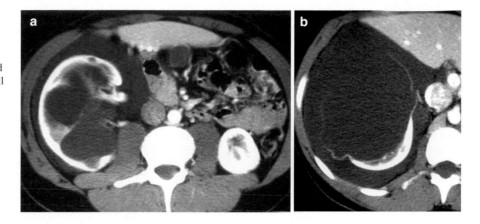

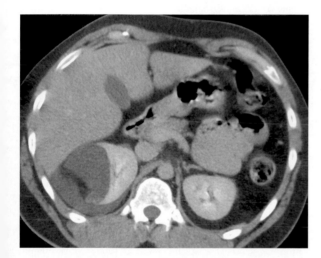

**Fig. 19.22** Renal cyst rupture. Blunt trauma has caused rupture of large renal cyst into adjacent perinephric fat

small series patients with renal artery thrombosis with the infarcted kidney left in situ no patient developed hypertension and all had normal creatinine levels at median 9 month follow-up (Jawas and Abu-Zidan 2008).

## 19.12  Conclusion

Renal injuries are commonly seen from both blunt polytrauma and penetrating torso trauma. Using primarily MDCT the extent of injury can be determined helping, with knowledge of other injuries and overall hemodynamic status, to determine immediate and long-term treatment requirements. The use of current CT technology has supported greater reliance on

nonoperative treatment in greater numbers of patients whose injuries are likely to remain stable. MDCT aids in detection of early complications of renal injury such as infection, urinoma, or delayed hemorrhage and can permit successful management of these without the need for surgical intervention.

## References

Armenakas N, Duckett CP, McAninch JW (1999) Indications for nonoperative management of renal stab wounds. J Urol 161:768–771

Baverstock R, Simons R, McLoughlin M (2001) Severe blunt renal trauma: a 7-year retrospective review from a provincial trauma centre. Can J Urol 8:1372–1376

Blankenship JC, Gavant ML, Cox CE et al. (2001) Importance of delayed imaging for blunt renal trauma. World J Surg 25:1561–1564

Bower P, Paul J, Brosman SA (1978) Urinary tract abnormality presenting as a result of blunt abdominal trauma. J Trauma 18:719–722

Cain M, Matsumoto JM, Husmann DA (1995) Retrograde filling of the renal vein on computerized tomography for blunt renal trauma: an indication of renal artery injury. J Urol 153:1247–1248

Cannon G, Polsky EG, Smaldone MC et al. (2008) Computerized tomography findings in pediatric renal trauma – indications for early intervention. J Urol 179:1529–1532

Cerva D, Mirvis SE, Shanmuganathan K et al. (1996) Detection of bleeding in patients with major pelvic fractures: value of contrast-enhanced CT. AJR Am J Roentgenol 166:131–136

Chedid A, Le Coz S, Rossignol P et al. (2006) Blunt renal trauma-induced hypertension: prevalence, presentation, and outcome. Am J Hypertens 19:500–504

Dowling JM, Lube MW, Smith CP et al. (2007) Traumatic renal artery occlusion in a patient with a solitary kidney: case report of treatment with endovascular stent and review of the literature. Am Surg 73:351–353

Dunfee B, Lucey BC, Soto JA (2008) Development of renal scars on CT after abdominal trauma: does grade of injury matter? AJR Am J Roentgenol 190:1174–1179

Federle M, Brown TR, McAninch JW (1987) Penetrating renal trauma: CT evaluation. J Comput Assist Tomogr 11: 1026–1030

Gourgiotis S, Germanos S, Dimopoulos N et al. (2006) Renal injury: 5-year experience and literature review. Urol Int 77: 97–103

Hardeman S, Husmann DA, Chinn HK et al. (1987) Blunt urinary tract trauma: identifying those patients who require radiological diagnostic studies. J Urol 138:99–101

Hoffman R, Stieper KW, Johnson RW et al. (1974) Renal ischemic tolerance. Arch Surg 109:550–551

Jawas A, Abu-Zidan FM (2008) Management algorithm for complete blunt renal artery occlusion in multiple trauma patients: case series. Int J Surg 6:317–322

Kantor A, Sclafani SJ, Scalea T et al. (1989) The role of interventional radiology in the management of genitourinary trauma. Urol Clin North Am 16:255–265

Kawashima A, Sandler CM, Corriere JN Jr et al. (1997) Ureteropelvic junction injuries secondary to blunt trauma. Radiology 205:487–492

Klink B, Sutherin S, Heyse P et al. (1992) Traumatic bilateral renal artery thrombosis diagnosed by computed tomography with successful revascularization: case report. J Trauma 32:259–262

Lang EK, Rudman E, Hanano A et al. (2009) Delayed interstitial renal contrast extravasation and vicarious excretion due to hypotension following blunt renal trauma. J Urol 181:1881

Lee Y, Oh SN, Rha SE et al. (2007) Renal trauma. Radiol Clin North Am 45:581–592

Lewis D, Mirvis SE, Shanmuganathan K (1996) Segmental renal artery infarction following blunt abdominal trauma: clinical significance and appropriate management. Emerg Radiol 3:236–240

Li WM, Liu CC, Wu WJ et al. (2007) Rupture of renal pelvis in an adult with congenital ureteropelvic junction obstruction after blunt abdominal trauma. Kaohsiung J Med Sci 23: 142–146

Matthews L, Spirnak JP (1995) The nonoperative approach to major blunt renal trauma. Semin Urol 13:77–82

Miller K, McAninch J (1995) Radiographic assessment of renal trauma: our 15-year experience. J Urol 154:352–355

Mirvis S (1989) Diagnostic imaging of the urinary system following blunt trauma. Clin Imaging 13:269–289

Mirvis S (1996) Trauma. Radiol Clin North Am 34:1225–1257

Mirvis S, Shanmuganathan K, Killeen K (2001) Injury to the urinary tract. In: Grainger RG, Allison D, Adam A, Dixon AK (eds) Diagnostic radiology: a textbook of medical imaging, 4th edn. Churchill Livingstone, London, Edinburgh, New York, pp 625–629

Moore EE, Shackford SR, Pachter HL et al. (1989) Organ injury scaling: spleen, liver, and kidney. J Trauma 29:1664–1666

Roberts R, Belitsky P, Lannon SG et al. (1987) Conservative management of renal lacerations in blunt trauma. Can J Surg 30:253–255

Sagalowsky A, McConnell JD, Peters PC (1983) Renal trauma requiring surgery: an analysis of 185 cases J Trauma 23: 128–131

Santucci R, McAninch JW, Safir M et al. (2001) Validation of the American Association for the Surgery of Trauma organ injury severity scale for kidney. J Trauma 50:195–200

Schmidlin F, Iselin CE, Naimi A et al. (1998) The higher injury risk of abnormal kidneys in blunt renal trauma. Scand J Urol Nephrol 32:388–392

Shariat S, Jenkins A, Roehrborn CG et al. (2008) Features and outcomes of patients with grade IV renal injury. BJU Int 102:728–733

Shariat S, Roehrborn CG, Karakiewicz PI et al. (2007) Evidence-based validation of the predictive value of the American Association for the Surgery of Trauma kidney injury scale. J Trauma 62:933–939

Shefler A, Gremitzky A, Vainrib M et al. (2007) The role of nonoperative management of penetrating renal trauma. Harefuah 146:345–348; 406–407

Stein J, Kaji DM, Eastham J et al. (1994) Blunt renal trauma in the pediatric population: indications for radiologic evaluation. Urology 44:406–410

Titton R, Gervais DA, Boland GW et al. (2002) Renal trauma: radiologic evaluation and percutaneous treatment of nonvascular injuries. AJR Am J Roentgenol 178:1507–1511

Thomason R, Julian JS, Mostellar HC et al. (1989) Microscopic hematuria after blunt trauma: is pyelography necessary? Am Surg 55:145–150

Wright J, Nathens AB, Rivara FP et al. (2006) Renal and extrarenal predictors of nephrectomy from the national data bank. J Urol 175:970–975

# Part IV

## Tumoral Pathology

## Contents

## Abstract

> Renal neoplasms histotypes have been recently reclassified by the World Health Organization. This chapter describes the fundamental imaging features of the most common benign solid renal tumors. The most common benign solid renal tumors are angiomyolipomas, and renal oncocytomas. The most typical imaging feature of renal angiomyolipoma is the evidence of macroscopic fat which can be identified by unenhanced CT and by fat-saturation MR sequences. Renal angiomyolipomas with minimal fat component may present the same imaging features of malignant renal masses . The most typical pattern of renal oncocytomas on contrast-enhanced CT consists in a spoke-wheel shaped or diffuse enhancement pattern, and a sharp, smooth rim. Stellate area of low attenuation may be found in 30–40% of large oncocytomas.

Benign solid renal tumors represent a frequent entity detected by imaging modalities, especially in the form of angiomyolipomas. The 2004 World Health Organization (WHO) classification scheme categorizes renal neoplasms on the basis of histogenesis (cell of origin) and histopathology (Eble et al. 2004). Renal neoplasms are thus classified into renal cell, metanephric, mesenchymal, nephroblastic, mixed epithelial and mesenchymal tumors, neuroendocrine tumors, hematopoietic and lymphoid tumors, germ cell tumors and metastatic tumors (Tables 20.1 and 20.2) (Prasad et al. 2006).

Recent advances in imaging technology, and in particular the wide use of ultrasonography (US) and

E. Quaia
Department of Radiology, Cattinara Hospital, University of Trieste, Strada di Fiume 447, 34149 Trieste, Italy
e-mail: quaia@univ.trieste.it

E. Quaia (ed.), *Radiological Imaging of the Kidney*,
Medical Radiology, DOI: 10.1007/978-3-540-87597-0_20, © Springer-Verlag Berlin Heidelberg 2011

**Table 20.1** World Health Organization (WHO) histological classification of benign neoplasms of the kidney

| Renal cell | Metanephric | Mesenchymal | Mixed epithelial and mesenchymal |
|---|---|---|---|
| Oncocytoma<br>Papillary adenoma | Metanephric adenoma<br>Metanephric adenofibroma<br>Metanephric stromal tumor | Angiomyolipoma<br>Leiomyoma<br>Hemangioma<br>Lymphangioma<br>Juxtaglomerular cell tumor[a]<br>Fibroma<br>Schwannoma | Cystic neproma<br>Mixed epithelial and stromal tumor |
| **Nephroblastic tumors** | | **Neuroendocrine** | |
| Nephrogenic rests[b] | | Somatostatinoma<br>VIPoma | |

Note: The histologic subtypes of benign tumors of the kidney

[a]Reninoma

[b]Nephrogenic rests are abnormally persistent foci of embryonal cells that are capable of developing into nephroblastomas. Nephroblastomatosis is defined as the presence of diffuse or multifocal nephrogenic rests

**Table 20.2** World Health Organization (WHO) histological classification of malignant neoplasms of the kidney

| Renal cell | Mesenchymal | Mixed epithelial and mesenchymal |
|---|---|---|
| Clear cell renal cell carcinoma[a]<br>Papillary renal cell carcinoma<br>Chromophobe renal cell carcinoma<br>Hereditary cancer syndromes<br>Multilocular cystic renal cell carcinoma<br>Collecting duct carcinoma of Bellini<br>Medullary carcinoma<br>Other forms[b] | *Occurring mainly in infants*<br>Clear cell renal cell sarcoma<br>Rhabdoid tumor<br>Congenital mesoblastic tumor<br>Ossifying renal tumor of infants<br><br>*Occurring mainly in adults*<br>Leiomyosarcoma<br>Angiosarcoma<br>Rhabdomyosarcoma 8900/3<br>Malignant fibrous histiocytoma<br>Hemangiopericytoma<br>Osteosarcoma<br>Renomedullary interstitial cell tumour<br>Solitary fibrous tumour | Synovial sarcoma |
| **Hematopoietic and lymphoid tumors** | **Neuroendocrine** | **Germ cell tumors** |
| Lymphoma<br>Leukemia<br>Plasmacytoma | Carcinoid<br>Neuroendocrine carcinoma<br>Primitive neuroectodermal tumor<br>Neuroblastoma<br>Phaeochromocytoma | Teratoma<br>Choriocarcinoma |

Note: The histologic subtypes of malignant tumors of the kidney

[a]Included the cystic variant multilocular clear cell renal carcinoma

[b]Including Xp11 translocation carcinomas, carcinoma associated with neuroblastoma-associated renal cell carcinoma, mucinous tubular and spindle cell carcinoma, and unclassified renal cell carcinoma. Renal metastatic tumors are not included

computed tomography (CT), have led to an increase in the numbers of incidentally discovered renal masses in seemingly asymptomatic patients. Although renal cell carcinoma (RCC) is by far the most lethal urologic malignancy, benign tumors constitute a significant proportion of incidental solid renal masses (Prasad et al. 2008b; Silverman et al. 2008). As benign solid renal masses are increasingly found, characterization of the lesion, especially as benign vs. malignant, as well as the decision of optimal treatment method, has been increased and become more important. In fact, a significant proportion of the surgically removed solid renal masses are histologically benign (Kutikov et al. 2006; Beland et al. 2007; Maturen et al.

2007; Vasudevan et al. 2006; Silverman et al. 2008) and unnecessary surgery is performed.

Anyway, the relatively high incidence of benign masses removed at surgery warrants a change in the management algorithm for patients with suspicious RCC, and proceeding to surgery, even with a minimally invasive approach such as partial nephrectomy, should be avoided whenever possible. Anyway, benign and malignant tumors may be impossible to differentiate by imaging. Moreover, pathologists advise caution when interpreting tumors, specifically those with oncocytic features or hybrid or collision tumors (Rowsell et al. 2007). Under these clinical circumstances, the need for less invasive and less extensive treatment strategies, such as careful follow-up with CT, US, or percutaneous biopsy, become critical treatment issues.

Different strategies have been proposed for the clinical management of enhancing renal masses. Percutaneous image-guided renal mass biopsy is suggested to preoperatively characterize renal masses and to establish definitive diagnoses (Silverman et al. 2006). Based largely on advances in cytological techniques, percutaneous biopsy can now be used to diagnose benign neoplasms and thus prevent them from being treated unnecessarily (Sahni and Silverman 2009). Percutaneous biopsy has been suggested also for renal masses without radiologic evidence of malignancy (Lebret et al. 2007). Minimally invasive management, such as partial nephrectomy, cryotherapy (Gill et al. 2000), or radiofrequency ablation (Fotiadis et al. 2007), should be considered for tumor removal, while conserving unaffected normal renal parenchyma.

Benign and malignant renal tumors may present a similar vascular architecture at color and power Doppler US and similar appearance on CT. In order to characterize a solid renal mass the contrast-enhanced CT examination should be multiphasic including the unenhanced scan, the corticomedullary phase scan to recognize the vascularization of the tumor, and the nephrographic phase scan to recognize the enhancement level and all the outline of the lesion. The most important aspect in analyzing a renal mass is to show the presence or absence of enhancement within it (Israel et al. 2006) even though it is not considered a sign of malignancy. An increase of 20 HU attenuation (Israel 2005) within a renal lesion after the intravenous administration of contrast agent has been generally accepted as a threshold for contrast enhancement. If the change in lesion density is between 10 and 20 HU (equivocal enhancement), or if the change in lesion density is <10 HU (absent enhancement) the lesion may be solid benign or malignant (typically papillary-cell carcinoma) or cystic.

In this case the renal lesion should be considered indeterminate and further evaluation with magnetic resonance (MR) imaging with image subtraction technique (Hecht et al. 2004) should be performed. MR imaging examinations are performed with a phased-array body coil. Each examination includes coronal or transverse T2-weighted half Fourier single-shot fast (or turbo) spin echo sequence (SSFSE, GE Healthcare; HASTE, Siemens Medical Solutions), T2-weighted turbo spin echo sequence with fat suppression including Spectral Presaturation with Inversion Recovery (SPIR), or spectral presaturation attenuated by inversion recovery (SPAIR), or short-tau inversion recovery (STIR) sequences, axial dual-echo in-phase and opposed-phase gradient echo (GRE) T1-weighted sequence, and axial or coronal 3D frequency-selective fat-suppressed fast spoiled GRE (SPGR) T1-weighted sequence obtained before and after the intravenous administration of contrast material. Dual-echo in-phase and opposed-phase GRE T1-weighted sequence are helpful in assessing for the presence of intratumoral fat. Images are obtained at specific echo times at which water and fat protons are in phase and out of phase with each other (at 1.5 T, 4.2 and 2.1 ms respectively). A loss of signal intensity on the opposed-phase images in comparison with the in-phase images occurs when both fat and water are present within a voxel as in the case of microscopic fat.

Except for angiomyolipoma, MR imaging sequences are not sensitive or specific in the characterization of renal masses as benign or malignant. In most cases, a renal solid enhancing mass corresponds to a malignancy, even though many benign lesions may present an hypervascular pattern after contrast administration. Image subtraction consists in the subtraction of the unenhanced from the gadolinium-enhanced fat-suppressed T1-weighted images and it represents a reliable method of showing enhancement within a renal mass (Hecht et al. 2004). If subtraction is not available or image misregistration is present, the percentage of enhancement can be calculated. If a renal mass or a portion of a renal mass enhances more than 15% after a scan delay of 2–4 min it is highly likely to be a solid mass (Ho et al. 2002). It is also possible to identify enhancement visually within a renal mass with a side-by-side comparison of the unenhanced and contrast-enhanced images (Israel et al. 2006). This is straightforward in hypervascular masses, while in hypovascular masses and in those masses that are hyperintense on unenhanced T1-weighted images, side-by-side comparison is usually not reliable.

In this chapter we will describe the most frequent benign renal tumors while the more rare histotypes are described on Chap. 22.

## 20.1 Angiomyolipoma

Angiomyolipomas are the most frequent mesenchymal benign neoplasms of the kidney with a prevalence of 0.3–3% and occurs more commonly in women than men. The other mesenchymal benign neoplasms are described in Chap. 22.

Angiomyolipomas, particularly when small, warrant no treatment, while they are resected only when over 4 cm or symptomatic due to risk of bleeding. Angiomyolipomas are rare in children as isolated lesions, but are found in up to 80% of children with tuberous sclerosis, then usually being bilateral, small and multifocal. The tumor appears usually as an expansive unifocal large mass which is yellowish on section when the fat component is prevalent, white if the muscular component is prevalent or red when the vascular component is prevalent which may present a hemorrhagic pattern. Angiomyolipoma rarely may become locally aggressive, with invasion into adjacent nodes or within the inferior vena cava. Angiomyolipoma contains smooth muscle, vascular, lipomatous, and myeloid elements in different proportions. When encountering an incidental solid renal mass, angiomyolipoma should be excluded (Silverman et al. 2008). To the pathologist, the most suggestive feature of angiomyolipoma are vessels. An interesting aspect of angiomyolipoma is the association with tuberous sclerosis, an autosomal dominant phakomatoses syndrome, and with lymphangioleiomyomatosis, a progressive disease which usually affects the lungs of young women and which is also related to tuberous sclerosis.

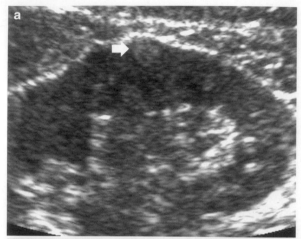

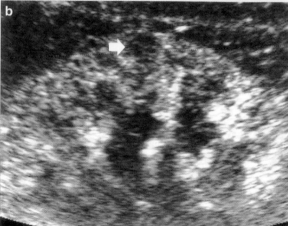

**Fig. 20.1** Small angiomyolipoma (*arrow*) scanned at unenhanced (**a**) and contrast-enhanced US (**b**). The angiomyolipoma typically appears as a small subcaspular tumor homogeneously hyperechoic at unenhanced US. After sulfur hexafluoride-filled microbubble injection (**b**) the small angiomyolipoma (*arrow*) appears persistently hypovascular in comparison to the adjacent renal parenchyma

- Small angiomyolipoma (<3 cm in diameter). Angiomyolipomas smaller than 3 cm appears typically as hyperechoic, sharply marginated, and homogeneous lesions at gray-scale ultrasound (US), with hypovascular appearance at contrast-enhanced US after microbubble contrast agent injection (Li et al. 2009) (Figs. 20.1 and 20.2). Presence of posterior acoustic shadowing may suggest angiomyolipoma. The CT diagnosis of angiomyolipoma is related to the identification of macroscopic (bulk) fat within the lesion in the absence of calcifications, and angiomyolipoma represents the most commonly imaged

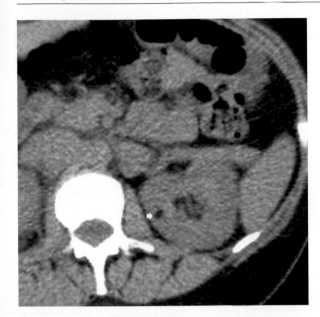

**Fig. 20.2** Small angiomyolipoma scanned by unenhanced CT. The lesion (arrow) appears hypodense with a fatty density.

renal tumor containing macroscopic fat (Fig. 20.2). Most angiomyolipomas can be diagnosed immediately by identifying regions of macroscopic fat (Fig. 20.2) frequently commixed with angiomatous enhancing component (Fig. 20.3) within a noncalcified renal mass at unenhanced CT (Bosniak et al. 1988; Silverman et al. 2008).

On MR imaging, the fatty and angiomyomatous solid components of angiomyolipoma appears respectively hyperintense and hypointense on T1-weighted sequences. On T2-weighted sequences the fat component appears hyperintense, with fat signal suppression on T1-weighted or T2-weighted sequences with fat saturation (Fig. 20.4). To establish the presence of macroscopic fat within a renal mass, obtaining fat-suppressed MR sequences such as STIR (Fig. 20.4) or frequency-selective fat-suppressed T1-weighted images and comparing them with nonfat-suppressed T1-weighted images is necessary (Israel et al. 2005).

- Large angiomyolipoma (≥3 in diameter. Large angiomyolipomas may reveal homogeneous (Fig. 20.5) or heterogeneous bright appearance at US due to solid, adipose and hemorrhagic components. Frequently large angiomyolipomas presents an extrinsic development and a wedge-shaped connection with the renal

parenchyma resulting in a parenchyma defect, also with evidence of posterior acoustic shadowing (Yamashita et al. 1993; Hélénon et al. 1997, 2001; Jinzaki et al. 1997). Color Doppler US reveals penetrating, peripheral or mixed peripheral and intratumoral vessel distribution, with a prevalence of mixed distribution in atypical hypervascular angiomyolipomas.

The evidence of a small amount of macroscopic fat is enough to suggest angiomyolipoma diagnosis. Angiomyolipomas larger than 3 cm prevalently reveal a prevalent hypodense macroscopic fat component at nonenhanced CT in varying proportions (Figs. 20.5 and 20.6), hypervascular soft tissue (Fig. 20.6), and intralesional aneurysms (Fig. 20.7). Contrast enhancement is heterogeneous on the solid peripheral or central component sparing the fat component after iodinated contrast agent injection. Thin-section CT may be needed for small angiomyolipomas and those angiomyolipomas that contain only small amounts of fat (Silverman et al. 2008). The identification of macroscopic fat is most reliable on unenhanced CT scan or by pixel map and represents the most important imaging features to diagnose renal angiomyolipomas. CT findings of more than 20 pixels with attenuation less than −20 HU and more than 5 pixels with attenuation less than −30 HU have a positive predictive value of 100% in detection of angiomyolipoma, but most angiomyolipomas with minimal fat cannot be reliably identified on the basis of an absolute pixel count (Simpfendorfer et al. 2009). Bilateral multiple renal angiomyolipomas are seen in patients who have tuberous sclerosis (Fig. 20.8). Simultaneous occurrence of angiomyolipoma with RCC and oncocytoma in the same kidney has been reported (Silpananta et al. 1984; Bahrami et al. 2007).

On MR imaging, the fatty portion of an angiomyolipoma is hyperintense to the renal parenchyma on T1-weighted images, while the angiomyomatous solid component is hypointense (Israel 2006). According to the prevalence of the different intratumoral components, frequently evident on angiomyolipomas ≥3 cm in diameter, renal angiomyolipomas may appear hyper-, iso- or hypointense to the adjacent renal parenchyma on T2-weighted sequences, and hypointense on T1- and T2-weighted sequences with fat saturation – SPIR, SPAIR, or STIR sequences – (Figs. 20.9–20.11). However, other renal masses, including hemorrhagic-proteinaceous cysts and RCCs that contain hemorrhage,

**Fig. 20.3** Small angiomyolipoma of the left kidney scanned by unenhanced and contrast-enhanced CT. (**a, b**) Unenhanced CT, and (**c, d**) contrast-enhanced CT on corticomedullary phase. The lesion (*arrow*) present an hypodense fatty component evident on unenhanced CT scan commixed with an enhancing angiomatous component

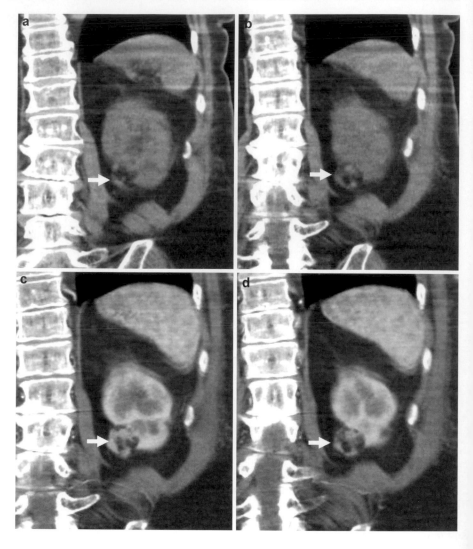

may have similar signal characteristics and may appear hyperintense on T1-weighted images (Israel et al. 2005). Therefore, to establish the presence of macroscopic fat within a renal mass, obtaining frequency-selective fat-suppressed T1-weighted images and comparing them with nonfat-suppressed T1-weighted images is necessary. The most reliable demonstration of macroscopic fat within an angiomyolipoma can be achieved by comparing images obtained with the same imaging parameters before and after applying a selective fat-suppression pulse (Pedrosa et al. 2008) (Figs. 20.9–20.11).

The use of in-phase and opposed-phase chemical shift MR imaging is helpful in the diagnosis of angiomyolipoma (Israel et al. 2005). The india-ink artifact can be recognized on opposed-phase MR images as a characteristic sharp black line at fat-water (fat-muscle or fat-solid organ) interfaces (Earls and Krinsky 1997) (Fig. 20.12). Because most angiomyolipomas contain macroscopic fat, the india ink artifact will appear at the interface of the angiomyolipoma with the kidney (Fig. 20.12) or at the interface of the fatty and nonfatty portions of the mass (Fig. 20.13). The india ink artifact is due to the presence of fat and water protons within the same imaging voxel, resulting in signal loss at the periphery of areas of macroscopic fat. It occurs along the entire border of fat-water interfaces and not only in the frequency-encoding direction because it is a result of fat and water proton phase cancelation in all directions.

Anyway, a signal intensity loss on out-of-phase MR images, indicative of microscopic intra-voxel fat, is not characteristic of angiomyolipomas, and a renal mass cannot be diagnosed as an angiomyolipoma

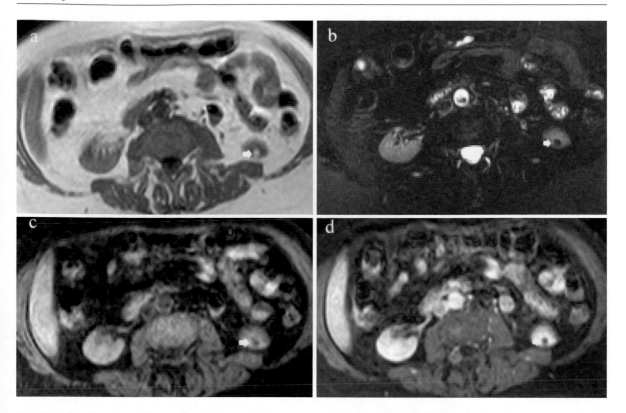

**Fig. 20.4** Small angiomyolipoma (*arrow*) scanned by unenhanced and contrast-enhanced MR imaging. (**a**) T1-weighted turbo spin echo sequence. A small hyperintense lesion is identified on the lower pole of the left kidney. (**b**) Short-tau inversion recovery (STIR). The same lesion appears hypointense with suppression of the signal related to macroscopic fat. (**c, d**) T1-weighted breath-hold spoiled gradient echo (SPGR) before (**c**) and after (**d**) gadolinium-based agent injection during nephrographic phase. The fat lesions does not present any contrast enhancement

solely on the basis of signal loss on out-of-phase MR images (Cohan et al. 2006; Pedrosa et al. 2008) since microscopic fat is present also in clear cell RCC. In fact, some renal cancers, particularly those of clear cell type, contain abundant intracellular lipid in addition to water which determines signal loss on out-of-phase (Outwater et al. 1997). However, by evaluating the location of the india ink artifact on opposed-phase chemical shift MR imaging, characterizing angiomyolipomas without the use of frequency-selective fat-suppressed T1-weighted images is possible (Israel et al. 2005). On opposed-phase chemical shift MRI, the presence of the india ink artifact at the interface of a renal mass with the renal parenchyma or within the renal mass is indicative of an angiomyolipoma while the evidence of india-ink at interface of mass with perinephric fat, indicating the absence of macroscopic fat, is more characteristic of RCC (Israel et al. 2005).

Opposed-phase chemical shift MRI has some advantages over frequency-selective fat-suppression techniques. At times, frequency-selective fat-suppressed sequences may have nonuniform fat suppression, and in this instance, the loss of signal within an angiomyolipoma may not be evident. In addition, at low field strengths, frequency-selective fat-suppressed sequences cannot be performed during a comfortable breath-hold. Opposed-phase chemical shift MRI can be performed at low field strengths without adding to the examination time and is not dependent on field homogeneity; therefore, an angiomyolipoma can still theoretically be diagnosed with confidence (Israel et al. 2005). Contrast enhancement after gadolinium-based contrast agent injection is heterogeneous on the solid peripheral or central component sparing the fatty component (Figs. 20.10 and 20.11).

• Atypical angiomyolipomas. Differential diagnosis between atypical angiomyolipomas from nonfatty renal tumors is not always solved even by CT and MR. Angiomyolipomas may have small intrarenal

**Fig. 20.5** Large angiomyolipoma with overt fat component on CT. (**a**) Baseline gray-scale US. Hyperechoic and homogeneous large renal mass (calipers). (**b**) Unenhanced CT. The same renal mass (*arrow*) appears hypodense with a fatty density. (**c**) Contrast material-enhanced CT, corticomedullary phase. Hypodense appearance of the lesion which maintains a fat-density appearance

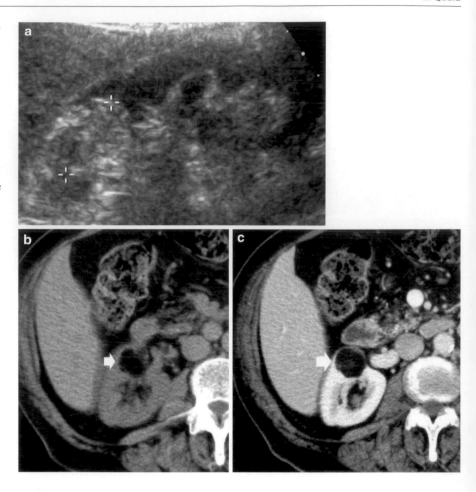

and large perinephric component. This is helpful in distinguishing angiomyolipoma from liposarcoma especially in large angiomyolipomas. Even though macroscopic fat component evident on CT and/or MR imaging represents the most suggestive feature of angiomyolipoma, not all solid renal masses with radiologically detectable fat are angiomyolipomas. The evidence of microscopic fat in renal angiomyolipoma evident is not a clue for diagnosis. Calcified (Helenon et al. 1993; Outwater et al. 1997; Lesavre et al. 2003) and noncalcified (Schuster et al. 2004) fat-containing renal masses have been reported to be RCCs.

Atypical angiomyolipomas with absent fat component are about 5% and usually appear iso or slightly hyperdense if compared to the adjacent kidney at unenhanced CT due to the smooth muscle components (Figs. 20.14 and 20.15), and homogeneously enhancing masses after contrast administration (Jinzaki et al. 1997; Kim et al. 2004; Prasad et al. 2008b; Silverman et al. 2008).

A similar pattern may be observed in complicated benign cysts (hemorrhagic, protein-rich or gelatinous), renal metastasis and RCC. The evidence of hyperdense and fat masses in the kidney at the same time is diagnostic of multiple angiomyolipoma. Moreover, atypical hypervascular angiomyolipomas present diffuse contrast enhancement after microbubble contrast agents (Figs. 20.16 and 20.17) (Quaia 2005; Li et al. 2009), or iodinated or paramagnetic contrast agent injection and complicated benign cysts may be excluded in this way.

When encountering a small (≤3 cm), hyperattenuating (at unenhanced CT), homogeneously enhancing renal mass, there is a strong possibility that the mass is benign and particularly it is an angiomyolipoma (Jinzaki et al. 1997; Kim et al. 2004). Rather than presume the mass is RCC and proceed directly to treatment, MR imaging, and if necessary, percutaneous biopsy are suggested (Silverman et al. 2008).

Renal angiomyolipoma should be differentiated also from fat surgical packing placed after partial nephrectomy (see chapter 32). In some cases, the surgeon

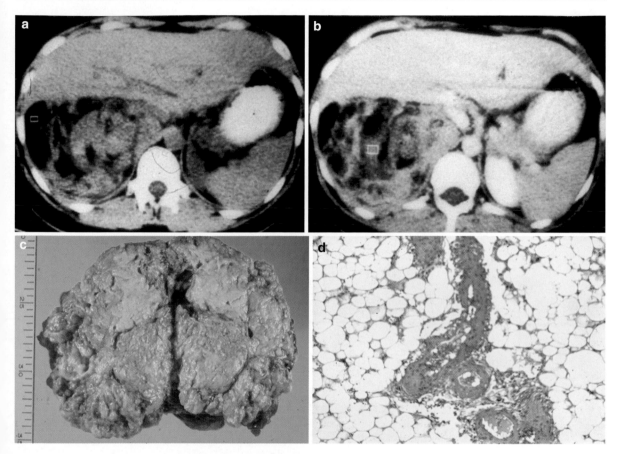

**Fig. 20.6** Giant angiomyolipoma with prevalent macroscopic fat and solid component at CT. Renal angiomyolipoma presents a prevalent macroscopic fat component hypodense at unenhanced CT (**a**) with heterogenous contrast enhancement at contrast material-enhanced CT (**b**). The gross specimen (**c**) reveals the adipose yellowish component (*arrows*). The microscopic specimen (**d**; hematoxylin and eosin, original magnification ×40) confirms the adipose component consisting of large foamy cells (*arrow*)

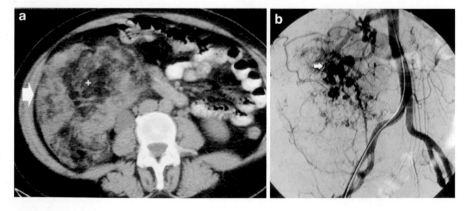

**Fig. 20.7** Giant angiomyolipoma. (**a**) Renal angiomyolipoma (*arrow*) presents a prevalent fat macroscopic component hypodense at nonenhanced CT. (**b**) Multiple intralesional aneurysms are evident on digital subtraction angiography

may pack perinephric fat into the surgical bed to help achieve hemostasis after partial nephrectomy for a small peripheral tumor, and a wedge-shaped defect in the renal parenchyma typically is visible at CT and MR imaging. The fatty packing material later may be mistaken for a fatty mass such as an angiomyolipoma. (Israel et al. 2006). Over time, the volume of fat used for surgical packing may decrease or remain unchanged. Biologically absorbable hemostatic agents also may be used to help control intraoperative bleeding but they

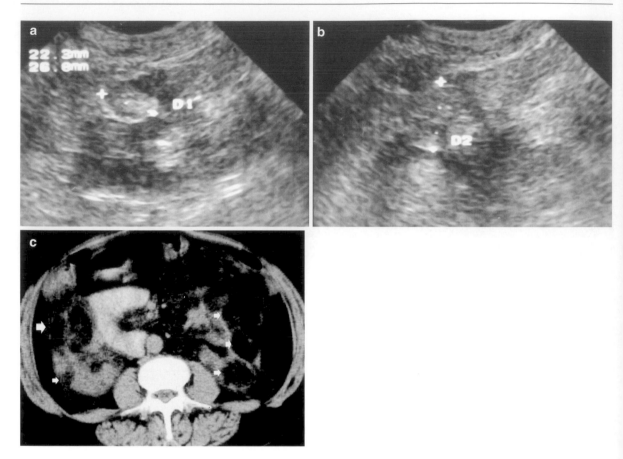

**Fig. 20.8** Bilateral angiomyolipomas (*arrows*) of different size in a 25-year old patient with sclerosis tuberosa. Gray-scale US, transverse (**a**) and longitudinal scan (**b**). Multiple hyperechoic lesions (calipers) are evident on both kidneys. (**c**) Contrast-enhanced CT. Multiple hypodense lesions (*arrows*) on both kidney with an evident fat density

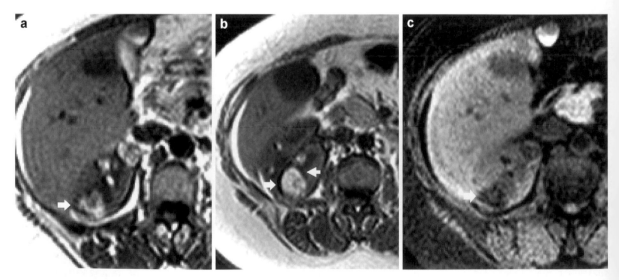

**Fig. 20.9** Large angiomyolipoma with macroscopic fat component on MR. (**a**) Axial T1-weighted turbo-spin echo sequence. A large hyperintense renal mass (*arrow*) is identified on the right kidney. (**b**) Axial opposed-phase T1-weighted MR image. India ink artifact (*arrows*) is present at interface of renal mass with kidney, diagnostic of angiomyolipoma. (**c**) Frequency-selective fat-suppressed T1-weighted sequence, spectral presaturation with inversion recovery (SPIR). The renal mass shows a clear decrease in signal intensity due to the suppression of the macroscopic fat component

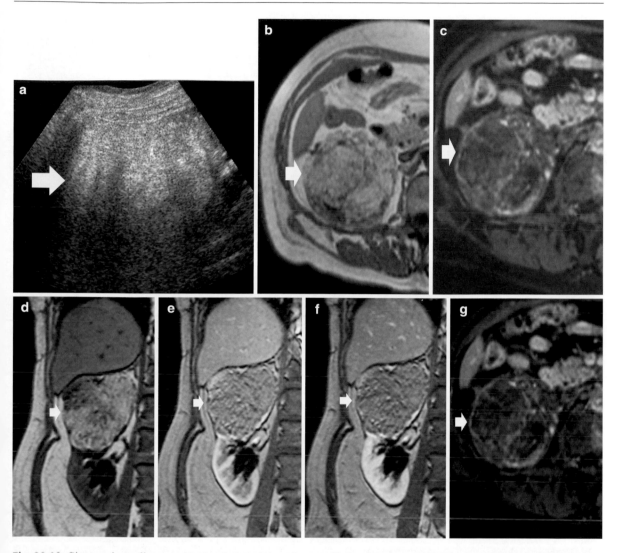

**Fig. 20.10** Giant angiomyolipoma with prevalent macroscopic fat component at MR imaging. (**a**) Gray-scale ultrasound shows an homogeneous hyperechoic renal mass on the upper pole of the right kidney; (**b**) T1-weighted turbo-spin echo sequence. Transverse plane. The renal mass appears hyperintense (*arrow*). (**c**) Frequency-selective fat suppressed T1-weighted SPIR sequence, spectral fat SPIR. The renal mass shows a clear decrease in signal intensity due to the suppression of the macro-scopic fat component. (**d–f**) Breath-hold frequency-selective fat-suppressed spoiled gradient echo (SPGR) T1-weighted sequence obtained before (**d**) and after Gd-based agent injection (**e**, **f**). Low contrast enhancement is identified. (**g**) T1-weighted SPIR sequence after Gd-based contrast agent injection. The renal mass shows a clear decrease in signal intensity due to the suppression of the macroscopic fat component with evidence of contrast enhancement in the vascular component

are easily differentiated from angiomyolipoma due to the absence of fat component and may contain air pockets or bubbles (see chapter 32).

- Complicated angiomyolipomas. Kidneys with underlying tumors are more susceptible to traumatic injury than are normal kidneys. Renal angiomyolipomas may be complicated by hemorrhage (Fig. 20.18), which can be spontaneous or associated with relatively minor or incidental trauma.

Bleeding may occur within the tumor (Fig. 20.18), in the adjacent renal parenchyma (Fig. 20.19), or may result in subcapsular or retroperitoneal bleeding (Fig. 20.20). These lesions may be treated surgically or by selective embolization (Fig. 20.21). Renal angiomyolipomas are benign but they can be locally invasive, extending into the perirenal fat or more rarely into a renal vein and even the inferior vena cava (Fig. 20.22) and right atrium. Involvement of the spleen and regional lymph nodes has been

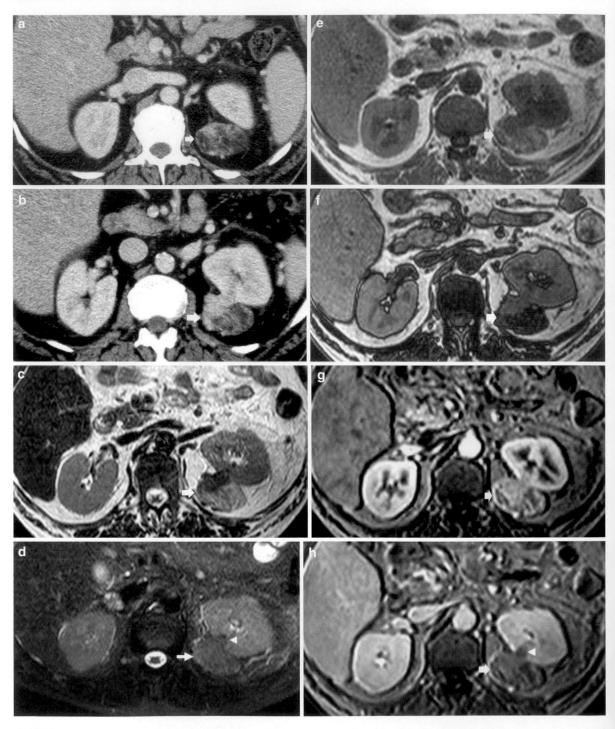

**Fig. 20.11** Large angiomyolipoma with fatty and solid tissue intra-tumoral components visible on CT and MR imaging. (**a**, **b**) Contrast-enhanced CT, nephrographic phase. A solid exophitic renal mass (*arrow*) is evident on the left kidney. The renal mass presents a prevalent fatty component, and a solid enhancing component. (**c–h**) MR imaging, axial plane. The signal of the macroscopic fatty component appears hyperintense on T2-weighted turbo spin echo sequence (**c**) and is suppressed on T2-weighted spectral presaturation attenuated by inversion recovery (SPAIR) sequence with fat suppression (**d**).

The microscopic fat component appears hyperintense on in-phase (**e**) and hypointense on opposed-phase (**f**) T1-weighted gradient recalled echo sequence. (**g**, **h**) Gadolinium-enhanced frequency-selective fat-suppressed spoiled gradient echo (SPGR) T1-weighted sequence during corticomedullary (**g**) and nephrographic phase (**h**). The solid component presents diffuse contrast enhancement while the fatty tissue component presents low contrast enhancement. There is also the evidence of wedge-shaped connection (*arrowhead*) of the renal mass with the renal parenchyma

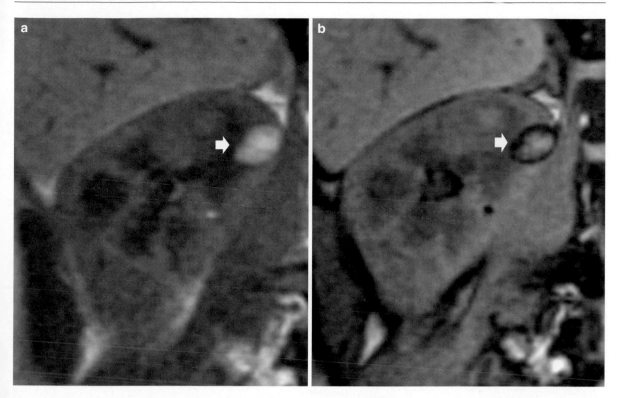

**Fig. 20.12** Evidence of india ink artifact on in-phase (**a**) and opposed-phase (**b**) chemical shift MR imaging in an angiomyolipoma with macroscopic fat component. The india ink artifact (*arrow*) appears at the interface of the angiomyolipoma with the kidney (courtesy of Nicolas Grenier, Bordeaux)

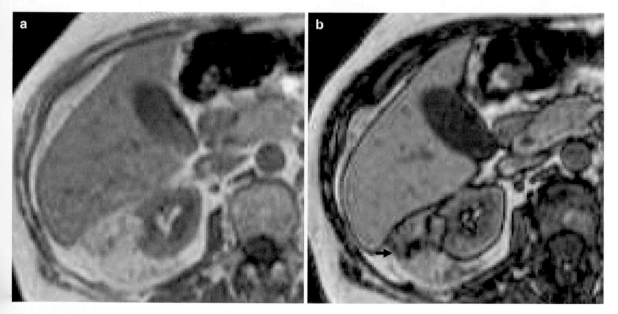

**Fig. 20.13** Evidence of india ink artifact on in-phase (**a**) and opposed-phase (**b**) chemical shift MR imaging in an angiomyolipoma with macroscopic fat component. The india ink artifact (*arrow*) appears at the interface of the fatty and nonfatty portions of the mass (courtesy of Catherine Roy, Strasburg)

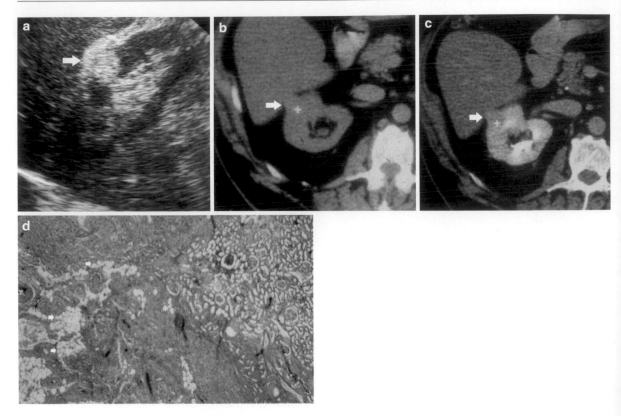

**Fig. 20.14** Small angiomyolipoma without macroscopic fat component detectable on CT. (**a**) Gray-scale US. Hyperechoic renal mass (*arrow*) on the right kidney. (**b**) Unenhanced CT. No evidence of fat component is identified. The renal mass appears slightly hyperdence (*arrow*) in comparison to the adjacent renal parenchyma. (**c**) Contrast-enhanced CT. No contrast-enhancement is identified inside the renal mass (*arrow*). (**d**) Histology, hematoxylin and eosin, original magnification ×40. Fat component (*arrows*) is visualized at the microscopic analysis

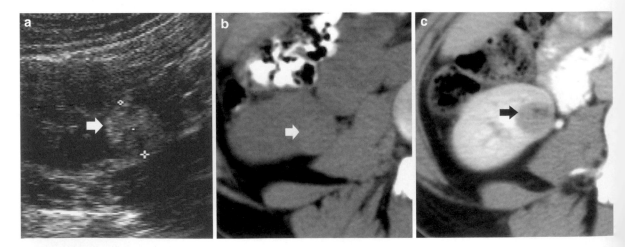

**Fig. 20.15** (**a–c**) Large angiomyolipoma without evidence of macroscopic fat component on CT. (**a**) Gray-scale US. Hyperechoic renal mass (*arrow*) on the right kidney. (**b**) Unenhanced CT. No evidence of fat component is identified. The renal mass appears slightly hyperdense (*arrow*) in comparison to the adjacent renal parenchyma. (**c**) Contrast-enhanced CT. No contrast-enhancement is identified inside the renal mass (*arrow*)

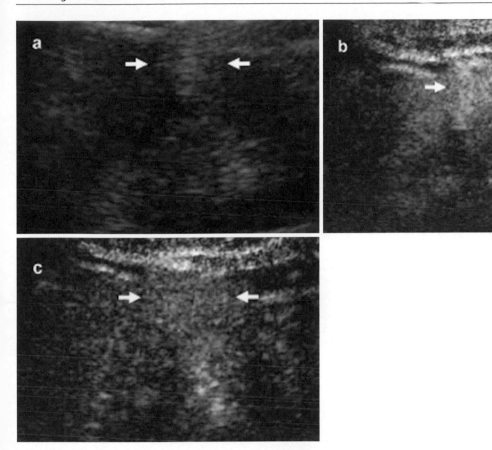

**Fig. 20.16** (**a–c**) Atypical hypervascular angiomyolipoma at contrast-enhanced US. Baseline US (**a**). Homogeneous hyperechoic lesion (*arrows*) with a wedge-shaped connection to the renal parenchyma. Contrast-specific mode (**b**, **c**) contrast-tuned imaging (Esaote, Genoa, Italy) with low acoustic power after sulfur hexafluoride-filled microbubble injection. The lesion reveals diffuse and homogeneous contrast enhancement at arterial phase (**b**) decreasing during late phase (**c**)

attributed to the multicentric primary nature of the tumor rather than to metastatic behavior and does not have adverse prognostic significance.

## 20.2 Renal Cell Neoplasms

### 20.2.1 Oncocytoma

Renal oncocytomas (2–5% of renal epithelial neoplasms in adults) are benign tumors arising from proximal tubular epithelial cells. Oncocytoma has an overall incidence of 3–7% among all renal tumors and is the second most common benign tumor after angiomyolipoma (Lieber 1993; Perez-Ordonez et al. 1997). The peak age of incidence is in the seventh decade; men are more likely to be affected than women (Prasad et al.

2008a, b). Most tumors occur sporadically in asymptomatic patients. It is now acknowledged that chromophobic RCC and renal oncocytoma arise from the intercalated cells of the collecting duct system. Some cases of coexistent chromophobic RCC and oncocytoma have been reported (Tickoo et al. 2000). Renal oncocytomas may be multicentric, bilateral, or methacronous in approximately 4–6% of oncocytomas, with coexistent RCC in 10% of cases (Dechet et al. 1999).

To consider a tumor as an oncocytoma the size is not important, only the cytological features, microscopic, ultrastructural, and immunohistochemically can help, but some chromosomal observations introduce some questions about its relation with the chromophobe RCC (Algaba 2008). Oncocytoma is characterized by large granular cells with small, uniform, round nuclei and an abundant eosinophilic cytoplasm. It appears brown on section for the lipocromic pigment of mitochondria with

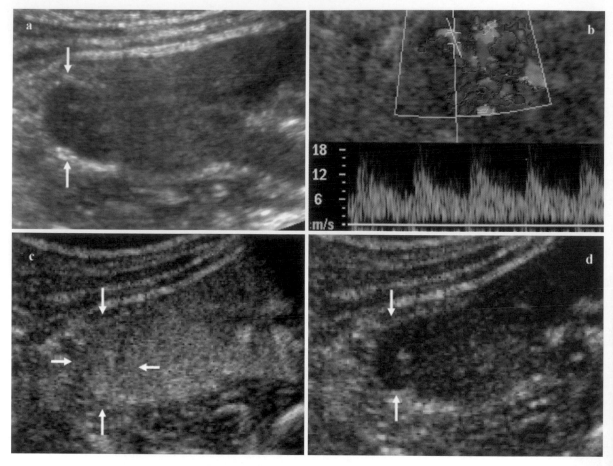

**Fig. 20.17** An AML with atypical pattern on conventional US and contrast-enhanced US. (**a**) Unenhanced gray-scale ultrasound. Inhomogeneous hypoechoic exophytic well-defined renal mass (*arrows*) in the lower pole of the right kidney. (**b**) Color Doppler ultrasound. Arterial intratumoral and penetrating vessels are identified. Renal mass (*arrows*) reveals intense contrast enhancement during early phase (**c**) after air-filled microbubble contrast agent injection, decreasing during late phase (**d**). Biopsy revealed AML with a prevalent vascular component

or without calcifications and, generally, without necrosis and hemorrhage and with a fibrotic stroma or hyalinized connective tissue with compressed blood vessels in the central scar. Microscopically, oncocytomas are composed of large dense cells with abundant highly granular eosinophilic cytoplasm due to mitochondria and arranged in solid, tubular, or trabecular rests. The cells are large in comparison with the other cell types. They commonly grow centrifugally from a central avascular scar. Calcifications may occur in the central scar.

Renal oncocytoma can be treated by local excision or heminephrectomy and their preoperative differentiation from RCC is very important. Although oncocytomas are considered to be benign, reports of recurrence and even metastases following resection of oncocytomas suggest that these neoplasms have the capability to become

malignant since they can contain chromophobe cells. Oncocytomas represent the most common benign lesions diagnosed after partial nephrectomy.

Oncocytoma diagnosis mostly rely on imaging features and on the histologic analysis of the surgical specimen. There have been advances in solid renal mass diagnosis on the basis of staining characteristics of the tissue obtained by biopsy. Nevertheless, even expertly performed percutaneous biopsy is limited by sampling error. This is especially problematic for oncocytoma, as RCC may have oncocytic features, and oncocytoma can be seen in association with these tumors (Neuzillet et al. 2005). Even though the presence of necrosis is helpful in distinguishing a benign from a malignant process, rarely necrosis can occur in an oncocytoma and is therefore available for sampling

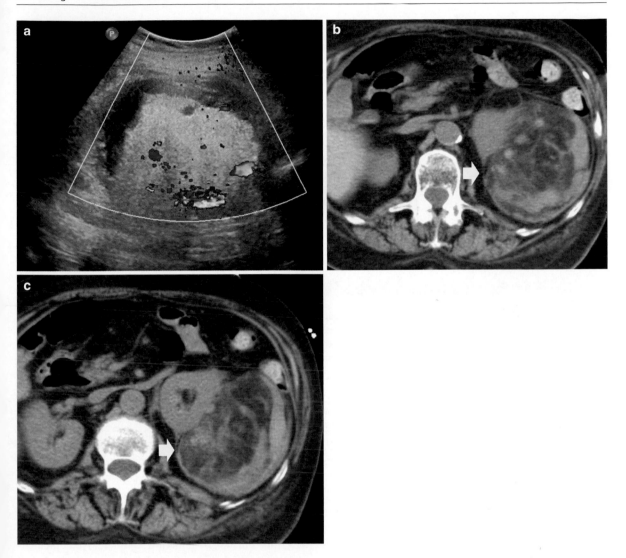

**Fig. 20.18** Angiomyolipoma of the left kidney with hemorrhage. (**a**) Gray-scale ultrasound shows an homogeneous hyperechoic renal mass on the upper pole of the left kidney; (**b, c**) unenhanced CT. The fat component present hyperdense striations (*arrow*) due to intratumoral hemorrhage

(Davidson et al. 1993). Although oncocytomas may show a central scar on CT or MR imaging in about 1/3 of patients, there are no available imaging features which allow a definite differentiation of renal oncocytomas from RCCs.

- Baseline and color Doppler US. Renal oncocytomas prevalently appear as hyperechoic or heterogeneous solid renal masses on gray-scale ultrasound (Figs. 20.23 and 20.24). The presence of a central scar appearing as a stellate hypoechoic area and absence of haemorrhage and necrosis are considered typical in renal oncocytoma (Hélénon et al. 2001). Large oncocytoma with stellate hypoechoic

central area may also reveal a central spoke-wheel shaped distribution of tumor vessels at color Doppler US (Hélénon et al. 2001). After microbubble-based contrast agent injection, renal oncocytoma shows persistent diffuse homogeneous contrast enhancement at early corticomedullary phase with a progressive reduction at late corticomedullary phase (Fig. 20.23).
- Computed tomography. A particularly important finding, a central sharply marginated stellate scar with a spoke-wheel configuration and low attenuation within an otherwise homogenous tumor (Quinn et al. 1984; Davidson et al. 1993) is frequently demonstrated after iodinated contrast agent

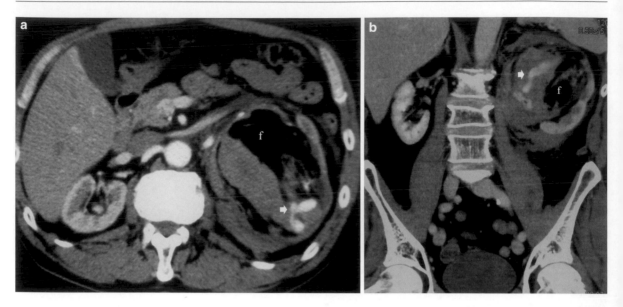

**Fig. 20.19** Giant angiomyolipoma of the left kidney with evidence of acute hemorrhage (*arrow*) on CT. (**a**) Contrast-enhanced CT, corticomedullary phase. (**b**) Contrast-enhanced CT, corticomedullary phase, coronal reformation. An intrarenal collection is visualized within the left kidney with active hemorrhage (*arrow*). The macroscopic fat component (*f*) is visualized suggesting the angiomyolipoma diagnosis

injection (Fig. 20.24) in 30–40% of large oncocytomas. The evidence of a central hypodense region without a spoke-wheel configuration (Fig. 20.25, 20.26, and 20.27) does not allow to differentiate renal oncocytoma from RCC. Moreover, uniform enhancement, and a sharp and smooth rim (Fig. 20.25) may be observed at contrast material-enhanced CT (Jasinski et al. 1985). Segmental enhancement inversion has been described as extremely specific for renal oncocytoma. It consists in different segmental enhancement in a solid mass with two segments showing different degrees of enhancement during corticomedullary phase and excretory phase, the relatively highly enhanced segment became less enhanced during excretory phase, whereas the less-enhanced segment during corticomedullary phase became highly enhanced during excretory phase (Kim et al. 2009). Anyway, areas of decreased attenuation different from stellate central area, which are usually found in RCC, may be observed in about 20–30% of oncocytoma, in particular if larger than 3 cm, and rarely in oncocytomas smaller than 3 cm. Rarely a fat component may be identified.

- Magnetic resonance imaging. The MR imaging appearance of oncocytoma is variable and nonspecific. Oncocytomas are typically spheric and

well-defined renal masses (Pedrosa et al. 2008). On T1-weighted sequences renal oncocytoma appears hypointense, while on T2-weighted sequences renal oncocytoma appears hypo- or hyperintense (Harmon et al. 1996) in comparison to the adjacent renal parenchyma. The central scar, present in about the 50% of cases, appears as a stellate area hypointense on T1-weighted sequences and hyperintense on T2-weighted sequences (Fig. 20.28) (Ball et al. 1986) sometimes with delayed enhancement after the administration of gadolinium-based contrast agents (Fig. 20.28) (Pedrosa et al. 2008). Prevalently, diffuse homogeneous enhancement (Fig. 20.29) is described at Gd-DTPA enhanced MR with hypointensity of the central scar during the corticomedullary phase. A well-defined psudocapsule (Figs. 20.27 and 20.29) can be seen surrounding the tumor in almost one-half of renal oncocytomas. However, the presence of a pseudocapsule is nonspecific and can be seen in up to 60% of RCCs as well.

Renal oncocytosis, defined as diffuse oncocytic nodules throughout the kidney, is a very rare entity which may be detected by imaging techniques (Ariaratnam et al. 2009). Chromophobe carcinoma is the type of RCC most commonly associated with renal

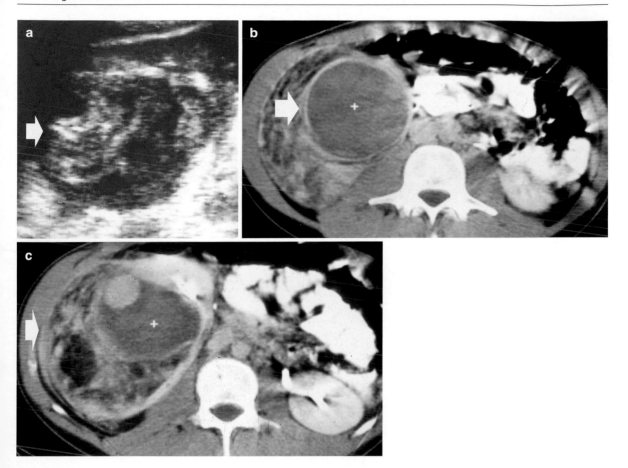

**Fig. 20.20** Giant angiomyolipoma of the right kidney with hemorrhage and pseudo-tumoral complex appearance. (**a**) Grayscale US reveals an heterogeneous mass on the right kidney simulating a renal tumor. (**b**) Unenhanced CT. A prevalent hypodense component is identified with peripheral macroscopic fat strands suggesting an angiomyolypoma nature. (**c**) Contrast-enhanced CT reveals heterogeneous contrast enhancement with a clear evidence of the peripheral fat component

oncocytosis (Tickoo et al. 1999). Patients with renal oncocytosis often present with abnormal renal function. Renal oncocytosis associated with Birt–Hogg–Dube syndrome (see Chap. 21) including skin papules, renal tumors, and pulmonary cysts has been reported (Pavlovich et al. 2002). The main imaging feature of renal oncocytosis is the bilateral renal involvement by at least one dominant mass and numerous smaller nondominant lesions (Fig. 20.30). Although the imaging features of the individual lesions vary and are not pathognomonic, the overall appearance of the involved kidneys is rarely encountered in other neoplastic or nonneoplastic process (Ariaratnam et al. 2009). The differential diagnosis may include lymphoma, meatastasis, tuberous sclerosis, Von Hippel–Lindau syndrome, and multifocal renal tumors such as RCCs and angiomyolipomas (Ariaratnam et al. 2009).

### 20.2.2 Renal Papillary Adenoma

Renal papillary adenomas are the most common renal epithelial neoplasms. The renal adenomas can be confused by imaging diagnosis with malignant renal tumors. The adenoma of clear cells is not accepted, instead it is considered that all the clear-cell tumors are carcinomas, with greater or lesser aggressiveness. Among the papillary neoplasms the WHO 2004 renal cell tumors classification are considered as papillary adenomas tumors with a maximum diameter of 5 mm and may represent a continuum biological process to papillary RCC (Algaba 2008). The papillary adenomas associated with endkidney and/or hemodialysis-associated acquired cystic disease may have a different pathogenesis.

According to autopsy series, approximately 40% of patients older than 70 years harbor renal adenomas.

**Fig. 20.21** A 45-years old female with a known left renal angiomyolipoma presenting with left flank and abdominal pain. (**a**) Contrast-enhanced axial CT. Corticomedullary phase. CT image shows a perinephric retroperitoneal collection with fat density anteriorly (**b**). Contrast-enhanced axial CT. Arterial phase. CT image shows contrast extravasation on the upper renal pole. (**c**) Selective left renal arteriogram reveals a vascular blush in the region corresponding to the upper renal pole mass (*arrow*). (**d**) Selective left renal arteriogram after transcatheter embolization of the bleeding arterial branch and placement of an occluding coil (Courtesy of Cristina Gius and Salvatore Sammartano, Department of Radiology, Santa Chiara Hospital, Trento, Italy)

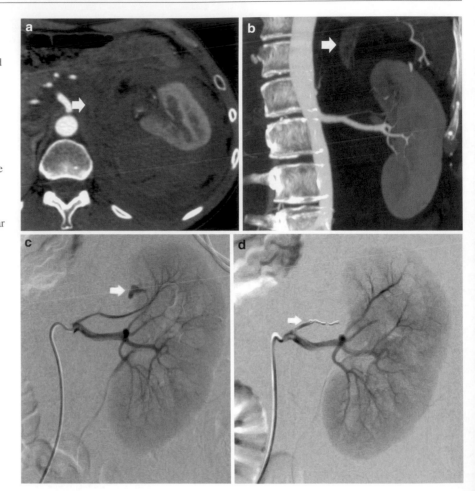

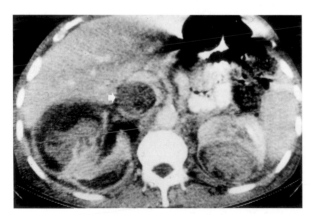

**Fig. 20.22** Contrast-enhanced CT. Nephrographic phase. Giant angiomyolipoma of the right kidney with extension to inferior vena cava and venous thrombosis (*arrow*)

Papillary adenomas are also commonly found in patients with hemodialysis-associated acquired renal cystic disease and in patients undergoing long-term hemodialysis. By definition, papillary adenomas measure 5 mm or less. They are usually subcapsular and solitary (Prasad et al. 2008a, b). Adenomas are histologically characterized by papillary or tubular cytoarchitecture and frequent psammoma bodies. Cytogenetic changes of papillary adenomas include loss of the Y chromosome and combined trisomy of chromosomes 7 and 17. Histologic and genetic abnormalities of renal adenomas are indistinguishable from papillary RCCs with a tubular, papillary, or tubulopapillary architectures.

Papillary adenomas are well circumscribed, yellow to grayish white nodules as small as less than 1 mm in diameter in the renal cortex. Most occur just below the renal capsule. The smallest ones usually are spherical, but larger ones sometimes are roughly conical with a wedgeshaped appearance in sections cut at right angles to the cortical surface (Eble et al. 2004). Usually, papillary adenomas are solitary, but occasionally they are

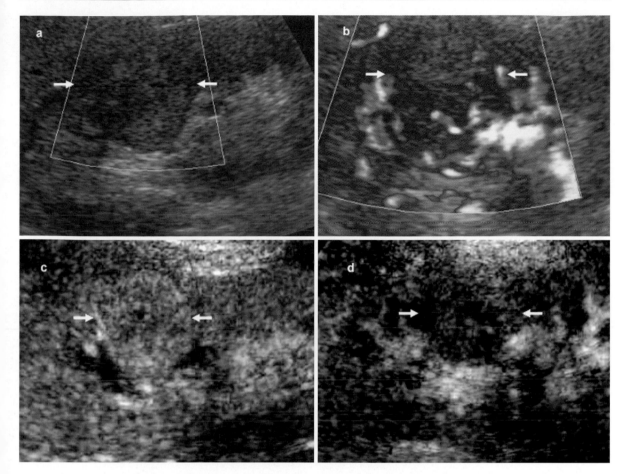

**Fig. 20.23** Oncocytoma on US and contrast-enhanced US. (**a**) Baseline gray-scale US. Baseline US (**a**) and color Doppler US (**b**). Longitudinal scan shows an heterogeneous and hypoechoic lesion (*arrows*) with peripheral and intratumoral ves- sels. Contrast specific mode (**c**, **d**) contrast tuned imaging with low acoustic power after sulfur hexafluoride-filled microbubble injection. Diffuse homogeneous contrast enhancement is identi- fied at arterial phase (**c**) decreasing during late phase (**d**)

multiple and bilateral. When they are very numerous, this has been called "renal adenomatosis." Papillary adenomas are extremely small and may not be distinguished from other renal tumors (particularly RCC) and pseudotumors on imaging studies.

## 20.3 Other Benign Solid Renal Tumors

### 20.3.1 Embryonal Metanephric Adenoma

Metanephric neoplasms are a heterogeneous group of benign renal neoplasms that include metanephric adenoma (epithelial tumor), metanephric stromal tumor (stromal neoplasm), and metanephric adenofibroma (mixed epithelial and stromal neoplasm) (Argani 2005; Prasad et al. 2008a, b). Embryonal meta- nephric adenoma (nephrogenic adenofibroma) is a rare benign renal tumor. The metanephric adenoma, a tumor with some morphological similarity with the nephroblastoma must be considered in the renal adenomas diagnosis. It is considered to originate from embryonic renal tissue and to be the benign counterpart of the Wilms tumor (Lerut et al. 2006). It accounts for 0.2% of adult renal epithelial tumors (Hwang and Choi 2004). The mean age at presenta- tion is 41 years with a wide age range (15–83 years) (Algaba 2008) with a female predominance. When symptomatic, patients have a flank mass, pain or hypertension. Blood analysis can show hypercalce- mia and polycythemia.

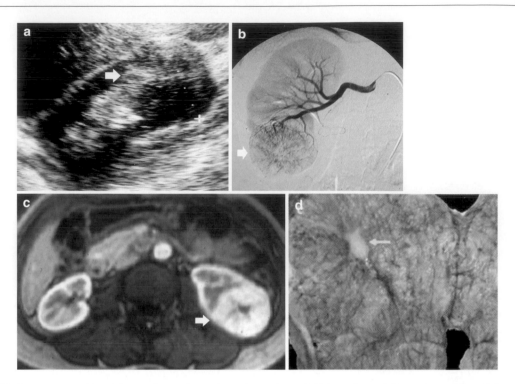

**Fig. 20.24** Oncocytoma with evidence of central scar (*arrow*) on CT. (**a**) Ultrasound, longitudinal scan. An heterogeneous lesion is visualized on the lower renal pole (*arrow*). (**b**) Digital subtraction angiography, selective right renal artery catheterization. The renal mass (*arrow*) appears hypervascular. (**c**) Contrast-enhanced CT, corticomedullary phase. The solid renal mass presents a diffuse contrast enhancement (*arrow*) with evidence of a central scar with septa radiating from the center towards the periphery. (**d**) The resected tumor reveals a central white scar (*arrow*)

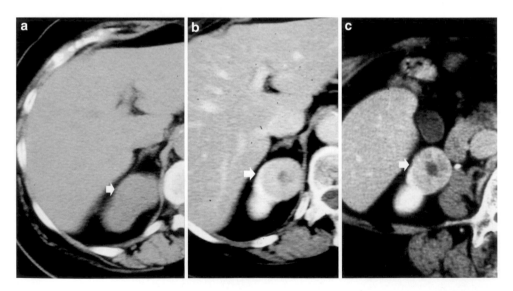

**Fig. 20.25** Renal oncocytoma. (**a**) Unenhanced CT. A solid renal mass (arrow) is identified on the upper pole of the right kidney. (**b**) Contrast-enhanced CT. Nephrographic phase. The solid renal mass (large arrow) appears hypodense in comparison to the adjacent renal parenchyma with evidence of central hypodense region (small arrow). Renal oncocytoma was diagnosed on the surgical specimen. (**c**) Renal cell carcinoma. Contrast-enhanced CT. Nephrographic phase. The same pattern of the previous oncocytoma is identified, showing as a central hypodense region without a spoke-wheel shape pattern does not allow to differentiate oncocytoma from RCC

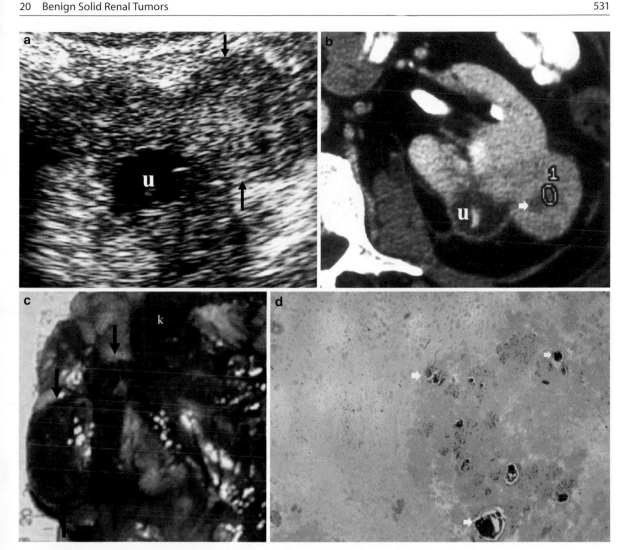

**Fig. 20.26** Renal oncocytoma with less evident central scar. (**a**) Ultrasound, transverse scan. A solid renal mass (*arrows*) is identified on the left kidney. An intra-renal urinoma (u) is also visualized. (**b**) Contrast-enhanced CT. Nephrographic-excretory phase. The solid renal mass (caliper) appears isodense to the adjacent renal kidney with a central hypodense area correspond-

ing to the central scar. An intra-renal urinoma (u) is also visualized. (**c**) Gross specimen with central section on the solid tumor (*arrows*) distinct from the kidney (k). (**d**) Histology, hematoxylin and eosin, original magnification ×40. Uniform fibromyxoid appearance at the microscopic analysis (**d**; with few vessels (*arrows*)

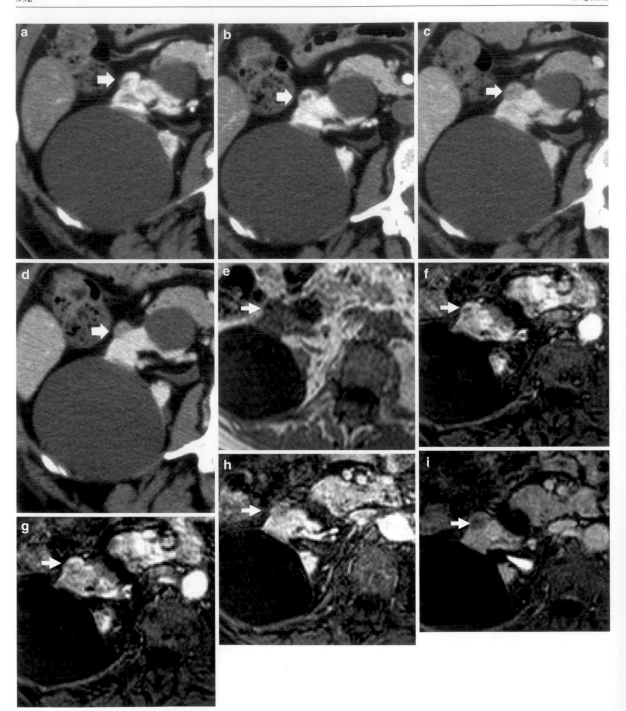

**Fig. 20.27** Small renal oncocytoma with central scar. (**a–d**) Contrast-enhanced CT. Corticomedullary phase. The solid renal mass (*arrow*) appears isodense to the adjacent renal kidney with a central hypodense area corresponding to the central scar. (**c, d**) Nephrographic phase. The same renal mass (*arrow*) appears homogeneous and hypodense in comparison to the adjacent renal parenchyma. (**e–i**) MR imaging. (**e**) Turbo spin-echo T1-weighted sequences; (**f–i**) Contrast-enhanced 3D T1-weighted high resolution isotropic volume examination (THRIVE) MR sequences. The renal mass presents diffuse contrast enhancement on arterial phase (**f, g**), initially sparing the central scar (**f**), and progressive contrast washout during nephrographic (**h**) and excretory phase (**i**) with evidence of a peripheral capsule. The right kidney presents also multiple cysts

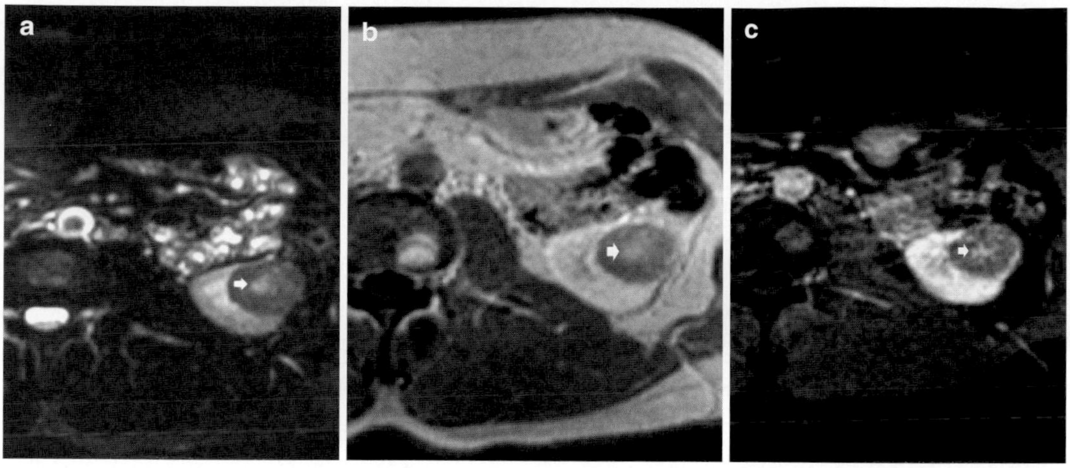

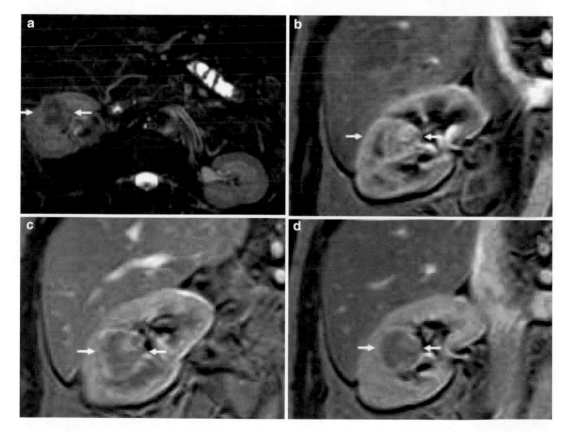

**Fig. 20.28** Oncocytoma on MR imaging. (**a**) Short tau inversion recovery (STIR) sequence. Transverse plane. A spheric and well-defined hypointense renal mass is identified on the left kidney. The central scar (*arrow*) appears hyperintense on T2-weighted sequences. (**b**) Contrast-enhanced T1-weighted spoiled gradient echo (SPGR) sequence, and (**c**) contrast-enhanced T1-weighted spectral fat SPIR sequence after Gd-DTPA injection during nephrographic phase. The central scar (*arrow*) presents a delayed enhancement after the administration of gadolinium-based contrast agents

**Fig. 20.29** Oncocytoma on MR imaging. (**a**) STIR sequence. Transverse plane. A spheric and well-defined renal mass (*arrows*) appearing slightly hyperintense and heterogeneous is identified on the right kidney. (**b–d**) Contrast-enhanced T1-weighted spoiled gradient echo (SPGR) sequence after Gd-DTPA injection during corticomedullary (**b**), nephrographic (**c**), and excretory phase (**d**). Diffuse homogeneous enhancement (*arrows*) is visualized during the corticomedullary phase. A well-defined peripheral pseudocapsule is evident during the nephrographic (**c**) and excretory phase (**d**)

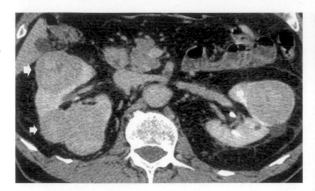

**Fig. 20.30** Renal oncocytosis. Contrast-enhanced CT, excretory phase. Bilateral renal involvement by one dominant mass and numerous smaller nondominant lesions (*arrows*) (Courtesy of Olivier Helenon, Paris)

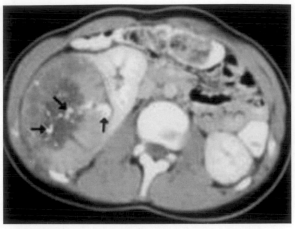

**Fig. 20.32** Embryonal metanephric adenoma in a 30-year-old woman. Axial images of a contrast-enhanced CT-scan in the parenchymal phase show a large, well-defined expansile mass located in the lateral part of the right kidney. The mass is heterogeneous with a hypoattenuating central portion. There are multiple calcifications (*arrows*) (Courtesy from Raymond Oyen, Leuven)

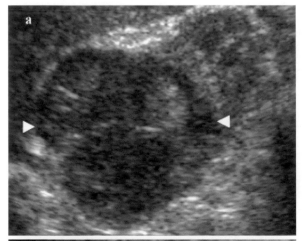

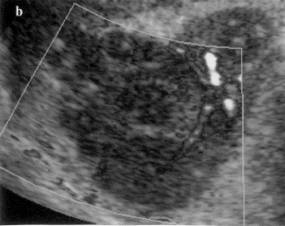

**Fig. 20.31** Embryonal metanephric adenoma. Ultrasound, longitudinal scan. The mass (*arrowheads*) appears heterogenous on gray-scale ultrasound (**a**), with some peripheral vessels at color Doppler analysis (**b**)

On imaging the adenoma presents as a well-defined unilateral solid mass. On US the mass can be hyper-or hypoechoic. Frequently, embryonal metanephric adenoma presents heterogeneous appearance at baseline US, with a mixed arterial vessels distribution at color Doppler US (Fig. 20.31). Sometimes the lesion is cystic with a mural nodule. On CT the mass can be iso-or hypodense (Fig. 20.32). Sometimes clusters of small calcifications can be present. The lesion shows mild contrast enhancement after iodinated contrast agent injection. On T1-weighted MR images metanephric adenoma appears hypointense and slightly hyperintense on T2-weighted MR images (Araki et al. 1998) while mild contrast enhancement is evident after gadolinium-based contrast agent injection (Fig. 20.33).

### 20.3.2 Benign Solid Tumors in Phakomatoses

Phakomatoses are inherited disorders (neurofibromatosis type 1, neurofibromatosis type 2, tuberous sclerosis or Bourneville's disease, Sturge–Weber syndrome, and neurocutaneous melanosis) have selective involvement of tissues of ectodermal origin (central nervous system, eye, and skin). All of these disorders, with the exception of Sturge–Weber syndrome, have an

**Fig. 20.33** (**a–d**) Embryonal metanephric adenoma in a 35-year old woman. A well-defined expansile mass is located in the inferior pole of the left kidney. Coronal 3D T1-weighted fast spoiled gradient echo (GRE) breath-hold sequence obtained before (**a**) and after gadolinium-based contrast agent injection during cortico-medullary (**b**), nephrographic (**c**), and excretory phase (**d**). The mass (*arrow*) presents only a mild contrast enhancement and appears persistently hypovascular in comparison to the adjacent renal parenchyma

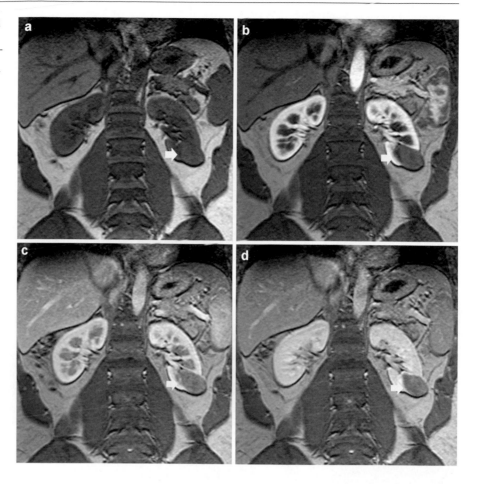

autosomal dominant inheritance pattern (Levy et al. 2005).

Tuberous sclerosis is a multisystem disorder characterized by hamartomas in various organs. It usually manifests itself during infancy or childhood with neurological features, including mental retardation and seizures. Renal angiomyolipomas are found in up to 80% of children with tuberous sclerosis (Fig. 20.34), usually being bilateral, small and multifocal (Khan et al. 1995). The brains of most tuberous sclerosis patients show tubers (hard, potato-like nodules in gyri) of the cerebral cortex and candle gutterings (irregular calcified nodules) in the lateral, third and fourth ventricles (Fig. 20.34). The face often shows angiofibromas on the cheeks and forehead, the heart may have rhabdomyomas.

Renal hemangioma is a very rare benign renal neoplasm, most often located in renal medulla and sinus. Most lesions are solitary, unilateral, and less than a centimeter in size. Hemangiomas may be of the capillary or cavernous type (Prasad et al. 2005; Vilanova

et al. 2004). Renal hemangiomas can be of the capillary or cavernous type, and may be part of a multiorgan syndrome including Sturge–Weber (encephalotrigeminal angiomatosis) and Klippel–Trenaunay–Weber syndrome. Patients usually present with intermittent hematuria (Prasad et al. 2005). Hemorrhage from these submucosal lesions is thought to occur as a result of thrombosis, infarction, or neoangiogenesis and subsequent mucosal erosion. On imaging they present as a solitary, small (often <1 cm) unilateral mass, hyperechoic on ultrasound and show intense arterial phase contrast enhancement (Fig. 20.35) in the arterial phase and can present persistent or delayed contrast enhancement on CT and MR imaging. On MRI hemangiomas are likely to be homogeneously T1-hypointense and T2-hyperintense. Imaging characteristics of renal hemangiomas are nonspecific and can be fairly similar to RCC and transitional cell carcinoma. The specific contrast enhancement may suggest the diagnosis preoperatively (Prasad et al. 2005; Surabhi et al. 2008).

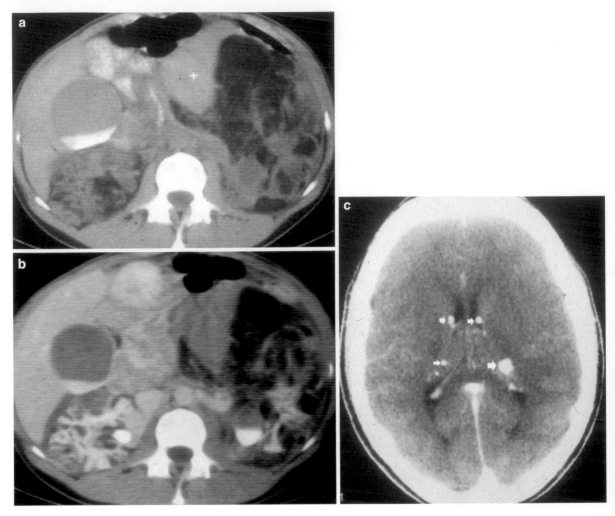

**Fig. 20.34** (**a–b**) Renal multiple angiomyolipomas in a patient with tuberous sclerosis syndrome. (**a**) Unenhanced CT. (**b**) Contrast-enhanced CT, nephrographic phase. Multiple lesions with evident fat component corresponding to multiple angio-myolipomas are evident on both kidneys. (**c**) CT of the brain. Contrast-enhanced scan. Evidence of multiple candle gutterings (irregular calcified nodules) in the lateral, third and fourth ventricles

Neurofibromas of the kidney are usually identified as part of neurofibromatosis type-1 (Levy et al. 2005). The most common abdominal locations for neurofibromas are the paraspinal and presacral regions in the distribution of the lumbosacral plexus. Rarely, plexiform neurofibromas can diffusely involve the periportal regions, retroperitoneum, and mesentery. In these cases, bulky soft-tissue masses are so extensive throughout the abdomen that they simulate malignancy. Renal neurofibromas appear as focal or diffuse soft-tissue attenuation lesions with iso- or hypovascular appearance after contrast agent injection (Fig. 20.36).

### 20.3.3 Arteriovenous Fistulas and Intra-Renal Vascular Malformations

Vascular anomalies and aneurysms are other renal lesions that can mimic an enhancing solid neoplasm (Bhatt et al. 2007; Silverman et al. 2008). In the case of arteriovenous malformations, the ipsilateral renal artery and/or vein are frequently enlarged (Fig. 20.37). Arteriovenous fistula is rare in native kidneys without the history of a biopsy or trauma. Color Doppler may show a large tortuous cluster of vessels with increased

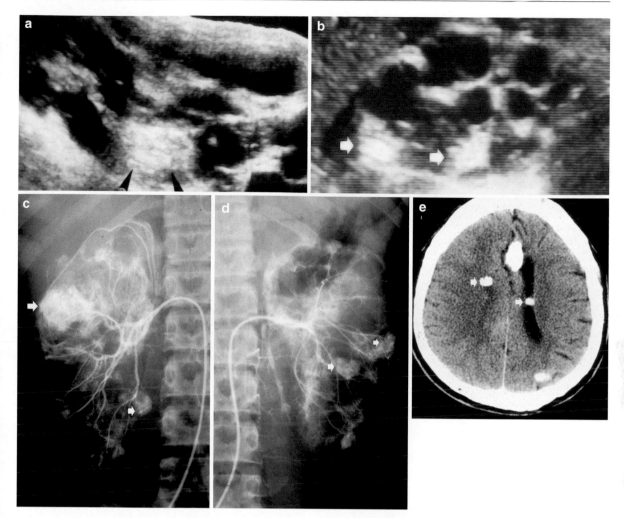

**Fig. 20.35** Renal multiple hemangiomas in a 29-years-old patient with Sturge–Weber syndrome. Ultrasound, transverse scan of the right (**a**) and left kidney (**b**). Multiple hyperechoic lesions (*arrows*), corresponding to renal hemangiomas, are evident on both kidneys presenting also multiple simple cysts. (**c, d**) Digital subtraction angiography. Multiple hypervascular lesions (*arrows*), corresponding to renal hemangiomas, are identified on both kidneys. (**e**) CT of the brain. Contrast-enhanced scan. Subependimal enhancing angiomatous malformation (*arrows*) and parenchymal venous anomalies

flow. Spectral Doppler waveforms of the renal arteries feeding the fistula will demonstrate high velocity and low resistance because the renal capillaries and glomeruli are bypassed by the fistulas. The main renal vein is often dilated, and it may have arterialized waveforms near the fistula. The appearance of an arteriovenous fistula on CT or MR imaging is similar to the sonographic findings. A cluster of dilated vessels will be present, and the renal vein may be dilated. Early filling of the ipsilateral vein is to be expected, and this may be shown depending upon the time of the contrast bolus. Multiplanar reformats of CT or MR imaging data may allow improved definition of the anatomy beyond the limits of ultrasound to aid in the surgical planning.

### 20.3.4 Rare Solid Benign Tumors

See Chap. 22.

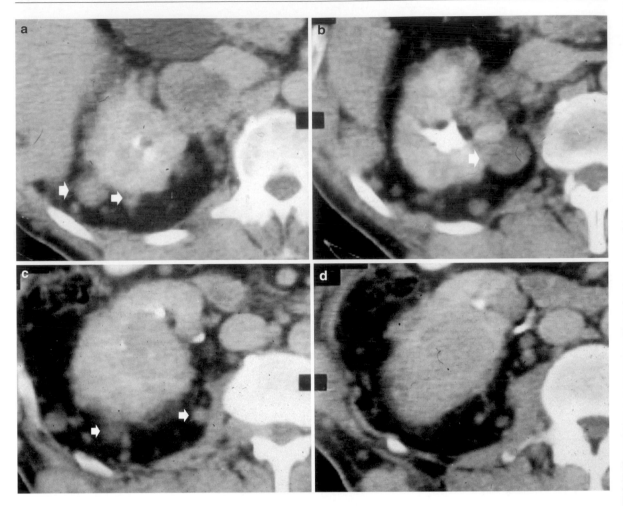

**Fig. 20.36** (**a–d**) Neurofibromatosis with renal involvement. Contrast-enhanced CT. Nephrographic phase. Multiple hypodense lesions (*arrows*) are identified in the renal subcapsu-lar parenchyma and in the perirenal space. Only some of the lesions are indicated

**Fig. 20.37** (**a–d**) Arteriovenous malformation. (**a**) Plain radiograph. Gross calcifications (*arrow*) are visualized in the left renal region. (**b**) Color Doppler ultrasound, longitudinal scan. Vascular signals (*arrow*) are visualized within the pelvis of the left kidney. (**c**) Unenhanced CT. Gross calcifications (*arrows*) are evident within the left renal pelvis. (**d**, **e**) Contrast-enhanced CT. Nephrographic phase. A dilated renal vein (v) is visualized in comparison to the left renal artery (a). Moreover, dilated vascular structures (*arrow*) with diffuse contrast enhancement are visualized within the renal pelvis

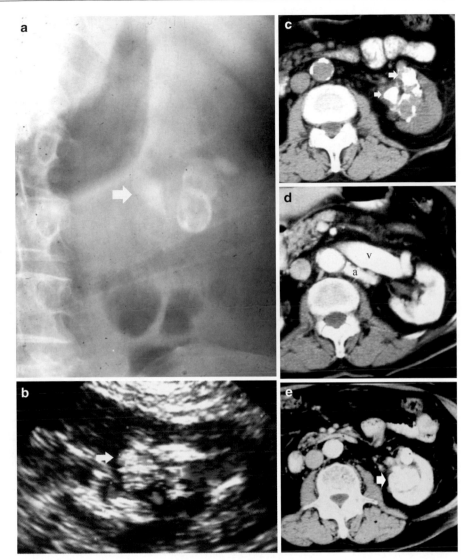

# References

Algaba F (2008) Renal adenomas: pathological differential diagnosis with malignant tumors. Adv Urol 2008:974848

Araki T, Hata H, Asakawa E et al. (1998) MRI of metanephric adenoma. J Comput Assist Tomogr 22(1):87–90

Argani P (2005) Metanephric neoplasms: the hyperdifferentiated, benign end of the Wilms tumor spectrum? Clin Lab Med 25:379–392

Ariaratnam N, Riedl C, Tickoo S et al. (2009) Renal oncocytosis: imaging consideration. Abdom Imaging 34:261–264

Bahrami A, Schwartz MR, Ayala AG et al. (2007) Concurrent angiomyolipoma and two oncocytomas in the same kidney. Ann Diagn Pathol 11(2):132–136

Ball DS, Friedman AC, Hartman DS et al. (1986) Scar sign of renal oncocytoma: magnetic resonance imaging appearance and lack of specificity. Urol Radiol 8:46–48

Beland MD, Mayo-Smith WW, Dupuy DE et al. (2007) Diagnostic yield of 58 consecutive imaging-guided biopsies of solid renal masses: should we biopsy all that are indeterminate? AJR Am J Roentgenol 188:792–797

Bhatt S, MacLennan G, Dogra V (2007) Renal pseudotumors. AJR Am J Roentgenol 188:1380–1387

Bosniak MA, Megibow AJ, Hulnick DH et al. (1988) CT diagnosis of renal angiomyolipoma: the importance of detecting small amounts of fat. AJR Am J Roentgenol 151: 497–501

Cohan RH, Cowan NC, Ellis JH (2006) Unknown ESUR cases 2004. Abdom Imaging 31:141–153

Davidson AJ, Hayes WS, Hartman DS et al. (1993) Renal oncocytoma and carcinoma: failure of differentiation with CT. Radiology 186:693–696

Dechet CB, Bostwick DG, Blute ML et al. (1999) Renal oncocytoma: multifocality, bilateralism, methacronous tumor development and coexistent renal cell carcinoma. J Urol 162:40–42

Earls JP, Krinsky GA (1997) Abdominal and pelvic applications of opposed-phase MR imaging. AJR Am J Roentgenol 169:1071–1077

Eble JN, Sauter G, Epstein JI, Sesterhenn IA (eds) (2004) World Health Organization classification of tumors: pathology and genetics of tumors of the urinary system and male genital organs. IARC Press, Lyon, France

Fotiadis NI, Sabharwal T, Morales JP et al. (2007) Combined percutaneous radiofrequency ablation and ethanol injection of renal tumours: midterm results. Eur Urol 52:777–784

Gill IS, Novick AC, Meraney AM et al. (2000) Laparoscopic renal cryoablation in 32 patients. Urology 56:748–753

Harmon WJ, King BF, Lieber MM (1996) Renal oncocytoma: magnetic resonance imaging characteristics. J Urol 155: 863–867

Hecht EM, Israel GM, Krinsky GA et al. (2004) MR imaging of renal masses: comparison of quantitative enhancement using signal intensity measurements versus qualitative enhancement with image subtraction. Radiology 232: 373–378

Helenon O, Chretien Y, Paraf F et al. (1993) Renal cell carcinoma containing fat: demonstration with CT. Radiology 188:429–430

Hélénon O, Correas JM, Balleyguier C et al. (2001) Ultrasound of renal tumors. Eur Radiol 11:1890–1901

Hélénon O, Merran S, Paraf F et al. (1997) Unusual fat-containing tumors of the kidney: a diagnostic dilemma. Radiographics 17:129–144

Ho VB, Allen SF, Hood MN et al. (2002) Renal masses: quantitative assessment of enhancement with dynamic MR imaging. Radiology 224:695–700

Hwang SS, Choi YJ (2004) Metanephric adenoma of the kidney. Abdom Imaging 29:309–311

Israel GM, Bosniak MA (2005) How I do it: evaluating renal masses. Radiology 236:441–450

Israel GM (2006) MRI of the kidneys and adrenal glands. In: Ho VB, Kransdorf MJ, Reinhold C (eds) Body MRI. Categorical course syllabus from the 2006 Annual Meeting of the American Roentgen Ray Society, pp 91–102

Israel GM, Hecht E, Bosniak MA (2006) CT and MR imaging of complications of partial nephrectomy. Radiographics 26: 1419–1429

Israel GM, Hindman N, Hecht E, Krinsky G (2005) The use of opposed-phase chemical shift MRI in the diagnosis of renal angiomyolipoma. AJR Am J Roentgenol 184:1868–1872

Jasinski RW, Amendola MA, Glazer GM et al. (1985) Computed tomography of renal oncocytomas. Comput Radiol 9: 307–314

Jinzaki M, Tanimoto A, Narimatsu Y et al. (1997) Angiomyolipoma: imaging findings in lesions with minimal fat. Radiology 205:497–502

Khan GA, Melman A, Bank N (1995) Renal involvement in neurocutaneous syndromes. J Am Soc Nephrol 5(7): 1411–1417

Kim JK, Park SY, Shon JH et al. (2004) Angiomyolipoma with minimal fat: differentiation from renal cell carcinoma at biphasic helical CT. Radiology 230:677–684

Kim JI, Cho JY, Moon KC et al. (2009) Segmental enhancement inversion at biphasic multidetector CT: characteristic finding of small renal oncocytoma. Radiology 252:441–448

Kutikov A, Fossett LK, Ramchandani P et al. (2006) Incidence of benign pathologic findings at partial nephrectomy for solitary renal mass presumed to be renal cell carcinoma on preoperative imaging. Urology 68:737–740

Lebret T, Poulain JE, Molinie V et al. (2007) Percutaneous core biopsy for renal masses: indications, accuracy and results. J Urol 178:1184–1188

Lerut E, Roskams T, Joniau S et al. (2006) Metanephric adenoma during pregnancy: clinical presentation, histology, and cytogenetics. Hum Pathol 37:1227–1232

Lesavre A, Correas JM, Merran S et al. (2003) CT of papillary renal cell carcinomas with cholesterol necrosis mimicking angiomyolipomas. AJR Am J Roentgenol 181:143–145

Levy AD, Patel N, Dow N et al. (2005) From the Archives of the AFIP: abdominal neoplasms in patients with neurofibromatosis type 1: radiologic-pathologic correlation. Radiographics 25:455–480

Li R, Zhang X, Hua X, Cai P, Zhong H, Guo Y, Ding S, Yan XC (2009) Real-time contrast-enhanced ultrasonography of resected and immunohistochemically proven hepatic angiomyolipomas. Abdom Imaging DOI: 10.1007/s00261-009-9592-x

Lieber MM (1993) Renal oncocytoma. Urol Clin North Am 20:355–359

Maturen KE, Nghiem HV, Caoili EM et al. (2007) Renal mass core biopsy: accuracy and impact on clinical management. AJR Am J Roentgenol 188:563–570

Neuzillet Y, Lechevallier E, Andre M et al. (2005) Follow-up of renal oncocytoma diagnosed by percutaneous tumor biopsy. Urology 66:1181–1185

Outwater EK, Bhatia M, Siegelman ES et al. (1997) Lipid in renal clear cell carcinoma: detection on opposed-phase gradient-echo MR images. Radiology 205:103–107

Pavlovich CP, Walther MM, Eyler RA et al. (2002) Renal tumors in the Birt-Hogg-Dube syndrome. Am J Surg Pathol 26:1542–1552

Pedrosa I, Sun MR, Spencer M et al. (2008) MR imaging of renal masses: correlation with findings at surgery and pathologic analysis. Radiographics 28:985–1003

Perez-Ordonez B, Hamed G, Campbell S et al. (1997) Renal oncocytoma: a clinicopathologic study of 70 cases. Am J Surg Pathol 21:871–883

Prasad SR, Humphrey PA, Catena FR et al. (2006) Common and uncommon histologic subtypes of renal cell carcinoma: imaging spectrum with pathologic correlation. Radiographics 26:1795–1810

Prasad SR, Humphrey PA, Menias CO et al. (2005) Neoplasms of the renal medulla: radiologic-pathologic correlation. Radiographics 25:369–380

Prasad SR, Dalrymple NC, Surabhi VR (2008a) Cross-sectional imaging evaluation of renal masses. Radiol Clic N Am 46:95–111

Prasad SR, Surabhi VR, Menias CO et al. (2008b) Benign renal neoplasms in adults: cross-sectional imaging findings. AJR Am J Roentgenol 190:158–164

Quaia E (2005) Characterization and detection of renal tumors. In: Quaia E (ed) Contrast media in ultrasonography: basic principles and clinical applications. Springer, Heidelberg, pp 224–244

Quinn MJ, Hartman DS, Friedman AC et al. (1984) Renal oncocytoma: new observations. Radiology 153:49–53

Rowsell C, Fleshner N, Marrano P et al. (2007) Papillary renal cell carcinoma within a renal oncocytoma: case report of an incidental finding of a tumour within a tumour. J Clin Pathol 60:426–428

Sahni VA, Silverman SG (2009) Biopsy of renal masses: when and why. Cancer Imaging 9:44–55

Schuster TG, Ferguson MR, Baker DE et al. (2004) Papillary renal cell carcinoma containing fat without calcification mimicking angiomyolipoma on CT. AJR Am J Roentgenol 183:1402–1404

Silpananta P, Michel RP, Oliver JA (1984) Simultaneous occurrence of angiomyolipoma and renal cell carcinoma. Clinical and pathologic (including ultrastructural) features. Urology 23(2):200–204

Silverman SG, Gan YU, Mortele KJ et al. (2006) Renal masses in the adult patient: the role of percutaneous biopsy. Radiology 240:6–22

Silverman SG, Israel GM, Herts BR et al. (2008) Management of the incidental renal mass. Radiology 249:16–31

Simpfendorfer C, Herts BR, Motta-Ramirez GA et al. (2009) Angiomyolipoma with minimal fat on MDCT: can counts of negative-attenuation pixels aid diagnosis. AJR Am J Roentgenol 192:438–443

Surabhi VR, Menias C, Prasad SR et al. (2008) Neoplastic and non-neoplastic proliferative disorders of the perirenal space: cross-sectional imaging findings. Radiographics 28:1005–1017

Tickoo SK, Lee MW, Eble JN et al. (2000) Ultrastructural observations on mitochondria and microvesicles in renal oncocytoma, chromophobe renal cell carcinoma, and eosinophilic variant of conventional (clear cell) renal cell carcinoma. Am J Surg Pathol 24:1247–1256

Tickoo SK, Reuter VE, Amin MB et al. (1999) Renal oncocytosis: a morphologic study of fourteen cases. Am J Surg Pathol 23:1094–1101

Vasudevan A, Davies RJ, Shannon BA et al. (2006) Incidental renal tumours: the frequency of benign lesions and the role of preoperative core biopsy. BJU Int 97:946–949

Vilanova JC, Barceló J, Smirniotopoulos JC et al. (2004) Hemangioma from head to toe: MR imaging with pathologic correlation. Radiographics 24:367–385

Yamashita Y, Ueno S, Makita O et al. (1993) Hyperechoic renal tumors: anechoic rim and intratumoral cysts in US differentiation of renal cell carcinoma from angiomyolipoma. Radiology 188(1):179–182

# Renal Cell Carcinoma

**21**

Nagaraj-Setty Holalkere, Daichi Hayashi, and Ali Guermazi

## Contents

N.-S. Holalkere, D. Hayashi, and A. Guermazi (✉)
Department of Radiology, Boston University School
of Medicine, 820 Harrison Avenue, FGH Building, 3rd Floor,
Boston, MA 02118, USA
e-mail: guermazi@bu.edu

E. Quaia (ed.), *Radiological Imaging of the Kidney*,
Medical Radiology, DOI: 10.1007/978-3-540-87597-0_21, © Springer-Verlag Berlin Heidelberg 2011

## Abstract

> Renal cell carcinoma (RCC) is the most common primary renal malignant neoplasm in adults. Approximately, 25–30% of cases present with metastatic disease and 2% of cases may have lesions in bilateral kidneys at the time of presentation. Extensive use of cross-sectional imaging in recent years has resulted in detection of such carcinoma incidentally at an early stage. Approximately 36% of RCCs are discovered incidentally. The radiologist should be aware of this and once a suspected mass is identified, further investigations should be instituted. Solid or complex cystic lesions are best characterized by computed tomography (CT) or magnetic resonance imaging (MRI) with contrast enhancement. These cross-sectional modalities are also indispensable in the staging and restaging of suspected RCC lesions. Other modalities including ultrasound and PET can also be utilized to play a complimentary role. Image-guided percutaneous renal biopsy is safe and accurate in sampling the lesion and reaching a final histopathological diagnosis. As the frequency of detection of renal masses increases and the utility of percutaneous biopsy and minimally invasive interventions including radiofrequency ablation (RFA), transarterial embolization (TAE) and nephron-sparing surgery (NSS) become more common, we are likely to see these procedures become more frequently employed in patient management.

## 21.1 Introduction

Renal cell carcinoma (RCC) is the most common primary renal malignant neoplasm in adults. RCC accounts for 3% of all cancer diagnoses in the United States (Jemal et al. 2007). In 2007 there were approximately 51,200 new cases of RCC, and an estimated 12,900 deaths. When compared with 1,971, these numbers represent a fivefold increase in new cases and a twofold increase in mortality (Silverberg and Holleb 1971). It accounts for approximately 85% of renal tumors and 2% of all adult malignancies. In United States roughly about $1.9 billion is spent each year on treatment of RCC (Provet et al. 1991). RCC is twice common in men than in women, and it most often occurs in patients aged 50–70 years. Approximately, 25–30% of cases present with metastatic disease and 2% of cases may have lesions in bilateral kidneys at the time of presentation. Risk factors include increased age; male sex; smoking; cadmium, benzene, trichloro-ethylene, and asbestos exposure; excessive weight; chronic dialysis use; and several genetic syndromes including von Hippel-Lindau syndrome, familial RCC, hereditary papillary RCC, and tuberous sclerosis. Bilateral multifocal renal tumors are present in approximately 5% of patients with sporadic renal tumors (Patel et al. 2003).

Extensive use of cross-sectional imaging in recent years has resulted in detection of such carcinoma incidentally at an early stage. Approximately 36% of RCCs are discovered incidentally (Leslie et al. 2003). The average size of RCC at the time of diagnosis has decreased significantly over the past two decades (Hollingsworth et al. 2006). At the same time, the proportion of early clinical stage (T1–T2) tumors have increased from 49 to 74%, while the percentage of patients with M1 disease decreased from 20 to 10% (Luciani et al. 2000).

## 21.2 Histopathological Subtypes

Several distinct histologic subtypes of RCC are recognized and are classified based on 2004 WHO classification (Table 21.1) into clear cell RCC, papillary RCC, chromophobe RCC, hereditary cancer syndromes, multilocular cystic RCC, collecting duct carcinoma, medullary carcinoma, mucinous tubular and spindle cell carcinoma, neuroblastoma-associated RCC, Xp11.2 translocation–*TFE3* carcinoma, and unclassified lesions. Each subtype carries a different prognostic profile (Prasad et al. 2008). For example, clear cell RCC has a less favorable prognosis (stage for stage) than do papillary RCC and chromophobe RCC. Similarly, collecting duct carcinoma and renal medullary carcinoma are associated with poor prognosis and aggressive clinical behavior (Storkel et al. 1997; Bruder et al. 2004).

**Table 21.1** Histological subtypes, prevalence and cell origin of renal cell carcinoma (RCC) based on 2004 WHO classification

| Histological subtype | Prevalence (%) | Putative cell of origin |
|---|---|---|
| Clear cell RCC | 70 | Epithelium of proximal convoluted tubule |
| Papillary RCC | 10 | Epithelium of proximal convoluted tubule |
| Chromophobe RCC | 5 | Cortical collecting duct, type B intercalated cell |
| Hereditary cancer syndromes | 5 | |
| Multilocular cystic RCC | <1 | |
| Collecting duct carcinoma | <1 | Medullary collecting duct |
| Medullary carcinoma | <1 | Medullary collecting duct |
| Mucinous tubular and spindle cell carcinoma | <1 | Possibly the loop of Henle |
| Neuroblastoma-associated RCC | <1 | |
| Xp11.2 translocation–TFE3 carcinoma | <1 | |
| Unclassified lesions | 4 | |

## 21.3 Imaging of Conventional (Clear Cell) Renal Cell Carcinoma

Clear cell RCC is also known as conventional RCC since it accounts for nearly 70% of all RCCs. Imaging manifestations are based on the contents of the tumor and typically have predominant soft tissue, adipose tissue, or cystic contents. However, RCCs may demonstrate significant tumor heterogeneity and may appear entirely cystic or necrotic, or may show a small proportion of macroscopic fat or areas of hemorrhage. Clear cell RCC originates from the renal cortex and typically exhibits an expansile growth pattern. Multicentricity and bilaterality are rare with clear cell RCC (Corica et al. 1999).

### 21.3.1 Plain Radiography

Plain radiographs were the mainstay of diagnosis before the advent of ultrasound or cross sectional imaging on computed tomography (CT) or MRI. Occasionally, RCC may be found on an abdominal or kidney-ureter-bladder (KUB) radiograph, usually appearing as an expansile lobulated mass extending from the kidney or as an ill-defined mass distorting the renal soft tissue outline. Approximately 15% of RCCs contain calcifications (Fig. 21.1) that can be detected

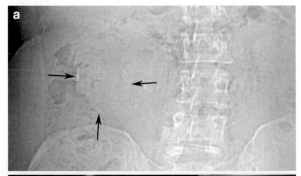
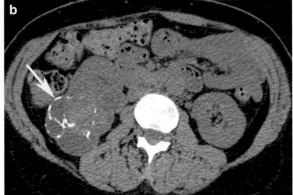

**Fig. 21.1** (**a**) Abdominal radiograph and (**b**) unenhanced axial abdominal computed tomography (CT) scan in a 46-year-old woman with hematuria demonstrates curvilinear calcification (*black arrows*) in the right renal region on radiograph that correlates to large exophytic solid right renal lower pole mass with peripheral calcification (*white arrow*)

on a plain abdominal radiograph. If the calcification is gross it is of significant importance indicating the high likelihood of RCC.

The patterns of calcification may vary from thin peripheral rim calcification to irregular central calcification, or a combination of both. Roughly 80% of the masses with thin, peripheral rim calcification are benign cysts, and 20% are cystic renal malignancies. In contrast, the renal masses that contain central, irregular calcification are more likely to be malignant (87% of lesions). Masses that have a combination of both central and peripheral calcification have a 50% chance of being malignant. Nearly 60% of renal masses that contain visible calcium on an abdominal radiograph, regardless of the pattern of calcification are RCCs (Bracken 1987).

Other plain radiographic findings that may be important are lytic skeletal abnormalities due to hematogenous metastases. The lesions are characterized by slow growth with bubbly appearance and focal expansion of the bone, mimicking other types of bone lesions, including primary bone neoplasms and myeloma. Finally, patients with tuberous sclerosis, a disease associated with RCC, can have multiple osteomas, which predominate in the skull and spine (Barker and Zagoria 2006).

### 21.3.2 Intravenous Urography

Intravenous urography (IVU) used to be the primary investigating modality in the past to determine the nature of a suspected lesion and the residual function of the involved kidney. Currently this technique is rarely utilized when other cross-sectional modalities such as CT and MRI are available.

IVU can be performed in the following way. A preliminary abdominal or KUB radiograph is followed by 100 mL of 30 mg% contrast administration over 30–60 s. The first minute coned radiograph of both kidneys and the nephrotomogram is followed by a 5-min coned radiograph of both kidneys with abdominal compression. Then, a 10-min coned radiograph of both kidneys with continued abdominal compression is taken and compression is released. A penultimate 15-min abdominopelvic plain radiograph, frontal and both obliques is followed by a final postvoid abdominopelvic plain radiograph. The scout radiograph is analyzed to detect any abnormal calcifications. RCC is typically an expansile lesion which can be a focal bulge extending from the kidney, deforming the normal contour and displacing the normal renal structures. These changes are optimally detected with nephrotomography. Large masses characteristically cause calyceal splaying, stretching, and draping. Occasionally, an exophytic RCC can spare the calyces with no detectable mass effect exerted on the calyceal system. However RCCs that extend solely in anterior or posterior direction from the kidney may be difficult to detect with IVU, because the mass contour can be obscured by superimposed normal kidney.

Other IVU signs of RCC include the renal pelvis notching or the ureteral notching from enlargement of ureteric and renal pelvic vessels (which are recruited to feed or drain a hypervascular RCC), obstruction or invasion of the collecting system, and diminished or absent renal function. Hydronephrosis, either focal or diffuse, occurs due to a large RCC compressing the major calyces, the renal pelvis, or the upper ureter. Less commonly, an RCC involves the adjacent structures by infiltration rather than by expansion, which can secondarily encase the ureter or invade the urothelium and cause its malignant constriction.

Limitations of excretory urography are that it lacks specificity and characterization of lesions and therefore requires further imaging with another technique such as ultrasound, CT or MRI.

### 21.3.3 Ultrasound

The most cost-effective imaging modality is renal ultrasound with Doppler. The ultrasound can easily differentiate approximately 80% of detected renal masses as simple cysts and avoid further diagnostic evaluation (Einstein et al. 1995). The remaining 20% of renal masses can be differentiated based on their characteristics of echogenicity, blood flow, extension into adjacent structures and calcification, but it does require further study with cross sectional (CT or MR) imaging (Barker and Zagoria 2006).

On ultrasound, RCCs appear as expansile, solitary renal masses and are typical but not diagnostic. They may appear hypoechoic, isoechoic, or hyperechoic in comparison with the renal parenchyma, with heterogeneous echo patterns in larger lesions with internal cystic areas (Barker and Zagoria 2006). Approximately one-third of small RCCs are markedly hyperechoic (Fig. 21.2), but many small RCCs are slightly

**Fig. 21.2** (**a–c**) Renal cell carcinoma (RCC) in a 66-year-old woman. (**a**) Longitudinal ultrasound image reveals markedly hyperechoic RCC (*arrow*) indistinguishable from angiomyolipoma (AML). (**b**) Axial contrast-enhanced CT scan reveals solid enhancing lesion (*arrow*) with no detectable fat. (**c**) Pathology specimen shows *yellow-orange* mass (*arrow*) with spongy consistency and areas of hemorrhage. Final diagnosis was conventional RCC. Images reproduced from Barker and Zagoria (2006), with permission

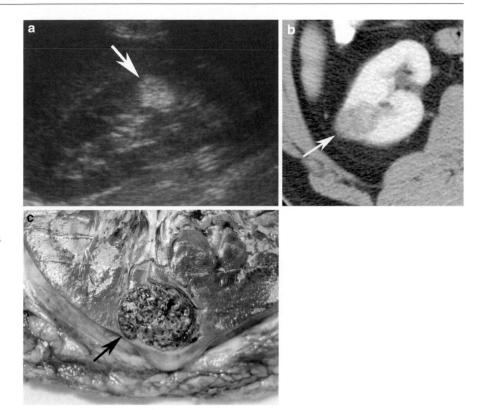

hyperechoic (Forman et al. 1993) and may mimic a benign angiomyolipoma (AML). Ultrasound finding of a mass lesion with anechoic perimeter or internal cystic areas strongly favors RCC, though CT or MRI is required for further evaluation (Yamashita et al. 1993). AML with intratumoral fat is easily detected on both CT and MRI (Takahashi et al. 1993) and excludes an RCC except in the rare case of a tumor with normal renal sinus or perirenal fat.

Another useful feature of ultrasound is the capacity to demonstrate the internal architecture of renal tumors. Ultrasound of lesions with an equivocal appearance (i.e., not clearly cystic, but not obviously malignant) on CT or MRI may demonstrate complexity of the architecture like internal septations, fronds of solid tissue lining the periphery of the mass or other evidence of malignancy. Ultrasound may also be useful to find the abnormalities secondary to infiltrating RCCs, including hydronephrosis and vascular encasement with diminished Doppler flow to the area of involvement. Alteration of the normal central sinus echo complex may be seen. An infiltrating RCC itself, however, may cause only subtle ultrasound abnormalities or none at all.

Staging of RCC with ultrasound is less accurate than either CT or MRI, and therefore ultrasound should not be used as the sole modality for staging RCC, but as an adjunct to other imaging techniques. The major limitations of ultrasound in staging RCC are the insufficient imaging of the renal vein and the subhepatic inferior vena cava and limited detection of abdominal lymphadenopathy. However ultrasound is more accurate than CT in evaluating the intrahepatic IVC for tumor thrombi with 95% sensitivity (Gupta et al. 2004).

### 21.3.4 Computed Tomography

The advent of multidetector-row computed tomography (MDCT) technology allows fast, multiphase, and high resolution imaging of the abdomen. Very short data acquisition times can be achieved because of short gantry rotation times (0.5 s) combined with multiple detectors providing increased coverage along the $z$ axis. Retrospective thin-section data reconstruction permits routine acquisition of isotropic data that can be displayed in a multitude of multiplanar and three dimensional (3D) formats, with minimal artifacts. Scanning through the entire kidney is possible in less than 10 s. Multiphase imaging of the kidney permits not only high-resolution imaging of the renal parenchyma but also that of its vasculature and collecting systems. 3D CT provides the urologist with an interactive road map of the relationships among the tumor, the major vessels, and the collecting system (Fig. 21.3). This information is particularly critical if the tumor extends into the inferior vena cava and if nephron-sparing surgery (NSS) is being planned.

A dedicated renal mass CT protocol (Fig. 21.4) consists of a precontrast, arterial (15–25 s delay), corticomedullary (35–85 s delay), nephrographic (85–180 s delay) and excretory (3 min or more) phases. An initial series of unenhanced scans through the kidneys should be part of every protocol for evaluation of a suspected renal mass. This provides a baseline to measure the enhancement within the lesion after the administration of intravenous contrast material. This enhancement characteristic is important in distinguishing hyperdense cysts from solid tumors. Because most RCCs have a rich vascular supply, they show significant contrast enhancement. Enhancement values of more than 12 Hounsfiled Unit (HU) are considered suspicious for malignancy. Most RCCs are solid lesions with attenuation values of 20 HU or greater at

unenhanced CT. Small (<3 cm) tumors usually have a homogeneous appearance, while larger lesions tend to be more heterogeneous owing to hemorrhage or necrosis. Calcifications are detected in up to 30% of cases of RCC (Fig. 21.1b).

Corticomedullary images are superior in the assessment of renal vascular anatomy, lesion vascularity, and venous involvement of the lesion. During this phase contrast resides in the cortical capillaries, peritubular cells, proximal convoluted tubules, and columns of Bertin. Optimal time delay for the corticomedullary phase depends on the rate of injection, the amount of contrast material administered, and the patient's cardiac output. Not all renal tumors are well delineated during the corticomedullary phase; small hypovascular lesions of the renal medulla (a low attenuation region during the corticomedullary phase) and small hypervascular tumors of the cortex (a high attenuation region during the corticomedullary phase) are difficult to detect. Small hypervascular cortical RCCs may enhance to the same degree as the normal cortex, whereas hypovascular tumors of the medulla may not enhance during this phase (Cohan et al. 1995; Birnbaum et al. 1996; Kopka et al. 1997; Szolar et al. 1997; Yuh and Cohan 1999; Schreyer et al. 2002; Zhang et al. 2007a). Images obtained during a later phase of enhancement (i.e., the nephrographic or excretory phase) must be included to facilitate the detection of such renal masses.

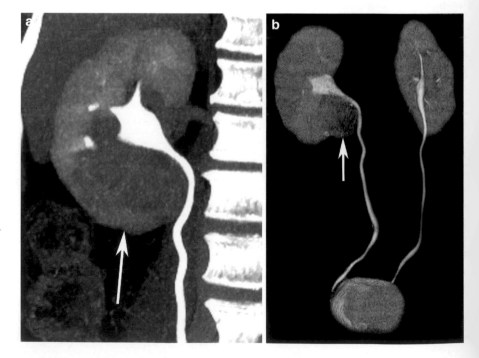

**Fig. 21.3** (**a**) CT urography with coronal three dimensional (3D) maximum intensity projection (MIP) of the right upper ureter and (**b**) 3D volume rendered display of bilateral ureters demonstrates a mass (*arrow*) in the lower pole of the right kidney with mass effect on pelvicalyceal system and right upper ureter

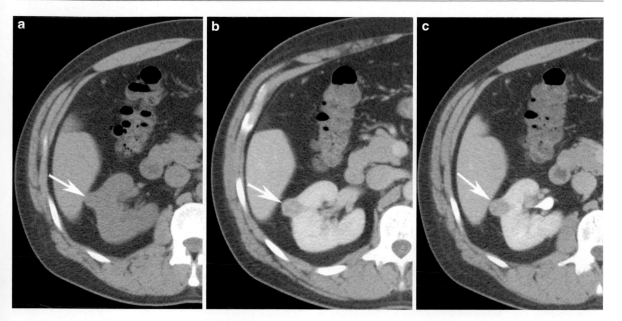

**Fig. 21.4** (**a–c**) Renal mass protocol CT evaluation in a 57-year-old man with hematuria demonstrates a 1.3 cm partially exophytic right renal lesion (*arrow*) that measures 32 HU on (**a**) nonenhanced CT, (**b**) enhances to 65 HU at nephrographic phase of enhancement and (**c**) de enhances to 37 HU at 10 min delayed scans. These enhancement features are highly suggestive of renal cell cancer. Patient subsequently underwent partial nephrectomy and pathology was consistent with clear cell renal cancer

The nephrographic phase is obtained during the passage of contrast material through the renal tubular system. During the nephrographic phase, the renal parenchyma enhances homogeneously. Although the duration of the nephrographic phase is not clearly defined, for practical reasons it may be divided into an early phase and a late phase, with the latter overlapping the excretory phase (Yuh and Cohan 1999; Schreyer et al. 2002). The nephrographic phase is considered the optimal phase for the detection and characterization of small renal masses (Cohan et al. 1995; Szolar et al. 1997; Yuh and Cohan 1999). In one study, 84 more renal masses smaller than 3 cm in diameter were seen on the nephrographic phase scans than were seen on the corticomedullary phase scans (Szolar et al. 1997).

The excretory phase begins when contrast material is excreted into the collecting system, 3–5 min after contrast administration. During this phase, the nephrogram remains homogeneous but its attenuation is diminished. This phase is occasionally helpful to better delineate the relationship of a centrally located mass with the collecting system and define potential involvement of the calices and renal pelvis. Delayed scanning can also be used in lieu of unenhanced scanning to characterize an incidental renal lesion detected on a routine contrast-enhanced CT scan.

In many cases, the pattern of enhancement within a renal neoplasm is dense and irregular, and in such cases, subjective assessment for enhancement is sufficient. Even if enhancement is not particularly dense but is irregular or nodular within the mass, the mass is most likely neoplastic. Conventional clear cell renal carcinoma is the most vascular type among all malignant renal cortical tumors, as shown by its greater degree of enhancement after administration of intravenous contrast material (Jinzaki et al. 2000; Kim et al. 2002; Sheir et al. 2005; Zhang et al. 2007b). A mixed enhancement pattern containing enhancing solid soft tissue and low-attenuation areas that may represent cystic or necrotic changes was most predictive of the clear cell type (Fig. 21.5). However, in cases of hypovascular masses, enhancement may be more subtle and uniform. In such cases, it is useful to compare attenuation measurements between the precontrast and each of the postcontrast phases.

One pitfall of CT is that attenuation measurements often drift upward slightly, even in a proven simple cyst, because enhancement of the adjacent normal renal parenchyma results in some degree of beam hardening. This drift is more pronounced with smaller, predominantly intrarenal lesions, because volume averaging and beam hardening have a higher statistical

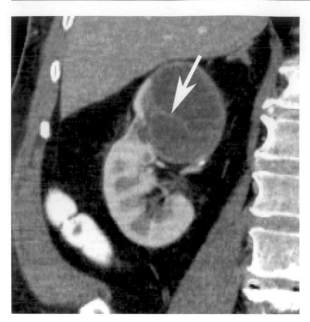

**Fig. 21.5** Contrast-enhanced coronal reformatted CT section of the right kidney depicts a large cystic mass in the upper pole with enhancing septations (*arrow*). Patient subsequently underwent total nephrectomy and on surgical pathology the lesion was proven to be a cystic clear cell RCC

impact on the measurement within small lesions, particularly those less than 2 cm in diameter (a phenomenon known as "pseudoenhancement"). As a rule, an increase in attenuation of 10 HU or more within a lesion between the pre- and post contrast images, in a lesion measuring at least 2 cm in diameter, indicates enhancement. However, because pseudoenhancement may occur, only conclusive evidence of enhancement should be accepted as diagnostic.

Although subtle areas of nodular enhancement can be convincing, lesions with no visual change that have an attenuation increase of 10–20 HU should be considered indeterminate, and further evaluation with ultrasound or MRI should be considered. It is often useful to use MRI to confirm the contrast enhancement, especially in small lesions. Because the enhancement of renal masses is transient, washout of contrast can be as useful as the initial enhancement. A study suggested that measurement of the washout of contrast material from a lesion at 15 min allows differentiation between hyperdense cysts and renal neoplasms (Macari and Bosniak 1999). In their study, there was no change in the attenuation of high-density cysts between the initial contrast-enhanced CT scan and the 15-min-delayed images. In comparison, all lesions that proved to be

neoplasms at surgery or follow-up studies showed a decrease in attenuation or "de-enhancement" of at least 15 HU at delayed CT, which was attributed to the washout of contrast material from the vascular bed of the tumor (Macari and Bosniak 1999). This may be useful if only a single phase scan of the abdomen was performed and the abnormality is detected before the patient leaves the department.

### 21.3.5 Magnetic Resonance Imaging

The single greatest advantage of MRI over ultrasound and CT is that MRI generates the highest intrinsic soft tissue contrast of any cross-sectional imaging modality. MRI can be used to stage renal malignancies and can serve as a guide to appropriate choice of therapy. Renal MRI is particularly useful for patients who should not receive iodine-based CT contrast agents, whether due to history of iodine allergy, renal insufficiency, or renal transplantation. It is also useful in follow-up imaging of patients who have had nephrectomy, partial nephrectomy, or percutaneous tumor ablation.

State-of-the-art MRI of renal masses includes the following breath hold sequences: (1) a T1-weighted in and out of phase gradient echo sequence, which is helpful in identification of macroscopic and microscopic fat in a renal tumor (Isralel et al. 2005); (2) a T2-weighted half-Fourier single-shot fast spin-echo sequence in axial or coronal planes, which is useful for evaluating the overall anatomy, renal collecting system, and complexity of a cystic renal lesion; and (3) a dynamic contrast-enhanced T1-weighted fat-suppressed sequence (Zhang et al. 2004). For dynamic contrast-enhanced images, three-dimensional fast spoiled gradient echo sequences are typically performed before and after contrast administration during the arterial, corticomedullary, and nephrographic phases for evaluation of the presence and pattern of enhancement in a renal mass. Multiplanar reconstruction may be performed if necessary to delineate better the spatial relationship of the renal mass to adjacent anatomic structures. If necessary, a dedicated MR angiography sequence during the arterial phase may be performed for better visualization of accessory renal vessels and facilitation of surgical planning. Coronal T1-weighted images may also be obtained during the excretory phase with administration of diuretics, from

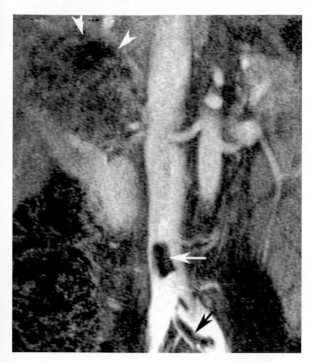

**Fig. 21.6** RCC in a 47-year-old woman. Coronal subtracted MIP image of contrast-enhanced magnetic resonance venography (MRV) examination (TR=3.7 ms, TE=1.4 ms) demonstrates bland, nonenhancing, nonocclusive thrombus of the inferior vena cava (*white arrow*) and left common iliac vein (*black arrow*). There is a large right-upper-pole-enhancing RCC (*arrowheads*)

which maximum intensity projection (MIP) images can be obtained to produce intravenous pyelography-like images, i.e., magnetic resonance venography (MRV). Presence of venous thrombi can be visualized with this technique (Figs. 21.6 and 21.7).

RCC has a highly variable appearance on MRI, due to the existence of multiple RCC histological types (Shinmoto et al. 1998), and to variability in internal necrosis, hemorrhage (John et al. 1997), and/or intratumoral lipid. On MRI, RCC most commonly appears hypointense or isointense to renal parenchyma on T1-weighted images, heterogeneously hyperintense on T2-weighted images, and enhances following gadolinium administration (Fig. 21.8). Variability is the rule, however, and lesions may be primarily hyperintense, hypointense, or isointense to normal renal parenchyma on both T1- and T2-weighted images. Although RCCs enhance with intravenous gadolinium administration, they tend to enhance less than normal renal parenchyma, and are often most easily identified on postcontrast dynamic T1-weighted gradient-recalled-echo (GRE)

images. Clear cell RCCs may lose signal on opposed-phase gradient-echo images, due to the presence of microscopic lipid in some of these neoplasms (Fig. 21.9; Outwater et al. 1997). The presence of intracellular lipid in a renal lesion should therefore not by itself be used to make the diagnosis of AML. The presence of macroscopic lipid within a renal lesion, however, remains very specific for AML, although very rare RCCs which have undergone osseous metaplasia may contain fat.

The MRI features of cystic neoplasms that have been shown to be highly associated with malignancy include mural irregularity, mural nodules, increased mural thickness, and intense mural enhancement. Cystic renal lesions with thicker septations, multiple septations or bulky calcifications are indeterminate, and should be excised (class III). Approximately 10–15% of RCCs display some cystic component. Lesions with enhancing mural solid nodules (class IV) should be excised, and the majority of these lesions will be cystic RCCs. Surgical cure rates for cystic RCC are very high (Corica et al. 1999).

### 21.3.6 Positron Emission Tomography

Oncological PET imaging with F-18 deoxyglucose (FDG) is used as an adjunct to CT and MRI and majority of the application involves the post therapy staging. It is based on the increased glucose utilization exhibited by tumor cells (Fig. 21.10) (Barker and Zagoria 2006). However its use in diagnosis of primary lesions is limited by physiological radiotracer uptake in the kidney in the background and modest uptake within the tumor itself. FDG-PET has 64–71% sensitivity in staging and restaging, but the overall sensitivity of in the detection of metastatic foci is limited (Jadvar et al. 2003; Majhail et al. 2003). FDG-PET plays a better complementary role in the restaging of RCC patients related to superior specificity and positive predictive value compared with conventional imaging (Kang et al. 2004).

### 21.3.7 Angiography

Renal angiography (Watson et al. 1968) is reserved for mapping vascular supply to the kidney with a renal

**Fig. 21.7** (**a–c**) Seventy-two-year-old woman with infiltrating clear cell carcinoma of the right kidney with tumor thrombosis of the right renal vein and IVC. (**a**) Contrast-enhanced coronal T1-weighted magnetic resonance imaging (MRI) at the level of the kidneys demonstrate heterogeneous enhancement of the entire right kidney (*white arrows*) as compared to the normal left kidney (*L*) suggestive of infiltrative tumor. (**b**) Contrast-enhanced coronal T1-weighted MRI of the IVC demonstrates large enhancing thrombus in the IVC (*white arrow*). (**c**) Coronal FDG-PET images demonstrate asymmetric uptake of F-18 deoxyglucose (FDG) in the right kidney (*arrowhead*) with enlarged and abnormal uptake in the region of IVC (*arrow*) suggestive of tumor thrombosis

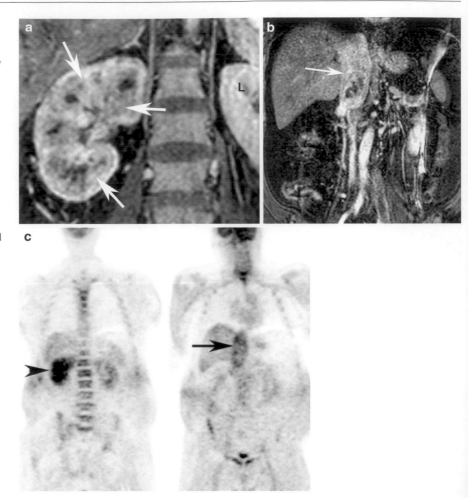

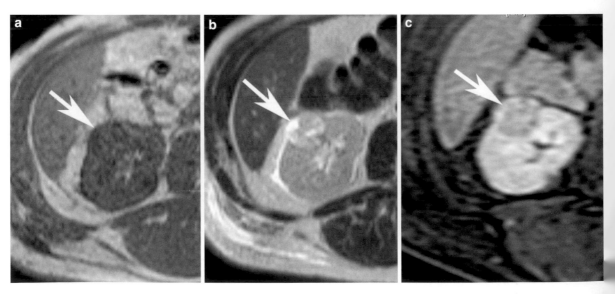

**Fig. 21.8** (**a–c**) Axial (**a**) unenhanced T1-weighted shows hypointense lesion (*arrow*) at the midpole of the right kidney, heterogeneously hyperintense on (**b**) T2-weighted with hetero-geneous enhancement on (**c**) contrast-enhanced T1-weighted fat-suppressed MRI. These are typical features of renal cancer on MRI

**Fig. 21.9** (**a**–**d**) Sixty-five-year-old man with proven clear cell cancer on surgical pathology specimen. (**a**) Axial T2-weighted MRI shows a left upper pole kidney lesion (*arrow*) with a minimal T2 hyperintensity. The lesion shows heterogenous enhancement on (**b**) contrast-enhanced T1-weighted MRI. (**c**) T1-weighted in-phase and (**d**) opposed-phase MRI show drop out of signal on opposed-phase images suggesting the presence of microscopic fat

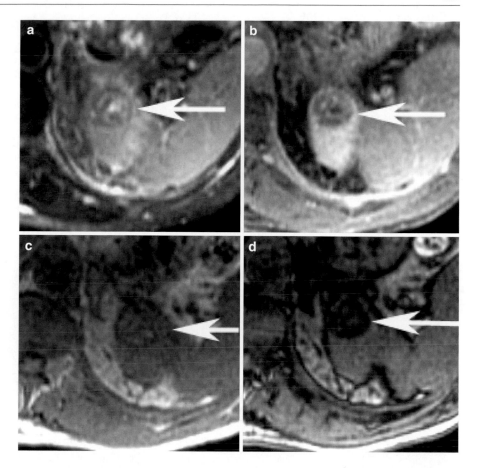

mass (Fig. 21.11) when a partial nephrectomy or NSS is contemplated. However, newer noninvasive techniques, such as CT or MR angiography, can derive similar information, and thus these techniques have largely replaced catheter angiography at most centers.

Nevertheless, renal arteriography is useful in embolization treatment of some RCCs. Tumor embolization aims to reduce intraoperative blood loss, or can diminish symptoms in inoperable patients. In some cases, angiography may be useful to distinguish among various renal masses. Angiography can be an alternative to open biopsy in the evaluation of infiltrating renal neoplasms, the differential diagnosis for which includes urothelial neoplasm, inflammatory lesion, infarct, or infiltrating RCC. These lesions except for infiltrating RCC are nearly always hypovascular or avascular, therefore an infiltrating renal mass that is hypervascular suggests an infiltrating RCC. It is important to differentiate among these lesions because treatment for each type of lesion is different: RCC is treated with

nephrectomy; transitional cell carcinoma is treated with nephroureterectomy; and many other infiltrating lesions are treated medically (Barker and Zagoria 2006).

## 21.4 Imaging of Uncommon Renal Cell Carcinoma

As described earlier in this Sect. 2, RCCs according to the pathologic tumor subtype are classified as papillary, chromophobe, collecting duct, medullary and sarcomatoid types. Radiological or pathological preoperative diagnosis of cyst-associated RCC (cystadenocarcinoma, multilocular cystic RCC, acquired cystic disease of the kidney, adult polycystic kidney disease) is difficult and it is especially so in cases of RCC originating in a cyst. RCCs with unusual infiltrative growth may mimic transitional cell carcinoma, with fatty component mimicking AML, and severe perinephric

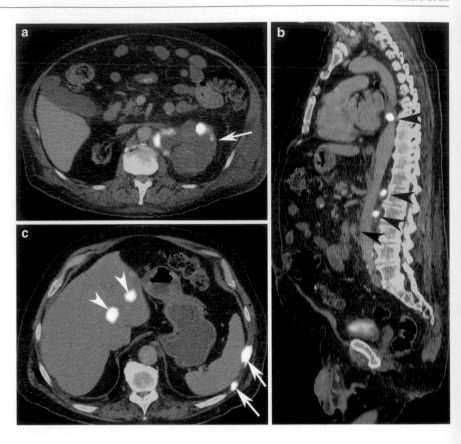

**Fig. 21.10** (**a–c**) Sixty-year-old woman with metastatic left renal cancer. (**a**) Axial FDG PET-CT image at the level of left kidney demonstrates peripherally FDG avid cystic left renal malignancy (*arrow*). (**b**) Sagittal FDG PET-CT image at the level of aorta show multiple FDG avid paraaortic lymph nodes (*black arrowheads*). (**c**) Axial FDG PET-CT image at the level of the right lobe of the liver shows bone lesions (*white arrows*) and liver lesions (*white arrowheads*) consistent with metastatic lesions

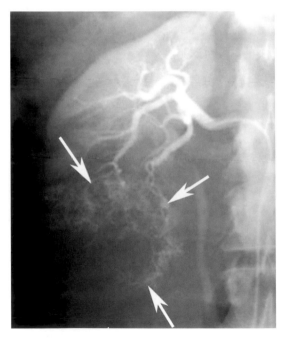

**Fig. 21.11** RCC in a 67-year-old man who presented with macroscopic hematuria. Anteroposterior selective right renal arteriography image demonstrates typical features of tumor vascularity, including large tortuous and meandering arteries and arterioles and numerous irregular branches (*arrows*), due to a lower pole RCC

infiltration and extensive calcifications mimicking inflammation or other tumor. Each subtype has a different prognosis and tumor behavior. A higher 5-year survival rate is seen in patients with papillary RCC or with chromophobe RCC than with conventional RCC of the same stage (Reuter and Presti 2000).

### 21.4.1 Papillary Type

Papillary RCCs present with variable size, and small tumors and true renal cortical adenomas must be distinguished. The classification of RCCs defines any papillary tumor larger than 0.5 cm as a carcinoma (Storkel et al. 1997). Grossly, the papillary type of RCC is well circumscribed and more than 80% of tumors are confined to the cortex and eccentrically situated within the renal capsule at the time of nephrectomy. Radiographic finding of reduced or absent tumor vascularity correlates with intratumoral hemorrhage and necrosis seen in 66% of cases (Press et al. 1984). They are often multiple and are associated with cortical adenomas.

CT features correlate with established clinico-pathologic and angiographic appearances. Papillary RCC presents at early stages in most cases (stages I or II), with a high frequency of calcification and less enhancement (i.e., diminished vascularity) than a typical RCC. Ultrasound pattern (Fig. 21.12a) is known to be inconsistent. On CT a prospective diagnosis of papillary RCC is reasonable. This is particularly important in NSS as a clinical consideration (Press et al. 1984). Homogeneity and low tumor-to-parenchyma enhancement ratios on the parenchymal-phase scans correlate with papillary RCC (Fig. 21.12b, c). Heterogeneity and tumor enhancement ratios do not correlate with the nuclear grade of the carcinoma (Herts et al. 2002).

## 21.4.2 Chromophobe Cell Type

This variant constitutes approximately 5% of renal neoplasms with distinctive histological and cytogenetic features, and needs to be distinguished from benign oncocytoma (Thoenes et al. 1988). The lesions are typically well-circumscribed and solitary. The cut surfaces mimic an oncocytoma and are pale yellow, tan, or brown. Histologically, there are two major patterns of growth, the classic and the eosinophilic types. Microvesicles may concentrate around the nucleus, producing a distinctive perinuclear halo, which is a distinguishing feature from oncocytoma (Murphy et al. 2004). The clinicopathologic characteristics of chromophobe RCC include hypovascularity/avascularity on

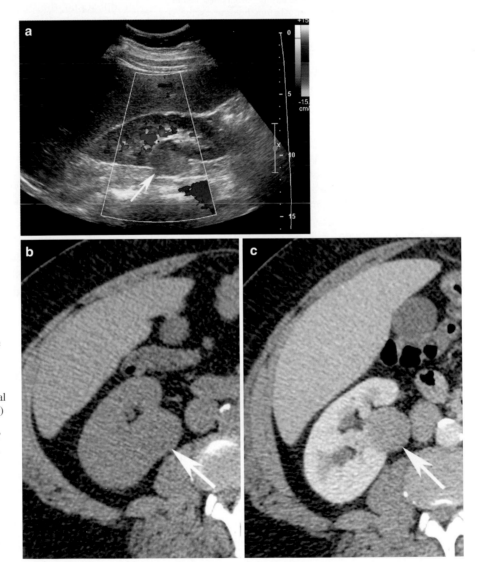

**Fig. 21.12** (a–c) Fifty-six-year-old man with right papillary renal cell cancer. (**a**) Sagittal ultrasound of the right kidney with color Doppler demonstrates well defined isoechoic rounded partially exophytic solid renal lesion in the midpole (*arrow*) with lack of vascularity. (**b**) On unenhanced axial CT scan the same lesion depicts a CT density of 23 HU and (**c**) measures 30 HU on post contrast image. Patient subsequently underwent nephrectomy which was diagnosed to be papillary renal cell cancer on surgical histopathology

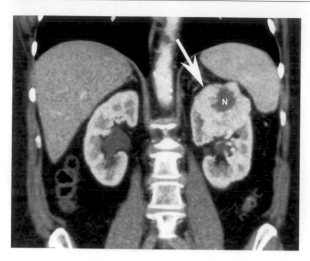

**Fig. 21.13** Contrast-enhanced coronal reformatted CT image shows a large heterogeneous peripherally enhancing lesion (*arrow*) with central necrosis (*N*). Histopathology discloses chromophobe RCC

angiography, low rate of laboratory abnormalities, low stage/low grade, and a favorable prognosis compared with the common types of RCC (Onishi et al. 1996).

On CT, the lesions are well circumscribed, solid, iso- to hypodense to renal parenchyma, with relatively low homogeneous contrast enhancement on early and delayed phase in 69% of cases (Fig. 21.13). There is neither venous nor lymph node involvement, and no distant metastases. The tumor stage is lower and the prognosis is better even where the nuclear grade is higher (Cho et al. 2002).

### 21.4.3 Collecting Duct Type

Collecting duct tumors are aggressively malignant, associated with an extremely poor prognosis, and account for less than 1% of malignant epithelial renal neoplasms in adults (Srigley and Eble 1998). In the WHO classification, the tumor is designated as carcinoma of the collecting ducts of Bellini, reflecting its presumed site of origin and is grouped with RCC (Eble et al. 2004). Grossly, collecting duct carcinomas are predominantly localized to the medulla but may invade the cortex distorting adjacent calyces and the renal pelvis, and infiltrate the adjacent renal parenchyma and produce a desmoplastic response. Hemorrhage, with or without necrosis, is typically present. Histologically, the classic collecting duct type of RCC is composed of a mixture of dilated tubules and papillae. Collecting duct carcinomas at presentation is metastatic to regional lymph nodes in approximately 80% of cases, to the lung or adrenal gland in 25% and to the liver in 20%. Median survival after nephrectomy has been reported to be 22 months (Dimopoulos et al. 1993).

On CT, collecting duct tumor may show minimum contrast enhancement (Fukuya et al. 1996). Medullary involvement is present in the majority of cases, but cortical involvement or an exophytic component may also be present. A cystic component may be present in the minority of cases. In large tumors, the features are frequently overshadowed by an exophytic or expansile component undistinguished from the more common cortical RCC (Pickhardt et al. 2001).

On ultrasound, the solid tumor component appears hyperechoic to normal renal parenchyma in most cases. On MRI, tumors are hypointense on T2-weighted imaging without a hypointense rim. On urography, lesions appear to show distortion of the intrarenal collecting system. On selective renal angiography, lesions are hypovascular compared with normal renal parenchyma.

### 21.4.4 Medullary Type

Medullary RCC is a distinctive entity occurring exclusively in patients with sickle cell hemoglobinopathies, mostly in patients with the sickle cell trait (Swartz et al. 2002). The tumor is not considered a subtype of collecting duct carcinoma despite its believed origin in the collecting ducts. At presentation renal medullary carcinoma has a dismal prognosis, with advanced metastatic disease and an overall mean survival after surgery of less than 4 months. Metastasis to regional lymph nodes, liver, and lung are common (Davis et al. 1995).

Radiologically, renal medullary carcinoma appears as a typical infiltrative lesion, with ill-defined mass in the renal medulla and extension into the renal sinus and cortex. Caliectasis may be seen as a result of the sinus invasion. Larger tumors expand the kidney but tend to maintain its reniform shape. The tumors show heterogeneous appearance on ultrasound and contrast enhanced CT, due to the presence of characteristic tumor necrosis (Davidson et al. 1995).

## 21.4.5 Sarcomatoid Type

Sarcomatoid RCC is present in 1.0–6.5% (Peralta-Venturina et al. 2001) of RCCs. It is large and invasive, represents high-grade transformation of different subtypes of RCC and is not a distinct histological entity. It has foci of high-grade spindle cells and reminisces a malignant fibrous histiocytoma (Eble et al. 2004). The presence of a sarcomatoid component in an RCC is a poor prognostic sign. The presence of a bulging, lobulated, soft, gray-white component indicates the possibility of a sarcomatoid element. Histologically, the sarcomatoid component is characterized by interlacing or whorled bundles or storiform pattern of spindle cells. The imaging features of sarcomatoid type RCC are not well characterized in the literature but can be similar to the subtype within which the sarcomatoid change has occurred, i.e., from well defined, circumscribed to ill-defined infiltrative lesion.

## 21.4.6 Hypovascular or Avascular Renal Cell Carcinoma

Majority of RCCs (up to 80%) are iso- and/or hypervascular with a typical distinguishing tumor blush after the arterial contrast injection on angiography (Weyman et al. 1980). This characteristic enables it to be differentiated from other renal tumors. Few of the remaining RCCs are hypovascular (Fig. 21.14) or avascular on imaging. Avascular tumors are difficult to diagnose as RCC, despite the fact that imaging modalities such as CT, MRI, and ultrasound have improved the accuracy of diagnosis of such lesions (London et al. 1989). Hypovascular or avascular RCCs can be categorized as nonclear cell carcinoma and some clear cell carcinoma accompanied by sarcomatoid changes. Papillary RCC was the most frequently observed hypovascular or avascular renal tumor (Onishi et al. 2002). The vascularity differs among the variants, with chromophobe cell type being the second most common hypovascular or avascular tumors. Cyst-associated RCC was the third most frequently observed hypovascular or avascular RCC. Sarcomatoid, spindle cell, and collecting duct carcinoma are the remaining less frequent variants with hypovascularity.

## 21.5 Hereditary Renal Cell Carcinoma

Hereditary renal carcinoma makes up approximately 4% of the total number of cases. These cancers include von Hippel-Lindau disease (VHL; Fig. 21.15), hereditary papillary renal cancer (HPRC), hereditary leiomyoma renal cell carcinoma (HLRCC), Birt-Hogg-Dubé syndrome (BHD), hereditary renal oncocytoma, familial renal oncocytoma, medullary carcinoma of the kidney, and tuberous sclerosis (TS) (Choyke et al. 2003).

Hereditary cancers are typically multifocal and bilateral, and the radiologists are often the first to

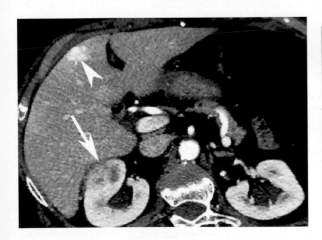

**Fig. 21.14** Contrast-enhanced axial CT scan at arterial phase shows heterogeneous mostly hypodense lesion of the anterior midpole of the right kidney (*arrow*) corresponding to RCC. There is also a hypervascular liver metastasis (*arrowhead*)

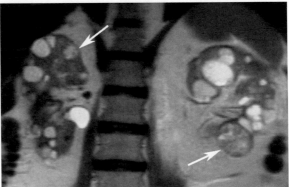

**Fig. 21.15** Coronal T2-weighted MRI of the upper abdomen in a patient with von Hippel-Lindau syndrome demonstrates bilateral solid small RCCs (*arrows*) and multiple renal cysts. Patient also had pancreatic cyst and cerebellar and cervical spinal cord hemangioblastomas (*not shown*)

raise the possibility of a hereditary cause for a particular renal cancer. It is therefore important to be familiar with the expanding list of diseases known to predispose to renal cancers (Miyazaki and Takahashi 2006). Imaging features of the above mentioned hereditary renal cancers are described below. Medullary carcinoma of the kidney has been described in Sect. 21.4.4.

## 21.5.1 von Hippel-Lindau Disease

About 40% of VHL patients develop radiologically evident renal cancers. Small tumorets are scattered throughout the renal parenchyma, but these are not visible to the naked eye. Only a few of many such lesions grow large enough to become apparent on CT (Fig. 21.16). This unusual feature is characteristic to VHL. Also, in VHL,

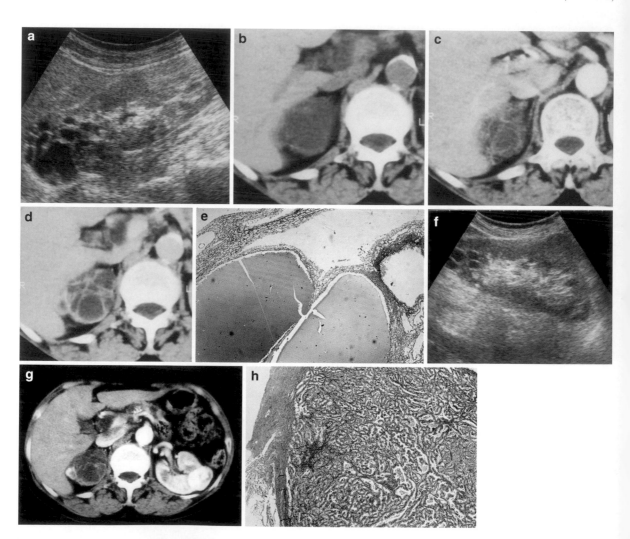

**Fig. 21.16** (**a–h**) Multilocular cystic RCC and solid RCC in a 65-year-old woman. (a) Longitudinal ultrasound image reveals a multilocular mass in the right kidney, approximately 4 cm in diameter. (**b**) Unenhanced axial and (**c, d**) dynamic contrast-enhanced CT scans through the tumor demonstrate slight enhancement and wall irregularity in the septa; however, there is no definite enhancement in the tumor parenchyma. Partial nephrectomy of the right kidney was performed. (**e**) Photomicrograph of the multilocular cystic tumor reveals an atypical hyperplastic layer, suggesting cystic clear cell renal carcinoma (hematoxylin and eosin stain; original magnification, ×25). (**f**) Longitudinal ultrasound image reveals a hypoechoic solid mass in the left kidney, approximately 3 cm in diameter. (**g**) Axial contrast-enhanced CT scan through the left renal tumor demonstrates mild enhancement; however, its surrounding rim is not visualized. Partial nephrectomy of the left kidney was performed. (**h**) Photomicrograph of the solid tumor shows a clear cell renal carcinoma with an alveolar configuration. Microcystic changes with hemorrhage are also seen (hematoxylin and eosin stain; original magnification, ×25). Images reproduced from Miyazaki and Takahashi (2006), with permission

bilateral tumors can take many forms, i.e., they can appear as cysts, cystic renal cancers and solid renal cancers (Choyke et al. 1995). Serial pre- and postcontrast CT imaging is recommended for patients with VHL. Patients with minimal disease can be scanned at 1–2-year intervals, whereas patients with active renal tumors need to be seen more frequently (every 6–12 months). In patients with lesions of borderline size (approximately 3 cm) even more frequent studies may be performed. MRI with gadolinium chelate administration is a viable alternative (Ho et al. 2002). Ultrasound is less accurate than other techniques for detecting and characterizing renal masses in VHL and should not be relied on exclusively (Jamis-Dow et al. 1996).

### 21.5.2 Hereditary Papillary Renal Cancer

The lesions of HPRC tend to be hypovascular and may show only slight enhancement on contrast-enhanced CT, and some lesions may be mistaken for cysts (Choyke et al. 1997). Both pre- and postcontrast helical CT are required. Enhancement on MRI after gadolinium chelate administration is often only modest (Choyke et al. 1997; Ho et al. 2002). Renal ultrasound can be misleading because the small lesions (<3 cm) are often isoechoic, and thus should not be used to monitor patients with HPRC (Choyke et al. 1997).

### 21.5.3 Hereditary Leiomyoma Renal Cell Carcinoma

The renal tumors in HLRCC are usually solitary, unilateral and hypovascular, but have a tendency to metastasize even when small. In addition to screening for renal cancer, patients should be screened for uterine leiomyomas and leiomyosarcomas. CT is used to screen for HLRCC and to assess the status of the uterus. MRI and ultrasound are suitable substitutes when contrast-enhanced CT is unavailable (Miyazaki and Takahashi 2006).

### 21.5.4 Birt-Hogg-Dubé Syndrome

The renal tumors seen in BHD are commonly, but not always, chromophobe carcinomas or oncocytomas.

Both clear cell and papillary tumors have also been seen in BHD (Pavlovich et al. 2002). The chromophobe or mixed-cell types typically demonstrate moderate uniform enhancement on CT. Imaging of BHD should always include scans of the lungs and abdomen, because multiple pulmonary cysts and asymptomatic pneumothoraces may be seen.

### 21.5.5 Familial Renal Oncocytoma

The diagnosis is based on the identification of multiple oncocytomas in one or more family members. On imaging, the lesions are indistinguishable from malignant renal cancers and must be treated as if they were renal cancers (Davidson et al. 1993). Renal function is frequently impaired and these patients are often scanned with MRI. Lifelong monitoring with imaging studies is recommended.

### 21.5.6 Tuberous Sclerosis

The most common manifestations of TS in the kidneys are cysts and AMLs. However, about one-third of AMLs may not contain fat visible on CT and are thus difficult to differentiate from cancer. Occasionally, renal cancers are the presenting sign of TS. Multifocality and bilaterality are characteristic to renal cancers associated with TS (Torres et al. 1997).

## 21.6 Staging of Renal Cell Carcinoma

Currently, the most commonly used staging system is the TNM system of the American Joint Committee on Cancer (Table 21.2). The patient's overall disease stage is determined by American Joint Committee on Cancer stage groupings (Table 21.3). Occasionally, the old Robson's classification of RCC is also used (Table 21.4).

### 21.6.1 Imaging Modalities for Staging

Current practice to stage RCC uses the well established MDCT or MRI. These modalities have their

**Table 21.2** The TNM classification

| Primary tumor (T) | Regional lymph nodes (N)[a] | Distant metastasis (M) |
|---|---|---|
| TX: primary tumor cannot be assessed | NX: regional lymph nodes cannot be assessed | MX: distant metastasis cannot be assessed |
| T0: no evidence of primary tumor | N0: no regional lymph node metastasis | M0: no distant metastasis |
| T1: tumor 7 cm or less in greatest dimension limited to the kidney | N1: metastasis in a single regional lymph node | M1: distant metastasis |
| T2: tumor more than 7 cm in greatest dimension limited to the kidney | N2: metastasis in more than one regional lymph node | |
| T3: tumor extends into major veins or invades adrenal gland or perinephric tissues but not beyond Gerota's fascia | | |
| T3a: tumor invades adrenal gland or perinephric tissues but not beyond Gerota's fascia | | |
| T3b: tumor grossly extends into the renal vein(s) or vena cava below the diaphragm | | |
| T3c: tumor grossly extends into the renal vein(s) or vena cava above the diaphragm | | |
| T4: tumor invades beyond Gerota's fascia | | |

[a]Laterality does not affect the N classification

**Table 21.3** American joint committee RCC stage grouping

| Stage | TNM |
|---|---|
| I | T1, N0, M0 |
| II | T2, N0, M0 |
| III | T1/T2, N1, M0<br>T3a, N0/N1, M0<br>T3b, N0/N1, M0<br>T3c, N0/N1, M0 |
| IV | T4, N0/N1, M0<br>Any T, N2, M0<br>Any T, Any N, M1 |

**Table 21.4** Robson's RCC classification

| Stage | Tumor spread |
|---|---|
| I | Confined to kidney |
| II | Through renal capsule but confined to Gerota's fascia |
| IIIA | Involvement of renal vein or IVC |
| IIIB | Involvement of local lymph nodes |
| IIIC | Involvement of vessel(s) and nodes |
| IV | Spread to local organs or distant metastases |

advantages, pitfalls and varying accuracies. The anatomic extent of the tumor (Fig. 21.17) is the important prognosticator of survival. The 5-year survival rate in tumors confined to organ is 60–90%, while it drops to 5–10% in tumors with distant metastases (Thrasher and Paulson 1993). Survival rates for RCC by T stage are summarized in Table 21.5. CT is the imaging modality of choice as it has staging accuracy of 91% (Catalano et al. 2003). Early stage RCC confined to the organ can be detected incidentally on cross-sectional imaging performed for other indications. Tumors less than 7 cm in diameter are staged as T1 and tumors >7 cm diameter as T2, reflecting the impact of tumor size on survival (Russo 2000).

The under- and over-staging of perinephric invasions is commonly seen in CT staging. The presence of an enhancing nodule in perinephric space is a specific finding of stage T3a, but has 46% sensitivity (Johnson et al. 1987). Tumor spread into the renal vein and inferior vena cava is seen in approximately 23% (Russo 2000) and 4–10% of the patients, respectively, commonly on the right side (Gill et al. 1994). This is stage T3b, the 5 year survival of which is 32–64% if the endoluminal thrombus is present without vessel wall invasion (Kallman et al. 1992). MDCT and electron beam CT have great capabilities to demonstrate the tumor spread into the venous channels with negative

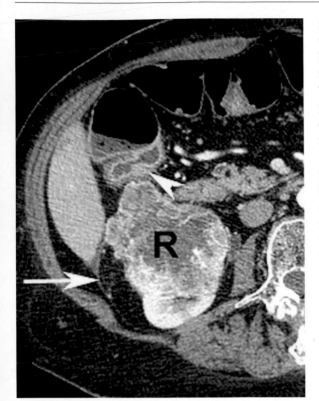

**Fig. 21.17** Contrast-enhanced axial CT image at the level of right kidney (*R*) demonstrates a large exophytic heterogeneously enhancing mass that extends beyond the gerota's fascia (*arrow*) with loss of fat planes between the mass and the right colon (*arrowhead*) consistent with colonic invasion

**Table 21.5** Survival rates for RCC by T stage

| Renal malignancy | Cancer-specific survival | |
|---|---|---|
| T stage | 5 years | 10 years |
| T1 | 95% | 95% |
| T2 | 88% | 81% |
| T3 | 59% | 43% |
| T4 | 20% | 14% |

predictive value of 97% and positive predictive value of 92%. This is best observed in the corticomedullary phase of enhancement (Birnbaum et al. 1996).

The tumor thrombus appears as a low attenuating filling defect on contrast-enhanced CT within the lumen. Associated changes in the vessel lumen caliber and collateral draining can be additional pointers to presence of thrombus (Welch and LeRoy 1997). The tumor thrombus reveals contrast heterogeneity indicating neovascularization and/or direct continuity with the mass, which differentiate it from bland thrombus (Zagoria et al. 1995). The superior level of tumor thrombi extension determines the surgical approach. The extension is best seen in the late corticomedullary phase. False positive diagnosis of intraluminal thrombi can be made due to streaming of unopacified blood returning from lower limbs (Sheth et al. 2001).

MRI is useful in detection, delineation and differentiation of solid and cystic renal lesions, and is also helpful in evaluating small lesions. MRI has a higher accuracy, but due to less availability of the scanner it remains to be the second choice. It is better than MDCT in its superior soft tissue resolution, multiplanar capabilities, and ability to delineate lesions at early stages. MRI is preferred for thrombus evaluation due to optimal venous opacification required for differentiating bland from tumor thrombus and accurate mapping of the extent of tumor thrombi (Hallscheidt et al. 2000). In particular, MRI plays a crucial role in determining the extent of caval thrombus because management of intracardiac extension requires the assistance of cardiac surgeons. Evaluation of perirenal lymphnode or distant metastases is preferred on MRI, but the evaluation of bowel loops and mesentery is better on CT. These capabilities make MRI an excellent staging modality that should be used when the CT findings are equivocal (Barker and Zagoria 2006).

### 21.6.2 Follow-Up Imaging

Follow up MDCT or MRI is performed for surveillance after surgery (Figs. 21.18 and 21.19) or ablation treatment. On follow-up imaging of ablation procedure, there should be no enhancement or interval increase in size. However, peri-ablational site enhancement (thin, symmetric, concentric enhancement) can be seen up to 6 months secondary to thermal injury associated with inflammation. Irregular peripheral nodular enhancement or residual enhancement within the tumor itself is concerning for residual or recurrent tumor. Most cases of incomplete treatment become manifest during the first year after therapy.

In addition, complications related to surgery or ablative therapies, such as hematoma, urinomas, and abscess formation can also be detected on follow-up imaging (Prasad et al. 2008).

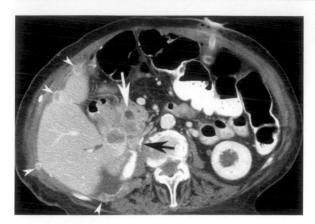

**Fig. 21.18** Contrast-enhanced axial CT scan 1 year after right nephrectomy shows local recurrence with large heterogeneous enhancing mass in the right kidney bed (*white arrow*). There are also multiple peritoneal seeding metastases (*arrowheads*). Note is made of surgical clips at the right kidney bed (*black arrow*)

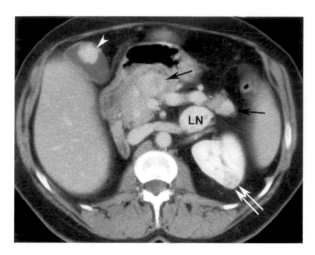

**Fig. 21.19** Contrast-enhanced axial CT scan shows multiple enhancing metastases to the gallbladder (*arrowhead*), pancreatic head and tail (*arrows*), and celiac trunk lymph node (*LN*) from a previously resected right kidney RCC. Note is made of a contralateral new RCC at the midpole of the left kidney (*double arrows*)

## 21.7 Imaging of Metastases and Recurrence

Nearly 20–60% of RCCs are diagnosed with distant metastases at the time of presentation, i.e., the metastasis is often diagnosed before the primary tumor (Skinner et al. 1971; Bohnenkamp et al. 1980; Takashi et al. 1995). The lungs (Fig. 21.20) followed by the osseous elements (Fig. 21.21) are the two most common sites, accounting

for about 20–40% of metastases (Bohnenkamp et al. 1980; Henriksson et al. 1992). Other sites of metastases include liver (Figs. 21.10, 21.14, and 21.22), peritoneum (Fig. 21.18), gallbladder (Fig. 21.19), pancreas (Fig. 21.19), pleura (Fig. 21.23), and muscle (Fig. 21.24). RCC must be considered among differential diagnoses for any metastatic bone tumor with an unknown primary tumor (Dorfman and Czerniak 1998).

For bone metastases, the most common sites of occurrence are the thoracolumbar spine, pelvic bone, ribs (Fig. 21.10c), and proximal humerus and femur. Solitary metastases are often found in the pelvis, spine, and long tubular bones (Saitoh 1981; Wilner 1982; Resnick and Niwayama 1995). Metastases in the small bones of the extremities are also reported (Forbes et al. 1977; Ghert et al. 2001). Most lesions develop in the metaphysis, but epiphyseal extension or diaphyseal lesions are also observed (Forbes et al. 1977). The predominant radiographic finding is osteolysis (Resnick and Niwayama 1995). The lesions are either purely osteolytic or predominantly osteolytic in about 90% of cases (Wilner 1982). Mixed osteolytic and osteosclerotic patterns are found in only a minority of lesions (Fig. 17.4) (Wilner 1982). Very occasionally, osteoblastic metastasis may occur (Neugut et al. 1981).

Distant metastases to liver (Fig. 21.14) and bone are generally easy to identify with CT or MRI. Organ-appropriate window settings of scans should be done to maximize the CT visualization of metastatic lesions. Since RCC metastases are often hypervascular, they are difficult to detect in the enhanced liver. CT images of the liver during the hepatic arterial phase of liver enhancement are therefore helpful in identifying many of these lesions. With MRI, hepatic metastatic deposits can be readily detected and distinguished from benign lesions such as hemangiomas and cysts. Splenic metastases can be very difficult to identify because of the MRI characteristics of the spleen, which can mask focal tumors. MRI may be more sensitive than CT in the detection of unsuspected bony metastases because of its exquisite bone marrow imaging capability (Barker and Zagoria 2006). Additional imaging modalities for metastases detection include bone scanning, which has been deemed superior to plain radiography, although a normal bone scan result does not exclude the possibility of bone metastases (Cole et al. 1975; Kim et al. 1983). PET can define metastatic disease in renal cancer (Hain and Maisey 2003) but its role in detection of bone metastasis in renal cancer remains to be clarified.

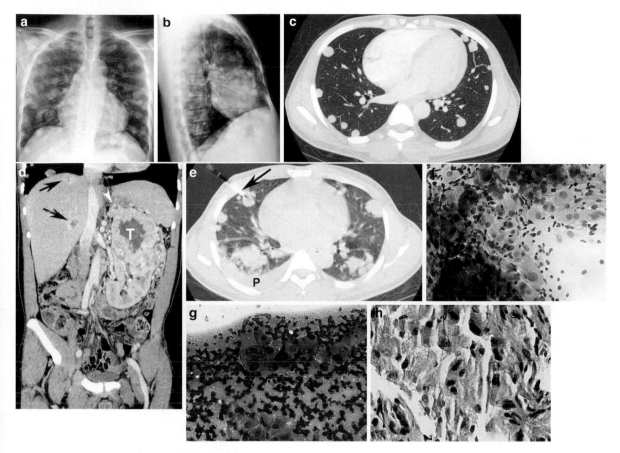

**Fig. 21.20** (**a–h**) Forty-five-year-old man presented with dyspnea without significant clinical history. (**a**) Anteroposterior and (**b**) lateral chest radiographs show innumerable lung nodules without pleural effusion or lymph node enlargement. (**c**) Axial chest CT scan confirms multiple bilateral lung nodules. (**d**) Coronal abdominal CT reformatted image shows a huge heterogeneous tumor at the upper pole of the left kidney (*T*) with central necrosis. There are several heterogeneously enhancing liver (*arrows*) and left adrenal gland (*arrowhead*) metastases. (**e**) Axial chest CT scan at the time of biopsy performed 4 days later shows the needle tip within of the middle lobe nodules (*arrow*) and new right pleural effusion (*P*). The tumor was vimentin and CD10 positive and CK7 and CK20 negative (*not shown*). (**f**) Papanicolau stain shows nuclear polymorphism. (**g**) Diff-Quick stain shows abundant cytoplasm vacuolated cytoplasm. (**h**) Photomicrograph of the tumor shows moderate degree of pleomorphism and cytoplasm clarity in keeping with clear RCC grade III (hematoxylin and eosin stain; original magnification, ×25)

## 21.8 An Overview of Role of Biopsy and Interventional Techniques

### 21.8.1 Percutaneous Biopsy of Renal Masses

A lot of benign renal masses are either incidentally discovered in asymptomatic patients at imaging or after surgery for presumed RCC. Many studies have also
found that 10–15% of solid renal masses are histologically benign. This differentiation of RCC from benign renal lesions is difficult on imaging studies alone. Percutaneous renal mass biopsy (Fig. 21.25) is being increasingly performed for definitive characterization of renal masses (Prasad et al. 2008). According to a study by Beland et al. (2007) imaging-guided biopsy was diagnostic in 90% of consecutive biopsies and the diagnosis of a benign lesion was made in 27% of diagnostic biopsies. In select cases, ultrasound or CT-guided

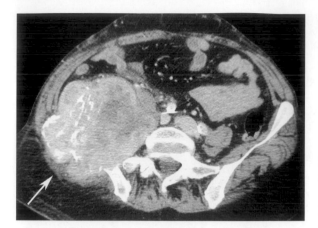

**Fig. 21.21** Fifty-eight-year-old man with previously resected right RCC. Contrast-enhanced CT scan of the abdomen shows a very large destructive bony lesion of the right iliac crest (*arrow*)

renal mass biopsy is a useful technique that can be performed with minimal morbidity and complications. For a more detailed discussion of renal mass biopsy, please see Chap. 9.

## 21.8.2 Radiofrequency Ablation

Radical nephrectomy used to be the standard treatment of RCC. However, the fact that small (<4 cm) indolent lesions with a slow growth rate (0.2–1.2 cm/year) occur frequently as asymptomatic tumors, particularly in elderly patients, has lead to the exploration of less invasive treatments. The introduction of laparoscopic radical and partial nephrectomy has lead to decreased recovery time, but they are technically difficult to perform. The interest in percutaneous ablation of RCC has increased as less invasive alternative to conventional or laparoscopic surgery or ablation. Since the first ablative therapy in 1997, ablative therapies under image-guidance are increasingly used to treat renal cancers (Fig. 21.25). The first percutaneous radiofrequency ablation (RFA) of a renal tumor was performed in 1998 (Gervais et al. 2000). The safety and short-term efficacy of RFA for routine clinical use have been acceptable in patients without co-morbid conditions and with life expectancies of longer than 10 years.

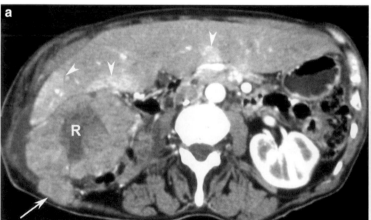

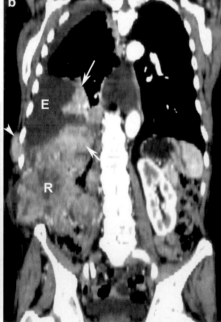

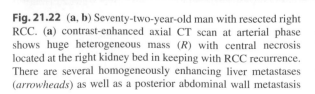

**Fig. 21.22** (**a, b**) Seventy-two-year-old man with resected right RCC. (**a**) contrast-enhanced axial CT scan at arterial phase shows huge heterogeneous mass (*R*) with central necrosis located at the right kidney bed in keeping with RCC recurrence. There are several homogeneously enhancing liver metastases (*arrowheads*) as well as a posterior abdominal wall metastasis

(*arrow*). (**b**) Coronal thoracic and abdominal CT reformatted images shows large diffuse right pleural metastases (*arrows*) with right pleural effusion (*E*), a right chest wall metastasis (*arrowhead*), and the large right RCC recurrence (*R*). The transition between the right pleural metastases and kidney recurrence is not well delineated

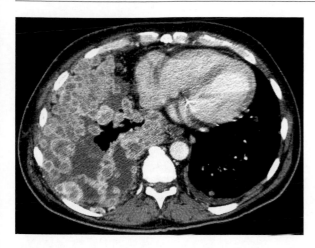

**Fig. 21.23** Fifty-six-year-old man with resected RCC. Contrast-enhanced CT scan of the chest shows innumerable heterogeneously enhancing right pleural metastases resulting in ipsilateral lung collapse

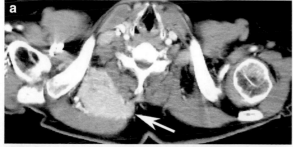

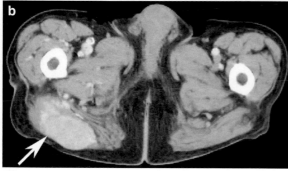

**Fig. 21.24** (**a**, **b**) Sixty-two-year-old man with RCC. Contrast-enhanced CT scans show large enhancing metastatic lesions to the region of right serratus anterior and rhomboid muscles (**a**, *arrow*) and gluteus maximus (**b**, *arrow*) muscles

The aims of RFA are twofold: (1) to treat patients with a high surgical risk and; (2) to preserve functional renal parenchyma in patients with limited reserve or have multifocal RCC (Schiller et al. 2005). RFA procedures can be performed under CT or ultrasound

guidance, under sedation or general anesthesia. Each RF generator kit includes an electrode, inflow tubing set, outflow tubing set, ground pads, and introducer (with cluster electrode only). The grounding pads are applied to the thighs, at an equal distance from the treatment site. The inflow and outflow tubing are responsible for the flow of iced water or saline to and from the electrode tip. The active tip of the electrodes is typically 2–3 cm in length and lies entirely inside the tumor to prevent damage to the surrounding tissues such as ureter or major vessels. After positioning the electrode tip in the tumor under image guidance, the tumor is ablated with one or more heating cycles lasting 12 min each. The current is pulsed in response to a rapid increase in impedance, which is caused by charring of tissue and subsequent inhibition of heat diffusion. As the geometry of the burn diameter may not cover the entire lesion, more than one overlapping treatments are frequently required.

After an RFA procedure, a tumor free margin of up to a centimeter around the tumor should be produced. A preablation biopsy at the same sitting or at an earlier session is commonly performed and may alter the treatment or follow-up of these patients. A benign diagnosis on biopsy precludes an unnecessary RFA procedure.

When US guidance is used, intense echoes spreading from the electrode tip can be seen. This appearance is secondary to the microbubbles produced by tissue ablation. This appearance is transient and the echogenicity of the focal renal lesion becomes heterogeneous after a few minutes (Singh et al. 2006).

When RFA is successful, lack of enhancement on follow-up CT or MRI is observed. Treated tumors are seen as a hypodense or hypointense defect in the renal parenchyma. The exophytic tumors retain the configuration of the original tumor with minimal decrease in size after RFA. The findings on follow-up CT or MRI also include fatty replacement at the interface with normal kidney and soft tissue stranding in fat around the tumor (Gervais et al. 2003; Matsumoto et al. 2004).

Although RFA is a low morbidity procedure, complications do occur and include hemorrhage, lumbar plexus damage, urinoma, ureteral stricture, and abscess. Postprocedural pain along the distribution of the lumbar plexus is known to occur in patients treated by the posterior approach where the psoas muscle is heated. Needle-track seeding after RFA of a renal mass has also been reported (Mayo-Smith et al. 2004).

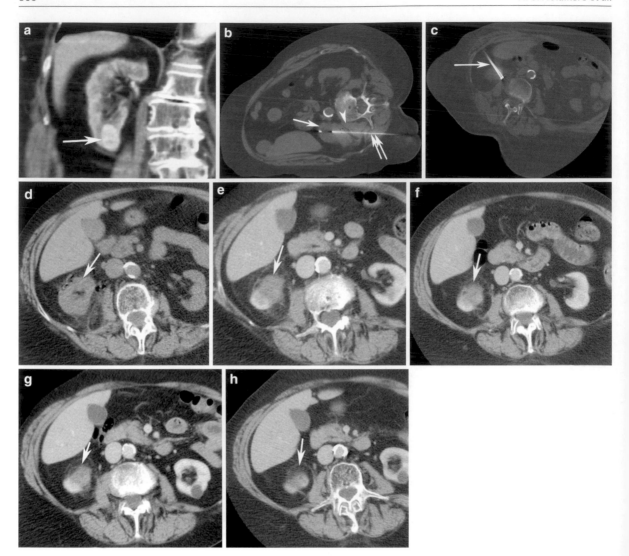

**Fig. 21.25** (**a**) Contrast-enhanced coronal reformat CT image shows an enhancing lesion (*arrow*) of the lower pole of the right kidney representing an RCC. (**b**) Lateral decubitus axial CT scan at the time of biopsy shows the tip of the needle within the previously described mass of the right kidney (*arrow*). Note is made of small hematoma (*arrowhead*) adjacent to the biopsy needle (*double arrows*) pathway. (**c**) Slightly left oblique decubitus axial CT scan during the RFA shows 15 cm cluster Radionics cool-tip electrode (*arrow*) with 2.5 cm active tip within the right lower pole RCC. (**d**) Unenhanced axial CT scan immediately post RFA shows self contained hypodense lesion (*arrow*) of the right lower pole synonym of successful treatment of the RCC. Follow-up in regular interval contrast-enhanced axial CT scans show stable self-contained hypodense lesion (*arrow*) without evidence of recurrence at (**e**) 1, (**f**) 3, (**g**) 6, and (**h**) 12 months post RFA

For a more detailed discussion of renal mass biopsy, please see Chap. 23.

## 21.8.3 Transarterial Embolization

Another minimally invasive therapy that has been utilized to treat RCC and its complications in surgically inoperable cases is transarterial embolization (TAE; Fig. 21.26). TAE is indicated: (a) to control symptoms related to the primary tumor in patients with advanced disease; (b) to provide an alternative to radical surgery and; (c) to be used as preoperative treatment. TAE is primarily used to control renal cancer-related symptoms such as hemorrhage from the tumor or after a biopsy, renal arteriovenous shunts or pseudoaneurysms (Albani and Novick 2003; Majhail et al. 2003), pain,

**Fig. 21.26** (**a**, **b**) Palliative embolization of a renal urothelial tumor invading the entire left kidney in a 58-year-old woman. (**a**) Selective angiogram shows a moderate tumoral hypervascularization. (**b**) The left renal artery appears completely occluded after palliative embolization using 300- to 500-μm microspheres and coils

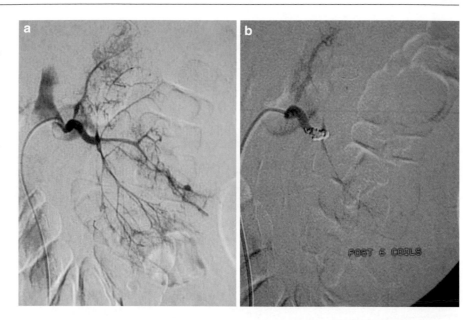

and compressive mass (McLean and Meranze 1985; Kuether et al. 1996). Cancer in a solitary kidney, bilateral tumors, and end-stage renal carcinoma are ideally treated by TAE as surgery is not preferred (Kalman and Varenhorst 1999). TAE can be combined with percutaneous RFA of renal tumor in a solitary kidney (Hall et al. 2000).

The embolic agents used are either temporary or permanent occlusion materials and the choice depends on the utility and duration of the occlusion required, and on the decision of desirable proximal or distal devascularization. The individual arterial anatomy and accessibility also determines the decision. Temporary embolic agent, such as gelatin sponge, is usually favored (Lanigan et al. 1992; Kalman and Varenhorst 1999) for emergency embolization in patients with intractable hematuria or for preoperative embolization. If a permanent and a more definitive embolization is desired then a nonabsorbable particles (such as nonspherical polyvinyl alcohol particles or calibrated microspheres) can be used to provide targeted tumoral devascularization.

TAE can also be used as a palliative therapeutic measure in patients with bone metastases, which are usually hypervascular (Chatziioannou et al. 2000), mainly to minimize pain and/or control bleeding in unresectable tumors or before surgery (Chuang et al. 1979). Successful renal TAE depends on selection of appropriate selective or super-selective catheterization and adequate operator experience.

Complication rates during renal TAE reported in the literature vary from 10 to 20%. Postembolization

syndrome is commonly encountered, along with constitutional symptoms such as fever, back pain in the embolized site, nausea, and/or vomiting for several days. This syndrome is a part of the process and is easily controlled with appropriate medication.

Reflux of liquid embolic materials into the proximal main renal artery may potentially occlude the main artery. A balloon-assisted occlusion of the main renal artery would potentially prevent this complication (Park et al. 2000). A super-selective coaxial microcatheter is used to target vessels distal to segmental arteries. Coaxial systems facilitate super-selective embolization with targeted tumoral devascularization sparing normal renal parenchyma (Beaujeux et al. 1995). Also, accidental embolization of nontarget vessels including visceral arteries, peripheral arteries of the lower extremities, and spinal cord branches are commonly seen complications of renal TAE. These may result in renal failure, colon infarction and spinal cord ischemia. A mortality rate of 3.3% and major morbidity of 9.9% is reported (Lammer et al. 1985).

### 21.8.4 Nephron-Sparing Surgery

NSS has established itself as a treatment option for RCC in recent times (Schlichter et al. 2000). NSS has replaced radical nephrectomy in treatment of RCC in patients who needs to preserve renal function, or to avoid anephric state in patients with a single kidney

**Table 21.6** Indications for nephron-sparing surgery (NSS)

| Imperative indications | | Elective indications |
|---|---|---|
| Absolute | Relative | |
| Anatomically or functionally solitary kidney | Future risk for dysfunction | Small, localized, often incidental RCC with a normal contralateral kidney |
| Past nephrectomy by contralateral RCC | Calculus disease | |
| Functionally solitary kidney due to benign renal disease | Chronic pyelonephritis | |
| Unilateral renal agenesis | Renal artery stenosis | |
| Bilateral synchronous RCC | Ureteral reflux | |
| Severe renal insufficiency | Systemic disease (i.e., diabetes mellitus) | |

and thus avoid dialysis (Grabstald and Aviles 1968). NSS has now being applied even in patients with a normal contralateral kidney due to good results of NSS over radical nephrectomy (Schiff et al. 1979). Indications for NSS are summarized in Table 21.6.

The success and preference of NSS is due to recent advancements in radiology and surgical techniques. Advances in radiological imaging techniques allow early detection of incidental RCC and detailed preoperative evaluation noninvasively. Also, improved surgical techniques minimize the risk of ischemic renal injury and hemorrhage. Furthermore, better postoperative management methods have reduced the risk of complications (Duque et al. 1998; Gacci et al. 2001). NSS has provided evidence of long-term functional advantage due to preservation of unaffected renal parenchyma, with satisfactory cancer control and patient satisfaction (Filipas et al. 2000; Fergany et al. 2000; Shinohara et al. 2001; Delakas et al. 2002). New minimally invasive experimental technologies such as laparoscopic partial nephrectomy and laparoscopic cryoablation are also being utilized to perform NSS.

Staging for nephron sparing surgeries requires delineation and detection of all lesions to ensure complete surgical resection while preserving maximum amount of functioning parenchyma. Three-dimensional

CT helps in precise localization of the mass and its relationship to renal surface, the collecting system and renal vessels (Zagoria et al. 1995). The arterial and venous anatomy of kidney is seen on three-dimensional CT angiography.

The complexity of NSS procedures leads to some avoidable complications such as postoperative mortality (1.5% or less), acute renal failure (6.0–17.1%) and urinary fistula (1.6–17.4%). These can be avoided by proper patient selection, thorough preoperative imaging, exacting surgical techniques and good postoperative management (Campbell et al. 1994; Polascik et al. 1995; Duque et al. 1998; Delakas et al. 2002; Ghavamian et al. 2002). Other reported complications are postoperative hemorrhage (2.4%), infection with or without retroperitoneal abscess (3.2%), injury to adjacent viscera such as the spleen (0.6%), and perioperative medical complications. The reoperative rate after NSS remains low, 0–3% in most series (Uzzo and Novick 2001). For a more detailed discussion of renal mass biopsy, please see Chap. 32.

## 21.9 Conclusion

Incidental detection of kidney cancers on imaging studies performed for another purpose is very common nowadays. The radiologist should be aware of this and once a suspected mass is identified, further investigations should be instituted. Solid or complex cystic lesions are best characterized by CT or MRI with contrast enhancement. These cross-sectional modalities are also indispensable in the staging and restaging of suspected RCC lesions. Other modalities including ultrasound and PET can also be utilized to play a complimentary role. Image-guided percutaneous renal biopsy is safe and accurate in sampling the lesion and reaching a final histopathological diagnosis. Image-guided renal mass biopsy is useful for avoiding unnecessary surgery for benign masses and in the diagnosis of renal malignancies. As the frequency of detection of renal masses increases and the utility of percutaneous biopsy and minimally invasive interventions including RFA, TAE and NSS become more common, we are likely to see these procedures become more frequently employed in patient management.

# References

Albani JM, Novick AC (2003) Renal artery pseudoaneurysm after partial nephrectomy: three case reports and a literature review. Urology 62:227–231

Barker DW, Zagoria RJ (2006) Renal cell carcinoma. In: Guermazi A (ed) Imaging of kidney cancer. Springer, Berlin, pp 103–124

Beaujeux R, Saussine C, al-Fakir A et al. (1995) Superselective endo-vascular treatment of renal vascular lesions. J Urol 153:14–17

Beland MD, Mayo-Smith WW, Dupuy DE et al. (2007) Diagnostic yield of 58 consecutive imaging-guided biopsies of solid renal masses: should we biopsy all that are indeterminate? AJR Am J Roentgenol 188:792–797

Birnbaum BA, Jacobs JE, Ramchandani P (1996) Multiphasic renal CT: comparison of renal mass enhancement during the corticomedullary and nephrographic phases. Radiology 200:753–758

Bohnenkamp B, Rhomberg W, Sonnentag W et al. (1980) Prognosis of metastatic renal cell carcinoma related to the pattern of metastasis (author's translation). J Cancer Res Clin Oncol 96:105–114

Bracken RB (1987) Renal carcinoma: clinical aspects and therapy. Semin Roentgenol 22:241–247

Bruder E, Passera O, Harms D et al. (2004) Morphologic and molecular characterization of renal cell carcinoma in children and young adults. Am J Surg Pathol 28: 1117–1132

Campbell SC, Novick AC, Streem SB et al. (1994) Complications of nephron sparing surgery for renal tumors. J Urol 151: 1177–1180

Catalano C, Fraioli F, Laghi A et al. (2003) High-resolution multidetector CT in the preoperative evaluation of patients with renal cell carcinoma. AJR Am J Roentgenol 180: 1271–1277

Chatziioannou AN, Johnson ME, Pneumaticos SG et al. (2000) Preoperative embolization of bone metastases from renal cell carcinoma. Eur Radiol 10:593–596

Cho KR, Park CM, Chung HH et al. (2002) Spiral CT findings of chromophobe renal cell carcinoma: correlation with pathologic features and prognosis. J Korean Radiol Soc 46: 57–62

Choyke PL, Glenn GM, Walther MM et al. (1995) von Hippe-Lindau disease: genetic, clinical, and imaging features. Radiology 194:629–642

Choyke PL, Glenn GM, Walther MM et al. (2003) Hereditary renal cell cancers. Radiology 226:33–46

Choyke PL, Watther MM, Glenn GM et al. (1997) Imaging features of hereditary papillary renal cancers. J Comput Assist Tomogr 21:737–741

Chuang VP, Wallace S, Swanson D et al. (1979) Arterial occulusion in the management of pain from metastatic renal carcinoma. Radiology 133:611–614

Cohan RH, Sherman LS, Korobkin M et al. (1995) Renal masses: assessment of corticomedullary-phase and nephrographic-phase CT scans. Radiology 195:445–451

Cole AT, Mandell J, Fried FA et al. (1975) The place of bone scan in the diagnosis of renal cell carcinoma. J Urol 114: 364–365

Corica FA, Iczkowski KA, Cheng L et al. (1999) Cystic renal cell carcinoma is cured by resection: a study of 24 cases with long-term follow-up. J Urol 161:408–411

Davidson AJ, Choyke PL, Hartman DS et al. (1995) Renal medullary carcinoma associated with sickle cell trait: radiologic findings. Radiology 195:83–85

Davidson AJ, Hayes WS, Hartman DS et al. (1993) Renal oncocytoma and carcinoma: failure of differentiation with CT. Radiology 186:693–696

Davis CJ, Mostofi FK, Sesterhenn IA (1995) Renal medullary carcinoma: the seventh sickle nephropathy. Am J Surg Pathol 19:1–11

Delakas D, Karyotis I, Daskalopoulos G et al. (2002) Nephron-sparing surgery for localized renal cell carcinoma with a normal contralateral kidney: a European three-center experience. Urology 60:998–1002

Dimopoulos MA, Logothetis CJ, Markowitz A et al. (1993) Collecting duct carcinoma of the kidney. Br J Urol 71: 388–391

Dorfman HD, Czerniak B (1998) Bone tumors. Mosby, St. Louis

Duque JL, Loughlin KR, O'Leary MO et al. (1998) Partial nephrectomy: alternative treatment for selected patients with renal cell carcinoma. Urology 52:584–590

Eble JN, Sauter G, Epstein JI et al. (2004) World Health Organization classification of tumours: pathology and genetics of tumours of the urinary system and male genital organs. IARC Press, Lyons

Einstein DM, Herts BR, Weaver R et al. (1995) Evaluation of renal masses detected by excretory urography: cost-effectiveness of sonography versus CT. AJR Am J Roentgenol 164:371–375

Fergany AF, Hafez KS, Novick AC (2000) Long-term results of nephron-sparing surgery for localized renal cell carcinoma: 10-year followup. J Urol 163:442–445

Filipas D, Fichtner J, Spix C et al. (2000) Nephron-sparing surgery of renal cell carcinoma with a normal opposite kidney: long-term outcome in 180 patients. Urology 56:387–392

Forbes GS, McLeod RA, Hattery RR (1977) Radiogrpahic manifestations of bone metastases from renal carcinoma. AJR Am J Roentgenol 129:61–66

Forman HP, Middleton WD, Melson GL et al. (1993) Hyperechoic renal cell carcinomas: increase in detection at US. Radiology 188:431–434

Fukuya T, Honda H, Goto K et al. (1996) Computed tomographic findings of Bellini duct carcinoma of the kidney. J Comput Assist Tomogr 20:399–403

Gacci M, Rizzo M, Lapini A et al. (2001) Imperative indications for conservative surgery for renal cell carcinoma: 20 years' experience. Urol Int 67:203–208

Gervais DA, McGovern FJ, Wood BJ et al. (2000) Radiofrequency ablation of renal cell carcinoma: early clinical experience. Radiology 217:665–672

Gervais DA, McGovern FJ, Wood BJ et al. (2003) Renal cell carcinoma: clinical experience and technical success with radio-frequency ablation of 42 tumors. Radiology 226: 417–424

Ghavamian R, Cheville JC, Lohse CM et al. (2002) Renal cell carcinoma in the solitary kidney: an analysis of complications and outcome after nephron sparing surgery. J Urol 168: 454–459

Ghert MA, Harrelson JM, Scully SP (2001) Solitary renal cell carcinoma metastasis to the hand: the need for wide excision or amputation. J Hand Surg [Am] 26:156–160

Gill IS, McClennan BL, Kerbl K et al. (1994) Adrenal involvement from renal cell carcinoma: predictive value of computerized tomography. J Urol 152:1082–1085

Grabstald H, Aviles E (1968) Renal cancer in the solitary or sole-functioning kidney. Cancer 22:973–987

Gupta NP, Ansari MS, Khaitan A et al. (2004) Impact of imaging and thrombus level in management of renal cell carcinoma extending to veins. Urol Int 72:129–134

Hain SF, Maisey MN (2003) Positron emission tomography for urological tumours. BJU Int 92:159–164

Hall WH, McGahan JP, Link DP et al. (2000) Combined embolization and percutaneous radiogrequency ablation of a solid renal tumor. AJR Am J Roentgenol 174:1592–1594

Hallscheidt P, Pomer S, Roeren T et al. (2000) Preoperative staging of renal cell carcinoma with caval thrombus: is staging in MRI justified? Prospective histopathological correlated study. Urologe A39:36–40

Henriksson C, Haraldsson G, Aldenborg F et al. (1992) Skeletal metastases in 102 patients evaluated before surgery for renal cell carcinoma. Scand J Urol Nephrol 26:363–366

Herts BR, Coll DM, Novick AC et al. (2002) Enhancement characteristics of papillary renal neoplasms revealed on triphasic helical CT on the kidneys. AJR Am J Roentgenol 178: 367–372

Ho VB, Allen SF, Hood MN et al. (2002) Renal masses: quantitative assessment of enhancement with dynamic MR imaging. Radiology 224:695–700

Hollingsworth JM, Miller DC, Daignault S et al. (2006) Rising incidence of small renal masses: a need to reassess treatment effect. J Natl Cancer Inst 98:1331–1334

Isralel GM, Hindman N, Hecht E et al. (2005) The use of opposed-phase chemical shift MRI in the diagnosis of renal angiomyolipomas. AJR Am J Roentgenol 184:1868–1872

Jadvar H, Kherbache HM, Pinski JK et al. (2003) Diagnostic role of [F-18]-FDG positron emission tomography in restaging renal cell carcinoma. Clin Nephrol 60:395–400

Jamis-Dow CA, Choyke PL, Jennings SB et al. (1996) Small (≤3cm) renal masses: detection with CT versus US and pathologic correlation. Radiology 198:785–788

Jemal A, Siegel R, Ward E et al. (2007) Cancer statistics, 2007. CA Cancer J Clin 57:43–66

Jinzaki M, Tanimoto A, Mukai M et al. (2000) Doublephase helical CT of small renal parenchymal neoplasms: correlation with pathologic findings and tumor angiogenesis. J Comput Assist Tomogr 24:835–842

John G, Semelka RC, Burdeny DA et al. (1997) Renal cell cancer: incidence of hemorrhage on MR images in patients with chronic renal insufficiency. J Magn Reson Imaging 7:157–160

Johnson CD, Dunnick NR, Cohan RH et al. (1987) Renal adenocarcinoma: CT staging of 100 tumors. AJR Am J Roentgenol 148:59–63

Kallman DA, King BF, Hattery RR et al. (1992) Renal vein and inferior vena cava tumor thrombus in renal cell carcinoma: CT, US, MRI and venacavography. J Comput Assist Tomogr 16:240–247

Kalman D, Varenhorst E (1999) The role of arterial embolization in renal cell carcinoma. Scand J Urol Nephrol 33:162–170

Kang DE, White RLJ, Zuger JH et al. (2004) Clinical use of fluorodeoxyglucose F 18 positron emission tomography for detection of renal cell carcinoma. J Urol 171:1806–1809

Kim EE, Bledin AG, Gutierrez C et al. (1983) Comparison of radionuclide images and radiographs for skeletal metastases from renal cell carcinoma. Oncology 40:284–286

Kim JK, Kim TK, Ahn HJ et al. (2002) Differentiation of subtypes of renal cell carcinoma on helical CT scans. AJR Am J Roentgenol 178:1499–1506

Kopka L, Fischer U, Zoeller G et al. (1997) Dual-phase helical CT of the kidney: value of the corticomedullary and nephrogenic phase for evaluation of renal lesions and preoperative staging of renal cell carcinoma. AJR Am J Roentgenol 169:1573–1578

Kuether TA, Nesbit GM, Barnwell SL (1996) Embolization as treatment for spinal cord compression from renal cell carcinoma: case report. Neurosurgery 39:1260–1263

Lammer J, Justich E, Schreyer H et al. (1985) Complications of renal tumor embolization. Cardiovasc Intervent Radiol 8:31–35

Lanigan D, Jurriaans E, Hammonds JC et al. (1992) The current status of embolization in renal cell carcinoma. Clin Rad 46:176–178

Leslie JA, Prihoda T, Thompson IM (2003) Serendipitous renal cell carcinoma in the post-CT era: continued evidence in improved outcomes. Urol Oncol 21:39–44

London NJ, Messions N, Kinder RB et al. (1989) A prospective study of the value of conventional CT, dynamic CT, ultrasonography and arteriography for staging renal carcinoma. Br J Urol 64:209–217

Luciani LG, Cestari R, Tallarigo C (2000) Incidental renal cell carcinoma-age and stage characterization and clinical implications: study of 1092 patients (1982–1997). Urology 56: 58–62

Macari M, Bosniak MA (1999) Delayed CT to evaluate renal masses incidentally discovered at contrast-enhanced CT: demonstration of vascularity with deenhancement. Radiology 213:674–680

Majhail NS, Urbain JL, Albani JM et al. (2003) F-18 fluorodeoxyglucose positron cmission tomography in the evaluation of distant metastases from renal cell carcinoma. J Clin Oncol 21:3995–4000

Matsumoto ED, Watumull L, Johnson DB et al. (2004) The radiographic evolution of radio frequency ablated renal tumors. J Urol 172:45–48

Mayo-Smith WW, Dupuy DE, Parikh PM et al. (2004) Imaging-guided percutaneous radiogrequency ablation of solid renal masses: techniques and outcomes of 38 treatment sessions in 32 consecutive patients. AJR Am J Roentgenol 180:1503–1508

McLean GK, Meranze SG (1985) Embolization techniques in the urinary tract. Urol Clin North Am 12:743–754

Miyazaki T, Takahashi M (2006) Hereditary kidney cancer. In: Guermazi A (ed) Imaging of kidney cancer. Springer, Berlin, pp 239–256

Murphy WM, Grignon DJ, Perlman EJ (2004) Tumor of the kidney, bladder, and related urinary structures, 4th series. Armed Forces Institute of Pathology Atlas of Tumor Pathology, Washington, DC

Neugut AI, Casper ES, Godwin TA et al. (1981) Osteoblastic metastases in renal cell carcinoma. Br J Radiol 54:1002–1004

Onishi T, Ohishi Y, Iizuka N et al. (1996) Clinicopathological study on patients with chromophobe cell renal carcinoma. Nippon Hinyokika Gakkai Zasshi 87:1167–1174

Onishi T, Oishi Y, Goto H et al. (2002) Histological features of hypovascular or avascular renal cell carcinoma: the experience at four university hospitals. Int J Clin Oncol 7: 159–164

Outwater EK, Bhatia M, Siegelman ES et al. (1997) Lipid in renal clear cell carcinoma: detection on opposed-phase gradient-echo MR images. Radiology 205:103–107

Park SI, Lee DY, Won JY et al. (2000) Renal artery embolization using a new liquid embolic material obtained by partial hydrolysis of polyvinyl acetate. Korean J Radiol 1:121–126

Patel MI, Simmons R, Kattan MW et al. (2003) Long-term follow-up of bilateral sporadic renal tumors. Urology 61:921–925

Pavlovich CP, Walther MM, Eyler RA et al. (2002) Renal tumors in the Birt-Hogg-Dubé syndrome. Am J Surg Pathol 26:1542–1552

Peralta-Venturina M, Moch H, Amin M et al. (2001) Sarcomatoid differentiation in renal cell carcinoma: a study of 101 cases. Am J Surg Pathol 25:275–284

Pickhardt PJ, Siegel CL, McLarney JK (2001) Collecting duct carcinoma of the kidney: Are imaging findings suggestive of the diagnosis? AJR Am J Roentgenol 176:627–633

Polascik TJ, Pound CR, Meng MV et al. (1995) Partial nephrectomy: technique, complications and pathological findings. J Urol 154:1312–1318

Prasad SR, Dalrymple NC, Surabhi VR (2008) Cross-sectional imaging evaluation of renal masses. Radiol Clin North Am 46:95–111, vi–vii

Press GA, McClennan BL, Melson GL et al. (1984) Papillary renal cell carcinoma: CT and sonographic evaluation. AJR Am J Roentgenol 143:1005–1009

Provet J, Tessler A, Brown J et al. (1991) Partial nephrectomy for renal cell carcinoma: indications, results and implications. J Urol 145:472–476

Resnick D, Niwayama G (1995) Tumors and tumor-like diseases. In: Resnick D, Niwayama G (eds) Diagnosis of bone and joint disorders. Saunders, Philadelphia, PA, pp 4019–4021

Reuter VE, Presti JCJ (2000) Comtemporary approach to the classification of renal epithelial tumors. Semin Oncol 27:124–137

Russo P (2000) Renal cell carcinoma: presentation, staging, and surgical treatment. Semin Oncol 27:160–176

Saitoh H (1981) Distant metastasis of renal adenocarcinoma. Cancer 48:1487–1491

Schiff M, Bagley DH, Lytton B (1979) Treatment of solitary and bilateral renal carcinomas. J Urol 121:581

Schiller JD, Gervais DA, Mueller PR (2005) Radiofrequency ablation of renal cell carcinoma. Abdom Imaging 30:442–450

Schlichter A, Wunderlich H, Junker K et al. (2000) Where are the limits of elective nephron-sparing surgery in renal cell carcinoma? Eur Urol 37:517–520

Schreyer HH, Uggowitzer MM, Ruppert-Kohlmayr A (2002) Helical CT of the urinary organs. Eur Radiol 12:575–591

Sheir KZ, El-Azab M, Mosbah A et al. (2005) Differentiation of renal cell carcinoma subtypes by multislice computerized tomography. J Urol 174:451–455; discussion 455

Sheth S, Scatarige JC, Horton KM et al. (2001) Current concepts in the diagnosis and management of renal cell carcinoma:

role of multidetector CT and three-dimensional CT. Radiographics 21:S237–S254

Shinmoto H, Yuasa Y, Tanimoto A et al. (1998) Small renal cell carcinoma: MR with pathologic correlation. J Magn Reson Imaging 8:690–694

Shinohara N, Harabayashi T, Sato S et al. (2001) Impact of nephron-sparing surgery on quality of life in patients with localized renal cell carcinoma. Eur Urol 39:114–119

Silverberg E, Holleb AI (1971) Cancer statistics, 1971. CA Cancer J Clin 21:13–31

Singh AK, Gervais DA, Hahn PF et al. (2006) Percutaneous biopsy and radiofrequency ablation. In: Guermazi A (ed) Imaging of kidney cancer. Springer, Berlin, pp 371–384

Skinner DG, Colvin RB, Vermillion CD et al. (1971) Diagnosis and management of renal cell carcinoma. A clinical and pathologic study of 309 cases. Cancer 28:1165–1177

Srigley JR, Eble JN (1998) Collecting duct carcinoma of the kidney. Semin Diagn Pathol 15:54–67

Storkel S, Eble JN, Adlakha K et al. (1997) Classification of renal cell carcinoma: Workgroup No. 1. Union Internationale Contre le Cancer (UICC) and the American Joint Committee on Cancer (AJCC). Cancer 80:987–989

Swartz MA, Karth J, Schneider DT et al. (2002) Renal medullary carcinoma; clnical, pathologic, immunohistochemical, and genetic analysis with pathogenetic implications. Urology 60:1083–1089

Szolar DH, Kammerhuber F, Altziebler S et al. (1997) Multiphasic helical CT of the kidney: increased conspicuity for detection and characterization of small (<3cm) renal masses. Radiology 202:211–217

Takahashi K, Honda M, Okubo RS et al. (1993) CT pixel mapping in the diagnosis of small angiomyolipomas of the kidneys. J Comput Assist Tomogr 17:98–101

Takashi M, Takagi Y, Sakata T et al. (1995) Surgical treatment of renal cell carcinoma metastases: progostic significance. Int Urol Nephrol 27:1–8

Thoenes W, Storkel S, Rumpelt HJ et al. (1988) Chromophobe cell renal cell carcinoma and its variants – a report on 32 cases. J Pathol 155:277–287

Thrasher JB, Paulson DF (1993) Prognostic factors in renal cancer. Urol Clin North Am 20:247–262

Torres VE, Zincle H, King BK et al. (1997) Renal manifestation of tuberous sclerosis complex. Contrib Nephrol 122:64–75

Uzzo RG, Novick AC (2001) Nephron sparing surgery for renal tumors: indications, techniques and outcomes. J Urol 166: 6–18

Watson RC, Fleming RJ, Evans JA (1968) Arteriography in the diagnosis of renal carcinoma. Review of 100 cases. Radiology 91:888–897

Welch TJ, LeRoy AJ (1997) Helical and electron beam CT scanning in the evaluation of renal vein involvement in patients with renal cell carcinoma. J Comput Assist Tomogr 21: 467–471

Weyman PJ, McClennan BL, Stabley RJ et al. (1980) Comparison of computed tomography and angiography in the evaluation of renal cell carcinoma. Radiology 137:417–424

Wilner D (1982) Radiology of bone tumors and allied disorders. Saunders, Philadelphia, PA

Yamashita Y, Ueno S, Makita O et al. (1993) Hyperechoic renal tumors: anechoic rim and intratumoral cysts in US

differentiation of renal cell carcinoma from angiomyolipoma. Radiology 188:179–182

Yuh BI, Cohan RH (1999) Different phases of renal enhancement: role in detecting and characterizating renal masses
during helical CT. AJR Am J Roentgenol 173:747–755

Zagoria RJ, Bechtold RE, Dyer RB (1995) Staging of renal adenocarcinoma: role of various imaging procedures. AJR Am
J Roentgenol 164:363–370

Zhang J, Isralel GM, Krinsky GA et al. (2004) Masses and
pseudomasses of the kidney: imaging spectrum on MR. J
Comput Assist Tomogr 28:588–595

Zhang J, Lefkowitz RA, Bach A (2007a) Imaging of kidney cancer. Radiol Clin North Am 45:119–147

Zhang J, Lefkowitz RA, Ishill NM et al. (2007b) Solid renal
cortical tumors: differentiation with CT. Radiology
244:494–504

# Rare and Secondary Tumors of the Kidney and Renal Pseudotumors

# 22

Annelies Rappaport and Raymond H. Oyen

## Contents

A. Rappaport (✉) and R.H. Oyen
Department of Radiology, University Hospitals Leuven,
Catholic University Leuven, Herestraat 49, 3000 Leuven,
Belgium
e-mail: annelies.rappaport@uzleuven.be
e-mail: raymond.oyen@uzleuven.be

**Abstract**

> As renal cell carcinoma and transitional cell carcinoma are by far the most common renal parenchymal tumoral lesions, less attention is paid to rare or secondary tumors of the kidney. Most of these lesions, benign or malignant, do not indeed have specific radiological features and differentiation from renal cell carcinoma, or transitional cell carcinoma based on imaging characteristics is often difficult or impossible. In cases lacking characteristics of renal cell carcinoma, biopsy may be required for histological diagnosis and decision on further therapeutic management. However, some imaging characteristics may be contributive to narrow the differential diagnosis, thereby enabling decisions on the therapeutic approach.

> In addition, the importance of identifying renal pseudotumors is underestimated. More pseudotumoral lesions are seen after nephron sparing surgery and thermal ablation. Knowledge of and recognizing all possible pseudotumoral renal lesions can help reducing false positive diagnosis and avoiding unnecessary invasive treatment or retreatment.

## 22.1 Secondary Tumors of the Kidney

Two types of secondary renal tumors are distinguished: renal involvement by an infiltrative tumor of an adjacent organ/structures and renal metastases.

E. Quaia (ed.), *Radiological Imaging of the Kidney*,
Medical Radiology, DOI: 10.1007/978-3-540-87597-0_22, © Springer-Verlag Berlin Heidelberg 2011

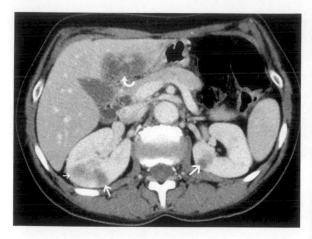

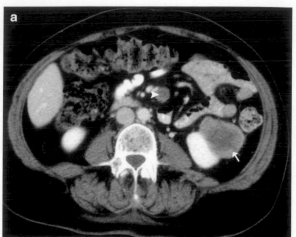

**Fig. 22.1** Liver and renal metastases from a lung carcinoma in a 52-year-old woman. Contrast-enhanced CT scan in the parenchymal phase shows bilateral small hypodense mass lesions (*arrows*) and a similar lesion posterior in the left liver lobe (*curved arrow*)

### 22.1.1  General Features

Necropsy reports estimate the frequency of renal metastasis in patients with known cancer between 2 and 20% (Abrams et al. 1950; Pascal 1980). With the routine use of CT in cancer staging, renal metastases are more frequently observed. Renal metastases are usually seen in patients with advanced disease. Most renal metastases remain asymptomatic (Choyke et al. 1987).

Primary tumors that are likely to spread to the kidney include bronchopulmonary carcinoma (Fig. 22.1), breast cancer, gastrointestinal cancers, and malignant melanoma (Fig. 22.2).

### 22.1.2  Imaging Features and Differential Diagnosis

Renal metastases are more likely to have an expansile growth pattern, while infiltrative growth pattern is highly uncommon (Pickhardt et al. 2000).

The most frequent imaging feature is that of multiple small bilateral, intracortical mass lesions, with a vascularity similar to the primary tumor. Less than 2% of renal cell carcinomas (RCC) have a similar imaging pattern. Furthermore, this resembles the most frequent presentation form of the rare renal malignant lymphoma (Choyke et al. 1987; Sheth et al. 2006).

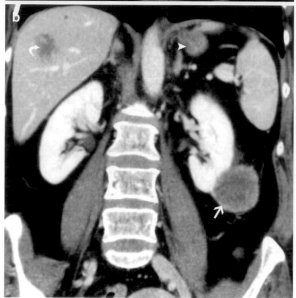

**Fig. 22.2** Renal, liver, and mesenterial metastases from a malignant melanoma in a 53-year-old woman. Axial (**a**) and coronal (**b**) images of a contrast-enhanced CT scan in the parenchymal phase show the well-delineated exophytic hypodense mass in the left kidney, extending in the perirenal space (*arrow*). Similar masses in liver (metastases – *curved arrow*) and in the mesentery (lymph node metastases – *arrowhead*)

The aspect of the lesions mostly depends on the aspect of the primary tumor. Most renal metastases are hypovascular at contrast-enhanced CT. Intravenous contrast administration is essential because on unenhanced CT, intracortical renal metastases may have similar attenuation as the parenchyma and often cause no deformation of the renal outline (Choyke et al. 1987). Metastases of colon carcinoma tend to be large and exophytic masses, while metastases of malignant melanoma and lung cancer tend to extend into the perirenal space (Choyke et al. 1987).

Both multifocal hypovascular RCC (papillary carcinoma) and renal lymphoma are rare. Especially in patients with a known primary tumor, multiple mass lesions are highly suspicious for renal metastases. If no primary tumor is known, imaging-guided biopsy is indicated to differentiate between surgical lesions (i.e., RCC) and nonsurgical lesions (renal metastases and lymphoma). This is a well-accepted indication for targeted percutaneous imaging-guided lesion biopsy.

High-density cysts may be difficult to differentiate from hypovascular mass lesions on routine staging CT. With dedicated techniques, including targeted renal ultrasonography, CT, or MRI, appropriate differentiation between high-density cysts and hypovascular masses can be achieved.

Diagnostic problems occur when metastases present as a solitary renal mass. In patients with advanced metastatic disease, a (newly discovered) solitary renal mass is more likely to be metastatic. In patients with tumoral remission, a solitary renal mass is problematic and percutaneous imaging-guided biopsy is required for further diagnostic and therapeutic management (Choyke et al. 1987).

## 22.2  Other Rare Renal Tumors

### 22.2.1  Medullary Tumors

Malignant medullary tumors account for 1–2% of malignant renal tumors (Pickhardt et al. 2000). They are classified in a separate subgroup than the primary malignant renal epithelial tumors of the renal cortex and pelvis. The pathogenesis of these tumors is uncertain and it is not yet obvious whether they are related (Srigley and Eble 1998).

#### 22.2.1.1  Collecting (Bellini) Duct Carcinoma (CDC)

General Features and Pathogenesis

Of all renal carcinomas, 0.6–1.3% are collecting duct carcinomas (CDC) (Chao et al. 2002). Old reports refer to these tumors as Bellini duct carcinoma as it

was hypothesized that they arose from the ducts of Bellini (Pickhardt et al. 2000). CDC was for a long time considered as a subtype of the RCC arising from the distal tubule/collecting duct, like chromophobic RCC and oncocytoma RCC (Störkel et al. 1997).

Because CDC's radiologic, clinical, and immunohistochemical appearance is completely different from RCC and, in addition, due to the resemblance with the behavior of urothelial carcinoma (transitional cell carcinoma, TCC), a recent study of Orsola et al. (2005) suggests an association of CDC with TCC. This can be explained by the common embryologic origin (branching of mesonephric duct) of collecting ducts and urothelial cells. This hypothesis is not yet confirmed since studies on CDC are limited due to their rarity.

The range of age at presentation is wide with a mean age of 55 years. There is a male predominance of 2:1 (Pickhardt et al. 2000).

Clinical presentation of CDC is similar to that of other renal carcinomas: hematuria, flank pain, and palpable mass. Prognosis is very poor as the tumor has an aggressive behavior with early metastases (Pickhardt et al. 2000). CDC spreads to regional lymph nodes (60–80%), lung or adrenal glands (25%), bone, and liver (Yoon and Rha 2006).

Imaging Features and Differential Diagnosis

CDC is somewhat arbitrarily classified into three types according to their predominant location: medullary location, medullary location with cortical extension, and medullary location with renal sinus extension (Yoon and Rha 2006).

At the time of discovery or presentation, the tumor is often bulky and usually cortical and sinus extension is present.

CDC has an infiltrative growth pattern, but sometimes presents with a concomitant expansile component (Fig. 22.3). On imaging studies, the tumor is ill-defined due to infiltrative growth pattern in some areas, while it can present as a well-defined mass in other areas due to the presence of a concomitant expansile component (Pickhardt et al. 2000).

Extension in the perirenal space and vascular invasion are not infrequent. Calcification is rarely present. Intralesional cyst-like areas are frequently encountered, sometimes due to tumor necrosis (Yoon and Rha

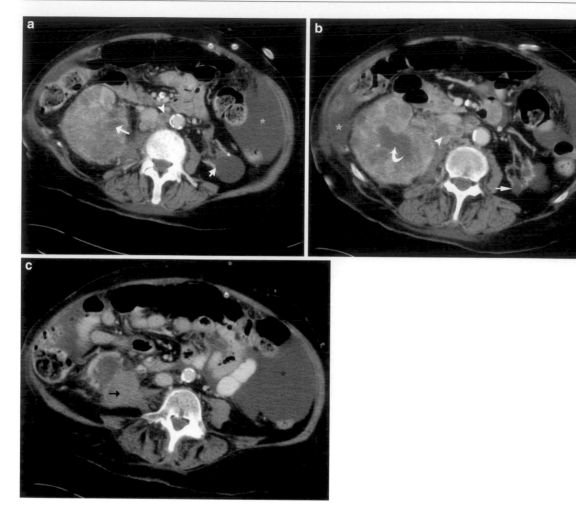

**Fig. 22.3** Collecting duct tumor in a 76-year-old woman. Axial images (**a, b, c**) of a contrast-enhanced CT scan in the parenchymal phase show a large infiltrative, centrally located right renal mass, with diffuse infiltration in the renal cortex and invasion in the renal sinus (*white arrow*). Presence of hypoattenuating areas (*curved arrow*) in the tumoral mass due to desmoplastic reaction. There is expansile growth in the right lower pole (*black arrow*). Note also the necrotic retroperitoneal lymphadenopathies (*arrowhead*), the wide spread ascites (*asterix*), and the left atrophic kidney (*short arrow*)

2006). Rarely, CDC presents with several satellite cortical nodules (Mejean et al. 2003).

On ultrasound, CDC is usually almost isoechoic to the renal parenchyma. On CT scan, the tumoral mass is hypovascular with avascular areas. These avascular areas are explained by the extensive desmoplastic reaction rather than necrosis.

On T2-weighted MRI, the tumoral mass is hypointense and isointense on T1-weighted images. T2 hypointensity combined with medullary location of the lesion favors the diagnosis of CDC (Yoon and Rha 2006). Similar to CT, the tumor is hypovascular with avascular desmoplastic areas.

Undifferentiated TCC may have an infiltrative growth pattern, and differential diagnosis can be impossible based on imaging studies.

More central location favors the diagnosis of CDC or invasive TCC. Distinguishing these tumors preoperatively is important as TCC requires a nephroureterectomy rather than a (radical) nephrectomy. If preoperative histologic analysis is uncertain, nephroureterectomy needs to be performed as TCC is much more frequent than CDC (Pickhardt et al. 2000).

Other differential diagnosis includes infiltrative forms of renal metastasis and lymphoma. Clinical history is contributive to resolve this differential diagnosis.

## 22.2.1.2 Renal Medullary Carcinoma

### General Features

By reviewing renal pelvic carcinomas of the database of the Armed Forces Institute of Pathology in 1995, this new variant of CDC associated with sickle cell trait (SCT) was described (Davis et al. 1995). Yet, sickle cell anemia (SCA) is surprisingly not associated with this subtype. SCT or sickle cell carrier (HbSA and HbSC) is much more common than sickle cell disease/anemia, but can be clinically occult (Pickhardt et al. 2000). Generally, six nephropathies were associated with SCT and SCA: macroscopic hematuria, papillary necrosis, nephrotic syndrome, renal infarction, failure to concentrate urine, and pyelonephritis. Renal medullary carcinoma is added as the seventh nephropathy by Davis et al. 1995, Warren et al. 1999.

The hypothesis for the relation between medullary carcinoma and SCT is that chronic hypoxia in the renal medulla secondary to the SCT may initiate transitional cell proliferation of the distal collecting ducts and papillary epithelium (Prasad et al. 2005).

This tumor occurs in young patients with an age span between 11 and 39 years. Between 11 and 24 years of age, there is a male predominance, and beyond 24 years of age, gender predominance is no longer present (Davis et al. 1995). The right kidney seems to be more often affected (Leitão et al. 2006).

Clinical presentation is similar to that of other renal carcinomas and includes hematuria, flank pain, and palpable mass (Pickhardt et al. 2000).

Gross hematuria is a common finding in patients with SCT and is usually self-limiting and painless. Even though it is commonly seen in patients with SCT without the presence of a tumor, this symptom should alert the clinician and radiologist to screen these patients for the presence of a renal tumor (Blitman et al. 2005).

The prognosis is very poor as in CDC, since the tumor has an extremely aggressive biological behavior with early metastases to regional lymph nodes, liver, and lung (Pickhardt et al. 2000).

### Imaging Features and Differential Diagnosis

Reported renal medullary carcinoma shows an infiltrative growth pattern. They are centrally located and can cause pelvic encasement. Sometimes smaller satellite lesions are present in cortex or hilum (Prasad et al. 2005). Hemorrhage and necrosis are frequently observed. Hydrocalyces (oncocalyces) without dilatation of the renal pelvis is an associated finding (Blitman et al. 2005; Pickhardt et al. 2000).

The differential diagnosis includes all invasive infiltrative tumoral lesions including TCC, RCC, renal metastases, lymphoma, and CDC (Davidson et al. 1995).

CDC is more often seen in adults and is not associated with a SCT. However, some pathologists suggest that renal medullary carcinoma is an aggressive form of CDC (Blitman et al. 2005).

Race (often black race), age (young patients), clinical presentation (aggressive tumor), and the presence of SCT are helpful to suggest the diagnosis. Other renal tumors at young age such as Wilms tumor and RCC usually have an expansile growth pattern (ball-shaped) and are located in the renal cortex (Davidson et al. 1995).

In conclusion, an infiltrative, right-sided renal tumor with necrosis, caliectasis, and regional lymph adenopathy in a young patient with SCT is to be considered as a renal medullary carcinoma until proven otherwise (Blitman et al. 2005).

## 22.2.2 Juxtaglomerular Cell Tumor (Reninoma)

Juxtaglomerular cell tumors are very rare benign renin-producing tumors with a female predominance. They occur in adolescence or early adulthood (Beaudoin et al. 2008). They are an extremely rare cause of secondary hypertension.

Symptoms are secondary to the renin-production and include moderate to severe headache (hypertension), polydipsia, polyuria, enuresis, and sometimes neuromuscular pains (hypokalemia).

On clinical examination, patients show moderate to severe hypertension. Elevated peripheral renin level with signs of secondary hyperaldosteronism is seen on blood analysis (Dunnick et al. 1983).

Tumorectomy or partial nephrectomy is the gold standard therapy with normalization of blood pressure soon postoperatively.

Histologically, reninoma has benign characteristics, but recent case reports have shown that vascular invasion and metastases may occur. Malignant behavior is observed in older patients with a large reninoma that has been present for many years (Beaudoin et al. 2008).

A reninoma most often presents as a small (2–3 cm) solitary mass on imaging studies, located subcapsularly. Occasionally, they can occur near the renal pelvis or in the perinephric space. The latter presumably occurs from perirenal embryonic rests (Dunnick et al. 1983).

They present rarely as a large mass which usually suggests the long-standing presence of this tumor.

Hemorrhage and necrosis can be present.

On ultrasound, a reninoma is homogeneously hyperechogenic; sometimes hypoechogenic areas are present due to hemorrhage or necrosis. On unenhanced CT scan, a reninoma is isodense to the renal parenchyma and hypovascular after intravenous contrast administration.

On MRI, a reninoma is T1-hypointense, T2-hypointense, and hypovascular after contrast administration (Pedrosa et al. 2008).

Imaging features are very nonspecific. Therefore, the notice of hypertension, hyperreninism in the absence of renal artery stenosis, and the presence of a renal mass should suggest a juxtaglomerular cell tumor.

Other differential diagnosis for hypertension and hyperreninism and secondary hyperaldosteronism are renal artery stenosis, incipient malignant hypertension, other renin-secreting tumors (renin-secreting Wilms tumor or RCC, very rare renin-secreting lung, pancreas, ovarian, liver, or orbital tumor) and other masses that compress the renal artery or parenchyma (larger than reninoma) (Dunnick et al. 1983; Garel et al. 1993).

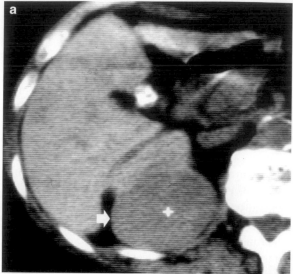

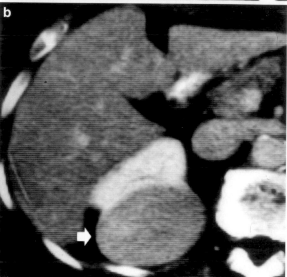

**Fig. 22.4** (**a**, **b**) Renal solitary fibrous tumor. (**a**) Well-defined, large, homogeneous, and relatively hypovascular mass (*arrow*) after iodinated contrast agent injection (**b**) with a slightly heterogeneous appearance (courtesy of Prof. Quaia)

### 22.2.3 Solitary Fibrous Tumor

A solitary fibrous tumor is a spindle cell tumor usually originating in the pleura. Extrapleural locations including the kidney are rarely reported. Renal solitary fibrous tumor arises from the renal capsule (Gelb et al. 1996). It is considered a benign tumor, but in rare occasions malignancy can be present (Gelb et al. 1996).

On imaging, they present as a well-defined, large, homogeneous and relatively hypovascular mass (Fig. 22.4). A typical cortical claw-sign is absent,

witnessing its extraparenchymal origin. Intralesional necrosis and cysts are infrequently encountered (Pedrosa et al. 2008).

On MRI, the lesion is predominantly T2-hypointense and homogeneous T1-isointense to the renal capsule (Johnson et al. 2005; Pedrosa et al. 2008). Contrast enhancement is limited in the arterial phase and heterogeneous in the delayed phase (Johnson et al. 2005; Pedrosa et al. 2008).

## 22.2.4 Leukemia, Plasmocytoma, Castleman Disease and Lymphoma

### 22.2.4.1 Leukemia

Leukemic involvement of the kidney is rare and is seen more frequently in acute lymphoblastic forms (Pickhardt et al. 2000; Surabhi et al. 2008). The real frequency of renal involvement is difficult to assess, because of the limited contribution of imaging in staging (Pickhardt et al. 2000). Renal involvement can present as bilateral diffuse renal infiltration; more rarely it presents as a focal expansile mass or a perirenal mass. Perirenal involvement is the result of extension of a renal mass in the perirenal space or more rarely as an isolated involvement (Pickhardt et al. 2000; Surabhi et al. 2008).

As imaging is nonspecific, clinical history may suggest the diagnosis, but percutaneous biopsy is required to achieve the diagnosis (Surabhi et al. 2008).

Granulocytic sarcomas (chloromas) are rare malignant tumors of granulocytic precursors that can present in up to 10% of patients with acute myelogenous leukemia and only rarely in acute lymphocytic leukemia. On imaging studies they present as focal hypovascular soft-tissue masses in one or both kidneys (Surabhi et al. 2008).

### 22.2.4.2 Plasmacytoma

Two subgroups are distinguished: solitary lesions (plasmacytoma) and multiple lesions (multiple myeloma or Kahler's disease). Extramedullary plasmacytoma is infrequent, but can involve the kidney.

On imaging plasmacytoma presents as a solitary infiltrative or expansile mass without specific radiologic features.

In isolated renal plasmacytoma, diagnosis is usually based on the occurrence of Bence-Jones proteinuria. In case of the absence of tumor-producing immunoglobulins, the diagnosis is only obtained by histopathologic analysis (Pickhardt et al. 2000).

### 22.2.4.3 Castleman Disease

Castleman disease is an infrequent idiopathic lymphoproliferative disorder which sporadically involves the retroperitoneum (Enomoto et al. 2007). Renal and perirenal involvement are rare. Unicentric and multicentric Castleman disease are distinguished. Multicentric Castleman disease is seen in association with Kaposi sarcoma and is frequently observed in patients with AIDS. Multicentric Castleman disease tends to be more aggressive and has a poor prognosis.

Imaging findings vary widely depending on the clinical presentation and histological subtype. Hepatosplenomegaly, lymphadenopathies, and ascites tend to be present.

Unicentric Castleman disease displays as a well-defined, homogeneous, solitary intra-abdominal mass (Surabhi et al. 2008).

### 22.2.4.4 Lymphoma

See Chap. 25

## 22.2.5 Sarcoma

See Chap. 25

## 22.2.6 Rare Benign Mesenchymal Tumors of the Kidney

### 22.2.6.1 Renal Leiomyoma

Renal leiomyomas are rare benign mesenchymal tumors originating from the renal capsule (Surabhi et al. 2008). Renal leiomyomas are divided into two groups: the more frequent, incidentally found and asymptomatic cortical leiomyomas smaller than 2 cm, and the large renal leiomyomas that generally become symptomatic.

The large leiomyomas appear more often in white women older than 20 years of age. In thin patients it may be palpable and cause flank pain and rarely hematuria (Tessler et al. 1998).

On imaging leiomyoma presents as a well-circumscribed mass lesion, either hyper or hypovascular. On ultrasound and CT, their appearance is variable: cystic, solid, and mixed form (Tessler et al. 1998).

Frequently, a distinct plane is distinguishable between the tumor and the kidney without parenchymal distortion, confirming the capsular origin of the tumor. Occasionally, the mass can be extremely exophytic or attached to the cortex by only a small stalk (Wagner et al. 1997). Calcifications and cystic appearance due to necrosis or cystic-myxoid involution can occur, especially in larger lesions (Tessler et al. 1998; Surabhi et al. 2008).

However, imaging findings are nonspecific: a peripheral, exophytic, well-demarcated, solid renal mass in a middle-aged woman should suggest the possibility of renal leiomyoma (Tessler et al. 1998).

The differential list includes leiomyosarcoma and RCC. Leiomyosarcomas tend to be larger and less encapsulated, but sometimes they mimic a leiomyoma. Biopsy may be an option for decision on further management (Roy et al. 1998).

### 22.2.6.2 Renal Lipoma

A primary renal lipoma is a very rare benign renal neoplasm. As in leiomyoma, small and large lesions are distinguished. When large, they may become palpable and cause flank pain and, rarely, hematuria. Renal lipoma contains more nonadipose components than subcutaneous lipomas. These nonadipose components are mesenchymal elements or areas of fat necrosis and present as nodular or globular regions on imaging.

On imaging, a renal lipoma presents as a well-circumscribed fatty mass. On CT this results in homogeneous negative density values. On MRI the mass is T1-hyperintense on in-phase images and hypointense on out-of-phase images, T2 weighted-images, and fat saturated images. In smaller lesions, chemical shifts characteristics allow the confirmation of subtle areas of fat more accurately compared to CT.

The differential diagnosis is angiomyolipoma. In lipoma other soft-tissue components, with the exception of feeding vessels, are less prominent than in angiomyolipoma.

Larger lipomas are more heterogeneous due to areas of fat necrosis. Thus, the differential diagnosis expands to liposarcoma. Biopsy may then be required (aimed at nodular and globular areas) (Chiang et al. 2006).

### 22.2.6.3 Renal Hemangioma

See Chap. 20

### 22.2.6.4 Renal Lymphangioma

Renal lymphangioma is a rare benign renal neoplasm, occurring uni or bilateral.

On imaging, a lymphangioma presents as a uni or multilocular cystic lesion, focal or diffuse. Contrast-enhanced imaging can sometimes show peripheral or septal enhancement.

The perirenal space can be affected and in the case of perirenal lymphangiomatosis, there are multiple cystic masses present bilateral in the perirenal mesenchyme (Surabhi et al. 2008).

## 22.2.7 Extraadrenal Myelolipoma

Myelolipoma is a rare benign monoclonal tumor containing a mixture of normal hematopoietic cells and mature lipomatous tissue (Kumar and Duerinckx 2004). Normally, this tumor is located in the adrenal gland. Extraadrenal myelolipomas are rare and occur mostly in perirenal or presacral area.

Age at presentation is the sixth decade in the extraadrenal form, while adrenal myelolipoma is most often found (incidentally) in the fifth decade. Extraadrenal myelolipomas show a female predominance.

On imaging an extraadrenal myelolipoma presents as a heterogeneous mass consisting of hypervascular soft-tissue and macroscopic fat. The aspect of the lesion depends on the dominating tissue component.

The differential diagnosis with other fat-containing lesions is very difficult. Biopsy may be required (Surabhi et al. 2008).

## 22.2.8 Mesoblastic Nephroma

Mesoblastic nephroma (fetal renal hamartoma or leiomyomatous hamartoma) is the most common solid renal tumor in the first 3 months of life. Sometimes it can be detected on prenatal ultrasound (Lowe et al. 2000).

A slight male predominance is noted (Lowe et al. 2000).

It is commonly located near the renal hilum (Prasad et al. 2005). It is usually detected on clinical examination as a palpable abdominal mass. Rarely, hematuria is present.

On imaging, mesoblastic nephroma presents as a solitary, relatively homogeneous solid mass in the renal sinus.

On ultrasound it presents homogeneously hypoechoic, on CT homogeneously hypodense, and on MRI T1- and T2 hypointense (Prasad et al. 2005). Hemorrhage and necrosis are uncommon.

Nephrectomy is the preferred therapy as mesoblastic nephroma has a relative benign behavior (Lowe et al. 2000).

## 22.2.9 Metanephric Adenoma (Nephrogenic Adenofibroma)

See Chap. 20

## 22.2.10 Multilocular Cystic Tumor

Multilocular cystic tumor consists of a spectrum from multilocular cystic nephroma to a cystic partially differentiated nephroblastoma (Lowe et al. 2000). They are rare, benign encapsulated lesions consisting of multiple noncommunicating cysts of varying size (Madewell et al. 1983). This tumor has a bimodal distribution, affecting boys between 3 months and 4 years of age and women over 40 years old (Madewell et al. 1983). They are usually detected incidentally (Lowe et al. 2000).

On imaging multilocular cystic tumors present as a unilateral, solitary, well-circumscribed mass consisting of multiple cysts of varying size. Herniation of this mass into the renal pelvis and ureter is frequently observed. Calcification, hemorrhage, and necrosis are infrequent (Prasad et al. 2005).

When the cystic spaces are small, the tumor may mimic a solid lesion.

Because multilocular cystic nephroma is extremely rare in adult males, a predominately cystic or multicystic mass lesion should be considered as a cystic RCC.

Ultrasound is the key modality to confirm the cystic nature of this lesion (Lowe et al. 2000).

On CT there is no secretion of contrast into the cysts (Lowe et al. 2000).

On MRI, the cyst fluid can be variable in signal intensity depending on its composition. The fibrous capsule is hypointense on every sequence.

The septations are usually regular and present a variable thickness. These septations enhance moderately on contrast-enhanced ultrasonography, CT, and MR.

Cystic nephroma and cystic partially differentiated nephroblastoma cannot be differentiated on imaging studies.

Multicystic dysplastic kidney (MCDK) can be differentiated from a multilocular cystic tumor by the absence of normally functioning renal parenchyma in MCDK. Sometimes in MCDK, there is a central core of solid dysplastic tissue that enhances, but this enhancement is different from the enhancement of normal renal parenchyma.

Segmental MCDK occurring in the obstructed part (generally the upper pole) in patients with complete ureteral duplication may be difficult to differentiate from multilocular cystic nephroma (Hopkins et al. 2004).

Nephrectomy is curative (Prasad et al. 2005). Tumorectomy should be complete, including the suburothelial component, to avoid local recurrence.

## 22.2.11 Neuro-Endocrine Tumor (NET) of the Kidney

In literature there are just a few cases reported of renal NET: renal somatostatinoma, renal VIPoma, renal carcinoid, and renal pheochromocytoma (Hamilton et al. 1980; Isobe et al. 2000; Melegh et al. 2002; Walsh et al. 1996). In the case report of the VIPoma, it was not clear if the lesion was a primary lesion or metastatic (Hamilton et al. 1980).

Primary carcinoid tumor of the kidney (Fig. 22.5) is extremely rare. Primary carcinoid tumor arising in horseshoe kidneys tends to be more benign than in orthotopic kidneys (Isobe et al. 2000).

If the NET is functional, symptoms depend on the type of hormone that is secreted.

In literature only limited information is available on the imaging characteristics of renal NET. It is expected that their general imaging features are independent on their location.

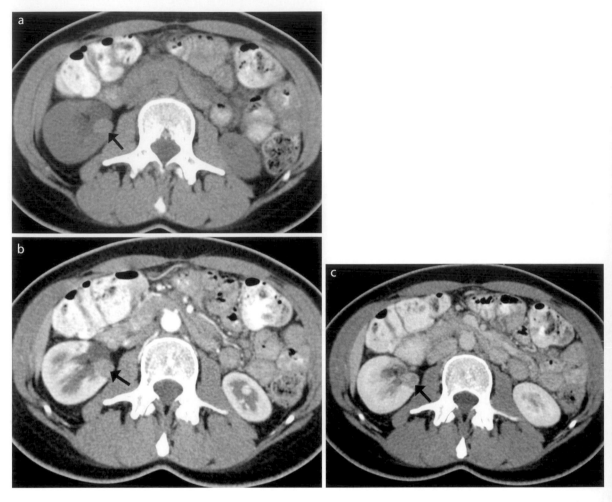

**Fig. 22.5** (**a–c**) Renal carcinoid tumor in a 39-year-old woman. (**a**) Axial images of unenhanced CT scan show a solitary, small, well-defined, spontaneous hyperdense lesion (*arrow*) in the posterior lip of the right kidney. (**b, c**) Axial images of contrast-enhanced CT scan in the corticomedullary (**b**) and parenchymal phase (**c**) show mild heterogeneous contrast enhancement of the lesion (*arrow*)

## 22.2.12 Extraintestinal GIST

The gastrointestinal stromal tumor (GIST) is a nonepithelial neoplasm that can arise from the c-KIT–positive interstitial cells of Cajal. These are the pacemaker cells of the gastrointestinal tract, where most GISTs are located. Primary extragastrointestinal stromal tumors are rare and mostly located in the omentum and mesentery (Takao et al. 2004). Extremely rare are reports of GIST in the perirenal area.

Perirenal extragastrointestinal stromal tumors appear as hypovascular soft-tissue masses. The imaging characteristics of extraintestinal GIST are nonspecific. Biopsy is required for correct diagnosis (Surabhi et al. 2008).

## 22.3 Renal Pseudotumors

Renal pseudotumoral lesions are included here to avoid the aggressive treatment.

## 22.3.1 Infection

### 22.3.1.1 Classical Presentation

Of course, pyelonephritis is a clinical diagnosis. Yet, often imaging is performed. Classical presentation of pyelonephritis on contrast-enhanced CT and MRI is the presence of wedge-shaped or striated areas of decreased contrast enhancement with contrast retention in these areas on delayed-phase studies. This can occur focal or multifocal, unilateral or bilateral.

In the presence of inflammatory symptoms and urinary tract infection, there is no diagnostic problem.

In the absence of typical symptoms of acute pyelonephritis, differentiation from solitary or multiple renal tumoral masses or renal infarction can be difficult. Diagnosis then can be achieved by the presence of an ill-defined demarcation between the lesion and the normal parenchyma, the presence of edema in the adjacent parenchyma, and of adjacent perinephric fat stranding (Israel and Bosniak 2008).

A subacute (Fig. 22.6) or chronic renal abscess may mimic a cystic renal neoplasm. The differentiation can be very difficult when the typical clinical findings are absent. Findings that suggest renal abscess are rim enhancement, the absence of central enhancement, and the possible concomitant pyelonephritis.

In case of doubt, imaging-guided needle aspiration should be performed. When pus is aspirated, the diagnosis of renal abscess is confirmed. In case blood or necrotic debris is aspirated, the diagnosis of abscess is less probable and surgical removal is usually required (Israel and Bosniak 2008).

Some specific forms of (chronic) renal infection need attention since they can mimic tumoral lesions.

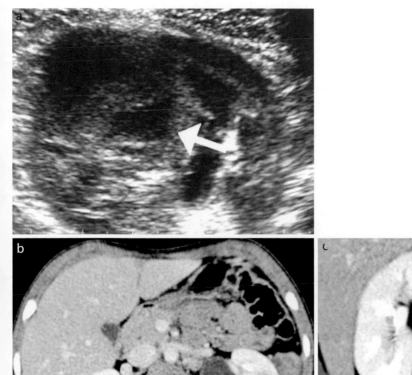
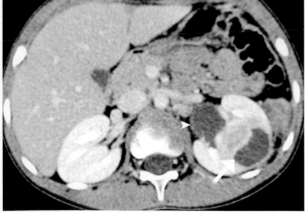
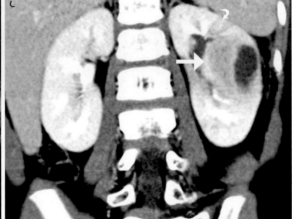

**Fig. 22.6** (a–c) Renal abscess and multifocal pyelonephritis in a 7-year-old boy. (a) Ultrasound shows a partially liquified nodular mass (*arrow*) posterolateral in the left kidney (b, c). Axial and coronal images of a contrast-enhanced CT in the parenchymal phase confirm the nodular lesion (*arrow*) in the left kidney. This nodular lesion contains liquified material in its lateral portion, while it appears solid in its medial portion soft-tissue. The liquified material was pus which was drained under ultrasound guidance. The medial soft-tissue component was edematous renal parenchyma bulging into the renal sinus secondary to edema and compression of the pus collection. Note the wedge-shaped unenhanced area in the upper pole of the left kidney (*curved arrow*) and the subtle enhancement of the wall of the excretory system (*arrowhead*) as CT features of pyelonephritis

### 22.3.1.2 Xanthogranulomatous Pyelonephritis

Xanthogranulomatous pyelonephritis (XGP) is a form of severe chronic infection, more often seen in women. Focal or diffuse renal destruction occurs with secondary replacement of the renal parenchyma by lipid-laden macrophages. The pathogenesis is not clear. Proteus species and Escherichia coli are frequently associated with XGP.

Several etiologic factors have been suggested (chronic urinary obstruction with or without calculus, inappropriate treatment of urosepsis, alteration of lipid metabolism, arterial insufficiency, venous occlusion, hemorrhage) (Hayes et al. 1991).

In 50% of the cases renal calculi or staghorn calculi are present (Pedrosa et al. 2008).

Presentation of the most frequent diffuse form includes (Fig. 22.7) nephromegaly, calculi, parenchymal calcifications, contracted pelvis as a sign of peripelvic fibrosis, parenchymal destruction, hydronephrosis, and lobulated masses replacing the normal parenchyma (Hayes et al. 1991). The inflammatory process may extend outside the kidney, into the perinephric fat (thickening Gerota's fascia) and the retroperitoneum, and even to the abdominal wall (Pedrosa et al. 2008).

Diagnostic problems occur when XGP presents as a focal mass. The differential diagnosis with renal tumor then becomes difficult. This focal form (Fig. 22.8), however, is rare.

On ultrasound it presents as a hypoechoic mass with an associated calculus.

On CT focal XGP presents as a hypodense mass with rim enhancement, frequently in association with a calculus in the underlying calyx (Hayes et al. 1991).

On MRI it presents as a T1-isointense and T2-hyperintense mass. Calculi are often difficult to detect on MRI, but can be seen as a signal void in the collecting system (Pedrosa et al. 2008).

When calculus and appropriate clinical presentation (i.e., chronic pyelonephritis in diabetic patients) are present, the diagnosis of XGP can be suggested (Pedrosa et al. 2008). However, in the absence, biopsy is often mandatory.

### 22.3.1.3 Renal Tuberculosis

The genitourinary system is one of the most common locations of extrapulmonary tuberculosis (Gibson et al. 2004). Renal tuberculosis results from hematogeneous spread of pulmonary *Mycobacterium tuberculosis*. Parenchymal involvement of TBC and calyceal

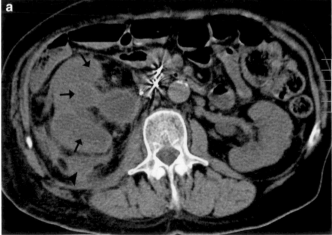
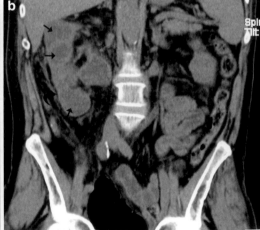
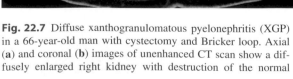

**Fig. 22.7** Diffuse xanthogranulomatous pyelonephritis (XGP) in a 66-year-old man with cystectomy and Bricker loop. Axial (**a**) and coronal (**b**) images of unenhanced CT scan show a diffusely enlarged right kidney with destruction of the normal parenchyma (*curved arrow*) and replacement by multiple low-attenuation masses (*arrows*). No renal calculus is present. Note also the presence of perirenal fat stranding and nodular pseudotumoral masses (*arrowhead*)

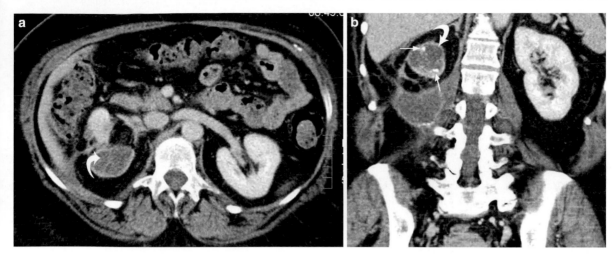

**Fig. 22.8** (**a**, **b**) Focal XGP in a 63-year-old woman. Axial (**a**) and coronal (**b**) images of contrast-enhanced CT scan show a well-defined hypodense mass with rim enhancement (*curved arrow*) in the upper pole of the right kidney. Note also the presence of a few calculi (*arrows*) in the excretory system and the retroperitoneal abscess collection (*arrowhead*)

strictures as result of TBC can mimic renal tumoral lesions (Fig. 22.9).

Parenchymal involvement (granulomas with or without cavitation) presents as an infiltrative mass and sometimes extends into the renal sinus. This presentation form is hard to differentiate from infiltrative tumoral masses (Zagoria 2004b). Cavitation within these lesions may be detected as irregular pools of contrast material (Engin et al. 2000).

Strictures are caused by the spread of the disease in the collecting system as a result of papillary necrosis.

The calyceal strictures and obliteration can mimic TCC (Zagoria 2004b).

In these cases of tumoral mimicking, clinical history and other classical imaging findings in renal TBC (medullary nephrocalcinosis, renal calcifications (sometimes extensive), calculi, and cicatricial retraction of the fibrotic parenchyma (Engin et al. 2000)) can suggest the diagnosis.

### 22.3.1.4 Renal Aspergillosis

Aspergillosis very rarely involves the kidney. Formation of aspergillomas, abscesses, and hemorrhagic masses due to vascular obstruction (invasive aspergillosis) can mimic renal tumoral lesions (Krishnamurthy et al. 1998; Rha et al. 2004). Clinical history, symptoms, and quick development of these masses can suggest the diagnosis.

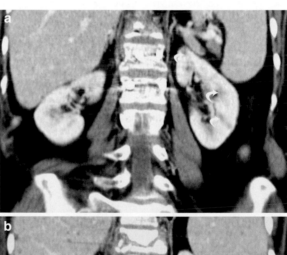
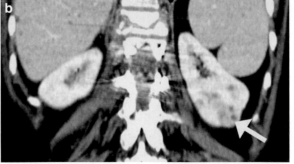

**Fig. 22.9** (**a**, **b**) Renal tuberculosis in a 43-year-old woman. Coronal images of a contrast-enhanced CT in the parenchymal phase show a nodular lesion with partial encapsulated liquified components (*arrow*) in the lower pole of the left kidney. This presents a multilocular abcedation or a caseous granuloma in the context of tuberculosis. Also, the presence of a few wedge-shaped nonenhancing areas (*curved arrows*) suggesting hematogeneous nephritis in the context of tuberculosis

### 22.3.1.5 Hydatid Cyst of the Kidney

Kidney involvement in echinococcosis is extremely rare (2–3% of cases). Kidney involvement becomes symptomatic when a hydatid cyst ruptures into the collecting system and causes colic pain.

Depending on the stage of the disease, multiple presentation forms are distinguished: unilocular cyst, presence of daughter cysts, and partially or completely calcified ("dead") cysts. When a solid component is present in the cysts, differentiation with malignant cystic lesions can be difficult.

The absence of significant contrast enhancement suggests the benign characteristics and allows the classification of hyperattenuating or hyperintense cystic lesions.

A cystic lesion with internal septations and sand, wall calcifications, or "wheel spoke" pattern in the appropriate clinical setting should suggest the diagnosis of echinococcosis (Volders et al. 2001).

## 22.3.2 Renal Malacoplakia

Malacoplakia is a type of granulomatous reaction which involves generally the genitourinary system. It is believed that abnormal macrophage function is responsible for the abnormal granulomatous reaction. Middle-aged women are most frequently affected. Malacoplakia is nearly almost associated with urinary tract infection (E. Coli).

Two types of renal malacoplakia are distinguished: the unifocal and the more frequent multifocal type.

On imaging the multifocal type presents as kidney enlargement with the presence of ill-defined cortical or medullar masses of variable size. These masses often cause renal contour bulging.

On imaging the unifocal type presents as a large mass (2.5–8 cm). Calcification is rarely present.

Renal malacoplakia is indistinguishable from malignant tumoral lesions.

Because of its rarity, renal malacoplakia is usually not diagnosed without histopathologic analysis. Therapy consists of treatment of the urinary tract infections and improving kidney function in case of renal failure. Nephrectomy is performed in case of unilateral renal involvement (Hartman et al. 1980).

## 22.3.3 Renal Hematoma

Intrarenal, subcapsular, and perirenal hematomas are distinguished. Hematoma in the kidney or perirenal space may be the consequence of either traumatic events (accidental or iatrogenic, i.e., renal biopsy, tumorectomy, ESWL) or can occur spontaneously (renal mass, vascular cause, end-stage renal disease) (Bechtold et al. 1996).

Sometimes (peri-)renal hematoma can mimic mass lesions when it presents as a nodular lesion (Fig. 22.10).

On unenhanced CT, subacute hematomas have higher attenuation numbers than a (peri)renal soft-tissue mass. If active bleeding is still present, these lesions can show heterogeneous enhancement by extravasation of contrast material.

Clinical history, the spontaneous hyperattenuating aspect, and the shrinking of the lesion in time suggest the correct diagnosis. Careful follow-up is mandatory whenever an underlying predisposing tumor cannot be excluded on initial imaging studies.

## 22.3.4 Renal Sarcoidosis

Renal involvement of sarcoidosis presents usually as nephrocalcinosis (hypercalcemia), as multiple low-attenuation nodules and less frequently as interstitial nephritis, glomerulonephritis, and diffuse granulomatous infiltration.

Granulomas can mimic tumoral lesions (Bhatt et al. 2007; Koyama et al. 2004).

## 22.3.5 Renal Amyloidosis

Amyloid is a complex protein that is deposited in certain locations in the body. Amyloidosis may be primary or secondary to a variety of disorders (rheumatoid arthritis, multiple myeloma, etc.). Amyloid is sometimes deposited in the kidney (Bechtold et al. 1996).

On imaging the presentation of renal amyloidosis is variable: enlarged kidneys (usually in the acute stage), small and cortical thinned kidneys (amyloid contracted kidney), amorphous calcifications, blood clots

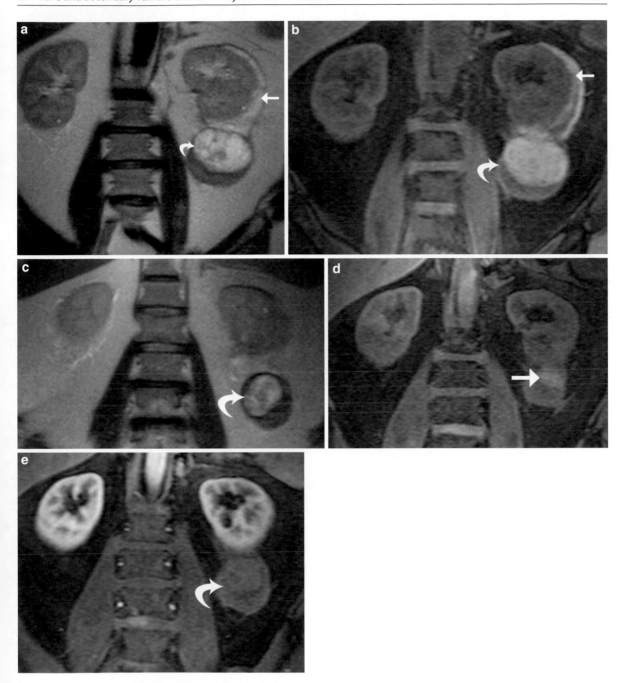

**Fig. 22.10** (**a–e**) Subcapsular and perirenal hematoma follow-ing ESWL in a 59-year-old man. (**a, b**) Coronal MRI shows mainly T2- (**a**) and T1- (**b**) hyperintense crescent-shaped sub-capsular collection (*arrow*) and a T1- and T2-hyperintense peri-renal nodule with a T1-and T2-hypointense crescent at the inferior pole of the left kidney (*curved arrow*). Three months later, a control MRI was performed. (**c**) Coronal MRI images show resorption of the subcapsular hematoma and a persistent perirenal hematoma with alteration of the signal characteristics in comparison with the first performed MR, caused by the

organization of this hematoma in time. This perirenal collection now presents as a T2-hypointense nodule with in its cranial por-tion, a mixed T2-hyper and hypointense nodular component (*curved arrow*). (**d**) Coronal T1-weighted images with fat sup-pression show a T1-isointense nodule with in its cranial portion, a T1 hyperintense nodular component (*arrow*). (**e**) After contrast enhancement, coronal T1-weighted images with fat suppression show no lesion enhancement (*curved arrow*). If no initial MRI was performed, this perirenal nodule could have been mistaken for a tumoral lesion or amyloid deposits in the renal pelvis, perirenal soft-tissue mass with calcifications, or focal parenchymal masses (Urban et al. 1993).

These last two presentation forms can be indistinguishable from tumoral lesions.

## 22.3.6 Renal Sinus Histocytosis

Sinus histocytosis is a lymphoproliferative disorder involving multiple organs (nodal and extranodal).

It presents more often in children or young adults. Symptoms depend on the organ involved. Fever and weight loss are regularly present. Blood analysis shows anemia, leukocytosis, and serum polyclonal hypergammaglobulinemia. Clinically, sinus histocytosis is considered a pseudolymphomatous disorder. Symptoms can persist for months, but usually regress spontaneously.

Kidney involvement is infrequent. On imaging renal involvement of sinus histocytosis can present as an infiltrative mass.

Sinus histocytosis can mimic leukemia or lymphoma, especially when lymphadenopathy is present.

The list of differential diagnosis includes malignant histocytosis, RCC, storage diseases, and tuberculosis.

When a young patient presents with a diffuse infiltrative mass in the kidney, the less common sinus histocytosis should be considered in the differential diagnosis. Unnecessary treatment must be avoided, because it is a benign disorder which may regress spontaneously (Bechtold et al. 1987).

## 22.3.7 Systemic Lupus Erythematosus

Renal involvement is usually present in systemic lupus erythematosus (SLE). Renal histopathologic findings in SLE are specific for entities such as membranous or proliferative glomerulonephritis.

However, imaging findings are generally nonspecific and present similar to other causes of medical renal disease.

On ultrasound the kidneys are generally hyperechoic and the size of the kidney depends on the onset of the renal involvement (Lalani et al. 2004).

Rarely, lupus nephritis leads to the formation of a pseudotumoral lesion (Fig. 22.11). Renal biopsy is frequently required for correct diagnosis.

## 22.3.8 Perirenal Fibrosis and Erdheim–Chester Disease

### 22.3.8.1 Perirenal Fibrosis

Retroperitoneal fibrosis is a fibrotic and inflammatory disorder of the central retroperitoneum. The fibrosis usually encompasses the aorta, inferior vena cava, and ureters and spreads in an ascending way (Bechtold et al. 1996).

Rarely, the process extends to the perinenal space where it simulates an infiltrative or nodal mass. It may also envelop the kidneys as a confluent mass that resembles the perirenal presentation form of lymphoma. When the renal hilum is involved, the fibrosis may cause obstruction of the excretory system, yet without dilatation. Renal failure may then be the presenting event, requiring ureteral stenting or percutaneous nephrostomy. The disease has three stages, ranging from chronic active inflammation to fibrous scarring (Surabhi et al. 2008).

If perirenal fibrosis occurs in combination with retroperitoneal fibrosis or multifocal fibrosclerosis, the diagnosis is usually obvious. However, when perirenal fibrosis is isolated (Fig. 22.12), imaging features are nonspecific and a biopsy may be required for correct diagnosis (Surabhi et al. 2008).

### 22.3.8.2 Erdheim–Chester Disease

Erdheim–Chester disease is a rare type of systemic non-Langerhans cell histocytosis of unknown etiology. It occurs in middle-aged persons, without gender predilection.

Skeletal (bilateral symmetric metadiaphyseal cortical thickening, a coarsened trabecular pattern, medullary sclerosis in the long bones of the appendicular skeleton) and extraskeletal involvement are distinguished. In 50% of the cases, extraskeletal involvement is present.

Perirenal involvement in Erdheim–Chester disease can occur. On imaging perirenal involvement presents as rindlike soft-tissue lesions enveloping the kidneys

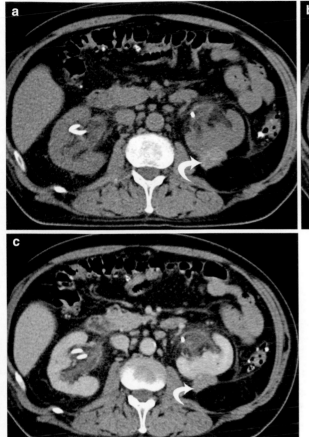

**Fig. 22.11** (a–c) Pseudotumoral lesion in a 63-year-old man with systemic lupus erythematosus (SLE). (a) Axial images of an unenhanced CT scan show the presence of a slightly lobulated, spontaneous hyperattenuating lesion (*curved arrow*) in the posterior lip of the left kidney. This lesion extends into the perirenal space. Bilateral ureteral double J stents. (b, c) Axial images of a contrast-enhanced CT scan in the corticomedullary and parenchymal phase show no contrast enhancement in the lesion (*curved arrow*)

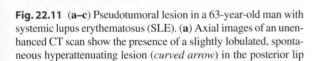

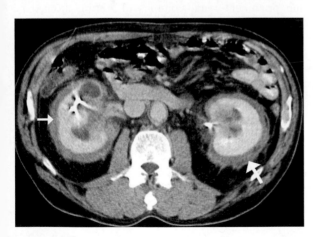

**Fig. 22.12** Perirenal fibrosis in a 57-year-old man. Axial image of a contrast-enhanced CT scan in the parenchymal phase shows a confluent soft-tissue mass enveloping both kidneys (*arrows*). Bilateral hydronephrosis is present secondary to the peripelvic fibrosis. Note the presence of bilateral ureteral stents

and ureters. This resembles the perirenal presentation form of lymphoma.

Secondary compression on the renal parenchyma and ureters leads to progressive renal failure.

Ureteral stent placement and systemic corticosteroid therapy are the standard therapy (Surabhi et al. 2008).

### 22.3.9 Inflammatory Pseudotumor

An inflammatory pseudotumor is a pseudoneoplastic lesion that most commonly involves the lung and the orbit, but it can occur in almost every site in the body, including the kidney. The pathogenesis is unknown. These pseudotumors can be locally aggressive, multifocal, and sometimes evolve into a malignant tumor.

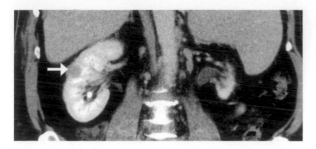

**Fig. 22.13** Inflammatory pseudotumor in a 55-year-old man. Coronal image of a contrast-enhanced CT scan in the parenchymal phase shows a solitary well-defined hypodense cortical nodule (*arrow*) in the interpolar region of the right kidney

The imaging appearances of this pseudotumoral mass can be variable (Fig. 22.13). Contrast enhancement can occur, but is limited and has a variable pattern. Larger lesions can have central necrosis.

Inflammatory pseudotumors and malignant tumors can be indistinguishable, and biopsy is often required (Narla et al. 2004).

## 22.3.10  Renal Sinus Lipomatosis

The normal renal sinus contains fat that envelops the renal vasculature and collecting system.

The quantity of fat in the renal sinus increases with age and obesity.

Sometimes there is an abnormal increase of fat in the renal sinus when there is destruction or atrophy of the renal parenchyma and when there is an increased presence of exogenous or endogenous steroids.

This abnormal increase is called renal sinus lipomatosis. The increased amount of fat causes compression on the collecting system, but rarely becomes symptomatic.

Replacement lipomatosis of the kidney is an extreme form of renal sinus lipomatosis. It usually occurs unilateral and with severe renal atrophy or destruction secondary to chronic calculus.

On imaging replacement lipomatosis may mimic focal fat-containing neoplasms of the renal sinus, such as angiomyolipoma, lipoma, or liposarcoma. But in neoplasms renal atrophy or staghorn calculus is usually lacking (Rha et al. 2004).

## 22.3.11  Extramedullary Hematopoiesis

Extramedullary hematopoiesis occurs when hematopoietic tissue develops outside the normal primary sites. This can be seen in hemolytic anemia, hemoglobinopathies, primary and secondary myelofibrosis, leukemia, lymphoma, or skeletal metastases. Rarely, renal involvement in extramedullary hematopoiesis is seen. It can be situated in the renal parenchyma, intrapelvic, and perirenal. Pelvic involvement can be an extension of parenchymal involvement or is isolated (Bhatt et al. 2007).

In imaging two patterns are seen: a diffuse infiltrative process in or around the kidneys or multiple small soft-tissue masses mixed with macroscopic fat (Surabhi et al. 2008).

These imaging findings may resemble those of other neoplasms.

The diffuse infiltrative type mimics lymphoma, whereas the fat-containing type mimics other fat-containing tumors.

Biopsy is usually required for the diagnosis (Surabhi et al. 2008).

## 22.3.12  Congenital and Acquired Pseudotumors

Congenital pseudotumors are normal variants including prominent renal columns of Bertin, dromedary humps, and hilar lips (Israel and Bosniak 2005).

*A prominent (or hypertrophied) column of Bertin* (Fig. 22.14) is hypertrophy of the septal cortex and

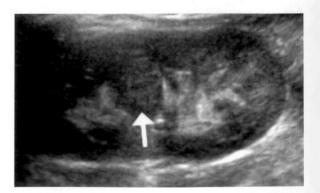

**Fig. 22.14** Ultrasound shows a hypertrophied column of Bertin in the left kidney of a 12-year-old boy (*arrow*)

extends from the outer cortex to the renal sinus. This is usually situated at the transition of upper and middle third of the kidney and is often associated with partial or complete duplication of the excretory system. It is also more often located at the left side. It may be erroneously mistaken for a tumoral lesion. Helpful in diagnosis is the fact that the column of Bertin enhances identically to the normal renal parenchyma (Bhatt et al. 2007; Zagoria 2004a) and shows similar vascularity at color Doppler ultrasound.

A *dromedary hump* (Fig. 22.15) is a prominent bulge on the superolateral border of the left kidney. It is believed to arise secondary to the molding of the upper pole of the left kidney by the spleen during development. There is a uniform thickness of the renal parenchyma between the bulge and the underlying normal calyces confirming that this is a normal variant (Bhatt et al. 2007; Zeman et al. 1986).

*Hilar lips* are areas of prominent renal tissue that occur in the medial part of the parenchyma surrounding the renal sinus. This is an area where complex lobar fusion took place during renal development. They occur more in the upper pole and on the left side. They can mimic tumoral lesions, but careful assessment in all imaging planes should resolve this problem (Bhatt et al. 2007; Zagoria et al. 2004a).

Sometimes the lobulation that is present in the fetal kidneys can persist in adulthood (*persistent fetal lobulation*). This can be misdiagnosed as a renal tumor or a scarred kidney. These indentations are centered at the base of the septal cortex, while renal scars are located in the cortex overlying the medullary pyramids (calyces) (Bhatt et al. 2007).

*Splenorenal fusion* is a rare benign entity. Splenorenal fusion is the presence of heterotopic splenic tissue in the renal capsule. It can originate from a developmental anomaly or secondarily acquired as result of splenosis after trauma or splenectomy. Splenorenal fusion is found almost exclusively in the left kidney. On CT or MRI it presents as a solid enhancing mass. 99mTc sulfur colloid-scan confirms the uptake by the splenic tissue. Sometimes biopsy is required (Bhatt et al. 2007).

An acquired pseudotumor is hypertrophied normal renal parenchyma adjacent to parenchymal scarring, mimicking a tumoral lesion. The "mass" enhances identically to the normal renal parenchyma. It is recommended to scan in the corticomedullary as the parenchymal phase to demonstrate the normal corticomedullary differentiation in the pseudomass (Israel and Bosniak 2005).

At present, pseudotumors are frequently seen after partial nephrectomy (tumorectomy) or radiofrequency ablation (RFA) of renal tumors.

### 22.3.13 Vascular Anomalies

Vascular anomalies, including renal artery aneurysm or arteriovenous fistula, can present as an enhancing parapelvic or peripelvic renal mass if a poor bolus of contrast material is administrated or scanning is performed in the excretory phase.

These lesions have the same attenuation of the vasculature. Also, enlargement of the feeding renal artery or draining renal vein may be apparent. In case of doubt, the exam has to be reperformed in ideal conditions or Doppler ultrasound can be performed to confirm the vascular origin of the lesion (Israel and Bosniak 2005; Rha et al. 2004).

### 22.3.14 Hemorrhagic Cysts

When a simple cyst hemorrhages, the imaging appearance varies and it may resemble a tumoral lesion.

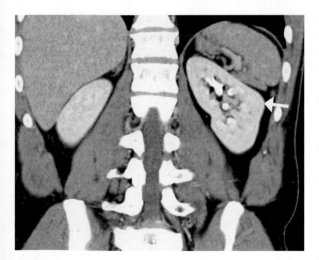

**Fig. 22.15** Dromedary hump in a 39-year-old man. Coronal image of a contrast-enhanced CT scan in the parenchymal phase shows the presence of focal bulge (*arrow*) on lateral border of left kidney

Sometimes the blood reabsorbs and the cyst regains its normal appearance. Sometimes the cyst wall may become thicker and may show contrast enhancement, which normally requires surgery. However, if previous imaging showed that a benign cyst was present or a history of trauma or anticoagulation treatment is known, the benign nature of this lesion is confirmed and less invasive therapy is needed (Israel and Bosniak 2008).

# References

Abrams HL, Spiro R, Goldstein N (1950) Metastases in carcinoma; analysis of 1000 autopsied cases. Cancer 3:74–85

Beaudoin J, Périgny M, Têtu B et al. (2008) A patient with a juxtaglomerular cell tumor with histological vascular invasion. Nat Clin Pract Nephrol 4:458–462

Bechtold RE, Dyer RB, Zagoria RJ et al. (1996) The perirenal space: relationship of pathologic processes to normal retroperitoneal anatomy. Radiographics 16:841–854

Bechtold RE, Wolfman NT, Karstaedt N et al. (1987) Renal sinus histiocytosis. Radiology 162:689–690

Bhatt S, MacLennan G, Dogra V (2007) Renal pseudotumors. AJR Am J Roentgenol 188:1380–1387

Blitman NM, Berkenblit RG, Rozenblit AM et al. (2005) Renal medullary carcinoma: CT and MRI features. AJR Am J Roentgenol 185:268–272

Chao D, Zisman A, Pantuck AJ et al. (2002) Collecting duct renal cell carcinoma: clinical study of a rare tumor. J Urol 167:71–74

Chiang IC, Jang MY, Tsai KB et al. (2006) Huge renal lipoma with prominent hypervascular non-adipose elements. Br J Radiol 79:e148–e151

Choyke PL, White EM, Zeman RK et al. (1987) Renal metastases: clinicopathologic and radiologic correlation. Radiology 162:359–363

Davidson AJ, Choyke PL, Hartman DS et al. (1995) Renal medullary carcinoma associated with sickle cell trait: radiologic findings. Radiology 195:83–85

Davis CJ Jr, Mostofi FK, Sesterhenn IA (1995) Renal medullary carcinoma. The seventh sickle cell nephropathy. Am J Surg Pathol 19:1–11

Dunnick NR, Hartman DS, Ford KK et al. (1983) The radiology of juxtaglomerular tumors. Radiology 147:321–326

Engin G, Acuna B, Acuna G et al. (2000) Imaging of extrapulmonary tuberculosis. Radiographics 20:471–488

Enomoto K, Nakamichi I, Hamada K et al. (2007) Unicentric and multicentric Castleman's disease. Br J Radiol 80: e24–e26

Garel L, Robitaille P, Dubois J et al. (1993) Pediatric case of the day. Reninoma of the left kidney. Radiographics 13:477–479

Gelb AB, Simmons ML, Weidner N (1996) Solitary fibrous tumor involving the renal capsule. Am J Surg Pathol 20:1288–1295

Gibson MS, Puckett ML, Shelly ME (2004) Renal tuberculosis. Radiographics 24:251–256

Hamilton I, Reis L, Bilimoria S et al. (1980) A renal vipoma. Br Med J 281:1323–1324

Hartman DS, Davis CJ Jr, Lichtenstein JE et al. (1980) Renal parenchymal malacoplakia. Radiology 136:33–42

Hayes WS, Hartman DS, Sesterbenn IA (1991) From the archives of the AFIP: xanthogranulomatous pyelonephritis. Radiographics 11:485–498

Hopkins JK, Giles HW Jr, Wyatt-Ashmead J et al. (2004) Best cases from the AFIP: cystic nephroma. Radiographics 24:589–593

Isobe H, Takashima H, Higashi N et al. (2000) Primary carcinoid tumor in a horseshoe kidney. Int J Urol 7:184–188

Israel GM, Bosniak MA (2005) How I do it: evaluating renal masses. Radiology 236:441–450

Israel GM, Bosniak MA (2008) Pitfalls in renal mass evaluation and how to avoid them. Radiographics 28:1325–1338

Johnson TR, Pedrosa I, Goldsmith J et al. (2005) Magnetic resonance imaging findings in solitary fibrous tumor of the kidney. J Comput Assist Tomogr 29:481–483

Koyama T, Ueda H, Togashi K et al. (2004) Radiologic manifestations of sarcoidosis in various organs. Radiographics 24:87–104

Krishnamurthy R, Aparajitha C, Abraham G et al. (1998) Renal aspergillosis giving rise to obstructive uropathy and recurrent anuric renal failure. Geriatr Nephrol Urol 8:137–139

Kumar M, Duerinckx AJ (2004) Bilateral extraadrenal perirenal myelolipomas: an imaging challenge. AJR Am J Roentgenol 183:833–836

Lalani TA, Kanne JP, Hatfield GA et al. (2004) Imaging findings in systemic lupus erythematosus. Radiographics 24:1069–1086

Leitão VA, da Silva W Jr, Ferreira U et al. (2006) Renal medullary carcinoma. Case report and review of the literature. Urol Int 77:184–186

Lowe LH, Isuani BH, Heller RM et al. (2000) Pediatric renal masses: Wilms tumor and beyond. Radiographics 20:1585–1603. [Erratum in: Radiographics 21:766]

Madewell JE, Goldman SM, Davis CJ Jr et al. (1983) Multilocular cystic nephroma: a radiographic-pathologic correlation of 58 patients. Radiology 146:309–321

Mejean A, Roupret M, Larousserie F et al. (2003) Is there a place for radical nephrectomy in the presence of metastatic collecting duct (Bellini) carcinoma? J Urol 169:1287–1290

Pascal RR (1980) Renal manifestations of extrarenal neoplasms. Hum Pathol 11:7–17

Melegh Z, Rényi-Vámos F, Tanyay Z et al. (2002) Giant cystic pheochromocytoma located in the renal hilus. Pathol Res Pract 198:103–106

Narla LD, Newman B, Spottswood SS et al. (2004) Inflammatory pseudotumor. Radiographics 23:719–729. [Erratum in: Radiographics 23:1702]

Orsola A, Trias I, Raventós CX et al. (2005) Renal collecting (Bellini) duct carcinoma displays similar characteristics to upper tract urothelial cell carcinoma. Urology 65: 49–54

Pedrosa I, Sun MR, Spencer M et al. (2008) MR imaging of renal masses: correlation with findings at surgery and pathologic analysis. Radiographics 28:985–1003

Pickhardt PJ, Lonergan GJ, Davis CJ Jr et al. (2000) From the archives of the AFIP. Infiltrative renal lesions: radiologic-pathologic correlation. Armed Forces Institute of Pathology. Radiographics 20:215–243

Prasad SR, Humphrey PA, Menias CO et al. (2005) Neoplasms of the renal medulla: radiologic-pathologic correlation. Radiographics 25:369–380

Rha SE, Byun JY, Jung SE et al. (2004) The renal sinus: pathologic spectrum and multimodality imaging approach. Radiographics 24(suppl 1):S117–S131

Roy C, Pfleger D, Tuchmann C et al. (1998) Small leiomyosarcoma of the renal capsule: CT findings. Eur Radiol 8:224–227

Sheth S, Ali S, Fishman E (2006) Imaging of renal lymphoma: patterns of disease with pathologic correlation. Radiographics 26:1151–1168

Srigley JR, Eble JN (1998) Collecting duct carcinoma of kidney. Semin Diagn Pathol 15:54–67

Störkel S, Eble JN, Adlakha K et al. (1997) Classification of renal cell carcinoma: Workgroup No. 1. Union Internationale Contre le Cancer (UICC) and the American Joint Committee on Cancer (AJCC) Cancer 80:987–989

Surabhi VR, Menias C, Prasad SR et al. (2008) Neoplastic and non-neoplastic proliferative disorders of the perirenal space: cross-sectional imaging findings. Radiographics 28:1005–1017

Takao H, Yamahira K, Doi I et al. (2004) Gastrointestinal stromal tumor of the retroperitoneum: CT and MR findings. Eur Radiol 14:1926–1929

Tessler FN, Tublin ME, Rifkin MD (1998) US case of the day. Renal leiomyoma. Radiographics 18:791–793

Urban BA, Fishman EK, Goldman SM et al. (1993) CT evaluation of amyloidosis: spectrum of disease. Radiographics 13:1295–1308

Volders WK, Gelin G, Stessens RC (2001) Best cases from the AFIP. Hydatid cyst of the kidney: radiologic-pathologic correlation. Radiographics 21 Spec No:S255–S260

Wagner BJ, Wong-You-Cheong JJ, Davis CJ Jr (1997) Adult renal hamartomas. Radiographics 17:155–169

Walsh IK, Kernohan RM, Johnston CF et al. (1996) Somatostatinoma in a horseshoe kidney. Br J Urol 78:958–959

Warren KE, Gidvani-Diaz V, Duval-Arnould B (1999) Renal medullary carcinoma in an adolescent with sickle cell trait. Pediatrics 103:E22

Yoon SK, Rha SH (2006) Collecting duct carcinoma. In: Guermazi A (ed) Imaging in kidney cancer. Springer, Berlin, pp 171–185

Zagoria RJ (2004a) The kidney and retroperitoneum: anatomy and congenital abnormalities. In: Genitourinary radiology: the requisites, 2nd edn. Mosby, Philadelphia, pp 62–63

Zagoria RJ (2004b) Renal masses. In: Genitourinary radiology: the requisites, 2nd edn. Mosby, Philadelphia, pp 118–120

Zeman RK, Cronan JJ, Rosenfield AT et al. (1986) Computed tomography of renal masses: pitfalls and anatomic variants. Radiographics 6:351–372

# Radiofrequency Ablation and Cryoablation for Renal Cell Carcinoma

## 23

Andrew Hines-Peralta and S. Nahum Goldberg

## Contents

**Abstract**

> Percutaneous tumor ablation has become one of the most prevalent treatment options for small renal cell carcinomas given continued favorable outcome, and is already a treatment of choice for selected patients. Currently, the most common indications are elderly patients with small incidental tumors of unclear metastatic potential, and high-risk surgical patients since this procedure has been shown to be safe in patients with multiple co-morbidities. This chapter describes the indications, applicators, procedure, outcomes, and complications of percutaneous tumor ablation of renal cell carcinoma. Importantly, the technologies are continuously improving and it is expected that patient selection and satisfaction will continue to expand and outcomes will continue to improve.

Radiofrequency ablation and cryoablation are treatments for focal malignancy where a needle applicator is advanced through the skin into the center of a tumor (guided by ultrasound, computed tomography, or magnetic resonance imaging) and then induces hot or cold cytotoxic temperatures that rapidly result in tumor death (Goldberg et al. 2000). Once reserved for nonsurgical patients, these minimally-invasive treatment options have now expanded to include a larger spectrum of patients, fueled by continued favorable outcome studies, scarce complications, lower immediate morbidity and mortality than surgery, lower cost, outpatient capacity, and importantly, patient satisfaction (McAchran et al. 2005; Onishi et al. 2007). These

A. Hines-Peralta (✉) and S.N. Goldberg
Department of Radiology, Beth Israel Deaconess Medical Center, 1 Deaconess Rd, Room CC308, Boston, MA 02215, USA
e-mail: ahines@bidmc.harvard.edu

E. Quaia (ed.), *Radiological Imaging of the Kidney*,
Medical Radiology, DOI: 10.1007/978-3-540-87597-0_23, © Springer-Verlag Berlin Heidelberg 2011

benefits must be balanced with the acknowledgement of the relative newness of these procedures which is accompanied by lack of long-term data and that there are challenges including the inability to treat large, centrally located tumors near the renal hilum and difficulties monitoring ablation. But even as initial outcome data is published, rapid technological advancements and improvements in technique evoke even greater promise for success going forward.

## 23.1 Indications

According to the American Cancer Association, there are approximately 50,000 new cases of renal cell carcinoma diagnosed each year in the United States, an incidence that has more than doubled since 1950 (Jemal et al. 2008). Most of these are incidentally detected on high-resolution diagnostic imaging for unrelated indications. Many of these incidentally noted RCCs are T1a tumors (less 4 cm in diameter limited to the kidney) and found in elderly patients who are generally poorer surgical candidates as they were imaged for other comorbid conditions (Jayson and Sanders 1998). In addition, the benefit of a total or partial nephrectomy (currently the most common treatment option) is unclear for these small, nonaggressive RCCs whose natural course may not affect patient longevity (Hollingsworth et al. 2006). Indeed, prior to the development of these minimally invasive procedures, conservative watchful waiting was often advocated, despite substantial patient anxiety (Chow et al. 1999). For these patients, percutaneous tumor ablation is an attractive option since it spares the significant morbidity of surgery while offering effective and potentially curative treatment option (Onishi et al. 2007). Lastly, from a public health perspective, tumor ablation is likely preferred over surgery for small RCC treatment at a societal willingness-to-pay threshold (Pandharipande et al. 2008).

Patients needing nephron-sparing treatment such as those with a single kidney, bilateral RCCs, or with genetic predisposition to multiple tumors are good candidates even if initially they are also candidates for partial nephrectomy (Goldberg and Dupuy 2001). For example, patients with von Hippel-Lindau syndrome are excellent candidates, as alternative treatments to multiple partial nephrectomies for recurring RCCs is important to save nephrons and prolong the time to dialysis. Patients already on dialysis are also at increased risk for renal cell carcinoma, and given their renal failure are often poor surgical candidates as well. Other risk factors for renal cell carcinoma which may lead to poor surgical candidacy include smoking and obesity (Cohen and McGovern 2005).

Other uses of ablation in the treatment of RCC have included local tumor recurrence after nephrectomy (McLaughlin et al. 2003), intractable tumor-related hematuria (Wood et al. 2001), palliation for lung and symptomatic bone metastases (Zagoria et al. 2001; Dupuy et al. 1998), and tumor debulking in conjunction with immunotherapy in patients with stage IV disease (Goldberg and Dupuy 2001). Again, each case should be reviewed on a case by case basis.

## 23.2 Patient Selection

Patients are usually jointly evaluated by a urologist and interventional radiologist, but practices may vary amongst different centers. Regardless, each practitioner must weigh best interests of the patient. Since one-quarter of patients with RCC will have metastatic disease at diagnosis which precludes local treatment and indicates a poor 5-year survival rate, the extent of disease should be well established with sufficient abdominal and nonabdominal imaging to verify the extent of local tumor and metastatic involvement (Cohen and McGovern 2005). In addition, pretreatment imaging is important for treatment planning which can be performed via ultrasound, magnetic resonance, or CT guidance (Goldberg et al. 2000). Important laboratory values include prothrombin time, partial prothrombin time, complete blood cell count, creatinine, and screening for intravenous sedation or anesthesia. A biopsy prior to the procedure is not imperative but should be strongly considered, because imaging does not always accurately differentiate benign from malignant disease (Silverman et al. 2006).

Tumor size and location are the two most important factors that govern whether RCCs can be successfully treated (Gervais et al. 2005a). Since heat exponentially decreases from the radiofrequency or cryo source, large tumors (>5 cm) pose a significant challenge, especially since a 0.5- to 1.0-cm "ablation margin" surrounding the tumor is also preferred (Goldberg and Dupuy 2001). In general, RCC tumors that are 4 cm in diameter or less are ideal for ablation, with highly favorable success rates (>90%) when performed by well-trained clinicians (Levinson et al. 2008). Most tumors smaller than 3 cm can also be successfully treated in a single session (Zagoria et al. 2004). Tumors between 3.0 and 4.0 cm in diameter can also be successfully treated with confidence, but multiple ablations and sessions may be required (Gervais et al. 2005b). Indeed, as implied above when describing therapy for VHL RCC, one of the benefits cited for RF ablation is the ability to perform minimally-invasive repeated treatments.

The location of the tumor also influences ablation results. The easiest tumors to treat are exophytic as they are surrounded by heat-insulating perirenal fat (Liu et al. 2006; Ahmed et al. 2004). As a result, even large exophytic tumors are almost always successfully treated, with 70% or more requiring only a single RF session (Hui et al. 2008). Parenchymal tumors may be more difficult to treat, but centrally located tumors represent a larger obstacle for successful ablation given with the surrounding vascular tissue which draws heat away from the tumor (i.e., the heat-sink effect) (Lu et al. 2002). As a result, central tumors larger than 3 cm have an increased risk of treatment failure (Ogan et al. 2002). Additional factors affecting ablation are the electrical and thermal conductivities of the tumor and surrounding tissues which influence the capacity for energy deposition and heat accumulation, respectively (Ahmed et al. 2008; Solazzo et al. 2005).

Contraindications may include a poor life expectancy of less than 1 year, multiple metastases, or difficulty for successful treatment due to size or location of tumor (Ahrar et al. 2005). In general, large tumors (>5 cm) or tumors in the hilum or central collecting system are not typically recommended for percutaneous tumor ablation (Atwell et al. 2007; Gervais et al. 2005b). In addition, tumors located so that thermal injury may occur to the proximal ureter, resulting in urine extravasation and urinoma production, are usually deferred until an intraureteral stent has been placed by a urologist (Johnson et al. 2003). However, the only absolute contraindications include irreversible coagulopathies or severe medical instability such as sepsis.

## 23.3  Procedure

Successful percutaneous tumor ablation is a balance between two objectives: first, kill all viable malignant cells within a designated area including an 5–10 mm "ablative" margin of surrounding tissue, if possible (Goldberg et al. 2000). The most well-studied techniques are radiofrequency ablation and cryoablation and receive most attention but some emerging energy sources such as microwave and high-intensity focused ultrasound show some promise, but are only available in controlled experimental situations.

### 23.3.1  Radiofrequency Ablation

RF delivers a high-frequency (460–500 kHz) alternating current into the tumor by means of an RF applicator, a single thin needle (usually 21–14 gauge) that is electrically insulated along all but the distal 1–3 cm of the shaft, or an array of multiple such tines extending from a central cannula. The current produces resistive friction in the tissue that is converted into heat, analogous to heat production from an electrical resister in a circuit. Heat, in turn, induces cellular destruction and protein denaturation. Cell death occurs at temperatures higher than 50°C with complete tumor necrosis being achieved at 60–100°C (Goldberg et al. 2000). Most RF systems used for the kidney are monopolar and the current is completed via grounding pads placed on the patient's thighs. Efforts to increase tumor ablation have led to the development of various RF applicators such as multitined applicators, cluster applicators, pulsed energy delivery, and others. Currently, there are three RF devices with 510-K Food and Drug Administration approval for soft tumor ablation (Valleylab Cool-tip™, Boulder, Colorado; Boston Scientific LeVeen®, Natick, Massachusetts; Angiodynamics Starburst™, Queensbury, New York). No study has yet demonstrated a clear advantage of any one device and new devices are sure to become available given increasing market demand.

### 23.3.2  Cryoablation

Cryoablation uses cooled cryoprobes to freeze and destroy tumor. Traditionally, given the large applicator size (up to 8 mm diameter, or 0.5 gauge) (Finley et al. 2008), it was almost always administered via laparoscopy, but smaller applicators now enable percutaneous image-guided application (17 gauge) (Finley et al. 2008). Liquid nitrogen or argon is introduced into the probe in a controlled fashion, resulting in freezing of the surrounding tissues. The formation of ice crystals and subsequent thawing within a cell disrupts the cell membrane and other intracellular activities leading to cell death. Additional cells which are not directly killed may undergo apoptosis. A typical cyroablation session involves freezing, thawing, and re-freezing which is particularly effective at mediating cellular disruption (Hoffmann and Bischof 2002; Rupp et al. 2002).

One cited benefit of cryoablation is the ability to visualize the iceball in real time via CT or MR which allows the extent of cell death to be more reliably predicted (Edmunds et al. 2000). It is thought that complete cell death occurs 3 mm inside the edge of the ice ball with most operators extending the ice ball at least 5 mm beyond the tumor margin (Warlick et al. 2006). However, for RF ablation performed under CT guidance, a postprocedural scan with contrast will also often enable gross visualization of enhancing residual tumor which can then be re-treated (Goldberg et al. 2000).

### 23.3.3  Emerging Technologies

Microwave energy is emerging as a potential source of heat for use in thermal ablation although the technology is still in its infancy with only small experimental series in patients (Liang et al. 2008; Clark et al. 2007). In contrast to radiofrequency, within the tip of the inserted microwave applicator is an antenna for externally applied energy at 1,000–2,450 mHz. The deposited microwave energy results in rotation of polar molecules that is opposed by frictional forces which are then converted to heat (Carrafiello et al. 2008). One potential advantage of microwave over RF is greater energy deposition and higher temperatures, especially since microwave is not impeded by peri-applicator tissue charring like RF. The higher energy may also be more resilient to the heat-sink effect which can be an important obstacle for RF (Brace et al. 2007). As such, the technology is deserving of further consideration, but requires further investigation as the efficacy and safety relative to more proven technologies are still to be determined (Liang et al. 2008).

High-intensity focused ultrasound is another emerging minimally invasive ablation tool with most research focused on fibroid treatment (Lenard et al. 2008). There has not yet been any well-documented investigation for the possible application for renal tumors. One theoretically attractive option is that cytotoxic heat accumulation is created via multiple high-intensity sound waves delivered by a transducer on the skin converge without any physical penetration of the skin surface (Klingler et al. 2008).

### 23.3.4  Difficulties Comparing Modalities and Approaches

There is currently no conventional acceptance as to which modality is superior given insufficient data for even the two most widely used procedures: radiofrequency ablation vs. cryoablation. Cryoablation is almost always performed with laparoscopy owing to the large size of most applicators, and there is insufficient follow-up data for the more recently developed percutaneous cryoablation to be useful for comparison. On the other hand, it has been used longer so there is potentially more experience with that technique. Recognizing these differences, meta-analyses indicate that a second treatment session is necessary more often for percutaneous radiofrequency ablation than for laparoscopic cryoablation (primary efficacy rates of 87.1% and 94.8%, respectively) (Kunkle and Uzzo 2008; Hui et al. 2008). However, the secondary efficacy rates after retreatment are similar (92% and 95%, respectively, $p > 0.05$) (Hui et al. 2008). There is also no significant difference between metastatic progression (2.5% and 1.0%, respectively, $p > 0.05$) (Kunkle and Uzzo 2008). However, meta-analysis does suggest that major complications may be lower in percutaneous radiofrequency ablation than laparoscopic cryoablation (3% vs. 7%, respectively) (Kunkle and Uzzo 2008). Additionally, other initial comparisons between percutaneous and laparoscopic cryoablation suggests that there may be higher overall complications, transfusion rates, analgesic use, and hospital stays with a laparoscopic approach compared to percutaneous treatment (40%, 28%, 17.8 mg, 3.1 days vs. 22%, 11%, 5.1 mg, 1.3 days, respectively, all $p < 0.05$) with similar failure rates at 1 year follow-up (4.2% and 5.3%, respectively) (Finley et al. 2008). Further validation with randomized prospective data is necessary as these studies are small retrospective studies that cannot control for factors that may have influenced the choice of approach. Analysis of 5- and 10-year follow-up data will be helpful when available.

Regardless, we adhere to the notion that less invasive approaches should be preferred over more invasive in the setting of similar outcomes.

In conclusion, in the setting of RCC, percutaneous ablation procedures can be considered over laparoscopic ones, saving partial nephrectomy for cases when the first two approaches are not advised. However, comparing the individual percutaneous modalities (i.e., radiofrequency ablation and cryoablation) for definite advantages over each other is challenging, as both are being presently refined. Thus, the most important factors will continue to be proper patient selection and meticulous technique by experienced clinicians.

## 23.3.5 Adjuvant Therapy

Recent studies have demonstrated that modification of tumor vessel density using antiangiogenic agents such as sorafenib (Nexavar®, Bayer HealthCare, Leverkusen, Germany) and sunitinib (Sutent®, Pfizer Labs, New York, New York) to increased RF coagulation. In one study, the administration of sorafenib prior to RF ablation markedly decreased microvascular density and led to significantly larger zones of RF-induced coagulation necrosis (Hakime et al. 2007). There is also the potential for combining treatment with radiation as has been examined in animal studies and in patients with lung cancer (Horkan et al. 2005; Dupuy et al. 2006). Although these methods are still in their investigational phase, there is promise for their rapid acceptance and adoption in standard clinical practice.

## 23.3.6 Biopsy Controversy

There is currently some debate about whether biopsy should be performed before ablation. For most institutions, pathologic confirmation of malignancy is a tacit or explicit requirement before any type of treatment is initiated, including thermal ablation, but some institutions are beginning to question whether a biopsy is always necessary (Beland et al. 2007). Additionally, ablation of the tumor will make pathologic examination of the tissue much more challenging if this is ever needed for future therapeutic considerations. The argument to not perform a biopsy is the need for two percutaneous procedures which are associated with increased costs and small but genuine procedural risks and that many tumors demonstrate imaging features that are highly suggestive of renal cell carcinoma perhaps making biopsy redundant (Herts and Baker 1995). In addition, even small amounts of hemorrhage associated with biopsy can potentially obscure the margins of the tumor which can increase the difficulty of the ablative procedure. Unlike laparoscopic surgery where port-site seeding is estimated to be 0.1%, percutaneous tumor tract seeding has only been reported in a single case report (Castillo and Vitagliano 2008; Bush et al. 1977; Tanaka et al. 2008). To minimize the risks and costs, a biopsy can be easily performed immediately prior to ablation, but pathologic analysis cannot be rendered before tumor ablation commences.

## 23.3.7 Day of the Procedure

Regardless of the energy source, the percutaneous procedure is usually an outpatient procedure unless comorbid conditions require hospitalization or closer observation. Only conscious sedation is typically necessary for anesthesia, although some physicians and patients prefer general anesthesia. The patient is placed prone, and after local anesthesia is applied, the applicator is percutaneous advanced into the center of the tumor under image guidance (CT, ultrasound, or MR). Heat or cold is then applied for approximately 10–20 min as dictated per manufacturer recommendations. Depending upon the size and location of the tumor, the applicator may need to be re-adjusted and additional treatments administered. After the procedure, the patient is monitored for several hours, and discharged home with oral analgesics for postprocedural pain with patients usually resuming to full activity in a couple of days. A laparoscopic approach is similar to other surgical laparoscopic procedures requiring general anesthesia, etc. Patients are hospitalized at least overnight and may have slightly higher postprocedural pain (Finley et al. 2008).

## 23.4 Outcomes and Complications

### 23.4.1 Imaging Follow-Up

The success of percutaneous tumor ablation is assessed by postprocedural imaging, typically by computed tomography or MR starting 1 month after treatment. Imaging immediately following the procedure can be difficult to interpret, because peripheral inflammation may mimic the appearance of viable tumor. On computed tomography, viable tumor is usually nodular and maintains its enhancement (>10-HU postcontrast injection) whereas successfully ablated tumor loses its attenuation, consistent with coagulation necrosis (Gervais et al. 2005a, b). It has also been noted that tumors usually decrease in size immediately after ablation by about 20% while many continue to involute over time (Ganguli et al. 2008). Very rarely does the zone of ablation enlarge because of liquefactive necrosis (Merkle et al. 2005). The area of nonenhancement itself may be larger than the original tumor as the zone of ablation is expected to be larger than the tumor to allow for an "ablative margin." Recurrent tumor will usually manifest as peripheral nodular or peripheral crescent enhancement (Gervais et al. 2005a, b). Subsequent follow-up imaging is usually performed at 3–6, 12, 18, and 24 months after ablation, and yearly thereafter.

Many patients who undergo percutaneous tumor ablation have renal insufficiency which is often a large contributing factor in deciding to undergo tumor ablation since it limits destruction to vital normal renal parenchyma. For these patients, follow-up imaging is often performed with MR to limit the toxicity of iodinated contrast administered with CT. Yet, unenhanced imaging is almost never sufficient for evaluation of recurrent tumor.

Current thinking is that even if the eGFR is estimated to be very low which may place the patient at risk for nephrogenic systemic fibrosis (Wertman et al. 2008), the risk-benefit ratio still usually favors proceeding with MR imaging with gadolinium rather than CT with iodine-based contrast agents (Geoffrey et al. 2007). Again, residual or recurrent tumor usually manifests as abnormal nodular or crescent enhancement with gadolinium. Immediate postablation MR imaging may demonstrates smooth rim peripheral enhancement secondary to surrounding hyperemia. Unenhanced T1 and T2 signal may be variable and complex due to hemorrhage, coagulated protein, and liquefactive necrosis (Merkle et al. 2005).

### 23.4.2 Imaging Pitfalls

During ablation, gas is formed without and about the tumor as a by-product of tissue coagulation (Fig. 23.1). This may be visualized on immediate postprocedural imaging and should not be mistaken for bowel injury. In addition, hydrodissection is occasionally employed prior to ablation to protect adjacent organs from heat injury. This involves infusing sterile water into the surrounding tissue to create a barrier between adjacent organs and the ablative zone (Fig. 23.2). This should not be mistaken for hemorrhage or bowel injury.

Follow-up imaging also commonly demonstrates inflammatory stranding within the surrounding perirenal fat which should not be confused with residual tumor. Over time, a thin soft tissue halo may also appear within the surrounding fat due to encapsulation of fat necrosis which should not be interpreted as recurrent tumor (Fig. 23.1) (Gervais et al. 2003). More recently, it has also been observed that enhancing inflammatory nodules do rarely appear (<2% of the time) after percutaneous ablation which may mimic tumor seeding of the applicator tract (Lokken et al. 2007). Real tumor tract seeding is exceeding rare and has only ever been reported once after radiofrequency ablation of RCC (Mayo-Smith et al. 2003). Instead, a new enhancing nodule within or adjacent to the applicator track is more likely to represent chronic inflammation containing histiocytes, granulation tissue, and fibrosis. These will usually appear as either a ring-enhancing nodule or ill-defined tram-tracking enhancement appearing 3–52 months after ablation (Lokken et al. 2007). Nodular enhancement along the ablated tumor margin, however, should be treated with suspicion for recurrence.

### 23.4.3 Outcomes

Results vary depending upon modality (cryoablation vs. radiofrequency), applicator type (single vs. multi-tine) but meta-analyses across all percutaneous

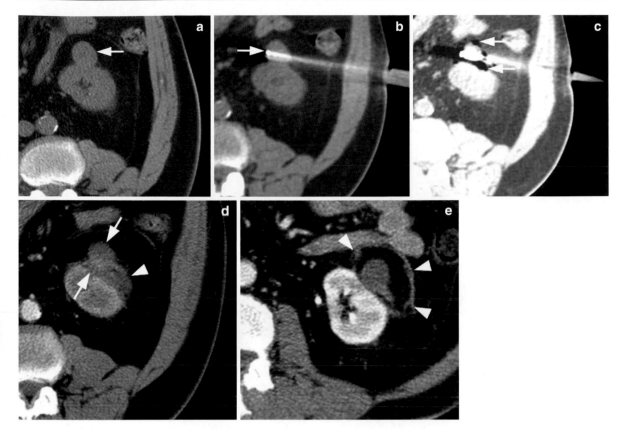

**Fig. 23.1** Successful radiofrequency ablation of renal cell carcinoma. (**a**) Noncontrast CT demonstrates exophytic 2.5 cm tumor (*arrow*), (**b**) positioning of RF applicator with tip at distal end of tumor (*arrow*), (**c**) gas (*arrows*) is produced during ablation secondary to high temperature coagulation (**d**) immediate contrast-enhanced CT demonstrates nonenhancement of the tumor with a small surrounding "margin" of nonenhancement of adjacent kidney (*arrows*) and small clinically insignificant peri-nephric hemorrhage (*arrowhead*), (**e**) 2 years after ablation, contrast enhanced CT follow up demonstrates continued nonenhancement of the tumor with a characteristic fat "halo" in the perirenal fat (*arrowheads*), suggesting complete treatment

approaches yields a secondary effectiveness rate (that is, no evidence of recurrence after multiple treatments is necessary) of greater than 90% for tumors smaller than 4 cm which does not significantly different than surgical treatment at 1 year (Hui et al. 2008).

### 23.4.3.1 Outcomes for Radiofrequency Ablation

Some mid-term data is becoming available demonstrating recurrence-free survival rate of approximately 90% at 5 years for tumors smaller than 4 cm (Levinson et al. 2008). Additionally, as technology and the learning curve have markedly progressed since treatment was performed for these initial survival data, future studies are expected to be as good or better. Again, treatment success is dependent upon size and location (exophytic vs. central) with near 100% recurrence-free disease possible with selected tumor sizes (<4 cm) with larger tumors associated with increased risk of recurrence.

### 23.4.3.2 Outcomes for Cryoablation

Data is very limited for percutaneous cryoablation but short-term success (1 year) also appears to also be excellent with success rates consistently above 95% (Atwell et al. 2008). In addition, technical success was achieved with tumors ranging up to 7 cm, though the same principle of selecting tumors less than 4 cm still applies for optimal results (Stein and Kaouk 2007). Again, 5- and 10-year follow-up outcome data will be helpful with the caveat that current treatments will likely be superior given continuously technological improvements.

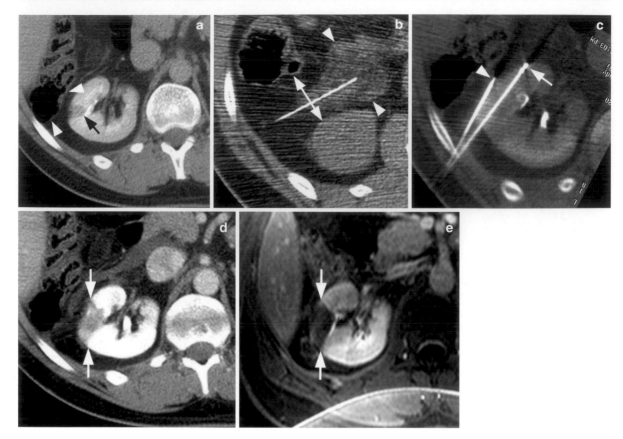

**Fig. 23.2** Use of hydrodissection in thermal ablation to protect adjacent structures in a patient with multiple RCCs. (**a**) The colon (*arrowheads*) is closely approximated to the 1.3 cm tumor in the right kidney (*black arrow*), risking thermal injury, (**b**) 5% dextrose in water (*arrowheads*) is injected into the perirenal fat which successfully separates the colon from the kidney (*double-headed arrow*), (**c**) applicator needle (*arrow*) is positioned into the tumor with aid of a guiding needle (*arrowhead*), (**d**) immediate postablation CT demonstrates the ablative zone about the tumor (*arrows*), (**e**) 6-month follow-up MR with gadolinium demonstrates no recurrent tumor enhancement (*arrows*). A second 1.5 cm RCC in the right lower pole was also successfully treated during the same session (not shown)

When comparing the outcomes of laparoscopic to percutaneous cryoablation at the same center, the procedural outcomes are demonstrably superior for percutaneous cryoablation including lower complications and transfusions (22% vs. 40%, respectively), shorter hospital stays (1.3 vs. 3.1 days, respectively), and lower narcotic use (5.1 vs. 17.8 mg, respectively). It should be noted that the complication rates reported in this series were higher than the accepted complication rate for percutaneous cryoablation (around 3%) (Hui et al. 2008). Regardless, in short-term follow-up (13 months), cancer specific survival is similar for percutaneous and laparoscopic cryoablation (100% and 100%, respectively) and initial treatment failure was also not significantly different at 5.3% (1/19) and 4.3% (1/24), respectively.

### 23.4.4 Complications

The average complication rate is less than 5% for both radiofrequency and cryoablation, but almost none result in long-term morbidity. Meta-analyses demonstrate a major complication rate of 3% for percutaneous treatment vs. 7% in the surgical treatment group (7%; $p < 0.05$) which is the accepted clinical understanding (Hui et al. 2008; Johnson et al. 2004). The most common complications include perinephric hematoma, pneumothorax, nerve injury, and pain. Central tumors and tumors within the lower pole also run the risk of ureteral or ureteropelvic injury. A few case reports have documented nephrectomies that were necessary after ureteral injury or obstruction, but again, this is compared to oncologic treatment that could have included nephrectomy itself.

It is also important to note that the very low complication rate associated with RF ablation is reported in patients who were already deemed too high risk for surgical intervention because of advanced age or medical co morbidities. Thus, even in high-risk patients, percutaneous tumor ablation is associated with a very low complication rate.

## 23.5 Conclusion

Minimally invasive treatments for renal cell carcinoma such as percutaneous tumor ablation will undoubtedly become more prevalent as outcomes continue to be favorable, and should be considered a viable treatment options for selected patients. Currently, the most common indications are elderly patients with small incidental tumors of unclear lethal potential, and for all high-risk surgical patients as this procedure has been shown to be safe in patients with multiple co-morbidities. Multiple modalities are available, but the most common are RF and cyroablation which are likely similar in efficacy but still lack sufficient long-term data. These technologies are continuously improving, and it is expected that as a result, patient selection and satisfaction will continue to expand.

## References

Ahmed M, Liu Z, Afzal KS et al. (2004) Radiofrequency ablation: effect of surrounding tissue composition on coagulation necrosis in a canine tumor model. Radiology 230(3):761–767

Ahmed M, Liu Z, Humphries S et al. (2008) Computer modeling of the combined effects of perfusion, electrical conductivity, and thermal conductivity on tissue heating patterns in radiofrequency tumor ablation. Int J Hyperthermia 24(7): 577–588

Ahrar K, Matin S, Wood CG et al. (2005) Percutaneous radiofrequency ablation of renal tumors: technique, complications, and outcomes. J Vasc Interv Radiol 16:679–688

Atwell TD, Farrell MA, Callstrom MR et al. (2007) Percutaneous cryoablation of large renal masses: technical feasibility and short-term outcome. AJR Am J Roentgenol 188(5): 1195–1200

Atwell TD, Farrell MA, Leibovich BC et al. (2008) Percutaneous renal cryoablation: experience treating 115 tumors. J Urol 179(6):2136–2140

Beland MD, Mayo-Smith WW, Dupuy DE et al. (2007) Diagnostic yield of 58 consecutive imaging-guided biopsies of solid renal masses: should we biopsy all that are indeterminate? AJR Am J Roentgenol 188(3):792–797

Brace CL, Laeseke PF, Sampson LA et al. (2007) Mircrowave ablation with multiple simultaneously powered small-guage triaxial antennas: results from an in vivo swine liver model. Radiology 244(1):151–156

Bush WH Jr, Burnett LL, Gibbons RP (1977) Needle tract seeding of renal cell carcinoma. AJR Am J Roentgenol 129(4): 725–727

Carrafiello G, Laganà D, Mangini M et al. (2008) Microwave tumors ablation: principles, clinical applications and review of preliminary experiences. Int J Surg 6(suppl 1):S65–S69

Castillo OA, Vitagliano G (2008) Port site metastasis and tumor seeding in oncologic laparoscopic urology. Urology 71(3): 373–378

Chow WH, Devesa SS, Warren JL et al. (1999) Rising incidence of renal cell cancer in the United States. JAMA 281: 1628–1631

Clark PE, Woodruff RD, Zagoria RJ et al. (2007) Microwave ablation of renal parenchymal tumors before nephrectomy: phase I study. AJR Am J Roentgenol 188(5):1212–1214

Cohen HT, McGovern FJ (2005) Renal-cell carcinoma. N Engl J Med 353:2477–2490

Dupuy DE, Safran H, Mayo-Smith WW et al. (1998) Radiofrequency ablation of painful osseous metastases. Radiology 209(P):389

Dupuy DE et al. (2006) Radiofrequency ablation followed by conventional radiotherapy for medically inoperable stage I non-small cell lung cancer. Chest 129(3):738–745

Edmunds TB, Schulsinger DA, Durand DB et al. (2000) Acute histologic changes in human renal tumors after cryoablation. J Endourol 14(2):139–143

Finley DS, Beck S, Box G et al. (2008) Percutaneous and laparoscopic cryoablation of small renal masses. J Urol 180(2): 492–498

Ganguli S, Brennan DD, Faintuch S et al. (2008) Immediate renal tumor involution after radiofrequency thermal ablation. J Vasc Interv Radiol 19(3):412–418

Geoffrey EW, Leyendecker JR, Krehbiel KA et al. (2007) CT and MR imaging after imaging-guided thermal ablation of renal neoplasms. Radiographics 27:325–339

Gervais DA, Arellano RS, McGovern FJ et al. (2005a) Radiofrequency ablation of renal cell carcinoma. II. Lessons learned with ablation of 100 tumors. AJR Am J Roentgenol 185:72–80

Gervais DA, McGovern FJ, Arellano RS et al. (2005b) Radiofrequency ablation of renal cell carcinoma. I. Indications, results, and role in patient management over a 6-year period and ablation of 100 tumors. AJR Am J Roentgenol 185:64–71

Gervais DA, McGovern FJ, Arellano RS et al. (2003) Renal cell carcinoma: clinical experience and technical success with radio-frequency ablation of 42 tumors. Radiology 226: 417–424

Goldberg SN, Dupuy DE (2001) Image-guided radiofrequency tumor ablation: challenges and opportunities – part I. JVIR 12:1021–1032

Goldberg SN, Gazelle GS, Mueller PR (2000) Thermal ablation therapy for focal malignancy: a unified approach to underlying principles, techniques, and diagnostic imaging guidance. Am J Radiol 174:323–331

Hakime A, Hines-Peralta AU, Peddy H et al. (2007) Combination of radiofrequency ablation with antiangiogenic therapy for tumor ablation efficacy: study in mice. Radiology 244(2): 464–470

Herts BR, Baker ME (1995) The current role of percutaneous biopsy in the evaluation of renal masses. Semin Urol Oncol 13(4):254–261

Hoffmann NE, Bischof JC (2002) The cryobiology of cryosurgical injury. Urology 60:40–49

Hollingsworth JM, Miller DC, Daignault S et al. (2006) Rising incidence of small renal masses: a need to reassess treatment effect. J Natl Cancer Inst 98:1331–1334

Horkan C et al. (2005) Reduced tumor growth with combined radiofrequency ablation and radiation therapy in a rat breast tumor model. Radiology 235(1):81–88

Hui GC, Tuncali K, Tatli S et al. (2008) Comparison of percutaneous and surgical approaches to renal tumor ablation: metaanalysis of effectiveness and complication rates. J Vasc Interv Radiol 19(9):1311–1320

Jayson M, Sanders H (1998) Increased incidence of serendipitously discovered renal cell carcinoma. Urology 51:203–205

Jemal A, Siegel R, Ward E et al. (2008) Cancer statistics, 2008. CA Cancer J Clin 58:71–96

Johnson DB, Saboorian MH, Duchene DA et al. (2003) Nephrectomy after radiofrequency ablation-induced ureteropelvic junction obstruction: potential complication and long-term assessment of ablation adequacy. Urology 62(2):351–352

Johnson DB, Solomon SB, Su LM et al. (2004) Defining the complications of cryoablation and radio frequency ablation of small renal tumors: a multi-institutional review. J Urol 172:874–877

Klingler HC, Susani M, Seip R et al. (2008) A novel approach to energy ablative therapy of small renal tumours: laparoscopic high-intensity focused ultrasound. Eur Urol 53(4):810–816

Kunkle DA, Uzzo RG (2008) Cryoablation or radiofrequency ablation of the small renal mass: a meta-analysis. Cancer 113(10):2671–2680

Lenard ZM, McDannold NJ, Fennessy FM et al. (2008) Uterine leiomyomas: MR imaging-guided focused ultrasound surgery – imaging predictors of success. Radiology 249(1): 187–194

Levinson AW, Su LM, Agarwal D et al. (2008) Long-term oncological and overall outcomes of percutaneous radio frequency ablation in high risk surgical patients with a solitary small renal mass. J Urol 180(2):499–504

Liang P, Wang Y, Zhang D et al. (2008) Ultrasound guided percutaneous microwave ablation for small renal cancer: initial experience. J Urol 180(3):844–848

Liu Z, Ahmed M, Weinstein Y et al. (2006) Characterization of the RF ablation-induced "oven effect": the importance of background tissue thermal conductivity on tissue heating. Int J Hyperthermia 22(4):327–342

Lokken RP, Gervais DA, Arellano RS et al. (2007) Inflammatory nodules mimic applicator track seeding after percutaneous ablation of renal tumors. AJR Am J Roentgenol 189: 845–848

Lu DS, Raman SS, Vodopich DJ et al. Effect of vessel size on creation of hepatic radiofrequency lesions in pigs: assessment of the "heat sink" effect. AJR Am J Roentgenol 178: 47–51

Mayo-Smith WW, Dupuy DE, Parikh PM et al. (2003) Imaging-guided percutaneous radiofrequency ablation of solid renal masses; techniques and outcomes of 38 treatment sessions in 32 consecutive patients. AJR Am J Roentgenol 180:1503–1508

McAchran SE, Lesani OA, Resnick MI (2005) Radiofrequency ablation of renal tumors: past, present, and future. Urology 66:15–22

McLaughlin CA, Chen MY, Torti FM et al. (2003) Radiofrequency ablation of isolated local recurrence of renal cell carcinoma after radical nephrectomy. AJR Am J Roentgenol 181:93–94

Merkle EM, Nour SG, Lewin JS (2005) MR imaging follow-up after percutaneous radiofrequency ablation of renal cell carcinoma: findings in 18 patients during first 6 months. Radiology 235:1065–1071

Ogan K, Jacomides L, Dolmatch BL et al. (2002) Percutaneous radiofrequency ablation of renal tumors: technique, limitations, and morbidity. Urology 60(6):954–958

Onishi T, Nishikawa K, Hasegawa Y et al. (2007) Assessment of health-related quality of life after radiofrequency ablation or laparoscopic surgery for small renal cell carcinoma: a prospective study with medical outcomes Study 36-Item Health Survey (SF-36). Jpn J Clin Oncol 37:750–754

Pandharipande PV, Gervais DA, Mueller PR et al. (2008) Radiofrequency ablation versus nephron-sparing surgery for small unilateral renal cell carcinoma: cost-effectiveness analysis. Radiology 248(1):169–178

Rupp CC, Hoffmann NE, Schmidlin FR et al. (2002) Cryosurgical changes in the porcine kidney: histologic analysis with thermal history correlation. Cryobiology 45:167–182

Silverman SG, Gan YU, Mortele JK et al. (2006) Renal masses in the adult patient: the role of percutaneous biopsy. Radiology 240(1):6–22

Solazzo SA, Liu Z, Lobo SM et al. (2005) Radiofrequency ablation: importance of background tissue electrical conductivity – an agar phantom and computer modeling study. Radiology 236(2):495–502

Stein RJ, Kaouk JH (2007) Renal cryotherapy: a detailed review including a 5-year follow-up. BJU Int 99:1265–1270

Tanaka K, Hara I, Takenaka A et al. (2008) Incidence of local and port site recurrence of urologic cancer after laparoscopic surgery. Urology 71(4):728–734

Thabet A, Kalva S, Gervais DA (2009) Percutaneous image-guided therapy of intra-abdominal malignancy: imaging evaluation of treatment response. Abdom Imaging 34(5): 593–609

Volpe A, Mattar K, Finelli A et al. (2008) Contemporary results of percutaneous biopsy of 100 small renal masses: a single center experience. J Urol 180(6):2333–2337

Warlick CA, Lima GC, Allaf ME et al. (2006) Clinical sequelae of radiographic iceball involvement of collecting system during computed tomography-guided percutaneous renal tumor cryoablation. Urology 67(5):918–922

Wertman R, Altun E, Martin DR et al. (2008) Risk of nephrogenic systemic fibrosis: evaluation of gadolinium chelate contrast agents at four American universities. Radiology 248(3):799–806

Wood BJ, Grippo J, Pavlovich CP (2001) Percutaneous radio frequency ablation for hematuria. J Urol 166:2303–2304

Zagoria RJ, Chen MY, Kavanagh PV et al. (2001) Radio frequency ablation of lung metastases from renal cell carcinoma. J Urol 166(5):1827–1828

Zagoria RJ, Hawkins AD, Clark PE et al. (2004) Percutaneous CT-guided radiofrequency ablation of renal neoplasms: factors influencing success. AJR Am J Roentgenol 183:201–207

# Upper Urinary Tract Tumors

# 24

## Emilio Quaia and Paola Martingano

## Contents

## Abstract

> The tumors of the upper urinary tract include tumors developing in the renal pelvis and ureter. Transitional cell carcinomas (TCCs) of the renal pelvis or renal calices are relatively rare tumors of the kidney. Multidetector CT urography is currently considered the most sensitive and comprehensive imaging modality for the evaluation of the entire urinary tract and the detection of TCCs. TCCs may manifest as single or multiple discrete filling defects, filling defects within distended calyces, calyceal obliteration (calyceal amputation), hydronephrosis with renal enlargement caused by tumor obstruction of ureteropelvic junction, or as reduced renal function – excluded kidney – without renal enlargement caused by long-standing tumor obstruction of the ureteropelvic junction and atrophy.

Urothelial tumors of the renal pelvis and ureters (upper urinary tract) are relatively rare. Transitional cell carcinoma (TCC) may be present in the bladder (90%), renal pelvis or calices (8%), or ureter and proximal two thirds of the urethra (2%). TCC accounts for up to 10% of neoplasms of the upper urinary tract (Browne et al. 2005; Kirkali and Tuzel 2003), while renal pelvic TCC corresponds to 15% of the renal tumors (Guinan et al. 1992; Wong-You-Cheong et al. 1998) and usually manifest as hematuria which may be frank or microscopic (Browne et al. 2005). Up to one third of patients present with flank pain or acute renal colic, symptoms more typically associated with calculi (Browne et al. 2005).

E. Quaia (⊠) and P. Martingano
Department of Radiology, Cattinara Hospital,
University of Trieste, Strada di Fiume 447,
34149 Trieste, Italy
e-mail: quaia@univ.trieste.it

E. Quaia (ed.), *Radiological Imaging of the Kidney*,
Medical Radiology, DOI: 10.1007/978-3-540-87597-0_24, © Springer-Verlag Berlin Heidelberg 2011

Occasionally, tumors may manifest with distant metastases or be discovered incidentally at radiologic examination.

Renal TCC most frequently arises in the extrarenal part of the pelvis, followed by the infundibulocaliceal region (Browne et al. 2005). The distribution is equal between the left and right kidneys, with 2–4% of cases occurring bilaterally. Twenty-five percent of the upper urinary tract tumors occur in the ureter, where 60–75% of cases are found in the lower third, with no side predominance. Tumor spread occurs by mucosal extension or local, hematogenous, or lymphatic invasion. The most common sites for metastases are the liver, bone, and lungs. The tumor stage at diagnosis influences the development of local recurrence and metastases, and hence, overall survival.

Multicentric TCC is common and associated with poor survival. Synchronous or metachronous tumor of the ipsilateral or contralateral collecting system is also common, necessitating urologic and radiologic follow-up. Metachronous multicentric upper urinary tract TCC corresponds to 11–13% of cases, while synchronous bilateral renal pelvic TCC accounts for 1–2% of cases. The upper urinary tract should also be evaluated carefully in patients with a history of bladder urothelial neoplasm, as 0–6% of these patients eventually develop methacronous upper tract urothelial neoplasms within approximately 6 years (Dillman et al. 2008; Leder and Dunnick 1990).

## 24.1 Pathology and Histology of Transitional Cell Carcinoma

Carcinomas of the renal pelvis or calices are relatively rare tumors of the kidney, and their incidence is reported to be 5–12% of all malignant tumors of the kidney (Grabstald et al. 1971; Nocks et al. 1982). It is commonly seen in older patients, usually between the sixth and eight decade of life with a mean age of 65 years (see Chap. 28). The incidence in men exceeds that in women and the usual sex ratio is between 2:1 and 4:1 (Nocks et al. 1982). TCC is divided into two histologic subtypes: papillary and nonpapillary. Both subtypes consist of transitional epithelium with varying degrees of cellular and architectural atypia, arranged on thin connective tissue cores in the papillary subtype and forming thickened urothelium in the nonpapillary subtype (Pedrosa et al. 2008).

The usual clinical manifestations are gross hematuria (about 80% of the patients), abdominal pain with or without acute flank pain (about 10% of patients). Hematuria may be intermittent or microscopic. Anyway, TCC may also be asymptomatic and incidentally identified during intravenous or CT urography. Rarely, the clinical presentation may be that of urinary retention following urinary tract obstruction by clots. The TCC of the renal pelvis may be experimentally induced by several agents, e.g., dibenzanthracene, methylcholanthrene, benzopyrene corresponding to the metabolites of benzidine, and lead salts. A relationship between TCC and Thorotrast used for retrograde pyelography, phenacetin, and tobacco smoke has been shown.

Renal TCC starts most frequently in the extrarenal pelvis and migrates next to the infundibulocaliceal region (Barentsz et al. 1996). Eighty-five percent of upper tract TCCs are low-stage, superficial, papillary neoplasms with a broad base and frondlike morphologic structure (Browne et al. 2005). Early tumors confined to the muscularis do not infiltrate and are separated from the renal parenchyma by sinus fat or excreted contrast material and have normal-appearing peripelvic fat. These tumors are usually small at diagnosis, grow slowly, and follow a relatively benign course. Pedunculated or diffusely infiltrating tumor is less common, accounting for approximately 15% of upper tract TCCs, but tends to behave more aggressively and be more advanced at diagnosis. Infiltrating tumors are characterized by thickening and induration of the ureteric or renal pelvic wall. If the renal pelvis is involved, there is often invasion into the renal parenchyma. However, this infiltrative growth pattern preserves renal contour and differs from renal cell carcinoma, which is typically expansile. Ureteral neoplasms are most commonly located in the distal third of the ureter (50–70% of cases), and more rarely in the middle (15–25% of cases) and proximal third of the ureter (10–12% of cases).

Typically, TCC is frequently multiple, affecting the renal pelvis, the ureter, and the bladder at the same time. The multiplicity of the site may be synchronous or metachronous. Synchronous bilateral TCC has been reported to occur in 1–2% of cases of renal lesions and 2–9% of cases of ureteric lesions. Eleven percent to 13% of patients with upper tract TCC subsequently develop metachronous upper tract tumors. Furthermore, 20–40% of patients initially presenting with upper tract TCC will develop metachronous tumors in the bladder, typically developing within 2 years of surgical treatment and seen more commonly with ureteric tumors than with renal tumors. Two percent of patients with bladder TCC also have synchronous upper tract tumors at presentation and 6% will develop metachronous upper tract disease (Browne et al. 2005).

Hematogenous spread is less common than with renal cell carcinoma, but lymphatic metastases occur early. High-grade tumors are more common in the upper urinary tract than in the bladder, even though stage, rather than tumor grade, is the main predictor of prognosis for urothelial tumors of the upper urinary tract (Ozsahin et al. 1999).

## 24.2 Imaging

### 24.2.1 Imaging of Upper Tract Urinary Tumors

The initial diagnosis of TCC is usually made on the basis of findings from urine cytology; the diagnostic yield is improved with selective lavage and collection and with brush biopsies performed at cystoscopy or retrograde pyelography. However, these techniques are invasive and technically demanding.

#### 24.2.1.1 Ultrasonography

Currently, renal US is frequently requested in the evaluation of patients with hematuria to assess for renal parenchymal masses. Calcification may be visualized on control radiographs but is uncommon, occurring in 2–7% of tumors, and when present, may mimic urinary tract calculi. Enlargement of the kidney may be seen with a large infiltrating tumor or a ureteric tumor causing prolonged obstruction. However, US is not as sensitive as CT in identifying or characterizing renal masses; as CT urography emerges as an initial imaging investigation for hematuria, US will likely play a limited diagnostic role in the future. US can be useful in patients with renal functional impairment or allergy to iodinated contrast material, although MR imaging is becoming established as the investigation of choice in these patients. US can also allow assessment of the degree of hydronephrosis and guide interventional procedures in the setting of acute obstruction.

At US, renal pelvic TCC typically appears as a central soft-tissue mass in the echogenic renal sinus (Fig. 24.1), with or without hydronephrosis. TCC is usually slightly hyperechoic relative to surrounding renal parenchyma; occasionally, high-grade TCC may show areas of mixed echogenicity. Infundibular tumors may cause focal hydronephrosis. Although lesions may extend into the renal cortex and cause focal contour distortion, TCC typically is infiltrative and does

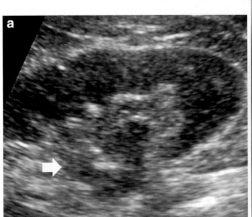
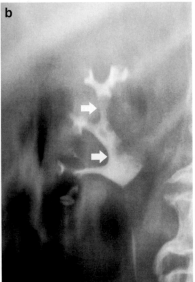

**Fig. 24.1** (**a**) Renal pelvic transitional cell carcinoma (TCC) (*arrow*) appearing as a central soft-tissue mass in the echogenic renal sinus at US. (**b**) The same case examined by intravenous excretory urography revealing multiple filling defects (*arrows*) on renal pelvis

not distort the renal contour. US has a limited role in the evaluation of ureteric TCC as the ureters are rarely visualized in their entirety, even if dilated. If visualized, these tumors are typically intraluminal soft-tissue masses with proximal distention of the ureter. US also allows limited assessment of periureteric tissues. Recent developments in high-resolution endoluminal US performed during ureterorenoscopy have shown promise in the evaluation of upper tract TCC, offering potential advantages over other imaging techniques, and may assume a more prominent role in future diagnosis.

### 24.2.1.2 Intravenous Excretory Urography

Intravenous excretory urography was traditionally considered the first imaging modality to identify upper urinary tract tumors. Intravenous excretory urography presents extremely high accuracy in the detection of upper urinary tract tumors, even though it cannot define the extraluminal extension of the tumor. Lowe and Roylance (1976) described five distinct patterns of upper urinary tract malignancies at intravenous excretory urography, which could be translated for CT urography: (a) single (Fig. 24.2)

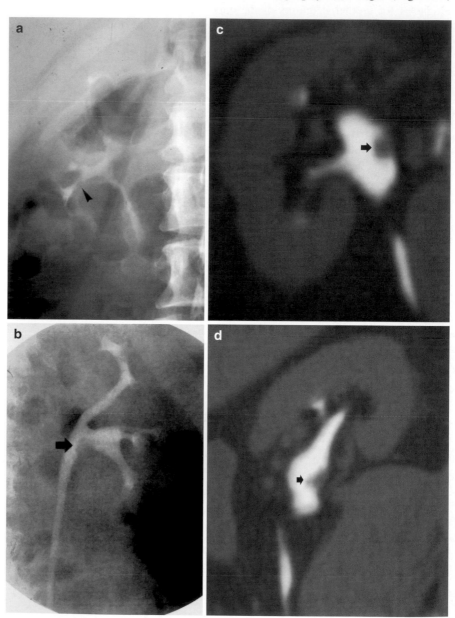

**Fig. 24.2** (**a–d**) The different morphologic patterns of urinary tract malignancies. A single filling defect at excretory urography (**a**, **b**) and CT urography (**c**, **d**). The filling defect may involve a calyx, the infundibulum (*arrowhead*) (**a**), or the renal pelvis (*arrow*) (**b–d**). The CT urography with maximum intensity projection (MIP) 3D images allows a better definition of the relationship between the urothelial tumor (*arrow*) and the renal pelvis with the possibility of multiple views

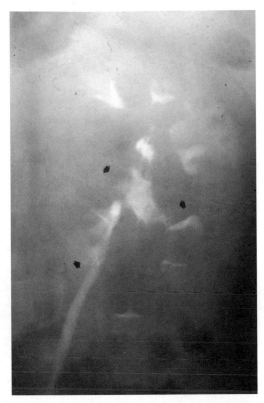

**Fig. 24.3** The different morphologic patterns of urinary tract malignancies. Multiple discrete filling defects (*arrows*) at intravenous excretory urography

or multiple (Fig. 24.3) discrete filling defects (35%); (b) filling defects within distended calyces (26%) (Fig. 24.4); (c) calyceal obliteration (calyceal amputation) (19%) (Fig. 24.5); (d) hydronephrosis with renal enlargement caused by tumor obstruction of ureteropelvic junction (6%) (Fig. 24.6); (e) reduced renal function – excluded kidney – without renal enlargement caused by long-standing tumor obstruction of the ureteropelvic junction and atrophy (13%) (Fig. 24.7).

Ureteric TCC classically appears as a solitary, polypoid filling defect with ureteric dilatation proximal to the lesion. The ureter itself may occasionally be fixed by diffuse ureteric wall infiltration from an intramural lesion. An "apple core" appearance may be observed with eccentric or encircling ureteric lesions. Malignant ureteric strictures may be circumferential or eccentric and can occasionally be confused with benign strictures, although ureteric fixation and nontapering margins are suggestive of malignancy.

### 24.2.1.3 Anterograde and Retrograde Pyelography

Intravenous excretory CT-urography is the primary examination for the evaluation of upper urinary tract neoplasms. However, if complete obstruction exists and the kidney is nonfunctioning, anterograde or retrograde pyelography or static-fluid MR urography (see Chap. 6) is necessary. Nowadays, both antegrade and retrograde direct pyelography are rarely performed.

Anterograde pyelography may be performed during percutaneous needle pyelography in a nonfunctioning hydronephrotic kidney due to a TCC of the upper urinary tract. The upper margins of the obstructing tumor are outlined by contrast (Fig. 24.8), while the inferior extension can be depicted only by retrograde pyelography. Antegrade pyelography presents the risk of potential tumor seeding in the needle tract (Huang et al. 1995; Vikram et al. 2009), even though the probability of extraluminal seeding by percutaneous manipulation is thought to be very small. Antegrade pyelography is generally used only if retrograde cannulation of the ureteral orifice cannot be performed or if a percutaneous nephrostomy has been placed.

Retrograde pyelography may be performed during cystoscopy or to further characterize abnormalities detected at intravenous excretory urography or multidetector CT urography, in inadequately excreting kidneys (O'Connor et al. 2008) or in cases of contrast material allergy. Although invasive, this procedure offers confirmation of the diagnosis by allowing collection of a sample for cytologic examination of localized urine collections. The findings suggestive of TCC, however, are similar to those seen on intravenous excretory urography (Vikram et al. 2009). As with intravenous excretory urography, on retrograde pyelography, renal TCC typically appears as an intraluminal filling defect, which may be smooth, irregular, or stippled. Opacification of a tumor-involved calix may show irregular papillary or nodular mucosa. If TCC involves an infundibulum, an "amputated" calix may be seen with or without focal hydronephrosis and calculi secondary to urinary stasis. Tumor-filled, distended calices are known as "oncocalices." Retrograde pyelography allows confirmation of the radiologic diagnosis while also facilitating ureteroscopy with biopsy or brushing and cytologic examination of localized urine collections. Anyway, it represents an invasive technique and it has been now almost completely replaced by CT urography.

**Fig. 24.4** (**a–c**) The different morphologic patterns of urinary tract malignancies. Multiple discrete filling defects (*arrows*) within calyx dilatation at excretory urography (**a, b**). The surgical specimen (**c**) confirms the presence of multiple urothelial tumors

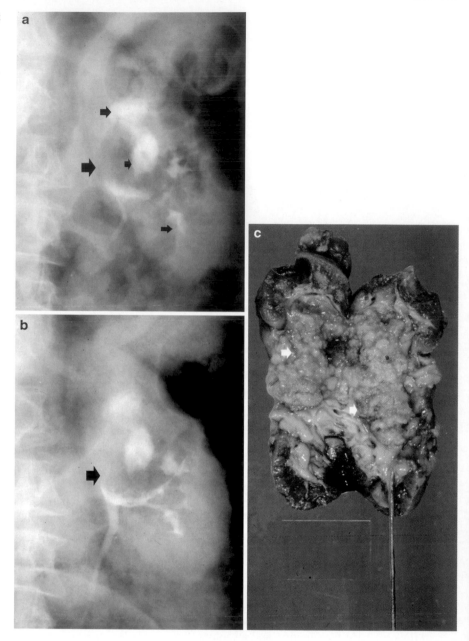

An additional indicator, the goblet sign (*Bergman sign*) is seen on retrograde pyelography when dilatation distal to the tumor is seen in addition to the filling defect caused by the lesion itself (Daniels 1999). The goblet sign corresponds to the cup-shaped collection of contrast material distal to the ureteral filling defect, occurs due to slow tumor growth with resultant lumen expansion, and is not characteristic of more acute

causes of obstruction. The goblet sign is a clue that the ureteral filling defect is a mass rather than a calculus (Daniels 1999). The slow expansion of a polypoid intraluminal tumoral mass from an uroepithelial carcinoma causes dilatation of the ureter distal as well as proximal to the mass. Propulsion of the mass distally during ureteral peristalsis further contributes to the dilatation of the ureter distal to the tumor and thus

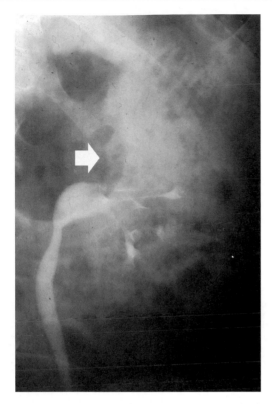

**Fig. 24.5** The different morphologic patterns of urinary tract malignancies. Calyceal obliteration (calyceal amputation-*arrow*-) at intravenous excretory urography

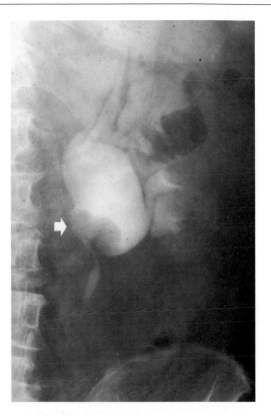

**Fig. 24.6** The different morphologic patterns of urinary tract malignancies. Hydronephrosis with renal enlargement caused by tumor obstruction of ureteropelvic junction (*arrow*) at intravenous excretory urography

causes the cup-shaped collection of contrast material (Daniels 1999). On the other hand, the ureteral lumen just distal to a mechanical obstruction caused by a calculus will have a narrowed appearance due to wall spasm, edema, or both. Dilatation proximal to either a tumor or calculus varies with the degree of obstruction.

### 24.2.1.4 Multidetector CT Urography

The upper urinary tract, including the intrarenal urinary tract, has been traditionally evaluated with excretory urography which presents a limited sensitivity due to the suboptimal contrast resolution. Intravenous excretory urography was used for a large variety of clinical indications, and its utilization decreased when each of these indications was shown not to be clinically

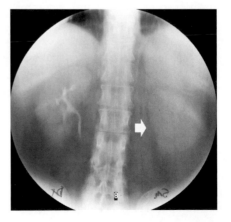

**Fig. 24.7** The different morphologic patterns of urinary tract malignancies. Functionally excluded kidney (*arrow*) without renal enlargement caused by long-standing urothelial tumor obstruction of the urinary tract

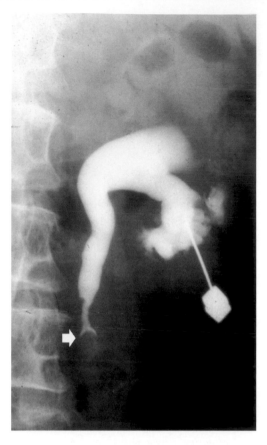

**Fig. 24.8** Anterograde pyelography. The upper margins of the obstructing tumor (*arrow*) are outlined by contrast

valid; cross-sectional imaging techniques have since proved superior to intravenous urography for most, if not all, remaining indications (Silverman et al. 2009). Even until the late 1990s, intravenous excretory urography was still considered the examination of choice for evaluating the urothelium (Silverman et al. 2009) since CT had a sensitivity of 50–68% for the detection of upper urinary tract neoplasms (McCoy et al. 1991; Scolieri et al. 2000). When unenhanced CT was shown to reliably detect urolithiasis, intravenous urography was pronounced dead in 1999 with the caveat that there might remain rare instances in which it is an appropriate examination (Amis 1999). These instances included untangling complicated congenital anomalies, depicting surgical reconstructions of the urinary tract, and surveillance of patients with a history of urothelial carcinoma.

Nowadays, the development of CT urography and MR urography has completely covered all the clinical indications previously addressed by excretory urography.

CT urography, with the use of multidetector CT (MDCT) allowing the acquisition of thinner axial images and an isotropic volumetric dataset, provided a comprehensive examination of the kidneys, collecting systems, ureters, and bladder. Newer 16 and 64-row multidetector CT scanners offer a thinner collimation (as this as 0.4 mm) with an improved z-axis spatial resolution allowing diagnostic reformatted images in any plane and faster imaging times which decrease motion-related artifacts. Some recent reports (Vrtiska et al. 2009) have shown that 64-MDCT technology with isotropic submillimeter spatial resolution allows coronal spatial resolution identical to that of traditional excretory urography using computed radiography (CR) detectors, and that the 64-MDCT scanner is able to detect the smallest filling defects (0.25 mm) in a phantom model, which closely approximated the smallest filling defects that have been traditionally detected by excretory urography, including pyeloureteritis cystica and TCC. Moreover, CT urography permits staging and assessment of the upper urinary tract in a single examination.

MDCT urography is currently considered the most sensitive and comprehensive imaging modality for the evaluation of the entire urinary tract (Caoili et al. 2002. The indications for CT are now expanded to include hematuria (Joffe et al. 2003; Lang et al. 2004; O'Malley et al. 2003), and CT urography has essentially replaced excretory urography in this clinical setting (Heneghan et al. 2001; McNicholas et al. 1998; McTavish et al. 2002; Noroozian et al. 2004). In general, MDCT urography can be tailored toward the clinical question based on clinical information. For benign indications where only the excretory phase will be relevant (variant urinary tract anatomy, ureteral pseudodiverticulosis, and iatrogenic ureter trauma), single-phase MDCT urography can suffice. Patients with more complex benign diseases and those with chronic symptomatic urolithiasis (complex infections, percutaneous nephrostolithotomy planning) may benefit from adding an unenhanced phase to the excretory phase. In chronic urolithiasis without complete obstruction, furosemide-assisted CT urography can demonstrate most ureteral stones within the enhanced urine. So for the evaluation of hydronephrosis due to obstruction by stones, the unenhanced phase may be safely deleted, whereas diagnosis of small nonobstructing stones may be done by an unenhanced phase limited to the kidneys.

It is difficult to obtain a single image of all urinary collecting system segments in an opacified and distended state and intravenous saline (250 mL) or furosemide injection improve the urinary tract and ureteral opacification and distension. It is not just about depicting anatomy, since opacification and distension help in the detection of small urothelial neoplasms. In addition to the evaluation of hematuria, MDCT urography can be useful in the surveillance of patients with suspected urothelial cancer (positive urine cytology), follow-up of urothelial cancers (Silverman et al. 2009), patients with obstructive uropathy (e.g., hydronephrosis, hydroureter of unknown etiology), or any time, a comprehensive evaluation of the urinary tract is warranted. MDCT urography can detect many different urinary tract abnormalities including tiny uroepithelial neoplasms (Caoili et al. 2002, 2005; Chow et al. 2007) with a sensitivity of 90–97% (Fritz et al. 2006; Cowan et al. 2007), even greater than on retrograde pyelography (McCarthy and Cowan 2002), with the possibility to employ coronal,

sagittal, and curved-planar reformatted images and 3D reconstructed images (Tsili et al. 2007; Dillman et al. 2008) in addition to axial reconstructed images.

On MDCT urography, the majority (55–60%) of renal TCCs present as wall thickening with a broad base and frondlike morphologic structure and manifest as sessile filling defects within the contrast-enhanced collecting system in the excretory phase. MDCT urography presents a sensitivity of 86–89% in detecting lesions with these features (Caoili et al. 2005) with high positive and negative predictive values. Postprocessing techniques including curved multiplanar reformations (MPRs) and 3D volume rendering (VR) are useful in urothelial tumor detection, while maximum intensity projection (MIP) 3D images do not detect urothelial tumor since they are less dense than contrast medium. Filling defects may be single (Figs. 24.2 and 24.9) or multiple (Fig. 24.10) and smooth, irregular (Fig. 24.11),

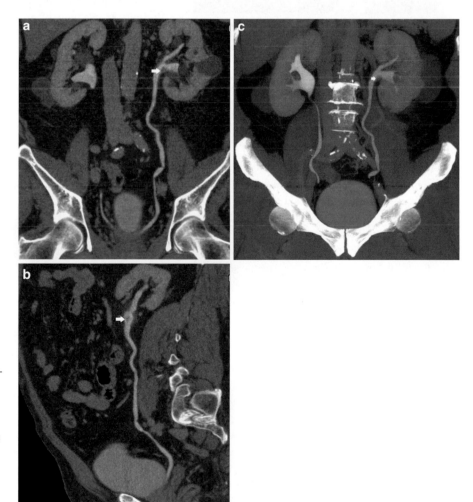

**Fig. 24.9** (**a–c**) Seventy-five-year-old male patient with persistent hematuria. Single TCC (*arrow*) at CT urography (**a**), curved-planar reformations (**b**), and volume rendering image (**c**). Small TCC (*arrow*) within the left renal collecting system with no sign of infiltration of the adjacent renal parenchyma

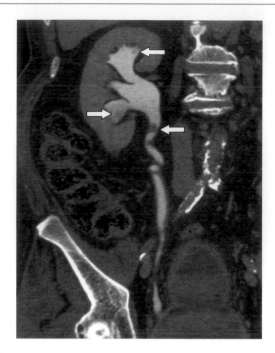

**Fig. 24.10** CT urography. Multiple filling defects (*arrows*) corresponding to TCC without infiltration of the adjacent renal parenchyma

or stippled and tend to expand centrifugally with compression of the renal sinus fat (Browne et al. 2005) (Fig. 24.12). These lesions present as central mass within the renal pelvis (Urban et al. 1997). The stipple sign (Fig. 24.13) refers to tracking of contrast material into the interstices of a papillary lesion. However, this sign may also be seen with blood clot and fungus balls and should be interpreted with caution. Stricture-like lesions of the pelvicaliceal system may be evident and, if multiple, may mimic renal tuberculosis. Filling defects within dilated calices may occur secondary to tumor obstruction of the infundibulum and may lead to caliceal "amputation." If calices fail to opacify with contrast material, they are known as "phantom calices." Other appearances include pelvicaliceal irregularity, oncocalyx (Fig. 24.14) (tumor-filled, distended calices), and focally obstructed calices. Early tumors confined to the muscularis are separated from the renal parenchyma by renal sinus fat or excreted contrast material and have normal-appearing peripelvic fat. Advanced TCC extends into the renal parenchyma in an infiltrating pattern that distorts normal architecture (Fig. 24.15). However, reniform shape is typically preserved (Fig. 24.16), unlike in renal cell carcinoma. About 15% of renal TCCs have a more aggressive

growth pattern, and they will appear as an infiltrative process in the renal parenchyma (Fig. 24.17), often with obliteration of the source collecting system structure (Baron et al. 1982), or as a focal or diffuse circumferential wall thickening (Fig. 24.18) (Caoili et al. 2005). Diffusely infiltrating TCC is characterized by thickening and induration of the wall of the renal pelvis or ureter (Fig. 24.18). Wall thickening of renal pelvis or ureter, or tumor extension into the renal pelvis presents as a hypodense filling defect that stands out against the contrast media within the lumen of the urinary tract.

Ureteric TCC is typically seen as single or multiple ureteric filling defects with or without surface stippling and proximal ureteric dilatation (Fig. 24.19). It is important to remember that long-standing tumor obstruction of the ureteropelvic junction or ureter may lead to generalized hydronephrosis and poor excretion. This is a major disadvantage of intravenous excretory urography when compared with CT urography, which allows assessment of nonfunctioning kidneys. Upper tract filling defects may be nonspecific at intravenous excretory urography, and obstruction of pelvicalyceal drainage may obscure distal synchronous ureteric tumors, meaning that retrograde pyelography is usually performed to further assess these patients.

### 24.2.1.5 CT

Contrast-enhanced CT is well established in the preoperative staging and assessment of upper tract TCC (Urban et al. 1997). CT has also been shown to be more sensitive than US in the detection of small renal mass lesions and urinary tract calculi. The recent advent of CT urography, offering single breath-hold coverage of the entire urinary tract, improved resolution, and the ability to capture multiple phases of contrast material excretion offers improved diagnostic potential over excretory urography and US in the assessment of patients with hematuria due to calculi or tumor. Recent studies have also shown higher detection rates for upper and lower tract urothelial malignancies with CT urography over excretory urography (Lang et al. 2003). Although the American College of Radiology still recommends intravenous excretory urography in the investigation of hematuria, as MDCT urography becomes more prevalent, it is likely to become the investigation of choice, as the urothelium, renal parenchyma, and perirenal tissues can be assessed at a single examination.

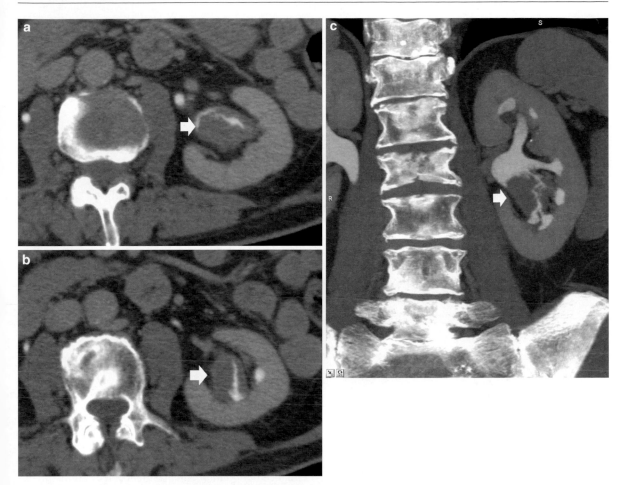

**Fig. 24.11** (**a–c**) TCC without infiltration of the adjacent renal parenchyma. CT urography (**a, b**) transverse plane and (**c**) reformations on the coronal plane. The urothelial carcinoma (*arrow*) determines a stricture-like lesion of the pelvicaliceal system with stenosis of the infundibulum and calyceal obliteration and slight compression of the renal sinus fat

**Fig. 24.12** (**a, b**) Single TCC without infiltration of the adjacent renal parenchyma. (**a**) Excretory urography, (**b**) contrast-enhanced CT excretory phase. (**a**) Multiple filling defects (*arrows*) on the intrarenal urinary tract with calyceal obliteration. (**b**) The urothelial carcinoma (*arrow*) presents a close proximity with the renal parenchyma without signs of parenchymal infiltration but with evident compression of the renal sinus fat

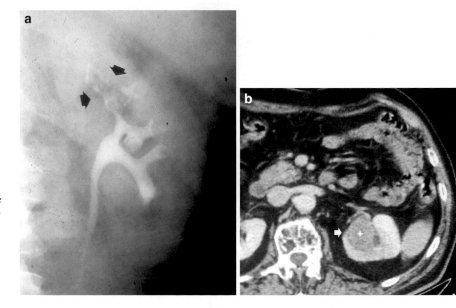

**Fig. 24.13** (a, b) CT urography. TCC of the right kidney. The filling defect (*arrow*) presents the stipple sign referring to tracking of contrast material into the interstices of a papillary lesion

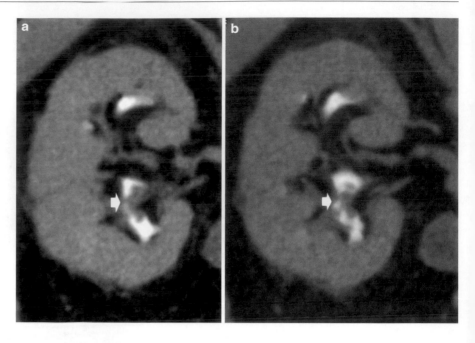

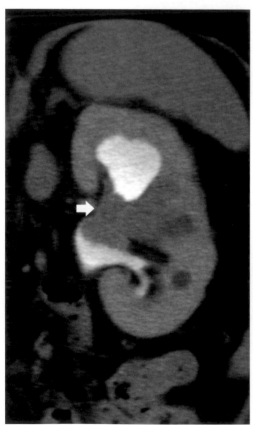

**Fig. 24.14** Multidetector CT (MDCT) urography. Filling defects (*arrow*) with dilatation of the upper calyces secondary to tumor obstruction of the infundibulum, and tumor-filled, distended calyces of the mesorenal region (oncocalyces)

The TCC manifests as isodense to slightly hyperdense (8–30 HU) mass relative to urine, sometimes with calcification on the surface or within the tumoral context, preserving the renal shape on nonenhanced CT and as an hypovascular infiltrative tumor with minimal enhancement (20–55 HU) on contrast-enhanced CT. Both TCC and renal cell carcinoma can show early enhancement and deenhancement after contrast material administration. Renal cell carcinoma, being hypervascular, tends to enhance more, although the two tumors often cannot be differentiated. Parenchymal invasion may be seen as a focal delay in all or part of the cortical nephrogram (Fig. 24.17), although superimposed pyelonephritis or obstruction alone can also have these appearances. A large infiltrating renal TCC may occasionally manifest with areas of necrosis and must be differentiated from lymphoma, metastases, and xanthogranulomatous pyelonephritis, which can have a similar appearance.

Hydronephrosis is the most frequent finding in ureteric TCC and hydroureter can often be seen to the point of obstruction, where Hounsfield unit values for attenuation and enhancement usually allow differentiation of TCC from calculus and clot. Ureteric wall thickening (eccentric or circumferential), luminal narrowing, or an infiltrating mass are other features of disease. A thickened enhancing ureteric wall with periureteric fat stranding is suggestive of extramural spread.

**Fig. 24.15** (**a–c**) Eighty-four-year-old woman presenting with hematuria. (**a**) Ultrasound. A renal mass (*small arrow*) is identified on the left kidney within the renal urinary tract with segmental dilatation of the upper urinary tract (*large arrow*). Contrast-enhanced CT during nephrographic phase (**b**). A hypodense mass (*arrow*) infiltrating the perirenal fat and renal parenchyma is visualized with dilatation of the intrarenal urinary tract. (**c**) Contrast-enhanced CT during nephrographic phase, curved reformations (**c**). A hypodense mass (*arrow*) is confirmed within the dilated intrarenal urinary tract with evidence of tumor-filled, distended calices (oncocalyces). Single TCC was diagnosed at histologic analysis

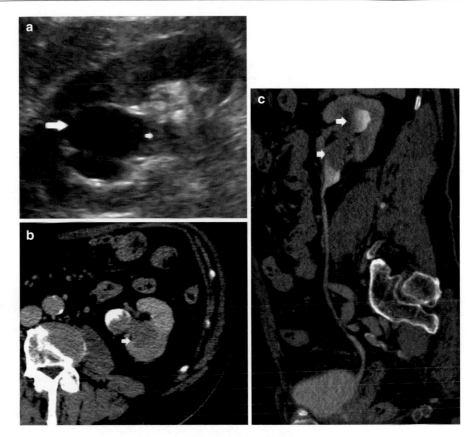

### 24.2.1.6 MR Imaging

MR imaging is infrequently used in the primary assessment of upper tract TCC, and the MR imaging characteristics of this tumor are not well described. In general, MR imaging has not played a leading role in renal tumor imaging due to limitations in image quality, time-consuming sequences, and susceptibility to artifacts. MR imaging offers inherently high soft-tissue contrast, is independent of excretory function, and allows multiplanar imaging, which permits direct image acquisition in the plane of tumor spread. The coronal plane is often advantageous because it allows evaluation of the kidneys, renal vessels, inferior vena cava, and spine in a small number of sections. As with CT, MR imaging can demonstrate tumor involvement of the renal parenchyma, perinephric tissues, or periureteric tissues and distant metastases (Pretorius et al. 2000).

TCC has lower signal intensity than the normally high-signal-intensity urine on T2-weighted images, permitting good demonstration of tumor in a dilated collecting system (Fig. 24.18). However, TCC is nearly isointense to renal parenchyma on T1- and T2-weighted images, and gadolinium contrast material is necessary for tumor identification and for the accurate assessment of tumor extent. Larger infiltrative tumors may obliterate the fat in the renal sinus, simulating the faceless kidney of possible identification in the duplicated collecting system (Pedrosa et al. 2008). Although TCC is a hypovascular tumor, moderate enhancement is seen with gadolinium contrast material, although not to the same degree as renal parenchyma. Enhancement of a focal filling defect in the renal collecting system is strongly suggestive of a TCC. Differentiation between blood clots and enhancing filling defects is best accomplished by reviewing subtracted data sets. Postcontrast imaging may be performed by using 3D sequences to allow dynamic evaluation of the kidney. This allows assessment of the renal vasculature in arterial and venous phases and of the renal parenchyma in cortico-medullary and nephrographic phases. Vascular invasion of the renal vein or inferior vena cava, although rare, may be demonstrated without gadolinium

**Fig. 24.16** (**a–d**) Eighty-year-old woman presenting with hematuria. (**a**) Ultrasound. A renal mass is identified on the left kidney. Unenhanced (**b**) and contrast-enhanced CT during nephrographic phase (**c**). A hypodense mass (*arrow*) infiltrating the renal sinus fat and renal parenchyma is visualized. (**d**) Gross surgical specimen. Single TCC was diagnosed at histologic analysis

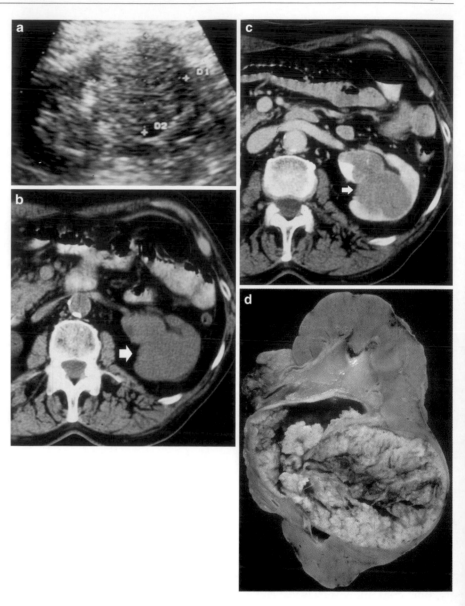

contrast material by using T2-weighted or gradient-echo flow-sensitive sequences.

MR imaging evaluation of upper tract TCC should include static or dynamic MR urography performed by using gadolinium contrast material (MR nephrography). Static MR urography performed by using heavily T2-weighted sequences can permit accurate localization of ureteric obstruction, although imaging of undilated systems may be suboptimal. Bright signal intensity due to urine in the collecting system on T2-weighted images provides excellent soft-tissue contrast for the detection of these tumors, which are characteristically seen as hypointense filling defects.

Infiltrative TCC can be seen on single-shot T2-weighted images as a hypointense soft-tissue mass infiltrating the renal parenchyma, which has intermediate signal intensity. Dynamic gadolinium-enhanced T1-weighted MR urography performed with or without a diuretic overcomes this problem and allows delayed acquisitions at various time intervals depending on the degree and level of obstruction. TCC appears as single or multiple filling defects within the distended calyces or renal pelvis (Fig. 24.20). Data postprocessing (e.g., MIPs) allows 3D rotation and evaluation of suspected areas of disease without superimposition of other structures. This can be performed for both vessels and

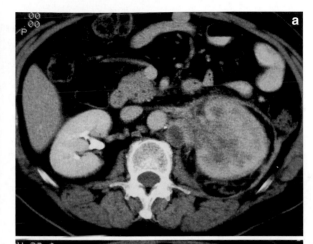

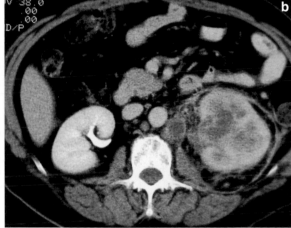

**Fig. 24.17** (**a**, **b**) TCC at CT urography with diffuse infiltration of the whole right kidney. Contrast-enhanced CT, excretory phase. Diffuse infiltration of the renal parenchyma in the left kidney by a TCC. No contrast excretion is evident on the left kidney which is functionally excluded

the collecting system. MR excretory urography is helpful in patients in whom urography with iodinated contrast material is not possible.

Tumor may extend into the renal parenchyma and appear as an infiltrating mass. Findings may be subtle, with only pelvic or ureteral wall thickening. Hydronephrosis proximal to the lesion is usually present unless the collecting system is completely filled by tumor. Occasionally, TCC may extend inferiorly within the periureteral fat, encasing the ureter without tumor involvement of the ureteral mucosa. The entire collecting system must be evaluated in patients with upper tract TCC because of the high prevalence of secondary foci of tumor. A cup-shaped dilatation of the ureter just distal to a focus of TCC of the ureter – also referred to as the goblet sign,

chalice sign, or Bergman sign – may be seen. This finding is secondary to distal propulsion of a slow-growing intraluminal polypoid mass during ureteral peristalsis (Pedrosa et al. 2008).

Ureteric TCC is isointense to muscle on T1-weighted images and slightly hyperintense on T2-weighted images (Rothpearl et al. 1995). At MR urography, ureteric TCC typically appears as an irregular mass, whereas calculi appear as sharply delineated filling defects, although differentiation between small calculi and tumor may be difficult. Tumor enhancement after administration of gadolinium contrast material can also help distinguish it from calculi. Soft-tissue stranding in the periureteric fat is suggestive of periureteric extension, although prior surgery, radiation, and inflammation can also give these appearances. MR imaging may help differentiate these entities, however, as fibrosis will appear hypointense on T2-weighted images, particularly in long-standing cases.

These comprehensive MR protocols can image all the anatomic components of the urinary tract in a single test and offer advantages over other techniques, including lack of iodinated contrast medium and radiation exposure. Although MR imaging remains second line to CT, it offers further noninvasive imaging of masses that are not adequately characterized with other imaging modalities. The main disadvantage of MR imaging is the inability to reliably detect urinary tract calcifications, calculi, and air, which limits its use as a first-line test in the investigation of hematuria. Although the sensitivity of renal parenchymal MR imaging with gadolinium for assessing renal masses and abnormalities of the nephrogram is considered similar to that of CT, spatial resolution is poor compared with that of intravenous urography or CT urography, making detection of subtle urothelial malignancies less likely. Furthermore, complete characterization of renal masses may require multiple time-consuming sequences before and after administration of gadolinium contrast material.

### 24.2.2 Imaging of Hematuria

Hematuria is a common urologic problem that accounts for 4–20% of all urologic visits. Hematuria is broadly divided into macroscopic and microscopic variants. Gross hematuria is determined by urologic cancer (including renal cell carcinoma and urothelial tumors)

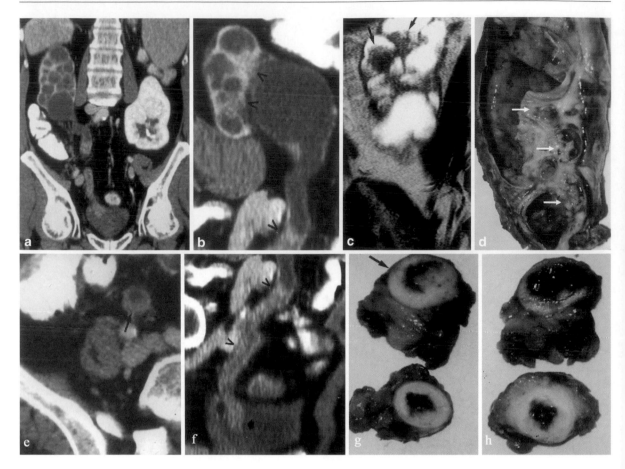

**Fig. 24.18** (**a–h**) Multicentric diffusely infiltrating TCC involving both the intra and extrarenal collecting system. (**a**) Contrast-enhanced CT. Coronal reformations. Dilatation of the intrarenal urinary tract with evidence of multiple mural noduleson the dilated renal pelvis and ipsilateral diffuse ureteral involvement by the tumor (*arrowheads*) (**b**) Contrast-enhanced CT. Coronal reformations. Dilatation of the intrarenal urinary tract with diffuse renal pelvis infiltration (*arrows*). (**c**) T2-weighted turbo spinecho MR sequence. Coronal plane. Multiple mural nodules (*arrows*) are evident on the dilated intrarenal urinary tract. (d) Gross surgical specimen. Multiple mural tumors on the renal pelvis (arrows) (**e, f**) Contrast-enhanced CT. Transverse plane (**e**) and coronal reformation (**f**). Diffuse ureteral infiltration by the TCC (*arrow* in **e**, and arrowheads in **f**). (**g, h**) Gross surgical specimen of the ureteral carcinoma with macroscopic whitish appearance of the tumor (*arrow*)

in about 25% of cases, while most of the other cases are due to urinary tract infections, urinary tract calculi, and renal parenchymal diseases. On the other hand, hematuria (particularly when microscopic) may not always signal the presence of serious disease, and therefore, has long been debated how aggressively to evaluate these patients. It must be underlined that hematuria may be determined by a plenty of causes many of which are insignificant (renal cyst, exercise, polyps, urethritis, urethrigonitis), some significant and require observation (benign prostatic hyperplasia, papillary necrosis, trauma, arteriovenous fistula), some other significant and require treatment (urolithiasis, vesicoureteral reflux, ureteropelvic junction obstruction, renal artery stenosis, renal vein

thrombosis, renal infections), and others are life-threatening (malignancies, abdominal aortic aneurysm).

In patients with hematuria, US represents a safe method of examination for urolithiasis, particularly in pediatric patients, thereby avoiding the use of radiation. US is employed to detect hydronephrosis, identify the stone, assess the renal size and renal parenchyma thickness, and detect complications. In nonhydrated patients US presents a sensitivity of 35–73% and a specificity of 74%, while the sensitivity becomes 85–100% and the specificity 83–100% in hydrated patients (Svedström et al. 1990; Haddad et al. 1992; Dalla Palma et al. 1993). In the detection of renal stones US has a low sensitivity (20–30%) and high

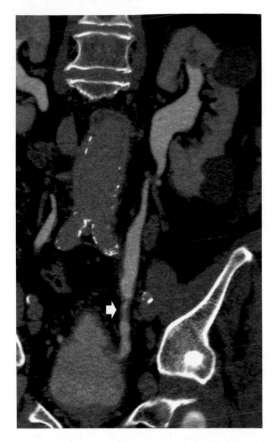

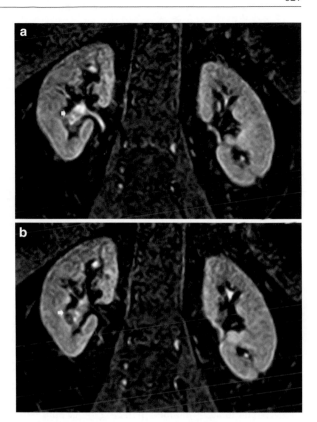

**Fig. 24.20** (**a**, **b**) MR excretory urography. Multiple filling defects (*arrows*) corresponding to multicentric TCC are identified within the upper urinary tract in the lower renal region

**Fig. 24.19** TCC of the distal ureter. CT urography. Curved planar reformat. An irregular thickening of the distal ureteral wall (*arrow*) is evident during the excretory phase

specificity (90%), while in the detection of ureteral stones US presents a moderate sensitivity (60–70%) and high specificity (90–95%) (Fowler et al. 2002). The detection of urinary stones and clarity of posterior shadowing are significantly improved by harmonic imaging (Ozdemir et al. 2008). US is limited in the detection of renal masses smaller than 2 cm (Warshauer et al. 1988), and CT represents the most sensitive imaging technique for the detection of renal masses (Jamis-Dow et al. 1996). US is useful in determining the internal architecture of renal masses detected by CT, especially in cystic renal masses in which US may be very effective to depict the peripheral wall thickening and internal septations. The main disadvantage of US as a screening test in patients with hematuria is its limited capability to thoroughly evaluate the urothelium for TCC. Moreover, US has poor sensitivity in detecting urothelial lesions in the pelvicaliceal system and also in the ureters (Browne et al. 2005).

Recently, the technique of MDCT urography (Joffe et al. 2003) has emerged as an alternative method of assessing patients with hematuria, offering superior detection of urinary calculi and renal parenchymal masses, and in some studies, improved detection of urothelial lesions of the upper urinary tract (Caoili et al. 2005). Because surrounding structures can also be assessed, CT urography is rapidly replacing excretory urography as the definitive study for these patients, potentially shortening the duration of diagnostic evaluation. The main advantage of MDCT urography in the evaluation of patients with hematuria is its ability to display and evaluate the entire urinary tract, including renal parenchyma, pelvicaliceal systems, ureters, and the bladder using a single imaging study.

Studies focusing on CT urography in patients with microscopic hematuria show that causes for hematuria are identified in 33.0–42.6% with overall CT urography sensitivity for identification of the cause of hematuria of

92.4–100% and specificity of 89.0–97.4% (Van Der
Molen et al. 2008). In studies on microscopic or unselected hematuria, upper tract TCC was present in
0.9–7.3%. In these populations, CT urography detection of upper tract TCC is high and significantly better
than intravenous urography. When applied to selected
high-risk groups of macroscopic hematuria, TCC tumor
prevalence may increase to 25–30% and it has been
shown that CT urography of the upper tract is equivalent to retrograde pyelography (Van Der Molen et al.
2008). CT may still have problems of correctly staging
advanced tumors. Thin-section ($\leq$3-mm) MDCT images
can be used to depict urothelial abnormalities just as
well, if not better than, contrast material-enhanced
radiographs (Caoili et al. 2005; Silverman et al. 2009).
Although radiographs have higher spatial resolution,
the higher contrast resolution and other inherent
advantages of cross-sectional imaging outweigh the
advantages of conventional radiography in intravenous urography. Radiography is a projectional imaging technique, and therefore, overlapping structures can
obscure important findings (Silverman et al. 2009).
Hence, there is a sound rationale for believing that thin-
section axial images obtained in the excretory phase are
more sensitive than contrast-enhanced radiographs for
the detection of urothelial abnormalities. As a result, it
is now generally accepted that CT urography is best
performed with MDCT alone (Silverman et al. 2009).
CT urography can also be powerful in the diagnosis of
bladder tumors, but results differ depending on the specific population studied. In a population of patients with
microscopic hematuria, CT urography sensitivity in
comparison with cystoscopy was only 40%, while in a
high-risk group with macroscopic hematuria, unequivocal CT urography results were 93% sensitive and 99%
specific for the detection of bladder cancer, which may
obviate the need for many flexible (diagnostic)
cystoscopies.

MR imaging, including the newer techniques of
MR angiography and MR urography, is also being
used, particularly in patients who cannot tolerate
iodinated contrast material and in whom multiplanar,
vascular, and collecting system imaging is required.
Because of the multifocal and metachronous nature
of TCC, thorough assessment of the entire urothelium is required before treatment. Therefore, evaluation of the upper tract with excretory urography (or

CT urography if equivalent) is indicated in those with
newly diagnosed bladder TCC; conversely, patients
with upper tract TCC should undergo cystoscopic
evaluation.

To date, there have been no randomized controlled
trials comparing different imaging modalities for
imaging of patients with hematuria (O'Regan et al.
2009). Therefore, current guidelines are based on
extensive literature searches and expert opinion.
Several different algorithms have been proposed, but
no single evidence-based algorithm currently exists
(O'Regan et al. 2009) and imaging protocols at individual centers vary greatly. In any diagnostic algorithm,
patients should be stratified according to the risk for
malignant disease. The American College of Radiology
Appropriateness Criteria recommends that some imaging examination, including intravenous urography or
CT urography with or without US, be performed in
almost all patients with hematuria excluding young
female patients with uncomplicated cystitis whose
hematuria resolves following treatment (Choyke et al.
2005). The European Society of Urogenital Radiology
(ESUR) has recently published guidelines on the use
of CT urography for investigation of painless hematuria (Van Der Molen et al. 2008). According to these
guidelines, patients are stratified according to malignancy risk into low-, medium-, and high-risk groups.
For low- and medium-risk patients, US and cystoscopy
are suggested with the recommendation to employ
intravenous excretory urography or CT urography if
both examinations are negative and symptoms persist.
In high-risk patients CT urography and cystoscopy are
advised.

The standard work-up for patients with hematuria
as recommended by the American Urological Association consists of urinalysis and cytologic analysis,
cystoscopy, and either intravenous urography or CT
urography (Grossfeld et al. 2001a, b). Microscopic
hematuria corresponds to >3 red blood cells/high
power microscopic field, and it is present in 9–18% of
normal patients. The prevalence of asymptomatic
microscopic hematuria varies 0.6–21% and is among
the most important clinical signs of a urologic malignancy. A cause for asymptomatic microscopic hematuria can be found in 32–100% of patients undergoing
a full urologic evaluation, with 3.4–56% of these
patients having either moderately or highly clinically

significant diagnoses. Patients with hematuria younger than 40 years represent the low-risk group for urologic disease, while patients with hematuria older than 40 years or smokers, or patients with gross hematuria or irritating voiding symptoms, urinary tract infections, or exposure to carcinogens (pelvic irradiation, analgesic abuse, cyclophosphamide, chemicals/dyes) represent the high-risk group (Grossfeld et al. 2001a, b). High-risk patients with one positive urine sediment (>3 red blood cells/high power microscopic field) should undergo urinary upper tracy imaging, cytology, and cystoscopy. If these examinations are negative, they should undergo further work-up every year for 3 year. Low-risk patients with two of three positive urine sediments should undergo upper tract imaging, cytology, and cystoscopy. If these examinations are negative, further work-up is considered optional (Grossfeld et al. 2001a, b). For lower risk groups, CT urography can be used as a problem-solving test if traditional work-up remains negative and significant undiagnosed symptoms persist. Symptomatic hematuria in patients younger than 40 years should be evaluated by unenhanced CT for the identification of calculi, while asymptomatic hematuria in patients older than 40 years should be evaluated by CT urography. In addition, relative to intravenous urography, CT urography can be used to depict structures outside the urinary tract and thus is useful in detecting unsuspected extraurinary disease. Nevertheless, a full urologic evaluation is recommended in many patients with asymptomatic microscopic hematuria.

## 24.3  Staging of Upper Urinary Tract Tumors

The TNM system is most frequently used for staging upper urinary tract tumors (Vikram et al. 2009). T1 indicates a tuor which invades the subepithelial connective tissue (lamina propria), T2 a tumor invading muscularis, T3 a tumor extending beyond the muscularis into the peripelvic fat (periureteric fat in the case of the ureteral carcinoma) or renal parenchyma, and T4 a tumor invading adjacent organs, the pelvic or abdominal wall, or through the kidney, the perinephric

fat. N1 corresponds to the presence of a metastasis to a single lymph node that is <2 cm in the greatest dimension, N2 metastasis to a single lymph node 2–5 cm in the greatest dimension or multiple lymph nodes ≤5 cm in the greatest dimension, N3 if the metastasis to a lymph node is >5 cm in the greatest dimension.

Conventional imaging methods such as intravenous excretory urography and retrograde pyelography cannot demonstrate extension into the peripelvic or periureteric fat or metastases. Cross-sectional imaging with CT or MR is now routinely employed in the presurgical work-up of these patients. These techniques can demonstrate intra and extrarenal local extension of tumor and the presence of nodal or distant metastases with a high degree of accuracy. They are used in conjunction with ureterorenoscopy and biopsy for staging before surgery.

CT has become routine in the further characterization of upper tract lesions demonstrated with other modalities and, despite varying reports on staging accuracy, is currently the preoperative imaging modality of choice. As studies show higher detection rates for urothelial malignancies with CT urography than with intravenous excretory urography, this technique is being advocated as a one-stop diagnostic and staging assessment of suspected urothelial malignancy. Although CT does not allow distinction between stage 0–II tumors, it does allow differentiation of early-stage TCC confined to the collecting system wall from advanced disease with local extension or distant metastases, which is important for defining surgical management. Early-stage tumors (stage 0–II) confined to the muscularis are separated from the renal parenchyma by renal sinus fat or excreted contrast material and have normal-appearing peripelvic fat.

More advanced tumors infiltrating beyond the muscularis into the peripelvic fat typically show increased inhomogeneous peripelvic attenuation, although this finding may also be seen with superimposed infection, hemorrhage, or inflammation and should be interpreted with caution to avoid overstaging. Metastatic spread via urinary or hematogenous routes usually manifests as multifocal mucosal nodules or wall thickening, whereas direct invasion produces a short or long stricture. Extrarenal spread can occur at or through the renal hilum, and common sites of metastases include the lungs, retroperitoneum, lymph nodes, and bones. Rarely, invasion of the renal vein or inferior vena cava is seen and can be well demonstrated with comprehensive CT urography protocols. The overall accuracy of CT in predicting the pathologic stage ranges from 36 to 83% in the literature, which means that ureterorenoscopy and biopsy remain essential additional tools.

As with CT, MR imaging can demonstrate tumor involvement of the renal parenchyma, perinephric fat, or periureteric fat and distant metastases. It, therefore, offers an alternative staging modality and has been shown to allow accurate staging of TCC lesions larger than 2 cm. As with CT, however, limitations exist in detecting superficial invasion of the renal parenchyma and small lesions may be missed because of motion artifacts. It is the preferred staging examination in patients who cannot tolerate iodinated contrast material and in whom multiplanar and vascular imaging is required for preoperative assessment.

The traditional treatment of upper tract TCC involves total nephroureterectomy with excision of the ipsilateral ureteric orifice and a contiguous cuff of bladder tissue. However, the development of endoscopic and minimally invasive surgical techniques allows renal preservation in selected patients, particularly those with a solitary kidney, bilateral tumor, poor renal function, low-grade tumor, or prohibitive surgical risk, with results comparable to those of radical surgery. Accurate radiologic detection and staging of tumor is, therefore, essential to determine appropriate surgical therapy, especially if conservative surgery is being considered, or the intensity of chemotherapy for advanced-stage tumors.

## 24.4 Follow-Up

There is still no widely accepted protocol for the radiologic follow-up of patients with primary TCC of the upper urinary tract. Current data suggest that routine follow-up imaging strategies should be individually tailored on the basis of primary tumor characteristics. Annual intravenous excretory urography, and nowadays CT urography, is recommended, especially in the first 2 years after initial diagnosis. Retrograde pyelography should be sought if intravenous excretory urography fails to depict or adequately distend the entire upper tract, especially if cystoscopy is being performed

to assess the bladder. This vigilance is justified in order to detect early recurrence after conservative surgery or, in patients who have only one remaining kidney, to detect contralateral lesions at an early stage when local excision may be feasible.

Owing to the high rate of metachronous tumor in the bladder, frequent cystoscopy should also be performed. At our institution this is performed every 3 months for the first year, every 6 months for the second year, and yearly thereafter. In the future, CT urography will likely become the primary radiologic method of TCC follow-up, allowing assessment of the entire urothelium and also facilitating virtual cystoscopy, although conventional cystoscopy is still necessary for direct visualization and biopsy.

## 24.5 Other Malignant Tumors of the Upper Urinary Tract

Epidermoid carcinoma (squamous epithelial carcinoma) is rare and occurs in patients with a long previous history of stones, urinary tract infections, and hematuria. Epidermoid carcinoma is responsible for 5–10% of renal pelvic, while it is rare in ureteral cancers. This tumor has a rapid growth and infiltrates and invades the ureter, the perirenal fat, and the lymph nodes and also metastatizes early. Macroscopically, the tumor presents as a mass inside the lumen, infiltrating both the wall and the renal parenchyma. The tumor is rarely multicentric, and due to its high grade of malignancy, the prognosis is poor. Radiographically, a stone is usually present on the plain film (Kawashima and Goldman 2000) and squamous cell carcinoma should be considered in patients in whom CT detects an infiltrating tumor associated with a calculus. Squamous cell carcinoma of the upper urinary tract may mimic xanthogranulomatous pyelonephritis on US and CT (Wimbish et al. 1983). When compared with TCC, squamous cell carcinoma of the upper urinary tract tends to appear with predominantly extraluminal tumor extension rather than purely intraluminal tumor growth on CT (Narumi et al. 1989; Kawashima and Goldman 2000).

Adenocarcinoma of the renal pelvis is very rare (less than 1% of urothelial carcinoma) and, as in the case of epidermoid carcinoma, is associated with

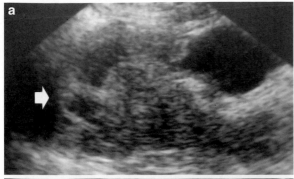

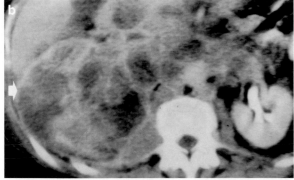

**Fig. 24.21** (**a**, **b**) Carcinosarcoma. (**a**) Gray-scale ultrasound. (**b**) Contrast-enhanced CT. A huge heterogeneous neoplasia (*arrow*) with diffuse involvement of the right kidney

a history of stones and urinary tract infections and probably originates from the glandular metaplasia following chronic irritation and repeated inflammatory disease.

Undifferentiated carcinoma has a variable histologic pattern, in some case similar to small cell carcinoma of the lung, while in others the degree of anaplasia is so high that classification is not possible. Other rare tumoral histotypes of possible observation on the upper urinary tract are the carcinosarcoma (Fig. 24.21) and small cell carcinoma.

## 24.6 Differential Diagnosis

When a lesion of the upper urinary tract presents the typical CT features described for TCC, it is highly suggested that the lesion is TCC as some benign lesions, such as blood clots and sloughted papillae, can be reliably ruled out due to no contrast enhancement (Fig. 24.22) and the high density of blood clots (Wang et al. 2009). However, a few rare lesions, including endometriosis, mycetomas, malacoplakia,

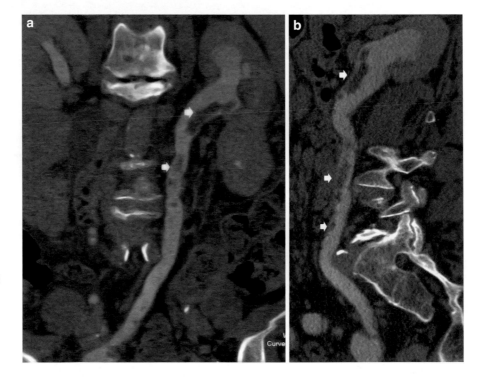

**Fig. 24.22** (**a**, **b**) CT urography. Patient with ileal neobladder and uretero-ileostomy. Multiple filling defects corresponding to coagula (*arrows*) within the extrarenal urinary tract simulating a diffuse TCC

**Fig. 24.23** (**a**, **b**) Retrograde cystography in a patient with chronic renal failure undergoing dialysis. Vesicoureteral reflux reveals multiple filling defects (*arrows*) in the upper urinary tract due to a cystic pyeloureteritis simulating multicentric TCC of the upper urinary tract

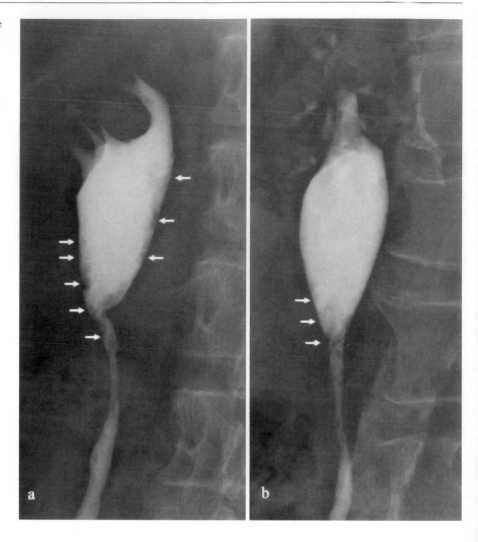

endometriosis, nephrogenic adenoma, and inflammatory pseudotumor (inflammatory myofibroblastic tumor), should be taken into account. Endometriosis, particularly of the upper urinary tract, is very rare. Nephrogenic adenoma results from the chronic irritation by calculi, infection, injury, or previous operation with consequent metaplasia of the urothelium which develops papillary and tubular growth (Wang et al. 2009).

Diffusely infiltrating TCC (Fig. 24.18) is characterized by thickening and induration of the wall of the renal pelvis or ureter. Some benign lesions also induce thickening of ureteral and renal pelvic wall, including complex urolithiasis, chronic ureteropelvic junction obstruction with superimposed infection, atypical pyelonephritis, and cystic pyeloureteritis (Fig. 24.23) and tuberculosis. Also, urothelial neoplasms and

inflammation can coexist in the same urinary tract (Wang et al. 2009). Urinary stone can lead to edema and thickening of the ureteral wall at its site of impaction. Calculi may be associated with pyelonephritis and may manifest with upper urinary tract wall thickening.

## 24.7 Benign Tumors of the Upper Urinary Tract

Benign urothelial tumors of the upper urinary tract include the inverted papillomas (Fig. 24.24), while benign tumors of mesodermal origin include fibroepithelial polyps (Fig. 24.25), hemangiomas,

**Fig. 24.24** (a–d)
Papillomatosis of the urinary
tract. Excretory urography.
Multiple filling defects
(*arrows*) are evident within
the intrarenal urinary tract,
the ureter, and the bladder

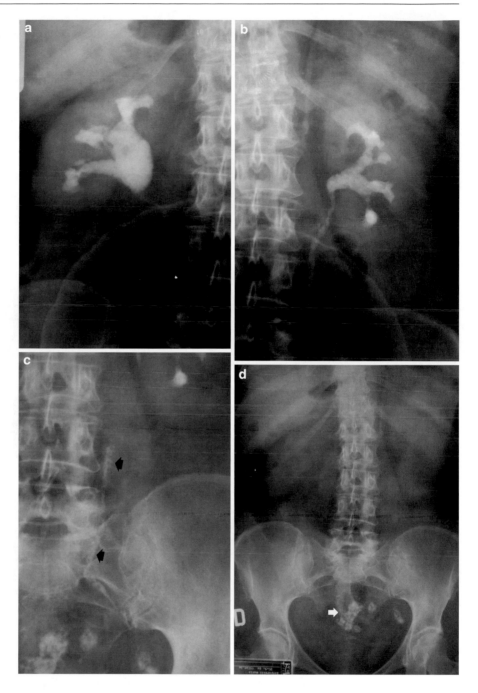

and leiomyomas. Renal papilloma is a rare tumor which determines the evidence of contrast defect on the dilated renal collecting system. The fibroepithelial polyps are rare tumors which manifest with hematuria and intermittent flank pain similar to a renal colic, and are frequently associated with upper urinary tract infections. Fibroepithelial polyp tends to be a low-grade malignant lesion with slow mural infiltration and late metastatization. The conservative treatment is possible, while follow-up is necessary when the histology pattern of the tumor is aspecific.

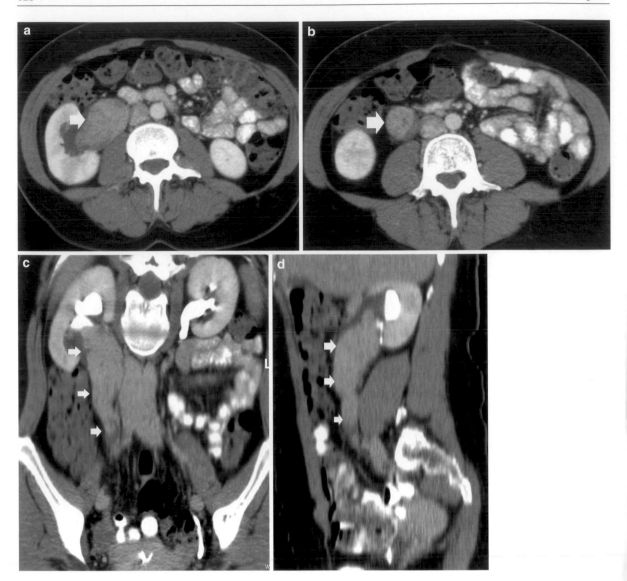

**Fig. 24.25** (**a–d**) Giant fibroepithelial polyp. Contrast-enhanced CT (**a**, **b**), and CT urography with coronal (**c**) and sagittal reformations (**d**). A huge soft-tissue mass (*arrows*) is evident within the renal and extrarenal urinary tract

# References

Amis ES Jr (1999) Epitaph for the urogram. Radiology 213: 639–640

Barentsz JO, Jager GJ, Witjes JA et al. (1996) Primary staging of urinary bladder carcinoma: the role of MRI and a comparison with CT. Eur Radiol 6(2):129–133

Baron RL, McClennan BL, Lee JK et al. (1982) Computed tomography of transitional-cell carcinoma of the renal pelvis and ureter. Radiology 144:125–130

Browne RF, Meehan CP, Colville J et al. (2005) Transitional cell carcinoma of the upper urinary tract: spectrum of imaging findings. Radiographics 25:1609–1627

Caoili EM, Cohan RH, Inampudi P et al. (2005) MDCT urography of upper tract urothelial neoplasms. AJR Am J Roentgenol 184:1873–1881

Caoili EM, Cohan RH, Korobkin M et al. (2002) Urinary tract abnormalities: initial experience with multi-detector row CT urography. Radiology 222:353–360

Chow LC, Kwan SW, Olcott EW et al. (2007) Split-bolus MDCT urography with synchronous nephrographic and excretory phase enhancement. AJR Am J Roentgenol 189:314–322

Choyke P, Bluth EI, Bush WH et al. (2005) American College of Radiology, ACR appropriateness criteria: hematuria. Version available at http://www.acr.org. Accessed 18 September 2009

Cowan NC, Turney BW, Taylor NJ et al. (2007) Multidetector computed tomography urography for diagnosing upper urinary tract urothelial tumour. Br J Urol 99(6):1363–1370

Dalla Palma L, Stacul F, Bazzocchi M et al. (1993) Ultrasonography and plain film versus intravenous urography in ureteric colic. Clin Radiol 47(5):333–336

Daniels RE (1999) The goblet sign. Radiology 210:737–738

Dillman JR, Caoili EM, Cohan RH et al. (2008) Detection of upper urinary tract urothelial neoplasms: sensitivity of axial, coronal reformatted, and curved-planar reformatted image-types utilizing 16-row multi-detector CT urography. Abdom Imaging 33:707–716

Fowler KAB, Locken JA, Duchesse JH et al. (2002) US for Detecting renal calculi with nonenhanced CT as a reference standard. Radiology 222:109–113

Fritz GA, Schoellnast H, Deutschmann HA et al. (2006) Multiphasic multidetector-row CT (MDCT) in detection and staging of transitional cell carcinomas of the upper urinary tract. Eur Radiol 16(6):1244–1252

Grabstald H, Whitmore WF, Melamed MR (1971) Renal pelvic tumors. JAMA 218:845–854

Grossfeld GD, Litwin MS, Wolf JS et al. (2001a) Evaluation of asymptomatic microscopic hematuria in adults: the American Urological Association best practice policy panel – part I. Definition, detection, prevalence, and etiology. Urology 57:599–603

Grossfeld GD, Litwin MS, Wolf JS et al. (2001b) Evaluation of asymptomatic microscopic hematuria in adults: the American Urological Association best practice policy panel – part II. Patient evaluation, cytology, voided markers, imaging, cystoscopy, nephrology evaluation, and follow-up. Urology 57:604–610

Guinan P, Vogelzang NJ, Randazzo R et al. (1992) Renal pelvic cancer: a review of 611 patients treated in Illinois 1975–1985. Cancer incidence and end results committee. Urology 40:393–399

Haddad MC, Sharif HS, Shahed MS et al. (1992) Renal colic: diagnosis and outcome. Radiology 184:83–88

Heneghan JP, Kim DH, Leder RA et al. (2001) Compression CT urography: a comparison with IVU in the opacification of the collecting system and ureters. J Comput Assist Tomogr 25:343–347

Huang A, Low RK, deVere White R (1995) Nephrostomy tract tumor seeding following percutaneous manipulation of a ureteral carcinoma. J Urol 153(3 pt 2):1041–1042

Jamis-Dow CA, Choyke PL, Jennings SB et al. (1996) Small (< or = 3 cm) renal masses: detection with CT versus US and pathologic correlation. Radiology 198(3):785–788

Joffe SA, Servaes S, Okon S et al. (2003) Multi-detector row CT urography in the evaluation of hematuria. Radiographics 23:1441–1455

Kawashima A, Goldman SM (2000) Neoplasms of the renal pelvis. In: Pollack HM, McClennan BL (eds) Clinical urography. Saunders, Philadelphia, PA, pp 1560–1641

Kirkali Z, Tuzel E (2003) Transitional cell carcinoma of the ureter and renal pelvis. Crit Rev Oncol Hematol 47:155–169

Lang EK, Macchia RJ, Thomas R et al. (2003) Improved detection of renal pathologic features on multiphasic helical CT compared with IVU in patients presenting with microscopic hematuria. Urology 61:528–532

Lang EK, Thomas R, Davis R et al. (2004) Multiphasic helical computerized tomography for the assessment of microscopic hematuria: a prospective study. J Urol 171:237–243

Leder RA, Dunnick NR (1990) Transitional cell carcinoma of the pelvicalices and ureter. AJR Am J Roentgenol 155:713–722

Lowe PP, Roylance J (1976) Transitional cell carcinoma of the kidney. Clin Radiol 27:503

McCarthy CL, Cowan NC (2002) Multidetector CT urography (MD-CTU) for urothelial imaging. Radiology 225(P):237

McCoy JG, Honda H, Reznicek M et al. (1991) Computerized tomography for the detection and staging of localized and pathologically defined upper tract urothelial tumors. J Urol 146:1500–1503

McNicholas MM, Raptopoulos VD, Schwartz RK et al. (1998) Excretory phase CT urography for opacification of the urinary collecting system. AJR Am J Roentgenol 170:1261–1267

McTavish JD, Jinzaki M, Zou KH et al. (2002) Multi-detector row CT urography: comparison of strategies for depicting the normal urinary collecting system. Radiology 225:783–790

Narumi Y, Sato T, Hori S et al. (1989) Squamous cell carcinoma of the uroepithelium: CT evaluation. Radiology 173:853–856

Nocks BN, Heney NM, Daly JJ et al. (1982) Transitional cell carcinoma of the renal pelvis. Urology 19:472–477

Noroozian M, Cohan RH, Caoili EM et al. (2004) Multislice CT urography: state of the art. Br J Radiol 77(suppl 1):S74–S86

O'Connor OJ, McSweeney SE, Maher MM (2008) Imaging of hematuria. Radiol Clin North Am 46:113–132

O'Malley ME, Hahn PF, Yoder IC et al. (2003) Comparison of excretory phase, helical computed tomography with intravenous urography in patients with painless haematuria. Clin Radiol 58:294–300

O'Regan KN, O'Connor OJ, McLoughlin P et al. (2009) The role of imaging in the investigation of painless hematuria in adults. Semin Ultrasound CT MRI 30:258–270

Ozdemir H, Demir MK, Temizöz O et al. (2008) Phase inversion harmonic imaging improves assessment of renal calculi: a comparison with fundamental gray-scale sonography. J Clin Ultrasound 36(1):16–19

Ozsahin M, Zouhair A, Villa S et al. (1999) Prognostic factors in urothelial renal pelvis and ureter tumours: a multicentre Rare Cancer Network study. Eur J Cancer 35:738–743

Pedrosa I, Sun MR, Spencer M et al. (2008) MR imaging of renal masses: correlation with findings at surgery and pathologic analysis. Radiographics 28:985–1003

Pretorius ES, Wickstrom ML, Siegelman ES (2000) MR imaging of renal neoplasms. Magn Reson Imaging Clin N Am 8:813–836

Rothpearl A, Frager D, Subramanian A et al. (1995) MR urography: technique and application. Radiology 194:125–130

Scolieri MJ, Paik ML, Brown SL et al. (2000) Limitations of computer tomography in the preoperative staging of upper tract urothelial carcinoma. Urology 56:930–934

Silverman SG, Leyendecker JR, Amis SE (2009) What is the current role of CT urography and MR urography in the evaluation of the urinary tract. Radiology 250:309–323

Svedström E, Alanen A, Nurmi M (1990) Radiologic diagnosis of renal colic: the role of plain film, excretory urography and sonography. Eur J Radiol 11(3):180–183

Tsili AC, Efremidis SC, Kalef-Ezra J et al. (2007) Multi-detector row CT urography on a 16-row CT scanner in the evaluation of urothelial tumors. Eur Radiol 17:1046–1054

Urban BA, Buckley J, Soyer P et al. (1997) CT appearance of transitional cell carcinoma of the renal pelvis. II. Advanced-stage disease. AJR Am J Roentgenol 169:163–168

Van Der Molen AJ, Cowan NJ, Mueller-Lisse UG et al. Urography Working Group of the European Society of Urogenital Radiology (2008) CT urography: definition, indications and techniques. A guideline for clinical practice. Eur Radiol 18:4–17

Vikram R, Sandler CM, Ng CS (2009) Imaging and staging of transitional cell carcinoma: part 2, upper urinary tract. AJR Am J Roentgenol 192:1488–1493

Vrtiska TJ, Hartman RP, Kofler JM et al. (2009) Spatial resolution and radiation dose of a 64-MDCT scanner compared with published CT urography protocols. AJR Am J Roentgenol 192:941–948

Wang J, Wang H, Tang G et al. (2009) Transitional cell carcinoma of upper urinary tract vs benign lesions: distinctive MSCT features. Abdom Imaging 34:94–106

Warshauer DM, McCarthy SM, Street L et al. (1988) Detection of renal masses: sensitivities and specificities of excretory urography/linear tomography, US, and CT. Radiology 169(2):363–365

Wimbish KJ, Sanders MM, Samuels BI et al. (1983) Squamous cell carcinoma of the renal pelvis: Case report emphasizing sonographic and CT appearance. Urol Radiol 5:267–269

Wong-You-Cheong JJ, Wagner BJ, Davis CJ (1998) Transitional cell carcinoma of the urinary tract: radiologic-pathologic correlation. Radiographics 18:123–142

# Renal Lymphoma and Renal Sarcoma

**25**

Annelies Rappaport and Raymond H. Oyen

## Contents

**Abstract**

> *Renal lymphoma* can present as a primary or secondary manifestation of lymphoma. Both are rare. At imaging studies, five different presentation forms of renal lymphoma can be distinguished: solitary or multiple renal masses, infiltrative lesions, perirenal lymphoma, and extension of a retroperitoneal lymphoid mass in the kidney.

> In general, diagnosis of renal lymphoma is not difficult as multisystemic disseminated disease is often present. Biopsy is recommended to avoid surgery. CT and PET-CT remain the modalities of choice for diagnosis and staging. MRI can be useful in patients with iodinated contrast allergy and renal insufficiency. Ultrasound has a roll in screening for renal mass in patients with flank pain or renal insufficiency and is the modality of choice in image-guided biopsy.

> *Renal sarcoma* can present as a primary or secondary manifestation of sarcoma. Both are very rare. Diagnosis on imaging is not straightforward because the imaging characteristics are extremely variable, depending on the nature and the degree of differentiation of the tumor components.

> There are no pathognomonic signs of a renal sarcoma, and frequently, imaging studies allow no differentiation from other primary epithelial renal parenchymal tumors.

> Some signs can suggest the preoperative diagnosis, such as a mass arising from the renal sinus or capsule and the absence of extension of the mass beyond its pseudocapsule. Some subtypes have specific characteristics. Histopathologic analysis is usually essential for the final diagnosis.

A. Rappaport (✉) and R.H. Oyen
Department of Radiology, Catholic University of Leuven,
Herestraat 49, 3000 Leuven, Belgium
e-mail: annelies.rappaport@uzleuven.be
e-mail: raymond.oyen@uz.kuleuven.ac.be

E. Quaia (ed.), *Radiological Imaging of the Kidney*,
Medical Radiology, DOI: 10.1007/978-3-540-87597-0_25, © Springer-Verlag Berlin Heidelberg 2011

## 25.1 Renal Lymphoma

### 25.1.1 General Features

Extranodal involvement of lymphoma is a common finding, occurring in approximately 40% of patients with lymphoma (Lee et al. 2008). "Extranodal" refers to sites other than lymph nodes including the spleen, thymus, tonsils, and Waldeyer ring, with the exception of non-Hodgkin's disease (malignant lymphoma), where the spleen is considered as an extranodal organ.

Every organ or structure can be involved by lymphoma. The kidney is the sixth most affected abdominal site after spleen, liver, gastrointestinal tract, pancreas, and abdominal wall (Lee et al. 2008). Extranodal involvement is more frequent in non-Hodgkin's lymphoma, patients with recurrent disease, and immune-suppressed patients (Guermazi et al. 2001; Lee et al. 2008; Leite et al. 2007). Recognition of extranodal involvement is crucial in initial staging (Cotswold-classification, Ann-Arbor-classification), since it is crucial for prognosis and therapy planning (Guermazi et al. 2001).

Imaging studies have an important role in diagnosis and staging.

### 25.1.2 Pathogenesis

Renal lymphoma is divided into primary and secondary forms. The existence of the very rare primary form is still controversial because the kidney does not harbor lymphoid tissue (Kandel et al. 1987; Stallone et al. 2000; Symeonidou et al. 2008).

In fact, renal lymphoma is a diagnosis of exclusion: the disease must be limited to the kidney and adjacent perirenal and perihilar lymph nodes. The pathophysiology of its development is unclear: many theories have been proposed, such as development as a result of chronic inflammatory processes, arising from perinephric lymphoid tissue or from the renal capsule, which is richly-embedded in lymph vessels (Pickhardt et al. 2000; Stallone et al. 2000).

More frequently, primary lymphoma is reported in immune-deprived patients and concerns a non-Hodgkin lymphoma.

Most patients with primary renal lymphoma quickly develop extrarenal disease and their prognosis is unfavorable (Kandel et al. 1987).

The more frequent secondary form of lymphoma is caused by hematogenous spread (causing, in general, bilateral involvement) of tumor cells, through sinus, perirenal, or capsular lymphatics or through direct extension from retroperitoneal lymphoma (Dyer et al. 2008; Leite et al. 2007).

Knowing the pattern of tumor growth and tumor spreading is essential in understanding the presentation of the tumor on imaging. Two patterns of tumor growth are distinguished: the infiltrative type and the expansile type.

In the less frequent *infiltrative growth pattern*, lymphoma proliferates along the normal interstitial structures, resulting in kidney enlargement and loss of internal architecture with initial preservation of the reniform shape (Pickhardt et al. 2000; Sheth et al. 2006; Urban and Fishman 2000). This appearance is also known as the "faceless kidney" (Zagoria 2004).

Formation of *expansile masses* is the result of spherical focal tumor proliferation (radial growth pattern), with compression or destruction of the adjacent renal parenchyma and formation of a pseudocapsule (Pickhardt et al. 2000; Urban and Fishman 2000).

### 25.1.3 Imaging Features and Differential Diagnosis

Lymphoma has five different appearances on imaging, depending partially on the growth pattern of the tumor: single and multiple masses, perirenal disease, infiltrative disease, and extension of retroperitoneal disease.

#### 25.1.3.1 Multiple Masses

This is the most frequent presentation pattern of renal lymphoma, seen in 50–60% of the cases (Cohan et al. 1990; Jafri et al. 1982; Sheth et al. 2006). They present typically bilateral, but unilateral forms have been reported. Size varies from 1 to 4.5 cm (Sheth et al. 2006). Renal contour bulging may be seen in eccentrically located or large masses (Cohan et al. 1990).

On unenhanced CT, the masses may have slightly higher attenuation numbers compared to the surrounding parenchyma; yet sometimes, these masses are hard to detect if no renal contour abnormalities are present. Intravenous contrast administration is indispensable for diagnosis and appropriate staging.

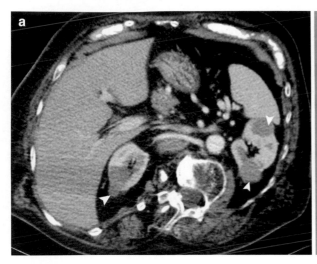

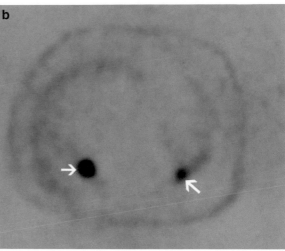

**Fig. 25.1** Diffuse large B-cell lymphoma in a 75-year-old woman. (**a**) Contrast-enhanced CT in the parenchymal phase shows multiple hypovascular masses in both kidneys (*arrow-* *heads*). (**b**) Axial FDG-PET-images in the same patient show foci of intense activity in both kidneys (*arrows*)

At contrast-enhanced CT, the masses are typically homogeneously hypovascular compared to the surrounding parenchyma, allowing easy detection (Fig. 25.1).

On MRI, the masses are hypointense on T1-weighted images and iso- or hypointense on T2-weighted images. The characteristics on contrast-enhanced MRI are similar to CT (Sheth et al. 2006).

Large retroperitoneal lymph adenopathies are present in less than 50% of the cases (Urban and Fishman 2000) and are the key feature for the diagnosis of lymphoma.

In the absence of large retroperitoneal adenopathies, differential diagnosis of bilateral multiple renal lymphoma includes renal metastases and papillary renal cell carcinoma. Clinical history is crucial in the diagnosis, but if there is no known primary malignancy present, biopsy needs to be performed to differentiate between surgical disease and disease processes where surgery must be avoided (Sheth et al. 2006).

From a theoretical point of view, other differential diagnoses include acute pyelonephritis, septic emboli, renal infarcts, and abscesses (Sheth et al. 2006). Their specific radiologic appearance and clinical presentation usually enable the differentiation with lymphoma.

### 25.1.3.2 Retroperitoneal Extension

Renal invasion from retroperitoneal extension is the second most frequent presentation pattern and accounts for 25–30% of the cases (Cohan et al. 1990).

Large confluent retroperitoneal masses encase the renal vasculature and invade the renal hilum with occasionally mild secondary hydronephrosis (Leite et al. 2007; Sheth et al. 2006; Symeonidou et al. 2008; Urban and Fishman 2000) (Fig. 25.2).

Occlusion or thrombosis of renal veins and arteries is rare despite the at times massive tumor burden (Sheth et al. 2006; Urban and Fishman 2000). Lateral displacement of the kidney is not infrequent.

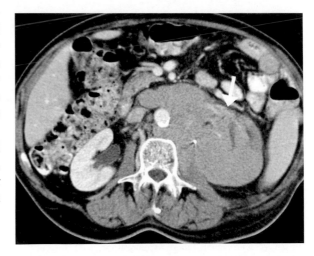

**Fig. 25.2** Follicular lymphoma in a 71-year-old man. Contrast-enhanced CT in the parenchymal phase shows a large hypovascular retroperitoneal mass extending into the renal hilum with encasement of the left renal vessels (*arrow*) and involving the kidney resulting in a hypoattenuating enlarged left kidney. Hydronephrosis is absent

Bulky lymphadenopathies can be seen in other tumors, even with extension into the kidney. Differential diagnosis is based on the aspect of the adenopathies, which tend to be softer in lymphoma. Lymphoma adenopathies encase vascular structures, whereas adenopathies from other primaries obstruct and invade vascular structures (Urban and Fishman 2000).

### 25.1.3.3 Infiltrative Disease

Infiltrative renal involvement presents as nephromegaly with disruption of the internal architecture and preservation of renal shape (Fig. 25.3). It occurs generally bilateral and is more commonly seen in Burkitt lymphoma (Sheth et al. 2006). It is observed in 20% of patients with renal lymphoma (Reznek et al. 1990).

Intravenous contrast administration is essential to appreciate enhancement characteristics, the focal ill-defined hypovascular areas, and the loss of cortico-medullary differentiation secondary to the infiltrative growth pattern. Encasement of the renal collecting system is often present.

Renal function is frequently moderately impaired.

Certainly, when this presentation is unilateral, the differential diagnosis includes other tumoral disease processes (renal cell carcinoma, medullary tumors, transitional and squamous cell carcinoma, renal sarcoma, leukemia, plasmocytoma, metastases, and infiltrative

pediatric tumors) and inflammatory diseases (bacterial and xanthogranulomatous pyelonephritis, renal parenchymal malakoplakia) with a predominately infiltrative pattern (Pickhardt et al. 2000).

### 25.1.3.4 Solitary Mass

A solitary mass is found in 10–20% of the cases (Cohan et al. 1990; Reznek et al. 1990). Solitary masses exhibit similar imaging characteristics as the multiple masses (Fig. 25.4). Solitary masses can be as large as 15 cm (Reznek et al. 1990).

Differential diagnosis with other solitary renal masses such as renal carcinoma has to be included, yet, the majority of renal cell carcinomas show hypervascular and heterogeneous enhancement. The presence of vascular invasion is also almost exclusively seen in renal cell carcinoma. Retroperitoneal adenopathy can be present in both cases, but tend to be much larger and confluent in lymphoma (Urban and Fishman 2000).

### 25.1.3.5 Perirenal Disease

Perirenal involvement is usually a part of retroperitoneal extension.

Isolated perirenal disease is very unusual (<10% of cases of perirenal lymphoma) and appears as a

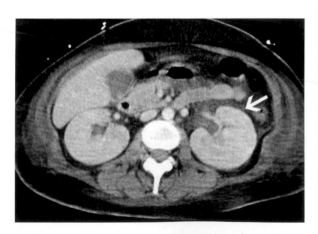

**Fig. 25.3** Large cell lymphoma in a 42-year-old woman who presented with renal failure. Contrast-enhanced CT in the parenchymal phase shows bilateral renal enlargement, loss of cortico-medullary differentiation, and homogeneously decreased enhancement of the renal parenchyma. Perirenal fat stranding (*arrow*) is seen at the left side. Diagnosis was achieved by percutaneous renal biopsy

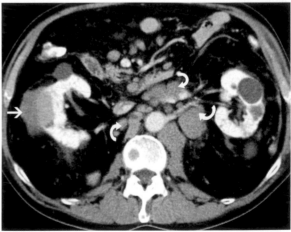

**Fig. 25.4** Posttransplant lymphoma in a 62-year-old man. Contrast-enhanced CT in the parenchymal phase shows a solitary, slightly irregular, delineated, hypovascular mass in the interpolar region of the right kidney (*arrow*). This mass extends in the perirenal space. Also note the multiple retroperitoneal adenopathies (*curved arrows*). Bilateral simple renal cysts

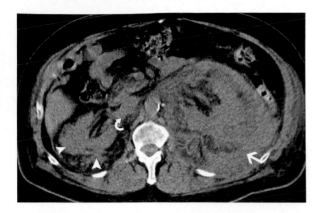

**Fig. 25.5** Posttransplant plasmoblastic lymphoma in a 68-year-old male heart transplant patient. Unenhanced CT (renal failure) shows an enlarged left kidney accompanied by perirenal fat infiltration and a band-like soft-tissue mass (*arrow*) more peripheral in the perirenal space. Note the subtle perirenal masses and nodular thickening in the right perirenal space (*arrowhead*) and the retrocaval adenopathy (*curved arrow*)

soft-tissue mass involving the perirenal space partially or completely, and compresses but not invades the kidney (Bechtold et al. 1996; Leite et al. 2007; Surabhi et al. 2008) (Fig. 25.5). The presentation of perirenal soft-tissue mass without renal invasion and functional impairment, is almost pathognomonic (Sheeran and Sussman 1998; Sheth et al. 2006; Urban and Fishman 2000). To differentiate the perirenal soft-tissue mass from the underlying parenchyma, contrast administration is crucial.

Findings can yet be more limited to plaques and nodules in the perirenal space and thickening of Gerota's fascia (Sheeran and Sussman 1998). These limited findings can cause a diagnostic problem since benign (perinephric hematoma, urinoma, extramedullary hematopoiesis, fibrosis, amyloidosis…) and malignant conditions (sarcoma, metastases, primary renal carcinoma) can cause minimal changes in the perirenal space (Sheth et al. 2006; Urban and Fishman 2000). Clinical history and secondary findings can help in further differentiation.

### 25.1.3.6 Atypical Findings

Although very unusual, atypical findings may be observed in each presentation form including calcification, necrosis, spontaneous hemorrhage, cyst formation, and heterogeneous enhancement (Heiken et al. 1983).

Heterogeneous or cystic appearance is rare and seen in larger masses and masses with tumor necrosis in the context of chemotherapy (Sheth et al. 2006; Urban and Fishman 2000).

### 25.1.4 Roll of Different Imaging Modalities

#### 25.1.4.1 Ultrasound

Ultrasound is widely accepted as the screening modality for renal mass lesions in patients with flank pain and functional renal impairment. Contrast-enhanced CT and MRI are superior to ultrasound in diagnosis (higher sensitivity and specificity) and in evaluating the extent of disease.

Ultrasound has a role in guiding percutaneous biopsies (Sheth et al. 2006; Törnroth et al. 2003) and is recommended because of the absence of radiation.

#### 25.1.4.2 Computed Tomography and Positron Emission Tomography-Computed Tomography (PET-CT)

Contrast-enhanced multidetector CT and PET-CT are the golden standard in detection, staging, and follow-up of lymphoma.

All presentation forms of renal lymphoma tend to be hypovascular and generally show a homogeneous enhancement. For optimal lesion detection, the CT must be performed in the nephrographic or parenchymal (venous) phase. In the venous phase, cortex and medulla enhance equivocally and the risk of missing medullar lesions is minimized. Unenhanced CT can be performed prior to contrast administration to objectivate the lesion enhancement.

Cortico-medullary or arterial phase is useful only in examining vascular involvement, and excretory phase in examining collecting system involvement.

CT further enables the evaluation of disease extension in adjacent structures and detection of other sites of nodal and extranodal involvement. This is important in initial staging and follow-up, because of the impact on therapy and prognosis.

In this respect, CT/PET-CT scan needs to be combined with thoracic and/or neck CT scan.

PET is more sensitive and specific than CT in detecting small tumor deposits (Moog et al. 1998).

Combination of PET and CT combines the advantages of both techniques, and at present, has become routine in disease follow-up.

CT can also be used in guiding percutaneous biopsy for lesions difficult to access with ultrasound.

### 25.1.4.3 MRI

On MRI, the lymphoid masses are like most renal masses, hypointense on T1-weighted images and iso- or hypointense on T2-weighted images. There is moderate enhancement on enhanced MRI.

Results in literature show that the MRI is equally reliable as CT in detection and characterization of lymphoid lesions (Lowe et al. 2000; Sheth et al. 2006).

Despite these good results, CT remains the golden standard because of its cost-effectiveness, ability to evaluate the chest, and availability.

MRI is useful in patients with iodinated contrast allergy or renal insufficiency (Sheth et al. 2006). MRI has perspectives in future for the evaluation of bone marrow involvement.

### 25.1.5 Diagnostic Approach

Usually, the radiological image is sufficient to establish the diagnosis of renal lymphoma. In most cases, the diagnosis is already known before imaging, due to nodal biopsy at initial presentation.

When a renal lesion has characteristics suggesting renal lymphoma, image-guided biopsy is recommended for diagnosis and further therapeutic management (Sheth et al. 2006).

## 25.2 Renal Sarcoma

### 25.2.1 General Features

Two subtypes are discriminated: primary and secondary sarcoma. The secondary form is further subdivided into renal metastases or direct extension of a retroperitoneal sarcoma. The secondary subgroup is more frequent (Pickhardt et al. 2000). The sarcomatoid type of RCC is not included.

Renal metastases from sarcoma are very rare and are often dependent on the location of the primary lesion. Extremity sarcomas tend to spread to the lungs, whereas retroperitoneal and gastrointestinal sarcomas often spread to the liver (Greene et al. 2006).

Primary renal sarcoma is a very rare presentation form of sarcoma. 1.1% of malignant renal tumors are sarcomas (Jenkins et al. 1971; Prasad et al. 2005; Shirkhoda and Lewis 1987).

Renal sarcoma affects patients in their fourth to seventh decade, with a slight male preponderance.

Patients often present with an abdominal mass, flank pain, hematuria, and sometimes weight loss. Occasionally, renal sarcoma is an incidental finding (Shirkhoda and Lewis 1987).

Sarcomas have high rates of local recurrence and metastases, and the prognosis is poor (Prasad et al. 2005; Shirkhoda and Lewis 1987). Invasive surgery and chemotherapy are usually indispensable.

### 25.2.2 Pathogenesis

Each type of mesenchymal cell in the kidney can develop into a different histologic type of sarcoma. About 11 histological subtypes are distinguished: liposarcoma, hemangiopericytoma, angiosarcoma, fibrosarcoma, malignant fibrous histiocytoma, leiomyosarcoma, rhabdomyosarcoma, Ewing sarcoma (ES), osteosarcoma, chondrosarcoma, and synovial sarcoma.

Leiomyosarcoma is considered to be the most frequent type of renal sarcoma and accounts for about 50% of the renal sarcomas. Liposarcoma and fibrosarcoma are also more frequently encountered (Pickhardt et al. 2000; Shirkhoda and Lewis 1987).

### 25.2.3 Imaging Features

Again, two growth patterns are seen in sarcoma: the expansile and the infiltrative growth pattern. Rhabdomyosarcoma and angiosarcoma present more often as an infiltrative lesion; leiomyosarcoma and the other sarcoma subtypes more often as an expansile mass (Pickhardt et al. 2000).

Imaging is variable and depends on the nature and the degree of differentiation of the tumor components. Sarcomas are rapid-growing, large tumors, but these are not specific features enabling the diagnosis. In general, renal sarcomas cannot be differentiated from renal cell carcinomas on imaging.

Some signs can suggest a preoperative diagnosis such as a mass that arises from the renal sinus or capsule, the absence of extension of the mass beyond its pseudocapsule, the highly vascularised areas, and the areas of necrosis (Shirkhoda and Lewis 1987). Some subtypes have specific characteristics.

The MRI appearance of renal sarcomas is rarely discussed in current literature. Sarcomas tend to be of intermediate to hypointense signal intensity on T1-weighted MR imaging and of intermediate to hyperintense signal intensity on T2-weighted MR imaging (Billingsley and Restrepo 2006).

### 25.2.3.1 Liposarcoma

Liposarcoma is the most common retroperitoneal malignant tumor (Surabhi et al. 2008). It arises from nonfat-containing areas in the kidney such as the capsule, and rarely, the parenchyma (Shirkhoda and Lewis 1987).

Their imaging appearance is strongly dependent on their histological subtype (well-differentiated, myxoid, round cell, pleomorphic, and dedifferentiated subtypes).

Well-differentiated liposarcomas contain mainly macroscopic fat. Round cell and pleomorphic liposarcomas present as a soft-tissue mass, the myxoid type has a cystic appearance, while dedifferentiated liposarcomas can present intralesional calcifications or ossifications (Secil et al. 2005; Surabhi et al. 2008). Liposarcomas tend to be hypovascular.

Differential diagnosis of angiomyolipoma with liposarcoma can be difficult if the angiomyolipomas are large and exophytic. The presence of large intratumoral vessels, intralesional hemorrhage, sharp parenchymal defect, and associated angiomyolipomas favor the diagnosis of an angiomyolipoma (Wang et al. 2002; Israel et al. 2002).

### 25.2.3.2 Hemangiopericytoma and Angiosarcoma

A *hemangiopericytoma* is a soft-tissue vascular tumor that originates from the Zimmerman pericytes. On imaging, it presents as a large, lobulated, well defined, hypervascular mass, usually with necrotic areas and calcifications. Differential diagnosis with renal cell carcinoma is difficult. Hemangiopericytoma often occurs in younger patients (fourth decade) than renal cell carcinoma (Brescia et al. 2008; Surabhi et al. 2008).

*Angiosarcoma* is a rare tumor that arises from endothelial cells. Renal involvement is mostly the result of metastases from primary dermal or visceral angiosarcoma. On imaging, it presents as a heterogeneous hypervascular infiltrative mass. Sometimes, hemorrhage can be observed on unenhanced CT or MRI. Calcification can be present. The role of carcinogens (arsenic, thorium dioxide, vinyl chloride exposure...) as in hepatic angiosarcoma has not been established in renal angiosarcoma (Leggio et al. 2006; Yu et al. 2008).

### 25.2.3.3 Malignant Fibrous Histiocytoma and Fibrosarcoma

*Malignant fibrous histiocytoma* arises from primitive mesenchymal cells which demonstrate both histiocytic and fibroblastic differentiation. They present as a large heterogeneous mass with areas of necrosis, hemorrhage, and local invasion (Kwak et al. 2003; Surabhi et al. 2008). Calcification or ossification can also be present (Secil et al. 2005).

*Fibrosarcoma* is thought to originate from the connective tissue in the renal capsule. On imaging, the tumor usually presents as a large, encapsulated, and hypovascular mass, but cannot be differentiated from leiomyosarcoma and (sarcomatoid) RCC. It can be differentiated only on immunohistochemical staining of appropriate biopsies. Invasion of the renal vein is seen in about 40% of the cases (Agarwal et al. 2008; Kansara and Powell 1980; Shirkhoda and Lewis 1987).

### 25.2.3.4 Leiomyosarcoma and Rhabdomyosarcoma

*Leiomyosarcoma* (Fig. 25.6) is the most frequent subtype of renal sarcoma. It arises from the smooth muscle cells in the inner layer of the renal capsule, from the smooth muscle cells in the tunica media of small vessels in the renal parenchyma or of the large renal vessels (renal vein, ..), or from the smooth muscle cells in the renal pelvis wall. Sometimes, leiomyosarcomas are the result

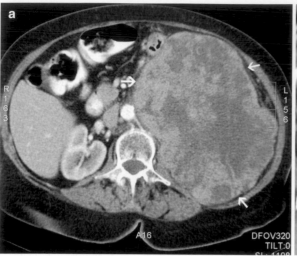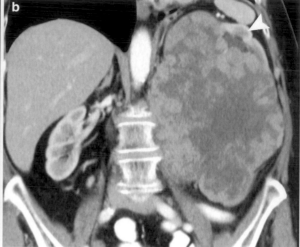

**Fig. 25.6** High-grade renal leiomyosarcoma in a 73-year-old woman. Axial (**a**) and coronal (**b**) images of a contrast-enhanced CT in the corticomedullar phase show a large heterogeneous, lobulated soft-tissue mass arising from and splaying the left kidney. Residual normal renal parenchyma (*arrowhead*) can be recognized at the upper pole. The mass is also well encapsulated (*arrows*)

of malignant transformation of an angiomyolipoma (Lowe et al. 1992).

On unenhanced CT, leiomyosarcomas are often hyperattenuating compared to the renal parenchyma and have almost equal attenuation values as the lumbar musculature. Tumor calcification is present in about 10% of the cases. Spontaneous ruptures have been reported (Billingsley and Restrepo 2006).

Leiomyosarcomas tend to be hypovascular on imaging, but exceptions have been reported. It is difficult to differentiate leiomyosarcoma with the benign renal leiomyoma. Most frequently, renal leiomyomas are well encapsulated, small cortical tumors of less than 2 cm, and originate most commonly from the renal capsule. Frequently, a plane is distinguishable between the tumor and the kidney without parenchymal distortion. Leiomyosarcomas are larger and less encapsulated, but sometimes, they have almost similar imaging characteristics as their benign counterpart. In that case, biopsy can be indispensable to obtain preoperative diagnosis (Roy et al. 1998).

*Renal rhabdomyosarcoma* arises from the embryonal mesenchyme that ultimately develops into striated skeletal muscle (Sola et al. 2007). It is generally found in young patients and rarely in adults. Rhabdoid tumor of kidney is considered as a different entity (Agrons et al. 1997; Schmidt et al. 1982). In literature, no specific imaging features have been assigned to renal rhabdomyosarcoma.

### 25.2.3.5 Osteosarcoma, Chondrosarcoma, Ewing Sarcoma, and Synovial Sarcoma

*Renal osteosarcoma* is believed to originate from undifferentiated renal mesenchymal cells.

Extraskeletal osteosarcoma is a rare aggressive tumor and accounts for 4% of osteosarcomas. The most frequent locations of extraskeletal osteosarcomas are the lower and upper extremities and retroperitoneum. Extraskeletal osteosarcoma occurs in older patients (fourth to sixth decade) than osteogenic osteosarcoma (Secil et al. 2005).

Imaging shows extensive intralesional ossification or calcification in a "sunburst" pattern (Fig. 25.7). This can be seen on plain abdominal radiography (O'Malley et al. 1991). The mass can show a variable grade of mineralization, but the calcification is frequently intense and amorphous. The nonmineralized areas have an attenuation that resembles muscle on CT scan and intermediate signal intensity on T1-weighted images (Secil et al. 2005). Renal osteosarcomas are frequently hypervascular.

Extensive intralesional ossification or calcification can also be seen in sarcomatoid renal cell carcinoma and metastatic lesion of osteogenic sarcoma (Micolonghi et al. 1984). Other renal sarcomas such as malignant fibrous histiocytoma and dedifferentiated liposarcoma can also undergo extensive calcification or ossification (Secil et al. 2005).

**Fig. 25.7** (**a–c**) Renal osteosarcoma in a 51-year-old woman. Axial (**a**) and coronal (**b, c**) images of a contrast-enhanced CT in the parenchymal phase show a large heterogeneous infiltrative mass occupying the left kidney with extensive intralesional calcification in a "sunburst" pattern. This mass infiltrates the kidney, with partial preservation of its bean-shaped configuration (curvilinear line form). On the other hand, the tumor also shows an expansile growth pattern with extension beyond Gerota's fascia (*arrowhead*). The tumor also extends in the renal sinus with calcified tumor thrombosis in the renal vein (*arrow*). Large heterogeneous/necrotic adenopathies are depicted in the left para-aortic region (*curved arrow*)

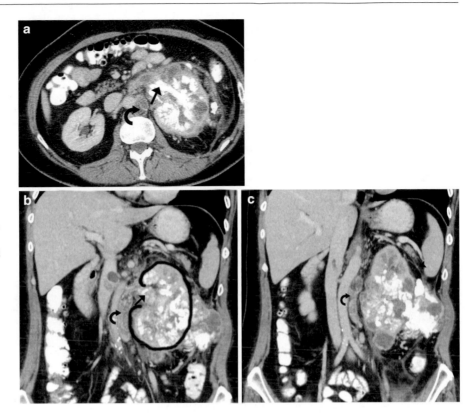

*Renal chondrosarcoma* is believed to originate from undifferentiated renal mesenchymal cells.

Extraskeletal chondrosarcoma occurs in young patients (second and third decade) with a female preponderance (Gomez-Brouchet et al. 2001).

The most frequent locations of extraskeletal chondrosarcoma are the brain, meninges, neck, trunk, retroperitoneum, and extremities (Malhotra et al. 1984).

They are generally slow-growing tumors, but late metastases can occur.

Imaging shows a large soft-tissue mass with central calcification (Nativ et al. 1985).

*Renal Ewing sarcoma (ES) and primitive neuroectodermal tumor (PNET)* are considered in the WHO-classification as one entity with a spectrum of differentiation (Ushigome et al. 2002).

Renal ES-PNET is supposed to originate from the neural cells in the kidney or the embryonic neural crest cells that migrate into the kidney (Clapp and Croker 1997).

Primary renal ES-PNET occurs more frequently in adolescents and young adults. They are aggressive tumors with invasion into the surrounding structures

(renal vasculature, spine) and early metastases to regional lymph nodes, bone, lung, and liver (Chu et al. 2008).

Imaging shows large heterogeneous tumors with sometimes ill-defined margins (Pickhardt et al. 2000). Figure 25.8 shows solitary renal metastasis of a primary Ewing sarcoma of the pelvic bone.

*Renal synovial sarcoma* is a very rare tumor. Primary synovial sarcoma of the kidney was first reported in 1999 (Faria et al. 1999). The knowledge about this type of sarcoma is limited as few case reports were published.

Imaging studies show a heterogeneous enhancing tumor with solid and cystic components (Fig. 25.9) (Erturhan et al. 2008; Mirza et al. 2008).

### 25.2.3.6 Granulocytic Sarcomas (Chloromas)

Granulocytic sarcomas (chloromas) are rare malignant tumors of granulocytic precursors that can present in up to 10% of patients with acute myelogenous leukemia and rarely in acute lymphocytic leukemia.

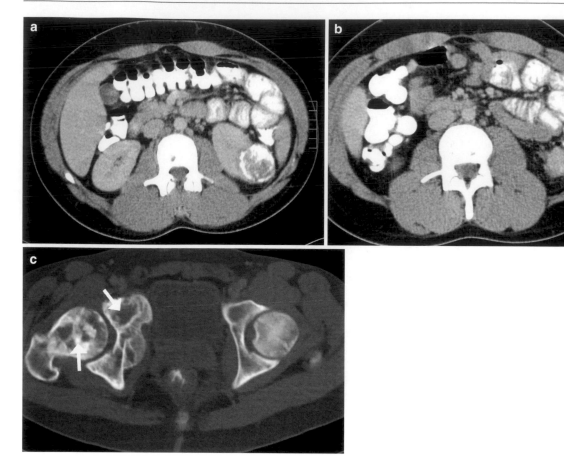

**Fig. 25.8** (**a**–**c**) Renal metastasis of a pelvic Ewing sarcoma in a 26-year-old woman. (**a**) Axial contrast-enhanced CT in the parenchymal phase shows a well circumscribed, heterogeneous, extensively calcified mass posterolateral in the inferior pole of the left kidney. (**b**) The mass lies in close relation with the ante- rior (*arrowhead*) and posterior renal fascia (*arrow*), which appear thickened. Note the thickening of the lateroconal fascia (*curved arrow*). (**c**) Primary site of the Ewing sarcoma in the right pelvic bone appearing as extended heterogeneous zones of osteolysis (*arrow*)

In imaging, they present as focal hypovascular soft-tissue masses in one or both kidneys (Surabhi et al. 2008).

Renal AIDS-related Kaposi sarcoma has been observed in autopsy reports, but rarely shows clinical or radiologic manifestations (Restrepo et al. 2006).

### 25.2.3.7 Kaposi Sarcoma

Kaposi sarcoma originates from the blood and lymphatic vessels.

Kaposi usually affects the skin, but can affect variable thoracic and abdominal organs.

It was a very uncommon type of tumor till the beginning of the AIDS epidemic.

## 25.2.4 Diagnostic Approach

If a large encapsulated renal mass with aggressive growth pattern arises from the renal sinus or capsule, renal sarcoma must be enclosed in your differential diagnostic list. Because of the lack of specific signs and high resemblance with the more frequent RCC, final diagnosis is usually made on histopathological analysis.

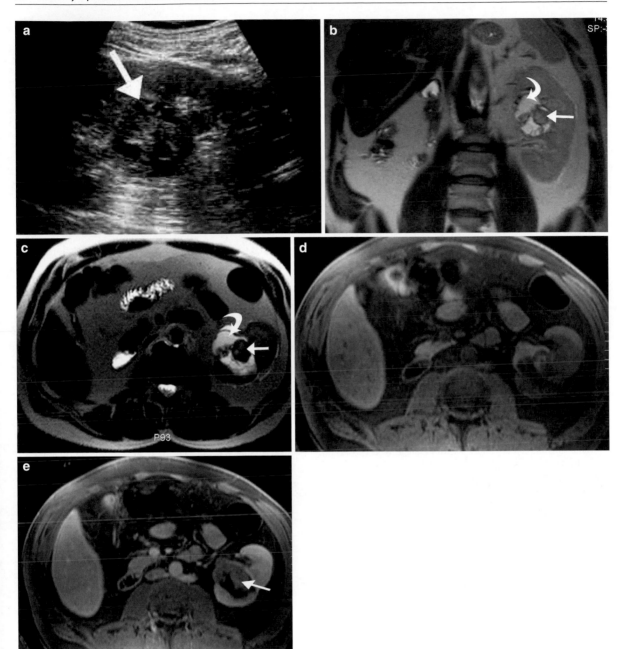

**Fig. 25.9** (a–e) Monophasic renal synovial sarcoma in a 47-year-old man. (**a**) Ultrasound shows a heterogeneous, partially cystic mass in the left renal sinus (*arrow*) with retro-acoustic intensification. Hydronephrosis is absent. MRI of the kidney was performed. (**b**) Coronal T2-weighted imaging and (**c**) axial late T2-weighted imaging show a left renal sinus mass with central T2-hypointense nodular component (*arrow*) and peripheral T2-hyperintense cystic component (*curved arrow*). (**d**) Axial T1-weighted imaging with fat saturation before contrast administration shows that the lesion has a mixed hyper- and hypointense signal intensity. (**e**) Contrast-enhanced axial T1-weighted imaging with fat saturation in the parenchymal phase shows an enhancing nodular soft-tissue component anteriorly in the lesion (*arrow*)

# References

Agarwal K, Singh S, Pathania OP (2008) Primary renal fibrosarcoma: a rare case report and review of literature. Indian J Pathol Microbiol 51:409–410

Agrons GA, Kingsman KD, Wagner BJ et al. (1997) Rhabdoid tumor of the kidney in children: a comparative study of 21 cases. AJR Am J Roentgenol 168:447–451

Bechtold RE, Dyer RB, Zagoria RJ et al. (1996) The perirenal space: relationship of pathologic processes to normal retroperitoneal anatomy. Radiographics 16:841–854

Billingsley ED, Restrepo S (2006) Kidney sarcomas. In: Guermazi A (ed) Imaging in kidney cancer. Springer, Berlin, pp 145–157

Brescia A, Pinto F, Gardi M et al. (2008) Renal hemangiopericytoma: case report and review of the literature. Urology 71:755.e9–12

Chu WC, Reznikov B, Lee EY et al. (2008) Primitive neuroectodermal tumour (PNET) of the kidney: a rare renal tumour in adolescents with seemingly characteristic radiological features. Pediatr Radiol 38:1089–1094

Clapp WL, Croker BP (1997) Adult kidney. In: Sternberg S (ed) Histology for pathologists, 2nd edn. Raven Press, New York, pp 799–834

Cohan RH, Dunnick NR, Leder RA et al. (1990) Computed tomography of renal lymphoma. J Comput Assist Tomogr 4:933–938

Dyer R, DiSantis DJ, McClennan BL (2008) Simplified imaging approach for evaluation of the solid renal mass in adults. Radiology 247:331–343

Erturhan S, Seçkiner I, Zincirkeser S et al. (2008) Primary synovial sarcoma of the kidney: use of PET/CT in diagnosis and follow-up. Ann Nucl Med 22:225–229

Faria P, Argani P, Epstein J (1999) Primary synovial sarcoma of the kidney: a molecular subset of so-called embryonal renal sarcoma. Mod Pathol 12:94A

Gomez-Brouchet A, Soulie M, Delisle MB et al. (2001) Mesenchymal chondrosarcoma of the kidney. J Urol 166:2305

Greene FL, Compton CC, Fritz AG et al. (2006) AJCC cancer staging atlas. Springer, New York, pp 191–194

Guermazi A, Brice P, de Kerviler E et al. (2001) Extranodal Hodgkin disease: spectrum of disease. Radiographics 21:161–179

Heiken JP, Gold RP, Schnur MJ et al. (1983) Computed tomography of renal lymphoma with ultrasound correlation. J Comput Assist Tomogr 7:245–250

Israel GM, Bosniak MA, Slywotzky CM et al. (2002) CT differentiation of large exophytic renal angiomyolipomas and perirenal liposarcomas. AJR Am J Roentgenol 179:769–773

Jafri SZ, Bree RL, Amendola MA et al. (1982) CT of renal and perirenal non-Hodgkin lymphoma. AJR Am J Roentgenol 138:1101–1105

Jenkins JD, Anderson CK, Williams RE (1971) Renal sarcoma. Br J Urol 43:263–267

Kandel LB, McCullough DL, Harrison LH et al. (1987) Primary renal lymphoma. Does it exist? Cancer 60:386–391

Kansara V, Powell I (1980) Fibrosarcoma of the kidney. Urology 26:419–421

Kwak HS, Kim CS, Lee JM (2003) MR findings of renal malignant fibrous histiocytoma. Eur Radiol 13 (suppl 6): L245–L246

Lee WK, Lau EW, Duddalwar VA et al. (2008) Abdominal manifestations of extranodal lymphoma: spectrum of imaging findings. AJR Am J Roentgenol 191:198–206

Leggio L, Addolorato G, Abenavoli L et al. (2006) Primary renal angiosarcoma: a rare malignancy. A case report and review of the literature. Urol Oncol 24:307–312

Leite NP, Kased N, Hanna RFB et al. (2007) Cross-sectional imaging of extranodal involvement in abdominopelvic lymphoproliferative malignancies. Radiographics 27:1613–1634

Lowe BA, Brewer J, Houghton DC et al. (1992) Malignant transformation of angiomyolipoma. J Urol 147:1356–1358

Lowe LH, Isuani BH, Heller RM et al. (2000) Pediatric renal masses: Wilms tumor and beyond. Radiographics 20:1585–1603

Malhotra CM, Doolittle CH, Rodil JV et al. (1984) Mesenchymal chondrosarcoma of the kidney. Cancer 54:2495–2499

Micolonghi TS, Liang D, Schwartz S (1984) Primary osteogenic sarcoma of the kidney. J Urol 131:1164–1166

Mirza M, Zamilpa I, Bunning J (2008) Primary renal synovial sarcoma. Urology 72:716.e11–2

Moog F, Bangerter M, Diederichs CG et al. (1998) Extranodal malignant lymphoma: detection with FDG PET versus CT. Radiology 206:475–481

Nativ O, Horowitz A, Lindner A et al. (1985) Primary chondrosarcoma of the kidney. J Urol 134:120–121

O'Malley FP, Grignon DJ, Shepherd RR et al. (1991) Primary osteosarcoma of the kidney. Report of case studies by immunohistochemistry, electron microscopy and DNA flow cytometry. Arch Pathol Lab Med 115:1262–1265

Pedrosa I, Sun MR, Spencer M et al. (2008) MR imaging of renal masses: correlation with findings at surgery and pathologic analysis. Radiographics 28:985–1003

Pickhardt PJ, Lonergan GJ, Davis CJ Jr et al. (2000) From the archives of the AFIP. Infiltrative renal lesions: radiologic-pathologic correlation. Armed Forces Institute of Pathology. Radiographics 20:215–243

Prasad SR, Humphrey PA, Menias CO et al. (2005) Neoplasms of the renal medulla: radiologic-pathologic correlation. Radiographics 25:369–380

Restrepo CS, Martínez S, Lemos JA et al. (2006) Imaging manifestations of Kaposi sarcoma. Radiographics 26:1169–1185

Reznek RH, Mootoosamy I, Webb JA et al. (1990) CT in renal and perirenal lymphoma: a further look. Clin Radiol 42:233–238. Erratum in: Clin Radiol 43(4):289

Roy C, Pfleger D, Tuchmann C et al. (1998) Small leiomyosarcoma of the renal capsule: CT findings. Eur Radiol 8:224–227

Schmidt D, Harms D, Zieger G (1982) Malignant rhabdoid tumor of the kidney. Histopathology, ultrastructure and comments on differential diagnosis. Virchows Arch A Pathol Anat Histopathol 398:101–108

Secil M, Mungan U, Yorukoglu K et al. (2005) Case 89: retroperitoneal extraskeletal osteosarcoma. Radiology 237:880–883

Sheeran SR, Sussman SK (1998) Renal lymphoma: spectrum of CT findings and potential mimics. AJR Am J Roentgenol 171:1067–1072

Sheth S, Ali S, Fishman E (2006) Imaging of renal lymphoma: patterns of disease with pathologic correlation. Radiographics 26:1151–1168

Shirkhoda A, Lewis E (1987) Renal sarcoma and sarcomatoid renal cell carcinoma: CT and angiographic features. Radiology 162:353–357

Sola JE, Cova D, Casillas J et al. (2007) Primary renal botryoid rhabdomyosarcoma: diagnosis and outcome. J Pediatr Surg 42:e17–20

Stallone G, Infante B, Manno C et al. (2000) Primary renal lymphoma does exist: case report and review of the literature. J Nephrol 13:367–372

Surabhi VR, Menias C, Prasad SR et al. (2008) Neoplastic and non-neoplastic proliferative disorders of the perirenal space: cross-sectional imaging findings. Radiographics 28:1005–1017

Symeonidou C, Standish R, Sahdev A et al. (2008) Imaging and histopathologic features of HIV-related renal disease. Radiographics 28:1339–1354

Törnroth T, Heiro M, Marcussen N et al. (2003) Lymphomas diagnosed by percutaneous kidney biopsy. Am J Kidney Dis 42:960–971

Urban BA, Fishman EK (2000) Renal lymphoma: CT patterns with emphasis on helical CT. Radiographics 20:197–212

Ushigome S, Machinami R, Sorensen PH (2002) World Health Organization classification of tumours: pathology and genetics: tumours of soft tissue and bone. IARC Press, Lyon, pp 298–300

Wang LJ, Wong YC, Chen CJ et al. (2002) Computerized tomography characteristics that differentiate angiomyolipomas from liposarcomas in the perinephric space. J Urol 167:490–493

Yu RS, Chen Y, Jiang B et al. (2008) Primary hepatic sarcomas: CT findings. Eur Radiol 18:2196–2205

Zagoria RJ (2004) Renal masses. In: Genitourinary radiology: the requisites, 2nd edn. Mosby, Philadelphia, pp 115–118

Zucca E (2008) Extranodal lymphoma: a reappraisal. Ann Oncol 19 (suppl 4):iv77–iv80

# Cystic Renal Masses

# 26

Olivier Hélénon, J. M. Correas, S. Merran,
E. Dekeyser, and A. Vieillefond

## Contents

O. Hélénon (✉), J.M. Correas, and E. Dekeyser
Service de Radiologie, Necker Hospital and Paris Descartes
University, 149 rue de Sèvres, 75743 Paris, Cedex 15, France
e-mail: olivier.helenon@nck.aphp.fr

S. Merran
Département d'imagerie médicale
Fédération Mutualiste Parisiene,
24 rue Saint Victor, 75008 Paris,
e-mail: smerran@gmail.com

A. Vieillefond
Service de pathologie, Cochin Hospital and
Paris Descartes University,
27 rue du faubourg saint Jacques, 75679 Paris, Cedex 14
e-mail: annick.vieillefond@cch.aphp.fr

## Abstract

> Cystic renal masses result from a wide spectrum of pathology including renal cysts, benign cystic lesions of nonepithelial origin, benign cystic neoplasms, and cystic carcinomas. Whereas the diagnosis of a simple renal cyst is easy, differentiation between complex cyst and cystic renal tumor can be difficult. Ultrasonography provides definitive diagnostic informations in most simple renal cysts that are incidentally screened. Computed tomography (CT) is the gold standard in detecting and characterizing cystic renal masses. The Bosniak classification system is based on specific CT criteria that rely on the cystic lesion enhancement properties and morphologic features. This classification scheme has been designed to separate cystic lesions requiring surgery (surgical categories III and IV) from those that can be left alone (nonsurgical categories I and II) or followed (nonsurgical category IIF). MRI is now considered at least equivalent to CT in the characterization of cystic lesions. It also plays a major role in the diagnosis of category IIF cystic renal masses and those that remain not categorizable at CT. Contrast-enhanced ultrasound has also been shown to improve the evaluation of complex cystic masses. It can be currently proposed as an alternative to CT in the follow-up of complex renal cysts and in patients with serious contraindication to contrast-enhanced CT or MRI.

E. Quaia (ed.), *Radiological Imaging of the Kidney*,
Medical Radiology, DOI: 10.1007/978-3-540-87597-0_26, © Springer-Verlag Berlin Heidelberg 2011

## 26.1 Introduction

The increasing use of ultrasonography (US) and computed tomography (CT) in conjunction with the high prevalence of renal cysts in adults has led to the frequent discovery of incidental cystic renal masses on routine abdominal imaging. Whereas the diagnosis of a simple renal cyst is easy, differentiation between complex cystic lesion and cystic renal tumor can be difficult. Such a diagnostic challenge is encountered by the radiologist in daily practice and requires a good knowledge of imaging findings and proper characterization of cystic lesions. The Bosniak classification system was first introduced in 1986 (Bosniak 1986), providing a practical approach in characterizing and determining the management of cystic renal masses. It has been widely accepted by radiologists and urologists as a diagnostic and communication tool.

The following paragraphs will deal with the diagnosis of cystic renal masses with the exception of renal cystic diseases (refer to Chap. 12). Imaging strategy and the differential diagnosis of cystic lesions will also be discussed.

## 26.2 Definition and Etiology of Cystic Renal Masses

### 26.2.1 Definition

A cystic renal mass is radiologically defined as a fluid-filled mass in which the major content exhibit water signal characteristics and/or a total lack of postcontrast enhancement indicating the absence of vascularity. Masses with intermediate or high internal attenuations without internal vascularity at CT should be viewed as cystic when they also exhibit postcontrast enhancing wall or septae or fulfill the criteria for a typical hyperdense cyst according to the Bosniak classification (refer to Sect. 26.4.2.2). Certain cases of solid renal tumors can exhibit some of these features, such as a water density on precontrast CT images or absence of significant enhancement on postcontrast images, and therefore, mimic a cystic lesion. The association of at least two of the above-mentioned criteria is therefore necessary to recognize the cystic nature of a renal mass. Identification of a cystic mass also requires adequate CT scanning, including at best, both unenhanced

and contrast-enhanced phases. However, abdominal contrast-enhanced CT with no preliminary unenhanced scanning provides sufficient information to distinguish between a simple cyst and complex cystic masses that require further appropriate imaging.

### 26.2.2 Etiologies

Cystic renal masses result from a wide sprectrum of pathology including renal cysts, benign cystic lesions of various nonepithelial origin, and cystic tumors.

#### 26.2.2.1 Benign Nonneoplastic Cystic Masses

The most common cause of a cystic renal mass is the renal cyst that occurs in up to 50% of individuals over the age of 50 years. The size and number of renal cysts tend to increase with age as well as its propensity to become complicated (Ravine et al. 1993; Terada et al. 2008). Renal cysts originate from the nephron and commonly arise within the renal cortex. The so-called simple cyst is a fluid-filled benign and asymptomatic unilocular lesion, with smooth thin wall lined by a monolayer of epithelial cells (Hill 1989). It contains straw-colored fluid with chemical composition similar to plasma. Complicated cysts manifest complex features resulting from infection, hemorrhage, or other causes of inflammation such as trauma, renal surgery, or percutaneous procedure. The so-called hyperdense cyst can result from various unusual contents including (Curry et al. 1982; Fishman et al. 1983; Sussman et al. 1984; Dunnick et al. 1984b) hemorrhagic debris, blood breakdown products, iron, protein, colloid, or iodine from prior contrast material administration.

Other causes of benign fluid-filled renal parenchymal masses include calyceal and pelvic diverticula; suppurative infectious processes; hydatid cyst; hydrocalix resulting from infundibular obstruction; and renal infarction with pseudocystic transformation.

#### 26.2.2.2 Benign Cystic Neoplasms (Fig. 26.1)

Among benign renal tumors, those presenting with a cystic pattern are multilocular cystic nephromas (MCN) and mixed epithelial and stromal tumors

**Fig. 26.1** (**a–f**) Cystic renal neoplasms. Gross anatomy of most common subtypes. (**a**) Multilocular cystic nephroma (consistent with Bosniak category III). (**b**) Multilocular cystic clear cell carcinoma (consistent with Bosniak category III). (**c**) Cystic RCC with multilocular cystic pattern (consistent with Bosniak category IV). Note the presence of *yellow* colored solid elements (*arrows*) composed of carcinomatous tissue. (**d**) Cystic RCC with unilocular cystic pattern (consistent with Bosniak category IV). Note the presence of a thick irregular wall with nodularity (*arrows*). (**e**) Pseudocystic RCC due to massive necrosis (consistent with Bosniak category IV). Note the presence of a mural solid nodule composed of tumor tissue (*arrow*). (**f**) Pseudocystic RCC due to massive necrosis (consistent with Bosniak category III). Note the absence of solid tumor tissue elements. The lesion is surrounded by a thick wall with slight irregularity

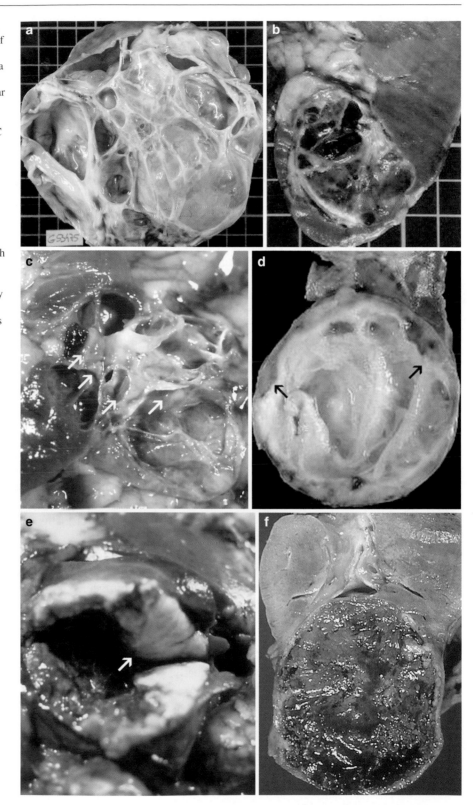

(MEST). Both tumors are deemed to represent opposite ends of the spectrum of the same entity. A unifying term "renal epithelial and stromal tumors" (REST) has been recently proposed to designate this group of neoplasms (Turbiner et al. 2007; Montironi et al. 2008).

MCN, also called cystic nephroma or multilocular cyst, is characterized by a multiseptated fluid-filled mass surrounded by a thick fibrous capsule. The fluid content of loculi consists of pale yellow serous fluid or, less commonly, myxomatous fluid. The cystic component is lined with a flattened unistratified cuboidal or hobnail-cell epithelium and septated by fibrous septa with ovarian type stroma. On gross inspection, solid or nodular elements are not found. MCN occurs most commonly in women over the age of 30 years.

MEST is characterized by an epithelial-lined tubular or cystic component combined with an abundant stroma of variable cellularity and growth patterns. The stromal proliferation is responsible for the presence of a solid component in a high proportion of cases. MEST also occur with a strong female predominance typically in perimenopausal women (Lane et al. 2008; Montironi et al. 2008).

Both entities are usually large and have the propensity to extend within the renal sinus and herniate into the renal pelvis unlike any other renal tumor (Alanen et al. 1987; Park et al. 2005). Such pattern has been reported to be highly suggestive of REST.

### 26.2.2.3 Malignant Cystic Neoplasms (Fig. 26.1)

Approximately 4–15% of RCCs show a cystic pattern. Cystic RCCs include one specific entity introduced in the 2004 WHO classification – the multilocular cystic renal cell carcinoma – and other variants of RCCs that can exhibit cystic changes due to various mechanisms (Hartman et al. 1986, 1987; Hartman 1990; Freire and Remer 2009; Lopez-Beltran et al. 2006). A recently introduced new entity – the tubulocystic carcinoma – is a rare malignant cystic neoplasm not yet included in the WHO classification of renal tumors.

#### Multilocular Cystic RCC of Low Malignant Potential

This uncommon (1–4% of RCCs) low-grade variant of clear cell carcinoma has an excellent prognosis. It is usually incidentally discovered in adults (mean age 51 years). Macroscopically it does not differ from MCN. The cysts are lined by a single layer of epithelial cells with clear to pale cytoplasm. A few small papillae can also be found but without any expansive solid nodules.

#### Clear Cell or Papillary RCCs with Cystic Changes

RCC of the clear cell type is the most common RCC accounting for about 75% of all RCCs. It is the most common subtype of RCC that can exhibit a cystic pattern either with a multilocular or unilocular presentation. Papillary RCC is a less aggressive variant characterized by a tubulo-papillary growth pattern with two cellular subtypes (types I and II) as described in the current WHO classification. The reported incidence of papillary RCC is 10%. Multicentric and bilateral papillary RCCs are not uncommon. Internal changes such as hemorrhage, necrosis, and cystic degeneration are frequently observed in large tumors.

RCCs (clear cell) with multilocular cystic pattern: The cystic component results from an intrinsic multilocular growth of the tumor. Macroscopically, the tumor is composed of thick-walled septate cysts that are filled with serous or hemorrhagic fluid. Grossly recognizable solid component such as irregular thick portions of septa or wall and soft tissue nodules can be found. Histopathologic analysis shows carcinomatous proliferation of malignant epithelial cells arranged in variable patterns.

RCCs (clear cell or papillary) with unilocular cystic pattern: Three mechanisms by which RCC exhibits a unilocular cystic pattern have been described (Silverman and Kilhenny 1969; Weitzner 1971; Varma et al. 1974; Sufrin et al. 1975; Levy et al 1999) : an intrinsic unilocular cystic growth of the tumor; a massive tumor necrosis; and carcinomas arising from the epithelium of a preexisting renal cyst.

#### Tubulocystic Carcinoma

Tubulocystic carcinoma has also been described under the term low-grade collecting duct carcinoma. This rare subtype of RCC is a new tumor entity not recognized in the WHO 2004 classification. It occurs in adults (mean age, 54 years) with a strong male predominance (7:1).

Grossly, the tumor exhibits a spongy or "bubble wrap" appearance reflecting the microscopic presence of variably sized cysts and dilated tubules separated by delicate septa (Sibony and Vieillefond 2008; Amin et al. 2009).

## 26.3 Imaging Techniques and Key Interpretation Criteria

### 26.3.1 Conventional Ultrasound

Because of the widespread use of US in routine examination of the abdomen (that include kidneys evaluation), the detection rate of renal masses in asymptomatic patients has dramatically increased. Fortunately, US provides definitive diagnostic information in most of the simple renal cysts that are incidentally screened.

Recent technical improvements of gray-scale imaging have increased US performance in the detection and characterization of cystic renal masses.

Nonlinear US technique (tissue harmonic imaging (THI), Differential THI, Pulse Inversion Imaging) is now a widely implemented modality that provides a better contrast resolution and less artifacts on gray-scale image enabling to eliminate "dirty echoes." Accuracy for classifying cystic masses has been reported to increase from 64 to 84% by using pulse inversion imaging (Schmidt et al. 2003). In addition to its better capabilities in characterizing cystic renal masses, this modality may help depict and characterize very small cysts.

Typically, the simple cyst exhibits anechoic content, enhanced through transmission of the US beam resulting in posterior acoustic enhancement, smooth and sharply defined margins without perceptible wall (Fig. 26.2).

Cystic renal masses that do not fulfill the criteria for a simple cyst remain indeterminate at US and require further contrast-enhanced imaging workup. However, there is some US criteria that can strongly suggest a cystic or pseudocystic renal neoplasm including (Hélénon et al. 2001) (Figs. 26.3 and 26.4a) a thick irregular peripheral wall or multiple thick septae; the presence of echoic mural nodules; and the demonstration of vascular flow signal within the solid component of the lesion at color Doppler US.

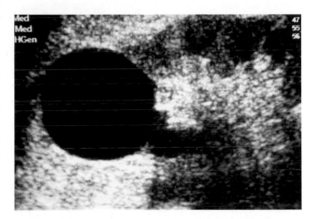

**Fig. 26.2** Ultrasonography (US) of a simple cyst. US shows an anechoic renal mass with posterior acoustic enhancement and homogeneous pattern without perceptible wall

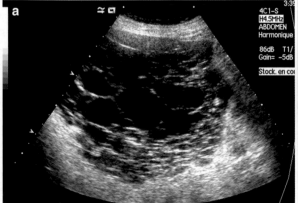
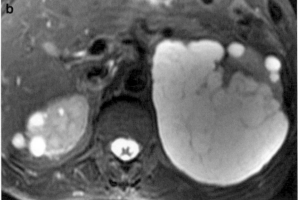

**Fig. 26.3** (**a, b**) US of a multilocular cystic renal mass. (**a**) US shows a septated multilocular cystic mass. (**b**) MRI (T2-weighted axial image) demonstrates the presence of multiple smooth septa with moderate enhancement (refer to Fig. 26.17e)

**Fig. 26.4** (**a–c**) Contrast-enhanced US of a cystic RCC. (**a**, **b**) Unenhanced color Doppler US (**a**) and postcontrast US (**b**) show a cystic renal mass with enhancing mural nodule (*arrow*) consistent with a cystic RCC. (**c**) Computed tomography (CT) confirmation of a complex cystic mass of Bosniak category IV. Note the slight enhancement of the solid component (*arrow*) after iodine contrast administration. The enhancing nodule is seen much better on contrast-enhanced US because of its higher sensitivity to microbubble signal enhancement

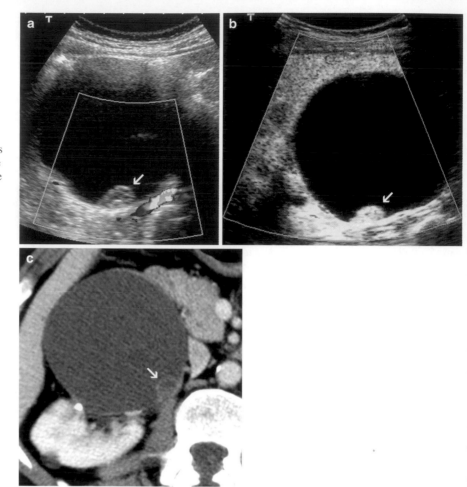

US may also provide additional diagnostic information over CT in selected cases among complex cystic renal masses that remain equivocal at CT (Hélénon et al. 2001). On the other hand, because of the higher sensitivity of US in detecting cyst septations, some cystic masses can appear more complex at US than at CT. Such discrepancy, however, should not be considered in the differentiation between surgical and nonsurgical complex cystic masses, although it can lead to the upgradation of a nonsurgical minimally complex cyst into a category that should be followed-up with CT or at best first reevaluated with MRI (refer to Sect. 26.5.4).

### 26.3.2 Contrast-Enhanced Ultrasound

Intravenous ultrasonography contrast agents (USCA) are useful in characterizing complex cystic masses since they improve the sonographic depiction of solid tissue vascularity. Real time contrast-enhanced US at low MI using second generation USCAs provides better resolution and longer persistence compared to first introduced dedicated US sequences and contrast agents (Correas et al. 2006). Contrast enhancement of the wall or septa, usually assessed by CT or MRI, is the key criteria in determining whether the lesion needs to be removed surgically or followed. The high sensitivity of contrast-enhanced US in detecting microbubble signal from the vascularized wall, septa, or solid nodules (Fig. 26.4) improve lesion classification and may change therapeutic options (Correas et al. 2006; Ascenti et al. 2007; Quaia et al. 2008). USCAs can therefore play a critical role in the characterization of complex cystic masses. However, contrast-enhanced US may be too sensitive as it can detect only a few microbubbles traveling in thin septations with a superior time and spatial resolution compared to any other imaging modalities. Such a finding may lead to over-classify certain cases of benign cysts.

The recently reported performance of the technique in evaluating complex cystic masses suggests that contrast-enhanced US is appropriate in the Bosniak classification system. In a recent study, Quaia et al. (2008) reported a better overall accuracy of CEUS compared to CT in the diagnosis of malignancy in complex cystic renal masses. CEUS can be currently proposed as an alternative to CT in the follow-up of complex renal cysts and in patients with serious contraindication to contrast-enhanced CT or MRI (Quaia et al. 2008). Moreover, it can be helpful in the follow-up of indeterminate cystic masses in order to reduce the radiation dose (Ascenti et al. 2007).

Some limitations of the technique including back-shadowing from wall calcification, bowel gas interposition, and US beam attenuation in cases of deep lesion location, can obscure contrast enhancement after microbubble injection. On the other hand, another pitfall can result from strong enhancement of the surrounding vessels or normal parenchyma that should not be confused with thick wall enhancement.

### 26.3.3 Computed Tomography

CT remains the gold standard in detecting and characterizing cystic renal masses (Warren and McFarlane 2004; Hartman et al. 2004; Israel and Bosniak 2005; Hélénon et al. 2008). The Bosniak classification

system is based on specific CT criteria that rely on the cystic lesion enhancement properties and morphologic features. This classification scheme will be discussed in more detail later.

Proper CT technique is needed for accurate categorization of cystic masses. Appropriate dedicated renal CT technique using multidetector row CT includes both unenhanced and contrast-enhanced scans with adequate bolus injection (at least 100 mL of a 300–350 mg iodinated contrast medium) delivered at a rate of 2–4 mL/s; multiple phasic acquisition including at least unenhanced, postcontrast arterial phase (approximately 30 s after the start of injection) and nephrographic phase (80–100 s) with additional delayed excretory phase in selected cases (for example, when contrast enhancement remains doubtful or in case of a suspected calyceal diverticulum); and thin section thickness (≤5 mm thick or at best 1–3 mm with 0.5–1.5 overlap).

Regarding interpretation technique and limitations, one should keep in mind that attenuation variation can result from volume averaging, motion, and beam-hardening artifacts. The latter can be responsible for pseudoenhancement that can reach up to +28 HU as assessed in a phantom model (Maki et al. 1999; Bae et al. 2000; Coulam et al. 2000; Heneghan et al. 2002; Gokan et al. 2002; Birnbaum et al. 2002; Abdulla et al. 2002) and +15 HU in vivo (Fig. 26.5). Imperfect placement of the ROI and evaluation of CT numbers on inadequate image acquisition, especially the early corticomedullary phase, can provide misleading information. Quantitative evaluation of attenuation variations

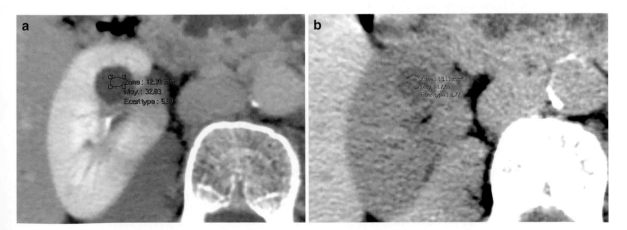

**Fig. 26.5** (**a**, **b**) Pseudoenhancement of a simple renal cyst at CT. (**a**) Contrast-enhanced CT (nephrographic phase) shows an increase in attenuation numbers of 15 HU compared to unenhanced evaluation (**b**)

between unenhanced and postcontrast images can also provide misleading information on masses that exhibit subtle enhancement of a limited internal portion not included within the ROI.

Some recommendations and general principles can therefore be made to avoid such pitfalls: attenuation values in very small lesions (i.e., <5–10 mm) should be considered unreliable to provide accurate characterization; accurate evaluation of enhancement need constant setting of exposure (kilovoltage and milliamperage), field of view, position in gantry and section thickness; measurements of ROI should be obtained in comparable portions of the lesion to assess enhancement; visual appreciation of attenuation variations using narrow window settings is also needed to identify enhancement within limited portions of the mass; the postcontrast images on which enhancement should be appreciated are those obtained at a nephrographic phase although all other contrast-enhanced images (depending on scanning protocol) need to be at least visually analyzed.

Analysis of CT features that lead to recognize and categorize cystic masses relies on internal attenuation values, enhancement properties, and morphologic features. Basic interpretation criteria are defined as follows:

- "Water" attenuation values are defined between −10 and +20 HU.
- A lack of enhancement usually indicating the absence of vascularity (except for some rare poorly vascularized solid tumors) if defined by attenuation variation less than +10 HU after the administration of contrast material.
- A significant enhancement indicating vascularity and therefore the solid nature of a mass is defined by a change in attenuation of more than +10HU after injection.
- Postcontrast attenuation variation assessed between +10 and +15 HU should be viewed as indeterminate and therefore prevent separate true cystic lesions and some solid neoplasms with poor vascularity.
- Enhancement characteristics of a known cystic mass is a major factor of evaluation and categorization. Wall and septa are generally appreciated only on postcontrast images because of their enhancement even in lesions categorized in minimally complicated benign cysts. The level of enhancement of soft tissue elements (wall, septa, or nodules) can be subjectively assessed as follows: minimal enhancement

that can be perceived (not measurable); significant measurable enhancement usually of grossly thickened wall or septa, or solid elements.

- "Thick wall" is a descriptive term that encompasses different degrees of thickening. The wall of a simple cyst is macroscopically smooth and thin (<1 mm) and should remain imperceptible at imaging (US, CT, or MRI). The different degrees of thickening, which are consistent with complex cystic masses, include (Fig. 26.6) minimal smooth wall thickening also described as "perceptible" (not measurable) or "hairline thin" (≤1 mm) wall; grossly thickened and uniform wall, slightly irregular thick wall, and marked irregular thick wall with solid elements (nodularity).
- Septations also can exhibit different degrees of thickening as mentioned above. The number of septa (few or multiple septa) is another important finding in complex renal cyst evaluation. MR imaging and US are more sensitive than CT in demonstrating septa within a lesion and therefore can cause a lesion to be upgraded (refer to Sect. 26.5.4).
- Calcification are morphologically described as thin and smooth or thick and irregular (Fig. 26.7). They can involve the cyst wall or septa.

### 26.3.4 MR Imaging

MRI plays an increasing role in evaluating cystic renal masses. It is now considered at least equivalent to CT in the characterization of cystic lesions (Israel and Bosniak 2004, 2005; Israel et al. 2004; O'Malley et al. 2009). It is commonly used as a substitute in patients with serious contraindication to CT (due to radiation exposure or iodinated contrast agent) and as a "problem-solving" modality especially in masses that remain indeterminate at CT. The increasing use of MRI in abdominal imaging has led to the frequent discovery of incidental cystic renal masses. Therefore, the radiologist should be able to provide accurate and definitive diagnosis in most cases of cystic renal lesions on the basis of MR findings and without the need for further imaging studies.

A high-quality examination is needed to accurately characterize a complex cystic renal mass. The MR examination of a complex cystic renal mass can be performed using a standard protocol dedicated to

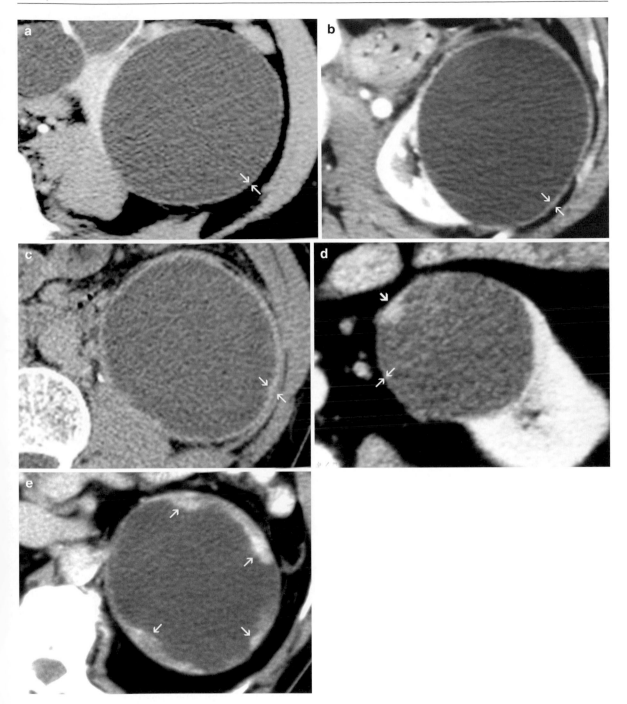

**Fig. 26.6** (a–d) Patterns of wall thickening in complex cystic masses. (a) Minimal "hairline thin" (≤1 mm) wall thickening (*arrows*). (b) Grossly thickened uniform and smooth wall (*arrows*). (c) Grossly thickened wall with slight irregularity (*arrows*). (d) Mural nodule (*arrowhead*) (here, arising from a minimally thickened wall) (*arrows*). (e) Marked irregular thick wall with solid elements (*arrows*)

renal "parenchymal" imaging which consists of fast or turbo spin echo T2-weighted imaging; T1-weighted spoiled gradient echo (GRE) sequence obtained in and out of phase; 3D fat-suppressed T1-weighted GRE before and after gadolinium complex administration (dynamic contrast-enhanced sequence) with

**Fig. 26.7** (**a, b**) Patterns of cystic calcifications. (**a**) Thin and smooth calcification of a cyst septum (*arrow*). (**b**) Thick irregular calcification of a "cyst" wall (cystic RCC)

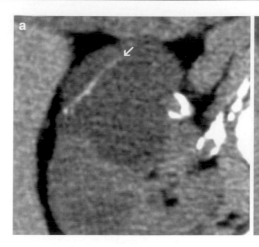

a scan delay of about 5 min including serial pre- and postcontrast corticomedullary, nephrographic, and excretory phases. Sequences should be performed using a torso phased-array coil. Whereas T1-weighted GRE sequences are necessarily obtained during breath-holding, the T2-weighted acquisition can also be performed with respiratory compensation that minimize motion artifact while providing better spatial resolution than with breath-held T2-weighted acquisition.

Advantages of MR imaging over CT in terms of imaging performance are its higher contrast resolution and higher sensitivity to detect even subtle contrast enhancement; the capability to better characterize the internal components of complex cystic masses including blood breakdown products and necrotic debris.

Contrast enhancement at MRI is usually appreciated subjectively by comparing side-by-side pre- and postcontrast images, since unquestionable enhancement is frequently apparent. In cases of subtle contrast enhancement, quantitative assessment is needed based on the relative percentage increase of signal intensity after contrast injection. A threshold of 15% is commonly used to define a significant contrast enhancement as reported in the study of Ho et al. (2002). Image subtraction which is now a widely implemented postprocessing technique can also be useful in assessing subtle postcontrast enhancement and enhancement characteristics of complex cystic lesions that show hyperintense signal intensity on precontrast images.

As recently reported by Gulani et al. (2008), artifactual thickening of the cyst wall can be observed on low resolution fat-saturated spoiled gradient echo (FS-SPGR) sequences. This apparent increase in the lesion wall thickness is seen in the phase-encoding direction. Image interpretation should therefore take into account the direction of the wall thickening. In case of suspected artifactual thick wall, higher resolution images (at best 512 × 512) can be acquired to rule out true thickening.

Specific indications of MRI in the diagnosis of complex cystic renal masses will be discussed later (refer to Sect. 26.5).

## 26.4 The Bosniak Classification System

In 1986, Morton Bosniak proposed a classification system of cystic renal masses designed to separate lesions requiring surgery from those that can be left alone or followed (Bosniak 1986). In this classification, cystic lesions were divided into four categories (nonsurgical categories I and II; surgical categories III and IV) by the analysis of specific CT criteria including morphological and enhancement characteristics.

During the following decade, M Bosniak first pointed out difficulties in classifying some cystic lesions using the original classification system (Bosniak 1991a) and finally introduced the category IIF (F for follow-up) in 1997 (Bosniak 1997a, b). This category consists of minimally complicated cysts that do not neatly fall into category II, but are not complex enough to fulfill the criteria of category III. In 2003, this follow-up approach of category IIF has been shown by Israel and Bosniak (2003a, b) to be appropriate and safe. It can prevent unnecessary surgery in more than 95% of complex cysts that belong to this category (Israel and Bosniak 2003a). It enables the identification of cystic neoplasms on the basis of the progression of imaging findings that lead to the upgradation of initial presentation into surgical category III or IV. In another retrospective study, Israel and Bosniak extended the category IIF to cysts with thick irregular or nodular calcifications provided no associated soft tissue or thickened wall or septa enhancement are present (Israel and Bosniak 2003b).

One year later, Israel et al. originated a new important step in the evaluation of cystic renal masses by introducing the role of MRI in the Bosniak classification system (Israel et al. 2004). It has been shown that the classification scheme can be applied to MRI and can benefit from MR informations especially in the characterization of category IIF complex cysts. Regarding the reliability of the Bosniak classification system, several studies have been reported between 1997 and the early 2000s (refer to Sect. 26.4.3). Among these, one major study by Curry et al. (2000) concluded that the Bosniak classification is reliable and requires adequate CT technique.

field of application of the Bosniak classification system. The latter has been designed to characterize renal cystic lesions including renal cysts and cystic neoplasms of nephron epithelial origin with the exception of cystic masses originating from the urinary tract (calyceal diverticulum or hydrocalix) or resulting from a chronic infectious process (chronic abscess or hydatid cyst) (Fig. 26.8). Such nonepithelial benign cystic lesions commonly exhibit a thickened wall, which reflects the urothelial wall or a fibrous pseudocapsule respectively, without suspicion of malignancy.

Moreover, the discovery of a complex cystic lesion that exhibits a uniformly thickened wall with contrast enhancement in the clinical context of an acute event such as hemorrhage, acute infection, renal trauma, or recent renal surgery should lead to specific imaging workup (Fig. 26.9). In this particular case, follow-up CT until clinical recovery is usually indicated to separate inflammatory cystic lesions from complex cysts with suspicion of neoplasm that require further management using the Bosniak classification. Percutaneous aspiration and drainage can also be mandatory in cases consistent with acute abscesses, infected cysts, or diverticula.

### 26.4.1  Field of Utilization

Utilization of the Bosniak classification system requires, first, previous identification of the cystic nature of a renal mass as defined earlier (refer to Sect. 26.2.1) with the exception of very small lesions (<5–10 mm), and second, to examine if the cystic lesion belongs to the

### 26.4.2  Bosniak Categories
(Fig. 26.10; Table 26.1)

The following paragraphs will describe the CT criteria that define each Bosniak category according to the

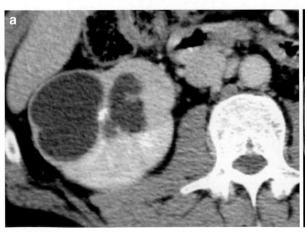
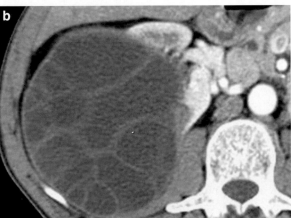

**Fig. 26.8** (**a**, **b**) Nonepithelial benign cystic renal masses that should not be categorized in the Bosniak classification system. (**a**) Cystic lesion due to renal tuberculosis (dilated calyces and caseous necrosis). (**b**) Hydatid cyst presenting as a multiseptated cystic renal mass at CT. Contrast-enhanced CT (not shown) showed absence of wall or septa enhancement

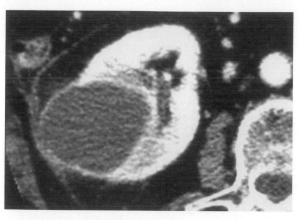

**Fig. 26.9** Acute complicated benign cyst that need specific imaging workup distinct from Bosniak classification scheme. Infected cyst with grossly uniform thick wall in a patient with acute pyelonephritis

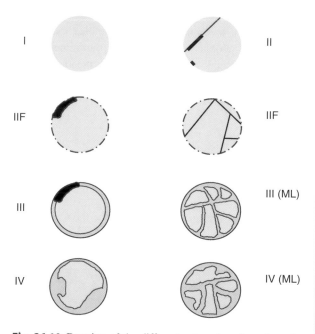

**Fig. 26.10** Drawing of the different categories of renal cystic masses according to Bosniak classification. *ML* multilocular

original classification system. With the exception of their water characteristics (low signal intensity on T1 and bright hypersignal on T2-weighted images with lack of postcontrast enhancement) (Fig. 26.11) and the appearance of calcifications (not depicted at MRI), the following morphologic features can be also applied to categorize cystic lesions at MRI (Levy et al. 1994;

**Table 26.1** Bosniak classification system of renal cystic masses

| Category | CT findings | Diagnosis |
|---|---|---|
| Cat I | Water attenuation (>−10, <20 HU) | Simple cyst |
| | Homogenous | |
| | Smooth margins without perceptible wall | |
| | Lack of enhancement (variation <+10HU) | |
| Cat II | Few thin septa (≤2 septa) no perceptible wall | Complicated cyst |
| | Fine calcification (wall or septum) | |
| | Lack of enhancement (variation <+10 HU) or minimal (perceptible) enhancement of septa | |
| Cat IIF | Thin septa (>2 septa) | Complicated cyst |
| | Minimal wall thickening (≤1 mm) (not measurable) | Multilocular cyst |
| | Thick or irregular calcification | Cystic tumor (cystic carcinoma or cystic nephroma) |
| | Hyperdense cyst[a] except for size (≥4 cm) or intraparenchymal location | |
| | Lack of enhancement (variation <+10 HU) or minimal enhancement (septa, wall) | |
| Cat III | Numerous thick septa | Complicated cyst |
| | Uniform grossly thick wall | Multilocular cyst |
| | Slightly irregular thick wall | Cystic tumor (cystic carcinoma, cystic nephroma) |
| | Thick or irregular calcification | |
| | Enhancement (septa and/or wall) | |
| Cat IV | Grossly thick and irregular wall | Cystic carcinoma |
| | Mural nodules or solid tissue component | Pseudocystic necrotic RCC |
| | Enhancement of the soft tissue elements | |

[a]Small (<3 cm) subcapsular cyst, with high attenuation values (50–90 HU), homogenous, with smooth margins, without any change after contrast administration

**Fig. 26.11** (**a**, **b**) Simple cyst. Typical appearance at MRI. (**a**, **b**) T2-weighted (**a**) and postcontrast T1-weighted gradient echo (FSPGR with fatsat) axial image (**b**). The lesion typically fulfill the morphologic criteria of a simple cyst in the Bosniak classification along with water characteristics and the lack of postcontrast signal enhancement

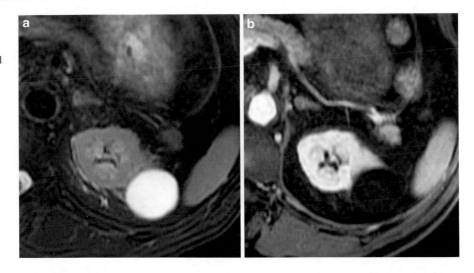

Israel and Bosniak 2004). The hyperdense category II cyst also reveals specific signal findings at MRI compared to CT (refer to Sect. 26.5.2).

### 26.4.2.1 Category I Lesions (Fig. 26.12)

Category I lesions are simple benign cysts that require no further imaging or intervention. They satisfy the following imaging criteria on both unenhanced and postcontrast images: homogeneous water density content (>−10 HU, <+20 HU); no enhancement (postcontrast attenuation variation <10 HU) and postcontrast

homogeneous pattern with sharp margins; unperceptible wall and no internal septa or solid components; absence of calcifications.

### 26.4.2.2 Category II Lesions (Figs. 26.13–26.15)

Category II lesions are minimally complicated benign cysts that are nonsurgical and do not require further imaging.

This group consists of three subtypes of complex cysts that fulfill the category I criteria except for some minimal changes:

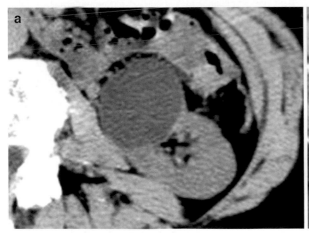
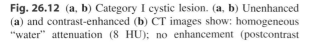
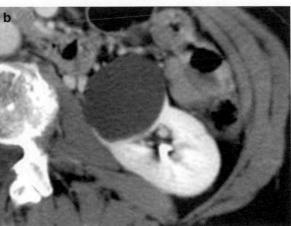

**Fig. 26.12** (**a**, **b**) Category I cystic lesion. (**a**, **b**) Unenhanced (**a**) and contrast-enhanced (**b**) CT images show: homogeneous "water" attenuation (8 HU); no enhancement (postcontrast attenuation 12 HU); homogeneous pattern with sharp margins; unperceptible wall and no internal septa or solid components; absence of calcifications

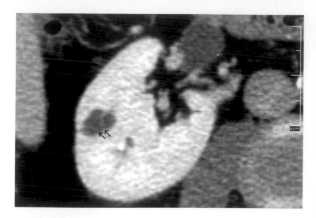

**Fig. 26.13** Category II septated cyst. Contrast-enhanced CT image. Small (20 mm) renal cyst containing two thin and smooth septa (*arrows*) with minimal "perceived" enhancement

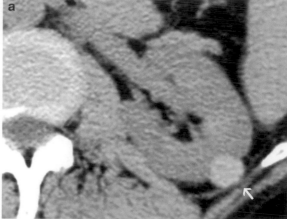

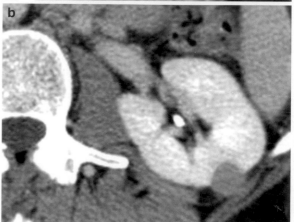

**Fig. 26.15** (**a**, **b**) Category II hyperdense renal cyst. (**a**) Unenhanced CT image shows a small subcapsular mass with homogeneous markedly hyperdense (>50 HU) content (*arrow*). (**b**) Contrast-enhanced CT image (nephrographic phase) shows unchanged pattern with total lack of contrast enhancement (variation in attenuation <+10 HU)

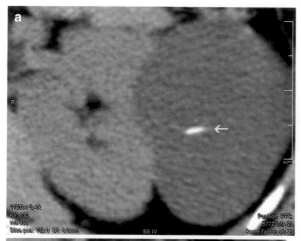

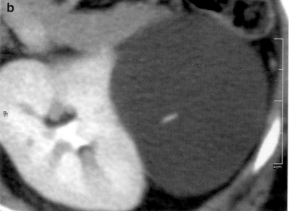

**Fig. 26.14** (**a**, **b**) Category II calcified and septated cyst. (**a**, **b**) Unenhanced (**a**) and contrast-enhanced (**b**) CT images. Large renal cyst with internal thin and smooth calcification (*arrow*) within a septation which is not seen and does not enhance

- *Minimally septated cysts* (Fig. 26.13) with one or few thin (<2 mm thick) and smooth septa in which perceived enhancement can be present (septa are usually visible only on postcontrast images), but without perceptible wall or any other solid elements.
- *Minimally calcified cysts* (Fig. 26.14) with one or few thin delicate calcifications within the wall or septa. Whereas the cyst wall should not be perceptible except for its calcification, septa can be visible in a minimally calcified-septated cyst.
- *Hyperdense cysts* (Fig. 26.15) that exhibit high attenuation values of at least 50 HU (50–90 HU) belong to category II provided the cyst diameter does not exceed 3 cm and that it is subcapsular

(with at least one quarter of the mass extending beyond the renal outline), so that the cyst margins can be accurately evaluated on postcontrast images to rule out wall thickening and poorly defined margins. The typical hyperdense cyst therefore fulfill all the characteristics of a simple cyst except for the high attenuation. The differential diagnosis include hyperdense solid neoplasms and cystic neoplasms with internal hemorrhagic debris that can mimic a hyperdense cyst (Coleman et al. 1984; Dunnick et al. 1984a; Hartman et al. 1992). A hyperdense lesion should be considered surgical or at least indeterminate (with the need for further imaging) if it shows at least one of the following features (Fig. 26.16): postcontrast enhancement, inhomogeneous texture on unenhanced or contrast-enhanced images, presence of calcification, poorly

defined and irregular contour or interface, and a solid appearance at other available imaging examinations (US, MRI).

### 26.4.2.3 Category IIF Lesions (Fig. 26.17)

This more recently introduced subtype is likely to be benign, but require follow-up CT examinations to show their stability over time and prove benignity.

Such lesions are not complicated enough to fall into category III, but too complicated for category II. They may contain multiple hairline-thin septa, but without wall thickening or have minimal smooth wall thickening resulting in a "perceptible" (not measurable) wall with "perceived" enhancement; they may also exhibit thick irregular calcification, but without associated

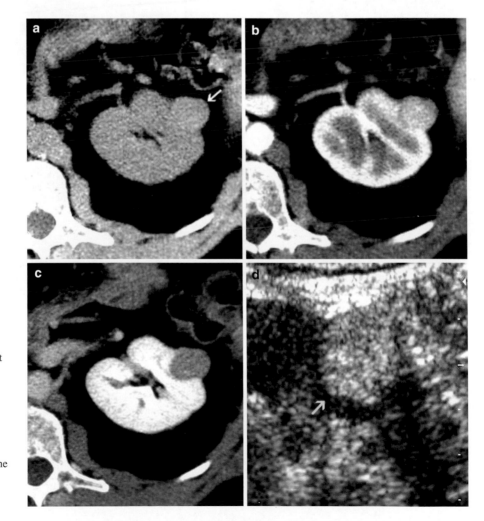

**Fig. 26.16** (**a–d**) Small hyperdense RCC. (**a**) Unenhanced CT shows a small hyperdense (50 HU) subcapsular mass of the left kidney (*arrow*). After contrast administration (**b, c**), the lesion exhibits unequivocal contrast enhancement (+62 HU) on early arterial phase image (**b**) with slightly heterogenous pattern. (**d**) At US, the tumor demonstrates a solid hyperechoic appearance (*arrow*)

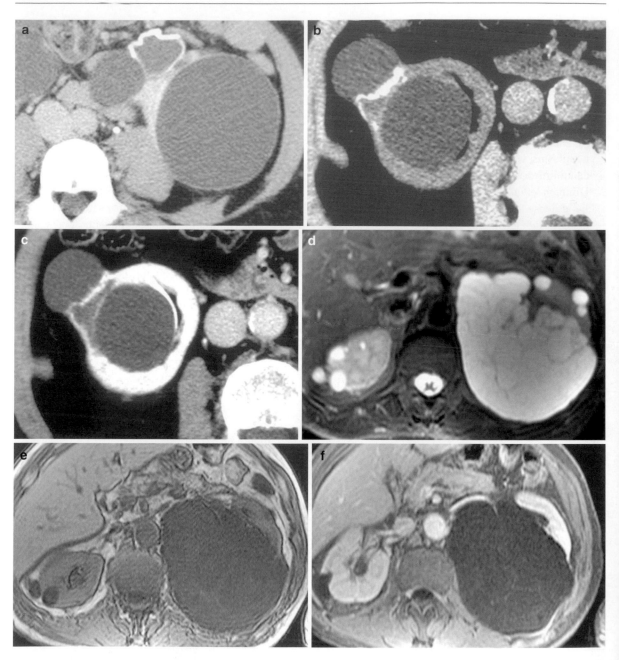

**Fig. 26.17** (a–f) Category IIF cysts. (a) Large uniloculated cyst with minimally thickened (not measurable) wall that otherwise fulfill the characteristics of a simple cyst. Note the presence of another complex calcified cyst and a simple cyst. (b, c) Grossly calcified cyst with total lack of enhancement after contrast administration. A simple cyst that develops within the renal sinus is also seen. (d, e) MRI of a multiloculated category IIF renal cyst in a patient with renal failure. T2-weighted (d), and contrast-enhanced (e), dynamic fat-saturated breath-held FSPGR sequence images. (f) Multiple hairline-thin septa with "perceived" enhancement are seen. The wall remains thin and nonperceptible

enhancing soft tissue component, thickened wall, or septa. Intrarenal (that do not extend outside the renal outline) and large (>3 cm) hyperdense cystic masses which otherwise fulfill the characteristics of a category II hyperdense cyst are also included in this category and require further follow-up.

### 26.4.2.4 Category III Lesions
(Figs. 26.18 and 26.19)

This category consists of "indeterminate" cystic renal masses that require surgery (nephron sparing surgery) because of a high risk of malignancy (between 30 and 60%). It can be divided into two subtypes depending on the presence of septa: multiloculated and uniloculated category III cystic masses. Multilocular cystic masses are consistent with multilocular cystic neoplasm including malignant and benign tumors (Madewell et al. 1983; Hartman et al. 1987; Levy et al. 1999) . Unilocular cystic lesions include benign complicated cysts and unilocular cystic renal carcinomas.

- Multiloculated category III (Fig. 26.18) is an encapsulated cystic mass that contains numerous thickened smooth or slightly irregular septa, uniform smooth or slightly irregular wall thickening. The cyst wall and septa which are grossly thickened (≥2 mm) demonstrate unequivocal enhancement after contrast administration, but no enhancing soft tissue components are present. Thick or irregular calcification can be present.
- Uniloculated category III (Fig. 26.19) demonstrates uniform, smooth, or slightly irregular wall thickening

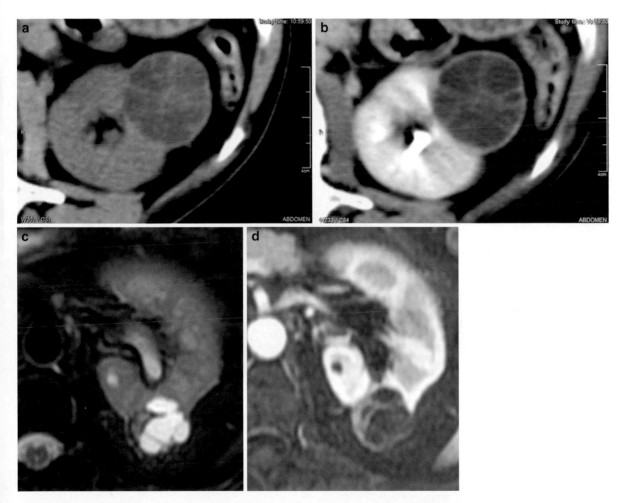

**Fig. 26.18** (**a–d**) Category III multilocular cystic lesions. (**a**, **b**) Unenhanced (**a**) and contrast-enhanced (**b**) CT images. Multiloculated cystic mass with multiple smooth septa and uniformly thickened wall. Postcontrast image shows moderate enhancement of the lesion wall and septa (cystic nephroma at pathologic examination). (**c**, **d**) T2-weighted (**c**) and contrast-enhanced (**d**) MR images show a multiloculated category III cystic renal mass with slightly irregular thick wall and septae. A multiloculated cystic RCC was found on pathologic examination

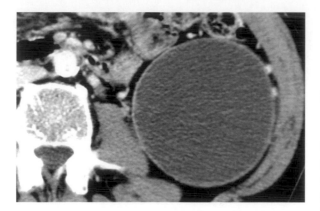

**Fig. 26.19** Category III unilocular cystic lesion. Contrast-enhanced CT shows a cystic renal mass with smooth grossly thickened enhancing wall. No solid tissue component is seen. Pseudocystic necrotic papillary RCC was found at surgery

with unequivocal enhancement after contrast administration. Thick or irregular calcification can be present.

### 26.4.2.5 Category IV Lesions
(Figs. 26.20 and 26.21)

Cystic masses that belong to this category are clearly malignant lesions which demonstrate nonuniform, enhancing, thick wall, or septa with nodularity and enhancing soft tissue elements. They can have findings similar to those seen in category III lesions including multiloculated and uniloculated masses, but also demonstrate solid components with unequivocal enhancement.

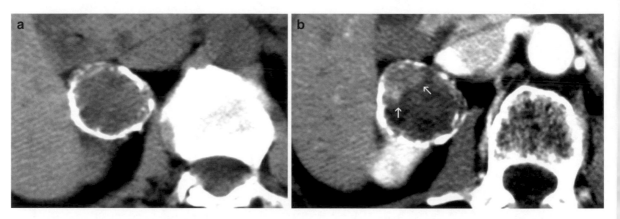

**Fig. 26.20** (**a, b**) Category IV cystic lesion. (**a, b**) Pre- (**a**) and postcontrast (**b**) CT images show a calcified cystic renal mass with enhancing solid tissue component (*arrows*). Cystic RCC was found at pathology

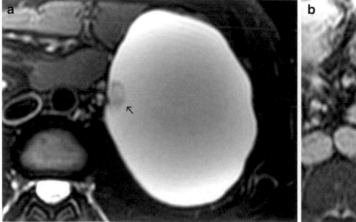

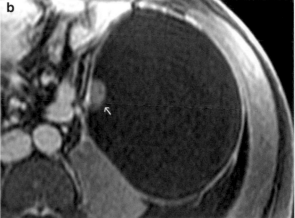

**Fig. 26.21** (**a, b**) Category IV cystic lesion. (**a, b**) MRI of a cystic RCC with minimal solid component. T2-weighted (**a**) and gadolinium-enhanced (**b**) images demonstrate a large cystic lesion that has a uniformly smooth, thickened, enhancing wall on which one small mural enhancing nodule is seen (*arrow*) consistent with a category IV lesion. Cystic RCC at pathology

### 26.4.3 Utility and Limitations of the Bosniak Classification System

Several studies have examined the validity of the Bosniak classification system (Aronson et al. 1991; Cloix et al. 1996; Wilson et al. 1996; Siegel et al. 1997; Koga et al. 2000; Curry et al. 2000; Israel and Bosniak 2003b) with somewhat discrepant results especially regarding the rate of malignancy in category II (assessed between 0 and 80% with a mean rate of 27%). Most of these however suffer from the limitations of retrospective studies and the small number of proven lesions (that do not exceed 40 cases in 5 of 7 studies). The role of the suboptimal CT technique and qualitative parameters of evaluation in such discrepancies has been emphasized.

The largest reported series reviewed 70 (Siegel et al. 1997) and 82 (Curry et al. 2000) surgically removed cystic masses that found to have good concordance with the Bosniak classification system. However, conflicting result still exists in the number of proven malignant lesions in category II and IV. Siegel et al. found 1 of 8 category II lesions to be malignant (12%) and 3 of 29 category IV to be benign (90%), whereas, Curry et al. reported a rate of malignancy of 0 and 100%, respectively as expected on the basis of the Bosniak classification scheme. It should be noticed that a significant number of lesions (about one half) has been inadequately scanned (e.g., without available unenhanced images or with 10 mm thick collimation) or interpreted (without available Hounsfield attenuation values) in the work of Siegel. Such limitations may increase the risk of misclassifying complex cystic lesions. Conversely, the study of Curry et al. has been designed with particular attention to CT technique since only patients with technically adequate scans were included to allow proper assignment of the lesion to a category. She concluded that the Bosniak classification system is useful and accurate in separating surgical from nonsurgical cystic lesions provided adequate CT technique is used. In category III lesions (indeterminate surgical), the risk of malignancy has been assessed at 59% in the study of Curry et al. and is approximatively 50% (range 25–100%) according to overall literature. With the exception of one reported series (Cloix) with suboptimal CT technique that may have caused misclassification of certain lesions, all reported category I

cysts were simple renal cysts. The risk for malignancy in the category IIF cystic lesion is approximately 5% as reported by Israel and Bosniak (2003a). The two cases that proved to be neoplasms were diagnosed at 1.5 and 3 years after initial imaging and were successfully removed. More recently, it has been shown that the introduction of the category IIF has increased the rate of malignancy in surgical lesions of the category III (from 50% to greater than 80%) (O'Malley et al. 2009).

One of the major limitation of the Bosniak classification system is that a large number of interpretation criteria are qualitative rather than quantitative. The employed terminology to describe the cyst wall or septa, calcifications or wall enhancement are somewhat confusing and often difficult to master and even teach. This lead to a high degree of interobserver disagreement especially in the differentiation of categories II and III (Siegel et al. 1997). It is also highly dependent on the reader's experience. In cases of indecision or discordance between radiologists in categorizing a cystic mass, the lesion should be placed in the higher category (Israel and Bosniak 2003b).

Although the Bosniak classification system provides a helpful guideline for the evaluation and management of a wide majority of renal cystic masses, atypical renal masses with equivocal CT features that cannot fall neatly into a Bosniak category are sometimes encountered in daily practice. These are called "indeterminate masses" until they prove to be cystic or solid, based on the result of specific imaging workup using US and MRI.

## 26.5 Indeterminate Renal Masses and Misclassified Cysts

Certain cases of cystic renal masses remain not categorizable at CT using the Bosniak classification scheme because of their small size or proper atypical attenuation characteristics or enhancement properties. The difficulties in characterizing such masses prevent their cystic nature to be clearly recognizable at CT and therefore to be categorized by using the Bosniak classification system. US and MRI play a major role in the evaluation of such renal masses by providing useful additional diagnostic information that help distinguish between atypical fluid fill masses and atypical solid neoplasms (Hélénon et al. 2008; Curry 1998). Among these, solid papillary renal cell carcinoma which usually shows poor vascularity, represents the differential diagnosis that is most often involved.

### 26.5.1 Very Small Renal Mass

As mentioned above, very small renal masses remain indeterminate at CT since attenuation measurements are unreliable to provide accurate characterization. In general population, very small lesions that are incidentally detected are usually not pursued because they are statistically likely to be cysts (Bosniak 1991b, 1997a, b; Curry 1995). On the other hand, in patients with genetic predisposition to renal neoplasm at risk of RCC (von Hippel Lindau disease, hereditary papillary carcinomas, Birt Hort Dubbe syndrome, etc.) or in those with an history of removed RCC or with synchronous RCC, very small lesions should be viewed as indeterminate and further imaged or followed-up. MRI can be useful in characterizing such extremely small cysts because of its higher contrast resolution compared to CT. Definitive diagnosis can be easily obtained on the basis of their T2-weighted signal characteristics alone (uniformly and markedly hyperintense and sharply marginated round mass) (Fig. 26.22).

### 26.5.2 Renal Mass with Indeterminate Attenuation

As previously mentioned, renal masses that exhibit attenuation values between 20 and 50 HU on unenhanced images with no significant enhancement on postcontrast images do not neatly fall into the typical profile of simple (category I) or hyperdense (category II) cysts. In these instances, it is not possible to securely differentiate an atypical hyperdense (with intermediate attenuation values) cyst from a poorly vascularized solid tumor (mostly papillary RCC) with no significant enhancement (variation of attenuation <10 HU) (Couvidat et al. 2008) (Fig. 26.23). Further imaging including US or MRI is therefore indicated to establish the true nature of these lesions. At US, hyperdense cysts are typically anechoic in about 30–50% of cases (Zirinsky et al. 1984; Foster et al. 1988). Contrast-enhanced US using microbubbles has been shown to demonstrate tumor vascularity with a high sensitivity (Correas et al. 2006); therefore, it has the potential to increase US performance in demonstrating the cystic nature of atypical hyperdense cysts (Fig. 26.24). Although this technique can be utilized for definitive characterization provided appropriate equipment and experienced operator are available, it is not yet considered in a routine practice, and further evaluation in this application is needed. When US fails to ensure the fluid characteristics of the mass, MRI is commonly used as a second step diagnostic modality (Hélénon et al. 2001;

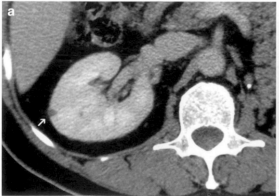
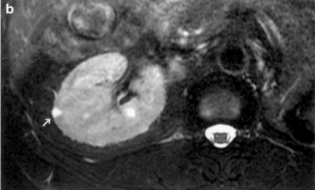

**Fig. 26.22** (**a**, **b**) Indeterminate very small renal mass. (**a**) Contrast-enhanced CT shows a very small mass (5 mm) (*arrow*) with indeterminate attenuation values and variation between unenhanced and postcontrast images. (**b**) T2-weighted MR image (fat-suppressed FSE) shows unequivocal water fluid characteristics consistent with a very small benign simple cyst (*arrow*)

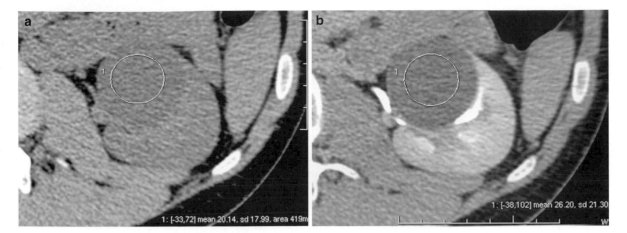

**Fig. 26.23** (**a**, **b**) Papillary RCC with no significant postcontrast enhancement. (**a**, **b**) Unenhanced (**a**) and delayed (excretory phase) postcontrast (**b**) CT images show a renal mass that exhibits borderline CT values (20 HU) on precontrast phase and absence of significant enhancement (maximum postcontrast density of 26 HU) after contrast material administration on arterial (not shown), nephrographic (not shown) and excretory (**b**) phases. With the exception of its density on unenhanced CT images, the tumor fulfill the criteria of a simple cyst (homogenous, sharply margined, lack of enhancement)

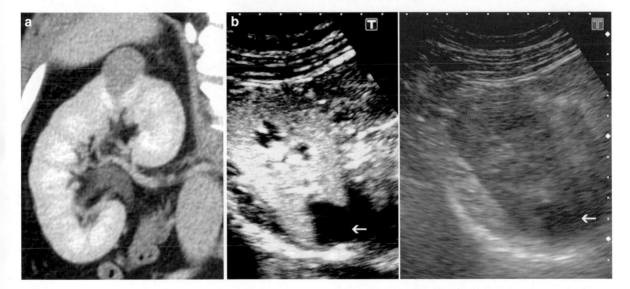

**Fig. 26.24** (**a**, **b**) Unenhanced renal mass with indeterminate attenuation. Contrast-enhanced CT (**a**) shows an upper polar renal mass that exhibits indeterminate attenuation (between 35 and 42 HU) on both unenhanced (not shown) and postcontrast images with no significant enhancement (variation of +7 HU). The lesion remains therefore indeterminate since it does not fulfill the criteria of a benign cystic lesion including simple cyst (category I) and typical hyperdense cyst (category II). Subsequent US examination failed to demonstrate either typical anechoic fluid or solid tissue content of the lesion which appeared hypoechoic (**b**, *right*) (*arrow*). Microbubble injection using dedicated US imaging modality (pulse inversion imaging at low mechanical index) (**b**, *left*) clearly demonstrated the total lack of contrast enhancement (*arrow*) which was consistent with a benign complex cyst (atypical hyperdense cyst)

Israel and Bosniak 2004). Typically, hyperdense cysts demonstrate a homogeneous bright signal or fluid-iron level pattern within the lesion on both T1 and T2-weighted images (Levy et al. 1994) (Fig. 26.25). Such pattern is encountered in about 50% of hyperdense cysts. The remaining half of these lesions can demonstrate a wide range of signal intensity often with heterogeneous pattern on T1 and T2-weighted images that prevent the differentiation of atypical hyperdense cyst from a solid neoplasm with intratumoral hemorrhage using morphologic and signal findings alone. Enhancement characteristics at best appreciated using

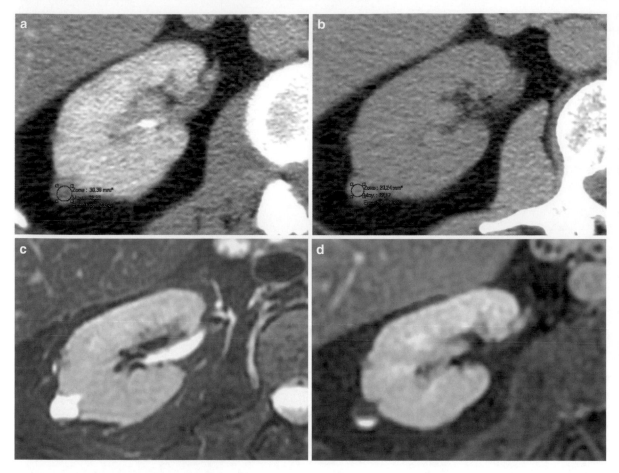

**Fig. 26.25** (**a–d**) Small indeterminate renal mass in a patient with a history of surgically removed papillary RCC of the left kidney. (**a, b**) CT shows a small right nonenhancing renal mass with indeterminate attenuation values (27 HU on unenhanced image). Hypoechoic pattern at US was nonconclusive (not shown). (**c, d**) MRI shows typical "hemorrhagic" cyst with fluid-iron level on both T2 and T1-weighted images

image subtraction (because of high signal intensity) are therefore critical in their proper characterization. Characterization of solid hypovascular neoplasms relies mainly on the ability of postcontrast MRI to clearly depict subtle tumor enhancement. It has been shown that masses with low signal intensity and homogenous pattern on T2-weighted images are highly suggestive of papillary renal cell carcinoma (Roy et al. 2007) (Fig. 26.26).

### 26.5.3  Renal Mass with Indeterminate "Enhancement"

With the advent of helical CT, it has been shown that pseudoenhancement can occur in simple cysts as a result of inadequate correction of the "beam hardening" effect (refer to Sect. 26.3.3). A change in attenuation values between 10 and 15 HU after contrast administration is therefore considered equivocal. Such a finding is consistent with pseudoenhancement phenomenon in a benign cyst or subtle nonsignificant (≤15 HU) enhancement of a hypovascular neoplasm (Herts et al. 2002; Couvidat et al. 2008). For these types of cases, appropriate imaging workup is similar to the one mentioned above. Even though such masses are indeterminate, it is sometimes possible to suggest whether the lesion is more likely cystic or solid. A small (less than 20 mm) intraparenchymatous water attenuating mass that exhibits borderline postcontrast increase in density at peak enhancement (i.e., nephrographic phase) is likely to be a benign cyst with pseudoenhancement. Conversely, findings suggestive of malignancy

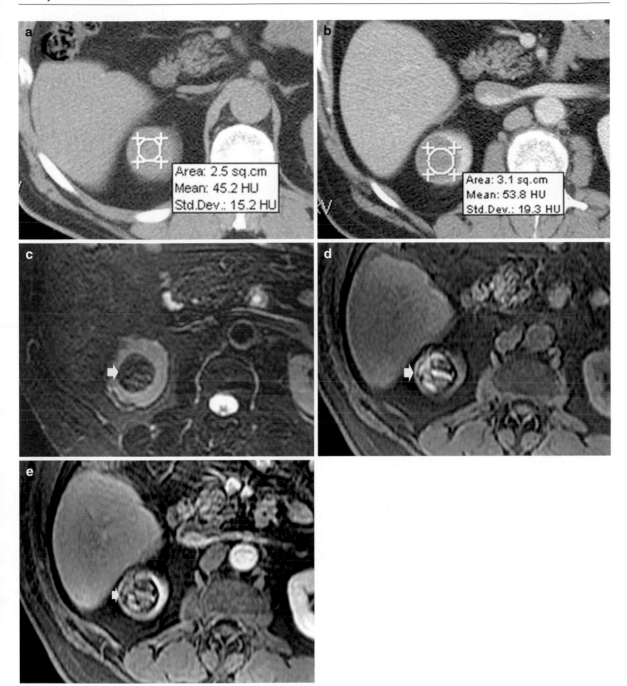

**Fig. 26.26** (**a–e**) Indeterminate nonenhancing renal mass. (**a**, **b**) CT shows a hyperdense renal mass with attenuation values of 45 HU and absence of enhancement (+9 HU) that does not fulfill the criteria for a typical hyperdense cyst. (**c–e**) MRI demonstrates hypointense pattern on T2-weighted image (**c**) and a

heterogenous appearance on T1-weighted images (**d**) with areas of bright signal intensity suggesting the presence of hemorrhagic debris. Subtle postcontrast enhancement was also demonstrated (**e**). Such signal characteristics are consistent with a RCC with intratumoral hemorrhagic changes

include inhomogeneous internal texture or slight variation of texture on postcontrast image; nonwater attenuation values (20–50 HU) on unenhanced

images; lack of sharp margins; atypical appearance (internal echoes, lack of posterior acoustic enhancement) at US examination; previous history of excised papillary cancer or multiple synchronous papillary tumors;and known hereditary papillary RCCs.

### 26.5.4 Renal Cyst with Discrepant Findings Between CT and Other Modalities

Some discrepancies between CT and US or MRI in renal cyst evaluation are sometimes encountered in routine practice. Such troublesome situations are in agreement with reported data, which suggest that intracystic details can be better seen on US and MRI making some cystic masses more complex than on CT. Septa within a complex cyst are often demonstrated with more sensitivity on US and MRI than on CT (Israel et al. 2004; Isracl and Bosniak 2004; Ascenti et al. 2007; Quaia et al. 2008). Such a finding would cause a complex cyst to be reclassified in a higher category than it would be with CT features alone. On the basis of the number of depicted septa, it is therefore possible to upgrade a renal cyst from category I or II to category II or IIF, respectively. Although upgrading a thin-walled cyst from category II to category IIF as a result of only the increased number of detected septa (with unperceptible wall) may affect patient management, the lesion is likely to be benign as initially suggested by CT. Another unusual

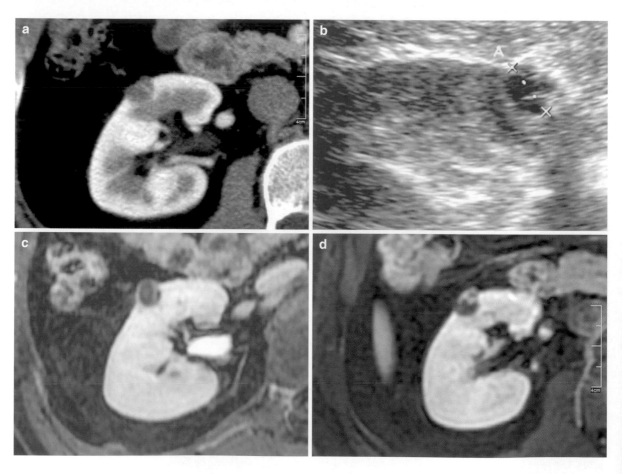

**Fig. 26.27** (a–d) Cystic renal mass with discrepant findings between CT, US, and MRI. Contrast-enhanced CT (a) shows a minimally septated cyst without enhancing thick wall. Findings were consistent with a Bosniak category II cyst lesion. At US (b), the lesion appeared more complex because of the presence of a thick wall (associated with few septa). Such discrepant findings cause the lesion to be upgraded to category IIF. Because of the lesion complexity MRI was performed. (c) Gadolinium-enhanced fat-suppressed T1-weighted MR image shows few smooth septa associated with a smooth minimally thickened enhancing wall. The lesion was therefore followed-up using MR imaging. One year later, MRI (d) (gadolinium-enhanced fat-suppressed T1-weighted) showed a more complex lesion with gross irregular thickening of the wall and septa typical of at least a category III lesion that need surgery

discrepant finding between imaging modalities has been reported in rare cases of microcystic multilocular cystic RCC (with cystic spaces smaller than 5 mm) that can exhibit a solid appearance at US and CT (Curry 1998), whereas it is expected to show a cystic pattern on T2-weighted MR images. We have recently reported two cases of tubulocystic renal carcinoma with a solid hyperechoic appearance at US that appeared as cystic lesions on both CT and MRI of category I and II respectively (Hélénon et al. 2005). Grossly, the tumors showed a spongy appearance related to a microcystic architecture.

MRI as well as contrast-enhanced US can also provide additional information on lesion vascularity and wall thickening compared to CT because of their highest sensitivity to contrast enhancement (Israel et al. 2004; Israel and Bosniak 2004; Ascenti et al. 2007; Quaia et al. 2008). It has been shown that MRI can lead to the upgradation complex cysts from category IIF to category III (in 3 of 10 cases) and from category III to category IV (in 2 of 9 cases) (Israel et al. 2004). Such data suggests that MRI can play a role in the management of cystic masses categorized by CT as IIF (lesions requiring follow-up CT), whereas in category III (lesion requiring surgery), it does not significantly affect patient management. It can therefore be recommended to add MRI in the imaging workup of category IIF as a first step evaluation before further follow-up. Depending on the results of MRI, the lesion can remain in the nonsurgical category IIF and be further followed-up or fall into category III that need to be removed surgically (Fig. 26.27). Contrast-enhanced US has also been shown to improve the evaluation of complex cystic masses (Ascenti et al. 2007; Quaia et al. 2008). It can therefore be proposed as an alternative to MRI and follow-up CT in the management of indeterminate category IIF cysts.

# References

Abdulla C, Kalra MK, Saini S et al. (2002) Pseudoenhancement of simulated renal cysts in a phantom using different multidetector CT scanners. AJR Am J Roentgenol 179:1473–1476

Alanen A, Nurmi M, Ekfors T (1987) Multilocular renal lesions: a diagnostic challenge. Clin Radiol 38:475–477

Amin MB, MacLennan GT, Gupta R et al. (2009) Tubulocystic carcinoma of the kidney: clinicopathologic analysis of 31 cases of a distinctive rare subtype of renal cell carcinoma. Am J Surg Pathol 33:384–392

Aronson S, Frazier H, Baluch JD et al. (1991) Cystic renal masses: usefulness of the Bosniak classification. Urol Radiol 13:83–90

Ascenti G, Mazziotti S, Zimbaro G et al. (2007) Complex cystic renal masses: characterization with contrast-enhanced US. Radiology 243:158–165

Bae KT, Heiken JP, Siegel CL et al. (2000) Renal cysts: is attenuation artifactually increased on contrast-enhanced CT images? Radiology 216:792–796

Birnbaum BA, Maki DD, Chakraborty DP et al. (2002) Renal cyst pseudoenhancement: evaluation with an anthropomorphic body CT phantom. Radiology 225:83–90

Bosniak MA (1986) The current radiologic approach to renal cysts. Radiology 158:1–10

Bosniak MA (1991a) Difficulties in classifying cystic lesions of the kidney. Urol Radiol 13:91–93

Bosniak MA (1991b) The small (≤ 3.0cm) renal parenchymal tumor: detection, diagnosis, and controversies. Radiology 179:307–317

Bosniak MA (1997a) Diagnosis and management of patients with complicated cystic lesions of the kidney. AJR Am J Roentgenol 168:819–821

Bosniak MA (1997b) The use of the Bosniak classification system for renal cysts and cystic tumors. J Urol 157:1852–1853

Cloix P, Martin X, Pangaud C et al. (1996) Surgical management of complex renal cysts: a series of 32 cases. J Urol 156:28–30

Coleman BG, Arger PH, Mintz MC et al. (1984) Hyperdense renal masses: a computed tomographic dilemma. AJR Am J Roentgenol 143:291–294

Correas JM, Claudon M, Tranquart F et al. (2006) The kidney: imaging with microbubble contrast agents. Ultrasound Q 22:53–66

Coulam CH, Sheafor DH, Leder RA et al. (2000) Evaluation of pseudoenhancement of renal cysts during contrast-enhanced CT. AJR Am J Roentgenol 174:493–498

Couvidat C, Eiss D, Merran S et al. (2008) Papillary renal cell carcinoma: spectrum of imaging findings with pathologic correlation. In: RSNA annual meeting. Chicago, USA

Curry NS (1995) Small renal masses (lesions smaller than 3 cm); imaging evaluation and management. AJR Am J Roentgenol 164:355–362

Curry NS (1998) Atypical cystic renal masses. Abdom Imaging 23:230–236

Curry NS, Brock G, Metcalf JS et al. (1982) Hyperdense renal mass: unusual CT appearance of a benign renal cyst. Urol Radiol 4:33–35

Curry NS, Cochran ST, Bissada NK (2000) Cystic renal masses: accurate Bosniak classification requires adequate renal CT. AJR Am J Roentgenol 175:339–342

Dunnick NR, Korobkin M, Clark WM (1984a) CT demonstration of hyperdense renal carcinoma. J Comput Assist Tomogr 8:1023–1024

Dunnick NR, Korobkin M, Silverman PM et al. (1984b) Computed tomography of high density renal cysts. J Comput Assist Tomogr 8:458–461

Fishman MC, Pollack HM, Arger PH et al. (1983) High protein content: another cause of CT hyperdense benign renal cyst. J Comput Assist Tomogr 7:1103–1106

Foster WL, Roberts L, Halvorsen RA et al. (1988) Sonography of small renal masses with indeterminate density characteristics on computed tomography. Urol Radiol 10:59–67

Freire M, Remer EM (2009) Clinical and radiological features of cystic renal masses. AJR Am J Roentgenol 192:1367–1372

Gokan T, Ohgiya Y, Munechika H et al. (2002) Renal cyst pseudoenhancement with beam hardening effect on CT attenuation. Radiat Med 20:187–190

Gulani V, Adusumilli S, Hussain HK et al. (2008) Apparent wall thickening of cystic renal lesions on MRI. J Magn Reson Imaging 28:103–110

Hartman DS (1990) Cysts and cystic neoplasms. Urol Radiol 12:7–10

Hartman DS, Choyke PL, Hartman MS (2004) A practical approach to the cystic renal mass. Radiographics 24:S101–S115

Hartman DS, Davis CJ Jr, Johns T et al. (1986) Cystic renal cell carcinoma. Urology 28:145–153

Hartman DS, Davis CJ, Sanders RC et al. (1987) The multiloculated renal mass: considerations and differential features. Radiographics 7:29–52

Hartman DS, Weatherby E III, Laskin WB et al. (1992) Cystic renal cell carcinoma: findings simulating a benign hyperdense cyst. AJR Am J Roentgenol 159:1235–1237

Hélénon O, Correas JM, Balleyguier C et al. (2001) Ultrasound of renal tumors. Eur Radiol 11:1890–1901

Hélénon O, Dekeyser E, Merran S et al. (2008) Kyste solitaire du rein. Classification de masses kystiques en imagerie. EMC (Elsevier Masson SAS, Paris). Radiodiagnostic–Urologie-Gynécologie 34-119-B-30:20

Hélénon O, Latourte S, Fabaron F et al. (2005). Le carcinome tubulokystique du rein: nouvelle entité radiologique? Séance scientifique de Société française de radiologie. Section Ile-de-France, Paris

Heneghan JP, Spielmann AL, Sheafor DH et al. (2002) Pseudo-enhancement of simple renal cysts: a comparison of single and multidetector helical CT. J Comput Assist Tomogr 26:90–94

Herts BR, Coll DM, Novick AC et al. (2002) Enhancement characteristics of papillary renal neoplasms revealed on triphasic helical CT of the kidneys. AJR Am J Roentgenol 178:367–372

Hill GS (1989) Cystic and dysplastic disease of the kidney. In: Hill GS (ed) Uropathology. Churchill Livingston Inc., New York

Ho VB, Allen SF, Hood MN et al. (2002). Renal masses: quantitative assessement of enhancement with dynamic MR imaging. Radiology 224:695–700

Israel GM, Bosniak MA (2003a) Follow-up CT of moderately complex cystic lesions of the kidney (Bosniak category IIF). AJR Am J Roentgenol 181:627–631

Israel GM, Bosniak MA (2003b) Calcification in cystic renal masses: is it important in diagnosis? Radiology 226:47–52

Israel GM, Bosniak MA (2004) MR imaging of cystic renal masses. Magn Reson Imag Clin N Am 12:403–412

Israel GM, Bosniak MA (2005) An update of the Bosniak cyst classification system. Urology 66:484–488

Israel GM, Hindman N, Bosniak MA (2004) Evaluation of cystic renal masses : comparison of CT and MR imaging by using the Bosniak classification system. Radiology 231:365–371

Koga S, Nishikido M, Inuzuka S et al. (2000) An evaluation of Bosniak's radiological classification of cystic renal masses. BJU 86:607–609

Lane BR, Campbell SC, Remer EM et al. (2008) Adult cystic nephroma and mixed epithelial and stromal tumor of the kid-ney: clinical, radiographic and pathologic characteristics. Urology 71:1142–1148

Levy P, Hélénon O, Melki P et al. (1994) Kystes atypiques du rein: aspects IRM. J Radiol 75:543–552

Levy P, Hélénon O, Merran S et al. (1999) Tumeurs kystiques du rein: corrélations radio-histopathologiques. J Radiol 80:121–133

Lopez-Beltran A, Scarpelli M, Montironi R et al. (2006) 2004 WHO classification of the renal tumors of the adults. Eur Urol 49:798–805

Madewell JE, Goldman SM, Davis CJ Jr et al. (1983) Multilocular cystic nephroma: a radiographic-pathologic correlation of 58 patients. Radiology 146:309–321

Maki DD, Birnbaum BA, Chakraborty DP et al. (1999) Renal cyst pseudoenhancement: beam-hardening effects on CT numbers. Radiology 213:468–472

Montironi R, Mazzucchelli R, Lopez-Beltran A et al. (2008). Cystic nephroma and mixed epithelial and stromal tumour of the kidney: opposite ends of the spectrum of the same entity? Eur Urol 54:1237–1246

O'Malley RL, Godoy G, Hecht EM et al. (2009) Bosniak category IIF designation and surgery for complex renal cysts. J Urol 182:1091–1095

Park HS, Kim SH, Kim SH et al. (2005) Benign mixed epithelial and stromal tumor of the kidney : imaging findings. J Comput Assist Tomogr 29:786–789

Quaia E, Bertolotto M, Cioffi V et al. (2008) Comparison of contrast-enhanced sonography with unenhanced sonography and contrast-enhanced CT in the diagnosis of malignancy in complex cystic renal masses. AJR Am J Roentgenol 191:1239–1249

Ravine D, Gibson RN, Donlan J et al. (1993) An ultrasounde renal cyst prevalence survey: specificity data for inherited renal cystic disease. Am J Kidney Dis 22:803–807

Roy C, Sauer B, Lindner V et al. (2007) MR Imaging of papillary renal neoplasms: potential application for characterization of small renal masses. Eur Radiol 17:193–200

Schmidt T, Hohl C, Haage P et al. (2003) Diagnostic accuracy of phase inversion tissue harmonic imaging versus fundamental B-mode sonography in the evaluation of focal lesions of the kidney. AJR Am J Roentgenol 180:1639–1647

Sibony M, Vieillefond A (2008) Non clear cell renal cell carcinoma. update in renal tumor pathology. Ann Pathol 28:381–401

Siegel CL, McFarland EG, Brink JA et al. (1997) CT of cystic renal masses: analysis of diagnostic performance and inter-observer variation. AJR Am J Roentgenol 169:813–818

Silverman JF, Kilhenny C (1969) Tumor in the wall of a simple renal cyst. Radiology 93:95–98

Sufrin G, Etra W, Gaeta J et al. (1975) Hypernephroma arising in wall of simple renal cyst. Urology 6:507

Sussman S, Cochran ST, Pagani JJ et al. (1984) Hyperdense renal masses: a CT manifestation of hemorrhagic renal cysts. Radiology 150:207–211

Terada N, Arai Y, Kinukawa N et al. (2008) The 10-year natural history of simple renal cysts. Urology 71:7–11

Turbiner J, Amin MB, Humphrey PA et al. (2007) Cystic nephroma and mixed epithelial and stromal tumor of kidney: a detailed clinicopathologic analysis of 34 cases and proposal for renal epithelial and stromal tumor (REST) as a unifying term. Am J Surg Pathol 31:489–500

Varma KR, Taimson E, Goldman SM et al. (1974) Papillary carcinoma in wall of simple renal cyst. Urology 3:762–765

Warren KS, McFarlane J (2004) The Bosniak classification of renal cystic masses. BJU Int 95:939–942

Weitzner S (1971) Clear cell carcinoma of the free wall of a simple renal cyst. J Urol 106:515–517

Wilson TE, Doelle EA, Cohan R et al. (1996) Cystic renal masses: reevaluation of the usefulness of the Bosniak classification system. Acad Radiol 3:564–570

Zirinsky K, Auh YH, Rubenstein WA et al. (1984) CT of the hyperdense renal cyst: sonographic correlation. AJR Am J Roentgenol 143:151–156

Part **V**

**Special Topics**

# The Pediatric Kidney

**27**

Michael Riccabona

## Contents

M. Riccabona
Department of Radiology, Division of Pediatric Radiology,
University Hospital, LKH Graz, Auenbruggerplatz,
8036 Graz, Austria
e-mail: michael.riccabona@meduni-graz.at

E. Quaia (ed.), *Radiological Imaging of the Kidney*,
Medical Radiology, DOI: 10.1007/978-3-540-87597-0_27, © Springer-Verlag Berlin Heidelberg 2011

## Abstract

> Children are not small adults. In the urinary tract, particularly, there are many conditions that are more or less specific to children which need early and reliable diagnosis in order to provide proper treatment to prevent renal damage and severe long-term sequalae such as hypertension or renal insufficiency. This is particularly important for all congenital urinary tract malformations and also for many other congenital renal conditions – these are often detected prenatally and, after birth, need prompt and reliable diagnostic workup at minimal invasiveness. Additionally, even in conditions that are the same or similar to adults, the specific needs and conditions in childhood require different imaging approaches and algorithms, partially because of each of the following reasons: the child's higher sensitivity to radiation, different physiology, different size and imaging appearance as well as different potential of the various imaging techniques. These differences are outlined, focusing on some important diseases and queries such as congenital hydronephrosis and obstructive uropathy, impact of vesicoureteral reflux on the kidney, imaging in infants with urinary tract infection, childhood urolithiasis and nephrocalcinosis, pediatric renal masses, as well as other miscellaneous renal conditions that may manifest in the child and indicate imaging. Additionally, specific needs for adapting and applying the various imaging techniques in childhood are discussed.

## 27.1 General Remarks on the Principles of Imaging Children and Radiation Protection Issues

There are a number of specific aspects that need to be considered when imaging the pediatric kidney. Some basic requirements and aspects are listed below:

- The lower body weight of infants and children demands for less contrast media and their relatively larger circulating blood volume necessitates a higher contrast media dose.

- The heart rate is faster and circulation times are shorter; therefore, delay times in computed tomography (CT) as well as Magnetic Resonance Imaging (MRI) are shorter and differ from adults.

- The faster respiration and the lack of cooperation particularly in the first years of life require faster imaging which can be challenging particularly for MRI.

- Their higher susceptibility to radiation demands the lowest possible radiation burden following the ALARA principle ("*As Low As Reasonably Achievable*" in terms of radiation exposure); thus, irradiating imaging techniques and particularly CT should be avoided in childhood whenever possible (Brenner et al. 2001; Kao et al. 2005; Brenner and Hall 2007). Additionally, as they are at far higher risk to experience a potential radiation-induced cancer than, for example, elderly patients, the accumulated dose must be kept as low as possible by trying to avoid repeated studies or multiphase CTs. If irradiating imaging must be performed, adapted techniques such as using only pulsed fluoroscopy, adequate filters and grids, proper use of shutters coning down the image to the field of interest (important for intravenous urography (IVU), radiographs of the kidney, ureter, and bladder (KUB), and voiding cystourethrography (VCUG)), age and size-adapted reduced device settings in terms of radiation dose, or careful use of scout views (avoid overranging!) must be followed.

- The smaller body circumference demands lower kilovolt and milliampere-seconds settings, as less tissue has to be penetrated, particularly for CT; note that the most CT-dose indices (CTDI) values provided by the various companies at the consoles are inaccurate for children and often underestimate the effective radiation significantly.

- Less body fat improves the potential of Ultrasound (US), but impairs the delineation of isodense soft tissue structures such as the ureter; thus, the rules for adult CT-urography and "stone-CT" do not always apply for particularly younger children. Additionally, as low tissue density differences are observed, proper tuning of low-dose CT protocols is challenging, as one will often need good soft tissue differentiation. Note that missing an important diagnosis due to too low dose is just as problematic as applying an unnecessarily high dose or performing a nonindicated CT.

- The smaller size, particularly of infants, demands higher imaging resolution techniques, e.g., the use of high-frequency US transducers or a smaller slice thickness in CT or MR.

- The different and mobile position of organs with less surrounding fat makes them more vulnerable (e.g., the kidney is not protected by the osseous thoracic cage leading to a higher risk of renal injury in trauma) or causes different trauma manifestations (e.g., intraperitoneal bladder rupture).

- Furthermore, the initially immature kidneys may also create problems. It is not only that they look different – the US appearance of a neonatal kidney resembles a severe nephropathy in an adult, but also a kidney with an adult-like US appearance in a neonate is highly indicative of renal disease (Fig. 27.1) (Jequier and Kaplan 1991). Additionally, IVU and scintigraphy as well as functional MR-urography (MRU) should not be performed in the first month(s) of life as they will deliver misleading results and inaccurate estimations of renal function and drainage (Gordon and Riccabona 2003).

- Finally, the entire environment as well as patient handling during an examination must be adapted: sick children are often afraid and in pain reducing their intrinsically restricted ability to cooperate in the hospital environment, communication may be difficult or even impossible, parents or other assisting persons are necessary as well as, sometimes, immobilization or sedation, and other practical needs such as pacifiers, swaddling facilities, a heater, blankets, and toys have to be provided. Note that due to these factors, all the investigations in children usually take considerably longer than the same study in adults!

- All these amounts to the evident necessity for specifically trained and experienced pediatric (uro) radiologists, child adapted environment and equipment, as well as different scheduling of investigations when imaging the child's urinary tract. Some basic procedural recommendations concerning the proper use of imaging in pediatric uroradiology have been published (Riccabona M, Avni FE, Blickman JG et al. 2008, 2009, 2010). The proper use of renal scintigraphy in children has been outlined by European association of nuclear medicine (Mandell et al. 1997; Piepsz 2002; Gordon et al. 2006; Piepsz and Ham 2006; Gordon 2008). The main messages of these recommendations are:

  - *US:* Use high-resolution (linear) high-frequency transducers; always perform a comprehensive study of the entire urinary tract and renal parenchyma in well-hydrated patients including a postvoid assessment (Riccabona M, Avni FE, Blickman JG et al. 2008). Try to exploit the

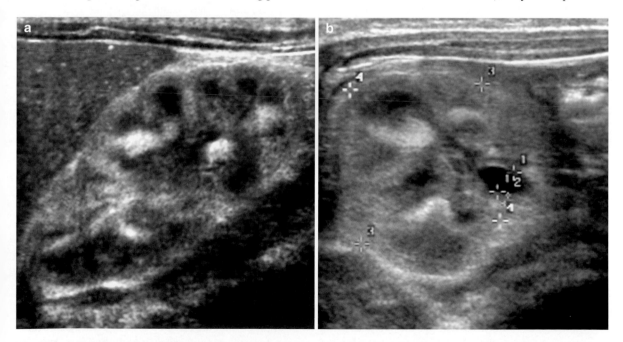

**Fig. 27.1** (**a**, **b**) Ultrasound (US) appearance of a normal neonatal kidney. US image – obtained using a high-resolution linear transducer – of a normal neonatal kidney in longitudinal (**a**) and axial (**b**) plane. Note the physiologic hyperechogenicity of the distal medullae and papillae, as well as the slight wall thickening (+...+[1]) of the nearly, though depictable, collapsed renal pelvis (+...+[2]). The axial diameters as used for volume calculations are marked (+...+[3,4]) in image (**b**)

potential of modern techniques such as (amplitude-coded) Color Doppler US or harmonic imaging (Riccabona et al. 2001; Bartram and Darge 2005; Riccabona 2002, 2009). Always use volume calculations and age-related growth charts – kidney length measurements are less reliable in children (Riccabona et al. 2002). Note that, particularly in the urinary bladder, the correction factor for the commonly used ellipsoid equation may vary depending on the bladder shape.

- *Radiographs of the KUB:* Age-adapted dose as well as the proper use of filters, grid, and shutters are mandatory; also consider the need for the adaptation of digital radiography equipment to pediatric needs (i.e., different electronic filters and postprocessing, sufficient spatial resolution of the detector).
- *IVU:* There are very few indications left. If necessary, use age-adapted CM and radiation dose as for KUB, and avoid multiple films – usually two or three well-timed films suffice for retrieving all therapeutically necessary information (Riccabona et al. 2002, 2010). To enable proper planning of the investigation and deciding on the optimal timing of films, a previous detailed US study is mandatory (Fig. 27.2).
- *VCUG:* It is an invasive investigation with relatively high radiation burden particularly to the ovaries, although modern equipment and skilled investigation technique help to bring down the effective applied dose significantly (Lebovic and Lebowitz 1980; Hernandez and Goodsitt 1996; Ward 2006; Ward et al. 2008). Always assure a reliable justification for this invasive and radiating study. Use only digital pulsed fluoroscopy with last image hold for documentation reducing spot films to the minimum. Try to fill the bladder at physiologic filling pressure, and perform cyclic VCUG in the first year(s) of life for the best yield, once you have decided to perform this study (Gelfand et al, 1999; Paltiel et al. 1992). Always dedicate your attention to the ureterovesical junction (oblique/lateral views mandatory!), the urethra (particularly in boys, lateral view!), the renal parenchyma (searching for intrarenal reflux), as well as the residual urine and the postvoid CM drainage dynamics (if refluxed) (Fernbach et al. 2000; Riccabona 2002; Riccabona et al. 2008).

- *Scintigraphy:* Select the method properly, depending on age, kidney function, and clinical query (static or dynamic diuretic renography). A previous detailed US study is mandatory, also for enabling a correct interpretation of scintigraphic findings. The method has been standardized and is considered essential or even the present gold standard for various queries (Prigent et al. 1999; Gorden et al. 2000; Piepsz 2002). Note that indirect cystoscopy should be performed only in toilet-trained patients. If you consider using single photon emission computed tomography (SPECT), adapt the technique in order to facilitate reliable results at the same dose; however, often – particularly in small children – this does not yield a lot of therapeutically relevant additional information.
- *CT:* The most important rule is: avoid CT whenever possible, and if indicated (e.g., no MRI available for tumor queries) avoid multiphase CTs (in the majority of cases, one adequate phase is sufficient for diagnosis) – or at least reduce their number! The adaptation of all other parameters such as CM dose, timing, tube settings, or scanning range vary with age, query, institution, and scanner (Tsapaki et al. 2006; Paterson and Frush 2007; Stöver and Rogalla 2008). Some orienting information can be retrieved from the recently published recommendation for uro-CT in children (Riccabona et al. 2010), and on the website of the image gently campaign in the USA (www.imagegently).
- *MRU:* At present, there are different approaches under evaluation – particularly, functional diuretic dynamic MRU is still considered "work in progress." For the use of contrast medium, the same rules apply as for CT or IVU, as prevention of nephrogenic systemic fibrosis has to be considered (Riccabona et al. 2008). Immobilization and sedation are often necessary in the first years of life; however, this also applies to CT (one should never "try a CT" and repeat it in case the child had moved during the critical acquisition phase, or use a field of view far larger than the targeted area to assure that everything is covered even if the child moves!). As MRI is a nonionizing imaging method that allows for simultaneous anatomic and functional

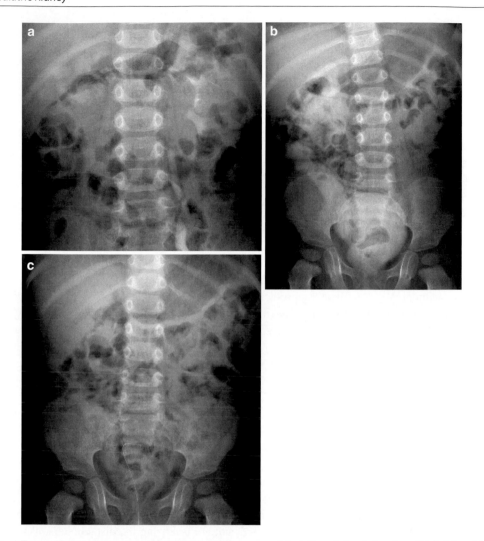

**Fig. 27.2** (**a–c**) Focused intravenous urography (IVU) in childhood urolithiasis. Focused IVU after ureteral reimplantation with sonographically suspected postoperative obstruction and huge dilatation of the right collecting system as well as the ureter: three well-timed exposures, defined according to the clinical query and the findings of the US examination: (**a**) An early kidney image at 7 min after contrast medium injection demonstrating delayed excretion into the operated and dilated right collecting system, but revealing all of the collecting tract anatomy of the left unobstructed system. (**b**) A delayed image showing the now homogeneously opacified dilated pelvocaliceal system and the diverted megaureter after ureterocutaneostomy on the right side, with complete drainage of CM from the unobstructed left kidney. (**c**) A final image after Furosemide i.v. and upright positioning (to allow for gravity-dependent drainage) demonstrating the complete washout of contrast medium from the dilated right system, thus proving a dilated, but not obstructed, right system obviating any further intervention

assessment, it has practically replaced IVU for most queries in childhood and is increasingly considered the ideal one-stop-shop investigation in the child's urinary tract; its implementation into routine diagnostics is strongly recommended and promoted, particularly for purely anatomic queries, where, in most instances, all relevant questions can be answered without the need for contrast administration.

## 27.2 Vesicoureteral Reflux and Reflux Nephropathy

### 27.2.1 General Considerations

One of the conditions that may potentially need early treatment to prevent long-term renal damage is vesicoureteral reflux. This very controversial topic is constantly under discussion; knowledge and insight into the natural course of the condition has grown and is constantly growing. New knowledge has been and is influencing the management and treatment strategies leading to a constantly changing role and task of imaging. Whereas, initially, vesicoureteral reflux was seen as a separate entity that needs to be treated in any way, today, only the consequences of vesicoureteral reflux such as bladder dysfunction and renal damage give reason for concern or treatment. Additionally, long-established treatment strategies such as antibiotic prophylaxis are under discussion, particularly, as most congenital vesicoureteral refluxes spontaneously decrease and eventually resolve without any long-term sequalae. With this, the present confusion becomes obvious – whom and how to image for a condition that probably will vanish without any treatment or problems without missing those who might and will suffer from vesicoureteral reflux and its sequalae? And is there an impact of vesicoureteral reflux on renal transplants?

In order to answer these difficult questions, we need to consider that there are many different forms of vesicoureteral reflux: various grades, congenital or acquired, primary or secondary, high or low pressure, with or without intrarenal reflux, uni- or bilateral, with normal ureteral anatomy or with pathologic changes such as a gaping ostium or a duplex and potentially ectopically inserting ureter, as an isolated finding or part of a more complex urinary tract malformation such as posterior ureteral valve, duplex systems, or in combination with obstructive uropathy, with or without renal parenchymal damage as in the typically newborn males with (bilateral) congenital high-grade vesicoureteral reflux and congenital renal dysplasia ("congenital reflux nephropathy") (Riccabona 2002, 2007). Additionally, one needs to acknowledge that vesicoureteral reflux itself probably does not cause renal damage, only early intrauterine high-grade high pressure vesicoureteral reflux (potentially causing renal damage based on the water hammer effect theory, in addition to the associated primary developmental renal dysplasia) or when associated with other factors such as compound papilla (enabling intrarenal reflux), bladder outlet obstruction, functional bladder disturbance, or urinary tract infection. This leads to an increasingly reluctant indication for the imaging assessment of vesicoureteral reflux in childhood. Generally accepted indications are significant neonatal hydronephrosis in baby boys or infants with complex urogenital tract or cloacal malformations (see Sect. 27.4), infants and children with (recurrent) upper urinary

tract infection (i.e., renal involvement and potential scaring in infection – see Sect. 27.3), for the differentiation of obstructive vs. refluxing dilatation, and with persisting bladder dysfunction (such as in neurogenic bladder, bladder outlet obstruction, or persistent dysfunctional voiding associated with recurrent urinary tract infection); additionally, vesicoureteral reflux into transplanted kidneys is increasingly becoming a major concern.

## 27.2.2 Methods for Vesicoureteral Reflux Assessment

### 27.2.2.1 Ultrasound

US is the workhorse in pediatric uroradiology. It has overcome its initial restrictions where it was considered just a rough initial orienting tool, and now offers many reliable options that may help in diagnosing and assessing vesicoureteral reflux. For this, it is important to have a state-of-the-art US device with a variety of transducers; particularly, in infants and neonates, high-resolution linear transducers (15–5 MHz) with color Doppler US option and ability for harmonic imaging are indispensable. Every investigation should be performed on a sufficiently filled bladder and include a postvoid assessment of not only potential residual urine, but also changes in upper tract dilatation that may indicate perimicturitional high pressure vesicoureteral reflux. And one should aim at visualizing the distal ureters, usually achievable in every sufficiently hydrated child. Important findings that may hint towards vesicoureteral reflux are a thickened or trabeculated bladder wall, an unusual ostium position or anatomy (asymmetric, lateralized, gaping, duplex ...), a dilated distal ureter – particularly with a thickened urothelium ("urothelial sign"), and changing width of the upper collecting system (Fig. 27.3). Other more advanced important options are color Doppler US (which may directly depict vesicoureteral reflux as soon as there are some reflecting particles in the urine), assessment of ureteric bladder inflow jet (which exhibit specific jet forms that are associated with vesicoureteral reflux, Fig. 27.4), and various bladder filling techniques for direct vesicoureteral reflux visualization after bladder catheterization. Air, (shaken) saline and – most commonly – sonographic contrast agents have been successfully used for reflux cystosonography; particularly, *contrast-enhanced voiding urosonography* (ce-VUS) has been established as a reliable and

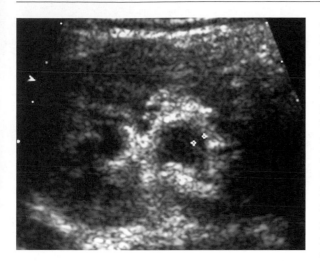

**Fig. 27.3** US image – thickened urothelium ("urothelial sign"). Axial section of the right kidney in a girl with vesicoureteral reflux and recurrent urinary tract infection demonstrating the thickened urothelium (+...+) of the slightly prominent renal pelvis, a nonspecific sign seen with vesicoureteral reflux, obstruction, or infection as well as other causes of pelvic wall edema, necessitating further workup and, today, included in the sonographic "extended US criteria" which indicate urinary tract pathology and rectify additional work-up

nonirradiating imaging modality for vesicoureteral reflux detection, with an even higher sensitivity for vesicoureteral reflux detection than conventional fluoroscopic VCUG, particularly using modern agent detection techniques (Bosio 1998; Darge et al. 1999, 2001; Kenda et al. 2000; Berrocal et al. 2001; Riccabona et al. 2003; Darge et al. 2005). Any contrast material detected in the ureter or the renal cavities indicates vesicoureteral reflux (Fig. 27.5). Recommendations on how to perform

ce-VUS and sonographically grade vesicoureteral reflux have been established (Darge and Tröger 2002; Claudon et al. 2008; Riccabona et al. 2008). The major setback of this technique is that, currently, no sonographic contrast agent is approved for pediatric use; furthermore, a panoramic display and the assessment of the entire ureter (if not dilated) is impossible, or bladder diverticula that briefly pose during voiding as well as short-lasting low-degree vesicoureteral reflux into a nondilated ureter may be missed; the latter, however, will not have much therapeutic consequences and thus may be less important. Finally, the assessment of the urethra during voiding is a little cumbersome and time consuming. However, *transperineal US* is capable of reliably visualizing the urethra and the pediatrically important urethral anomalies (Good et al. 1993; Teele and Share 1997; Schöllnast et al. 2004). Additionally, US allows for early and noninvasive assessment of the inner genitalia that may also be affected in urogenital or cloacal malformations, particularly important in baby girls with some urinary tract malformations such as single kidneys (Gassner and Geley 2004; Geley and Gassner 2008).

The other important aspect in suspected vesicoureteral reflux is imaging of the renal parenchyma – US is the established imaging tool that reveals information on renal size, parenchymal structure, and focal lesions such as dysplastic cysts or large scars, particularly if associated with scared and clubbed calices (Fig. 27.6). Power Doppler sonography (= amplitude-coded color Doppler sonography) additionally allows for the assessment of peripheral renal perfusion and vasculature, improving the depiction of diffuse or focal perfusion disturbances associated with diffuse

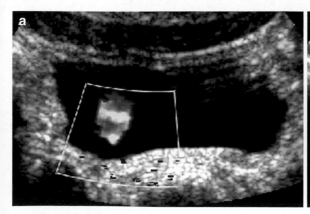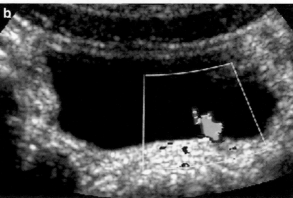

**Fig. 27.4** (**a, b**) Ureteric inflow jet. Ureteric inflow jet using color Doppler US. Asymmetric jet with a lateralized ostium on the right side (**a**) in a child that then showed medium degree vesicoureteral reflux on the right side. The blue color of the jet from the normal positioned left ostium (**b**) is due to aliasing

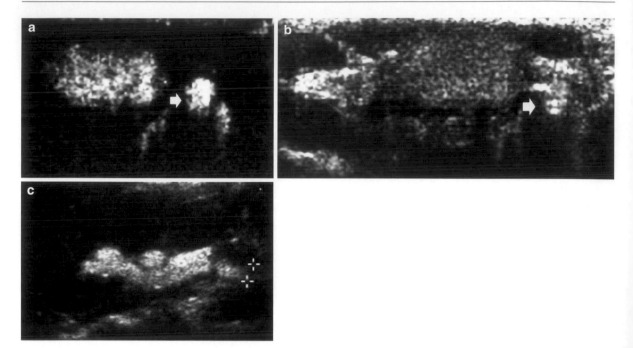

**Fig. 27.5** (a–c) Contrast-enhanced voiding urosonography (ce-VUS) in dilating vesicoureteral reflux: (**a, b**) Urinary bladder (axial plane) filled with the microbubble contrast agent, using a dual image-specific contrast imaging technique (**a**) and an orienting baseline gray scale B-mode image (**b**). Note the excellent depiction of the contrast-filled, dilated, and refluxing left ureter (*small arrow*) on the contrast image. (**c**) Longitudinal image of the left kidney using the same technique and contrast harmonic imaging showing the dilated ureter (+…+) and pelvocaliceal system, filled by the echogenic microbubble contrast agent consistent with vesicoureteral reflux IV°

renal parenchymal damage or focal scaring. Again, restrictions have to be acknowledged – small or minor and diffuse scaring may be missed by US; thus, additional renal assessment by static Tc$^{99m}$DMSA scintigraphy is presently considered essential and the gold standard in children after 3–6 months of age. In future, MRI may play a bigger role also for this query (Chan et al. 1999; Thoeny et al. 2005). US remains the routine imaging for regular follow-up of children with symptomatic vesicoureteral reflux and reflux

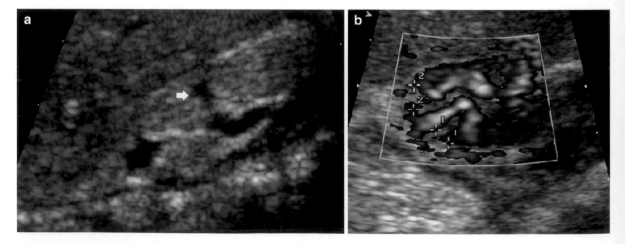

**Fig. 27.6** (**a, b**) US image of a scarred kidney ("reflux nephropathy"). Longitudinal scan of a small, echogenic, nondifferentiated kidney with clubbed calices (*arrow*) (**a**) and focal perfusion defects demonstrating scars depicted by amplitude coded Power Doppler US (+…+) in an axial section of the upper pole area of the right kidney (**b**)

nephropathy (an old term that is used more reluctantly for postnatally acquired renal scaring after urinary tract infection, even in children with vesicoureteral reflux).

### 27.2.2.2 Voiding Cystourethrography

VCUG is considered the gold standard of vesicoureteral reflux imaging. It is invasive and burdening as it requires bladder catheterization or suprapubic puncture and uses radiation. On the other hand, it offers a panoramic overview, allows for exquisite anatomical display of the urethra and the bladder, and – if refluxing – the entire ureter as well as the renal collecting system, also enabling the depiction of intrarenal reflux. With modern fluoroscopic techniques using age-adapted grids, pulsed fluoroscopy, last image hold for documentation, and skilled device handling that allows for short fluoroscopy time, the effective radiation burden can be significantly reduced, even when performing

cyclic investigation as recommended in the first years of life (Lebovic and Lebowitz 1980; Gelfand et al. 1992; Paltiel et al. 1992; Hernandez and Goodsitt 1996; Ward 2006; Ward et al. 2008). The entire procedure as well as grading (I°–V°) have been standardized, recommendations exist and have been published (Lebowitz et al. 1985; Fernbach et al. 2000; Riccabona 2002a, b, 2005; Riccabona et al. 2008) (Fig. 27.7; Table 27.1). VCUG was and is the base for most international vesicoureteral reflux studies, also with less investigator dependency than US. Furthermore, modified protocols that use a physiologic filling pressure of the contrast infusion – which is monitored to detect the phases of increased bladder pressure with consecutive infusion stops that guide fluoroscopy – have enabled a simultaneous functional assessment (Fotter et al. 1986). This is increasingly important, as functional bladder disturbances are being recognized as an important aspect in dealing with patients who have vesicoureteral reflux and recurrent urinary tract infection (Fotter 2008) – unrecognized and untreated bladder dysfunction will

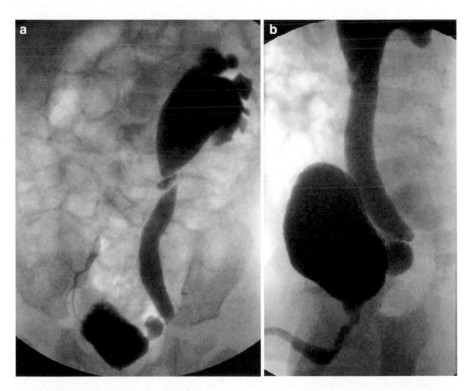

**Fig. 27.7** (**a**, **b**) Vesicoureteral reflux shown on voiding cystourethrography (VCUG). Cyclic VCUG in an infant after urinary tract infection with US signs of a left-sided megaureter and hydronephrosis III° taken as last image hold without the need for additional exposures: Image (**a**) demonstrates a dilating high-degree vesicoureteral reflux (vesicoureteral reflux IV°) on the left side with a kink at the ureteropelvic junction, and a low-degree vesicoureteral reflux into the distal right ureter (vesicoureteral reflux I°) that had occurred only during previous voiding. Image (**b**) during voiding (lateral oblique projection) demonstrates the diverticula at the ureterovesical junction of the left side, nicely posing during voiding (due to the perimicturitional higher intravesical pressure)

**Table 27.1** Grading of vesicoureteral reflux according to international radiographic reflux grading system (Lebowitz et al. 1985)

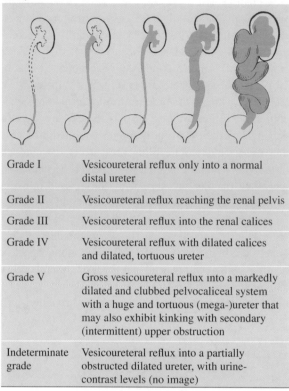

| Grade I | Vesicoureteral reflux only into a normal distal ureter |
|---|---|
| Grade II | Vesicoureteral reflux reaching the renal pelvis |
| Grade III | Vesicoureteral reflux into the renal calices |
| Grade IV | Vesicoureteral reflux with dilated calices and dilated, tortuous ureter |
| Grade V | Gross vesicoureteral reflux into a markedly dilated and clubbed pelvocaliceal system with a huge and tortuous (mega-)ureter that may also exhibit kinking with secondary (intermittent) upper obstruction |
| Indeterminate grade | Vesicoureteral reflux into a partially obstructed dilated ureter, with urine-contrast levels (no image) |

not only perpetuate urinary tract infection and clinical symptoms, but may also lead to the reoccurrence of operated vesicoureteral reflux. On the other hand, successful treatment of bladder dysfunction will often result in the resolution of vesicoureteral reflux, without the need of cystoscopic treatment or open surgery.

### 27.2.2.3 Radionuclide Cystography (RNC)

RNC is another option for VUR diagnosis.

*Direct RNC* uses – instead of radiopaque contrast – a Tc[99m] labeled tracer that is directly instilled into the bladder via a catheter; any activity observed in the projection on the ureter or the kidney is indicative of vesicoureteral reflux. The radiation dose is slightly lower than in VCUG, and – partially due to the longer observation period – the yield is higher. The disadvantage is lack of anatomical details, especially of the urethra (Mandell et al. 1997; Piepsz 2002; Gordon 2008).

*Indirect RNC* consists of the delayed phase of a dynamic renography using intravenously applied

Tc[99m] MAG3 that is excreted by the renal tubular cells into the collecting and draining system – thus it avoids catheterization and offers a more physiological approach (Gordon et al. 2000; Piepsz 2002; Gordon 2008). After the activity has passed into the bladder during the early phases of the investigation, any reoccurrence of activity in the upper collecting system indicates vesicoureteral reflux, particularly during and after voiding. However, it can be performed only in toilet-trained patients, and anatomical resolution is low too.

### 27.2.3 Imaging Algorithm – When to Perform What in Whom

It is difficult to propose an imaging algorithm for children with suspected vesicoureteral reflux; in general, VCUG is preferred in male neonates and for preoperative assessment as well as in complex malformations, particularly with suspected (additional) obstruction. If available, ce-VUS is recommended for screening conditions, vesicoureteral reflux assessment in girls, as well as for bed-side or follow-up investigations. RNC is used for screening purposes and for following up children with symptomatic vesicoureteral reflux as well as postoperatively. Renal imaging in children with significant vesicoureteral reflux should start with US and a baseline static renal scintigraphy (usually after the age of 6 months, except for severe reflux nephropathy or malformations); follow-up usually relies on US, with a repeated scintigraphic study in case of deterioration or equivocal US findings, if these results potentially impact further patient management. In future, MRI may become an alternative imaging tool to assess split renal function (dynamic diuretic contrast-enhanced MRU, see Sect. 27.4) or to visualize scars, particularly on T2*-weighted inversion recovery sequences.

### 27.3 Childhood Urinary Tract Infection, Including (Acute) Pyelonephritis

Importance and management of, and thus also imaging for, childhood urinary tract infection are different from adults, particularly in early childhood. As with vesicoureteral reflux, the imaging in childhood urinary tract infection has changed. Initially, vesicoureteral reflux was considered the major condition that endangered the kidney and caused infection and scaring; therefore, aggressive search for vesicoureteral reflux was performed in all infants and children with urinary tract infection. Today we know that there are many factors that cause urinary tract infection as well as renal involvement, and that vesicoureteral reflux itself is harmless and regresses spontaneously in the majority of cases; even high-grade vesicoureteral reflux may spontaneously regress. Thus, today, vesicoureteral reflux is considered as just one other point in a long list of risk factors that cause renal harm in children with urinary tract infection. The focus of imaging has moved towards the kidney, as only diffuse or segmental renal involvement in urinary tract infection causes long-term sequalae, particularly during the first 2 years of life, when the still somewhat immature kidney is prone to severe scaring, also affecting the kidney's growth potential and thus endangering renal function, particularly if bilateral. Today, the task of imaging in pediatric urinary tract infection is to diagnose or rule out upper urinary tract infection (i.e., acute pyelonephritis or diffuse renal involvement) and to assess for potentially endangering preexisting urinary tract conditions or malformations. This new approach has impacted the imaging algorithms for children with urinary tract infection, with some age as well as local variations; in the United Kingdom, for example, the "NICE guidelines" suggest not to perform any imaging at all in children with urinary tract infection as long as they respond well to antibiotic treatment.

## 27.3.1 Which Imaging Modalities are Available and How Do Things Look Like?

Again, the major imaging tool is US. It is easily available, nonirradiating, relatively inexpensive, and quite reliable if performed with professional skills by specifically trained, experienced, and knowledgeable investigators. US always includes the assessment of the entire well-hydrated urinary tract; an additional "sonoscopic" overview of the entire abdomen for other potential reasons of the child's symptoms is recommended (Riccabona et al. 2008; Riccabona 2009). The aim of this initial US investigation in urinary tract infection is to find signs that enable the differentiation of "upper" from "lower" urinary tract infection, to detect potentially undiagnosed preexisting urinary tract malformations early, to search for potential complications such as abscess formation or pyonephrosis, or to depict unusual disease such as infected urolithiasis or xanthogranulomatous pyelonephritis. US findings that indicate renal involvement are (Fig. 27.8):

- Kidney enlargement – they often become more spherical; therefore, volume calculations using the ellipsoid equation and comparison with age/size correlated growth charts are mandatory.
- Focally or diffusely altered renal parenchymal echogenicity, with impaired corticomedullary differentiation.
- Increased peripyelonal echoes and/or thickened urothelium/pelvic wall ("urothelium sign") (Alton et al. 1992; Sorantin et al. 1997; Riccabona and Fotter 2004).
- Echoes within the upper collecting system.
- Focal or diffuse perfusion impairment on Color and/or Power Doppler Sonography US (Dacher et al. 1996; Riccabona et al. 2001)
- Potential remnants of old infections with scaring such as clubbed calices and parenchymal narrowing.

Note that these changes only gradually decrease after successful treatment even without any scaring – reestablishment of a normal US appearance can take up to 8 weeks.

Typical complications are necrosis and abscess formation: US will visualize the focal hypoechoic patchy destruction of the renal parenchyma with the gradual development of complicated fluid in an unphysiologic cavity; US may also depict edema and hyperemia of the perirenal tissue, and (amplitude-coded) Color Doppler US will help visualizing the necrotic nature of the abscess (Fig. 27.9). Usually, these abscesses resolve under antibiotic treatment; rarely, US-guided drainage may become indicated. Note that, sometimes, infected or hemorrhaged cysts/tumors or obstructed calices/caliceal diverticula may mimic abscesses. Chronic pyelonephritis and particularly xanthogranulomatous pyelonephritis are

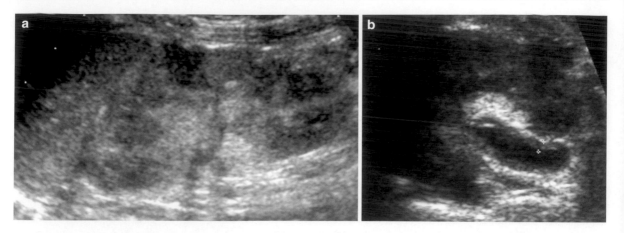

**Fig. 27.8** (**a**, **b**) Renal US findings in upper urinary tract infection: (**a**) Longitudinal display of an enlarged, swollen, diffusely and inhomogenously echogenic kidney with irregular echotexture; the cortical echogenicity is partially interrupted by focal hypoechoic regions that eventually became necrotic and scars.

(**b**) Axial view of a slightly distended renal pelvis in a swollen kidney with increased echogenicity and hazy differentiation demonstrating a gross thickening of the pelvic urothelium (+...+) due to upper UTI. Note some sludge-like echoes in the collecting system

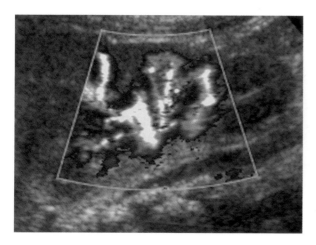

**Fig. 27.9** Power Doppler in acute Pyelonephritis: Same kidney as in Fig. 27.8a – Power Doppler US depicts the focal perfusion defect in acute pyelonephritis well

rare; however, when observing the key diagnostic features such as more centrally located complex cystic masses that may be confluent, with a more or less destructed renal parenchyma in the presence of a central, stag horn-shaped stone, the diagnoses can be assumed sonographically (Fig. 27.10). A special entity is fungal infection: in the pediatric population, it typically occurs in children with dilated or obstructed cavities under antibiotic prophylaxis and

in preterm infants or other immuno-compromised children. The typical US features are echogenic (floating) masses in the collecting system that may cause dorsal shadowing and can cause obstruction (Fig. 27.11). All other features do not differ significantly from any other urinary tract infection manifestations. Although these fungus balls cannot be reliably differentiated from urolithiasis, the history, the urine findings, and the clinical details will enable the assumption of this condition. The signs of and findings in other complicating conditions in conjunction with urinary tract infection such as obstructive uropathy, urolthiasis, or tumors will be described in the respective chapters.

On the other hand, lower urinary tract infection (i.e., cystitis) can be assumed when changes are seen only in the bladder such as a hypervascular thickened bladder wall or floating echoes in the bladder without alteration of the renal collecting system or parenchyma (Fig. 27.12). Note that cystitis can sometimes produce impressive changes such as fibrous clots (e.g., in hemorrhagic cystitis) that may be difficult to be differentiated from bladder tumors such as rhabdomyosarcoma, or a very pronounced echogenic wall thickening as observed in schistomatosis. And also consider that since renal changes may take some time to develop, early US, particularly, may sometimes miss the developing upper UTI.

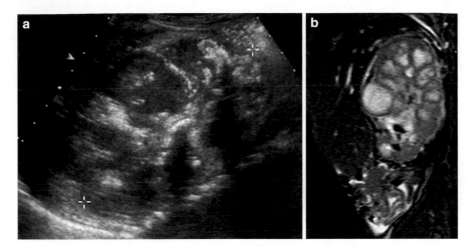

**Fig. 27.10** (**a**, **b**) US and magnetic resonance imaging (MRI) appearance of chronic xanthogranulomatous pyelonephritis. (**a**) Longitudinal US section through a grossly distorted and enlarged kidney (+…+) with irregularly dilated calices, destructed medullary parenchyma, only rim-like residual cortical parenchyma, atypical echoes within the collecting system, and a central hyperechoic structure (= concrement in the pelvis) with acoustic shadowing in a child with xanthogranulomatous pyelonephritis. (**b**) A sagittal MRI image (SSFP sequence) of the same child as in Fig. 27.10a demonstrates similar findings; even urolithiasis/calcifications can be discriminated as patchy areas with signal void in the lower calices (*arrows*)

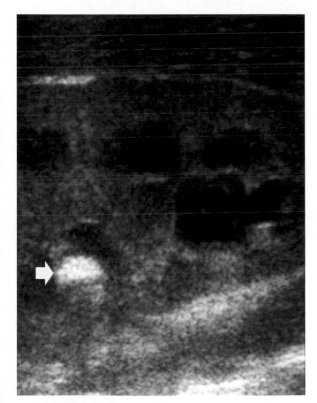

**Fig. 27.11** Fungus ball – US appearance. Sagittal US image demonstrating an echogenic clot-like material (*arrow*) within the dilated collecting system of an enlarged and swollen kidney in a preterm neonate – without acoustic shadowing – in renal candidas infection after long-time antibiotic treatment

The major alternative imaging tool is static renal $Tc^{99m}$ *DMSA* scintigraphy (Piepsz et al. 1999; Piepsz et al. 2000; Craig et al. 2000). Though it may also be false positive and negative in rare cases, static renal scintigraphy is considered the gold standard for the assessment of renal involvement. Note that for differentiating reversible impaired parenchymal function in acute inflammatory involvement from persisting scars, a delayed scan 6–9 months after the infection is necessary. Furthermore, due to the restricted anatomic resolution of scintigraphy, some sort of anatomic study (usually US) is necessary for differentiating other focal lesions such as cysts or dysplastic moieties from focal infectious defects.

In future, DMSA may be increasingly replaced by *MRI* which demonstrates reduced contrast uptake and diffusion disturbances in acute pyelonephritis well (Lonergan et al. 1998; Kavanagh et al. 2005). However, today, due to sedation needs, restricted availability, as well as high costs, MRI is used rather reluctantly for this query.

Note that IVU – which was the major imaging requisite for decades – does not any longer play a role in the assessment of urinary tract infection and scaring in children, as it applies considerable radiation and needs intravenous contrast media with far less information than alternative modern imaging by US and scintigraphy or MRI.

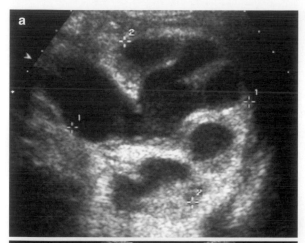

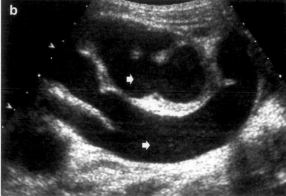

**Fig. 27.12** (**a, b**) US in pyonephrosis. (**a**) Axial US image of a pyonephrosis seen as echogenic sedimentations in the grossly dilated pelvicaliceal system with narrow, echogenic residual parenchyma in a child with known hydronephrosis IV and megaureter. (**b**) Same child as in Fig. 27.12a: longitudinal US section demonstrating diffuse floating inflammatory particles (*arrows*) on the ureter and the collecting system

### 27.3.2 Imaging Algorithm in Pediatric Urinary Tract Infection

In our experience, comprehensive US in conjunction with clinical and laboratory information can reliably establish the diagnosis of lower or upper urinary tract infection in the majority of cases, thus obviating the need for further investigations in a large number of children (Brader et al. 2008).

In patients where US is not clear, no high-end US or amplitude-coded color Doppler sonography is available or performable, or US findings do not match clinical and laboratory results, additional imaging by acute renal scintigraphy or MRI for establishing the

diagnosis or ruling out upper urinary tract infection will become necessary, particularly if only those with proven renal involvement will undergo further studies (for the assessment of vesicoureteral reflux and scarring, the latter by delayed renal scintigraphy), as suggested by many local and international recommendations (Riccabona and Fotter 2004; Riccabona et al. 2008).

At present, MRI is recommended for assessing urinary tract infection complications in patients with equivocal US findings and has practically replaced CT for this indication in children, as CT is a highly irradiating modality and should be avoided in children whenever possible. If you need to perform a CT in a child with complicated urinary tract infection, use age-adapted protocols at lower radiation and contrast dose and avoid multiphase acquisitions – in the majority of children a single scan is sufficient for diagnosis.

After the resolution of the acute infection, all those with (persisting) renal involvement will need vesicoureteral reflux assessment (see Sect. 27.1) and clinical as well as US follow-up (further renal development, scaring, development of hypertension). As US has limitations in diagnosing particularly small scars with little anatomical changes, a delayed DMSA scan is often recommended to prove scaring. But one has to acknowledge that what we see today is far more than what the original work of Smellie – who used IVU for the assessment of scars when establishing the importance of renal scaring for long-term outcome – was based upon; therefore, we, at present, do not know the long-term implication of small peripheral scars, and whether these already justify more invasive imaging.

Increasingly, the importance of bladder dysfunction is recognized as a major contributing factor to childhood urinary tract infection particularly in slightly older children, mostly girls. Therefore, bladder function assessment is becoming very important, and imaging is urged to provide information on potential bladder dysfunction. This can be achieved by observing bladder shape and bladder neck form and activity as well as potential residual urine on US, and doing voiding protocols in infants; in older toilet-trained children, uroflow measurements and pelvic floor electromyography are the first additional test. If VCUG is performed, the modified protocol will reveal most of the necessary functional information similar to video-VCUG (simultaneous fluoroscopy with bladder manometry and pelvic floor EMG) (Fotter 2008).

## 27.4 Congenital Hydronephrosis and Urinary Tract Obstruction

### 27.4.1 Congenital Hydronephrosis

Congenital disorders and urinary tract malformations which often present with prenatally diagnosed hydronephrosis are addressed in Chap. 11. Due to prenatal US (screening), there are many infants submitted for the assessment of prenatally recognized hydronephrosis. It is important to understand the history of the term hydronephrosis and its implications: this expression derives from early days when any distension of the renal central echo complex detectable on obstetric US suggested pathology. Today, the resolution of modern US has significantly increased and the normal distension of the physiologic renal cavities can routinely be visualized. This implies that not every fetally visible pelvocaliceal system needs postnatal assessment. An axial diameter of the fetal pelvis of 5–9 mm has been suggested as cut-off value, with some variance depending on the gestational age and bladder filling. Furthermore, fetal and, accordingly, neonatal hydronephrosis has been graded; low-degree hydronephrosis (i.e., hydronephrosis 0°–II°, with no or only little pelvic distension less than 7–10 mm pelvic diameter, and normal caliceal configuration) is considered normal; only moderate (hydronephrosis III°, with rounded calices) or severe (hydronephrosis IV°, with parenchymal narrowing) and gross dilatation (sometimes also called hydronephrosis V°, when with only a thin residual parenchymal rim) indicate further postnatal assessment (Fernbach et al. 1993; Riccabona et al. 2008).

### 27.4.2 Imaging Algorithm for Congenital Hydronephrosis

The postnatal imaging algorithm depends on these prenatal findings, with a delayed US investigation (after at least 1 week after birth) only in moderate degree hydronephrosis, and early comprehensive imaging workup in particularly bilateral high-grade hydronephrosis. Only those patients with low to moderate degree of fetal hydronephrosis who exhibit persisting sonographic abnormalities as defined by "extended US criteria" (i.e., pelvic dilatation ≥10/12 mm, hydronephrosis ≥III°, renal parenchymal or bladder wall abnormalities, urothelial sign …) need further assessment (Alton et al. 1992; Sorantin et al. 1997; Riccabona et al. 2008). Note that high-grade hydronephrosis is usually associated with obstructive uropathy, posterior urethral valve, or severe vesicoureteral reflux – in some of these patients, an early urinary tract infection may have devastating effects justifying early diagnosis by comprehensive US and VCUG (Riccabona et al. 2008a, b, c, 2009). Renal scintigraphy can be used to estimate residual renal function early in the most severe cases; otherwise, scintigraphy or MRU should always be postponed until at least after the sixth week of life, better the third month of life, as the immature kidney will not provide reliable results (Gordon and Riccabona 2003). Note that today there is no indication for IVU for these queries.

### 27.4.3 Obstructive Uropathy

The most common form of obstructive uropathy is ureteropelvic junction obstruction. This is usually a congenital condition often recognized in utero by high grade fetal hydronephrosis; there are cases of late manifestation detected only during childhood ("juvenile type" of ureteropelvic junction obstruction). The other important entity is (primary/obstructive) megaureter. Additionally, there are acquired forms of obstruction by space occupying lesions and after surgery or trauma. Acute secondary obstruction as in urolithiasis will be described in Sect. 27.5. Posterior urethral valve, prune-belly syndrome, and megazystis-microcolon-hypoperistalsis syndrome are conditions primarily of the lower urinary tract and ureters which – although potentially impacting the kidney as mentioned in Sect. 27.1 – will not be discussed, as the renal consequences primarily are dysplasia, hydronephrosis, and secondary infection, with the same renal pathology and imaging aspects as detailed above, or discussed in Chap. 11.

There are different definitions of urinary tract obstruction. While, initially, obstruction was defined as "*any stenosis that impairs urinary drainage from the pelvo-caliceal system and leads to increased pressure and reduced urine flow rate*" (Whitaker et al. 1982), already in the same year, the importance of future renal function was highlighted by defining obstruction as "*any restriction to urine flow, that left untreated will cause progressive renal deterioration*" (Koff 1982). The most recent and presently generally accepted definition is the modification that defines urinary tract obstruction as "*any condition that, left untreated, endangers renal functional and growth potential*" (Peters 1995). The role of imaging in obstructive uropathy is to assess the degree of obstruction and to help decide on which kidney needs treatment, and which will maintain function and growth even if left untreated. This a very difficult task, as, by today, there is no imaging tool that allows a decisive a-priori pro-futuro assessment that can reliably identify those kidneys that will benefit from treatment and thus may be protected against deterioration of function or loss of growth potential. This inability to prospectively grade obstructive uropathy induces serial investigations to monitor renal development (Riccabona 2010).

The major initial imaging modality, usually, is *US*. Initially, in ureteropelvic junction obstruction, any gross dilatation detected by US was operated. Today, this is considered rather urinary tract cosmetics – we learned that dilatation does not equal obstruction, and that US is only able to demonstrate dilatation, but has severe restrictions in assessing function and drainage even when observing US prerequisites such as good hydration and standardized (axial) measurements. Furthermore, dilatation varies with position, hydration, bladder filling, and kidney function – sometimes, constantly diminishing dilatation does not indicate improvement of obstruction, but is due to the deterioration of renal function with reduced urine production. The US intrinsically lacks the fundamental need to observe and quantify renal excretion and drainage, though modern US approaches such as Doppler sonography (i.e., asymmetrically elevated resistive indices in acute deterioration), diuretic US (serial investigations after diuretic stimulation by Furosemide to observe and monitor renal response to diuretic stress based on pelvocaliceal dilatation and Doppler sonography findings), and 3D-US (enabling reliable relative renal parenchymal size assessment even in gross hydronephrosis) have improved the US potential (Riccabona et al. 2003, 2005).

Additional functional imaging is needed which is usually provided by *dynamic diuretic Tc$^{99m}$MAG3 scintigraphy*. Here, an intravenously applied radioactive tracer is taken up and excreted by the kidney; thus, renal perfusion and uptake (function) can be measured, and split/relative renal size can be calculated (Prigent et al. 1999; Gordon et al. 2000a, b; Piepsz 2002; Gordon 2008). Urinary drainage is assessed after diuretic stimulation using standardized drainage patterns to divide disturbances into normal, nonobstructive dilatation, and partial- or complete obstruction (O'Reilly et al. 1978, 1979, 1981). The major restriction of this technique is that the immature neonatal kidney with a very elastic (extrarenally) dilated pelvis creating a "wind kettle" effect does not allow accurate grading during the first months of life, often exhibiting equivocal results; sometimes, even a persisting normal and symmetrical renal function is observed in spite of a (initially) completely obstructive drainage pattern (Gordon 2001). This leads to repeated investigations with consecutive radiation burden. Furthermore, indications for surgery vary – some (particularly in America) focus in renal function and operate when split renal functions has deteriorated; in Europe, one more often relies on drainage patterns trying to indicate surgery before renal functional impairment occurs, and some even reject to operate infants under 1 year of age. And scintigraphy lacks anatomic details as sometimes necessary, e.g., for planning surgery; therefore, other anatomic imaging is usually required.

For decades, this additional anatomic imaging has been *IVU* – however, today, IVU has been replaced by ("anatomic") MRU wherever available (see below). If IVU needs to be performed, adapted pediatric protocols with reduced number of well-timed and properly focused films should be applied. It should be avoided before 6 weeks of age, and contrast amount as well as radiography dose settings needs to be adapted to the patient's age and weight (Riccabona et al. 2010).

There is no role for *CT* in infants and children with obstructive uropathy due to its high radiation burden, particularly if multiphase acquisitions are necessary because of the delay in the opacification of the collecting system.

Over the last years, *MRU* has been introduced into pediatric imaging. Using fast heavily T2-weighted (3D) sequences with breathhold or diaphragmatic triggering, the (dilated) plevocaliceal system and ureter can be exquisitely demonstrated; note that previous hydration as well as the administration of Frusemide is essential for an optimal filling (Sigmund et al. 1991; Nolte-Ernsting et al. 2001, 2003, Borthne et al. 2000,

2003, Grattan-Smith and Jones 2006). Additionally, Gadolinium (Gd) can be administered intravenously which then allows the assessment of renal and vascular anatomy, renal parenchymal contrast uptake, as well as excretion and drainage of Gd in a single nonionizing investigation; this investigation has practically replaced IVU for most pediatric queries (Avni et al. 2002; Riccabona et al. 2002; Perez-Brayfield et al. 2003 Rohrschneider et al. 2003; Riccabona et al. 2004; Boss et al. 2006). A further refinement of this technique is diuretic dynamic functional Gd-enhanced MRU which now allows assessing renal perfusion, function, and drainage (see Chap. 34). This offers an ideal "one-stop-shop" imaging approach which – using dedicated software and protocols – enables quantification of (split and overall) renal function and (to a certain extent) urinary drainage as well as ureteral peristalsis (Rohrschneider et al. 2000a, b; Grattan-Smith et al. 2003; Jones et al. 2004; Vivier et al. 2009). The base for this assessment is continuously and repeatedly acquired T1-weighted 3D gradient-echo sequences that need to have signal linearity with contrast concentration. The calculations are based on similar models as scintigraphy ("area under the curve technique" – also applicable for drainage assessment) (Rohrschneider et al. 2000a, b, 2002). Alternatively, the equation is based on an unidirectional 2-compartment model, using the abdominal aorta as the reference to define perfusion and thus defining parenchymal Gd handling after the deduction of the intravascular component ("Patlok plot" – restricted for drainage assessment) (Hackstein et al. 2003, 2005; Grattan-Smith et al. 2008a, b). However, availability of these methods is still restricted, they are not standardized or homogenized and have not spread out yet, and infants as well as small children will need sedation for the MR-study. Currently, efforts are undertaken to overcome some of these restrictions; software is being distributed on the internet, and recommendations for standardization are being prepared (Darge et al. 2009; Riccabona et al. 2010). Therefore, many envision MRU to be the major imaging tool for pediatric uroradiology – still, a comprehensive initial US and the differentiation of reflux-ive vs. obstructive disease (particularly, also in patients with megaureter) will remain indispensable. Due to its restrictions and availability, MRU is at present often used only for complex cases with complicated disease or scintigraphically equivocal findings with repeated follow-up examinations.

## 27.4.4 Imaging Algorithm in Obstructive Uropathy

In *megaureter*, US and ce-VUS or VCUG usually constitute the initial assessment. MAG3 scintigraphy is then used for the quantification of renal function and urinary drainage. Usually, these conditions do not need early intervention; thus, scintigraphy should be delayed until reliable values can be obtained (third to sixth month of life). Follow-up heavily relies on US – all investigations however need to be performed under standardized hydration (enabling conclusive comparisons). Besides measuring ureteral and pelvo-caliceal width with full and empty bladder and assessing potential renal parenchymal changes (such as parenchymal narrowing, cystic/dysplastic areas, increased parenchymal echogenicity, lack/vanishing of corticomedullary differentiation), observation of ureteral peristalsis can be crucial for therapy decisions (Fig. 27.13). Video-clip cine-loop documentation or m-mode US improves the comparison of peristalsis during follow-up and thus improves the detection of impairment or deterioration (i.e., increasing hyperperistalsis in the aggravation of stenosis, lack of peristalsis in adynamic-dysplastic megaureter segments or in ureteral exhaustion) (Riccabona et al. 1998). In complex conditions (e.g., duplex kidney, ectopic insertion), MRU is the modality of choice for additional imaging of (preoperative) anatomic and – by additional delayed acquisitions – drainage details (Avni et al. 1997; Gylys-Morin et al. 2000; Avni et al. 2001, 2002; Riccabona et al. 2004). Only rarely – in infected systems that do not respond to intravenous antibiotic treatment or in bilateral obstruction with renal failure – percutaneous nephrostomy under US-guidance needs to be performed (Riccabona et al. 2002). This access can then (after successful treatment) be used for antegrade pelvi-ureterography sometimes helping to decide between primary ureteral reinsertion or temporary diversion via ureterostomy. Conditions such as ureteroceles, segmental dysplasia, or severe cystic dysplastic kidneys that resemble multicystic dysplastic kidneys (MCDK) and are sometimes difficult to differentiate from chronically decompensated high-grade obstructive uropathy (and probably are just the other end of the same spectrum) are addressed in Chap. 11 (Fig. 27.14).

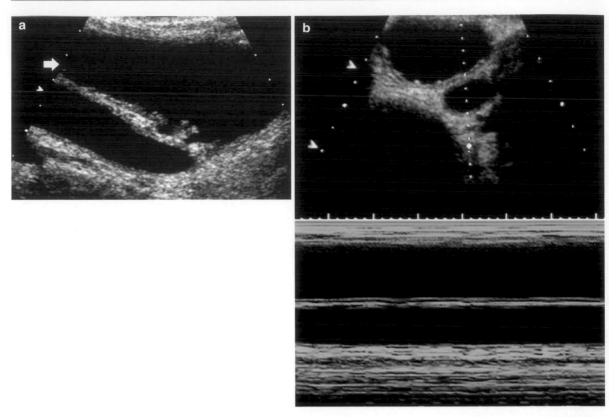

**Fig. 27.13** (**a**, **b**) US image of a megaureter with m-mode trace. US demonstrates a parasagittal view of a megaureter behind the grossly trabeculated (neurogenic) bladder (*arrow*) (**a**), without any sign of peristalsis as documented by the m-mode trace (**b**) obtained through the megaureter on an axial view through the bladder

**Fig. 27.14** (**a–c**) Imaging in multicystic dysplastic kidneys (MCDK). (**a**, **b**) Longitudinal (**a**) and axial (**b**) US image of a MCDK, with some dysplastic residual parenchyma and many cysts of varying size. (**c**) MR-urography (MRU) (maximum intensity rendering of a heavily T2-weighted 3D-sequence with additional editing) of an atypical MCDK with depictable ectopically inserting dysplastic megaureter draining into the partially fluid-filled vagina (*arrow*)

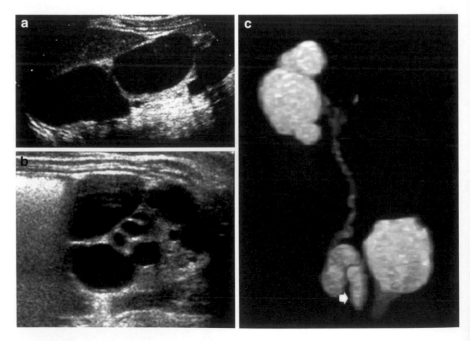

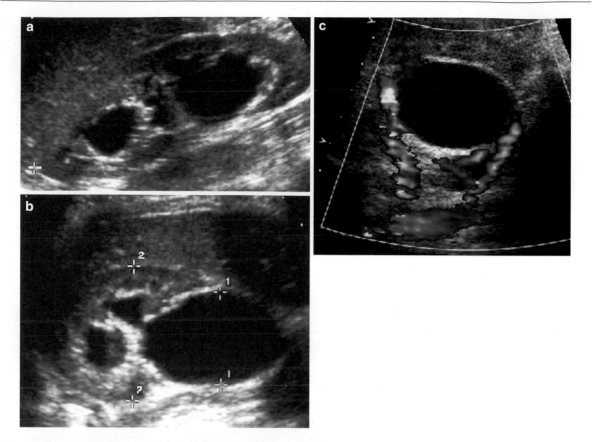

**Fig. 27.15** (**a–c**) US in ureteropelvic junction obstruction. Longitudinal and axial US section of the right kidney (**a, b**) in a 10-year-old boy demonstrates a hydronephrosis IV° with dilated pelvis and calices as well as some parenchymal narrowing. CDS (**c**) in the same kidney reveals an additional renal artery, crossing the ureteropelvic junction causing this "juvenile" extrinsic pelvi-ureteric junction obstruction

In ureteropelvic junction obstruction, US again is the workhorse of routine imaging, as detailed above (Fig. 27.15). VCUG (or ce-VUS) is recommended as a part of the initial workup. However, due to the intrinsic methodical restrictions of US, additional functional imaging by MAG3 scintigraphy or diuretic MRU is mandatory – initially for establishing the final diagnosis (if possible, avoid functional studies before the third month of life) (Fig. 27.16). Thereafter, during follow-up, particularly if US shows deterioration or other significant unexplainable changes, repeated functional studies may become necessary. A basic imaging algorithm has been recommended recently trying to address this common query (Riccabona et al. 2009). The necessity for preoperative imaging depends on the surgeon and the provided US quality – in many centers, high-end US that reliably answers important questions such as the existence of an additional crossing vessel or a small upper duplex system suffices, and only in complex anatomy, additional anatomic imaging is deemed necessary – preferably by MRU.

## 27.5 Childhood Urolithiasis and Nephrocalcinosis
(see also Chap. 15)

### 27.5.1 Urolithiasis

Urolithiasis is a less common complaint in children, with a strong geographic variation. It is defined as

**Fig. 27.16** MRU in ureteropelvic junction obstruction. (**a**) 3D-maximum intensity rendering of a heavily T2-weighted sequence demonstrating the anatomy of the collecting and draining urinary system, particularly, the dilated pelvocaliceal system of the right kidney with mild ureteropelvic junction obstruction and the urine filled ureters and urinary bladder after Furosemide i.v.; other fluid structures such as the spinal fluid are also visualized and not subtracted or edited. (**b**) Dynamic MRU (fast T1-weighted gradient-echo sequence (T1-GRE) after Gadolinium (Gd) application) – early phase: This arterial phase can be used for angiographic reconstruction of the major vessels, i.e., the abdominal aorta and the renal arteries. (**c**) Dynamic MRU (T1-GRE) – 10 min after Gd: The left system including the entire left ureter is well contrasted, whereas, there is filling of only the right dilated renal pelvis and no contrast drainage into the right ureter. (**d**) Dynamic MRU (T1-GRE) – after intermittent emptying of the bladder, 20 min after Gd application and 10 min after diuretic stimulation: The normal left system has drained, whereas, the right kidney exhibits increasing dilatation, ballooning of the renal pelvis, and insufficient contrast drainage into the right ureter in this girl with severe UPJO (the corresponding MAG3 study showed complete obstruction)

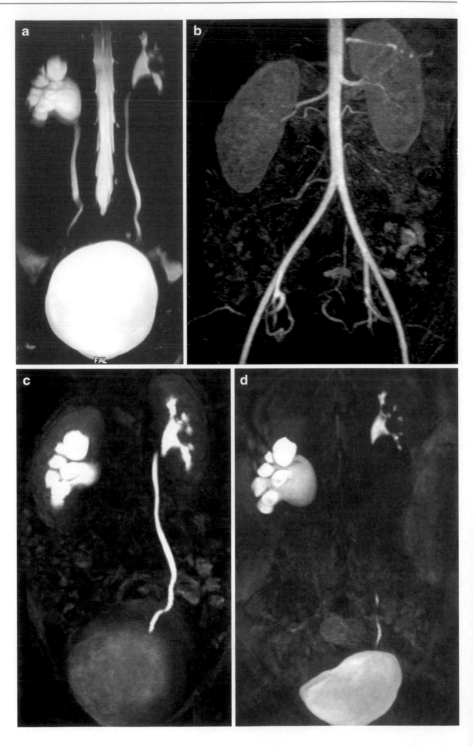

macroscopic calcification in the collecting system. Urinary stones consist of crystal agglomerations, sometimes mixed with proteins. In children, common causes are infection, hypercalciuria, cystinuria or oxaluria, as well as low citrate excretion, drugs, and metabolic disorders (e.g., Bartter syndrome). They form in the kidney, the ureter, and the bladder, the latter becoming increasingly uncommon due to the early detection of the underlying conditions. Symptoms can be unspecific particularly in infants; therefore,

US as the first imaging step is used generously. The vast majority of urinary calculi can be detected by US, particularly at the most common sites of obstruction – i.e., the ureteropelvic and the vesicoureteric junction, provided a sufficiently filled bladder and appropriate scanning technique and equipment are available (Fig. 27.17).

The typical *US* appearance is a hyperechoic focus with dorsal shadowing and upstream dilatation of the collecting system; particularly, infectious or proteinaceous "stones" may also be less echogenic or have less shadowing, whereas echogenic papillae may cause shadowing-like appearance without calcification (i.e., marginal shadowing artifact). Stones in the bladder and the kidney can be differentiated from other echogenic structures by positioning maneuvers. An acutely obstructed kidney usually exhibits little distension of the pelvocaliceal system, potentially echoes within due to hematuria, and sometimes, a thickened and edematous wall can be observed. The kidney is swollen and enlarged, may have an asymmetrically increased echogenicity, and a diffusely altered corticomedullary differentiation. On Doppler US, there may be peripheral vessel rarefaction and elevated resistive index values. Furthermore, color Doppler US will show sparkling undirectional color signals at the concrement known as the "twinkling sign," particularly useful for finding distal ureteral stones (Darge and Heidemeier 2006). Note that not all stones twinkle, and that not everything that twinkles is a stone – other reverberation artifacts from gas or noncalcified deposits may also cause a similar color Doppler US phenomenon. The most important aspect, however, is the proper visualization of the crucial parts, i.e., the distal ureter through the full bladder, the area of the ureteral crossing of the iliac vessel, and the pelvi-ureteral junction (Fig. 27.18).

An *abdominal radiograph* (KUB) often completes the assessment, though, particularly, poorly calcified small stones in the distal ureter may be missed.

*IVU* is hardly necessary for urolithiasis in children; sometimes, a focused and adapted IVU (only two or three well-timed films) may become necessary for the assessment of coexisting anatomic variations or for planning lithotripsy (Riccabona et al. 2010).

The unenhanced "stone uro-CT" as commonly used in adults is reserved for complicated cases, where all other imaging cannot sufficiently reveal all therapeutically necessary aspects (Smergel et al. 2001; Strouse et al. 2002; Maudgil and McHugh 2002; Akay et al. 2006). This is not only for radiation protection but also, because the small concrements with little calcification (as more often observed in children) and less fat surrounding the child's ureter (thus reducing contrast and obviating ultralow-dose CT protocols) may not be visualized. Follow-up depends on the initial findings – preferably US is applied. Contrast-enhanced 3D-MRU can be used to provide the necessary anatomic information for planning percutaneous lithoapraxy, and in future, *MRI* may probably become more important also for this condition.

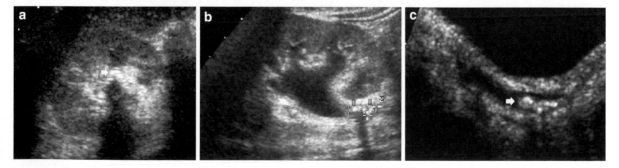

**Fig. 27.17** (**a–c**) US demonstration of urolithiasis (**a**) Axial US image with echogenic material (*arrow*) filling the renal pelvis with dorsal shadowing. (**b**) A longitudinal image demonstrates urolithiasis in the proximal ureter at the pelvi-ureteric junction with acoustic shadowing (+…+) and dilated collecting system as well as thickened pelvic wall. (**c**) Parasagittal US of the dilated distal ureter acquired through the sufficiently filled urinary bladder depicts echogenic intraureteral material (*arrow*) with only little shadowing in after lithotripsy

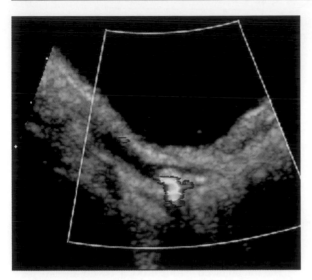

**Fig. 27.18** Twinkling sign in urolithiasis. Same patient as in Fig. 27.17c: Color Doppler US reveals moderate "twinkling" of the distal ureteral concrement

## 27.5.2 Nephrocalcinosis

Nephrocalcinosis is a (microscopic) renal tubular or interstitial renal calcification. Depending on the location, a medullary, cortical, or diffuse type is differentiated. In a variety of diseases, urolithiasis and nephrocalcinosis occur simultaneously, and then, usually urolithiasis is a sequalae of the underlying disease. There is a long list of conditions causing nephrocalcinosis; for cortical nephrocalcinosis, the most important causes are chronic hypercalcemia, primary hyperoxaluria, sickle cell disease (also medullar, called "sickle cell nephropathy"), acute cortical necrosis, and intoxication. Important causes for medullary nephrocalcinosis are ACTH therapy, adrenal insufficiency, hypercalciuria and hyperoxaluria, hyperparathyroidism or hyper-/hypothyroidism, drugs (furosemide, dexamethasone), medullary sponge kidney, long-time parenteral nutrition or ascorbic acid supplementation, various syndromes (Bartter, Cushing, Lesch–Nyhan, Lowe, William, Wilson disease) and distal renal tubular acidosis, granulomatous diseases, Tyrosinemia, Vitamin D or A intoxication, as well as neoplasms (with bone metastasis). It may also occur (or just manifest as urolithiasis) in chronic malabsorption syndromes such as celiac disease or cystic fibrosis (Jequier and

Kaplan 1991; Benz-Bohm and Hoppe 2008; Karlowicz and Adelman 1998).

*US* is the major imaging tool that is very sensitive to early changes and also allows staging and classification of nephrocalcinosis, although with some interobserver variations (Dick et al. 1999) (Table 27.2). The striking (early) finding is an increased echogenicity of the corticomedullary bounder or the medullae; sometimes small tubular deposits may be seen (Fig. 27.19). US shows these findings much earlier than they show on radiographs. When nephrocalcinosis progresses, parenchymal echogenicity increases and shadowing of calculi and calcified medullae may obscure the deeper kidney compartments, potentially needing CT or MRI for the assessment of treatable conditions of the collecting system (e.g., chronic infection in obstructed calices, xanthogranulomatous pyelonephritis, etc.). In neonates, it may be difficult to differentiate early nephrocalcinosis from the physiologically increased echogenicity of the (prepapillary) medullae due to proteinous deposits that usually clear by the end of the second month of life; if additional medication or intensive care treatment and parenteral nutrition or diuretics are needed, these transient findings may become permanent and even cause papillary obstruction and necrosis (Fig. 27.20) (Haller et al. 1982; Hufnagel et al. 1982; Jacinto et al. 1988; Perale et al. 1988; Nakamura et al. 1999). Other most important differential diagnoses are all conditions that may cause an increased renal echongenicity such as dehydration, acute pyelonephritis, renal vein thrombosis, (chronic) glomerulonephritis, hemolytic-uremic syndrome, acute transplant rejection, hypodysplasia as in Alport syndrome, or the physiologically higher echogenicity of the medullae in neonates (Riebel et al. 1993; Katz et al. 1994; Karlowicz and Adelman 1998; Riccabona and Fotter 2006; Riccabona et al. 2008; Riccabona and Ring 2008).

**Table 27.2** US grading of nephrocalcinosis (Dick et al. 1999)

| Grade I | Mild increase in echogenicity around the border of the medullary pyramids |
|---|---|
| Grade II | Mild diffuse increase in echogenicity of the medullary pyramids |
| Grade III | Greater, more homogeneously increased echogenicity of the entire medulla |

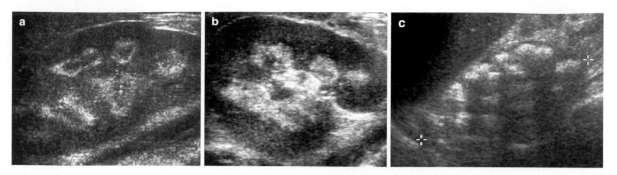

**Fig. 27.19** (**a–c**) US appeerence of nephrocalcinosis. US images of nephrocalcinosis: initial stage with increased echogenicity at the corticomedullary border (stage I, **a**), with a completely echogenic medulla (stage II, **b**), or with echogenic medullae and adjacent cortex, with, practically, only a small parenchymal rim left uncalcified (in a child with oxaluria, stage II–III, **c**)

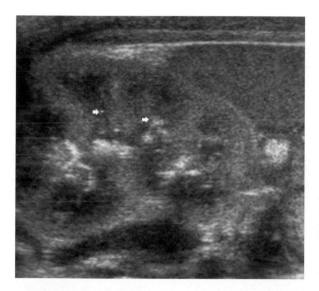

**Fig. 27.20** US: Echogenic papilla in a neonate after furosemide therapy. Note the partially longitudinal, partly patchy echogenicities in the distal prepapillary tubules (*arrows*) in the preterm neonate after long-term intensive care, consistent with clacification after furosemide

## 27.6 Pediatric Renovascular Disorders (General Renovascular Disorders) (see Chap. 18)

### 27.6.1 Pediatric Renal Artery Stenosis

There are a few major entities that are specifically important in children – (neonatal) renal vein thrombosis, traumatic or iatrogenic injuries to the renal vasculature, and hemolytic-uremic syndrome. All other entities are very similar to adult conditions. In children, *renal artery stenosis* is usually caused by vasculopathy and not arteriosclerosis, often being situated intrarenally, often multiple and peripheral, and thus less accessible to noninvasive imaging such as US or MR angiography/CT angiography (MRA/CTA). This necessitates a (slightly) different approach to imaging children with suspected renal hypertension that starts with a comprehensive US, includes a detailed Doppler study of extrarenal and major intrarenal arteries, and then – in profound suspicion, particularly if an interventional treatment by balloon angioplasty is anticipated – directly goes to conventional catheter angiography, thus often avoiding Captopril scintigraphy and CTA – their role as well as the value of MRA in childhood hypertension is currently under debate.

### 27.6.2 The Hemolytic-Uremic Syndromes

The *hemolytic-uremic syndromes* are a heterogeneous group of similar entities with variable severity (Riccabona 2008). Pathogenetically, renal endothelial cell injury leads to platelet activation and intravascular coagulation resulting in hemolytic anemia with fragmented erythrocytes, thrombocytopenia, and renal failure. The typical form of shiga toxin-associated hemolytic-uremic syndromes occurs mainly in childhood by infection with entero-hemorrhagic strains of *Escherichia coli* or *Shigella dysenteriae* and is the most common cause of acute renal failure in this age (Repetto 1997; Rondeau and Peraldi 1996). Extrarenal symptoms are quite common, too. Other causes of "atypical" hemolytic-uremic syndromes are familial or genetic, often the result of coagulopathies, vasculopathies, or complement deficiencies (e.g., systemic lupus erythematosus, lupus anticoagulant syndrome, cancer, glomerulonephritis, pregnancy, vonWillebrand factor deficiency, thrombotic thrombocytopenic purpura). Imaging relies on *US*. It usually shows (in the full stage) enlarged echogenic kidneys with small medullae, accentuated corticomedullary differentiation, ascites, and possibly, signs of enterocolits. On Doppler US, the renal perfusion alterations are depicted by reduced (peripheral) vasculature on power Doppler US (corresponding to the degree of renal failure) and increased resistive index values on spectral Doppler flow analysis that indicate the severity of renal involvement (Garel et al. 1983; Hoyer 1996;

Platt et al. 1990, 1991; Riccabona 2006, 2008). Improvement of Doppler findings may predict relapse or improvement before laboratory parameters change and may even serve for prognostic considerations (Scholbach 1999).

### 27.6.3  Renal Vein Thrombosis

(Neonatal) *renal vein thrombosis* may start peripherally; the central renal vein may still be patent in early stages. Then only focal changes may occur; before the kidney starts to increase due to congestive changes and will exhibit diffusely increased echogenicity, the resistive index is then increased, with better identification of these changes by high-frequency transducers (Wright et al. 1996). One may find venous flow disturbances such as increased flow velocity and spectral broadening in partially thrombosed veins. In central renal vein thrombosis, no venous flow can be

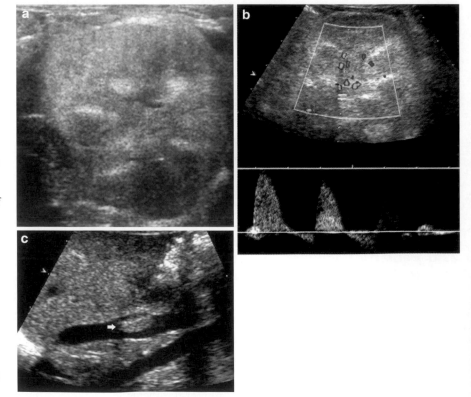

**Fig. 27.21** (**a–c**) Typical US appearance of (neonatal) renal vein thrombosis. (**a**) An axial US image shows the swollen and enlarged echogenic kidney with loss of corticomedullary differentiation. (**b**) The Doppler study depicts a reversed diastolic arterial flow, confirmed by spectral duplex Doppler US analysis. (**c**) The renal vein thrombus (*arrow*) is visualized reaching into the inferior vena cava as demonstrated by the echogenic mass within the inferior cava vein in this coronal US image at the level of the renal vein entrance

visualized; sometimes, the thrombus may extend into the inferior cava vein (Fig. 27.21). Doppler US can then demonstrate regression of the thrombus and improvement of arterial perfusional waveforms during treatment, much earlier than clinical improvement or regression of gray scale findings occur (Hoyer 1996; Bökenkamp et al. 2000).

### 27.6.4 Other Pediatric Vascular Conditions

Other conditions deal with usually congenital vascular variations that may cause or be associated with renal sequalae:

- *An accessory renal artery* is quite common, and only in part associated with ureteropelvic junction obstruction (depending on its course relative to the pelvi-ureteric junction). Using modern US equipment, Color Doppler US depicts most of them and usually allows following them till their origin from the abdominal aorta, with adequate scanning technique and dedicated search.
- *Venous drainage problems* may occur in conjunction with cava vein anomalies or obstruction, but are rare, and additional renal veins usually do not cause problems.
- A *retroaortal left renal vein* can cause nutcracker syndrome if the left renal vein is compressed significantly. Venous congestion of the left kidney then causes intermittent hematuria, proteinuria, and pain (Fig. 27.22). The left kidney is asymmetrically enlarged, the left renal vein exhibits marked changes in diameter at the aortal crossing and elevated velocity of the turbulent flow, with arterialized pulsatility due to the propagation of the pulsation of the abdominal aorta. If the left renal vein crosses in normal preaortal position, but has to pass through a narrow gap between the superior mesenteric artery and the aorta and then may exhibit similar findings as detailed above, this phenomenon is called "renal superior mesenteric artery syndrome" (Scholbach 1999). If venous drainage is impaired too much, it may become directed towards the ovarian vein and the deep pelvic vessels causing the pelvic congestion syndrome.

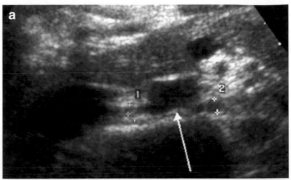

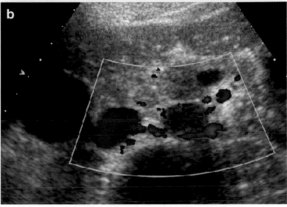

**Fig. 27.22** (**a**, **b**) Retroaortal left renal vein – US with color Doppler US. Axial middle abdominal scan on gray-scale US (**a**) and color Doppler US (**b**) showing a retroaortal crossing (*arrow*) of the left renal vein (+...+[1,2]) and its drainage into the inferior cava vein

## 27.7 Renal Neoplasms in Childhood (see also Chaps. 20–26)

The role of imaging in the query "renal tumor" in children has changed. Initially, imaging was just a tool to discover tumors, mostly using US and IVU. Today, imaging has evolved and plays a major role also in childhood neoplasms, for classification and staging, or by offering all preoperatively necessary information – particularly for modern surgical approaches such as nephron-sparing surgery. Though modern imaging by MRI (or CT) offers information regarding tumor entity, histology remains irreplaceable to establish the final diagnosis.

There are many different pediatric renal tumors – benign conditions (such as harmatoma and angiomyolipoma, mesoblastic nephroma, ossifying renal tumor of infancy, metanephric adenoma, or juvenile reninoma), pre- or semimalignant neoplasms such as nephroblastomatosis or cystic nephroma. Wilms' tumor and its precursors are the most common renal neoplasm in children and thus the most important entity in childhood (Riccabona 2003). There is a long list of other malignant renal tumors including clear cell sarcoma, malignant rhabdoid tumor, renal cell or renal medullary carcinoma, and lymphoma or leukemia. Renal PNET, renal metastasis, or renal transitional cell carcinoma as well as renal rhabdomyosarcoma are extremely rare in infancy, do not exhibit any specific imaging features, and therefore, shall not be discussed in detail.

For all oncology imaging, a close collaboration between pediatric radiologists, pediatricians, and pediatric/oncologic surgeons is essential, and international oncologic protocols provide guidelines for imaging workup allowing an interinstitutional comparison not only for research, but also for second opinion statements as well as multicenter therapy evaluation; these have to be considered when planning imaging for pediatric renal tumor conditions. US, including Doppler sonography, remains the first modality for investigating suspected renal masses, MRI is presently considered the gold standard for further workup, with a limited role of CT in staging and when MRI is not available or contraindicated. Increasingly, modern MRI applications such as perfusion studies, diffusion weighted imaging, whole body MRI, and MR-spectroscopy will become important for initial assessment as well as for follow-up of renal masses, e.g., for the assessment of chemotherapy response or metastasis (Humphries et al. 2008; Darge et al. 2008; Avni and Riccabona 2010).

### 27.7.1  Imaging Benign Renal Tumors in Children

*Angiomyolipoma* is rare in children as isolated hamartomatous lesions, but very common in children with tuberous sclerosis. In tuberous sclerosis, there are usually bilateral, small, and multifocal lesions. Angiomyolipoma consists of fat, smooth muscle, and vessels, and have a tendency to aneurysm formation and spontaneous bleeding, particularly when larger than 3 cm (Steiner et al. 1993). On US they appear hyperechoic. On CT, a specific diagnosis of the often cortical heterogeneous lesions can be made if the mass

contains fat (then measuring <20 HU on a 120 KV scan). Vascular elements within may enhance after i.v. contrast medium injection making density measurements less reliable, as well as different kilovolt settings as they impact HU measurements. Therefore – if an angiomyolipoma is suspected – an unenhanced CT scan or an MRI usually suffices; today, MRI should be the modality of choice for imaging and follow-up. The appearance on MRI varies with the composition – fatty components can be identified using fat suppression or chemical shift imaging techniques. Note that in children with known angiomyolipoma, any acute abdominal pain with hematuria should prompt an urgent US (or/and contrast-enhanced CT) to evaluate possible hemorrhage which can and needs to be treated by emergency intraarterial selective embolization, which may also be performed prophylactically in a large angiomyolipoma (Riccabona et al. 2002).

The most common renal neoplasm in neonates is *mesoblastic nephroma*, 60% of which are diagnosed during the first 3 months of life. Histologically, it predominantly consists of immature myofibroblasts. A more aggressive form, the "cellular variant," is considered a separate entity and characterized by dense fibroblastic proliferation; it also carries a 12–15 translocation identical to infantile fibrosarcoma (Chan et al. 1987). Usually, the tumor is detected prenatally or presents as a large abdominal mass; only rarely is it diagnosed secondary to unspecific symptoms such as hypertension or hypercalcemia. On US, the tumor is a large solid renal mass with low or mixed echogenicity; the residual renal parenchyma may present like a pseudocapsule (Fig. 27.23). On CT, it appears as a large uniform soft tissue mass replacing the majority of the renal parenchyma. It may extend beyond the capsule, but does not invade the renal vein, and generally enhances less than the renal parenchyma, although focal areas of strong enhancement may be present – then the tumor is indistinguishable from Wilms' tumor even on MR, particularly if areas of necrosis, fluid collections, or hemorrhage are present (Hartman et al. 1981; Christmann et al. 1990). Although it is considered a benign tumor with a generally excellent prognosis, nephrectomy is suggested as the appropriate radical treatment, and often just a preoperative US is needed without the need for any further imaging. Only the more aggressive subtype may develop local recurrence or metastases, thus prompting further imaging and follow-up (Schlesinger et al. 1995).

**Fig. 27.23** (a–c) US image of a nephroblastic nephroma. (**a, b**) Axial and longitudinal US section using a high-resolution linear transducer of the right kidney in a neonate demonstrating the mesoblastic nephroma (+...+[1,2]):the gas nearly replaced the entire kidney, with some residual parenchyma that appears like a pseudocapsule (+...+[3]). (**c**) Color Doppler US shows the renal vessels and their course along the tumor (+...+), also with some color signal within the tumor

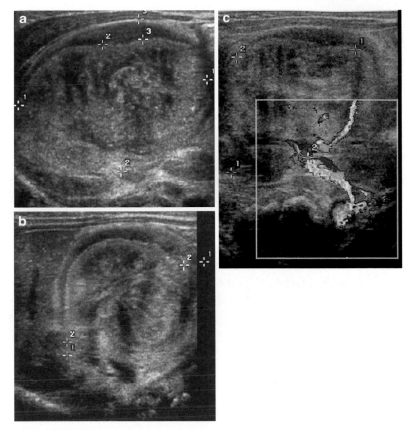

All other benign tumors are rare in infancy, but, particularly, later on need to be considered for the differential diagnosis of renal masses. They are often unspecific on imaging, and treated by enucleation or partial nephrectomy. *The ossifying renal tumor of infancy* occurs during the first year of life and appears as a (partially) calcified renal hamartomatous soft tissue mass arising from the renal medulla; it commonly occupies parts of the collecting system causing obstruction and hematuria (Riccabona 2002). Histologically, it consists of osteoid elements, osteoblasts, and spindle cells. As US is restricted by the calcified mass, abdominal plain film and CT are necessary for diagnostic workup. *Metanephric adenoma* is another rare benign pediatric renal tumor with a female predominance, but it observed at any age (Davis et al. 1995; Navarro et al. 1999). It is composed of tubular and glomeruloid structures similar to embryonal epithelium. It is often discovered incidentally or by nonspecific signs, but has a high association with polycythemia. There are only few reports of imaging appearance. The sonographically well-circumscribed hypo- or hyperechoic mass is hyperdense on unenhanced CT – sometimes with punctuate calcifications – with less intense enhancement than the renal parenchyma. On MRI it appears isointense on T1- and T2-weighted sequences. *Reninoma (=juxtaglomerular cell tumor)* occur mainly in the second decade of life with hypertension and hyperaldosteronism. CT or MRI (combined with CTA/MRA) may be performed to appreciate the tumor's anatomic relation to the renal artery, as arterial compression is an important preoperative information (Agrawal et al. 1995). *Oncocytoma* – arising from the tubular cells – is very rare in childhood. On any imaging (US with Doppler, CT, or MRI), they exhibit a typical central scar with radiating vasculature, sometimes causing problems in differentiation against renal carcinoma which may present with central necrosis resembling that central scar. *Renal teratoma* is an extremely rare, usually benign entity found in adolescents and young adults. The well-defined tumor presents all the more or less typical features of any teratoma and may include mesenchymal or endothelial tissue, fat, calcifications, osseous structures, and cystic parts. As fat or calcifications may also occur in other tumors (even in Wilms' tumor), imaging-based differentiation may be difficult. Teratoma may undergo malignant transformation; thus, a thorough tumor enucleation or (partial) nephrectomy is recommended. *Renal lymphangiomatosis* is located either centrally around the pelvocaliceal system or in the periphery, at the renal capsule and perirenal space. It is a multiloculated connected cystiform mass compressing and distorting the adjacent structures, but not invasive or destructive. Treatment often consists of partial resection and unroofing to reduce the local compression of adjacent structures. Other benign renal and pararenal masses (lipoma, fibroma, mesenchymal or hemangiomatous tissue …) may occur in conjunction with syndromatic disease or genetic predisposition (e.g., von Hippel Lindau, tuberous sclerosis, neurofibromatosis, prune-belly syndrome, megazystis-microcolon-hypoperistalsis syndrome). The role of imaging in these conditions is detection and follow-up, and to rule out malignancy – which sometimes is achievable only by biopsy or surgery.

## 27.7.2 Indeterminate Renal Masses

*Multilocular cystic nephroma* often occurs in male children less than 4 years of age (and adult females);

they can be completely benign or even very malignant (Agrons et al. 1995). The histological subtypes as well as other cystic renal lesion, even cystic nephroblastoma, are indistinguishable on imaging. Characteristically, the multiloculated cystic mass has a capsule on MRI, CT, or US, and may involve the entire organ or just part of the kidney (="segmental" cystic nephroma) (Fig. 27.24). There may be solid tissue stripes or thickened septae with atypical echogenicity and irregular borders as well as some minimal atypical vasculature on (a) Color Doppler US that may show enhancement on MRI or CT and thus may indicate a more malignant lesion. Nephrectomy is recommended because of the lesion's possible malignant potential.

*Nephroblastomatosis* is defined as the presence of multiple nephrogenic rests (persisting embryonic renal parenchyma = metanephric blastema) and are thought to represent maturation failure of fetal tissue. It is seen in 25% of children with unilateral, and in all with bilateral Wilms' tumors, and occurs as uni- or multifocal as well as diffuse forms (Lonergan et al. 1998a, b). Other associations are hemihypertrophy, sporadic aniridia, Denis Drash and Beckwith–Wiedermann or Perlman syndrome which all are also associated with Wilms' tumors.

US may usually depict cortical ovaloid to spherical areas with subtle changes in echogenicity and echostructure, disrupting the regular corticomedullar differentiation or cortical echo, sometimes with only little

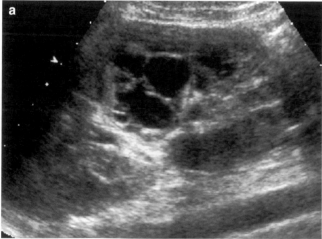
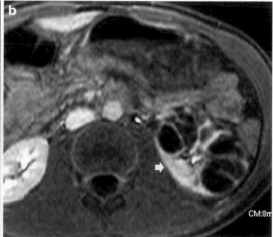
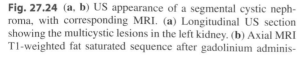

**Fig. 27.24** (**a**, **b**) US appearance of a segmental cystic nephroma, with corresponding MRI. (**a**) Longitudinal US section showing the multicystic lesions in the left kidney. (**b**) Axial MRI T1-weighted fat saturated sequence after gadolinium administration demonstrates the multicystic lesions with small septae and residual parenchyma (*arrow*), histologically proven to be a segmental cystic nephroma

mass effect; particularly, small lesions are easily missed. Doppler sonography and contrast-enhanced US improve sonographic depiction by demonstrating areas with atypical vessel architecture and reduced vascularity (Fig. 27.25). On CT and MRI, the abnormal tissue appears as homogeneously less-enhancing compared to the avidly enhancing normal kidney, and in most cases, may be differentiated from the typically heterogeneous and variably enhancing necrotic Wilms' tumors (Gylys-Morin et al. 1993). CT is better than US; however, MRI is probably the best tool for demonstrating these lesions that typically exhibit low signal relative to the renal cortex on T1-weighted sequences and are iso- to hyperintense on T2-weighted sequences (Rohrschneider et al. 1998; Schenk 2008). Small superficial plaques of nephroblastomatosis may be imperceptible, and differentiation against renal lymphoma may be difficult. Small metanephric rests are followed closely; if they grow or show signs of transformation, they may receive chemotherapy. Every doubtful entity should undergo either biopsy or enucleation.

### 27.7.3 Malignant Tumors

Imaging of malignant tumors usually uses a range of imaging modalities. Usually, US is the first modality and can often answer many questions on tumor location and size, local affected nodes, residual renal parenchyma, or urinary drainage obstruction; Doppler sonography provides a powerful tool to assess for renal vein thrombosis. However, for further staging MRI is generally preferred and widely accepted. CT would be more readily available, quicker, and easier to perform in small children (as the shorter duration of the examination reduces the need for sedation) and also will enable the evaluation of lung metastasis; but these children will undergo repeated investigations that add up to a considerable radiation burden over years. As MRI has become easier accessible for pediatric radiology, offers exquisite multiplanar multiphase imaging with superb visualization of all involved compartments (vessels, collecting system…), has improved imaging potential for tumor response assessment during follow-up, and is constantly improving also in the lung and as a whole body imaging modality, it has, in many places, replaced CT and is now considered the ideal imaging modality in imaging these conditions. The necessity of chest plain films is controversial. Skeletal metastasis is usually assessed by bone scintigraphy.

*Wilms' tumor (nephroblastoma)* is the commonest malignant abdominal neoplasm in children under the age of 9 years, with a peak at 2–3 years. It accounts for 12% of childhood cancers and 90% of pediatric renal tumors. It has a good prognosis due to efficient, well-

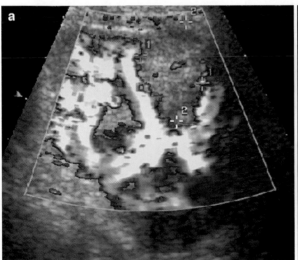
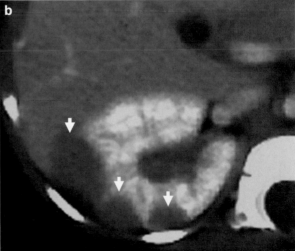

**Fig. 27.25** (**a**, **b**) Nephroblastomatosis. (**a**) Color Doppler US delineating conspicuously a focal hypovascular area (in relation to the normal renal parenchyma) consistent with a nephroblastomatotic focus (+…+) in a child with contralateral Wilms' tumor and bilateral nephroblastomatosis. (**b**) The nephrographic phase of a ce-CT delineates multiple cortical nephroblastomatotic foci (*arrows*)

established treatment strategies. At presentation, they are typically large and spherical, usually spare but compress and distort the collecting system. There are many different subtypes and forms – adult-mature, rhabdoid, teratoid. anaplastic, or cystic and necrotic (Schenk 2008). Prognosis varies with histology. They may be atypical; there are pre-and neonatal Wilms' tumors, and the tumor is associated with syndromes or genetic links (see above). In these risk patients, US-screening for Wilms' tumor is suggested until school age at approximately 6–12 months intervals, based on the hypothesis that tumor detection may decrease morbidity and permit curative nephron-sparing surgery.

US is excellent in depicting the solid, fairly well-defined tumor and its pseudocapsule, identifying the invasion of the adjacent organ (using real time) and the tumor thrombus extension into the renal vein or inferior cava vein (Bilal and Brown 1997; Riccabona 2003) (Fig. 27.26). US may show areas of hemorrhage, necrosis, or cysts. On MRI (or CT), Wilms' tumor appears heterogeneous, with slightly lower attenuation and hypointense on T1- as well as T2-weighting compared to the uninvolved renal cortex; it may exhibit different changes due to cystic components, hemorrhage, or necrosis. On T2-weighted sequences, it often has a hypointense (pseudo-)capsule. Contrast enhancement is heterogeneous and less than the normal parenchyma. Some tumors contain (usually curvilinear) calcifications, compared to the stippled calcification of neuroblastoma. CT and particularly MRI usually permit differentiation against nephroblastomatosis (Lowe et al. 2000; Ritchey et al. 1995; Babyn et al. 1995) and also

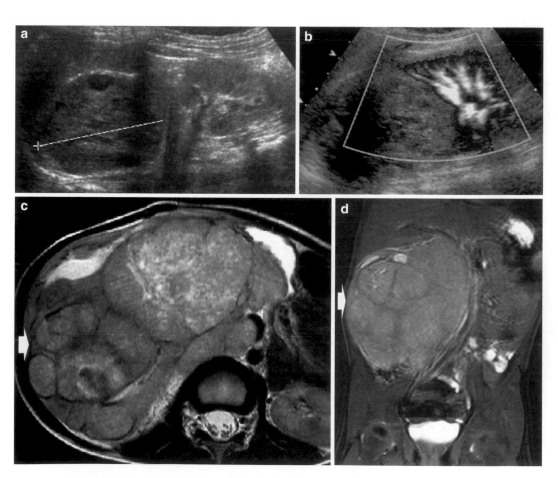

**Fig. 27.26** (a–d) US and MRI in Wilm's tumor. (a, b) Sagittocoronal extended view US of the left kidney documenting a partially cystic renal upper pole tumor (a), with the corresponding aCDS image (b) demonstrating the border between the Wilm's tumor and the residual unaffected renal parenchyma. (c, d) Axial (c) T2-weighted and coronal (d) SSFP sequence demonstrating a large Wilm's tumor (*arrow*), with its typical, but not specific appearance

against other common important tumors in this body region such as neuroblastoma. A definite classification, however, cannot be provided and histology is needed for final diagnosis. In the United States, surgery precedes chemo- and radiotherapy obviating initial biopsy. In Europe chemotherapy precedes surgery; thus chemotherapy is partially started without histology. However, biopsy before starting treatment is recommended in any case with doubt (clinically or by imaging features) concerning the tumor's histological entity (atypical age, invasion or destruction of adjacent organs, atypical calcifications …) – the indications for early biopsy as well as the biopsy technique (open vs. percutaneous) differ in various centers.

Staging is based on tumor extent and performed by imaging – in terms of lung assessment, there are some controversies whether chest films suffice or lung CT (or in the future, MRI of the lung) should be performed (Cohen 1996; Delemarre et al. 1996; Brisse 2009). Stage I tumors are restricted to the kidney, while stage II describes tumors that grow outside the kidney, but are confined. Local metastatic spread defines grade III. Stage IV includes tumors with systemic metastasis (usually to the lung), intraperitoneal rupture, or inferior cava vein thrombus. Stage V is reserved for patients with bilateral tumors.

*Clear cell sarcoma* occurs in 3–5-year-old children, and accounts for 4% of childhood renal neoplasms. It has a high metastatic potential, involving the skeleton, brain, lungs, or liver; thus, these patients require bone imaging (i.e., bone scintigraphy, complemented by MRI and plain films) (Geller et al. 1997). The bone metastases may be osteolytic, osteoblastic, or mixed. On sectional imaging, it appears as a solid mass with no specific imaging features, potentially with necrotic and cystic areas making it essentially indistinguishable from Wilms' tumor.

The extremely aggressive *malignant rhabdoid tumor* in infants accounts for 3% of pediatric renal neoplasms. Often, there is metastases to the lungs, the liver, the brain, and the skeleton at diagnosis; synchronous or metachronous neuroectodermal brain tumors may be associated. Imaging is unspecific except for a commonly observed (subcapsular or perinephric) peripheral crescentic fluid collection in the peritumoral space (representing subcapsular hemorrhage or peripheral tumor necrosis), and a thickened "pseudo-"capsule around the heterogeneous mass (Agrons et al. 1997).

*Renal cell carcinoma* accounts for less than 1% of pediatric renal tumors, occurs in slightly older patients (mean age 9 years, often girls), and otherwise does not differ from adult manifestation (see Chap. 21). On imaging, it is difficult to be distinguished from Wilms' tumor (Fig. 27.27a). Definitive diagnosis requires biopsy. Note that patients with Von Hippel Lindau disease and sickle cell anemia have an increased risk of developing renal cell carcinoma or pheochromocytoma.

*Renal medullary carcinoma* is an aggressive tumor of adolescents or young adults with sickle cell trait that carries an unfavorable prognosis due to poor response to treatment. Symptoms are hematuria, abdominal pain, weight loss, or fever. Usually, it is located centrally, invading the renal sinus. Imaging shows a

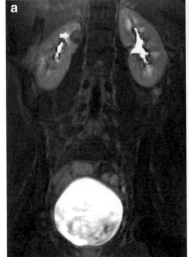
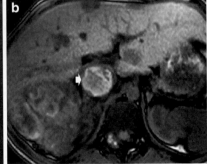

**Fig. 27.27** (**a**, **b**) Childhood renal carcinoma. (**a**) Coronal T1-weighted, contrast-enhanced MR image with fat saturation, late urographic phase: Note the relatively small, less-enhancing, slightly exophytic mass (*arrow*) in the median aspect of the upper third of the right kidney that proved to be a renal cell carcinoma in a 13-year-old girl. (**b**) Axial T1-weighted, contrast-enhanced MR image: A large, inhomogenously enhancing renal cell carcinoma with a nearly homogenously enhancing large tumor thrombus (*arrow*) in the inferior cava vein in a 16-year-old girl with renal cell carcinoma

heterogeneous mass with caliectasis and adjacent nodes; there may also be renal vein invasion (Fig. 27.27b).

The kidneys may also be affected by *lymphoma* which does not differ significantly from adults. The kidney may actually be a sanctuary site during the remission of lymphoma and *leukemia*. Renal leukemic involvement may present as multiple nodules of varying size, as diffuse renal infiltration, or as retroperitoneal infiltration with encasement of the kidney – the latter is difficult to be differentiated from retroperitoneal fribrosis by US, but usually distinguishable by MRI or CT. Typical US signs for the involvement are bilateral renal enlargement and loss of corticomedullary differentiation, sometimes inhomogeneous parenchymal pattern or slightly hypoechoic nodules; sometimes, nodular lesions may be depictable only by color Doppler US.

In conclusion, it becomes obvious that – though most of pediatric malignant renal tumors will be Wilms tumors – there are many entities that, at present, cannot be reliably differentiated by imaging; thus, histology remains irreplaceable. Imaging can serve for tumor detection, staging, and follow-up, and as a tool to provide preoperative anatomic information or image-guided biopsy.

## 27.8 Other Renal Parenchymal Disease and Miscellaneous Renal Disorders

There are many other renal conditions where imaging may vary from adult appearance and algorithm. All these conditions such as cystic renal diseases as well as other renal parenchymal diseases such as glomerulonephritis, nephrotic syndrome, renal involvement in systemic disease, or renal failure and renal transplant imaging are discussed in separate chapters and will not be addressed in detail (see Chaps. 12, 13, 26, 29, and 30). Some basic remarks concerning specific pediatric aspects in some of these conditions are provided here.

### 27.8.1 Pediatric Cystic Renal Disease

- A single cyst in a child should always prompt a follow-up and a family assessment, as this may be the manifestation of a familiar or syndromal cystic renal disease that may need surveillance and treatment.

- Any sonographically complicated cyst (i.e., large, multiple, septated, with echoes and sedimentations, nodular wall components, changing size or growing=Bosniak type ≥III) needs to be assessed for unusual entities such as a cystic tumor or caliceal diverticula, particularly if associated with clinical symptoms. The additional sectional imaging is preferably performed by contrast-enhanced MRU also including delayed postcontrast sequences.

- Not all cystic renal diseases exhibit cysts that can be visualized by imaging; particularly, neonatal autosomal recessive polycystic kidney disease creates an enlarged kidney with diffusely disturbed architecture due to the multiple microcysts (sonographically called the "salt and pepper" appearance) (Riccabona 2008). Similarly, no cysts are seen in glomerulocystic kidney disease or early stages of (segmental) medullary sponge kidneys.

## 27.8.2 Pediatric Renal Parenchymal Disease

Imaging appearance of glomerulonephritis and nephritic syndrome is often unspecific, and particularly Doppler findings often rather reflect the degree of renal insufficiency and systemic perfusion disturbance (partially treatment-related) than the specific underlying kidney disease. In most of these conditions, US is sufficient for imaging; sometimes MRI can be helpful (Riccabona 2008). IVU is not used for these queries any longer. Uro-CT should be used reluctantly in children not only due to radiation protection issues, but also because of potential contrast medium nephrotoxicity that could cause deterioration of an already impaired or endangered renal function (see Chap. 33).

Particularly in infants and young children, *renal biopsies* can cause *arteriovenous fistula*; when performed with large core-cut needles, we found arteriovenous fistulas in 12% of patients (Riccabona et al. 1998a, b). A smaller needle size of 20–16 gauge that is usually sufficient for nontumorous conditions helps to reduce the arteriovenous fistula incidence; rarely, a second or third pass is needed to harvest enough material. Proper pre-, peri-, and postinterventional imaging and management is advisable, not only to plan and monitor the procedure avoiding large vessels and a risky needle path, but also to detect potentially dangerous conditions. Furthermore, this management can either help prevent arteriovenous fistulas or support spontaneous resolution by avoiding medication that affects the renin-angiotensin-system, by good blood pressure management, as well as by prolonged immobilization and monitoring. A dedicated search for arteriovenous fistulas that may manifest hours and days after the intervention by Color Doppler sonography (with skilful setting of the various Doppler parameters to allow for the visualization of focal flow disturbances or acceleration, and thereafter confirmation of suspected findings by spectral Doppler analysis) is necessary to reliably depict or rule out any significant arteriovenous fistula, obviating other imaging (Fig. 27.28). If the arteriovenous fistula stays or becomes symptomatic, percutaneous transarterial embolization is the treatment of choice; in rare cases, preinterventional imaging by MRA may become necessary for supporting treatment decisions (see also Chaps. 7 and 9).

### 27.8.3  Acute and Chronic Renal Failure

As in adults, different forms of renal failure or insufficiency have to recognized (see also Chap. 29), per-, intra-, and postrenal, depending on its cause. The role of imaging is to help differentiating these entities by depicting specific changes such as bilateral high-grade obstruction (i.e., postrenal), systemic perfusional disturbance (i.e., prerenal), or signs for nephropathy such as an enlarged and swollen, echogenic kidney (also seen secondarily to severe acute hypoxic-ischemic injury) or bilateral cirrhotic kidneys (i.e., intrinsic or intrarenal). This is usually achieved by a detailed US study that always must include Doppler US assessment (Riccabona 2006). Specific pediatric conditions are perfusional impairment due to congenital cardiac malformations or a persisting ductus arteriosus of Botalli with high left to right shunt, the bilateral renal vein thrombosis (which in neonates may start peripherally and segmentally, and will grow only

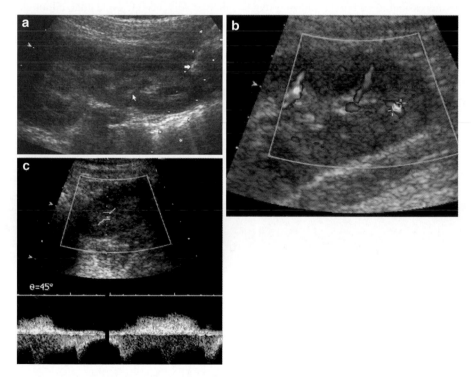

**Fig. 27.28** (**a–c**) Renal biopsy and Doppler US of a postbiopsy arteriovenous fistula. (**a**) Renal biopsy as documented by a sagittal still-frame image of the video loop of the procedure demonstrating the entrance of the core-cut needle (*arrows*) into the lower pole of the left kidney as indicated by the *dotted line* using a biopsy gun and the systems' biopsy guide device with the systems tracing software indicating the needle path by *two dotted lines*. (**b**) Color Doppler US image of the same area after biopsy depicting a relatively small arteriovenous fistula (+…+, arteriovenous fistula) as shown by the aliasing color signals in relation to the other renal vessels without aliasing. (**c**) Duplex Doppler trace at the arteriovenous fistula demonstrating relatively high flow velocities, particularly, a relatively high diastolic flow in the feeding artery, and a turbulent, slightly arterialized, and grossly accelerated venous flow in the draining vein

gradually and then eventually exhibit the typical thrombus in the main renal vein, and may be associated with adrenal gland hemorrhage), systemic hypoxia with renal involvement after birth asphyxia, severe bilateral congenital obstructive uropathy, or neonatal onset of infantile polycystic kidney disease or neonatal nephrotic syndrome ("finish type") and glomerulonephritis/glomerulocystic disease. Rarely, other imaging is necessary (only for the workup of congenital malformations or for the diagnosis of the underlying systemic disease), sometimes US-guided biopsy may become necessary to histologically establish the final diagnosis or prognosis. In some conditions, repeated US and Doppler follow-up studies help to predict renal recovery, as for example, in hemolytic-uremic syndrome, Doppler findings improve before clinical improvement can be noted. Basically, management of children with chronic renal failure does not differ from adults; however, particular notice has to be given to all the aspects that involve the growth potential and the child's nutritional needs for future unimpaired development, sometimes necessitating additional imaging (e.g., wrist radiograph).

### 27.8.4  Imaging in Childhood Renal Trauma

As in adults, severe renal and multiple trauma is imaged by (spiral MD-)CT after the "F.A.S.T." US examination

in the emergency room (see Chap. 19). All other situations are primarily addressed by a detailed US study that must always include Doppler sonography for the depiction of renal vascular impairment. Note that even a completely devascularized kidney (e.g., due to dissection of the main artery) will initially look normal on gray scale US, only Doppler US will reveal the lack of perfusion (Fig. 27.29). Power Doppler helps to depict focal renal lesions or perirenal hematoma, as in the early posttraumatic phase, the hemorrhage may still have the same echogenicity as the cortex making gray scale depiction more difficult. Always try to assess ureteral patency (by observing the ureteral jet into the bladder). As most of these conditions are managed conservatively, regular follow-up investigation are mandatory – unexplainable increase of particularly clear perirenal fluid may raise the suspicion of urinoma after caliceal or pelvic rupture. Then, with equivocal findings or results that are inconsistent with the child's clinical course, additional imaging becomes indicated – preferably by Gd-enhanced MRU, alternatively ce-CT. Note that although children stay, clinically, perfectly stable for a long time even with severe blood loss and substantial injury, all of a sudden they may deteriorate dramatically. Therefore, the initial US study should thoroughly assess all the relevant aspects and compartments to deliver all necessary information for deciding on further management needs and monitoring intensity. Joint European recommendations for imaging children after urinary tract trauma are just being developed and hopefully will be available next year.

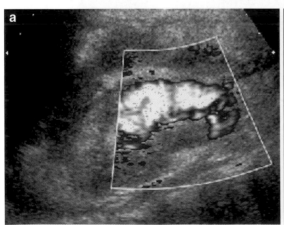
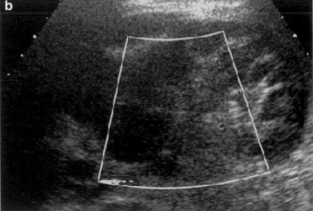
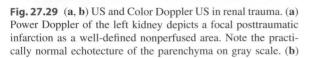

**Fig. 27.29** (**a**, **b**) US and Color Doppler US in renal trauma. (**a**) Power Doppler of the left kidney depicts a focal posttraumatic infarction as a well-defined nonperfused area. Note the practically normal echotecture of the parenchyma on gray scale. (**b**) Color Doppler US of the right kidney: no depictable color signals in the morphologically normal-looking kidney in a 14-year-old boy after a bicycle accident, consistent with a hilar disruption of a completely devascularised right kidney

## 27.9 Conclusion

In general, it is important to remember that children are not small adults, but are different: organs may be physiologically immature; congenital malformations are a common query; the normal findings are different from adults; and many diseases manifest differently, look differently, and may additionally impair renal growth potential, thus being more devastating than similar conditions in adults. They have a high radiation risk, need dedicated handling as well as equipment, and potential as well as practical application of the various imaging modalities differ. All these aspects impact imaging algorithms and procedural recommendations. US is the most commonly used (initial) imaging modality that can answer most queries. Additional imaging then depends on the clinical query and US findings. VCUG, scintigraphy, and MRI are the most important methods, while IVU is practically outdated for most situations and uro-CT is restricted to trauma conditions, acute hemorrhage, or – if MRI is unavailable – difficult queries such as complications or tumors. All these need special knowledge and training to naturally deliver the same high level of imaging quality that we all expect for ourselves and the general adult population. This can be acheived only if professionals with profound knowledge and training are made available for the care of pediatric patients.

## References

Agrawal R, Jafri SZ, Gibson DP et al. (1995) Juxtaglomerular cell tumor. MR findings: a case report. J Comput Assist Tomogr 19:140–142

Agrons GA, Kingsman KD, Wagner BJ et al. (1997) Rhabdoid tumor of the kidney in children: a comparative study of 21 cases. Am J Roentgenol 168:447–451

Agrons GA, Wagner BJ, Davidson AJ et al. (1995) Multilocular cystic renal tumor in children: radiologic-pathologic correlation. Radiographics 15:653–669

Akay H, Akpinar E, Ergun O et al. (2006) Unenhanced multi-detector. CT evaluation of urinary stones and secondary signs in pediatric patients. Diagn Interv Radiol 12:147–150

Alton DJ, LeQuesne GW, Gent R et al. (1992) Sonographically demonstrated thickening of the renal pelvis in children. Pediatr Radiol 22:426–429

Avni F, Bali MA, Regnault M et al. (2002) MR urography in children. Eur J Radiol 43:154–166

Avni FE, Matos C, Rypens F et al. (1997) Ectopic vaginal insertion of an upper pole ureter: demonstration by special sequences of MR imaging. J Urol 158:1931–1932

Avni FE, Nicaise N, Hall M et al.(2001) The role of MR imaging for the assessment of complicated duplex kidneys in children: preliminary report. Pediatr Radiol 31:215–223

Avni F, Riccabona M (2010) MR-imaging of the pediatric abdomen. In: Gourtsoyiannis N (ed) Clinical MRI of the abdomen. Springer, in press

Babyn P, Owens C, Gyepes M et al. (1995) Imaging patients with Wilms tumor. Hematol Oncol Clin North Am 9:1217–1252

Bartram U, Darge K (2005) Harmonic versus conventional ultrasound imaging of the urinary tract in children. Pediatr Radiol 35:655–660

Benz-Bohm G, Hoppe D (2008) Urolithiasis and nephrocalcinosis. In: Fotter R (ed) Pediatric uroradiolgy. Springer, Berlin, pp 281–286

Berrocal T, Gaya F, Arjonilla A et al. (2001) Vesicoureteral reflux: diagnosis and grading with echoenhanced cystosonography versus voiding cystourethrography. Radiology 221:359–365

Bilal MM, Brown JJ (1997) MR imaging of renal and adrenal masses in children. Magn Reson Imaging Clin N Am 5: 179–197

Bluemke DA, Breiter SN (2000) Sedation procedures in MR imaging: safety, effectiveness, and nursing effect on examinations. Radiology 216:645–652

Bökenkamp A, von Kries R, Nowak Göttl U et al. (2000) Neonatal renal venous thrombosis in Germany between 1992 and 1994: epidemiology, treatment and outcome. Eur J Pediatr 159:44–48

Borthne A, Pierre-Jerome C, Nordshus T et al. (2000) MR urography in children: current status and future development. Eur Radiol 10:503–511

Borthue AS, Pierre Jerome C, Gjesdal KI et al. (2003) Pediatric excretory MR urography: comparison study of enhanced and non enhanced techniques. Eur Radiol 13. 1423–1427

Bosio M (1998) Cystosonography with echocontrast: a new imaging modality to detect vesico-ureteric reflux in children. Pediatr Radiol 28:250–255

Boss A, Schaefer JF, Martirosian P et al. (2006) Contrast-enhanced dynamic MR nephrography using the TurboFLASH navigator-gating technique in children. Eur Radiol 16: 1509–1518

Brader P, Riccabona M, Schwarz T et al. (2008) Value of comprehensive renal ultrasound in children with acute urinary tract infection for assessment of renal involvement: comparison with DMSA scintigraphy and clinical diagnosis. Eur Radiol 18:2981–2989

Brenner DJ, Elliston CD, Hall EJ et al. (2001) Estimated risks of radiation-induced fatal cancer from pediatric CT. AJR 176:289–296

Brenner DJ, Hall EJ (2007) Computed tomography – an increasing source of radiation exposure. NEJM 357:2277–2284

Brisse HJ (2009) Staging of common paediatric tumors. Pediatr Radiol 39(suppl):S482–S490

Caldair AD, Hiorus MP, Abbuyantar A et al. (2007) CE-MRA for the detection of crossing vessels in children with symptomatic UPJ obstruction. Pediatr Radiol 37:356–361

Chan HS, Cheng MY, Mancer K et al. (1987) Congenital mesoblastic nephroma: a clinico-radiologic study of 17 cases representing the pathologic spectrum of the disease. J Pediatr
111:64–70

Chan Y, Chan K, Yeung G et al. (1999) Potential utility of MRI
in the evaluation of children at risk of renal scanning. Pediatr
Radiol 29:816–862

Christmann D, Becmeur F, Marcellin L et al. (1990) Mesoblastic
nephroma presenting as a haemorrhagic cyst. Pediatr Radiol
20:553

Claudon M, Cosgrove D, Albrecht T et al. (2008) Guidelines
and good clinical practice recommendations for contrast
enhanced ultrasound (CEUS) – update. Ultraschall Med 29:
28–44

Cohen MD (1996) Commentary: imaging and staging of Wilms'
tumor: problems and controversies. Pediatr Radiol 26:
307–311

Craig JC, Wheeler DM, Irwig L et al. (2000) How accurate is
DMSA scintigraphy for the diagnosis of acute pyelonephritis? A meta-analysis of experimental studies. J Nucl Med
41:986–993

Dacher JN, Pfister C, Monroc M et al. (1996) Power Doppler
sonographic pattern of acute pyelonephritis in children:
comparison with CT. Am J Roentgenol 166:1451–1455

Darge K, Grattan-Smith JD, Riccabona M. Pediatric uroradiology: state of the art. Pediatr Radiol 2010, in press

Darge K, Heidemeier A (2006) US diagnosis of urinary tract
calculi in children using the "Twinkling Sign". Ultrasound
14:167–173

Darge K, Jaramillo D, Siegel MJ (2008) Whole body MRI in
children: current status and future applications. Eur J Radiol
68:289–298

Darge K, Moeller RT, Trusen A et al. (2005) Diagnosis of vesicoureteric reflux with low-dose contrast-enhanced harmonic
ultrasound imaging. Pediatr Radiol 35:73–78

Darge K, Tröger J, Duetting T et al. (1999) Reflux in young
patients: comparison of voiding US of the bladder and the
retrovesical space with echo enhancement versus voiding
cystourethrography for diagnosis. Radiology 210: 201–207

Darge K, Troeger J (2002) Vesicoureteral reflux grading in contrast-
enhanced voiding urosonography. Eur J Radiol 43:122–128

Darge K, Zieger B, Rohrschneider W et al. (2001) Contrast-
enhanced harmonic imaging for the diagnosis of vesicoureteral
reflux in pediatric patients. Am J Roentgenol 177:1411–1415

Davis CJ Jr, Barton JH, Sesterhenn IA et al. (1995) Metanephric
adenoma. Clinico-pathological study of fifty patients. Am J
Surg Pathol 19:160–164

Delemarre JF, Sandstedt B, Harms D et al. (1996) The new SIOP
(Stockholm) working classification of renal tumours of
childhood. International Society of Paediatric oncology.
Med Pediatr Oncol 26:145–146

Dick PT, Shuckett BM, Tang B, Daneman A, Kooh SW (1999)
Observer reliability in grading nephrocalcinosis on ultrasound examinations in children. Pediatr Radiol 29:68–72

Fernbach SK, Feinstein KA, Schmidt MB (2000) Pediatric voiding cystourethrography: a pictorial guide. Radiographics
20:155–168

Fernbach SK, Maizels M, Conway JJ (1993) Ultrasound grading
of hydronephrosis: introduction to the system used by the
Society for Fetal Urology. Pediatr Radiol 23:478–480

Fotter R (2008) Nonneurogenic bladder sphincter dysfunction
("voiding dysfunction"). In: Fotter R (ed) Pediatric uroradiology, 2nd edn. Springer, Berlin, pp 271–294

Fotter R, Kopp W, Klein E et al. (1986) Unstable bladder in children: functional evaluation by modified VCUG. Radiology
161:811–813

Garel L, Habib R, Babin C et al. (1983) Hemolytic uremic syndrome. Diagnosis and prognostic value of ultrasound. Ann
Radiol 26:169–174

Gassner I, Geley T (2004) Imaging femal genital anomalies. Eur
Radiol 14(suppl 4):L107–L122

Geley TE, Gassner I (2008) Lower urinary tract anomalies of
urogenital sinus and female genital anomalies. In: Fotter R
(ed) Pediatric uroradiology, 2nd edn. Springer, Berlin,
pp 137–163

Gelfand MJ, Koch BL, Elgazzar AH et al. (1999) Cyclic cystography: diagnostic yield in selected pediatric populations.
Radiology 213:118–120

Geller E, Smergel EM, Lowry PA (1997) Renal neoplasms of
childhood. Radiol Clin North Am 35:1391–1413

Good CD, Vinnicombe SJ, Minty IL et al. (1993) Posterior urethral valves in male infants and newborns: detection with US
of the urethra before and during voiding. Radiology
198:387–391

Gordon I (2001) Diuretic renography in infants with prenatal
unilateral hydronephrosis: an explanation for the contro-
versy about poor drainage. BJU Int 87:551–555

Gordon I (2008) Diagnostic procedures: nuclear medicine.
In: Fotter R (ed) Pediatric uroradiology. Springer, Berlin,
pp 37–52

Gordon I, Colarinha P, Fettich J et al. (2000) Guidelines for indirect radionuclide cystography in children. Eur J Nucl Med
28:BP16–BP20

Gordon I, Colarinha P, Fettich J et al. (2000) Guidelines for standard and diuretic renogram in children. Eur J Nucl Med
28:BP21–BP30

Gordon I, Riccabona M (2003) Investigating the newborn kidney – update on imaging techniques. Semin Neonatol 8:
269–278

Grattan-Smith JD, Jones RA (2006) MR urography in children.
Pediatr Radiol 36:1119–1132

Grattan-Smith JD, Little SB, Jones RA (2008) MR urography in
children: now we do it. Pediatr Radiol 38(suppl 1):S3–S17

Grattan-Smith JD, Little SB, Jones RA (2008) MR urography
evaluation of obstructive uropathy. Pediatr Radiol 38(suppl 1):
S49–S69

Grattan-Smith JD, Perez-Bayfield MR, Jones RA et al. (2003)
MR imaging of kidneys: functional evaluation using F-15
perfusion imaging. Pediatr Radiol 33:293–304

Gylys-Morin V, Hoffer FA, Kozakewich H et al. (1993) Wilms
tumor and nephroblastomatosis: imaging characteristics at
Gadolinium-enhanced MR imaging. Radiology 188:
517–521

Gylys-Morin VM, Minevich E, Tackett LD et al. (2000)
Magnetic resonance imaging of the dysplastic renal moiety
and ectopic ureter. J Urol 164:2034–2039

Hackstein N, Heckrodt J, Rau WS (2003) Measurement of single-kidney glomerular filtration rate using a contrast-enhanced
dynamic gradient-echo sequence and the Rutland-Patlak plot
technique. J Magn Reson Imaging 18: 714–725

Hackstein N, Kooijman H, Tomaselli S et al. (2005) Glomerular filtration rate measured using the Patlak plot technique and contrast-enhanced dynamic MRI with different amounts of gadolinium-DTPA. J Magn Reson Imaging 22:406–414

Haller JO, Berdon WE, Friedman AP (1982) Increased renal cortical echogenicity: a normal finding in neonates and infants. Radiology 142:173–174

Hartman DS, Lesar MS, Madewell JE et al. (1981) Mesoblastic nephroma: radiologic-pathologic correlation of 20 cases. Am J Roentgenol 136:69–74

Hernandez RJ, Goodsitt MM (1996) Reduction of radiation dose in pediatric patients using pulsed fluoroscopy. AJR 167: 1247–1253

Hoyer PF (1996) Niere. In: Hoffmann V, Deeg KH, Weitzel D (eds) Ultraschall in Pädiatrie und Kinderchirurgie. Thieme, Stuttgart-New York, pp 340–381

Hufnagel KG, Khan SN, Penn D et al. (1982) Renal calcifications: a complication of long term furosemide therapy in preterm infants. Pediatrics 70:360–363

Humphries PO, Sebire NJ, Siegel MJ et al. (2008) Tumors in pediatric patients at diffusion-weighted MR imaging: apparent diffusion coefficient and tumor cellularity. Radiology 245:848–854

Jacinto JS, Modanlou HD, Crade MC et al. (1988) Renal calcification incidence in very low birth weight infants. Pediatrics 81:31–35

Jequier S, Kaplan BS (1991) Echogenic renal pyramids in children. J Clin Ultrasound 19:85–92

Jones RA, Perez-Brayfield MR, Kirsch AJ et al.(2004) Renal transit time with MR urography in children. Radiology 233:41–50

Kao SCS, Huda W, Frush DP (2005) Radiation and medical imaging in children. In: Carty H, Brunelle F, Stringer D et al. (eds) Imaging children, 2nd edn, vol I. Elsevier Science Publisher, New York, pp 3–44

Karlowicz MG, Adelman RD (1995) Renal calcification in the first year of life. Pediatr Clin North Am 42:1397–1413

Karlowicz MG, Adelman RD (1998) What are the possible causes of neonatal nephrocalcinosis? Semin Nephrol (US) 18:364–367

Katz ME, Karlowicz MG, Adelman RD et al. (1994) Nephrocalcinosis in very low birth weight neonates: sonographic patterns, histologic characteristics, and clininal risk factors. J Ultrasound Med 13:777–782

Kavanagh EC, Ryan S, Awan A et al. (2005) Can MRI replace DMSA in the detection of renal parenchymal defects in children with urinary tract infections? Pediatr Radiol 35: 275–281

Kenda RB, Novljan G, Kenig A et al. (2000) Echo-enhanced ultrasound voiding cystography in children: a new approach. Pediatr Nephrol 14:297–300

Koff SA (1982) Ureteropelvic junction obstruction: role of newer diagnostic methods. J Urol 127:898–900

Koff SA, Thrall JH, Keyes JW Jr (1979) Diuretic radionuclide urography: a non-invasive method for evaluating nephro-ureteral dilatation. J Urol 122:451–454

Lebowitz RL, Olbing H, Parkkulainen KV et al. (1985) International Reflux Study in children: International system of radiographic grading of vesico-ureteric reflux. Pediatr Radiol 15:105–109

Lebovic SJ, Lebowitz RL (1980) Reducing patient dose in voiding cystourethrography. Urol Radiol 2:103–107

Lonergan GJ, Martinez-Leon MI, Agrons GA et al. (1998) Nephrogenic rests, nephroblastomatosis, and associated lesions of the kidney. Radiographics 18:947–968

Lonergan GJ, Pennington DJ, Morrison JC et al. (1998) Childhood pyelonephritis: comparison of gadolinium-enhanced MR imaging and renal cortical scintigraphy for diagnosis. Radiology 207:377–384

Lowe LH, Isuani BH, Heller RM et al. (2000) Pediatric renal masses: Wilms tumor and beyond. Radiographics 20: 1585–1603

Mandell GA, Eggli DF, Gilday DL et al. (1997) Procedure guideline for radionuclide cystography in children. Society of Nuclear Medicine. J Nucl Med 38:1650–1654

Maudgil DD, McHugh K (2002) The role of computed tomography in modern paediatric uroradiology. Eur J Radiol 43: 129–138

Nakamura M, Yokota K, Chen C et al. (1999) Hyperechoic renal papillae as a physiological finding in neonates. Clin Radiol 54:233–236

Navarro O, Conolly B, Taylor G et al. (1999) Metanephric adenoma of the kidney: a case report. Pediatr Radiol 29: 100–103

Nolte-Ernsting CC, Adam GB, Gunther RW (2001) MR urography: examination techniques and clinical applications. Eur Radiol 11:355–372

Nolte-Ernsting CCA, Straty G, Tacke J et al. (2003) MR urography today. Abdom Imaging 28:191–209

Oguzkurt L, Karabulut N, Haliloglu M et al. (1997) Medullary nephrocalcinosis associated with vesicoureteral reflux. Br J Radiol 70.850–851

O'Reilly PH, Lawson RS, Shields RA et al. (1979) Idiopathic hydronephrosis – the diuresis renogram: a new non-invasive method of assessing equivocal pelvioureteral junction obstruction. J Urol 121:153–155

O'Reilly PH, Lupton EW, Testa HJ et al. (1981) The dilated non-obstructed renal pelvis. Br J Urol 53:205–209

O'Reilly PH, Testa HJ, Lawson RS et al. (1978) Diuresis renography in equivocal urinary tract obstruction. Br J Urol 50: 76–80

Paltiel H, Rupich R, Kiruluta G (1992) Enhanced detection of VUR in infants and children with use of cycling VCUG. Radiology 184:753–755

Paterson A, Frush DP (2007) Dose reduction in paediatric MDCT: general principles. Clin Radiol 62:507–517

Patriquin H, Robitaille P (1986) Renal calcium deposition in children: sonographic demonstration of the Anderson-Carr progression. AJR 146:1253–1256

Perale R, Talenti E, Lubrano G (1988) Ultrasound for the diagnosis of the uric acid nephropathy in children. Pediatr Radiol 18:265–268

Perez-Brayfield MR, Kirsch AJ, Jones RA et al. (2003) A prospective study comparing ultrasound, nuclear scintigraphy and dynamic contrast enhanced magnetic resonance imaging in the evaluation of hydronephrosis. J Urol 170:1330–1334

Peters CA (1995) Urinary tract obstruction in children. J Urol 154:1874–1883; discussion 1883–1884

Piepsz A (2002) Radionuclide studies in paediatric nephro-urology. Eur J Radiol 43:146–153

Piepsz A, Blaufox MD, Gordon I et al. (1999) Consensus on renal cortical scintigraphy in children with urinary tract infection. Semin Nucl Med 29:160–174

Piepsz A, Colarinha P, Gordon I et al. (2000) Guidelines on Tc-99m DMSA scintigraphy in children. Eur J Nucl Med 28:BP37–BP41

Piepsz A, Ham HR (2006) Pediatric applications of renal nuclear medicine. Semin Nucl Med 36:16–35

Platt JF, Ellis JH, Rubin JM et al. (1990) Intrarenal arterial Doppler sonography in patients with non-obstructive renal diseases: correlation of resistive index with biopsy findings. Am J Radiol 154:1223–1227

Platt JF, Rubin JM, Ellis JH (1991) Acute renal failure: possible role of duplex Doppler US in distinction between acute prerenal failure and acute tubular necrosis. Radiology 179:419–423

Platt JF, Rubin JN, James HE (1997) Lupus nephritis: predictive value of conventional and Doppler US and comparison with serologic and biopsy parameters. Radiology 203:82–86

Prigent A, Cosgriff P, Gates GF et al. (1999) Consensus report on quality control of quantitative measurements of renal function obtained from renogram. International Consensus Committee from the Scientific Committee of Radionuclides in Nephrourology. Semin Nucl Med 29:146–159

Repetto HA (1997) Epidemic hemolytic-uremic syndrome in children. Kidney Int 52:1708–1719

Riccabona M (2002) Cystography in infants and children – a critical appraisal of the many forms, with special regard to voiding cystourethrography. Eur Radiol 12:2910–2918

Riccabona M (2002) Potential of modern sonographic techniques in paediatric uroradiology. Eur J Radiol 43:110–121

Riccabona M (2003) Imaging of renal tumours in infancy and childhood. Eur Radiol 13:L116–L129

Riccabona M (2004) Interventional uroradiology in paediatrics: a potpourri of diagnostic and therapeutic options. Minerva Pediatr 56:497–505

Riccabona M (2004) Pediatric MRU – its potential and its role in the diagnostic work-up of upper urinary tract dilatation in infants and children. World J Urol 22:79–87

Riccabona M (2005) Vesico-ureteral reflux (VUR). In: Carty H, Brunelle F, Stringer D et al. (eds) Imaging children, 2nd edn, vol I. Elsevier Science Publisher, New York, pp 671–690

Riccabona M (2006) (Acute) Renal failure in neonates, infants, and children – the role of ultrasound, with respect to other imaging options. Ultrasound Clin 1:457–469

Riccabona M (2009) Urinary tract maging in infancy. Pediatr Radiol 39(suppl 3):S436–S445

Riccabona M, Avni FE, Blickman JG et al.; ESUR Paediatric Guideline Subcommittee and ESPR Paediatric Uroradiology Work Group (2008) Imaging recommendations in paediatric uroradiology: minutes of the ESPR workgroup session on urinary tract infection, fetal hydronephrosis, urinary tract ultrasonography and voiding cysto-urethrography ESPR-Meeting, Barcelona/Spain, June 2007. Pediatr Radiol 38:138–145

Riccabona M, Avni FE, Blickman JG et al.; Members of the ESUR Paediatric Recommendation Work Group and ESPR Paediatric Uroradiology Work Group (2009) Imaging recommendations in paediatric uroradiology, Part II: urolithiasis and haematuria in children, paediatric obstructive uropathy, and postnatal work-up of foetally diagnosed high grade hydronephrosis. Minutes of a mini-symposium at ESPR annual meeting, Edinburg, June. Pediatr Radiol 39: 891–898

Riccabona M, Avni FE, Dacher JN et al. (2010) ESPR uroradiology task force and ESUR paediatric working group: Imaging and procedural recommendations in paediatric uroradiology, Part III. Minutes of the ESPR uroradiology task force mini-symposium on intravenous urography, uro-CT and MR-urography in childhood. Pediatr Radiol 40(7):1315–1320

Riccabona M, Fotter R (2004) Urinary tract infection in infants and children: an update with special regard to the changing role of reflux. Eur Radiol 14(suppl 4):L78–L88

Riccabona M, Fotter R (2006) Radiographic studies in children with kidney disorders: what to do and when. In: Hogg R (ed) Kidney disorders in children and adolescents. Taylor and Francis, Birmingham, pp 15–34

Riccabona M, Fritz GA, Schollnast H et al. (2005) Hydronephrotic kidney: pediatric three-dimensional US for relative renal size assessment – initial experience. Radiology 236: 276–283

Riccabona M, Fritz G, Ring E (2003) Potential applications of three-dimensional ultrasound in the pediatric urinary tract: pictorial demonstration based on preliminary results. Eur Radiol 13:2680–2687

Riccabona M, Lindbichler F, Sinzig M (2002) Conventional imaging in paediatric uroradiology. Eur J Radiol 43: 100–109

Riccabona M, Mache CJ, Lindbichler F (2003) Echo-enhanced Color Doppler Cystosonography of vesico-ureteral reflux in children: improvement by stimulated acoustic emission. Acta Radiol 44:18–23

Riccabona M, Mache CJ, Ring E (2008) Renal parenchymal disease. In: Fotter R (ed) Pediatric uroradiology, 2nd edn. Springer, Berlin, pp 355–384

Riccabona M, Olsen OE, Claudon M et al. (2008) Gadolinium and nephrogenic systemic fibrosis. In: Fotter R (ed) Pediatric uroradiology, 2nd edn. Springer, Berlin, pp 515–517

Riccabona M, Riccabona M, Koen M et al. (2004) Magnetic resonance urography: a new gold standard for the evaluation of solitary kidneys and renal buds? J Urol 171: 1642–1646

Riccabona M, Ring E (2008) Renal agenesis, dysplasia, hypolplasia and cystic diseases of the kidney. In: Fotter R (ed) Pediatric uroradiology, 2nd edn. Springer, Berlin, 2008, pp 187–210

Riccabona M, Ruppert-Kohlmayr A, Ring E et al. (2004) Potential impact of pediatric MR urography on the imaging algorithm in patients with a functional single kidney. Am J Roentgenol 183:795–800

Riccabona M (2010) Obstructive diseases of the urinary tract in children: lessons from the last 15 years. Pediatr Radiol 40(6): 947–955

Riccabona M, Schwinger W, Ring E (1998) Arteriovenous fistula after renal biopsy in children. J Ultrasound Med 17:505–508

Riccabona M, Schwinger W, Ring E et al. (2001) Amplitude coded color Doppler sonography in pediatric renal disease. Eur Radiol 11:861–866

Riccabona M, Simbrunner J, Ring E et al. (2002) Feasibility of MR-urography in neonates and infants with abnormalities of the upper urinary tract. Eur Radiol 12:1442–1450

Riccabona M, Sorantin E, Fotter R (1998) Application of functional m-mode sonography in pediatric patients. Eur Radiol 8:1457–1461

Riccabona M, Sorantin E, Hausegger K (2002) Imaging guided interventional procedures in paediatric uroradiology – a case based overview. Eur J Radiol 43:167–179

Riebel TW, Abraham K, Wartner R et al. (1993) Transient renal medullary hyperechogenicity in ultrasound studies of neonates: is it normal phenomenon or what are the causes? J Clin Ultrasound 21:31–35

Ritchey ML, Azizkhan RG, Beckwith JB et al. (1995) Neonatal Wilms tumor. J Pediatr Surg 30:856–859

Rohrschneider WK, Becker K, Hoffend J et al. (2000) Combined static-dynamic MR urography for the simultaneous evaluation of morphology and function in urinary tract obstruction. II. Findings in experimentally induced ureteric stenosis. Pediatr Radiol 30:523–532

Rohrschneider WK, Haufe S, Clorius JH et al. (2003) MR to assess renal function in children. Eur Radiol 13:1033–1045

Rohrschneider WK, Haufe S, Wiesel M et al. (2002) Functional and morphologic evaluation of congenital urinary tract dilatation by using combined static-dynamic MR urography: findings in kidneys with a single collecting system. Radiology 224:683–694

Rohrschneider WK, Hoffend J, Becker K et al. (2000) Combined static-dynamic MR urography for the simultaneous evaluation of morphology and function in urinary tract obstruction. I. Evaluation of the normal status in an animal model. Pediatr Radiol 30:511–522

Rohrschneider WK, Weirich A, Rieden K et al. (1998) US, CT and MR imaging characteristics of nephroblastomatosis. Pediatr Radiol 28:435–443

Rondeau E, Peraldi M-N (1996) Escherichia coli and hemolytic-uremic syndrome. N Engl J Med 335:660–662

Schenk JP (2008) Renal tumours. In: Troeger J, Seidenstricker P (eds) Paediatric imaging manual. Springer, Heidelberg, pp 97–99

Schlesinger AE, Rosenfield NS, Castle VP (1995) Congenital mesoblastic nephroma metastatic to the brain: a report of two cases. Pediatr Radiol 25:S73–S75

Scholbach Th (1999) Prognostische Bedeutung der farbduplex-sonographischen Nierenperfusionsmessung beim hämolytisch-urämischen Syndrom. Ultraschall Med 20:S33

Schöllnast H, Lindbichler F, Riccabona M (2004) Ultrasound (US) of the urethra in infants: comparison US versus VCUG. J Ultrasound Med 23:769–776

Sigmund G, Stöver B, Zimmerhackl LB et al. (1991) RARE-MR-urography in the diagnosis of upper urinary tract abnormalities in children. Pediatr Radiol 21:416–420

Smergel E, Greenerg BS, Crisci KL et al. (2001) CT urograms in pediatric patients with ureteral calculi: do adult criteria work? Pediatr Radiol 31:720–723

Sorantin E, Fotter R, Aigner R et al. (1997) The sonographically thickened wall of the upper urinary tract: correlation with other imaging methods. Pediatr Radiol 27:667–671

Steiner MS, Goldman SM, Fishman EK et al. (1993) The natural history of renal angiomyolipoma. J Urol 150: 1782–1786

Stöver B, Rogalla P (2008) CT examinations in children. Radiologe 48:243–248

Strouse PJ, Bates DG, Bloom DA et al. (2002) Non-contrast thin-section helical CT of urinary tract calculi in children. Pediatr Radiol 32:326–332

Teele RL, Share JC (1997) Transperineal sonography in children. Am J Roentgenol 168:1263–1267

Thoeny HC, Keyzer FD, Oyen RH et al. (2005) Diffusion weighted MRI of kidneys volunteers and patients with parenchymal disease. Radiology 235:911–917

Tsapaki V, Aldrich JE, Sharma R et al. (2006) Dose reduction in CT while maintaining diagnostic confidence: diagnostic reference levels at routine head, chest, and abdominal CT–IAEA-coordinated research project. Radiology 240:828–834

Vivier PH, Blondiaux E, Dolores M et al. (2009) Functional MR urography in children. J Radiol 90:11–19

Ward VL (2006) Patient dose reduction during voiding cystourethrography. Pediatr Radiol 36(suppl 2):168–172

Ward VL, Strauss KJ, Barnewolt CE et al. (2008) Pediatric radiation exposure and effective dose reduction during voiding cystourethrography. Radiology 249:1002–1009

Whitaker RH, Bullock KN, Buxton-Thomas MS et al. (1982) Role of modern radiological investigations in obstructive uropathy. Br Med J (Clin Res Ed) 285:211–212

Wright NB, Blanch G, Walkinshaw S et al. (1996) Antenatal and neonatal renal vein thrombosis: new ultrasonographic features with high frequency transducers. Pediatr Radiol 26:686–689

# The Kidney in the Elderly

## Emilio Quaia and Marco Cavallaro

## Contents

**Abstract**

> The aims of this chapter are to illustrate the typical imaging findings of the kidney in elderly patients and the typical features of the main renal pathologies in the elderly patient. The kidneys present some important morphologic changes according to the patient's age, which can be detected first by gray-scale ultrasound (US) and color Doppler US, and second, by all the other imaging modalities. These changes have an impact on patient management, particularly with respect to drug therapy. The landmark is diffuse irregular margins due to nephronangiosclerosis of the intrarenal arteries. The fundamental alterations of renal morphology in elderly patients include size reduction, parenchymal thickness reduction, margin irregularities, and increased corticomedullary differentiation. The main renal pathologies, including vascular and tumoral diseases, present some peculiar features in the elderly patient.

Population aging is taking place throughout the world, and about 13% of the 76 million persons in the United States were aged 65 years and older (Ferrucci et al. 2008). In Europe, there is the oldest population in the world, with almost 25% of European projected to be aged 65 years or older by 2030. In particular, Italy and Germany are estimated to have the oldest population in Europe. The progressive increase in the proportion of a population that is elderly depends on changes in the survival of older persons and in the birth rate (Ferrucci et al. 2008). The increasingly greater life expectancy of

E. Quaia (✉) and M. Cavallaro
Department of Radiology, Cattinara Hospital, University of Trieste, Strada di Fiume 447, Trieste 34149, Italy
e-mail: quaia@univ.trieste.it

E. Quaia (ed.), *Radiological Imaging of the Kidney*,
Medical Radiology, DOI: 10.1007/978-3-540-87597-0_28, © Springer-Verlag Berlin Heidelberg 2011

the population has been mainly determined by the reduced mortality at older ages. The five leading causes of death, including heart disease, cancer, stroke, chronic lower respiratory tract disease, and Alzheimer's disease, account for 69.5% of all death (Ferrucci et al. 2008). The renal causes of death account only for 2% of all deaths and for 4% of chronic conditions in persons aged >65 years, even though these represent an important cause of disability and comorbidity in the older patients.

Due to the progressive increase in the mean age of the population, it is very important to know the morphologic changes of the kidney according to the aging. As a matter of fact, older individuals, often with a compromised renal reserve and substantial comorbidities, are the norm in the hospitalized population (Dagher et al. 2003). The functional alterations of the aged kidney are characterized principally by a progressive reduction of renal blood flow from about 600 to 300 mL/min/1.73 m$^2$ and of glomerular filtration rate (GFR) from 130 to 60–80 mL/min. An accurate quantitation of the GFR should always be performed in the elderly patient before injection of iodinated and gadolinium-based contrast agents. Moreover, when exposed to iodinated contrast agents, nonsteroidal anti-inflammatory drugs, aminoglycosides, or emodynamic challenges (e.g., surgery and anesthesia, sepsis, volume depletion), this at-risk patient population often develops an abrupt decline in GFR.

The kidneys undergo involutional changes with age. There is a gradual decline in kidney weight starting after the age of 50 years, with the most marked decrease occurring between the seventh and eight decade. The progressive loss of kidney mass appears to affect the renal cortex more than renal medulla (Faubert and Porush 1998). Microscopically, there is a reduction in the number of glomeruli and an increase in glomerular sclerosis with increasing age (Davison 1998). The glomerular sclerosis in the elderly is different from the diabetic intercapillary diffuse sclerosis and focal glomerulosclerosis and corresponds to a progressive glomerular hyalinization, such that glomeruli become shrunken, eosinophilic, and hypocellular masses. The increase in the percentage of sclerotic glomeruli has been attributed to the protein-rich diet characteristic of modern society which probably determines a state of chronic glomerular hyperfiltration and hyperperfusion. A further cause would be the glomerual ischemia secondary to the changes of the renal

blood flow occurring with ages. The presence of atherosclerosis increases the incidence of glomerular sclerosis, raising the possibility that the glomerular sclerosis in the elderly is nothing other than a reflection of vascular disease and thus should be considered a secondary phenomenon. On electron microscopic analysis, there is an increase in focal thickening of both glomerular and tubular basement membranes, probably due to the accumulation of type IV collagen (Faubert and Porush 1998). The loss of glomerual mass is proportional to the loss of tubular mass, so that the tubular balance is well-preserved. The outer cortical glomeruli are more extensively involved than the deeper glomeruli. Moreover, in addition to glomerular sclerosis, there is a gradual increase in the interstitial fibrosis.

Although most would agree there is a decrease in the total number of glomeruli, there is a very wide scatter in the data, and many elderly people seem to retain the same number of glomeruli as expected in younger persons (Davison 1998). The average thickness of the glomerular basement membrane increases with age, but this does not appear to be associated with any change in function. The volume of the mesangium increases, but as this is accompanied by a decrease in glomerular volume, it is difficult to draw any significant conclusion. The most significant changes appear in the juxtamedullary glomeruli. Changes also take place in the tubules where there may be irregular thickening of the basement membrane and, particularly in the distal tubule, the formation of diverticula. There is overall reduction in the tubular volume, and this seems to parallel the reduction in glomerular volume. The interstitium may contain areas of tubular atrophy and fibrosis. Renal arteries develop intimal thickening and reduplication of the elastic lamina. Increasing tortuosity and tapering of the interlobular arteries have been reported. Changes have been recognized in afferent arterioles, and there is evidence that there are differences between those arterioles supplying juxtaglomerular glomeruli and more cortical glomeruli. It would appear that with increasing age, shunts develop between the afferent and efferent arterioles in the juxtamedullary glomeruli, whereas in the cortical glomeruli the vessels become obliterated. The significance of these findings are unclear, as it is difficult to separate out changes which may have been engendered by hypertension and those due to aging alone (Davison 1998).

## 28.1 Morphologic Alterations in the Kidney of an Elderly Patient

Aging induces in the kidney a progressive, functional, and anatomic decay that does not have a particular clinical impact. The fundamental alterations of renal morphology in the elderly patients include size reduction, parenchymal thickness reduction, margin irregularities, and increased cortico-medullary differentiation. In particular, the most important morphologic alteration of the aged kidney is the volume reduction, approximately 20–30% in 80-year-old man, and a loss

of weight that decreases from 250–270 to 180–200 g after age 65 (Mulder and Hillen 2001).

In the elderly patients, the kidneys appear frequently reduced in their largest dimension (within the range of 9–9.5 cm) on gray-scale US, with reduction in the renal parenchymal thickness due to chronic reduction of the renal parenchyma perfusion from nephroangiosclerosis. The renal capsule becomes thicker and there is an increase of the renal sinus fatty tissue, in particular at the level of the renal hilum (Figs. 28.1 and 28.2). Typically, there is evidence of irregular margins (Figs. 28.3 and 28.4a), frequently with a pseudolobular

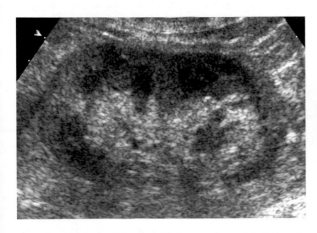

**Fig. 28.1** Fundamental morphologic alterations of the kidney in the elderly patient. Gray-scale ultrasound (US), longitudinal scan. Reduction of renal cortical thickness and increase of the renal sinus fatty tissue, in particular evident at the renal hilum

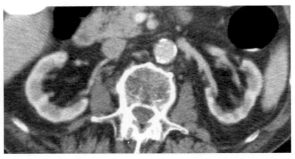

**Fig. 28.2** Contrast-enhanced CT, cortico-medullary phase. Reduction of renal cortical thickness and increase of the renal sinus fatty tissue evident on both kidneys

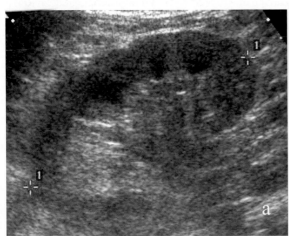

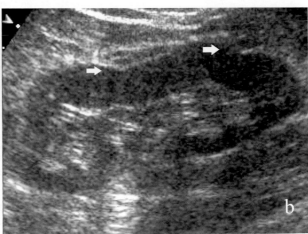

**Fig. 28.3** (**a, b**) Sixty-six-year-old patient with normal creatinine levels. Longitudinal gray-scale US scan of the right (**a**) and of the left kidney (**b**). Increased cortico-medullary differentiation due to the increased echogenicity of the renal cortex (**a, b**) with clear marginal irregularities (*arrows*) in the left kidney

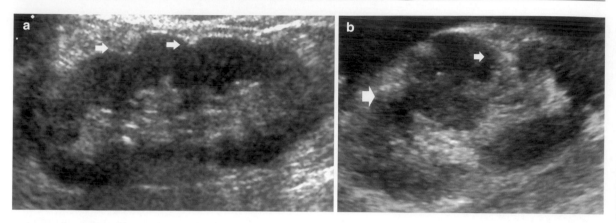

**Fig. 28.4** (**a**, **b**) Different grades of renal margin irregularities. Longitudinal gray-scale US scan. (**a**) Reduction of the renal parenchyma thickness with renal contour irregularities (*arrows*), and increased cortico-medullary differentiation. (**b**) Diffuse renal margin irregularities also with evidence of renal parenchymal scars (*arrows*) due to previous regional infarctions. The interposed renal parenchyma presents a pseudolobar appearance

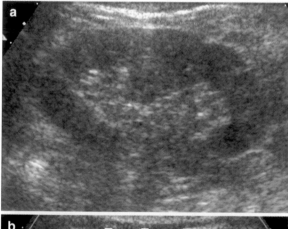

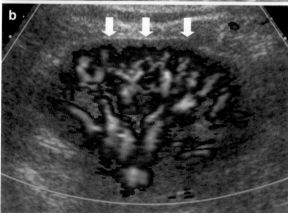

**Fig. 28.5** (**a**, **b**) Fundamental morphologic alterations of the kidney in the elderly patient. (**a**) Gray-scale US. Increased echogenicity of the renal parenchyma with reduced cortico-medullary differentiation. (**b**) Power Doppler US. Reduced renal parenchyma vascularization at the level of the subcapsular region (*arrows*)

appearance (Fig. 28.4b) and/or coexisting with renal parenchyma scars due to previous renal cortical infarctions (Fig. 28.4b). The cortico-medullary differentiation appears usually increased due to the relative higher echogenicity of the renal cortex compared to medulla due to nephroangiosclerosis (Figs. 28.1 and 28.3). Anyway, less frequently, the cortico-medullary differentiation may also be reduced (Fig. 28.5). On color/power Doppler US, the renal peripheral vessels are usually not visualized in the subcapsular renal parenchyma (Fig. 28.5).

On contrast-enhanced CT a typical diffuse irregularity of margins is identified (Fig. 28.6), often associated to a reduced cortical thickness or to renal parenchyma scarring due to previous renal infarcts (Fig. 28.7). Renal parenchymal retention cysts (Fig. 28.8) and renal sinus cysts (Fig. 28.9) are frequently identified and probably develop because of inflammatory reactions and infections that occur in the distal tract of the tubuli (Pozzi Mucelli et al. 2008). On CT-urography these fundamental morphological changes are frequently associated with calyceal alterations with narrowing of the first-order calyces and multiple cysts of the renal sinus (Fig. 28.10).

## 28.2 Nephrosclerosis

Nephrosclerosis is the term used for the renal pathology associated with sclerosis of renal arterioles and small arteries due to medial and intimal thickening as

**Fig. 28.6** (**a, b**) Fundamental morphologic alterations of the kidney in the elderly patient. Contrast-enhanced CT, excretory phase. Coronal reformation. Diffuse reduction of the renal cortical thickness with overt focal irregularities of renal margins (*arrows*)

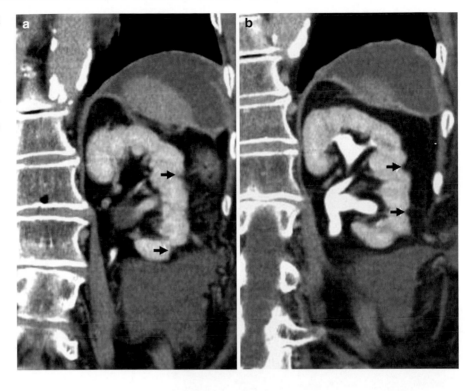

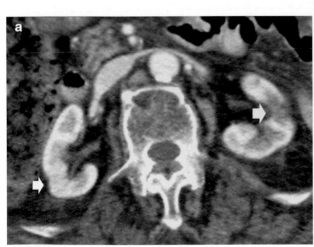

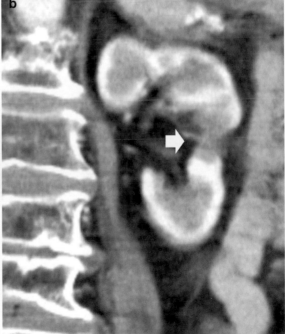

**Fig. 28.7** (**a, b**) Multiple renal scarring due to previous vascular infarcts in the kidneys of an 80-year-old patient. Contrast-enhanced CT, cortico-medullary phase. (**a**) Transverse plane. Both kidneys present irregular margins due to underlying neph-rosclerosis and overt renal parenchyma scarring due to previous renal infarctions (*arrows*). (**b**) Coronal reformation. The left kidney presents overt parenchymal scarring (*arrow*)

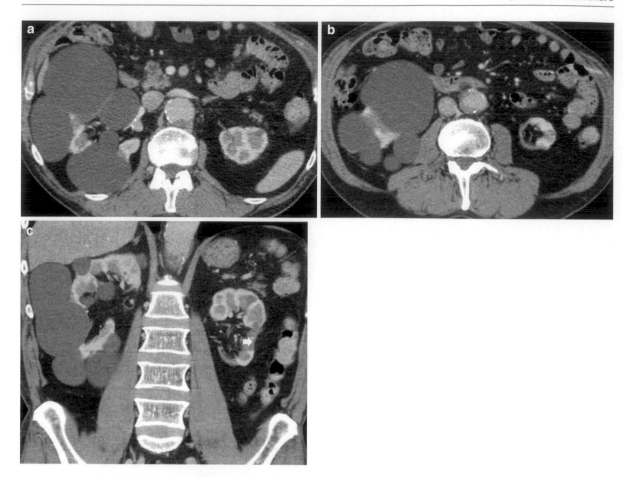

**Fig. 28.8** (**a–c**) Fundamental morphologic alterations of the kidney in the elderly patient. Contrast-enhanced CT. (**a**, **b**) Multiple renal cortical cysts are evident on the right kidney with a reduced cortical thickness of the left kidney. (**c**) The left kidney presents also a cortical scar (*arrow*) due to a previous vascular infarct

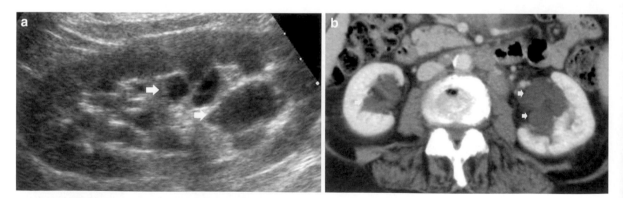

**Fig. 28.9** (**a**, **b**) Fundamental morphologic alterations of the kidney in the elderly patient. (**a**) Gray-scale US. Longitudinal scan of the left kidney. Multiple cysts of renal sinus (*arrows*). (**b**) Contrast-enhanced CT, nephrographic phase. Multiple renal sinus cysts (*arrows*) are evident on both kidneys

**Fig. 28.10** (a, b) Fundamental morphologic alterations of the kidney in the elderly patient. Contrast-enhanced CT, excretory phase. Coronal reformation. Multiple cysts of renal sinus (*arrows*) with narrowing of the renal calyces, associated to irregular margins due to underlying nephrosclerosis and previous renal infarctions

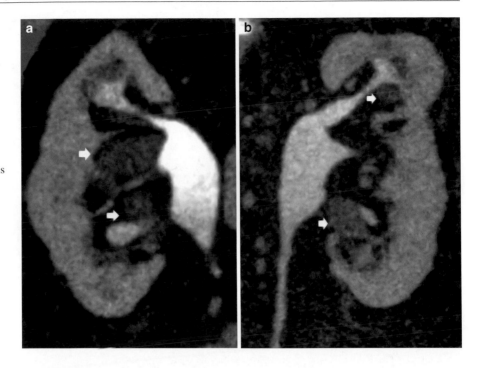

a response to hemodynamic changes, aging, genetic defects, or some combination of these and to hyaline deposition in arterioles (Alpers 2005). The resultant effect is focal ischemia of the renal parenchyma supplied by vessels with thickened walls and consequent narrowed lumen (Alpers 2005). Some degree of nephrosclerosis is present at autopsy with increasing age preceding or in the absence of hypertension. Hypertension and diabetes mellitus increase the incidence and severity of the lesions. In nephrosclerosis, there is a general hardening of the kidney due to overgrowth and contraction of interstitial connective tissue. Nephrosclerosis may be compared to the arteriosclerosis of the small renal arteries and it is due to renovascular disease, mainly chronic hypertension. The renal vascular alterations of hypertension depend on the severity of the blood pressure elevation and whether the process accelerates to malignant hypertension. Arteriolosclerosis of small cortical renal arteries, interlobar, arcuate, and interlobular, is a common feature of kidney in patients with systemic arterial hypertension and particularly in elderly patients (Quaia and Bertolotto 2002).

In nephroangiosclerosis both kidneys are usually symmetrically reduced in their diameters with cortical scars. Cortical echogenicity is increased with increased or reduced cortico-medullary differentiation according to the grade of echogenicity of renal medulla. Color and power Doppler US reveals nonspecific reduction of vascularization (Fig. 28.11). If compared to the younger population, renal RIs are typically increased (>0.7 and frequently around 0.8) (Figs. 28.12 and 28.13). Renal perforating arteries and veins (Bertolotto et al. 2000) are much more visible in kidneys of nephroangiosclerotic patients in comparison with normal subjects, since they enlarge in nephroangiosclerosis and present normally directed flows from the kidney toward renal capsule. Renal RIs are increased with values ranging from 0.8 and 0.98.

## 28.3  Renovascular Disease

The geriatric population is affected by many vascular diseases, since the incidence of atherosclerosis increases with age. Generally, the imaging of vascular diseases in the elderly is complicated by the presence of coexisting diseases, while the image quality is degraded due to obesity and limited patient compliance. Renovascular hypertension accounts for 0.5–5% of patients who have hypertension. The renovascular disease may manifest as asymptomatic renal artery stenosis, intractable or uncontrollable hypertension requiring multiple medications, or ischemic nephropathy with progressive loss

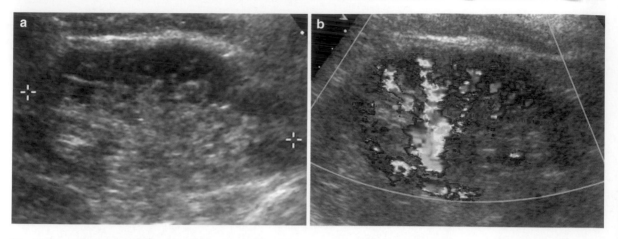

**Fig. 28.11** (**a, b**) Fundamental morphologic alterations of the kidney in the elderly patient. Renal morphological changes due to nephrosclerosis. (**a**) Gray-scale US, longitudinal scan. Reduction of renal cortical thickness with diffuse irregularities of renal margins. (**b**) Color Doppler. Reduction of renal cortical vascularization at color Doppler analysis due to nephrosclerosis

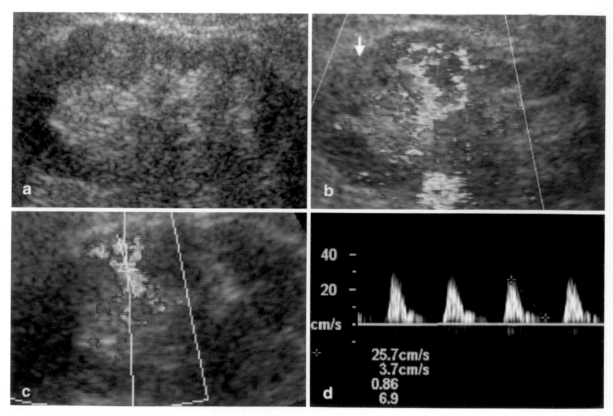

**Fig. 28.12** (**a–d**) Fundamental morphologic alterations of the kidney in the elderly patient. Reduction of the renal parenchyma thickness reduction, margin irregularities, and increased cortico-medullary differentiation are evident on gray-scale US (**a**). (**b**) Color Doppler US, longitudinal scan. Reduction of renal cortical vascularization. (**c, d**) Doppler interrogation of the intra-renal segmental arteries with increased arterial resistive indices

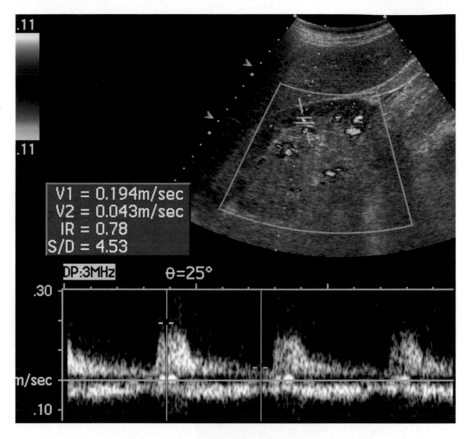

**Fig. 28.13** Fundamental morphologic alterations of the kidney in the elderly patient. Color Doppler US with Doppler interrogation of renal segmental artery. Increased arterial resistive index measured at the level of one renal segmental artery of the lower renal pole

of renal function (Kalva and Mueller 2008). In the young patient the most common cause of renovascular hypertension is fibromuscolar dysplasia, while in the elderly the most common cause is atherosclerosis mainly localized in the ostial or proximal tract of the renal artery.

Color Doppler US, helical computed tomographic (CT) angiography, angiotensin converting enzyme (ACE) inhibitor scintigraphy with captopril, and magnetic resonance (MR) angiography have been assessed in the diagnosis of renal artery stenosis (see Chap. 18). Digital subtraction angiography remains the gold standard for the diagnosis of renal artery stenosis, and it is part of any endovascular intervention. Contrast-enhanced CT and MR imaging angiographic techniques have improved in their detection of renal artery stenosis and MR angiography is generally considered more sensitive for renal artery stenosis than US (Zhang and Prince 2004). Anyway, kidney disease limits the use of contrast agents during CT and MR imaging examinations, and this is particularly true in the elderly patients. Moreover, coexistent cardiopulmonary diseases, such

as congestive heart failure, arrhythmias, and chronic obstructive lung diseases, limit the ability of the elderly to hold breath during image acquisition (Kalva and Mueller 2008). Additionally, the cardiopulmonary diseases may preclude the use of some of the imaging modalities because of the inherent contraindications, such as pacemakers in MR examinations. Consequently, color Doppler US is the principal imaging technique employed in the elderly for renovascular disease diagnosis.

The velocitometric analysis of Doppler trace derived from renal arteries is of primary importance to identify renal artery stenosis. Direct Doppler criteria have been proposed for the detection of renal arterial stenosis, including an increased peak systolic velocity (>150–180 cm/s) (Fig. 28.14) and end-diastolic velocity at the level of the stenosis (Correas et al. 1999; Grant and Melany 2001), poststenotic flow disturbance resulting in spectral broadening and reversed flow (Correas et al. 1999), increased ratio (≥3.5) of peak systolic velocity in renal artery and aorta (renal-aortic ratio), and the presence of turbulence within the renal artery (Desberg

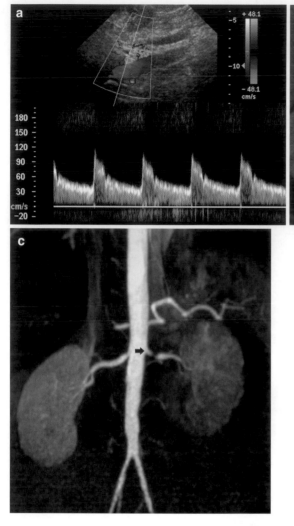

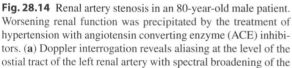

**Fig. 28.14** Renal artery stenosis in an 80-year-old male patient. Worsening renal function was precipitated by the treatment of hypertension with angiotensin converting enzyme (ACE) inhibitors. (**a**) Doppler interrogation reveals aliasing at the level of the ostial tract of the left renal artery with spectral broadening of the Doppler trace. (**b**) CT angiography (CTA). Stenosis of the left renal artery is confirmed (*arrow*). (**c**) MR angiography. 3D maximum intensity projection. Stenosis of the left renal artery is confirmed (*arrow*)

et al. 1990; Helenon et al. 1995). Although this technique is easy to perform, its accuracy is questionable because the lack of an early systolic peak has a low sensitivity for moderate stenoses, and the waveform is dependent on the maintenance of vessel compliance, which limits its effectiveness in elderly patients and patients with atherosclerosis (Bude et al. 1994; Bude and Rubin 1995).

Downstream hemodynamic repercussions of renal artery stenosis in the distal intrarenal arterial bed may be identified by Doppler US and may provide an indirect diagnosis of renal artery stenosis. Numerous parameters are still debated (Correas et al. 1999), except in cases of critical stenosis (>80%). In fact, even though intraparenchymal arteries examination is technically easier than the evaluation of the main renal artery, Doppler US findings in interlobar-arcuate renal cortical arteries are less reliable than Doppler US findings on stenotic site, since downstream repercussions are absent in 20% of principal renal artery tight stenosis (>80%), for a well-developed collateral blood supply. In the presence of a hemodynamically significant renal artery stenosis, the Doppler trace reveals a "tardus et parvus" profile at poststenotic or intrarenal tract of renal artery (Stavros et al. 1992; Bude et al. 1994), consisting in an increased time to reach the peak of the trace (acceleration time >70 ms) with loss of early systolic peak and decreased acceleration index (<300 cm/s$^2$). Poststenotic pulsus tardus is caused by the compliance of the poststenotic vessel wall in conjunction with the stenosis, which produces the tardus effect by damping the high-frequency components of the arterial waveform. This information allows to identify those conditions, which may produce false-positive or false-negative results when the tardus phenomenon is used to predict hemodynamically significant upstream stenosis (Bude et al. 1994). This is the case of the loss of vascular compliance in severe diffuse atherosclerosis or elderly patients, which may prevent the tardus-parvus phenomenon decreasing the sensitivity of color Doppler US (Grant and Melany 2001). Other findings that may be observed in the intraparenchymal arteries in the presence of renal artery stenosis is a decreased resistive indices in interlobar-arcuate renal cortical arteries with increased side difference higher than 10% (Correas et al. 1999).

Contrast-enhanced CT angiography (CTA) and MR imaging angiography (MRA) CTA is also very sensitive and specific for the demonstration of renal artery occlusion. Additional views provided by CTA allow for display of the renal arteries in multiple planes and projections, often necessary for the depiction of stenosis (Fig. 28.14). Calcified plaques limit the CT evaluation of luminal narrowing. In particular, in cases with extensive calcification, as is frequently observed in elderly patients, renal artery stenosis can be obscured by MIP technique and requires careful evaluation with the volume-rendered images. CTA can also depict secondary signs of renal artery stenosis, including poststenotic dilatation and renal parenchymal changes of atrophy and decreased cortical enhancement. CTA is also very helpful in the posttreatment evaluation of renal stent grafts and can usually delineate between the highly attenuating graft material and the intraluminal contrast material.

MRA is well suited for the evaluation of renal artery stenosis in the elderly. Calcified atheromatous plaques do not hamper the assessment of the arterial lumen. MR angiography provides information about the size of the kidney, collateral vessels, and poststenotic dilatation. Contrast-enhanced axial MR imaging can directly show the narrowing of the stenosis, and reformatted multiplanar imaging is often used. Both MIP and volume rendering are useful and complimentary in the evaluation of renal artery stenosis. Axial images alone are not sufficient for the evaluation of renal artery stenosis because the renal arteries often have a tortuous course especially in the elderly patient. Multiplanar reformations are very useful, in particular to show renal artery occlusion (Fig. 28.14).

## 28.4 Renal Infarction

Nontraumatic acute renal infarction may present the same symptoms of stone colic or acute pyelonephritis. Renal infarction may be caused by tight stenosis or occlusion of segmental or of the main renal artery, or by renal artery embolization due to renal angioplasty, atrial fibrillation, and cardiac valvular defects. Other causes of renal infarction are vasculitis, systemic lupus erythematosus, drug-induced vasculitis, paraneoplastic syndrome, hypercoagulable state, or acute venous occlusion (Kawashima et al. 2000). Fever and leucocytosis are common and the volume of infarcted renal parenchyma is substantial. Both CT and angiography are reference imaging techniques in renal infarcts detection, whereas US presents a lower sensitivity. Even though large renal infarcts may be hypoechoic in comparison with the viable renal parenchyma, segmental renal infarcts are usually isoechoic or rarely hyperechoic if haemorrhagic component is present.

Even though large renal perfusion defects or infarcts may be hypoechoic in comparison with the viable renal parenchyma, segmental renal infarcts are usually isoechoic or rarely hyperechoic if haemorrhagic component is present. Renal infarcts often reveal a wedge shape with capsular base. Even though baseline color Doppler US and power Doppler US present overt limitations to detect renal perfusion defects due to the low sensitivity to low-velocity and low-amplitude flow states, they may increase diagnostic capabilities of US in detecting renal infarcts, especially in elderly or obese patients and in patients with renal diseases.

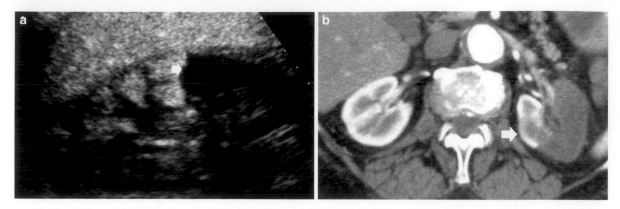

**Fig. 28.15** (**a**) Contrast-enhanced US after sulfur hexafluoride-filled microbubble injection. (**b**) Contrast-enhanced CTA, cortico-medullary phase. The left kidney shows partial parenchyma infarction (*arrow*) in a 72-year-old woman with atrial fibrillation

In renal infarct, color Doppler US and power Doppler US reveal absolute absence of renal cortical flows, even though it is very difficult to differentiate renal segmental infarct from areas which appear poorly perfused due to underlying parenchymal disease, deep renal position, and artifacts. Moreover, color Doppler US presents a low accuracy in the detection of small renal infarcts in the subcaspular region for limited spatial resolution and in the superior renal pole for the high Doppler angle and for the depth position (Correas et al. 2003).

Recent advances in microbubble-based contrast agents, and dedicated contrast-specific modes, have determined the achievement of increased image contrast in tissues. By transmitting at the fundamental frequency and receiving selectively harmonic frequencies, the background signal from stationary tissues is markedly suppressed resulting in a greater signal-to-noise ratio and a better visibility of renal infarcts. Blooming and flash artifacts are eliminated, shadowing artifacts are lessened, both spatial and temporal resolutions are improved, and the brightness of gray-scale pixel does not depend on angle-dependent frequency shift estimates. Differently from iodinated contrast agent and gadolinium-based contrast agents, microbubbles are pure intravascular agents which are not excreted in renal tubules and may be safely employed in patients with advanced chronic renal failure, which is frequently observed in the elderly. Microbubble-based contrast agents and contrast-specific imaging techniques improve significantly the diagnostic confidence level in identifying nonperfused renal parenchymal zones and allow a reliable depiction of renal

perfusion defects (Fig. 28.15). Renal perfusion defects due to renal parenchyma infarction appear as single or multiple focal wedge-shaped areas of absent, diminished, or delayed contrast enhancement in comparison to the adjacent renal parenchima after microbubble injection (Bertolotto et al. 2008).

Contrast-enhanced CT is the reference imaging technique in renal infarcts detection. The parenchymal appearance of renal perfusion defects depends on the site of arterial occlusion, if segmental (Fig. 28.15) or the main renal artery are involved (Fig. 28.16), and on thrombus age (Kawashima et al. 2000). Contrast material-enhanced CT shows the absence of enhancement in the affected renal tissue. Acute renal infarctions typically appear as wedge-shaped areas of decreased attenuation, while after the acute phase of renal infarction, atrophy begins and the infarcted tissue contracts, leaving a cortical scar. Chronic renal artery stenosis with persistent renal parenchyma hypoperfusion led to progressive shrinkage of the parenchyma with absent residual function (Fig. 28.17).

## 28.5 Atheroembolic Renal Disease

Atheroembolic renal disease (renal artery atheroembolization) is a complication of severe ulcerative atheromatosis of the abdominal aorta (Cohen 1992) or may be due to renal angioplasty, atrial fibrillation, and cardiac valvular defects. Atheroemboli localize in vessels smaller than interlobular arteries, so that renal

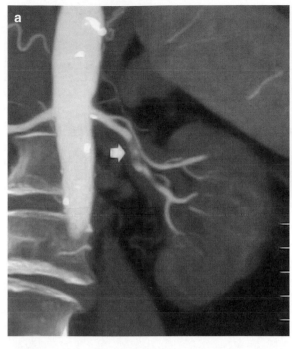

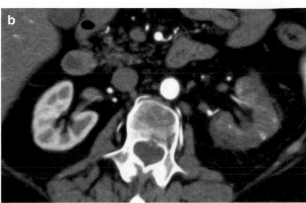

**Fig. 28.16** (**a**, **b**) Renal artery thrombosis in a 75-year-old male patient. (**a**) Contrast-enhanced CTA. Coronal reformation. The left renal artery is occluded by a complex thrombus (*arrow*) with relative avascularity of the left kidney. (**b**) Contrast-enhanced CT. Cortico-medullary phase shows a complete renal infarction

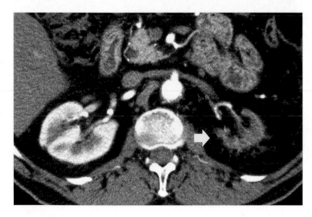

**Fig. 28.17** Renal shrinkage due to chronic vascular hypoperfusion due to the tight stenosis of the left renal artery. Contrast-enhanced CT. Cortico-medullary phase. The left kidney (*arrow*) appears small and without any sign of function (contrast excretion)

infarction does not occur and clinical picture is frequently bland (Cohen 1992) even though acute renal failure is the mode of presentation in most cases. Atheroembolic renal disease with acute renal failure may develop during or immediately after intravascular surgical intervention, intravascular interventional procedures (e.g., renal angioplasty), or anticoagulation due to atheroemboli detached from the renal artery wall. The most common clinical manifestation is the sudden onset of flank or back pain with or without hematuria, proteinuria, fever, and leukocytosis.

Color and power Doppler US is a first-line imaging procedure to detect renal perfusion defect, but present clear limitations due to the relative insensitivity to low-velocity and low-amplitude flow states (Taylor et al. 1996). Coley et al. (1991) found a global accuracy of color Doppler US for the detection of partial renal infarction of 20%. Contrast-enhanced color and power Doppler US is limited by blooming and flash artifacts, which may be attenuated by reducing the instrument gain settings, also diminishing the detection of focal abnormalities in renal blood flow (Taylor et al. 1996). Contrast-enhanced CT (Fig. 28.18) is the reference imaging technique to identify renal perfusion defects (Kawashima et al. 2000). Contrast-enhanced US (Fig. 28.19) represents a very sensitive and reliable imaging technique in revealing the renal parenchyma

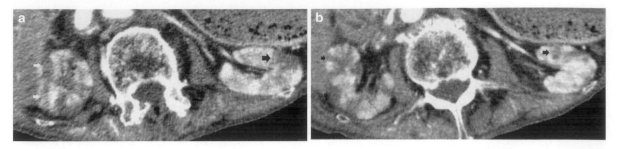

**Fig. 28.18** (**a**, **b**) Contrast-enhanced CT. Multiple renal parenchyma perfusion defects (*arrows*) due to diffuse septic embolization are evident on both kidneys of a 85-year-old patient

perfusion defects due to renal artery embolization (Bertolotto et al. 2008). Renal perfusion defects may appear as multiple focal wedge-shaped areas of absent, diminished, or delayed contrast enhancement in comparison to the adjacent renal parenchima after microbubble injection (Bertolotto et al. 2008).

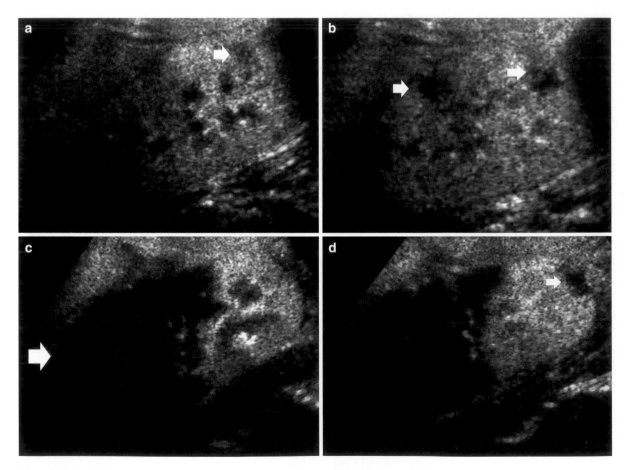

**Fig. 28.19** (**a–h**) Renal artery embolization in a 82-year-old male patient presenting at the emergency unit with acute flank pain on right side. (**a–d**) Contrast-enhanced US after sulfur hexafluoride-filled microbubble injection. (**e–h**) Contrast-enhanced CT, nephrographic phase. Multiple bilateral renal parenchyma perfusion defects (*arrows*), involving mainly the right kidney, due to embolization of an ulcerated plaque of the thoracic aorta

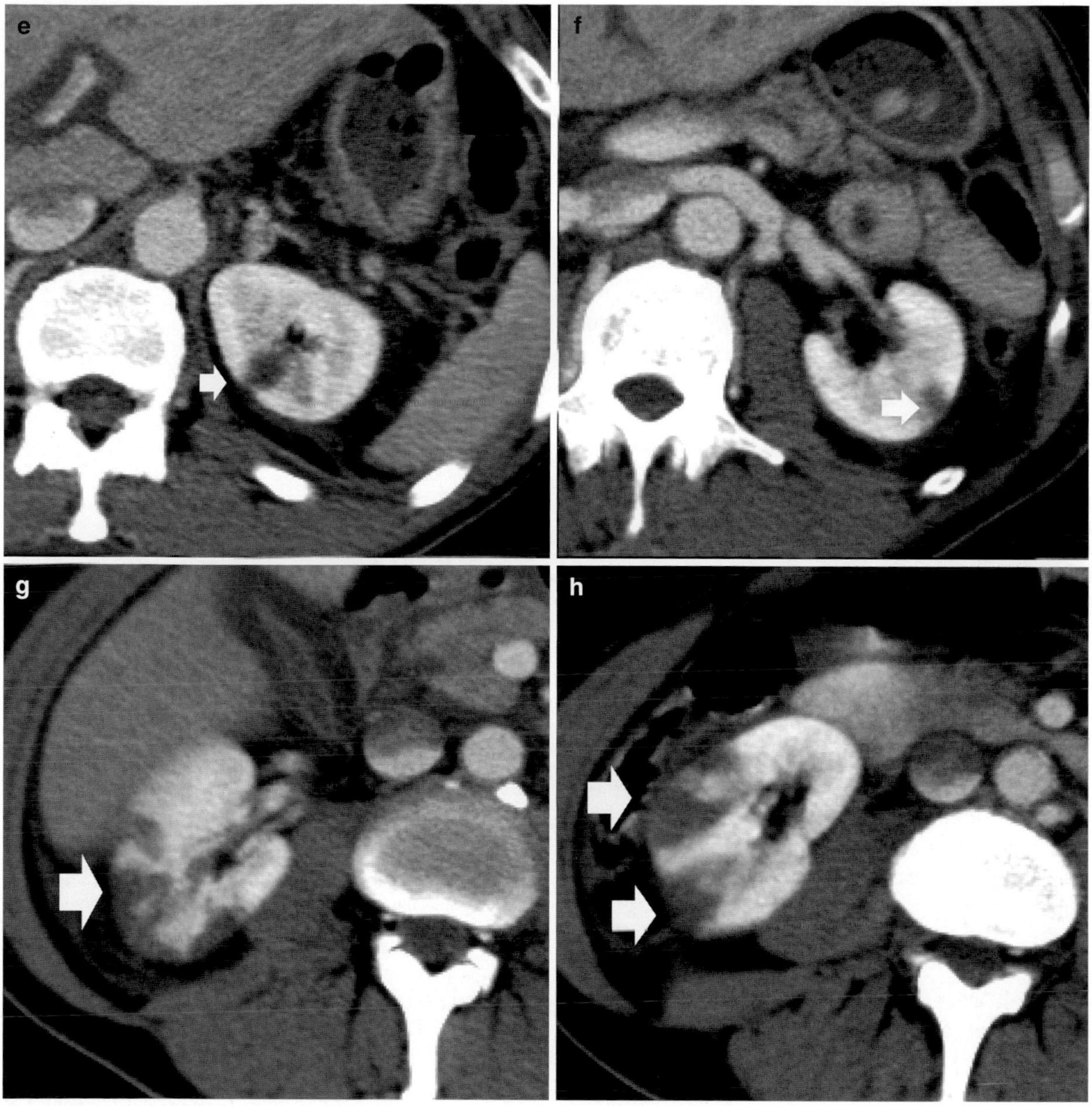

**Fig. 28.19** (continued)

## 28.6 Renal Vein Thrombosis

Renal vein thrombosis in elderly patients, as in adults and differently from infants, is typically of insidious onset and is almost always overimposed on an established disease (Cohen 1992). Causes of renal vein thrombosis in the elderly patients include idiopathic nephrotic syndrome, especially that due to membranous glomerulonephritis, volume loss due to dehydratation (often aggravated by diuretic therapy) with altered renal blood flow, hypercoagulable states (malignancy), renal cell carcinoma, or extrinsic compression of the renal vein (retroperitoneal fibrosis, lymphoma, etc.). The process may progress without any clinical sign. Mild abdominal or back pain may be present, but severe pain is uncommon. Pulmonary emboli occur during the course of approximately 50% of patients with chronic renal vein thrombosis and are frequently the first manifestation of this condition (Cohen 1992).

Diagnosis of renal vein thrombosis relies on the visualization of an echogenic thrombus within a dilated renal vein devoid of flow signals on CD evaluation. Both kidneys are usually enlarged with reduced cortical–medullary differentiation on gray-scale US. Doppler spectral analysis of renal arteries may reveal slightly increased RIs and normal parenchymal venous flows, since collateral venous supplies open after renal vein thrombosis. Absent or reversed end-diastolic flow in renal interlobar–arcuate arteries has been described in transplanted kidney which lack collateral venous supply. US contrast agents facilitate identification of renal vein patency and thrombosis in cases of technical failure and enhance detection of collateral venous blood supply. A mass is evident in the renal vein with renal enlargement and delayed renal function.

CTA and MRA show complete occlusion of the renal vein (Kawashima et al. 2000) which appears dilated and heterogenous, while the infracted kidney appears enlarged and with a diffuse alteration of the nephrographic phase (Fig. 28.20). Renal vein involvement by tumor (Fig. 28.21) is frequently identified in elderly patients and it is crucial in the determination of surgical options for removing a renal tumor. The renal veins are well depicted on CT during the cortico-medullary or nephrographic phase of contrast enhancement.

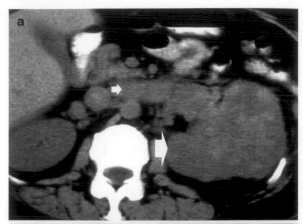

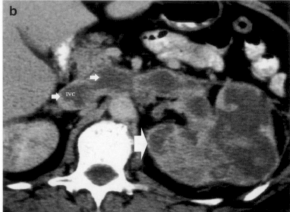

**Fig. 28.21** (**a**, **b**) Thrombosis of the left renal vein due to infiltrating papillary renal cell carcinoma. (**a**) Unenhanced CT. (**b**) Contrast-enhanced CT. Contrast-enhanced CT. Nephrographic phase. The renal vein appears dilated and heterogenous (*small arrow*), while the left kidney (*large arrow*) appears enlarged and with diffuse alteration of the nephrographic phase. The inferior vena cava (IVC) is also involved and appears occluded by a tumoral thrombus

## 28.7 Renal Failure

### 28.7.1 Acute Renal Failure

In the elderly, the kidneys are more vulnerable when other pathologies occur, in particular, atherosclerosis, arterial hypertension, diabetes mellitus, bacterial infections, and malnutrition. Most cases of acute renal failure in the elderly patients are caused by drugs or are secondary to dehydratation, especially in patients with hypertensive intrarenal nephrosclerosis. In elderly patients, the differentiation between renal and prerenal cause of acute renal failure may be difficult because

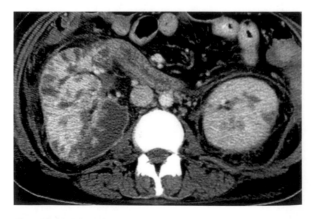

**Fig. 28.20** Thrombosis of the right renal vein. Contrast-enhanced CT. Nephrographic phase. The renal vein appears dilated and heterogenous, while the right kidney appears enlarged and with diffuse alteration of the nephrographic phase

the RIs are usually elevated for the preexisting renal parenchyma disease. Moreover, an elderly patient with severe and prolonged prerenal acute renal failure leading to acute tubular necrosis may present increased RIs.

The acute renal failure is a common complication of hypertensive nephrosclerosis in elderly patients with mild chronic renal failure (Pozzi Mucelli et al. 2001). Worsening renal function may be precipitated by the treatment of hypertension, mainly with ACE inhibitors or by other cause such as nephrotoxic drug or dehydration (Fig. 28.14). The evidence of acute renal failure without an apparent cause following therapy with ACE inhibitors highly suggests renal artery stenosis in well-hydrated elderly patients. Other possible causes of acute renal failure in these patients are renal artery thrombosis or atheroembolic renal disease. Doppler US examination is the first imaging modality to be employed in these patients to rule our renal artery stenosis. Identification of kidneys of two different sizes is suggestive of ischemic disease.

The demonstration of increased flow velocity at the level of renal artery stenosis is diagnostic. Anyway, the Doppler evaluation of intrarenal and renal perforating arteries can be useful in these patients since the direct assessment of the main renal artery may be difficult due to bowel gas interposition and incomplete patient compliance. The intrarenal vessels may show an altered waveform morphology-defined pulsus tardus and parvus consisting in an increased time to reach the peak of the trace (acceleration time >70 ms) with loss of early systolic peak and decreased acceleration index (<300 cm/s²). Perforating arteries are vessels connecting the capsular plexus with the interlobar and interlobular arteries, which became hypertrophic in those pathologic conditions that reduce the blood flow through the renal artery. Perforating arteries with flow toward the kidney have been detected and interrogated in about 60% of kidneys with renal artery stenosis of hypertensive elderly patients with acute renal failure. On the other hand, in the kidneys with no ischemic arterial lesions, only perforating arteries with flow toward the renal capsule were identified (Bertolotto et al. 2000).

Acute cortical necrosis is a rare cause of acute renal failure, usually occurring in extremely ill individuals, often as a result of obstetric complications, hemorrhagic shock, disseminated intravascular coagulation, severe trauma, sepsis, shock, or burns. Contrast-enhanced US or CT (Fig. 28.22) has been shown to be diagnostic of acute cortical necrosis showing necrosis of the renal cortex with sparing of the renal medulla appearing as enhancing renal medulla, nonenhancing renal cortex and a thin rim of subcapsular tissue, and absent renal excretion of iodinated contrast agent (Jordan et al. 1990). Necrosis results from constriction of small intracortical blood vessels with preferential flow of blood away from the renal cortex. The likelihood that normal renal function will return is low. Usually, the involved kidney becomes shrunken and scarred. Cortical nephrocalcinosis may then develop (Cohan et al. 2006).

Cholesterinic renal embolization represents an acute diffuse renal vessel embolization, frequently manifesting with acute renal failure. Clinical diagnosis includes the presence of livedo reticularis due to distal embolization in the lower extremities and cholesterol crystals on the eye fundus examination. Color Doppler US examination is not useful to diagnose this pathologic entity due to the small size of renal perfusion defects. In cholesterinic renal embolization, the identification of small renal perfusion defects in the renal subcapsular region is penalized by the limited spatial resolution of US which cannot identify renal perfusion defects smaller than 5 mm since in this clinical situation the renal perfusion defects are often very small to be detected by contrast-enhanced US. Anyway, if larger or equal to 5 mm, renal perfusions defects may be identified on contrast-enhanced US after microbubble injection (Fig. 28.23). Microbubble-based agents should be always employed to exclude renal infarcts in every old patient presenting with a renal colic-like pain in the flank region.

## 28.7.2 Chronic Renal Failure

The proportion of elderly individuals is growing rapidly in all societies and the incidence of chronic kidney disease among elderly people increases constantly (Fliser 2008). Therefore, the accurate monitoring of kidney function, that is, GFR in elderly people is of considerable clinical interest in order to detect individuals who are at risk for developing chronic kidney disease. The management of end-stage renal failure in the elderly should not be significantly different from that in younger patients and should be based on the capacity for rehabilitation rather than any arbitrary age.

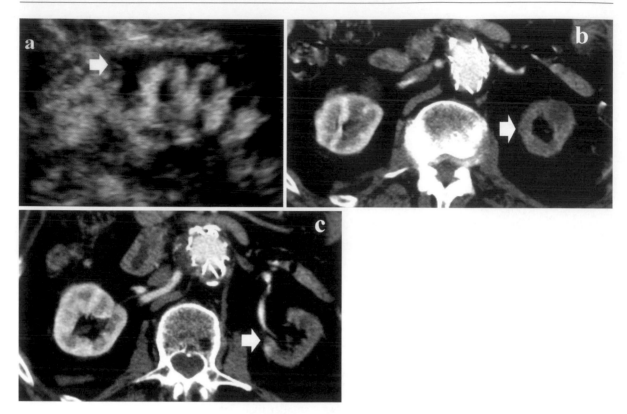

**Fig. 28.22** (**a–d**) Renal acute cortical necrosis. Eighty-year-old patient with aortic encoprosthesis was admitted to the emergency unit with acute renal failure. Absence of contrast enhancement in the superficial cortex of the left kidney (*arrow*) is identified after microbubbles injection (**a**). (**b, c**) Contrast-enhanced CT confirmed the existence of diffuse renal cortical necrosis in the left kidney (*arrow*).

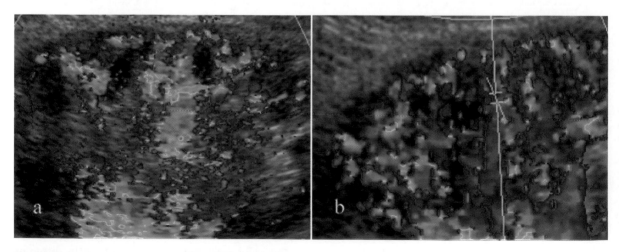

**Fig. 28.23** (**a–d**) Cholesterinic renal embolization in a 70-year-old female patient presenting with acute renal failure. Baseline color Doppler US (**a, b**) does not allow the identification of renal perfusion defects. Contrast-enhanced US (**c, d**) allows a reliable depiction of renal perfusion defect (*arrow*)

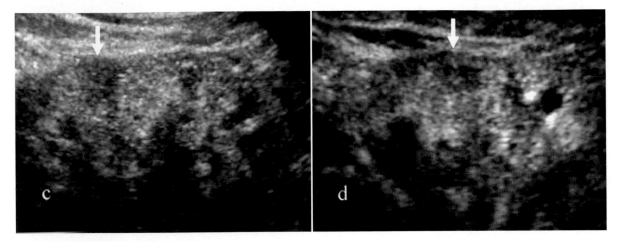

**Fig. 28.23** (continued)

Chronic kidney disease is an important problem in the elderly and is associated with a high risk of kidney failure, cardiovascular disease, and death (Stevens and Levey 2005). The disorder is indicated either by a GFR of less than 60 mL/min/1.73 m² of body-surface area or by the presence of kidney damage, assessed most commonly by the finding of albuminuria for three or more consecutive months (National Kidney Foundation 2002; Levey et al. 2005; Stevens ct al. 2006). Among persons 60–69 years of age, approximately 18% have albuminuria and 7% have an estimated GFR of less than 60 mL/min/1.73 m². In persons 70 years of age or older, those percentages increase to 30 and 26, respectively (Stevens and Levey 2005).

Risk factors for chronic kidney disease include an age of more than 60 years, hypertension, diabetes, cardiovascular disease, and a family history of the disease. According to a recent series, diabetic nephropathy, obstructive uropathy, and hypertensive nephrosclerosis were the major causes of chronic renal failure and accounted for 80% of total chronic renal failure in the elderly (Prakash et al. 2001). Recommendations for evaluating people at increased risk are to measure urine albumin to assess kidney damage and to estimate the GFR with an equation based on the level of serum creatinine (Stevens et al. 2006). Older adults who suffer an acute injury to the kidneys – from trauma, surgery, or illness – are at dramatically increased risk of later end-stage renal disease.

Special care should be used in patients with chronic renal failure when the i.v. injection of iodinated or gadolinium-based agents is planned. Iodinated contrast agents should be employed in patients with chronic renal failure only before and after proper hydratation (see Chap. 33), while gadolinium-based contrast agents should not be employed in patients with a GFR value below 30 mL/min. Differently from iodinated contrast agent and gadolinium-based contrast agents, microbubbles may be safely employed in patients with advanced chronic renal failure, especially in the evaluation of renal masses and perfusion defects.

US reveals reduced renal length and cortical thickness and an hyperechoic renal parenchyma with a poor visibility of renal pyramids and of renal sinus. Doppler US reveals a reduced parenchymal perfusion and increased resistive indices (RIs) values. In the elderly patients with mild chronic renal failure, the acute renal failure represents a common complication of hypertensive nephrosclerosis (Pozzi Mucelli et al. 2001). Worsening renal function may be precipitated by the treatment of hypertension, mainly with ACE inhibitors, or by other causes such as nephrotoxic drug or dehydration.

Elderly patients with mild chronic renal failure may easily develop acute renal failure as a common complication of hypertensive nephrosclerosis. Worsening renal function may be precipitated by the treatment of hypertension, mainly with ACE inhibitors or by other cause such as nephrotoxic drug or dehydration. The evidence of acute renal failure without an apparent cause following therapy with ACE inhibitors highly suggests renal artery stenosis in well-hydrated patients. Doppler US examination is the first imaging modality to be employed in these patients to rule out renal artery stenosis. Other possible causes of acute renal failure in patients with mild chronic renal failure are renal artery thrombosis or atheroembolic renal disease. Many urological interventions can precipitate or exacerbate chronic kidney disease, most notably radical nephrectomy which is greatly overused.

## 28.8 Obstructive Uropathy

In the elderly patient acute urinary tract obstruction can occur anywhere in the urinary tract from the renal papilla to the urethral meatus and may be determined by a plenty of causes (see Chap. 14). As in younger patients, obstruction may be completely asymptomatic even though, most frequently, it manifests with clear clinical symptoms.

Due to nephrosclerosis or dehydratation frequently present in the elderly patients, hydronephrosis may also be absent in the acute obstruction of the urinary tract (see Chap. 14) principally due to hypovolemia, dehydratation, or nephrosclerosis. The most important causes of urinary tract obstruction in the elderly patients are urinary stones, tumors of the urinary tract and ureter, and benign prostatic hyperplasia (Fig. 28.24).

The obstruction of the urinary tract, if not treated, usually determines a progressive atrophy of the renal parenchyma which is frequently observed in the elderly patient. Chronic obstructive uropathy (Fig. 28.25) may be determined by the tumoral infiltration of the ureteral wall, or by chronic incomplete obstruction of the ureter, which may be suddenly complicated by an acute event such as infection.

## 28.9 Renal Infections

Acute pyelonephritis is an infectious disease involving both renal parenchyma and renal pelvis mucosa which can be diffuse or focal. Diffuse pyelonephritis is an infection involving the entire kidney, even though the severity of the process may vary in extension (in one or both kidneys). Focal pyelonephritis is a localized infection of the kidney appearing as a wedge or round-shaped parenchymal lesion, which

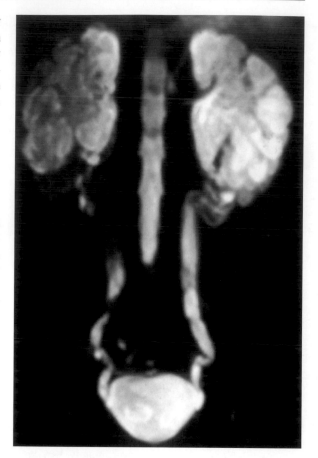

**Fig. 28.24** Static-fluid MR urography in an 85-year-old man patient with benign prostatic hyperplasia. Bilateral fourth-grade hydronephrosis

can regress if well-treated or evolve to a collection extending toward the peri and pararenal spaces. Focal and diffuse pyelonephritis may resolve with the evidence of normal renal parenchyma or scarring or may evolve with liquefaction and formation of nephric or perinephric abscesses. A detailed description of the imaging features of acute renal infections is present in Chap. 16.

Pyelonephritis is the most common cause of gram-negative bacteremia in elderly patients admitted to a community hospital. Acute pyelonephritis can be severe in the elderly as in people who are diabetic or immunosuppressed with frequent evidence of renal abscesses (Fig. 28.26). Appropriate antibiotic therapy and, of equal importance, a lack of serious associated

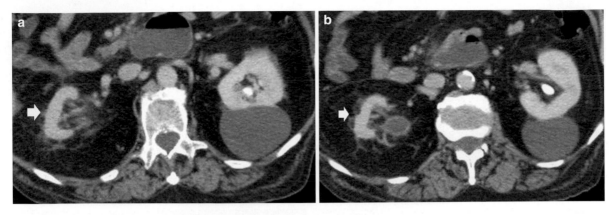

**Fig. 28.25 (a, b)** Contrast-enhanced CT, excretory phase. Chronic urinary tract obstruction of the right kidney (*arrow*) due to tissue scarring of the lower ureter. The kidney appears small and without any sign of function (contrast excretion). Perirenal strands with dilatation and wall thickening of the renal pelvis are also evident on the right kidney

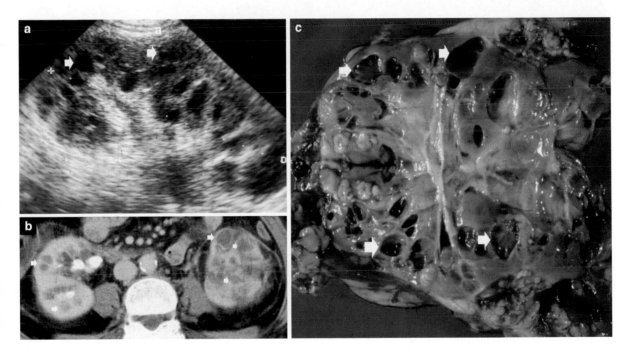

**Fig. 28.26** Pyelonephritis with diffuse abscessual evolution in a 70-year-old diabetic women presenting with septic shock (**a**) Gray-scale US. Longitudinal scan. The left kidney appears increased in dimension with a multiple cystic lesions (*arrows*). (**b**) Contrast-enhanced CT during the nephrographic phase after iodinated contrast injection. Both kidneys appear involved by multiple abscessual lesions (*arrows*). (**c**) Gross autopsy specimen confirming multiple renal abscesses (*arrows*)

medical illnesses contributed to the 97% survival. An increased incidence of bacteremia and septic shock distinguish acute, symptomatic, and bacterial pyelonephritis in the elderly from that in young patients, and particularly in women (Gleckman et al. 1982).

Pyonephrosis is the most common complication of pyelonephritis in the elderly patient when ureteral obstruction is present. Urinary tract obstruction due to a urinary stone is the most common cause of pyonephrosis (Fig. 28.27).

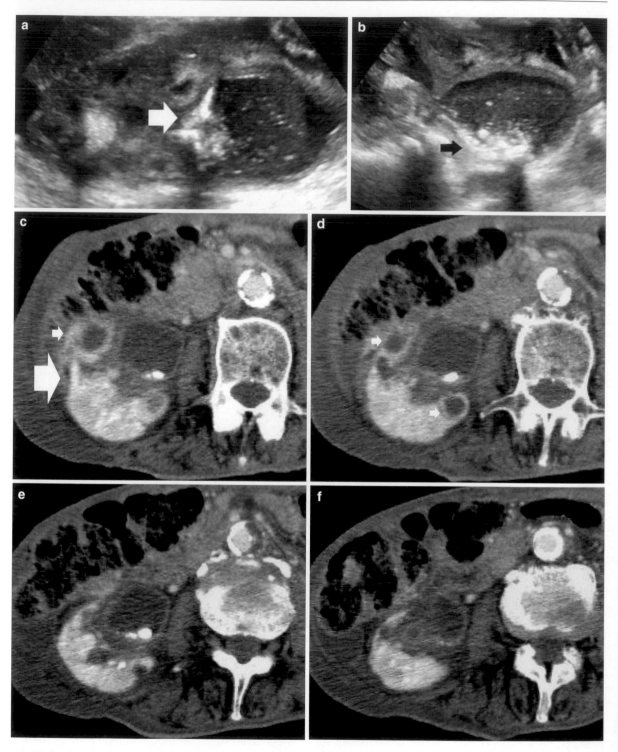

**Fig. 28.27** (a–f) Pyonephrosis in an 82-year-old women presenting with acute right flank pain. Gray-scale US, longitudinal (**a**) and transverse scan (**b**). The right kidney presents dilatation of the lower urinary tract (*white arrow*) with diffuse corpuscular echogenic content, and evidence of renal stones (*black arrow*) lying in the renal pelvis with posterior acoustic shadowing.

(**c–f**) Contrast-enhanced CT, nephrographic phase. The right kidney (*large arrow*) presents increased dimensions, multiple renal stones lying in the renal pelvis, and dilatation and diffuse thickening of the renal pelvis. Renal parenchyma presents also some abscesses (*small arrows*) due to infection diffusion to the renal parenchyma

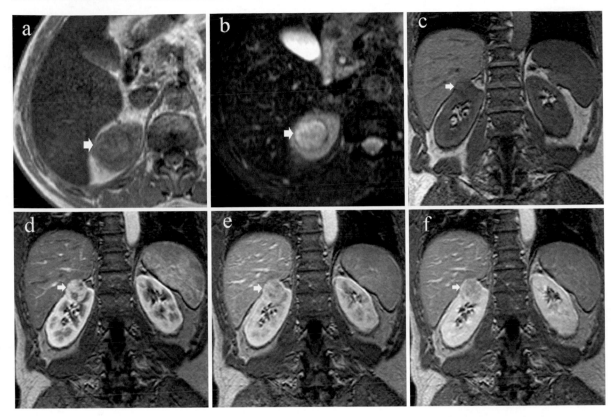

**Fig. 20.28** (**a–f**) Small renal tumor incidentally found in a 67-year-old male patient during US examination of the abdomen. T2-weighted (**a**), and spectral fat-saturated T2-weighted MR sequences (**b**) identify a solid mass (*arrow*) on the right kidney. Unenhanced (**c**) and contrast-enhanced (**d–f**) T1-weighted MR sequences reveal heterogeneous contrast enhancement with progressive washout during the nephrographic phase. Clear cell type renal cell carcinoma is identified after partial nephrectomy

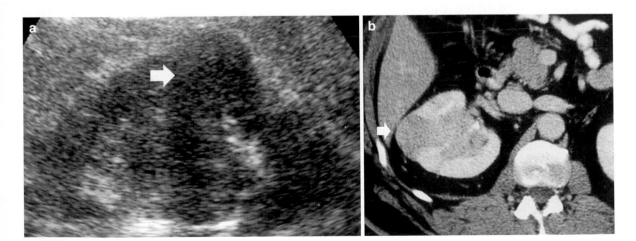

**Fig. 28.29** (**a–d**) Clear cell type renal cell carcinoma in a 75-year-old man with hematuria. Local tumoral invasiveness. (**a**) Grayscale US. A solid renal mass (*arrow*) is identified on the right kidney. (**b**, **c**) Contrast-enhanced CT. Nephrographic phase shows a renal mass (*arrow*) on the right kidney with invasion of the renal pelvis. (**d**) Photograph of gross specimen. Evidence of invasion of the renal pelvis which justified the presenting symptom hematuria

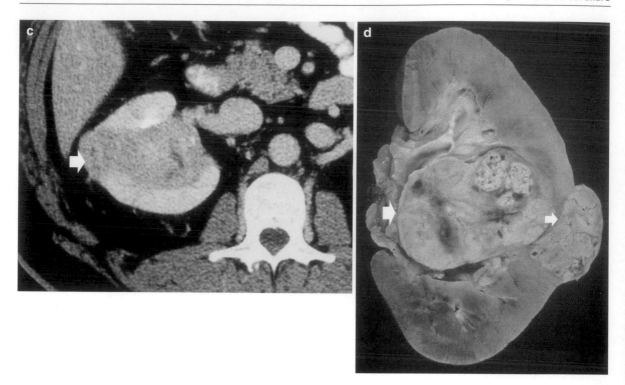

**Fig. 28.29** (continued)

## 28.10 Neoplastic Pathologies

Frequently, the urologists are confronted with an elderly patient (≥75 years of age) with a renal mass seeking treatment. As the population ages, comorbidities become more confounding in predicting patient outcome to therapy and may influence the application of surgical therapy with curative intent to elderly patients (Berdjis et al. 2006). Epidemiological studies show an increasing incidence of renal cell carcinoma over the past two decades, and interestingly, this increase has included a larger proportion of elderly people. The presentation of renal cancer has evolved. There has been an increase in the incidence of cases in the USA and several European countries, and at the same time, a shift to incidentally diagnosed, smaller, localized tumors in a slightly older population (Linehan and Nguyen 2009).

Generally, in the elderly patients there is an increase in neoplastic disorders including clear cell type renal carcinoma and transitional cell carcinoma (see Chaps. 21 and 24). The median age of presentation of renal cell carcinoma is in the sixth decade of life. On the other hand, transitional cell carcinoma of the upper urinary tract is commonly seen in older patient, usually between the sixth and eight decade of life. This increased incidence is mainly due to the more widespread use of imaging technology (Jayson and Sanders 1998). Most renal tumors are completely asymptomatic and are found incidentally in the elderly patients during imaging of the upper abdomen mainly by US (Fig. 28.28). There is a great variance of growth rate with the majority of small renal tumors (≤3 cm in diameter) in the elderly, with a prevalence of low growth rate (0.35 cm/year with a median range of 0–10 cm), and a low incidence of distant metastases (Bosniak et al. 1995). On the other hand, the majority of larger renal tumors usually present local invasiveness (Figs. 28.29, 28.30 and 28.31) and distant metastases (Figs. 28.32 and 28.33). A "wait and see" observational approach for renal masses 1.5 cm or smaller in the elderly can be suggested (Silverman et al. 2008).

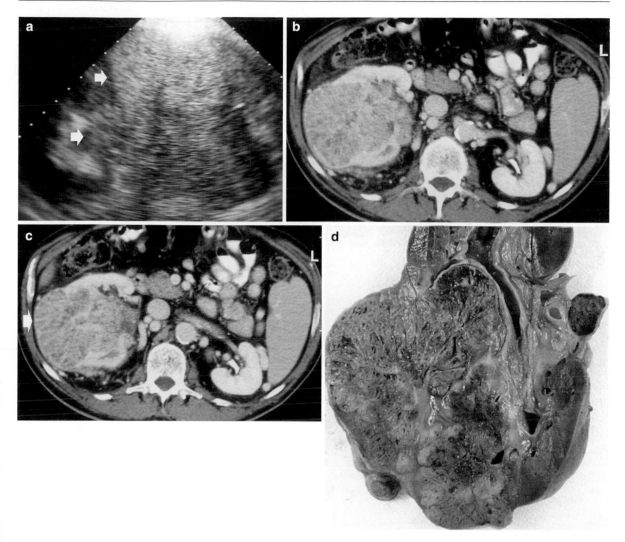

**Fig. 28.30** (**a–d**) Clear cell type renal cell carcinoma in a 70-year-old man. Local tumoral invasiveness. (**a**) Gray-scale US. A huge renal mass (*arrow*) is identified on the right kidney. (**b, c**) Contrast-enhanced CT. Nephrographic phase shows the large renal mass (*arrow*) on the right kidney with invasion of the renal pelvis and of the perirenal fat. (**d**) Photograph of gross specimen with evidence of invasion of the renal pelvis and extrarenal growth of the tumor

**Fig. 28.31** (**a, b**) Clear cell type renal cell carcinoma in an 82-year-old man. Local tumoral invasiveness. Contrast-enhanced CT. (**a**) Transverse plane. (**b**) Sagittal plane. Cortico-medullary phase shows a large solid renal mass of the right kidney invading the adjacent liver parenchyma (*arrow*)

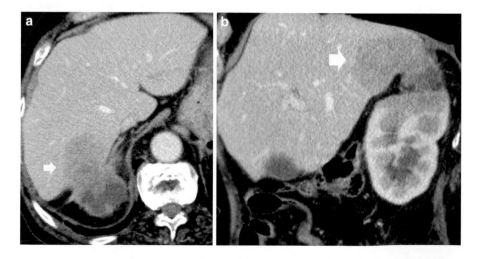

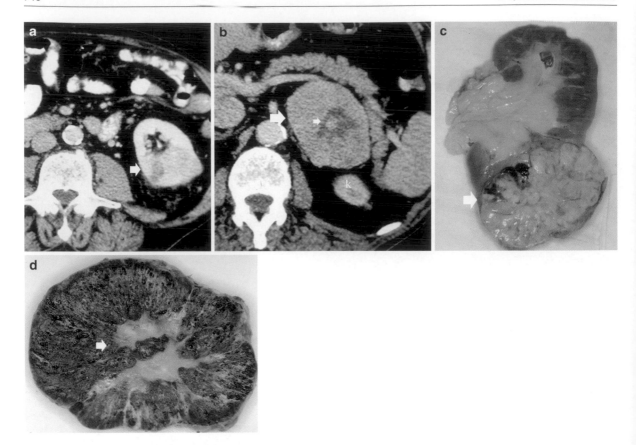

**Fig. 28.32** (**a–d**) Clear cell type renal cell carcinoma in a 73-year-old man with hematuria. (**a**) Contrast-enhanced CT. Nephrographic phase shows a renal mass (*arrow*) on the lower pole of the left kidney. (**b**) A large adrenal metastasis is identi- fied on CT (*large arrow*) with a central necrotic component (*small arrow*). *k* = kidney, upper pole. (**c**) Macroscopic specimen of the tumor. (**d**) Macroscopic specimen of the adrenal metasta- sis with the central necrosis (*arrow*)

Transitional cell carcinomas are relatively rare tumors of the kidney, while they are commonly seen in the older patient usually between the sixth and eight decade of life with a mean age of 65 years. Transitional cell carcinomas (see Chap. 24) of the renal pelvis or calices present an incidence of 5–12% of all malignant tumors of the kidney and 5% of all urothelial tumors (Grabstald et al. 1971; Nocks et al. 1982). The incidence in men exceeds that in women and the usual sex ratio is between 2:1 and 4:1 (Nocks et al. 1982). Over 85–90% of upper urinary tract tumors are TCCs, with the renal pelvis (Fig. 28.34) being more commonly involved than the ureter (Wong-You-Cheong et al. 1998).

Renal lymphoma occurs in all age groups, even though the disease usually affects adults (average age: 60 years) and frequently the elderly patient. Renal involve- ment with lymphoma occurs much more commonly with non-Hodgkin disease, the majority of patients having intermediate or high-grade lymphomas including Burkitt and histiocytic types (Urban and Fishman 2000). Lymphoma that is isolated to the kidney as a primary site of involvement is quite rare, whereas additional sites of extranodal involvement are common and are seen in most patients at the time of diagnosis. Lymphoma typi- cally involves the kidney in one of several recognizable patterns including multiple renal masses, solitary masses, diffuse renal infiltration, renal invasion from contiguous retroperitoneal disease (Fig. 28.35), perirenal disease, or atypical patterns of renal involvement with invasion of the renal pelvis (Fig. 28.36).

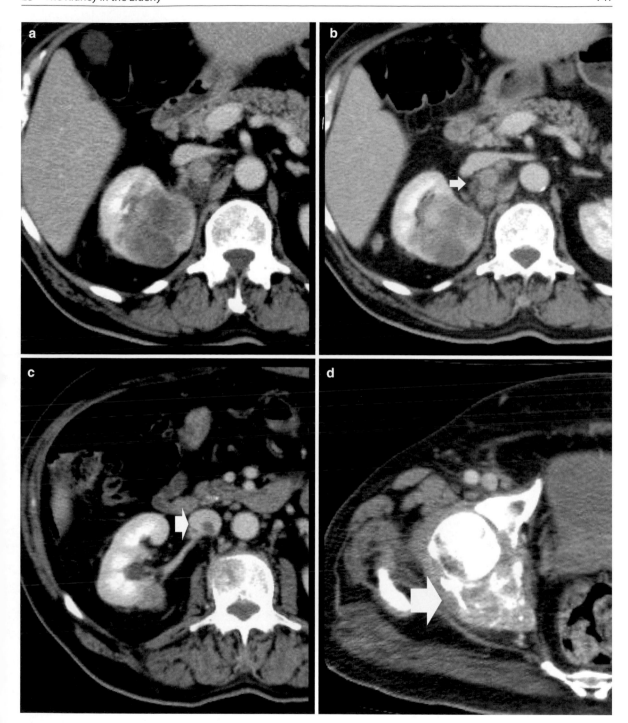

**Fig. 28.33** (**a–d**) Clear cell type renal cell carcinoma in a 77-year-old man. (**a**) Contrast-enhanced CT. Nephrographic phase shows a heterogeneous large renal mass on the lower pole of the right kidney. (**a, b**) Multiple enlarged lymph-nodes (*small white arrow*) are identified in the retrocaval nodal site. (**c**) Floating thrombus (*large white arrow*) in the inferior vena cava is also present. (**d**) Distant bone metastasis is visualized on the right acetabulum (*large arrow*)

**Fig. 28.34** (**a**, **b**)
Transitional renal cell
carcinoma in a 70-year-old
man with hematuria. (**a**)
Contrast-enhanced CT.
Coronal (**a**) and sagittal
reformations (**b**). A solid
endoluminal tumor (*arrow*) in
the left kidney pelvis

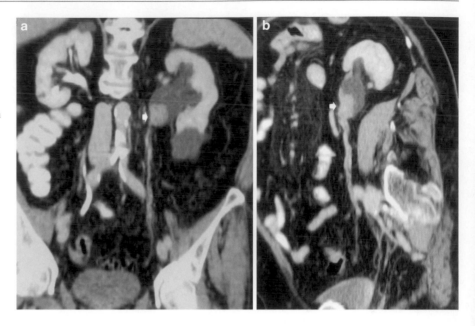

**Fig. 28.35** (**a**, **b**) Renal
lymphoma in a 67-year-old
male patient with a known
non-Hodgkin disease
retroperitoneal disease.
(**a**) Contrast-enhanced CT,
transverse plane. Direct and
extensive renal parenchyma
invasion from contiguous
retroperitoneal disease.
(**b**) Photograph of gross
specimen from autopsy.
Gross pathologic examination
reveals *yellow/gray* tumor
with extensive renal
parenchyma invasion

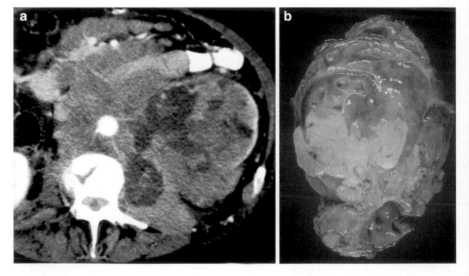

**Fig. 28.36** (**a, b**) Renal lymphoma in a 75-year-old male patient with acute right flank pain. (**a**) Contrast-enhanced CT, transverse plane. (**b**) Coronal reformations. Perirenal lymphoma expressing as ab initio peripheral invasion of the right renal pelvis (*arrows*) with encasement of the intrarenal urinary tract

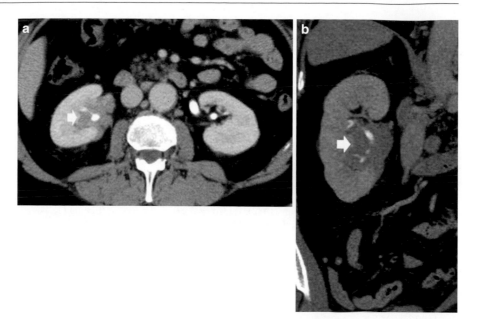

# References

Alpers CE (2005) The kidney. In: Kumar V, Abbas AK, Fausto N (eds) Robbins and Cotran pathologic basis of disease. Elsevier Saunders, Philadelphia, pp 955–1021

Berdjis N, Hakenberg OW, Novotny V et al. (2006) Treating renal cancer in the elderly. BJU Int 97:703–705

Bertolotto M, Martegani A, Aiani L et al. (2008) Value of contrast-enhanced ultrasonography for detecting renal infarcts proven by contrast-enhanced CT. A feasibility study. Eur Radiol 18(2):376–383

Bertolotto M, Quaia E, Galli G et al. (2000) Color Doppler sonographic appearance of renal perforating vessels in subjects with normal and impaired renal function. J Clin Ultrasound 28:267–276

Bosniak MA, Birnbaum BA, Krinsky GA et al. (1995) Small renal parenchymal neoplasms: further observations on growth. Radiology 197(3):589–597

Bude RO, Rubin JM (1995) Detection of renal artery stenosis with Doppler sonography: it is more complicated than originally thought (editorial). Radiology 196:612–613

Bude RO, Rubin JM, Platt JF et al. (1994) Pulsus tardus: its cause and potential limitations in detection of arterial stenosis. Radiology 190:779–784

Cohan RH, Cowan NC, Ellis JH (2006) Unknown ESUR cases 2004. Abdom Imaging 31:141–153

Cohen JJ (1992) Vascular disorders of the kidney. In: Wyngaarden JB, Smith LH, Bennett JC (eds) Cecil textbook of medicine. Saunders, Philadelphia, pp 598–599

Coley BD, Mattrey RF, Roberts A et al. (1991) Potential role of PFOB enhanced sonography of the kidney. II. Detection of partial infarction. Kidney Int 39:740–745

Correas JM, Claudon M, Tranquart F et al. (2003) Contrast-enhanced ultrasonography: renal applications. J Radiol 84:2041–2054

Correas JM, Helenon O, Moreau JF (1999) Contrast enhanced ultrasonography of native and transplant kidney diseases. Eur Radiol 9 (suppl 3):394–400

Dagher PR, Herget-Rosenthal S, Ruehm SG et al. (2003) Newly developed techniques to study and diagnose acute renal failure. J Am Soc Nephrol 14:2188–2198

Davison AM (1998) Renal disease in the elderly. Nephron 80:6–16

Desberg AL, Paushter DM, Lammert GK et al (1990) Renal artery stenosis: evaluation with color Doppler flow imaging. Radiology 177:749–753

Faubert PF, Porush JG (1998) Renal disease in the elderly, 2nd edn. Marcel Decker, Basel, Switzerlad

Ferrucci L, Giallauria F, Guralnik JM (2008) Epidemiology of aging. Radiol Clin N Am 46:643–652

Fliser D (2008) Assessment of renal function in elderly patients. Curr Opin Nephrol Hypertens 17 (6):604–608

Gleckman R, Blagg N, Hibert D et al. (1982) Acute pyelonephritis in the elderly. South Med J 75(5):551–554

Grabstald H, Whitmore WF, Melamed MR (1971) Renal pelvic tumors. JAMA 218:845–854

Grant EG, Melany ML (2001) Ultrasound contrast agents in the evaluation of the renal arteries. In: Goldberg BB, Raichlen JS, Forsberg F (eds) Ultrasound contrast agents. Basic principles and clinical applications, 2nd edn. Martin Dunitz, London, pp 289–295

Helenon O, Rody EL, Correas JM et al (1995) Color Doppler US of renovascular disease in native kidneys. Radiographics 15:833–854

Jayson M, Sanders H (1998) Increased incidence of serendipitously discovered renal cell carcinoma. Urology 51:203–205

Jordan J, Low R, Jeffrey RB (1990) CT findings in acute renal cortical necrosis. J Comput Assist Tomogr 14(1):155–156

Kalva SP, Mueller PR (2008) Vascular imaging in the elderly. Radiol Clin N Am 46:663–683

Kawashima A, Sandler CM, Ernst RD et al. (2000) CT evaluation of renovascular disease. Radiographics 20:1321–1340

Levey AS, Eckardt KU, Tsukamoto Y et al. (2005) Definition and classification of chronic kidney disease: a position statement from Kidney Disease: Improving Global Outcomes (KDIGO). Kidney Int 67:2089–2100

Linehan JA, Nguyen MM (2009) Kidney cancer: the new landscape. Curr Opin Urol 19(2):133–137

Mulder WJ, Hillen HF (2001) Renal function and renal disease in the elderly: part I. Eur J Intern Med 12(4):327–333

National Kidney Foundation (2002) K/DOQI clinical practice guidelines for chronic kidney disease: evaluation, classification, and stratification. Am J Kidney Dis 39(suppl 1):S1–S266

Nocks BN, Heney NM, Daly JJ et al. (1982) Transitional cell carcinoma of the renal pelvis. Urology 19:472–477

Pozzi Mucelli R, Bertolotto M, Quaia E (2001) Imaging techniques in acute renal failure. In: Ronco C, Bellomo R, La Greca G (eds) Blood purification in intensive care. Contrib Nephrol, Basel, Karger, pp 76–91

Pozzi Mucelli R, Faccioli N, Manfredi R (2008) Imaging findings of genitourinary tumors in the elderly. Radiol Clin N Am 46:773–784

Prakash J, Saxena RK, Sharma OP (2001) Spectrum of renal disease in the elderly: single center experience from a developing country. Int Urol Nephrol 33(2):227–233

Quaia E, Bertolotto M (2002) Renal parenchymal diseases: is characterization feasible with ultrasound? Eur Radiol 12:2006–2020

Silverman SG, Israel GM, Herts BR et al. (2008) Management of the incidental renal mass. Radiology 249:16–31

Stavros AT, Parker SH, Yakes WF et al (1992) Segmental stenosis of the renal artery: pattern recognition of tardus and parvus abnormalities with duplex sonography. Radiology 184:487–492

Stevens LA, Coresh J, Greene T et al. (2006) Assessing kidney function – measured and estimated glomerular filtration rate. N Engl J Med 354:2473–2483

Stevens LA, Levey AS (2005) Chronic kidney disease in the elderly – how to assess risk. N Engl J Med 352:2122–2124

Taylor GA, Ecklund K, Dunning PS (1996) Renal cortical perfusion in rabbits: visualization with color amplitude imaging and an experimental mircobubble-based US contrast agent. Radiology 201:125–129

Urban BA, Fishman EK (2000) Renal lymphoma: CT patterns with emphasis on helical CT. Radiographics 20:197–212

Wong-You-Cheong JJ, Wagner BJ, Davis CJ (1998) Transitional cell carcinoma of the urinary tract: radiologic-pathologic correlation. Radiographics 18:123–142

Zhang II, Prince MR (2004) Renal MR angiography. Magn Reson Imaging Clin N Am 12:487–503

# Renal Failure

## 29

Emilio Quaia

## Contents

### Abstract

> Renal failure is a common clinical situation in which imaging modalities, and especially gray-scale ultrasound (US) with color/power Doppler US and Doppler interrogation of renal vessels may be essential for the diagnosis and characterization of the type of acute renal failure, especially to differentiate the renal from the postrenal forms. In the postrenal forms of acute renal failure, gray-scale US is accurate in detecting hydronephrosis, even though it may reveal false-negative results, such as obstructive ARF with nondilated urinary tract, or false-positive results such as dilation of the urinary tract in nonobstructed patients. In chronic renal failure, both kidneys present typical imaging features, which can be identified by US and color Doppler US.

Renal failure is the reduction of renal function expressed by a reduction, rapid or progressive, respectively, in the acute or chronic form, of the glomerular filtration rate (GFR) with consequent retention of nitrogenous waste products. The extent of decline in GFR is known to correlate with the appearance of oliguria, and patients with the most impaired renal hemodynamics, such as older individuals, have the least long-term potential for recovery of renal function (Dagher et al. 2003).

All major organ systems are affected by renal failure. Prevalence of symptoms is a function of the GFR, which averages 120 mL/min in a healthy adult. As the GFR falls to less than ~20% of normal, symptoms of uremia may begin to occur. They almost are invariably

E. Quaia
Department of Radiology, Cattinara Hospital, University of Trieste, Strada di Fiume 447, 34149 Trieste, Italy
e-mail: quaia@univ.trieste.it

E. Quaia (ed.), *Radiological Imaging of the Kidney*,
Medical Radiology, DOI: 10.1007/978-3-540-87597-0_29, © Springer-Verlag Berlin Heidelberg 2011

present when the GFR decreases to less than 10% of normal. Signs and symptoms of renal failure are due to overt metabolic derangements resulting from inability of failed kidneys to regulate electrolyte, fluid, and acid-base balance; they are also due to accumulation of toxic products of amino acid metabolism in the serum. Malaise, weakness, and fatigue are very common. Gastrointestinal disturbances include anorexia, nausea, vomiting, and hiccups. Peptic ulcer disease and symptomatic diverticular disease are common in patients with chronic renal failure. Peripheral neuropathy and restless legs syndrome are the most common neurologic complications of chronic renal failure. Anemia is inevitable in chronic renal failure because of loss of erythropoietin production. Abnormalities in white cell and platelet functions lead to increased susceptibility to infection and easy bruising. Pruritus is a common dermatologic complication assumed to be secondary to accumulation of toxic pigments (urochromes) in the dermis.

Ultrasound (US) with Doppler US examination of intrarenal vessels is the imaging modality of choice to be employed in patients with renal failure and is commonly performed early in the clinical course. The generally accepted value of gray-scale US in the evaluation of acute renal failure (ARF) is largely to exclude renal obstruction, which accounts for only 5–25% of patients with ARF in the common clinical practice. Another important field of application of US is the differentiation between an acute condition affecting previously normal kidneys and a preexisting chronic renal disease that has rapidly worsened.

The first issue to be considered for preventing contrast-media induced nephropathy is the identification of patients at risk, above all, patients with eGFR < 60 mL/min/1.73 m² (see chapter 32). In patients with renal failure, imaging tests that do not require the use of intravenous contrast material should be considered first; these include US, unenhanced CT, and unenhanced MR. If the procedure requiring iodinated contrast is deemed necessary, a number of strategies to reduce the risk of contrast media-induced nephropathy can be considered, namely hydration, use of pharmacologic agents, withdrawal of nephrotoxic drugs, hemodialysis and hemofiltration, choice of contrast material type, and dose. All contrast media, iodinated and gadolinium, can be removed by hemodialysis or peritoneal dialysis, even though there is no evidence that hemodialysis protect patients with impaired renal

function from contrast media induced renal failure or nephrogenic systemic fibrosis (ESUR guidelines to contrast media 2008).

Patients with acute or chronic renal insufficiency remain a problem for both CT urography and MR urography (Silverman et al. 2009). Computed tomography (CT) with administration of iodinated contrast agents is not justified because these agents are potentially nephrotoxic, especially in patients with preexisting renal failure, with the consequent development of contrast-induced nephropathy (Gleeson and Bulugahapitiya 2004). Magnetic resonance (MR) imaging with the administration of gadolinium-based contrast agents should be used with caution in patients with renal failure (Kanal et al. 2007; Thomsen et al. 2007), while they must be avoided in patients with severely compromised renal function (GFR < 30 mL/min/1.73 m²) for the high risk of nephrogenic systemic fibrosis (Shabana et al. 2008)".

The role of nonenhanced functional MR imaging in the ARF is described in Chap. 34.

Nuclear Medicine has an important role in the diagnostic work-up of patients with ARF. The diagnostic capabilities of nuclear medicine, and particularly, of single photon emission tomography (SPECT) are described on Chap. 8.

## 29.1 Acute Renal Failure

ARF is a clinical entity characterized by rapid decline in the GFR and retention of nitrogenous waste products. The precipitous decline in the GFR usually takes place over hours or days and may be attended by either oliguria (urine output <400 mL/day) or anuria (urine output <50 mL/day), but may also manifest with more copious urine flow (Clive and Cohen 1991). An accurate estimation of GFR in ARF may be of prognostic importance. This knowledge would also help in stratifying patients into mild, moderate, and severe ARF, which has significance for clinical studies (Dagher et al. 2003). ARF may affect patients with previously normal-functioning kidneys or may develop in patients with preexisting chronic renal disease.

Table 29.1 shows the principal causes of ARF. ARF may be determined by renal hypoperfusion (prerenal ARF), renal parenchymal diseases (renal ARF), or by

**Table 29.1** Principal causes of acute renal failure

| *Prerenal* |
| Reduced cardiac output |
| Dehydratation |
| Hypovolemia |
| Hemorrhagic shock |
| Systemic vasodilatation |
| Anaphylactic shock |
| Intrarenal vasoconstriction |
| Sepsis |
| Liquid sequestration (e.g., acute pancreatitis) |
| *Renal* |
| Acute cortical necrosis |
| Glomerular diseases |
| Papillary necrosis |
| Renal vascular diseases |
| *Postrenal* |
| Urinary obstructive disease |
| Renal vein thrombosis |

The principal causes of acute renal failure

acute obstruction of the urinary tract (postrenal ARF). Prerenal ARF is essentially functional and reversible if the underlying causes are corrected and results from kidney hypoperfusion due to hypovolemia, low cardiac output, systemic vasodilatation or intrarenal vasoconstriction. Prerenal ARF can exist in the absence of intrinsic renal disease or may be superimposed on preexisting renal disease (Clive and Cohen 1991). Renal ARF is caused mostly by acute tubular necrosis (ATN) or by other causes including acute glomerular

nephritis, acute interstitial nephritis, severe acute pyelonephritis, renal vasculitides including systemic lupus erythematosus, papillary necrosis, acute ischemia due to renal artery or vein thrombosis, lymphoma, or nephrotoxic agents. Postrenal ARF is caused by urinary tract obstruction.

## 29.1.1 Prerenal and Renal Acute Renal Failure

Morphological evaluation of the kidney is now more reliable by more recent US equipment and tissue harmonic techniques. Morphological alterations in renal parenchyma are observed in almost 10% of ARF patients. Renal dimensions are usually normal in prerenal ARF, may be increased in acute renal disease, such as ATN, tubulo-interstitial nephritis, and acute glomerulonephritis, and are reduced in renal failure complicating chronic nephropathy (Table 1). Most patients with ARF have normal renal echogenicity, even though acute and diffuse renal parenchymal diseases may show hyperechogenicity, increased parenchymal thickness, and increased cortico-medullary differentiation (Table 29.2). A hypoechoic band surrounding the kidney is considered a typical feature of cortical necrosis.

There are no specific features regarding kidney size of patients with ARF (Table 29.2). However, the renal size is usually normal in prerenal ARF and it may

**Table 29.2** Differential diagnosis of renal failure based on US

|  | Renal dimension | Renal echogenicity | Cortico-medullary differentiation | Parenchyma thickness | Resistive Indices |
|---|---|---|---|---|---|
| Prerenal acute renal failure | Normal | Normal | Normal | Normal | Normal |
| Acute tubular necrosis | Increased | Increased | Increased | Increased | Increased |
| Interstitial nephritis | Increased | Increased | Increased | Normal or increased | Increased |
| Acute glomerulonephritis | Increased | Increased or normal | Increased or normal | Normal or increased | Normal |
| Diabetic nephropathy | Increased | Increased | Increased | Increased | Increased |
| Ischemic nephropathy | Reduced | Normal | Normal | Reduced | Normal |
| Chronic renal failure | Reduced | Increased | Increased | Reduced | Increased |

The different features of the kidney on US scanning which may differentiate different cause of acute renal failure

increase in acute renal diseases such as ATN, interstitial nephritis, and acute glomerular nephritis. The finding of large, smooth kidneys with nondilated calyces should indicate that ARF is probably due to primary acute renal disease and that the process is potentially reversible. On the other hand, detection of kidneys of reduced size suggests a complicated underlying chronic nephropathy and worse prognosis.

In prerenal ARF, RIs values lower than 0.7 are related to complete recovery after fluid restoration, whereas resistive indices (RIs) higher than 0.7 indicate a progression toward ischemic ATN and worse prognosis. In renal ARF, RIs values are usually higher than 0.7. An RI value of 0.75 is reported as optimal in attempting differential diagnosis between renal and prerenal ARF (Platt et al. 1991). Differential diagnosis between renal and prerenal ARF is difficult if ARF is determined by drug abuse or dehydration in elderly patients with hypertensive nephrosclerosis, since RIs are usually elevated for the preexisting renal parenchymal disease. Doppler US is unable to distinguish among various causes of renal ARF and ATN, since similar changes in renal RIs may be seen in septicemia, hypovolemia, rhabdomyolysis, nephrotoxic drug intake, and multiple-organ failure. On Doppler US evaluation, most patients with prerenal ARF have normal parenchymal flow, whereas patients with renal ARF reveal reduced renal parenchyma vascularity on color/power Doppler US (Fig. 29.1) with high RIs (Figs. 29.2 and 29.3). Renal parenchyma vascularity may appear even absent at the automatic color signal optimization

(Fig. 29.1) due to slow arterial flow suppression from wall filters. The threshold values of renal RI for renal impairment and/or values prognostic of poor renal outcome range from 0.70 to 0.79 (Platt et al. 1994, 1997; Petersen et al. 1997; Radermacher et al. 2002). Anyway, the diastolic component of the Doppler trace may appear very much reduced or even inverted (Figs. 29.2 and 29.3).

On the other hand, Doppler US is a useful tool in the follow-up of prerenal and renal ARF during medical treatment, and normalization of renal RIs frequently advances recovery of renal function. Color and power Doppler US may identify a global reduction of intraparenchymal flow signal intensity in diffuse renal parenchyma disease, or focal reduction of renal perfusion in renal infarction, severe acute pyelonephritis, or embolic disease. Recently, contrast-enhanced US has been proposed as a potential technique to quantify the reduction of renal perfusion in ARF (Wei et al. 2001).

Prolonged or severe prerenal ARF may lead to ATN, which designates any form of ARF not due to obstruction, vascular disorders, or glomerular or interstitial disease (Finkel 2009). ATN is a reversible renal lesion and represents the most common presentation of ARF in hospitalized patients affecting 5–7% of all hospitalized patients, and it may be determined by ischemia-reperfusion injury, nephrotoxic injury or rhabdomyolysis, nephrotoxic drugs (aminoglycosides, antibiotics, iodinated contrast agents, heavy metals, or myoglobin), inflammation, or sepsis. In a significant number of

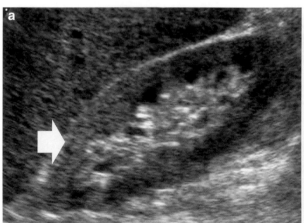
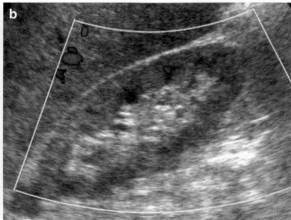

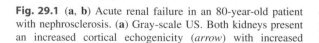

**Fig. 29.1** (**a**, **b**) Acute renal failure in an 80-year-old patient with nephrosclerosis. (**a**) Gray-scale US. Both kidneys present an increased cortical echogenicity (*arrow*) with increased cortico-medullary differentiation. (**b**) Color Doppler. The renal parenchyma vascularity appears reduced on color Doppler analysis with no evidence of parenchymal arterial vessels

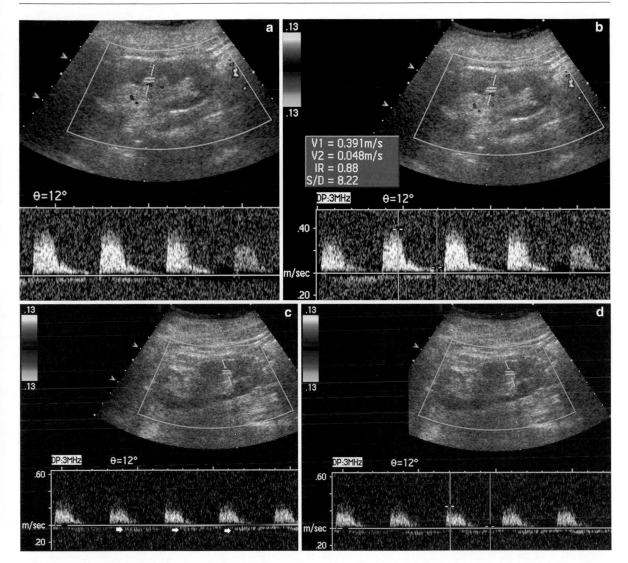

**Fig. 29.2** (**a–d**) Acute renal failure (ARF) with nephrotic syndrome in a 65-year-old man. Color Doppler US with pulsed Doppler interrogation of intrarenal arteries. Both kidneys present hyperechogenicity in the renal cortex with increased cortico- medullary differentiation. (**a, b**) Right kidney; (**c, d**) left kidney. High resistive indices (RIs) are registered in the intrarenal arteries even with inversion of the diastolic component (*arrows*) of the Doppler trace on the left kidney

patients, ATN is multifactorial. The mortality rate in intensive care unit patients with ATN approaches 60% when renal replacement therapy is required. Chronic dialysis therapy is needed by 5–30% of surviving patients and tubular occlusion by casts. ATN is characterized histologically by destruction of tubular cells with rupture of basement membrane. US is usually employed to rule out postrenal ARF due to urinary tract obstruction from renal and prerenal ARF usually due to ATN. ATN may not determine any morphological renal alteration.

In renal ARF both kidneys frequently appear enlarged and with increased cortical echogenicity and cortico-medullary differentiation (Fig. 29.4) and with increased values of RIs. The clinical course of the parenchymal disease determining the ARF may be monitored with Doppler US by using serial measurements of renal RIs with a progressive decrease of RIs (Fig. 29.5), which can precede the recovery of renal function, or with an increase of RIs in case of complications leading to a further deterioration of Doppler waveforms (Platt et al. 1991).

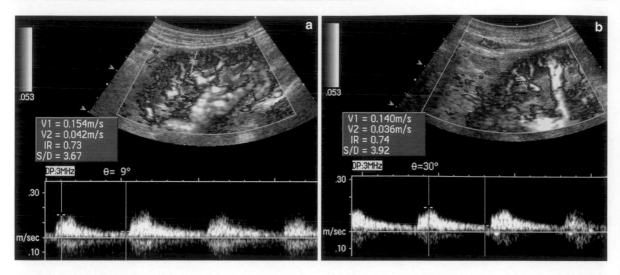

**Fig. 29.3** (**a, b**) ARF due to glomerulonephritis in a 55-year-old man. Power Doppler US with pulsed Doppler interrogation of intrarenal arteries. Both kidneys present hyperechogenicity in the renal cortex with increased cortico-medullary differentiation. High RIs (from 0.75 to 0.8) are registered in the intrarenal arteries

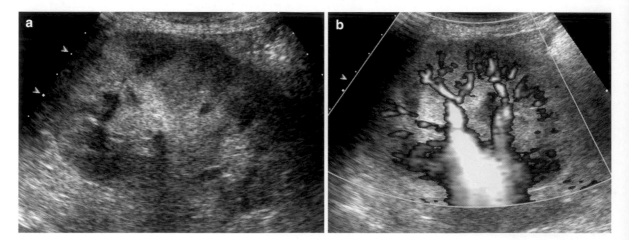

**Fig. 29.4** (**a, b**) ARF due to acute tubular necrosis in a 60-year-old man with a progressive increase in the creatinine levels. (**a**) On gray-scale US, kidneys appear enlarged and reveal increased cortical echogenicity and cortico-medullary differentiation. (**b**) Power Doppler US revealed reduced renal cortical perfusion

## 29.1.2 Postrenal Acute Renal Failure

In postrenal ARF urinary tract obstruction must be bilateral or unilateral in patients with a solitary kidney as in patients with renal agenesis or with renal transplantation or with preexisting impaired renal function. It may be due to various pathological conditions such as pelvic malignancies or prostatic disease (Fig. 29.6). In clinical practice, this condition accounts for approximately 5–25% of cases of ARF. US is accurate in detecting hydronephrosis, even though it may reveal false-negative results, such as obstructive ARF with nondilated urinary tract, or false-positive results such as dilation of the urinary tract in nonobstructed patients (Quaia and Bertolotto 2002). The employing of tissue harmonic imaging modality has improved the detection of dilated urinary tract and of small perirenal urinomas due to the increased signal-to-noise ratio and spatial and contrast resolution, and reduction of artifacts. The clinically important distinction of renal obstruction from nonobstructive dilatation cannot in general be resolved by gray-scale US. The accuracy of US to rule out obstruction increases in patients with an high pretest probability of urinary

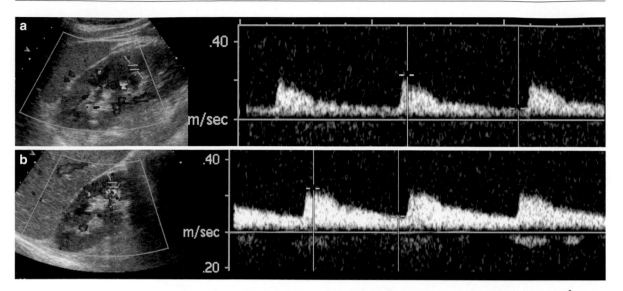

**Fig. 29.5** (**a**, **b**) ARF due to glomerulonephritis in a 66-year-old woman. (**a**) Color Doppler US with Doppler interrogation of the intrarenal arterial vessels. Both kidneys appear enlarged with increased RIs. (**b**) The clinical course of glomerulonephritis is monitored with Doppler US 7 days after the beginning of the corticosteroid therapy. There is a progressive decrease of the RIs due to a progressive increase of the diastolic component of the arterial Doppler trace

tract obstruction such as patients with a history suggestive for obstruction like pelvic malignancy, palpable abdominal or pelvic mass, suspected renal colic, and recent pelvic surgery.

Doppler US may provide unique data not available from conventional US in postrenal ARF. Renal vasoconstriction is the key factor in the pathophysiological course of acute and chronic obstruction and increased RIs values result. A mean RI > 0.7 and a difference of > 0.06–0.08 between the average RI of the two kidneys are considered diagnostic of obstruction. Demonstration of high RI in patients with ARF and hydronephrosis increases the diagnostic confidence for a diagnosis of obstruction. RIs elevation occurs by

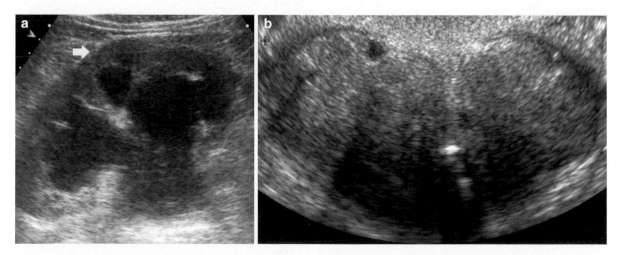

**Fig. 29.6** (**a**, **b**) Acute postrenal renal failure. Gray-scale US shows upper urinary tract dilatation in a 70-year-old man with benign prostatic hyperplasia. (**a**) Gray-scale US reveals third-grade hydronephrosis on both kidneys with clear reduction of the renal cortical thickness (*arrow*). (**b**) Benign prostatic hyperplasia with urethral obstruction was the cause of the whole urinary tract obstruction

6 h of clinical acute renal obstruction and may precede pyelocaliectasis. A significant fall in RIs values appears after the removal of the urinary obstruction (Fig. 29.7) or after nephrostomy. In general, there should be a rapid return to normal RIs if obstruction is relieved within 5 h, whereas RIs may take days or even weeks to return to baseline levels if obstruction is present for at least 18–24 h.

The static-fluid MR urography with relaxation enhancement (RARE) or half-Fourier acquisition single-shot turbo spin echo (HASTE) heavily T2-weighted pulse sequences is effective in demonstrating urinary tract dilatation or obstruction (Fig. 29.8). On the heavily T2-weighted images, the urinary tract is hyperintense because of its long relaxation time, independent of the excretory renal function. This technique is ideally suited for patients with dilated or obstructed collecting system.

## 29.1.3 Clinical Scenarios Related to ARF

Detection of multiple perfusion defects with color or power Doppler in patients with ARF may suggest the diagnosis of infarction, severe acute pyelonephritis, or embolic renal disease.

ARF is common in elderly patients with hypertensive nephrosclerosis and mild chronic renal failure where ARF is usually determined by angiotensin converting enzyme (ACE) inhibitors, drug abuse, dehydration, renal artery thrombosis, or atheroembolic renal disease. ARF following therapy with ACE inhibitors highly suggests renal artery stenosis in well-hydrated elderly patients, and Doppler US is the modality of choice in patients with ARF to rule out renal artery stenosis since iodinated contrast agents are nephrotoxic (Fig. 29.9).

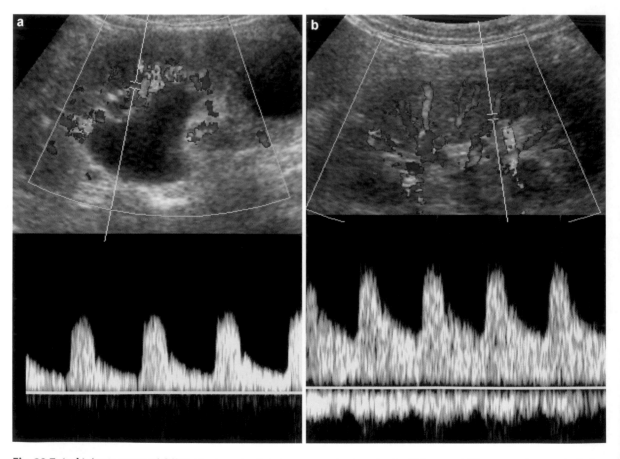

**Fig. 29.7** (**a**, **b**) Acute postrenal failure due to ureteral obstruction from a urinary stone. Gray-scale US with Doppler interrogation of the intrarenal arterial vessels. (**a**) Dilatation of the renal urinary tract with increased RIs measured on renal arteries. (**b**) Dilatation of the urinary tract is reduced with normalization of the RIs after removal of the ureteral stone

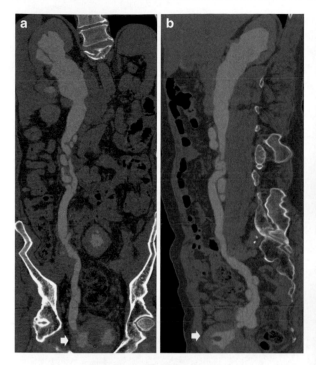

**Fig. 29.8** Urinary tract obstruction due to benign prostatic hypertrophy in a patient with a previous left nephrectomy. CT urography, curved planar reformations on the coronal (**a**) and sagittal plane (**b**). Third-grade hydronephrosis and hydroureter due to benign prostatic hypertrophy with bladder wall hypertrophy (*arrow*)

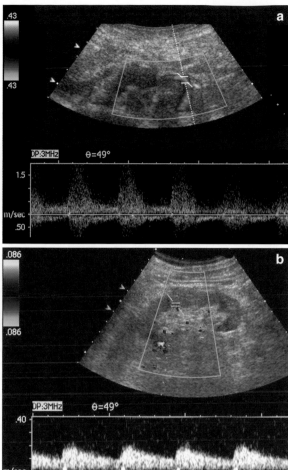

**Fig. 29.9** (**a, b**) Seventy-five-year-old patient with mild chronic renal failure due to hypertensive nephrosclerosis with ARF after treatment of hypertension by angiotensin converting enzyme. (**a**) Demonstration of increased flow velocity at the level of left renal artery due to a tight stenosis. (**b**) The Doppler evaluation of intrarenal arteries shows a pulsus tardus and parvus pattern with increased time to reach the peak of the trace (acceleration time 80 ms) and decreased acceleration inde250 cm/s$^2$)

Hepatorenal failure (HRF) is a well-recognized cause of ARF in patients with liver disease characterized by early renal vasoconstriction. Although most patients are cirrhotic, they may have other liver pathologies such as fulminant hepatitis or hepatic tumors. HRF is generally considered to be a functional renal disease since there are no histological findings and ARF reverses after liver transplantation. HRF is reported to develop in 26% of subjects with elevated values of RIs and only in 1% of those with normal RIs. Virtually all patients with clinically overt HRF have markedly elevated RIs (Fig. 29.10).

Hemolytic uremic syndrome (see also Chap. 27) is a form of ARF that occurs mainly in children and consists in a thrombotic microangiopathy. This disease presents some overlap with thrombotic thrombocytopenic purpura, and clinically manifest with microangiopathic hemolytic anemia, thrombocytopenia, and in certain conditions, renal failure. The renal failure is associated with platelet or platelet-fibrin thrombi in the interlobular renal arteries, arterioles, and glomeruli (Alpers 2005). US examination reveals an increased echogenicity of the renal cortex, with sharp delineation of swollen hypoechoic pyramids and increased cortico-medullary differentiation. RIs are markedly increased (Patriquin et al. 1989).

Acute renal cortical necrosis is a rare form of ARF characterized by total or partial necrosis of the renal cortex of both kidneys which is observed with a variety of pathologic conditions, the most common of which are pregnancy associated (Pozzi Mucelli et al. 2001). It may also occurs in extremely ill individuals, often as a result of obstetric complications, hemorrhagic shock,

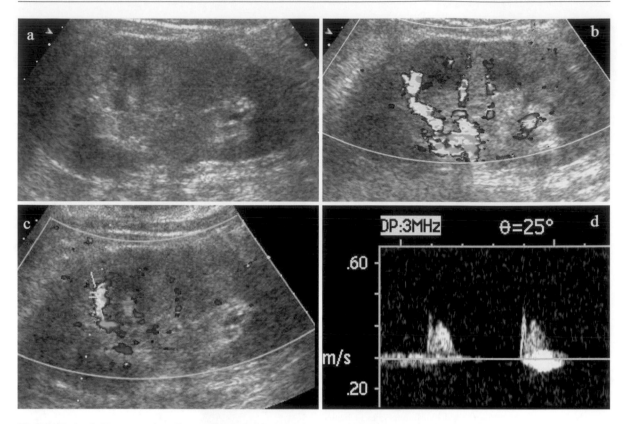

**Fig. 29.10** (**a–d**) Hepatorenal syndrome. Seventy-six-year-old woman with liver cirrhosis and progressive increase of serum creatinine (4.4 mg/dL). (**a**) Gray-scale US. Both kidneys present an increased cortical echogenicity with reduced renal cortex vascularization on color Doppler US (**b**). (**c**) Doppler interrogation of segmentary renal arteries reveals a markedly increased resistive index with the absence of diastolic component on the speed trace (**d**)

disseminated intravascular coagulation, severe trauma, sepsis, shock, or burns (Cohan et al. 2006). Necrosis results from constriction of small intracortical blood vessels with preferential flow of blood away from the renal cortex. The likelihood that normal renal function will return is low. Usually, the involved kidney becomes shrunken and scarred. Cortical nephrocalcinosis may then develop. US and color/power Doppler are non-specific. Contrast-enhanced CT has been shown to be diagnostic of acute cortical necrosis showing enhancing renal medulla, nonenhancing renal cortex, and a thin rim of subcapsular tissue (Jordan et al. 1990). However, due to nephrotoxicity of iodinated contrast media in the context of ARF, contrast-enhanced CT is performed rarely.

A particular form of ARF is that caused by multiple myeloma. Multiple myeloma is characterized by plasma cell dyscrasia with multiple masses throughout the skeleton and soft tissues. In patients with multiple myeloma, renal failure is a major cause of death only second to infections and occurs in up to 50% of patients (Kim and Kim 1990). Bence Jones proteinuria is present in three fourths of these patients. Renal failure is caused either by blockage of the tubules with waxy casts due to proteinuria or by hypercalcemia and hyperuricemia. Intratubular obstruction results in tubular atrophy and fibrosis with diffusely enlarged kidneys with smooth surface (Kim and Kim 1990).

ARF in the HIV population may be due essentially to renal intrinsic causes. Intrinsic renal causes include ATN secondary to nephrotoxic agents used to treat opportunistic infections, such as pentamidine, amphotericin B, and foscarnet (Symeonidou et al. 2009). Other causes include interstitial nephritis and crystal deposition. Causes of prerenal failure include hypovolemia or sepsis, while causes of postrenal failure include tumors or obstruction.

**Fig. 29.11** (**a, b**) The reduction of renal size associated to chronic renal failure. The different morphological appearances of the kidney during the reduction in the renal size occurring during months (**a**) or years (**b**)

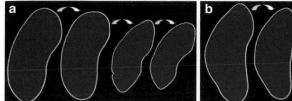

## 29.2 Chronic Renal Failure

Chronic renal failure – or chronic kidney disease – is a functional diagnosis defined as a progressive and generally irreversible reduction in the GFR (Levey et al. 2005; Stevens et al. 2006) corresponding to a loss of more than half of kidney function. In chronic renal failure, beside a progressive loss of renal function, there is also a progressive reduction of the renal size over a period of months or years (Fig. 29.11) through different stages according to the GFR value, which is associated with a high risk of kidney failure, cardiovascular disease, and death (Stevens and Levey 2005). Chronic renal failure can result from numerous diseases (Table 29.3), the most common being glomerulonephritis (Murphey et al. 1993), diabetes, hypertension, and polycystic kidney disease. Diabetes and hypertension are now recognized as the leading causes of chronic renal failure in the United States (Warnock 1992). In the initial phases of advancing renal failure, most organs function normally, so that the patient often seeks medical attention only when the disease has progressed to the uremic stage. Normally, the adult patient is unaware of advancing renal failure until the GFR has decreased to less than 15 mL/min, namely end-stage renal disease (Warnock 1992).

### 29.2.1 Classification

Recommendations for evaluating people at increased risk are to measure urine albumin to assess kidney damage and estimate the GFR with an equation based on the level of serum creatinine (Stevens et al. 2006). Once chronic kidney disease is detected, identification of the cause, coexisting conditions, and stage is essential for further evaluation and management. Serum creatinine is an unreliable indicator of GFR especially in elderly people, particularly in those who are sick or malnourished or both. The differing accuracy of current estimating equations in people with and those without the disease may make it difficult to interpret GFR estimates that are near 60 mL/min/1.73 m$^2$. In this range, the interpretation of GFR estimates depends on the clinical context. Patients with markers of kidney damage such as proteinuria or abnormalities on imaging studies or on kidney biopsy have chronic renal failure, even though GFR estimates are 60 mL/min/1.73 m$^2$ or greater (Stevens et al. 2006). Patients without markers of kidney damage who have GFR estimates of 60 mL/min/1.73 m$^2$ or greater are unlikely to have chronic renal failure. There is some uncertainty with respect to patients without markers of kidney damage who have GFR estimates just below 60 mL/min/1.73 m$^2$ (Stevens

**Table 29.3** Principal causes of chronic renal failure

| |
|---|
| *Prerenal* |
| Untreated renal artery stenosis |
| Chronic dehydration |
| Congestive heart failure |
| Liver cirrhosis |
| *Renal* |
| Diabetic nephropathy |
| Nephrosclerosis due to hypertension |
| Polycystic kidney disease |
| Glomerulonephritis |
| Congenital metabolic disease (oxalosis, tubular acidosis, cystinosis, etc.) |
| Drugs |
| Systemic disease (goiter, AIDS, Wegener granulomatosis, scleroderma, etc.) |
| *Postrenal* |
| Obstructive nephropathy |
| Ureteropelvic junction obstruction |
| Vesicoureteral reflux |
| Ureteral stenosis (stones, tumors) |
| Bladder neck obstruction (benign prostatic hypertrophy, neurologic bladder) |

The principal causes of chronic renal failure

et al. 2006). Some of these patients may have a measured GFR above 60 mL/min/1.73 m², and therefore, would not be considered to have chronic renal failure.

The National Kidney Foundation (2002) currently recommends using a creatinine-based estimate of GFR (e.g., *Modification of Diet in Renal Disease Study Group–MDRD*–(Levey et al. 1999) and has advocated a standardized classification for chronic renal failure. The severity of chronic renal failure is described by six stages: stage 0: normal kidney function – GFR above 90 mL/min/1.73 m² and no proteinuria; stage 1: GFR above 90 mL/min/1.73 m² with evidence of kidney damage; stage 2 (mild): GFR of 60–89 mL/min/1.73 m² with evidence of kidney damage; stage 3 (moderate or early stage of disease): GFR of 30–59 mL/min/1.73 m²; stage 4 (severe): GFR of 15–29 mL/min/1.73 m²; stage 5 (kidney failure: dialysis or kidney transplant needed): GFR less than 15 mL/min/1.73 m².

The most severe 3 stages (stages 3–5) are strictly defined by the estimated GFR value, while the first 3 (stages 0–3) also depend whether there is other evidence of kidney disease (e.g., proteinuria). An estimated GFR of less than 60 mL/min/1.73 m² is associated with a graded increase in the risk of each of the major adverse outcomes of chronic kidney disease, which are impaired kidney function, progression to kidney failure, and premature death caused by cardiovascular disease.

Chronic renal failure is associated to a reduction of renal size (Fig. 29.11), which develops over months (Fig. 29.11a) or years (Fig. 29.11b). Renal length does not correlate with renal reduced function, whereas it correlates, as does cortical echogenicity, with severity of pathological changes, such as global sclerosis, focal tubular atrophy, and numerous hyaline casts per glomerulus. There is no correlation between chronic renal failure and the type of renal disease since kidneys lose peculiar US features of original renal disease. US reveals reduced renal length and cortical thickness and a hyperechoic renal parenchyma with a poor visibility of renal pyramids and of renal sinus (Fig. 29.12). Color Doppler US reveals a reduced parenchymal perfusion and increased RIs values (Petersen et al. 1995, 1997) according to the stage of chronic renal failure (Figs. 29.13–29.16). The capability of the renal RI to aid prediction of progression of renal dysfunction has been demonstrated (Splendiani et al. 2002). US

follow-up of native scarred kidneys is indicated in patients with chronic renal failure treated with dialysis or renal transplantation, because they develop acquired polycystic kidney disease with a significantly increased risk of solid and cystic malignancies. CT confirms the US findings by revealing reduced renal length and cortical thickness (Fig. 29.17). Polycystic kidney disease, one of the leading causes of chronic renal disease, presents typical pattern on US and cross-sectional imaging (see Chap. 12) (Fig. 29.18).

Chronic unilateral obstructive uropathy with long-term blockage of the ureter usually occurs when ureteral or kidney stones, ureteral tumors (Fig. 29.19), or extrinsic ureteral compression from tumors arise in the surrounding anatomical structures (uterus, cervix, or lymph nodes) with obstructive uropathy.

## 29.2.2 Clinical Scenarios Related to Chronic Renal Failure

In patients with mild chronic renal failure, especially elderly patients (Fliser 2008), the ARF represents a common complication of hypertensive nephrosclerosis (Pozzi Mucelli et al. 2001). Worsening renal function may be precipitated by the treatment of hypertension, mainly with ACE inhibitors, or by other cause such as nephrotoxic drug or dehydration. The evidence of ARF without an apparent cause following

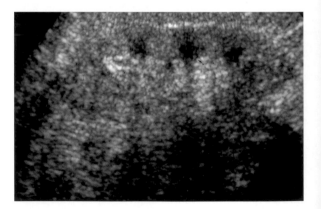

**Fig. 29.12** Chronic renal failure. Gray-scale US. Both kidneys reveal a short length and diffuse reduction of cortical thickness, irregular margins, and low cortico-medullary differentiation

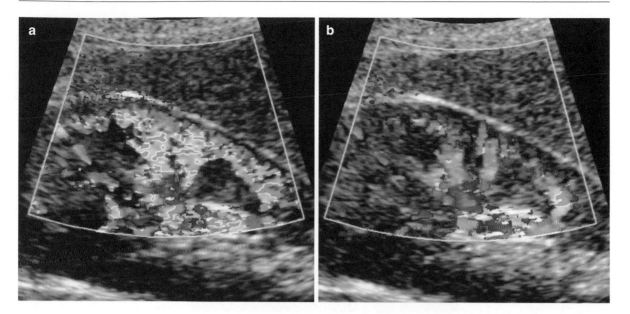

**Fig. 29.13** (**a**, **b**) Color Doppler US. (**a**) Normal renal parenchyma perfusion; (**b**) Renal vascularization in a patient with chronic renal failure at an early stage with a progressive reduction of renal vessels on the renal cortical surface

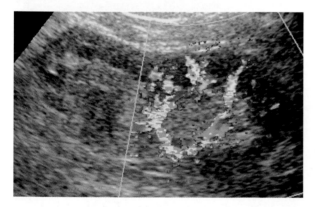

**Fig. 29.14** Color Doppler US. Renal vascularization in a patient with chronic renal failure at an advanced stage with clear reduction of renal vessels on the renal cortical surface with deformation of renal margins

therapy with ACE inhibitors highly suggests renal artery stenosis in well-hydrated patients (Fig. 29.9). Doppler US examination is the first imaging modality to be employed in these patients to rule our renal artery stenosis. The demonstration of increased flow velocity at the level of renal artery stenosis is diagnostic. Anyway, the Doppler evaluation of intrarenal and renal perforating arteries can be useful in these patients since the direct assessment of the main renal artery may be difficult due to bowel gas interposition and incomplete patient compliance. The intrarenal vessels may show an altered waveform morphology defined pulsus tardus and parvus consisting in an increased time to reach the peak of the trace (acceleration time >70 ms) with loss of early systolic peak and decreased acceleration index (<300 cm/s$^2$). Perforating arteries with flow toward the kidney have been detected and interrogated in about 60% of kidneys with renal artery stenosis of hypertensive elderly patients with ARF. On the other hand, in the kidneys with no ischemic arterial lesions, only perforating arteries with flow toward the renal capsule were identified (Bertolotto et al. 2000).

Other possible causes of ARF in patients with mild chronic renal failure are renal artery thrombosis or atheroembolic renal disease (see Chaps. 18 and 28). Many urological interventions can precipitate or exacerbate chronic kidney disease, most notably radical nephrectomy which is greatly overused.

In HIV population chronic renal failure may be caused by HIV-associated nephropathy, immune complex disease, and microangiopathies such as thrombotic thrombocytopenic purpura (Symeonidou et al. 2009).

**Fig. 29.15** Color Doppler US. Renal vascularization in a patient with chronic renal failure at an advanced stage with reduced parenchymal perfusion and increased RIs at duplex Doppler interrogation

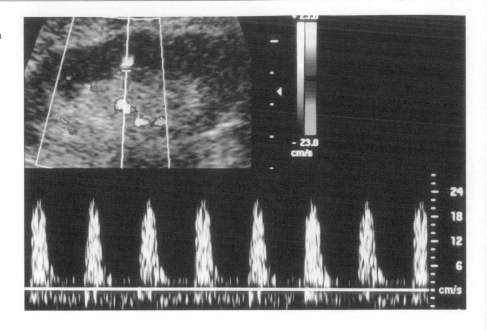

**Fig. 29.16** (**a–c**) Chronic renal failure, in a patient undergoing renal dialysis. (**a**) On gray-scale US, kidneys reveal a short length and diffuse reduction of cortical thickness, irregular margins and poor cortico-medullary differentiation. (**b**) On CD a reduced parenchymal perfusion is visualized, whereas (**c**) duplex Doppler reveals increased resistive index values (0.74)

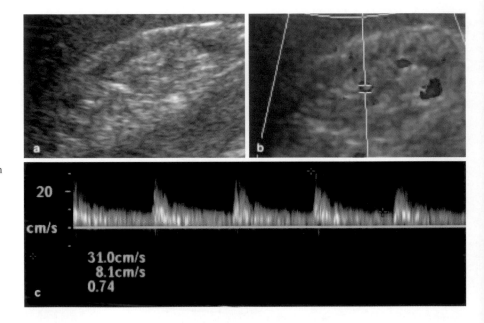

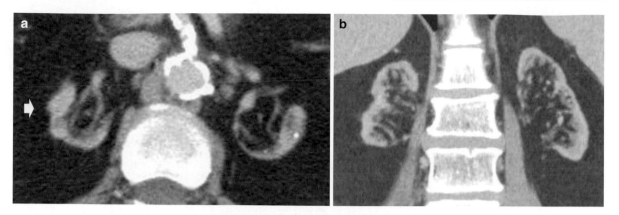

**Fig. 29.17** (**a**, **b**) Chronic renal failure, in a patient undergoing renal dialysis. Contrast-enhanced CT performed before dialysis. (**a**) Transverse plane, and (**b**) coronal plane. Kidneys reveal diffuse reduction of cortical thickness and irregular margins

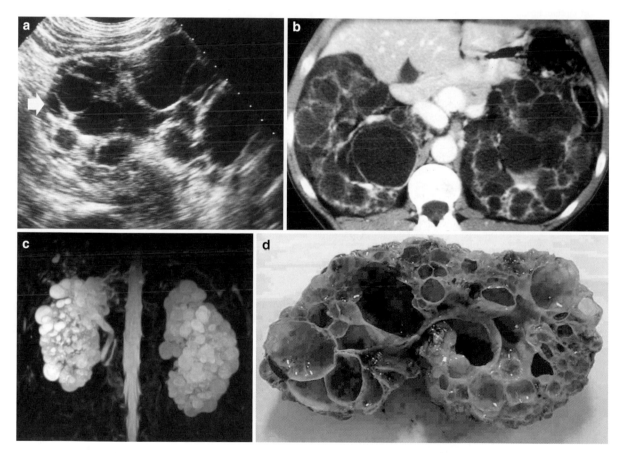

**Fig. 29.18** (**a–d**) Autosomal dominant polycystic kidney disease in a patient with end-stage chronic renal disease undergoing emodyalysis. (**a**) US. Longitudinal scan, right kidney. (**b**) Contrast-enhanced CT. (**c**) Static-fluid MR urography sequence. (**d**) Gross specimen

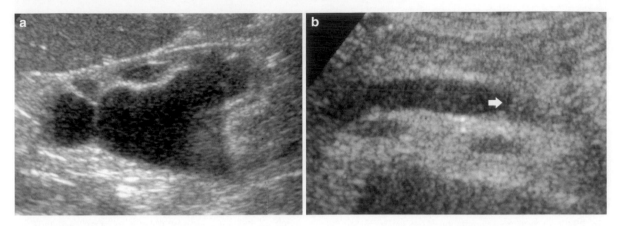

**Fig. 29.19** (**a**, **b**) Chronic renal failure due to chronic urinary obstruction in a patient with a solitary kidney. On gray-scale US, longitudinal scan. (**a**) The kidney reveals chronic dilatation of the intrarenal urinary tract (hydronephrosis) with a strongly reduced renal cortical thickness. (**b**) The extrarenal urinary tract appears dilated due to obstruction (*arrow*) of the distal tract of the ureter due to transitional cell carcinoma

# References

Alpers CE (2005) The kidney. In: Kumar V, Abbas AK, Fausto N (eds) Robbins and Cotran pathologic basis of disease. Elsevier Saunders, Philadelphia, pp 955–1021

Bertolotto M, Quaia E, Galli G et al. (2000) Color Doppler sonographic appearance of renal perforating vessels in subjects with normal and impaired renal function. J Clin Ultrasound 28:267–276

Clive DM, Cohen AJ (1991) Acute renal failure. In: Rippe JM, Irwin RS, Alpert JS, Fink MP (eds) Intensive care medicine. Little, Brown and Company, Boston, pp 764–774

Cohan RH, Cowan NC, Ellis JH (2006) Unknown ESUR cases 2004. Abdom Imaging 31:141–153

Dagher PR, Herget-Rosenthal S, Ruehm SG et al. (2003) Newly developed techniques to study and diagnose acute renal failure. J Am Soc Nephrol 14:2188–2198

ESUR guidelines on contrast media. European Society of Urogenital Radiology. ESUR Contrast Media Safety Committee 2008

Finkel KW (2009) Acute tubular necrosis. In: Ronco C, Bellomo R, Kellum JA (eds) Critical care nephrology. Saunders Elsevier, Philadelphia, pp 351–354

Fliser D (2008) Assessment of renal function in elderly patients. Curr Opin Nephrol Hypertens 17 (6): 604–608

Gleeson TG, Bulugahapitiya S (2004) Contrast-induced nephropathy. AJR Am J Roentgenol 183:1673–1689

Jordan J, Low R, Jeffrey RB (1990) CT findings in acute renal cortical necrosis. J Comput Assist Tomogr 14:155–156

Kanal E, Barkovich AJ, Bell C et al. (2007) ACR guidance document for safe MR practices: 2007. AJR Am J Roentgenol 188: 447–1474

Kim SH, Kim B (1990) Renal parenchyma disease. In: Pollack HM, McClennan BL, Dyer R, Kenney PJ (eds) Clinical urography. Saunders, Philadelphia, pp 2652–2687

Levey AS, Bosch JP, Lewis JB et al. (1999) A more accurate method to estimate glomerular filtration rate from serum creatinine: a new prediction equation. Modification of Diet in Renal Disease Study Group. Ann Intern Med 130(6):461–470

Levey AS, Eckardt KU, Tsukamoto Y et al. (2005) Definition and classification of chronic kidney disease: a position statement from Kidney Disease: Improving Global Outcomes (KDIGO). Kidney Int 67:2089–2100

Murphey MD, Sartoris DJ, Quale JL et al. (1993) Musculoskeletal manifestations of chronic renal insufficiency. Radiographics 13:357–379

National Kidney Foundation (2002) K/DOQI clinical practice guidelines for chronic kidney disease: evaluation, classification, and stratification. Am J Kidney Dis 39(suppl 1):S1–S266

PatriquinHB, O'Regan S, Robitaille P et al. (1989) Hemolytic-uremic syndrome intrarenal arterial Doppler patterns as useful guide to therapy. Radiology 172:625–628

Petersen LJ, Petersen JR, Ladefoged SD et al. (1995) The pulsatility index and the resistive index in renal arteries in patients with hypertension and chronic renal failure. Nephrol Dial Transplant 10:2060–2064

Petersen LJ, Petersen JR, Talleruphuus U et al. (1997) The pulsatility index and the resistive index in renal arteries: associations with long-term progression in chronic renal failure. Nephrol Dial Transplant 12:1376–1380

Platt JF, Rubin JM, Ellis JH (1991) Acute renal failure: possible role of duplex Doppler US in distinction between acute prerenal failure and acute tubular necrosis. Radiology 179:419–423

PlattJF, Ellis JH, Rubin JM et al. (1994) Renal duplex Doppler ultrasonography: a noninvasive predictor of kidney dysfunction and hepatorenal failure in liver disease. Hepatology 20:362–369

Platt JF, Jonathan M, Rubin JF et al. (1997) Lupus nephritis: predictive value of conventional and Doppler US and comparison with serologic and biopsy parameters. Radiology 203:82–86

Pozzi Mucelli R, Bertolotto M, Quaia E (2001) Imaging techniques in acute renal failure. In: Ronco C, Bellomo R, La Greca G (eds) Blood purification in intensive care. Contrib Nephrol, Basel, Karger, pp 76–91

Quaia E, Bertolotto M (2002) Renal parenchymal diseases: is characterization feasible with ultrasound? Eur Radiol 12: 2006–2020

RadermacherJ, Ellis S, Haller H (2002) Renal resistance index and progression of renal disease. Hypertension 39:699–703

Shabana WM, Cohan RH, Ellis JH et al. (2008) Nephrogenic systemic fibrosis: a report of 29 cases. AJR Am J Roentgenol 190:736–741

Silverman SG, Leyendecker JR, Amis SE (2009) What is the current role of CT urography and MR urography in the evaluation of the urinary tract. Radiology 250:309–323

Splendiani G, Parolini C, Fortunato L et al. (2002) Resistive index in chronic nephropathies: predictive value of renal outcome. Clin Nephrol 57:45–50

Stevens LA, Levey AS (2005) Chronic kidney disease in the elderly – how to assess risk. N Engl J Med 352:2122–2124

Stevens LA, Coresh J, Greene T et al. (2006) Assessing kidney function – measured and estimated glomerular filtration rate. N Engl J Med 354:2473–2483

Symeonidou C, Hameeduddin A, Hons B et al. (2009) Imaging features of renal pathology in the huma immunodeficiency virus-infected patients. Semin Ultrasound CT MRI 30: 289–297

Thomsen HS, Marckmann P, Logager VB (2007) Enhanced computed tomography or magnetic resonance imaging: a choice between contrast medium–induced nephropathy and nephrogenic systemic fibrosis? Acta Radiol 48:593–596

Warnock DG (1992) Chronic renal failure. In: Wyngaarden JB, Smith LH, Bennett JC (eds) Cecil textbook of medicine. Saunders, Philadelphia, pp 533–541

Wei K, Le E, Bin JP et al. (2001) Quantification of renal blood flow with contrast-enhanced ultrasound. J Am Coll Cardiol 37:1135–1140

# Renal Transplantation

## Nicolas Grenier

**30**

## Contents

N. Grenier (✉)
Service d'Imagerie Diagnostique et Interventionelle de
l'Adulte, Groupe Hospitalier Pellegrin,
Place Amélie Raba-Léon, 33076 Bordeaux Cedex, France
e-mail: nicolas.grenier@chu-bordeaux.fr

**Abstract**

> Renal transplantation represents the treatment of choice for chronic renal insufficiency. The first year after transplantation is special, as it is characterized by the highest rates of acute rejection and opportunistic infections, but the principal cause of graft loss after the first year is chronic allograft nephropathy. Imaging is particularly useful in evaluating the graft recipient and the kidney donor to adequately plan the graft implantation. After transplantation, noninvasive techniques (mainly ultrasound and MR imaging) play a major role in characterizing the causes of renal dysfunction, separating surgical causes (urological and vascular) and medical causes, and lately, in detecting tumors in both, recipients and grafts.

## 30.1 Epidemiology

Renal transplantation represents the treatment of choice for chronic renal insufficiency. It not only improves patients' quality of life, but significantly prolongs their survival compared to those remaining on hemodialysis (Wolfe et al. 1999). The advances made in immunosuppressive therapies have provided constant improvement of short-term graft survival, which now exceeds 90% 1 year after transplantation (Cecka 2002). In contrast, graft half-life had improved very little, remaining around 7.5–9.5 years until the early 1990s. Over the past 10 years, this situation has changed, with significantly prolonged graft survival for large cohorts of renal graft recipients. The half-life

E. Quaia (ed.), *Radiological Imaging of the Kidney*,
Medical Radiology, DOI: 10.1007/978-3-540-87597-0_30, © Springer-Verlag Berlin Heidelberg 2011

of engrafted cadaveric kidneys increased from 7.5 years in 1988 to 13.8 years in 1996 (Hariharan et al. 2000), with progressively improved renal function over time (Gourishankar et al. 2003).

The first year after transplantation is special, as it is characterized by the highest rates of acute rejection and opportunistic infections, such as cytomegalovirus. The principal cause of graft loss after the first year is chronic allograft nephropathy (CAN), followed by patient death, late acute rejections, nephropathy recurrence, and polyomavirus infection (Hariharan 2001). However, prolongation of graft survival also means extended exposure of the patient to side effects associated with immunosuppressive therapies, mainly infections and cancers, and other late-onset cardiovascular, bone, and/or metabolic complications. In this review, we successively address the presurgical evaluation of the patient, the operation itself, and its possible complications, then the early (first year) and late (after the first year) medical complications.

## 30.2 Presurgical Evaluations

### 30.2.1 Evaluation of the Graft Recipient

The pretransplantation work-up is aimed at determining whether the patient's general condition can tolerate the surgical intervention and whether local conditions permit graft implantation, and the latter orients the choice of the technique to be used. The local status of the lower urinary tract and blood vessels to be attached to the graft is evaluated essentially through imaging explorations.

#### 30.2.1.1 The Lower Urinary Tract

Retrograde cystography is mandatory to assess bladder morphology and function. The bladder capacity must be assessed because it is often decreased, depending on the degree of urine output before transplantation. Bladder diverticulum and vesicoureteral reflux must be excluded because they could facilitate urinary infection during the posttransplantation period. Such abnormalities should be treated during or before the transplantation. Finally, bladder-output function and urethral

morphology during voiding can be examined during cystouretrography.

#### 30.2.1.2 Status of the Vasculature

For young recipients (<50 years old) who have not been on dialysis for a prolonged period and thus have a low probability of developing arterial lesions, Doppler examination of the lower limbs suffices. If the Doppler examination appears abnormal, contrast-enhanced imaging should be performed; the choice between computed tomography angiography (CTA) and magnetic resonance angiography (MRA) depends on residual renal function. However, after 50 years old and, at any age after several years of dialysis, a precise evaluation of arterial status is critical. Prolonged dialysis may induce extensive arterial calcifications, mainly in the lower aorta and iliac vessels, sometimes rendering arterial anastomosis extremely difficult. The site, the severity, and the degree of extension of these calcifications, and the presence of arterial stenoses directly influence the choice of the implantation site. Today, the best technique to determine arterial wall status is nonenhanced multidetector-row CT (MDCT) with axial sections and coronal reformations. For lumen patency assessment, the choice between contrast-enhanced CTA and MRA, as above, depends on residual renal function.

### 30.2.2 Evaluation of the Donor

Examination of the kidney to be engrafted depends on the donor's status, that is, either being maintained in a state of brain death (cadaveric) or living. We are concerned here exclusively with the renal morphology explorations obtained with different imaging techniques.

#### 30.2.2.1 Evaluation of Cadaveric Donor Kidneys

No consensus has been reached for the assessment of the renal status of cadaveric donors: it can be based on simple abdominal ultrasonography (US) or contrast-enhanced CT. As the diagnosis of cerebral death moves toward cerebral contrast-enhanced CT angiography, helical CT now plays an increasing role for that purpose.

### 30.2.2.2 Evaluations of Living-Donor Kidneys

The aim of these evaluations is the assessment of kidney anatomy, volume and function, determination of the number of renal arteries and veins, and overall examination of the anatomy of the entire excretory system. MDCT scanners offer short image-acquisition time and thin collimation and better spatial resolution with a precise anatomical coverage, increased contrast enhancement of the arteries, and greater longitudinal spatial resolution. The MDCT protocol includes unenhanced acquisitions to detect urolithiasis, followed by acquisitions after iodine enhancement; during the vascular phase (25–30 s), to assess the number and location of renal arteries; during the tubular phase (65–75 s), to assess the number and length of renal veins, renal morphology and volume; and during the excretory phase (2–10 min), to assess the morphology of the upper excretory system. In a recent study based on 94 renal donors, MDCT's overall accuracy rates were 94, 97 and 99%, for the identification of variant anatomy of renal arteries, veins, and ureters, respectively (Sahani et al. 2005). MDCT seems more accurate than MRA for assessing the anatomy of renal arteries and veins (Bhatti et al. 2005).

## 30.3 Current Surgical Techniques

### 30.3.1 Graft Preservation

The usual kidney storage solutions use an impermeant solute, such as phosphate, lactobionate, glucose, sucrose, or raffinose. At present, the best known solutions are University of Wisconsin (UW), histidine-tryptophan ketoglutarate (HTK, Custodiol®), or Celsior®. Two methods are described for kidney preservation: the most common is an initial flushing followed by ice storage and the second is continuous hypothermic pulsatile perfusion, mainly used for nonheart–beating donors. In all cases, the period of cold ischemia should be as short as possible, especially with marginal donors or elderly kidneys.

### 30.3.2 Transplantation

Some teams systematically implant the first graft on the right because of the more superficial iliac vessels; others prefer implanting a right kidney on the left and left kidney on the right so that the renal pelvis and ureter are placed anteriorly, thereby facilitating subsequent nephrostomy should it be necessary.

In most cases, the renal vein is attached to the external iliac vein. The arterial anastomosis is more variable: end-to-side to the external iliac, or to the primary iliac artery (Fig. 30.1); sometimes end-to-end to the hypogastric artery, when taken from a living donor, because the graft's artery does not have an aortic patch.

The type of ureterovesical anastomosis chosen depends on the initial radiological images, the condition of the graft's ureter, and intraoperative observations. As a general rule, the ureterovesical anastomosis is made using the Lich–Gregoir technique, with an extravesicular approach. The Leadbetter–Politano technique, which corresponds to an intravesicular reimplantation with the creation of a submucosal tunnel, is preferred when the bladder is small.

## 30.4 Radiological Assessment of the Graft

US is the most useful technique for early and late transplant follow-up. Implantation of the graft within the iliac fossa improves its accessibility and makes possible the use of high-frequency probes, which provide high resolution and high Doppler sensitivity. On gray-scale US, the normally functioning grafted kidney shows the same corticomedullary differentiation (CMD) as a native kidney (Fig. 30.2a,b). High-frequency probes (10–15 MHz) show clear separations of all the kidney compartments: the cortex, the outer medulla, and the inner medulla, with a decreasing echogenicity gradient from the capsule to the papilla (Fig. 30.2c). Color Doppler is now essential for the detection of intra or extrarenal arterial or venous abnormalities. The entire graft, venous and arterial anastomoses, can be imaged with a 3.5–5 MHz probe (Fig. 30.3). A high frequency (7.5–14 MHz) probe allows examination by generating high-resolution images of the anterior distal intrarenal vasculature

**Fig. 30.1** Vascular and ureterovesical anastomoses. The renal vein is attached to the external iliac vein. The arterial anastomosis is variable: end-to-side to the primary iliac artery (**a**), or to the external iliac artery (**b**), most often above the venous implantation

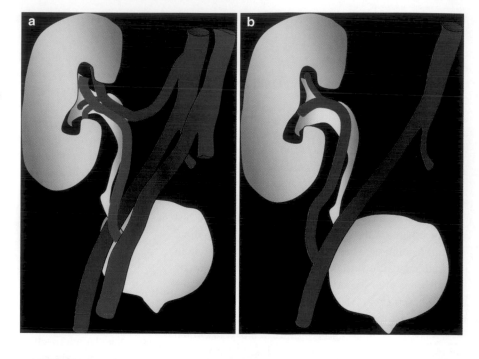

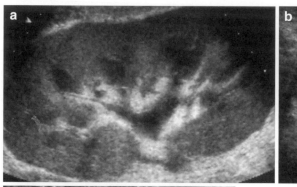

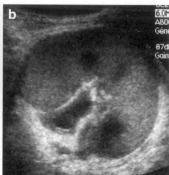

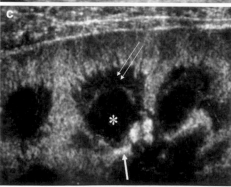

**Fig. 30.2** Gray-scale ultrasonography of a normal transplant. Low frequency probes show the normal corticomedullary differentiation on the long (**a**) and short axes (**b**) and the wall of pyelocaliceal system within sinus. Using high-frequency probes (**c**), differentiation between outer medulla (*double arrow*) and inner medulla (*asterisk*) above the papilla (*thick arrow*) becomes possible

(interlobular and arcuate arteries), which are better delineated with the power mode. Spectral sampling of renal artery flow and interlobar arteries at two or three levels of the graft is also mandatory in all cases. The renal artery velocity profile is analyzed and the peak systolic velocity, after angle correction, is measured. Flow sampling of interlobar arteries enables calculation of the resistivity index (RI).

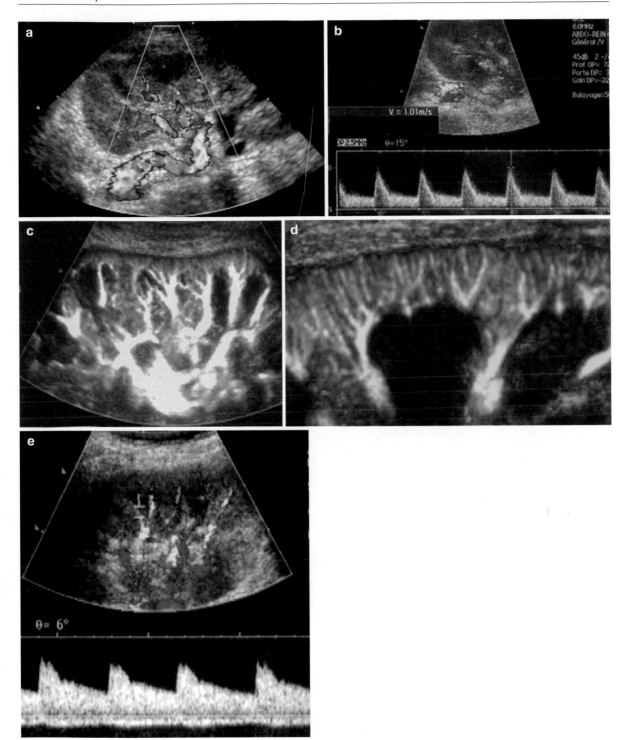

**Fig. 30.3** Color flow ultrasonography of normal transplant: the renal pedicle with a unique renal artery implanted on the primary iliac artery (**a**). The flow is characterized by low resistance and systolic velocities between 80 and 120 cm/s (**b**). Using a low frequency probe (**c**), intrarenal vasculature must be harmo- nious, without any defect. With a high-frequency probe (**d**), the cortical interlobular vessels must be visualized until the capsule. Spectral sampling of interlobar arteries shows a low resistivity of the flow (**e**)

MRI of the renal graft is performed with body phased-array coils, using adequate sequences for visualizing successively the renal parenchyma and its environment, the vascular tree, and the excretory system (Figs. 30.4 and 30.5). On T1-weighted (T1w) (spin-echo or gradient-echo) sequences, the normal CMD is visible on normally functioning kidneys: the medulla generates a lower signal intensity (SI) than the cortex. On T$_2$-weighted (T2w) sequences (usually obtained with a fast spin-echo technique), the medulla generates a higher SI. Gadolinium (Gd) injection gives an accurate delineation of perfused, and nonperfused areas of

the graft and high-resolution 3D-MR angiograms can be obtained for the entire arterial tree – from the iliac axis to the third or fourth order branches. However, the distal vascular tree (from interlobar to interlobular arteries) cannot be visualized. The same 3D sequence must be repeated 5 min after Gd injection (or later if necessary) to obtain MR-urograms and furosemide injection is generally not necessary for that purpose.

CT has always played a minor role in kidney transplant-imaging because it requires normal renal function for the analysis of the renal parenchyma or renal vessels.

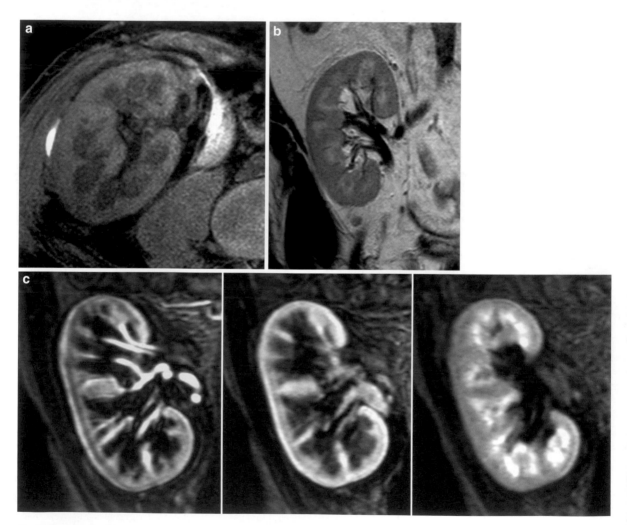

**Fig. 30.4** MR imaging of normal transplant with fat saturated T1-weighted (**a**) and T2-weighted (**b**) sequences. Postgadolinium renal enhancement can be demonstrated dynamically with gradient-echo T1-sequences (**c**)

**Fig. 30.5** 3D contrast-enhanced MR angiography (**a**) showing renal arteries and anastomotic site, and at a later phase (**b**), showing upper excretory system (MR urography)

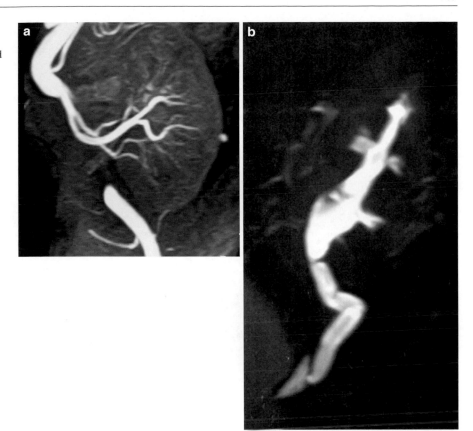

## 30.5 Early Graft Complications (First Year)

### 30.5.1 Urological Complications

Urological complications, often of technical origin, can be a source of morbidity and sometimes mortality after kidney transplantation. The current urological complication rate ranges from 4 to 7% (Gogus et al. 2002; Kocak et al. 2004) and death is highly unusual.

#### 30.5.1.1 Urinary Fistulas

The urinary fistula frequency ranges from 1 to 5%, the most common early complication, occurring during the first 2 weeks after transplantation. The majority of urinary leaks are attributed to ureteral ischemia. The other causes of urinary leaks are failure of ureterovesical anastomosis or a missed ureteral duplication. Leakage may be suspected when increasing volumes

of a clear liquid are collected by drains, while diuresis tends to decline during the days following surgery. Determination of fluid electrolytes, ingestion of methylene blue thereafter found in the fluid collected and US showing a perirenal fluid collection can confirm the diagnosis. US usually finds a well-defined anechoic collection at the lower pole of the kidney (Fig. 30.6). This fluid appears hypointense on unenhanced MR T1w and hyperintense on T2w sequences. T2w-MR urography shows the collection and the entire dilated excretory system. The differential diagnosis includes lymphoceles, which usually occur later. Chemical analysis of the fluid may suggest the diagnosis, if the creatinine concentration is higher than that in blood. However, the definitive diagnosis of urinoma is based on the demonstration of an extravasation of contrast medium into the collection after intravenous injection. This can be obtained with Gd-enhanced MRI, iodine-enhanced CT or radionuclides. Urine collection contamination by the contrast agent or the radiotracer often requires delayed imaging (5–15 min after injection) (Fig. 30.6d,e).

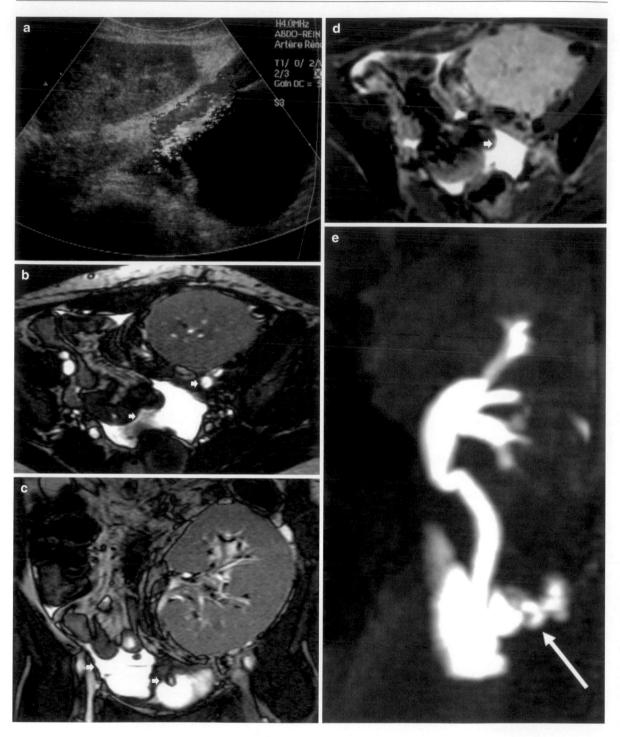

**Fig. 30.6** Urinary leak secondary to ureteral ischemia. Ultrasonography (**a**) shows a fluid collection between the lower pole of the transplant and the bladder. On T2-weighted axial (**b**) and coronal (**c**) images, fluid (*short arrow*) is noted below the graft and within the peritoneal cavity. The pelvic fluid collection enhances at a late phase (**d**) after injection of contrast medium. The MR urographic image shows the leak (*long arrow*) at the uretero-bladder junction (**e**)

Whereas the treatment of most of these leaks is surgical, small ones can be treated by nephrostomy and/or ureter stenting. Open surgery consists of reimplanting the ureter, with the technique to be used chosen as a function of its remaining healthy length.

### 30.5.1.2 Ureteral Stenosis

This complication develops later (several months) and its frequency tends to increase with time, 5% at 1 year and 10% at 5 years. In 80% of the cases, it is the consequence of progressive fibrosis of the ureterovesical anastomosis, but it can also result from inflammatory infiltration of the ureter wall during rejection. The differential diagnosis includes intraluminal causes of obstruction, such as lithiasis or blood clot, and extraluminal compression by perigraft fluid collections.

The diagnosis is suspected when decreased renal function is associated with dilatation of the collecting system on US (Fig. 30.7a,b). Differentiation between obstructive and nonobstructive pyelocaliectasis remains difficult and Doppler RI measurement is neither sensitive nor specific in transplanted kidneys (Platt et al. 1991). Renal scintigraphy may characterize the obstruction when the tracer accumulates within the collecting system on delayed images and by measuring increased clearance time after furosemide injection.

When obstruction is suspected, visualization of the entire upper urinary tract is mandatory to determine its exact location and cause. The least invasive method for that purpose is MR urography because most of these patients have decreased renal function (Fig. 30.7). Both types of sequences (T2w and Gd-enhanced T1w) have to be obtained. When dilatation is sufficient, T2w sequences demonstrate the entire collecting system up to the anastomosis or the site of obstruction. If not, T1w Gd-enhanced sequences, with delayed acquisitions, usually do.

### 30.5.1.3 Graft Infection

Urinary infections are common during the first month following transplantation. They are usually nosocomial bacterial infections, sometimes facilitated by the presence of catheters, which can lead to real pyelonephritis of the graft or the development of renal or perirenal abscesses. Sometimes, perigraft abscesses may be secondary to bacterial contamination of a preexisting fluid collection (hematoma, lymphocele, or urinoma).

US, using B-mode and Doppler techniques, should be performed first and will show a perigraft collection (Fig. 30.8), often extending toward superficial planes, which, in this context, must always be considered infected. Thin or coarse echoes, sediment, septa and a thickened hypervascularized peripheral wall are evocative of infection. When infection of a perigraft collection is suspected, contrast-enhanced MRI or CT will help to assess their exact extension before treatment. Fluid aspiration from these collections, under US control, may be necessary for confirmation of the diagnosis, and optimal treatment combines percutaneous or surgical drainage and systemic antibiotic therapy.

Renal parenchyma infection may be seen as an increased graft volume and/or areas of decreased or increased echogenicity with decreased flow on color Doppler examination (Fig. 30.9). Gd-enhanced MRI and enhanced CT are able to distinguish between infection and infarction in most of cases, because enhancement is observed in the former and not in the latter, except for a thin peripheral capsular rim.

Urinary infections with Corynebacterium urealyticum is uncommon, but can expose the transplant to complications, such as ureteral obstruction, renal abscess formation, or progressive destruction of the graft (Dominguez-Gil et al. 1999). Color Doppler US detects these urothelial calcifications that produce a twinkling artifact within the bladder and/or the upper urinary tract (Fig. 30.10).

### 30.5.1.4 Perigraft Fluid Collections

In addition to those associated with fistulas and perigraft abscesses discussed above, these fluid build-ups can be constituted of blood and/or lymph. Postsurgical lymphorrhea causing a lymphocele remain the most frequent cause of perigraft collections, occurring in 1–20% of renal graft recipients, usually after the fourth week posttransplantation. Sometimes, their volume may cause ureteral or venous compression. On ultrasonograms, a lymphocele appears as a well-defined anechoic

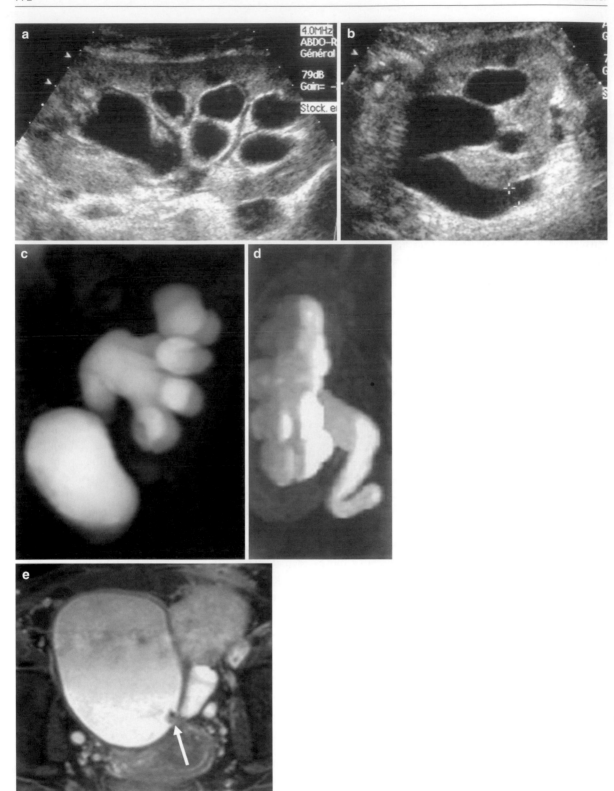

**Fig. 30.7** Urinary obstruction at the level of the uterovesical anastomosis. Sonography shows a dilatation of pyelocaliceal system (**a**) and ureter (**b**) of renal graft. Ureteropyelectasis is well visualized on 3D T2w (**c**) and Gd-enhanced T1w (**d**) MR images. T2w axial section (**e**) shows a thickened anastomosis due to fibrotic tissue (*arrow*)

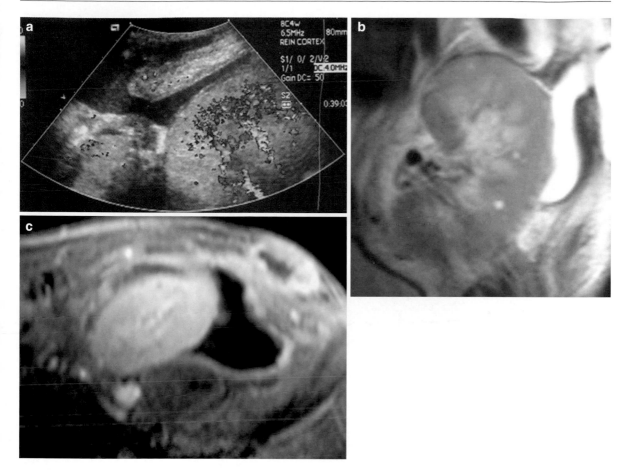

**Fig. 30.8** Perirenal abscess in a patient with graft tenderness and fever. A fluid collection is seen around the graft on color flow sonography, extending through the disrupted abdominal wall to subcutaneous tissues (**a**). This fluid collection is con-firmed by MR imaging on coronal (**b**) T2w sequence. Peripheral wall of the collection and superficial soft tissue are enhancing after Gd injection (**c**)

collection (Fig. 30.11a). CT density values and SI on MR sequences (Fig. 30.11) are typical of simple fluids, without any enhancement after contrast injection. When a lymphocele is responsible for ureteral or venous compression, radical therapy is essential. Simple aspiration and drainage are ineffective because they do not prevent lymph leakage. Therefore, percutaneous drainage must be combined with sclerosis of the cavity by repeated instillations of doxycycline, tetracycline, acetic acid, alcohol, or povidine–iodine. Multiple sessions until daily drainage falls below 10 mL are necessary for larger ones (Karcaaltincaba and Akhan 2005).

Hematomas account for approximately 9% of peri-transplant collections and usually occur during the immediate postoperative period, due to surgery. The other main causes are: (1) early renal biopsy complicated by a cortical pseudoaneurysm, which may increase in size and subsequently rupture in the perirenal space; this complication occurs immediately (24–48 h) or several weeks after biopsy; (2) graft rupture secondary to severe acute rejection, which occurs in 3–6% of renal transplants and during the first 2 weeks after transplantation. During the early postoperative period, hematomas are echogenic collections without flow on US images and are hyperattenuated on unenhanced CT images (Fig. 30.12). MRI is more specific, showing high intensity on both T1w and T2w sequences (Neimatallah et al. 1999).

**Fig. 30.9** Pyelonephritis of the transplant. A hypoechoic triangular area is detected at the upper pole of the graft with a hypoperfusion on the color Doppler mode (**a**). Contrast-enhanced CT (**b**, **c**) shows two foci of parenchymal infection

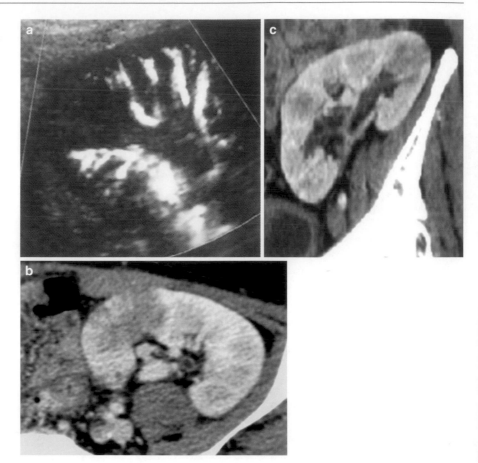

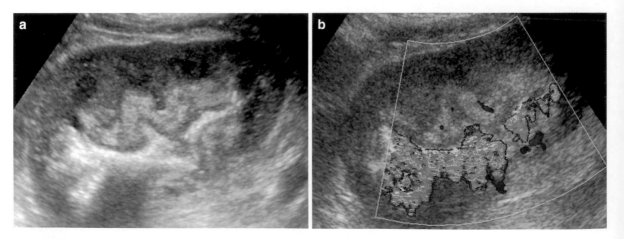

**Fig. 30.10** Corynebacterium infection of the transplant. On the B-mode image, the pyelocaliceal system appears as a hyperechoic linear structure within the sinus fat, without acoustic shadowing (**a**). The color Doppler mode shows a twinkling artifact along this linear structure (**b**). (courtesy of Dr. Derchi, Genoa)

**Fig. 30.11** Perigraft lymphocele responsible for urinary obstruction. On sonography, the pyelocaliceal system (**a**) and the ureter (**b**) are dilated due to a pelvic fluid collection showing thin septas. On T2w axial (**c**) MR images, the collection seats below and in front of the lower pole of the kidney, compressing the ureter. The lymphocele and the obstructed excretory cavities are superimposed on the T2w MR urographic image (**d**), whereas only the later appear on the Gd-enhanced T1w MR urographic image (**e**)

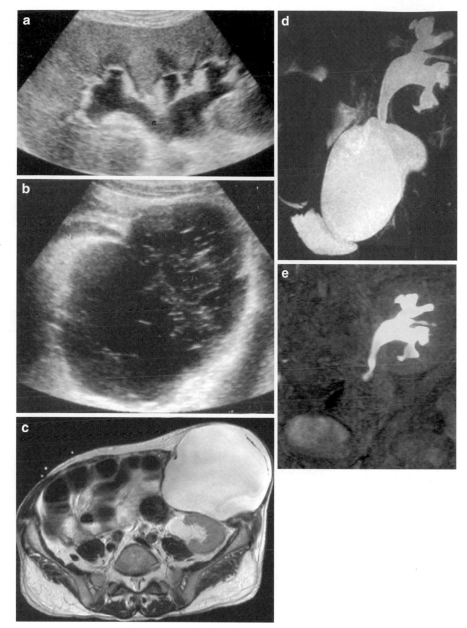

## 30.5.2 Vascular Complications

### 30.5.2.1 Renal Artery Thrombosis

Arterial thrombosis is very unusual, occurring in <1% of renal graft recipients, but is extremely severe, leading in most cases to graft loss. It occurs early, caused by a hypercoagulable state, hypotension, hyperacute rejection, immunosuppressive therapy, or a surgical complication: anastomotic occlusion, arterial dissection, renal artery kinking when it is too long or torsion of the renal artery when implanted intraperitoneally. Its diagnosis is suspected soon after transplantation, when severe renal impairment is associated with anuria. Confirmation is easily obtained with color flow Doppler US (Fig. 30.13) showing arterial flow in the iliac artery, absence of flow within the entire graft, which is swollen and hypoechoic, and a persistent "to-and-fro" flow pattern within renal veins (Grenier et al. 1991, 1997). If confirmation is necessary, Gd-enhanced MRI examination can demonstrate

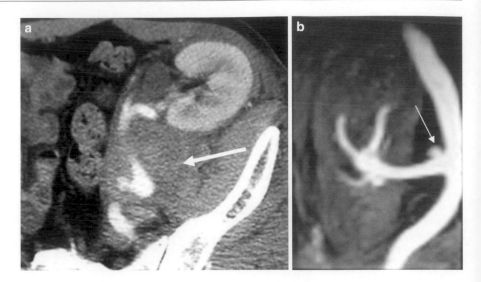

**Fig. 30.12** Perigraft hematoma secondary to the rupture of a mycotic aneurysm. (**a**) Contrast-enhanced CT shows a dense collection (*arrow*) at the lower pole of the transplant surrounding the renal artery. (**b**) Gd-enhanced MR angiography shows the aneurysm (*arrow*) close to the arterial anastomosis (Reprinted with permission from Trillaud et al. 1998)

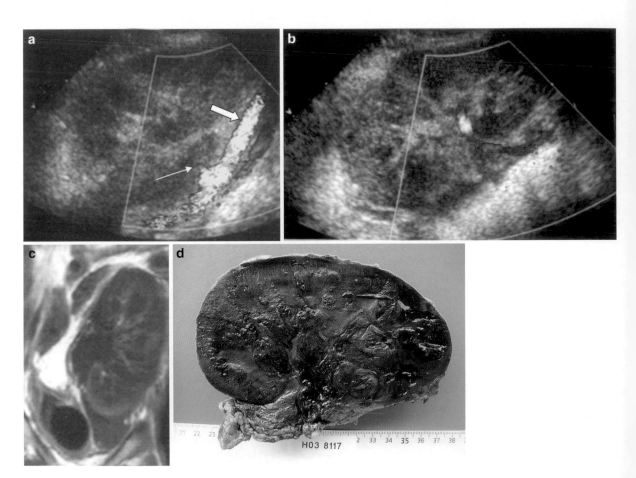

**Fig. 30.13** Renal artery thrombosis. (**a**) The iliac artery appears patent (*thick arrow*) on the sagittal section with color flow sonography, whereas no flow is detected within the graft. The stump of the occluded renal artery is visible (*thin arrow*). (**b**) More medially, the renal vein is also patent with a to-and-fro flow (with successive *blue* and *red* encoding). The contrast-enhanced MR image (**c**) shows an absence of enhancement within the entire graft. Complete necrosis of the graft was confirmed by the macroscopic examination (**d**)

the complete devascularization of the graft (Helenon et al. 1992). Only rapid reintervention, within 12 h for surgical thrombectomy, can save the graft and does so in half of the cases. Percutaneous endovascular revascularization has been described for allograft salvage, but only for late thrombosis (Juvenois et al. 1999).

### 30.5.2.2 Infarctions

Segmental infarcts can also be due to segmental or reimplanted accessory renal artery thrombosis or be associated with acute rejection. They are usually asymptomatic and renal function impairment depends on their size. Doppler US is not specific, showing wedge-shaped areas of decreased or increased echogenicity without flow (Dodd et al. 1991; Grenier et al. 1997) (Fig. 30.14). Injection of ultrasound contrast agents may help differentiate with infection (Lefevre et al. 2002). Similarly, contrast-enhanced MR images demonstrate the absence of enhancement within the infarcted segments, except for the subcapsular cortex corticis (Neimatallah et al. 1999; Sebastia et al. 2001).

### 30.5.2.3 Renal Artery Stenosis

The frequency of renal artery stenosis (RAS) in transplanted kidneys varies from 1 to 23%, and they may represent around 75% of all posttransplant vascular complications (Bruno et al. 2004). It develops most often during the first year following surgery. Their origin is multifactorial: atherosclerotic plaque in the donor's renal artery or in the recipient's iliac artery; dissection, kinking or twisting of the renal artery (due to excessive vessel length); malpositioning of the graft; flow turbulences generating intimal hyperplasia; graft perfusion catheter during cannulation causing intimal damage; wall ischemia due to excessive dissection with destruction of vasa vasorum. It is also possible that prolonged cold ischemia may play a role through ischemia–reperfusion injury (Halimi et al. 1999; Patel et al. 2001).

Severe hypertension with or without allograft dysfunction is the most frequent clinical symptom. Hypertension is a common feature in transplant recipients (up to 80%). Therefore, RAS is suspected when hypertension develops suddenly, rapidly becomes more severe and resistant to medical therapy, and is associated with graft dysfunction without any other cause or when associated with an audible bruit over the graft (Palleschi et al. 1980; Rijksen et al. 1982). It may account for around 1–5% of posttransplant hypertension.

US is able to detect renal artery stenoses (Figs. 30.15 and 30.16). Both velocity-profile changes, responsible for spectral broadening and perivascular color artifact, and systolic acceleration must be observed to make this diagnosis. A systolic velocity threshold of

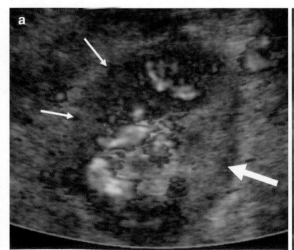
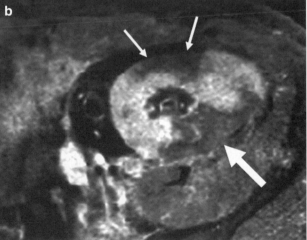

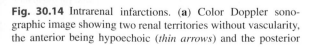

**Fig. 30.14** Intrarenal infarctions. (**a**) Color Doppler sonographic image showing two renal territories without vascularity, the anterior being hypoechoic (*thin arrows*) and the posterior hyperechoic (*thick arrow*), at the upper pole of the kidney. Same pattern is visible on contrast-enhanced T1-weighted MR image (**b**)

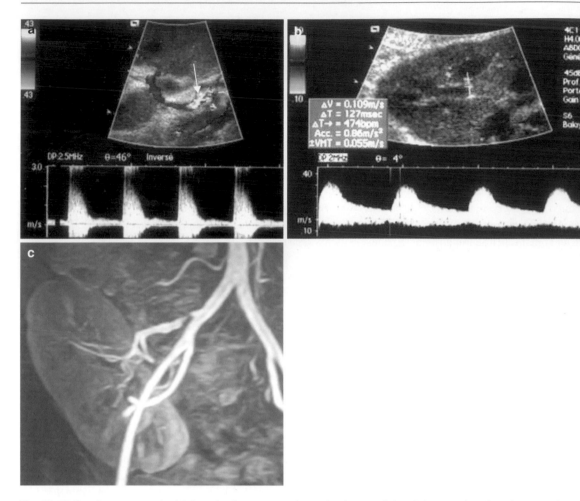

**Fig. 30.15** Renal artery stenosis. (**a**) On color flow sonography, an aliasing phenomenon is present at the proximal portion of the renal artery (*arrow*). The spectral waveform shows an increased peak systolic velocity (2.8 m/s) with frequency broadening. On the intrarenal interlobar arteries (**b**), the ascension time is increased at 127 ms. (**c**) Gd-enhanced MR angiography confirms the postostial renal artery stenosis

190–200 cm/s (Grenier et al. 1991; Loubeyre et al. 1997) or a systolic velocity ratio between renal and external iliac arteries of 1.5 (Loubeyre ct al. 1997) has been proposed for significant stenoses. When the renal artery is too long, kinking is easily demonstrated on the color display, but only spectral sampling is able to confirm the presence of a stenosis (Fig. 30.17). As described for native kidneys, intrarenal sampling of interlobar arteries and looking for dampened waveforms may help detect severe proximal stenosis (Gottlieb et al. 1995). However, these intrarenal features are less useful in transplanted kidneys because the proximal changes are more easily accessible than in native kidneys.

MRA is the most suitable to confirm this diagnosis. 3D Gd-enhanced acquisitions were recommended (Fang and Siegelman 2001, Ferreiros et al. 1999) (Figs. 30.15c and 30.16a), using body phased-array coils and a parallel imaging technique. But today, noncontrast techniques allow to avoid injection of contrast agent in patients with severely impaired function. The sensitivity and specificity of MRA in detecting significant stenoses were 100 and 98%, respectively, and interobserver kappa concordance values exceeded 0.85 (Ferreiros et al. 1999).

Percutaneous transluminal angioplasty, with or without stent placement, is the preferred primary treatment of RAS, when medical therapy can no

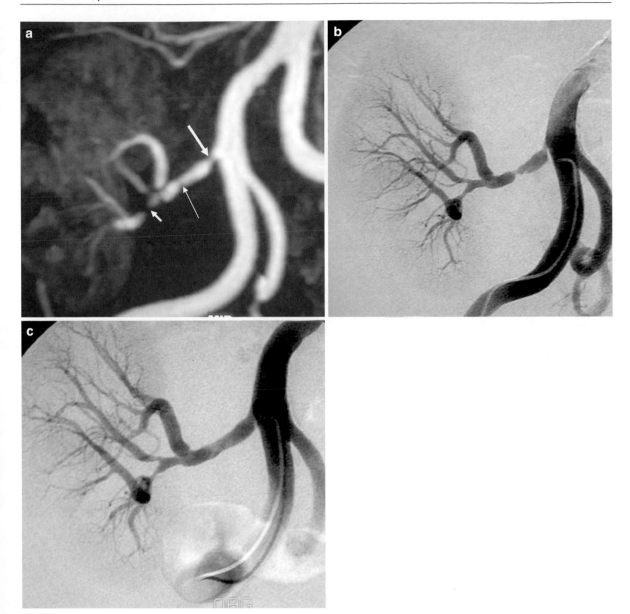

**Fig. 30.16** Renal artery stenosis. (**a**) Gd-enhanced MR angiography shows a significant stenosis immediately after the ostium (*thick arrow*), a moderate stenosis on the trunk (*thin arrow* and a tight stenosis on the lower polar artery (*short arrow*). (**b**) DSA confirms the three stenoses, but the stenosis of the trunk appears more severe than on MR angiography. (**c**) The two proximal stenoses were successfully dilated

longer control blood pressure and/or renal function progressively deteriorates (Fig. 30.16c). Artery stenting is an effective method for recurrent stenosis (Sierre et al. 1998). The clinical success rate varies from 82 to 94% (Beecroft et al. 2004; Patel et al. 2001) and the reported midterm patency (mean of 30 months) reached 100% (Beecroft et al. 2004; Sierre et al. 1998).

### 30.5.2.4  Renal Vein Thrombosis

Acute venous thrombosis occurs in approximately 1–4% of renal transplant recipients and usually during the early postoperative period. When it is complete and abrupt, graft pain and swelling are observed, associated with oliguria and proteinuria. Acute venous thrombosis is often due to faulty surgical technique,

**Fig. 30.17** King-king of the renal artery on color Doppler sonography with a narrowing at the site of plicature (**a**). Spectral waveform shows a spectral broadening with a high peak systolic velocity. MR angiography (**b**) confirms the king-king phenomenon with a significant stenosis

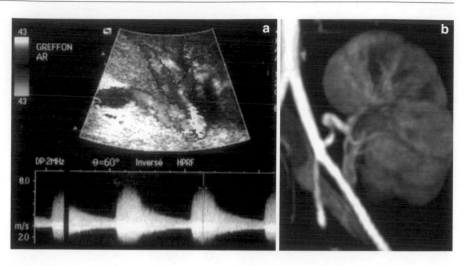

with hypovolemia, hypercoagulation state, or renal vein compression by a perigraft fluid collection as predisposing factors. It may also be a complication of postoperative lower limb or iliac vein thrombosis extending into the renal vein.

Diagnosis of renal vein thrombosis is difficult. On Doppler images, no venous flow is present and arterial flow appears decreased and highly resistive, showing protodiastolic or holodiastolic reflux (Fig. 30.18). On B-mode, the kidney is often enlarged and sometimes heterogeneous. When seen later, transcapsular collaterals may have developed that drain venous flow toward the iliac veins (Fig. 30.19). In difficult cases, using either unenhanced "white blood" axial gradient-echo or Gd-enhanced T1w MRI sequences may help visualize the venous thrombus.

In the case of partial venous thrombosis, anticoagulants administration is usually sufficient. However, when confronted with early complete thrombosis, rapid surgical revascularization is required. Percutaneous thrombectomy, associated with anticoagulation, has also been proposed (Melamed et al. 2005).

### 30.5.2.5 Vascular Complications of Biopsy

Intrarenal arteriovenous fistulas and pseudoaneurysms occur in approximately 1–18% of the grafts after percutaneous transplant biopsies. Most of them are asymptomatic and resolve spontaneously. But they may be responsible for severe perirenal hemorrhage or hematuria.

Pseudoaneurysms present as localized vessel dilations, anechoic on B-mode US, with a rotative flow

inside on color-encoded images (Dodd et al. 1991) and, when isolated, with a to-and-fro flow pattern of the spectral waveform in the neck (Fig. 30.20). Shunts are responsible for enlargement of the supply artery and draining vein associated with high-grade turbulence (Fig. 30.21a) responsible for a perivascular artifact (Grenier et al. 1991; Middleton et al. 1989). On arterial spectral waveforms of feeding arteries, the flow profile is severely altered, with increased velocities and decreased RI (Hubsch et al. 1990) (Fig. 30.21b, c). Venous flow resembles arterial flow with systolic enhancement.

When a clinical complication occurs, they can be treated by transcatheter embolization, using microcoils and providing a 95% technical success rate (Perini et al. 1998) (Fig. 30.22).

### 30.5.2.6 Parenchymal Necrosis

Allograft necrosis is a rare and extremely severe covmplication. It results from defective distal perfusion occurring immediately after graft implantation (primary nonfunction) or as a consequence of severe acute tubular necrosis (ATN) or acute rejection. It is most often limited to the cortex (cortical necrosis) or extends into the medulla (total necrosis).

In cortical necrosis, the graft may appear normal on gray-scale ultrasonograms, when imaged early, or show a hypoechoic cortex. Using a high-frequency probe on the anterior cortex, the cortex on power Doppler ultrasonograms appears to be partially or entirely devascularized (Fig. 30.22). Gd-enhanced MRI confirms the diagnosis and clearly shows the

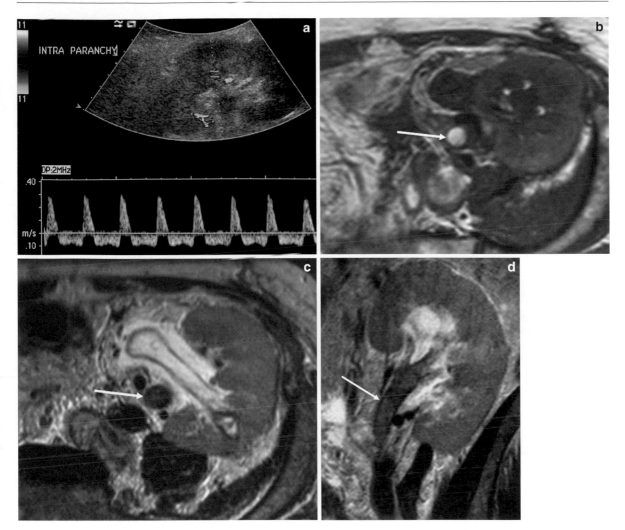

**Fig. 30.18** Renal vein thrombosis, characterized by a spectral waveform with a holodiastolic reflux (**a**). MR imaging shows the thrombosed venous content of renal vein (*arrow*) with a high-signal intensity on T1-weighted sequence (**b**) and a low-signal intensity on T2-weighted sequences (**c**, **d**)

in-depth extension of the parenchymal devascularization (Helenon et al. 1992) (Figs. 30.22c and 30.23a).

## 30.5.3 Medical Complications

### 30.5.3.1 Clinical Considerations

Different causes can be responsible for the failure or deterioration of renal graft function:

- Primary nonfunction, characterized by immediate anuria without subsequent improvement. It is favored by elderly donor, hypertension, prolonged ischemia, kidneys from children implanted into adults.

- ATN, characterized by delayed recovery of renal function. It becomes manifest 12–24 h after revascularization as anuria or renal insufficiency with preserved diuresis. It is favored by the donor's age and vascular history, intensive care of the donor (hemodynamic status) and drugs used, difficulties encountered during organ excision (multiple organs), perfusion and cooling fluids used, and duration of cold ischemia. It resolves spontaneously over the first 2 weeks.

- Acute rejection remains the primary cause of graft loss in the short term and represents a major risk factor for the development of chronic graft dysfunction. Its rate is 10–15%. Clinical signs are few in number

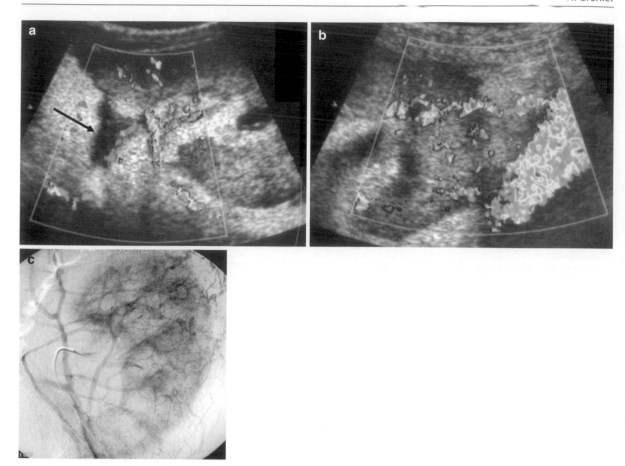

**Fig. 30.19** Renal vein thrombosis. Color flow sonography shows thrombosed segmental veins within the renal sinus (*arrow*) (**a**) and transcapsular venous drainage, toward the external iliac vein, at the lower pole of the kidney (**b**). The venous phase of renal DSA (**c**) shows the absence of venous drainage through the normal renal vein and a heterogeneous renal parenchyma

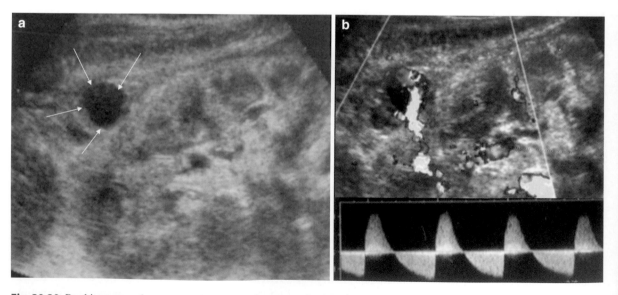

**Fig. 30.20** Postbiopsy pseudoaneurysm. On gray-scale sonography (**a**), an anechoic area appears at the anterior aspect of the graft (*arrows*). The color flow sonography shows that this lesion is circulating (**b**) with a typical "to and fro" spectral pattern

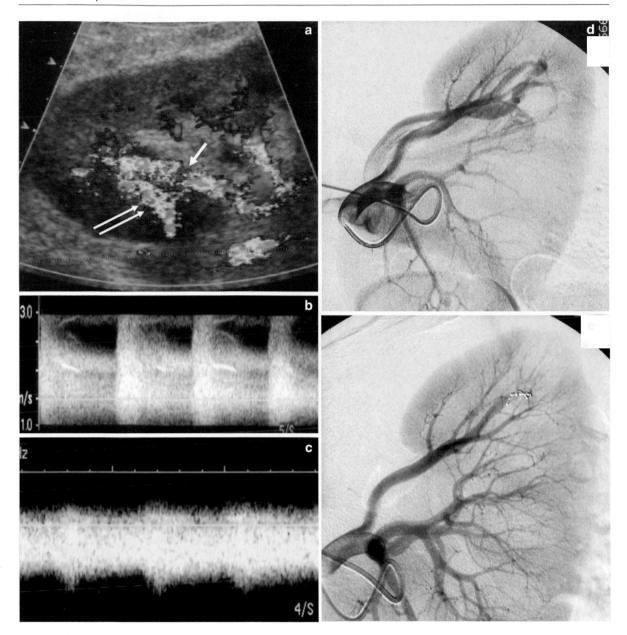

**Fig. 30.21** Postbiopsy arteriovenous fistula. At the upper pole of the kidney graft, two vessels appear enlarged with high velocities on color flow sonography (**a**). Spectral sampling allows separating the afferent artery (*arrow*) and the efferent vein (*double arrow*). Arterial waveform shows increased velocities, spectral broadening, and low resistance (**b**). Venous waveform shows increased flow and arterial modulation (**c**). The angiogram (**d**) shows the shunt with a small pseudoaneurysm and an early venous return. After embolization with microcoils (**e**), the shunt was closed without any significant parenchymal infarction

and become manifest late, with a painful and enlarged graft, markedly diminished diuresis and febricula. Notably, a serum creatinine rise of >20% is an important warning signal. The definitive diagnosis and the severity of the episode are provided by a renal biopsy. First-line therapy consists of high-dose corticosteroids and, in the case of corticoresistant rejection, administration of antilymphocyte globulins or monoclonal antibody OKT3. Acute cellular rejection is reversible in the majority of cases.

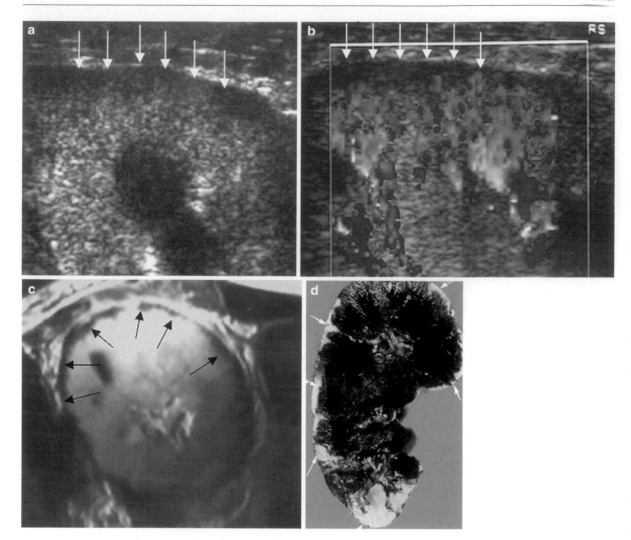

**Fig. 30.22** Partial cortical necrosis. The outer cortex (*arrows*) of this graft appears hypoechoic on gray-scale image (**a**) and devascularized on color flow sonography (**b**), using a high-frequency probe. The Gd-enhanced MR sequence confirms the absence of enhancement within the outer cortex (**c**). (**d**) Macroscopic specimen of a similar case of outer cortical necrosis from another patient (Fig. 29b reprinted with permission from Hélénon et al., Radiographics 1992,12:21-33)

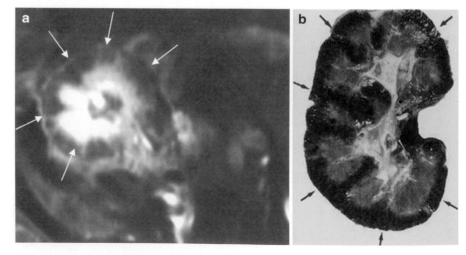

**Fig. 30.23** Complete cortical necrosis. On this transverse Gd-enhanced TIw image (**a**) the medulla is enhancing normally, whereas the cortex remains unenhanced (*arrows*). (**b**) Macroscopic specimen of a similar case of cortical necrosis from another patient (Fig. 28b reprinted with permission from Hélénon et al., Radiographics 1992,12:21-33)

- *The possibility of drug nephrotoxicity* has to be excluded, either directly caused by calcineurin inhibitors (cyclosporin A, tacrolimus) or more indirectly amplified by drug interactions. Again, the definitive diagnosis is provided by the biopsy.

### 30.5.3.2 Imaging

Distinguishing between these medical entities may be difficult and, unfortunately, imaging techniques have not yet played a major role in alleviating that difficulty, thereby still justifying renal biopsies. Many US features have been described as being highly suggestive of acute rejection: enlarged graft, effacement of the central sinus–echo complex, enlargement of pyramids, increased or decreased cortex echogenicity, loss of CMD (Fig. 30.24), and thickened collecting system walls. Unfortunately, these features are subjective and not specific and have low reproducibility (Frick et al. 1981; Fried et al. 1983; Hoddick et al. 1986; Hricak et al. 1987; Kelcz et al. 1990; Linkowski et al. 1987).

Duplex Doppler RI >0.75 or >0.80 can be observed in each of these medical complications (Allen et al. 1988; Don et al. 1989; Genkins et al. 1989; Kelcz et al. 1990; Linkowski et al. 1987). However, the extent of RI increase directly reflects the degree of cortical hypoperfusion (Fig. 30.25). Thus, it seems that the degree of RI increase might be associated with the clinical outcome: in the most severe cases, protodiastolic or even holodiastolic reverse flow, evocative of severe acute rejection, severe ATN, or renal vein

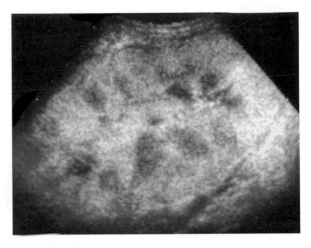

**Fig. 30.24** B-mode sonographic features of acute rejection: increased transverse diameter with effacement of the central sinus–echo complex and increased cortex echogenicity

thrombosis, is associated with a poor functional prognosis (Kaveggia et al. 1990).

Power Doppler US using high-frequency transducers to delineate cortical blood flow visualizes the dense cortical interlobular pedicles all the way to the cortex cortices (Martinoli et al. 1996). In renal grafts with impaired function, focal or diffuse absence of interlobular signals can be observed (Fig. 30.26). These changes can be reversed with treatment and are associated with a prediction of poor functional recovery at 12 months (Trillaud et al. 1998).

Findings on MR T1w-sequences detecting these entities overlap too. Initially, decreased CMD on T1w sequences was considered specific to acute rejection

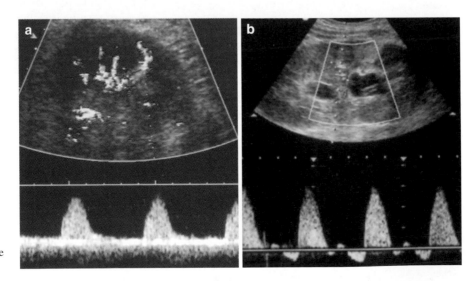

**Fig. 30.25** Increase of intrarenal resistances with a absence of telediastolic flow in an acute rejection episode (**a**) and a proto- and telediastolic reflux in a severe acute tubular necrosis (**b**)

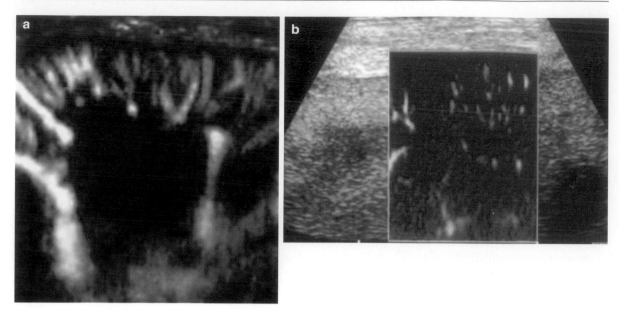

**Fig. 30.26** Progressive alteration of the cortical vasculature (interlobular vessels) in acute rejection episodes, using high-frequency probes and power Doppler mode: presence of a moderate (**a**) and a severe (**b**) decreased cortical vessel density

(Hricak et al. 1986; Rholl et al. 1986). Now, this feature is considered nonspecific for any nephropathy (Neimatallah et al. 1999).

## 30.6 Long-Term Follow-Up

### 30.6.1 Chronic Allograft Nephropathy (CAN)

CAN can be defined as a progressive deterioration of renal function appearing several months after transplantation, independently of acute rejection, another nephrotoxicity phenomenon or recurrence of the initial nephropathy with a suggestive histological appearance (Halloran et al. 1999). Different scores have been devised to classify CAN according to its severity. The mechanism leading to CAN development is complex and poorly understood, bringing together causes dependent on and independent of the allogeneic reaction. Its natural history shows that it comprises two very distinct phases: an early phase (first year), with an exponential increase of fibrotic interstitial lesions and tubular atrophy; and a late phase (after the first year), during which lesions caused by the nephrotoxicity of

anticalcineurins predominate and play a major role after 3 years posttransplantation.

Kidneys suffering from CAN are decreased in size and have poorer CMD and, sometimes, mild dilatation of the renal calices and pelvis. Most imaging techniques focus on the loss of parenchymal vascularity in the cortex to recognize this entity. However, neither RI measurement nor evaluation of intrarenal vessel density with power Doppler mode help to identify transplants developing CAN. Although RI measurements have no value for this diagnosis, they could have a prognostic value for long-term allograft outcomes: Radermacher et al. (Radermacher et al. 2003) showed that renal arterial RI ≥0.80, measured at least 3 months after transplantation was associated with poor subsequent allograft performance and death.

### 30.6.2 Recurrence of the Initial Nephropathy

Glomerular nephropathies represent the primary cause of chronic renal insufficiency (CRI) and are the principal entities that recur in the graft. According to the type of glomerulonephritis, the risk of recurrence ranges from 6 to 19% (Hariharan et al. 1999), which corresponds to the third cause of graft loss (after CAN and patient death with a functional graft), and it rises with the duration of the transplant.

### 30.6.3 Calculus Disease

The incidence of urolithiasis is 0.11% for males and 0.15% for females (Abbott et al. 2003). The stones can be transplanted from cadaveric or living donors or develop de novo, favored either by metabolic disorders (tertiary hyperparathyroidism, hypercalciuria, hypocitraturia) or infection (*Proteus mirabilis*), or the presence of a foreign body in the urinary tract (double-J stent) (Crook and Keoghane 2005). Stones can be easily detected by US, when located in the pyelocaliceal system or within the ureter, or when they have migrated, facilitated by the subsequent dilatation. In difficult cases, unenhanced CT may help (Fig. 30.27).

### 30.6.4 Solid Tumors

Most renal cancers developing in renal graft recipients are clear-cell carcinomas, with 90% occurring in native

kidneys and 10% in renal allografts (Fig. 30.28). They become apparent 2–258 (average 75) months after transplantation. Many renal carcinomas developing in native kidneys result from underlying kidney disease. Two predisposing causes have been identified: analgesic nephropathy and acquired cystic disease (ACD) of the recipients' native kidneys (Heinz-Peer et al. 1995). Patients presenting with micro or macrohematuria should undergo exploratory procedures to actively search for cancer at the level of native and transplanted kidneys, looking for a renal or urothelial tumor. US and CT, when renal function is normal, or US and MRI, when it is impaired, can provide the necessary information about the renal parenchyma and the entire excretory system. Radical nephrectomy or nephroureterectomy is recommended for native kidney tumors. Conservative percutaneous radiofrequency (RF) techniques should be considered for tumors developing within the graft (Goeman et al. 2006).

### 30.6.5 Lymphoproliferative Disorders/PTLD

PTLD are the third most common cancer in graft recipients in Europe. For renal transplant recipients, their frequency is 1–2%, or 30–50 times higher than that for

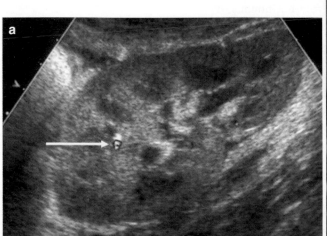
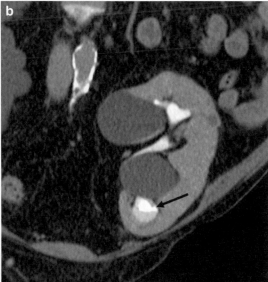

**Fig. 30.27** Examples of intracaliceal stones: (**a**) color Doppler image showing a tiny calculus with a twinkling artifact (*arrow*). (**b**) Contrast-enhanced CT of an old renal transplant shows a stone in a posterior calice (*arrow*); note the presence of two cortical cysts

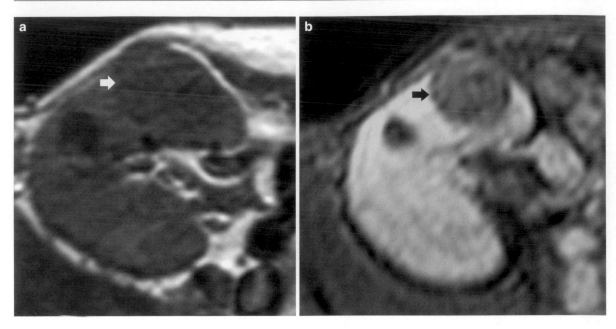

**Fig. 30.28** MR T1-weighted sequences, before (**a**) and after (**b**) injection of contrast agent showing a papillary renal cell carcinoma (*arrow*) developed on the renal graft

the general population, and they represent 21% of the malignancies, as opposed to 5% for the general population. These pathologies cover a large spectrum of hematological proliferations, ranging from benign hyperplasia to undifferentiated lymphoma. They are very often induced by Epstein–Barr virus (EBV), whose infection is favored by the immunosuppressive therapy.

The principal sites of involvement are the liver, brain, lymph nodes, lung, and gastrointestinal tract. The renal graft itself can also be involved. Most of the time, the lesion develops within the renal hilum, infiltrating the perirenal fat and encasing renal arteries and veins (Fig. 30.29). The tumor tissue may spread into the sinus, then into the renal parenchyma or toward the perirenal fat. Less often, renal involvement resembles multiple renal nodules. Involvement of the native kidneys and the bladder is also possible (Bellin et al. 1995).

These locations are difficult to assess ultrasonographically at the early phase and only dilatation of the collecting system may be seen. When visible, they appear as hypoechoic masses with hyperechoic components within the hilum and sinus. Color Doppler is able to identify encasement of renal vessels.

On CT scans, the lymphomatous tissues show low attenuation (20–30 HU) and moderate enhancement after iodine contrast-medium injection. On MR

images, they exhibit a relatively typical signal intensity pattern: a hilar mass hypointense on T1w and T2w sequences, traversed by renal vessel with minimal enhancement (Ali et al. 1999). Sometimes, a hyperintensity is seen on T2w images and the enhancement may be more prominent during the early phase after Gd injection (Claudon et al. 1998). Other sites include retroperitoneal nodes, liver, and spleen. The definitive diagnosis is based on image-guided percutaneous biopsy, which can be difficult if the mass is limited to the hilum.

## 30.7 Conclusion

The culmination of more than a century of trials and errors, renal transplantation, as it is practiced today, is a relatively simple intervention that gives excellent results as long as a rather strict procedure is respected. It requires a multidisciplinary approach to the patient, harmoniously combining the competencies of the nephrologist, radiologist, and urologist. This close-knit association and the contribution of each specialist before and after surgery should optimize the chances of successful transplantation and limit perioperative complications. Development of noninvasive imaging

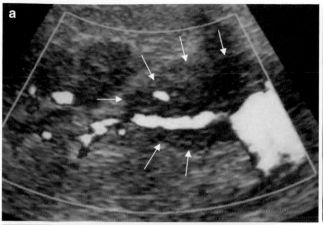

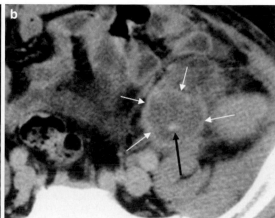

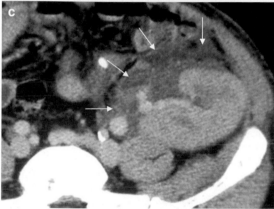

**Fig. 30.29** Pelvic lymphoma. A hypoechoic infiltration around the renal artery is shown by color flow sonography. Enhanced CT shows this low density tissue infiltration (*white arrows*) below the kidney surrounding the renal artery (*black arrow*) (**b**) extending upward into the sinus (**c**)

techniques has already transformed the diagnosis of many of these complications, by rapidly providing complete useful morphological information. Emerging methods, once they have found their place, will soon further enhance that knowledge by adding functional data obtained during the same imaging sessions.

## References

Abbott KC, Schenkman N, Swanson SJ et al. (2003) Hospitalized nephrolithiasis after renal transplantation in the United States Am J Transplant 3: 465–470

Ali MG, Coakley FV, Hricak H et al.(1999) Complex posttransplantation abnormalities of renal allografts: evaluation with MR imaging. Radiology 211:95-100

Allen KS, Jorkasky DK, Arger PH et al. (1988) Renal allografts: prospective analysis of Doppler sonography. Radiology 169:371–376

Beecroft JR, Rajan DK, Clark TW et al. (2004) Transplant renal artery stenosis: outcome after percutaneous intervention. J Vasc Interv Radiol 15:1407–1413

Bellin MF, Fuerxer F, Bitker MO et al. (1995) Tumors of the genito-urinary tract in renal transplant recipients: clinical and radiological findings. Eur Radiol 5:26–32

Bhatti AA, Chugtai A, Haslam P et al. (2005) Prospective study comparing three-dimensional computed tomography and magnetic resonance imaging for evaluating the renal vascular anatomy in potential living renal donors. BJU Int 96: 1105–1108

Bruno S, Remuzzi G, Ruggenenti P (2004) Transplant renal artery stenosis. J Am Soc Nephrol 15:134–141

Cecka JM (2002) The UNOS Renal Transplant Registry. Clin Transpl: 1-20

Claudon M, Kessler M, Champigneulle J et al. (1998) Lymphoproliferative disorders after renal transplantation: role of medical imaging Eur Radiol 8:1686–1693

Crook TJ, Keoghane SR (2005) Renal transplant lithiasis: rare but time-consuming. BJU Int 95:931–933

Dodd GD IIIrd, Tublin ME, Shah A et al. (1991) Imaging of vascular complications associated with renal transplants AJR Am J Roentgenol 157:449–459

Dominguez-Gil B, Herrero JC, Carreno A et al. (1999) Ureteral stenosis secondary to encrustation by urea-splitting Corynebacterium urealyticum in a kidney transplant patient. Nephrol Dial Transplant 14:977–978

Don S, Kopecky KK, Filo RS et al.(1989) Duplex Doppler US of renal allografts: causes of elevated resistive index Radiology 171:709–712

Fang YC, Siegelman ES (2001) Complications of renal transplantation: MR findings. J Comput Assist Tomogr 25:836–842

Ferreiros J, Mendez R, Jorquera M et al. (1999) Using gadolinium-enhanced three-dimensional MR angiography to assess arterial inflow stenosis after kidney transplantation. AJR Am J Roentgenol 172:751–757

Frick MP, Feinberg SB, Sibley R et al. (1981) Ultrasound in acute renal transplant rejection. Radiology 138:657–660

Fried AM, Woodring JH, Loh FK et al. (1983) The medullary pyramid index: an objective assessment of prominence in renal transplant rejection. Radiology 149:787–791

Genkins SM, Sanfilippo FP, Carroll BA (1989) Duplex Doppler sonography of renal transplants: lack of sensitivity and specificity in establishing pathologic diagnosis. AJR Am J Roentgenol 152:535–539

Goeman L, Joniau S, Oyen R et al. (2006) Percutaneous ultrasound-guided radiofrequency ablation of recurrent renal cell carcinoma in renal allograft after partial nephrectomy. Urology 67:199

Gogus C, Yaman O, Soygur T et al. (2002) Urological complications in renal transplantation: long-term follow-up of the Woodruff ureteroneocystostomy procedure in 433 patients. Urol Int 69:99–101

Gottlieb RH, Lieberman JL, Pabico RC et al. (1995) Diagnosis of renal artery stenosis in transplanted kidneys: value of Doppler waveform analysis of the intrarenal arteries. AJR Am J Roentgenol 165:1441–1446

Gourishankar S, Hunsicker L, Jhangri G et al. (2003) The stability of the glomerular filtration rate after renal transplantation is improving. J Am Soc Nephrol 14:2387–2394

Grenier N, Claudon M, Trillaud H et al. (1997) Noninvasive radiology of vascular complications in renal transplantation. Eur Radiol 7:385–391

Grenier N, Douws C, Morel D et al.(1991) Detection of vascular complications in renal allografts with color Doppler flow imaging. Radiology 178:217–223

Halimi JM, Al-Najjar A, Buchler M et al.(1999) Transplant renal artery stenosis: potential role of ischemia/reperfusion injury and long-term outcome following angioplasty. J Urol 161:28–32

Halloran P, Melk A, Barth C (1999) Rethinking chronic allograft nephropathy: the concept of accelerated senescence. J Am Soc Nephrol 10:167–181

Hariharan S (2001) Long-term kidney transplant survival. Am J Kidney Dis 38:S44–S50

Hariharan S, Adams MB, Brennan DC et al. (1999) Recurrent and de novo glomerular disease after renal transplantation: a report from Renal Allograft Disease Registry (RADR). Transplantation 68:635–641

Hariharan S, Johnson C, Breshnahan B et al. (2000) Improved graft survival after renal transplantation in the united states, 1988 to 1996. N Engl J Med 342:605–612

Heinz-Peer G, Maier A, Eibenberger K et al. (1998) Role of magnetic resonance imaging in renal transplant recipients with acquired cystic kidney disease. Urology 51:534–538

Heinz-Peer G, Schoder M, Rand T et al. (1995) Prevalence of acquired cystic kidney disease and tumors in native kidneys of renal transplant recipients: a prospective US study. Radiology 195:667–671

Hélénon O, Attlan E, Legendre C et al. (1992) Gd-DOTA-enhanced MR imaging and color Doppler US of renal allograft necrosis. Radiographics 12:21–33

Hoddick W, Filly RA, Backman U et al. (1986) Renal allograft rejection: US evaluation. Radiology 161:469–473

Hricak H, Terrier F, Demas BE (1986) Renal allografts: evaluation by MR imaging. Radiology 159:435–441

Hricak H, Terrier F, Marotti M et al.(1987) Posttransplant renal rejection: comparison of quantitative scintigraphy, US, and MR imaging. Radiology 162:685–688

Hubsch PJ, Mostbeck G, Barton PP et al. (1990) Evaluation of arteriovenous fistulas and pseudoaneurysms in renal allografts following percutaneous needle biopsy. Color-coded Doppler sonography versus duplex Doppler sonography. J Ultrasound Med 9:95–100

Juvenois A, Ghysels M, Galle C et al. (1999) Successful revascularization for acute renal allograft thrombosis after 32 hours of ischaemia. Nephrol Dial Transplant 14:199–201

Karcaaltincaba M, Akhan O (2005) Radiologic imaging and percutaneous treatment of pelvic lymphocele. Eur J Radiol 55:340–354

Kaveggia LP, Perrella RR, Grant EG et al. (1990) Duplex Doppler sonography in renal allografts: the significance of reversed flow in diastole. AJR Am J Roentgenol 155:295–298

Kelcz F, Pozniak MA, Pirsch JD et al. (1990) Pyramidal appearance and resistive index: insensitive and nonspecific sonographic indicators of renal transplant rejection. AJR Am J Roentgenol 155:531–535

Kocak T, Nane I, Ander H et al. (2004) Urological and surgical complications in 362 consecutive living related donor kidney transplantations. Urol Int 72:252–256

Lefevre F, Correas JM, Briancon S et al. (2002) Contrast-enhanced sonography of the renal transplant using triggered pulse-inversion imaging: preliminary results. Ultrasound Med Biol 28:303–314

Linkowski GD, Warvariv V, Filly RA et al. (1987) Sonography in the diagnosis of acute renal allograft rejection and cyclosporine nephrotoxicity. AJR Am J Roentgenol 148:291–295

Loubeyre P, Abidi H, Cahen R et al. (1997) Transplanted renal artery: detection of stenosis with color Doppler US. Radiology 203:661–665

Martinoli C, Crespi G, Bertolotto M et al. (1996) Interlobular vasculature in renal transplants: a power Doppler US study with MR correlation. Radiology 200:111–117

Melamed ML, Kim HS, Jaar BG et al. (2005) Combined percutaneous mechanical and chemical thrombectomy for renal vein thrombosis in kidney transplant recipients. Am J Transplant 5:621–626

Middleton WD, Kellman GM, Melson GL et al. (1989) Postbiopsy renal transplant arteriovenous fistulas: color Doppler US characteristics. Radiology 171:253–257

Neimatallah MA, Dong Q, Schoenberg SO et al. (1999) Magnetic resonance imaging in renal transplantation. J Magn Reson Imaging 10:357–368

Palleschi J, Novick AC, Braun WE et al. (1980) Vascular complications of renal transplantation. Urology 16:61–67

Patel NH, Jindal RM, Wilkin T et al. (2001) Renal arterial stenosis in renal allografts: retrospective study of predisposing factors and outcome after percutaneous transluminal angioplasty. Radiology 219:663–667

Penn I (2000) Post-transplant malignancy: the role of immunosuppression. Drug Saf 23:101–113

Perini S, Gordon RL, LaBerge JM et al. (1998) Transcatheter embolization of biopsy-related vascular injury in the transplant kidney: immediate and long-term outcome. J Vasc Interv Radiol 9:1011–1019

Pickhardt PJ, Siegel MJ (1999) Posttransplantation lymphoproliferative disorder of the abdomen: CT evaluation in 51 patients. Radiology 213:73–78

Platt JF, Ellis JH, Rubin JM (1991) Renal transplant pyelocaliectasis: role of duplex Doppler US in evaluation. Radiology 179:425–428

Radermacher J, Mengel M, Ellis S et al. (2003) The renal arterial resistance index and renal allograft survival. N Engl J Med 349:115–124

Rholl KS, Lee JK, Ling D et al. (1986) Acute renal rejection versus acute tubular necrosis in a canine model: MR evaluation. Radiology 160:113–117

Rijksen JF, Koolen MI, Walaszewski JE et al. (1982) Vascular complications in 400 consecutive renal allotransplants. J Cardiovasc Surg (Torino) 23:91–98

Sahani DV, Rastogi N, Greenfield AC et al. (2005) Multidetector row CT in evaluation of 94 living renal donors by readers with varied experience. Radiology 235:905–910

Sebastia C, Quiroga S, Boye R et al. (2001) Helical CT in renal transplantation: normal findings and early and late complications. Radiographics 21:1103–1117

Sierre SD, Raynaud AC, Carreres T et al. (1998) Treatment of recurrent transplant renal artery stenosis with metallic stents. J Vasc Interv Radiol 9:639–644

Trillaud H, Merville P, Tran Le Linh P et al. (1998) Color Doppler sonography in early renal transplantation followup: resistive index measurements versus power Doppler sonography. AJR Am J Roentgenol 171:1611–1615

Wolfe RA, Ashby VB, Milford EL et al. (1999) Comparison of mortality in all patients on dialysis, patients on dialysis awaiting transplantation, and recipients of a first cadaveric transplant [see comments]. N Engl J Med 341:1725–1730

# Imaging of Dialysis

**31**

Emilio Quaia and Salvatore Sammartano

## Contents

**Abstract**

> Electrolyte alterations and extrarenal disorders are quite frequent in patients undergoing hemodialysis or peritoneal dialysis. Also the native kidneys may be the site of important pathologics in patients undergoing dialysis, especially in the form of acquired renal cystic disease with frequent malignant transformation. Renal neoplasms represent an important complication of hemodialysis-associated acquired kidney cystic disease and imaging surveillance is suggested. Other important fields in which imaging techniques may provide important information are arteriovenous fistula and graft complications. Renal neoplasms represent an important complication of hemodialysis-associated acquired kidney cystic disease and imaging surveillance is suggested.

End-stage renal disease occurs when chronic renal failure progresses to the point at which the kidneys are permanently functioning at less than 10% of their capacity, namely, the GFR is permanently less than 15 mL/min/1.73 m². End-stage renal disease was a lethal condition until the advent of long-term hemodialysis and renal transplantation. Dialysis is the exchange of solutes and waste products via either an extracorporeal membrane (hemodialysis) or a peritoneal membrane (continuous ambulatory or cycling peritoneal dialysis). In the United States, diabetic nephropathy, hypertension, and glomerulonephritis cause approximately 75% of all adult cases (Warnock 1992).

In hemodialysis, solute removal depends primarily on passive diffusion across a semipermeable membrane. Blood and dialysate flow rates are adjusted to replenish

E. Quaia (✉)
Department of Radiology, Cattinara Hospital, University of Trieste, Strada di Fiume 447, 34149 Trieste, Italy
e-mail: quaia@univ.trieste.it

S. Sammartano
Department of Radiology, Santa Chiara Hospital, Trento, Italy

E. Quaia (ed.), *Radiological Imaging of the Kidney*,
Medical Radiology, DOI: 10.1007/978-3-540-87597-0_31, © Springer-Verlag Berlin Heidelberg 2011

the supply of incoming solute available for diffusion (Cohen and Alfred 1991). The dialytic removal of protein-free water (ultrafiltration) is the result of hydrostatic pressure gradient applied across the membrane. The efficiency of ultrafiltration depends on device water permeability and surface area (Cohen and Alfred 1991). The dialysis machine delivers blood and dialysate to the artificial kidney consisting of a blood pump, a dialysate delivery system, and a number of safety devices. The speed of the blood pump can be used to adjust blood flow rate. Dialysate that is diluted with water from concentrate to a ratio of 34:1 is mixed by an online proportioning system, which provides a continuous supply of fresh dialysate to the artificial kidney. Like hemodialysis, peritoneal dialysis relies on diffusion of solute down a concentration gradient. The ability of a solute to diffuse through the peritoneal membrane depends on its molecular weight and protein binding. Hemodialysis has a higher clearance rate for small-molecular-weight substances such as urea, but peritoneal dialysis is equally effective for the clearance of middle molecules in the weight range of inulin (Cohen and Alfred 1991). The decision of which modality to choose depends on local availability, patient preference, type of renal failure (acute or chronic), and clinical conditions of the patient. Anyway, there are two basic circumstances in which hemodialysis is definitely preferred: when rapid solute removal is important and when peritoneal dialysis cannot be safely performed (e.g., colostomy, or localized intraabdominal infections). Peritoneal dialysis should be performed in infants and in patients with relative contraindications to hemodialysis such as severe vascular disease, active bleeding, hemorrhagic diathesis, or cardiovascular instability.

The clinical constellation of signs and symptoms of end-stage renal disease is known as uremic syndrome. Patients with end-stage renal disease are commonly encountered with problems related to the metabolic complications of their renal disease or dialysis complications. Various problems related to vascular access in patients on hemodialysis and to abdominal catheters in patients taking continuous ambulatory peritoneal dialysis are also common since peritoneal dialysis catheter leads to the risks of peritonitis and local infection. Patients in end-stage renal failure are prone to all of the complications of any underlying condition, such as diabetes and hypertension, and other metabolic and physiologic derangements. In addition, chronic immunosuppression makes patients with end-stage renal disease prone to infection.

## 31.1 Uremic Syndrome

Uremic syndrome (uremia) refers to the final stages of progressive renal insufficiency and results from functional derangements of many organ systems, although the prominence of specific symptoms may vary from patient to patient (Warnock 1992).

### 31.1.1 Electrolyte Alterations

Iatrogenic complications related to fluid administration (fluid overload) or medications are frequently encountered in patients with renal failure. Volume overload, a common cardiovascular complication of chronic renal failure, occurs when salt and water intake exceeds losses and excretion. Hyperkalemia is the most common immediately life-threatening metabolic complication of chronic renal failure and the most common cause of sudden death in patients with end-stage renal disease. Hyperkalemia is often encountered in patients who have missed dialysis or commit dietary indiscretion.

Metabolic acidosis develops when exogenous intake and endogenous production of acid exceed renal net acid excretion. In uremic acidosis there is a progressive fall in plasma bicarbonate concentration when the urinary net acid excretion rate cannot keep up with endogenous production of acid. Initially, extrarenal buffering mechanisms are involved, including bone salts and intracellular buffers, and allow for maintenance of relatively stable, but reduced, blood bicarbonate concentration. Loss of bone buffer stores contributes to the development of osteomalacia and renal osteodystrophy. This chronic metabolic acidosis is well tolerated by most patients due to its slow development and respiratory compensation. Ketoacidosis or sepsis may determine acute worsening of metabolic acidosis.

Chronic renal failure results in the inability of the kidneys to adequately excrete phosphate, leading to hyperphosphatemia. This causes hyperplasia of the parathyroid chief cells and increased levels of parathyroid hormone (PTH). PTH is also increased because of the reduced degradation that normally occurs in the kidney. PTH enhances the absorption of calcium and magnesium and inhibits the absorption of phosphate and bicarbonate in the proximal tubule. Excess PTH affects the development of osteoclasts, osteoblasts, and osteocytes. Hypocalcemia is potentially life-threatening and results from the loss of vitamin D and increased PTH levels. Hypermagnesemia may also occur.

## 31.1.2 Extrarenal Disorders

No organ system is spared from involvement in patients with chronic renal failure. Patients with end-stage renal disease frequently have central nervous system abnormalities, some related to end-stage renal disease itself and others related to problems secondary to hemodialysis (Brouns and De Deyn 2004).

Cardiovascular complications are common in patients with chronic renal failure and are related to atherosclerosis and hyperlipidemia, hypertension due to sodium retention and alterations in the renin-angiotensin axis, myocardial dysfunction, and pericarditis. In particular, accelerated atherosclerosis is one of the major factors limiting the longevity of patients with chronic renal failure (Warnock 1992). Patients undergoing dialysis present a higher risk of atherosclerosis (Fig. 31.1), also for the underlying diabetes mellitus and/or hypertension as the causes of end-stage renal disease. Atherosclerosis involve the main arteries and all the peripheral arteries including the intrarenal arteries.

Patients with chronic renal failure may present several abnormal findings on chest radiography and CT, due to changes in the phosphorus and calcium metabolism, changes in hemostasis, arterial hypertension, fluid retention, or due to dialysis. The most frequent abnormalities include interstitial and alveolar edema and cardiomegaly, pleural effusion, metastatic pulmonary calcifications and calcifications of the bronchial walls, pleura, and chest wall vessels.

Hematologic abnormalities are among the most consistent manifestations of uremia (Warnock 1992). These abnormalities include anemia, bleeding, and granulocyte and platelet dysfunction. The primary causes of anemia in chronic renal failure are a deficiency of erythropoietin, which is a glycoprotein normally produced by the kidney, and iron deficiency due to reduced iron intake and frequent blood sampling. Erythropoietin therapy has improved the general status of patients with chronic renal failure. In patients with uremic syndrome, the fat bone marrow is progressively replaced by hematopoietic marrow content

(Ito et al. 1994) with prolonged T1 relaxation time in various anatomical regions (especially the spine and the upper and lower limb bones). A hemorrhagic diathesis is common in patients with chronic renal failure. Spontaneous nontraumatic bleeding may affect the perinephric and subcaspular spaces, the renal parenchyma, or the collecting system. Gastrointenstinal bleeding is also common in uremic patients.

The most common neurologic complications in this patient group include focal white matter lesions, cerebral atrophy, osmotic demyelination syndrome, dialysis encephalopathy, hypertensive encephalopathy, intracranial hemorrhage, infarction, sinus thrombosis, and infection. Peripheral neuropathy is also common in patients with chronic renal failure.

Abnormalities involving the musculoskeletal system are numerous and frequent in patients with chronic renal insufficiency (Murphey et al. 1993). Chronic renal insufficiency, hemodialysis, peritoneal dialysis, renal transplantation, and administration of different medications provoke complex biochemical disturbances of the calcium–phosphate metabolism with wide spectrum of bone and soft tissue abnormalities termed renal osteodystrophy (Jevtic 2003). By the time dialysis is initiated, nearly all patients are affected. Renal osteodystrophy is a global term applied to all pathological features of bone in patients with chronic renal failure and it comprises osteomalacia or rickets according to patient age, secondary hyperparathyroidism with bone resorption (Figs. 31.2 and 31.3), periosteal reaction, and brown tumors, osteosclerosis (Fig. 31.4), osteoporosis, and soft tissue and vascular calcifications. Bone resorption typically manifests along the radial aspects of the middle phalanges of the index and middle fingers (Fig. 31.2), beginning in the proximal metaphyseal region. Additional sites of subperiosteal bone resorption include the upper medial tibia, humerus, and femur, the superior and inferior ribs, and lamina dura (Murphey et al. 1993). The irregular cortical surface may create a false appearance of periosteal reaction (pseudoperiostitis). Subchondral bone resorption affects single distal interphalangeal joint (most frequently the fourth and fifth fingers), the metacarpophalangeal joint and the proximal interphalangeal joints, the distal clavicle, the acromioclavear joint, sacroiliac joint, sternoclavicular joint, symphysis pubis, and posterior patella (Murphey et al. 1993). Subligamentous bone resorption include the inferior surface of the calcaneus and clavicle (coracoclavicular ligaments), greater and lesser femoral

**Fig. 31.1** (**a**, **b**) Contrast-enhanced angio-TC. (**a**) Diffuse calcifications of the abdominal aorta and ileofemoral arteries with bilateral obstruction of the distal tract of the superficial femoral artery in a patient undergoing chronic hemodialysis. (**b**) Magnification of the proximal tract of the superficial femoral artery showing diffuse atherosclerosis with calcific plaques

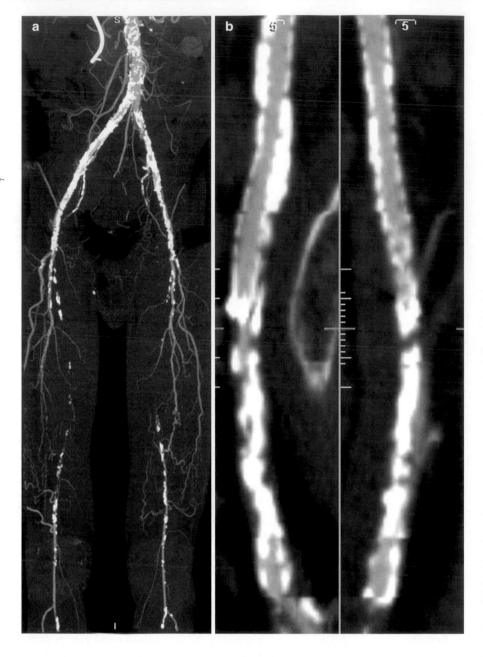

trochanters, anterior inferior iliac spine region, humerus near the insertion of the rotator cuff, ischial tuberosities, and elbow at the level of the extensor surface of the ulna and posterior olecranon (Murphey et al. 1993). Osteoclastomas or brown tumors are caused by localized replacement of bone by vascularized fibrous tissue (osteitis fibrosa cystica) resulting from PTH-stimulated osteoelastic activity. The fibrous tissue contains giant cells, and the lesions may become cystic following necrosis and liquefaction. Radiographically, brown tumors are well-defined lytic lesions, often eccentric

or cortical, that may cause endosteal scalloping and osseous expansion (Murphey et al. 1993).

Others abnormalities related to biochemical disturbance of chronic renal failure include soft tissue/vascular calcifications (Fig. 31.5) and crystalline arthropathies. Musculoskeletal sequelae predominantly related to dialysis include aluminum toxicity manifesting as osteomalacia from ingestion of aluminum salts in phosphate-binding antiacids used to control hyperphospatemia, amyloidosis with carpal tunnel syndrome, and destructive spondyloarthropathy (Murphey et al.

**Fig. 31.2** (**a, b**) Plain hand radiograph of a male patient undergoing hemodialysis from 2 years. (**a**) Normal view; (**b**) magnification of the fifth finger. Secondary hyperparathyroidism with bone resorption along the radial aspects of the middle phalanges of the fingers (*arrow*)

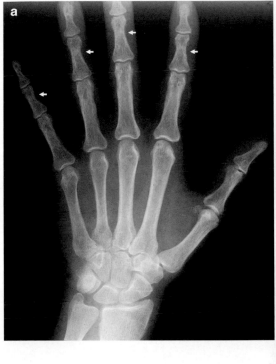

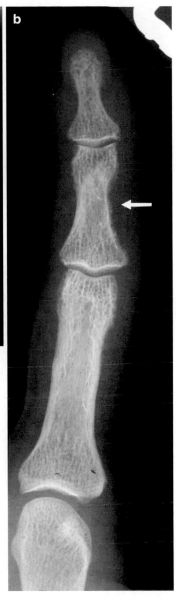

1993). Avascular necrosis, osteomyelitis, septic arthritis, tendinosis/tendon rupture, and bursitis/synovitis are caused by a combination of chronic renal failure, steroid/immunosuppressants, and dialysis (Katz et al., 2007).

## 31.2  Acquired (Dialysis-Associated) Cystic Kidney Disease

Acquired (dialysis-associated) cystic kidney disease (ACKD) was first described by Dunnill et al. (1977) and is characterized by the development of numerous fluid-filled cysts in patients with end-stage renal disease who have undergone prolonged dialysis, but without a history of hereditary cystic disease (Fig. 31.6). The cysts measure 0.5–2 cm in diameter, contain clear fluid, are lined by either hyperplastic or flattened tubular epithelium, and often contain calcium oxalate crystals (Fig. 31.6). They probably form as a result of obstruction of tubules by interstitial fibrosis or by oxalate crystals (Alpers 2005). Frequently, some cysts may develop a hemorrhagic pattern causing hematuria (Fig. 31.7). The likelihood of the development of ACKD increases with the duration of hemodialysis and is increased in men and older patients (Heinz-Peer

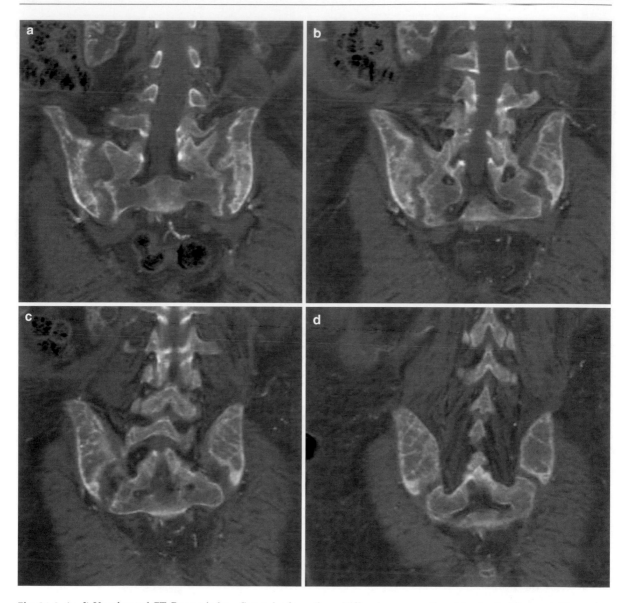

**Fig. 31.3** (**a–d**) Unenhanced CT. Bone window. Coronal reformations. Diffuse bone resorption at the level of the sacro-iliac region in a patient undergoing hemodialysis with secondary hyperparathyroidism

et al. 1995). Other factors, such as the underlying renal insufficiency and serum creatinine level, have no significant influence on the development of ACKD (Heinz-Peer et al. 1995). After 1–3 years of hemodialysis, 10–20% of patients have ACKD, 40–60% at 3–5 years of hemodialysis, and more than 90% after 5–10 years of hemodialysis. ACKD and neoplasia can develop in those patients who have undergone long-term hemodialysis (Scanlon and Karasick 1983).

The development of renal cell carcinoma (Figs. 31.8–31.10) in the wall of the cysts is the most serious

complication of ACKD (Truong et al. Truong et al. 1995). In patients with dialysis-associated ACKD undergoing long-term hemodialysis, the prevalence of renal cell carcinoma is increased being in the range of 3–6% (Gardner 1984). The prevalence is similar in patients with ACKD undergoing renal transplantation (Heinz-Peer et al. 1995). A comprehensive review of the pertinent literature shows that there is up to 50-fold increased risk of renal cell carcinoma in ACKD compared to the general population (Truong et al. 1995). ACKD-associated renal cell carcinoma accounts for

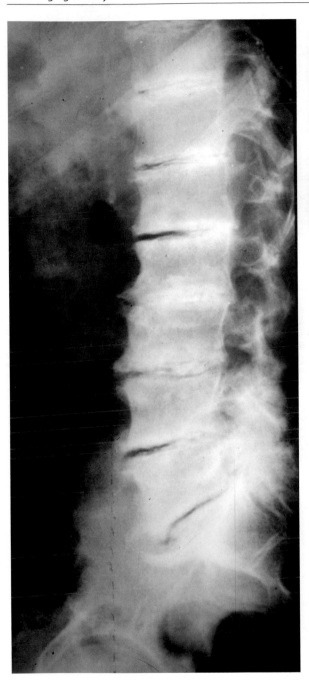

**Fig. 31.4** Plain radiography of the spine. Diffuse osteosclerosis of the spine in patient undergoing chronic hemodialysis. Diffuse sub-endplate densities at multiple contiguous levels, a pattern knwon as "rugger-gersey spine"

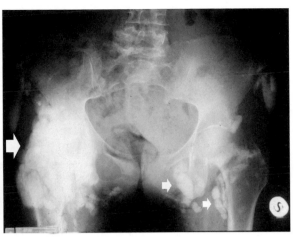

**Fig. 31.5** Renal osteodystrophy of a male patient undergoing hemodialysis from 2 years. Plain radiograph of the hip. Diffuse soft tissue calcifications (*arrows*)

approximately 2% of deaths in renal transplant patients. A median length of survival of approximately 14 months and a 5-year survival rate of 35% are comparable to the same data for renal cell carcinoma in the general population. Successful renal transplant probably decreases the risk of renal cell carcinoma in ACKD patients, but this preliminary observation needs confirmation. The development of ACKD-associated renal carcinoma is a continuous process with evolving phenotypic expression, including damaged renal tubule, simple cyst, cyst with atypical lining, adenoma, and finally, carcinoma. The pathogenesis of this continuous process is not entirely known, but growth factor-induced compensatory growth of tubular epithelium initiated by the changes of end-stage kidney disease, and probably perpetuated by activation of proto-oncogenes, seems to be the most significant factor. The ACKD-associated renal cell carcinoma is seen predominantly in males, occurs approximately 20 years earlier than in the general population, and is frequently bilateral (9%) and multicentric (50%). Acquired cystic kidney disease-associated renal cell carcinoma is frequently asymptomatic (86%), but may be associated with bleeding, abrupt changes in hematocrit, fever, and flank pain or rarely with hypoglycemia, hypercalcemia, or metastases at presentation (Truong et al. 1995).

CT seems to provide a better diagnostic yield than US or MR imaging. It is generally agreed that there is a need for regular surveillance of symptomatic ACKD patients for early detection of renal cell carcinoma (Scandling 2007; Schwarz et al. 2007). Screening kidney transplant candidates for ACKD and kidney cancer is recommended by the North American and European professional transplantation societies, but the guidelines as to who should be screened are vague. The guideline of the American Society of

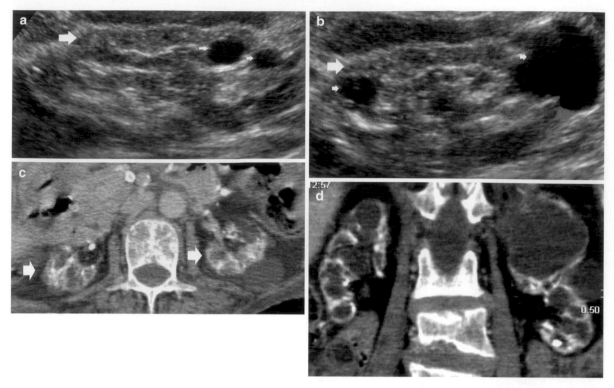

**Fig. 31.6** (**a–d**) (**a, b**) Baseline gray-scale ultrasound. 57-year-old male patient with acquired cystic kidney disease under dialysis treatment from 5 years. Diffuse reduction of the renal cortex thickness (*large arrows*) with evidence of multiple parenchymal cysts (*small arrows*). (**c, d**) 71-year-old female patient with acquired cystic kidney disease under dialysis treatment from 10 years. Diffuse calcifications at the level of intrarenal arteries and multiple parenchymal cysts with diffuse reduction of the renal cortical thickness

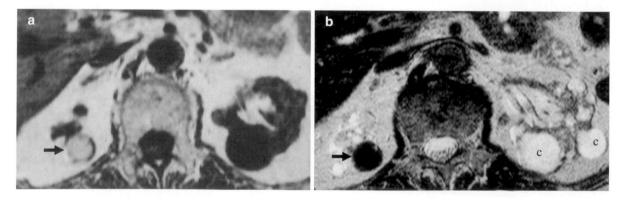

**Fig. 31.7** (**a, b**) Hemorrhagic renal cyst (*arrow*) in the right kidney in a patient with acquired cystic kidney disease, appearing hyperintense on T1-weighted MR sequences (**a**) and hypointense on T2-weighted MR sequences (**b**)

Transplantation recommends screening patients who are at high risk for renal cell carcinoma, but does not define high risk (Kasiske et al. 2001). The guideline of the EBPG Expert Group on Renal Transplantation, European Renal Association-European Dialysis and Transplant Association (2000) recommends screening of candidates who have been long-term dialysis patients but does not define long term. Schwarz et al. (2007) recommend a screening and management protocol in transplant recipients, incorporating the Bosniak renal cyst classification system (Israel and Bosniak 2005). All renal transplant recipients should undergo a yearly

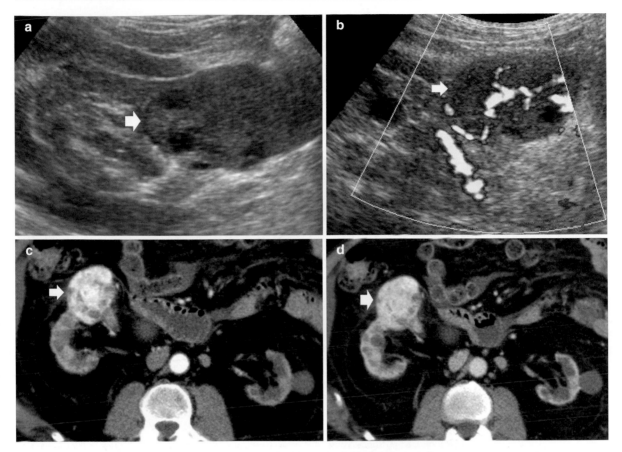

**Fig. 31.8** (**a–d**) Clear cell renal cell carcinoma in a patient undergoing hemodialysis from 2 years and evidence of initial acquired renal cystic disease. (**a**) Gray-scale ultrasound. (**b**) Power Doppler ultrasound. Contrast-enhanced CT during corticomedullary (**c**) and nephrographic phase (**d**). Both kidneys present reduced dimensions and diffuse marginal scars. The left kidney presents some parenchymal cysts. (**a, b**) Evidence of a solid renal tumor (*arrow*), with some cystic intratumoral areas on the right kidney. The renal tumor presents intratumoral vessels on power Doppler ultrasound (**b**). After iodinated contrast agent administration (**c, d**) the solid renal tumor (*arrow*) presents diffuse contrast enhancement and reveals infiltration of the anterior renal fascia

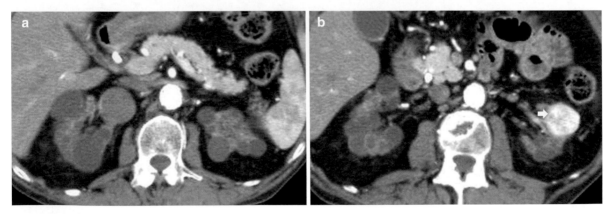

**Fig. 31.9** (**a, b**) Clear cell renal cell carcinoma complicating advanced acquired renal cystic disease in a patient undergoing hemodialysis from 10 years. Unenhanced (**a**) and contrast-enhanced (**b**) CT. Both kidneys present multiple cysts with a liquid density on unenhanced CT scan (**a**). After contrast administration (**b**) a solid enhancing lesion is evident on the left kidney (*arrow*)

**Fig. 31.10** (**a–f**) Renal solid neoplasm complicating acquired renal cystic disease in a patient undergoing hemodialysis from 10 years. Unenhanced (**a**) and contrast-enhanced (**b**) MR imaging. Both kidneys present multiple cysts with a liquid density on unenhanced CT scan (**a**). After contrast administration (**b**) a solid enhancing lesion is evident on the left kidney (*arrow*)

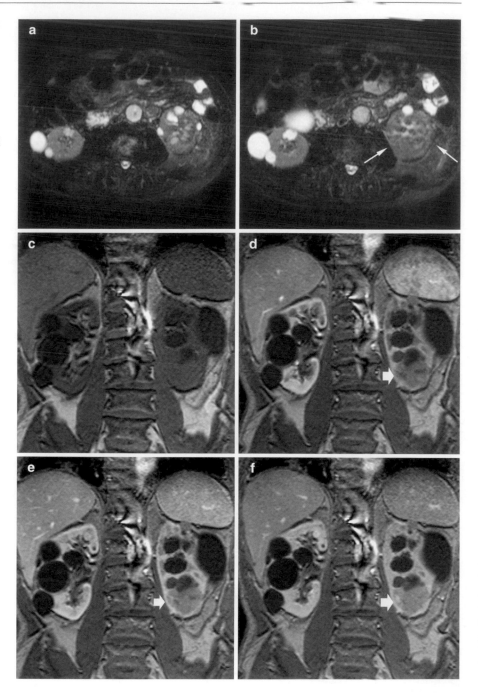

ultrasound screening of the native kidneys. In patients with ACKD and Bosniak category I or II cysts (benign simple cysts), twice yearly US screening and CT scan if progression is evident are suggested. In patients with ACKD and Bosniak category IIF (F for follow-up) cysts (moderately complex cysts), a quarterly US screening and yearly CT or MR imaging scan are suggested. Nephrectomy is suggested if progression is evident, even if not reaching category III or IV. In patients with ACKD and Bosniak category III ("indeterminate" cystic masses) or IV (clearly malignant cystic masses), nephrectomy is suggested.

## 31.3 Dialysis Access Complications

Repeated access to the circulation is essential to perform adequate maintenance hemodialysis. End-stage renal failure patients requiring long-term hemodialysis need a durable vascular access and maintenance of acceptable vascular access is an important issue for patients with renal failure. Hemodialysis is usually performed with an internal arteriovenous fistula (AV fistula) with the side of the radial artery anastomosed to the side of the cephalic vein at the wrist on the nondominant side, or with a polytetrafluoroethylene (PTFE, Teflon) graft known also as prosthetic bridge graft (PBG) consisting in a relatively bioinert material, when an internal fistula is no longer feasible. Surgically constructed arteriovenous (AV) fistulas (radio- or brachiocephalic) and synthetic AV grafts (Fig. 31.11) or venous catheter positioned in a central vein are common means of establishing vascular access for long-term hemodialysis.

Vascular stenoses are the major cause of access failure, and stenosis development at or near the venous anastomosis of bridge grafts and at the AV anastomosis of AV fistulas represents the most common cause of late-access thrombosis; however, more than one third of stenoses are located in the venous outflow tract of the accesses. Treatment of stenoses with percutaneous intervention, angioplasty or endoluminal vascular stents, or thombolysis, as an alternative to surgery, has been shown to increase survival of patients with dialysis AV fistulas and PBGs (van der Linden et al. 2002). Several surveillance techniques may be used in the timely detection of access stenosis development. Color Doppler US (Doelman et al. 2005) and digital subtraction angiography (Froger et al. 2005) are most widely used for the detection of access stenoses, while contrast-enhanced multidetector CT (Rooijens et al. 2008) or MR angiography of shunts (Pinto et al. 2006) has recently been introduced. Color Doppler US should be the initial imaging modality of dysfunctional shunts, but complete access should be depicted at digital subtraction angiography, with arterial or venous contrast injection, to detect all significant stenoses eligible for intervention. Contrast-enhanced CT or MR angiography should be considered only if digital subtraction angiography is inconclusive (Doelman et al. 2005). Angiographic evaluation, via puncture of the brachial artery, is indicated when interventional procedure is planned.

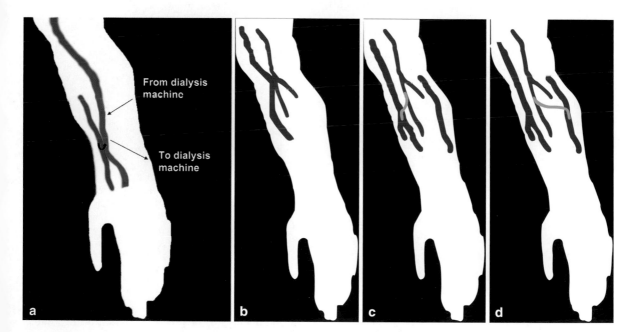

**Fig. 31.11** (**a–d**) (**a**, **b**) Scheme describing the essential feature of (**a**) wrist and (**b**) arm arteriovenous fistula in a patient undergoing chronic hemodialysis (see text). (**c**, **d**) Arteriovenous graft – prosthetic bridge graft – consisting of a synthetic catheter inserted and sutured into the radial artery, 5 cm distally to its origin, and the cephalic vein (**c**) or the basilic vein (**d**). red = artery; blue = vein; curved arrow = blood flow direction; green = prosthetic bridge graft

## 31.3.1 Arteriovenous Fistulas

The AV fistula is considered the best long-term vascular access for hemodialysis because it provides adequate blood flow, lasts a long time, and has a lower complication rate than other types of access. An AV fistula requires advance planning because a fistula takes a while after surgery to develop – in rare cases, as long as 24 months. But a properly formed fistula is less likely than other kinds of vascular access to form clots or become infected. Also, properly formed fistulas tend to last many years – longer than any other kind of vascular access. A nephrologist or a surgeon creates an AV fistula by connecting an artery directly to a vein, frequently in the forearm or the wrist. The nondominant forearm is preferred. The most employed vessels are: (1) distal site, the distal portion of the radial artery and the cephalic vein at the level of the wrist: the side of the radial artery is anastomosed to the side of the cephalic vein and the fistula is allowed to mature for several weeks (Fig. 31.11a); (2) proximal site, the radial artery immediately after its origin from the brachial artery and a nearby vein, usually the median cubital branch of the cephalic vein (Fig. 31.11b). As a result, the vein grows larger and stronger, making repeated needle insertions for hemodialysis treatments easier. As complications occur within the original AV fistula, more proximal fistulas are created, but the incidence of distal ischemia and motor neuropathy increases the more proximally the fistula is placed.

An AV fistula (Fig. 31.12) provides superior access survival relative to the AV graft and inferior incidence of complications. Anyway, dysfunction of fistulae is the most common reason for a second intervention and recurrent hospitalization. The rate of AV fistula complications increases with age, erythropoietin weekly dose, with proximal elbow and right-side AV fistulas, and also among patients with a history of a previous failed shunt (Salahi et al., 2006). The clinical symptoms include poor flow with loss of thrill in the graft, enlarging pseudoaneurysm, or ipsilateral limb swelling. AV fistula complications are seen less frequently and are also less severe than in the AV graft. However, AV fistulas present some disadvantages including the incomplete maturation of the vein and that a period of 1–4 months may be required before the AV fistula may be used.

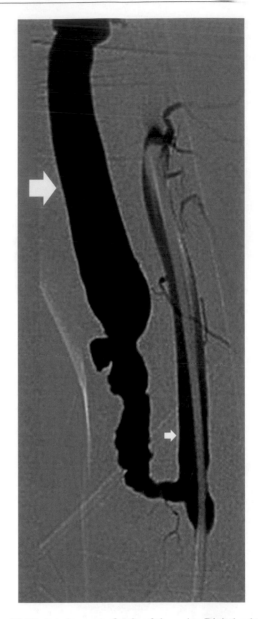

**Fig. 31.12** Arteriovenous fistula of the wrist. Digital subtraction angiography. The side of the radial artery (*small arrow*) is anastomosed to the side of the cephalic vein (*large arrow*). Dilatation and arterialization of the venous component (*arrow*) of the arteriovenous fistula

The principal complications of the AV fistula include thrombosis with occlusion or stenosis of the venous outflow and aneurysms or pseudoaneurysm of the venous tract near or distally the anastomosis with the radial artery (Rodriguez et al. 2005). In particular, venous

**Fig. 31.13** (a–c) Arteriovenous fistula of the forearm. Seventy-year-old male patient with chronic renal failure under dialysis. The radial artery immediately after its origin from the brachial artery is anastomosed to the median cubital branch of the cephalic vein. (**a**) Tight stenosis (*arrow*) of the venous outflow proximal to the anastomosis with the radial artery. The stenosis is treated by angioplasty and a wall stent (*arrow*) (**b**) with restoration of the normal patency (**c**)

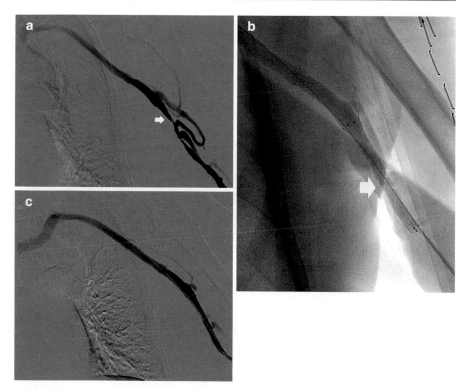

**Fig. 31.14** Arteriovenous fistula of the forearm. Eighty-two-year-old patient with chronic renal failure under dialysis. Two psudoaneurysms (*arrows*) of the venous tract of the arteriovenous fistula, respectively, proximal and at the level of the anastomosis with the radial artery

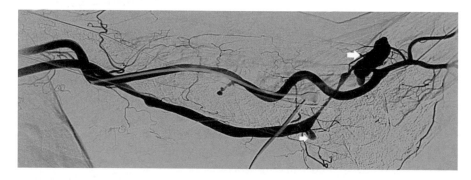

outflow obstruction (Fig. 31.13) is the most common cause of AV fistula thrombosis and poor dialysis. Most typically, pseudoaneurysms (Fig. 31.14) are found in areas of repeated puncture or surgical anastomosis.

The complications of the arterial tract of AV fistulas are rare. Proximal arterial disease or occlusion or an arterial anastomotic stenosis are readily demonstrated by digital subtraction angiography. Arterial stenosis appears as a narrowed area adjacent to or between areas of graft ectasia. Radial artery laceration may determine a hematoma with compression of the nervous structures in the carpal tunnel (Fig. 31.15).

## 31.3.2 Arteriovenous Grafts

The AV fistula with its long patency rate and low complication profile is usually the first choice for vascular access creation. However, when superficial veins are not suitable for AV fistula creation or all have been exhausted as a result of repeated AV fistula procedures, AV grafts using expanded PTFE are an alternative (Nikeghbalian et al. 2006). The PTFE graft – PBG – consists of a synthetic catheter inserted and sutured into the artery, usually the radial, and vein, usually the cephalic – Fig. 31.11c – or the basilic vein – Fig. 31.11d.

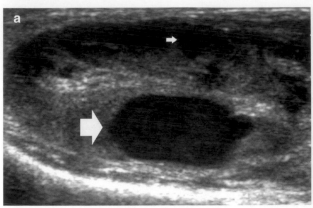
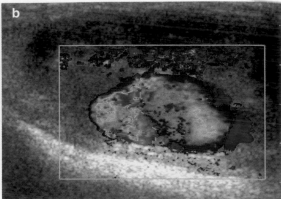

**Fig. 31.15** (**a**, **b**) Arteriovenous fistula complication. Eighty-two-year-old patient with chronic renal failure under dialytic treatment from 15 years presenting a painful swelling on the right wrist and carpal tunnel syndrome. (**a**) Ultrasound of the right wrist, transverse scan. A anechoic collection (*arrow*) is evident below the level of flexor muscle tendons (*small arrow*). (**b**) Color Doppler analysis of the collection reveals a turbulent flow with evident aliasing due to radial artery laceration compressing the radial nerve in the carpal tunnel

Generally, the graft is anastomosed to the side of the radial artery approximately 5 cm distal to its origin. To avoid narrowing during flexion of the elbow, the venous anastomosis is created with the basilic vein below the elbow joint. Again, the nondominant forearm is preferred (Becker et al. 1990).

Unlike the AV fistula used for chronic hemodialysis, the AV graft can be used immediately. Successful creation of a vascular access using prosthetic material requires good arterial inflow and venous outflow. Several graft configurations have been developed for dialysis. Just as in natural AV fistula, the nondominant arm should be used first (Nikeghbalian et al. 2006). The graft becomes an artificial vein that can be used repeatedly for needle placement and blood access during hemodialysis. A graft does not need to develop as a fistula does, so it can be used sooner after placement, often within 2 or 3 weeks. Compared with properly formed fistulas, grafts tend to have more problems with clotting and infection and need replacement sooner. However, a well-cared-for graft can last several years.

The overall complication rate for the AV graft is twice as that of AV fistulas (Becker et al. 1990). The most common complication associated with the AV graft is venous outflow obstruction with graft thrombosis, which accounts for 85–90% of problems with hemodialysis. PBGs have a shorter mean patency than native AV fistulas. The most common causes of failure include surgical twisting or kinking of the graft during implantation, an arterial plug, a stenosis of the venous anastomosis, or an unsuspected venous stenosis. Venous stenosis results in problems that have the net effect of inadequate dialysis. Stenosis occurs most frequently at the venous anastomosis, but may occur anywhere within the system composed by the graft, the anastomosis, and its draining veins. Complete thrombosis is easily identified when it involves the graft or the entire venous limb. Moreover, AV grafts may produce complications related to arterial inflow stenosis, arterial anastomotic stenosis, intragraft stenosis, graft pseudoaneurysm, and graft degeneration. Treatment options are surgical revision or endovascular stent graft placement.

### 31.3.3 Dialysis Access Catheters

High thrombosis rate of AV fistula and PBGs and the high recurrence rates after thrombolysis and angioplasty have led to a consideration of performing hemodialysis with percutaneous inserted venous catheters. Nowadays, venous catheters are often considered for a long-term solution for hemodialysis due to the developments in the biomaterials available for catheters. Percutaneous venous catheters present the advantage that they are placed on an outpatient basis, they do not require maturation period, and they avoid the repeated punctures of AV fistula. Disadvantages are represented by the fact that venous catheters are cosmetically less acceptable and that the peak achievable flow rates are lower than those with AV fistulas and PBGs.

A venous catheter positioned in a central vein (usually the right internal jugular vein or less frequently the femoral or subclavian veins) through the subclavian vein for a temporary access has two chambers to allow a two-way flow of blood. Once a catheter is placed, needle insertion is not necessary. Catheters are not ideal for permanent access, and this patency is maintained by heparin-saline infusion by flushing the catheter twice daily (every 12 h) with 2 or 3 mL of heparin (2,000–3,000 units). They can clog, become infected, and cause stenosis (Fig. 31.16) or complete thrombosis (Fig. 31.17) of the central vein in which they are placed. But if you need to start hemodialysis immediately, a catheter will work for several weeks or months while your permanent access develops.

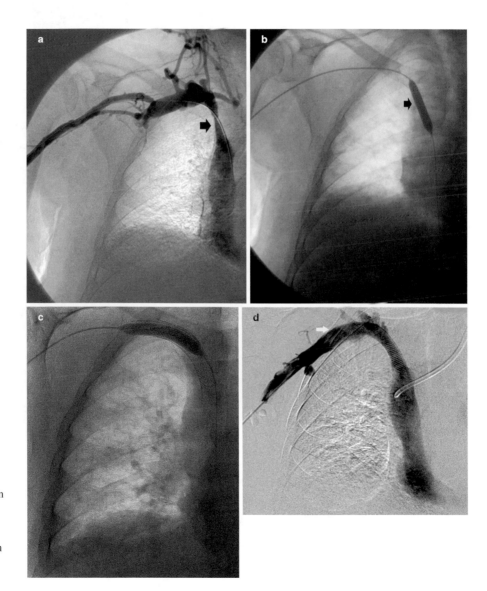

**Fig. 31.16** (**a–c**) Vascular complication in patients undergoing dialysis. (**a**) Digital subtraction venography. Stenosis (*arrow*) of the anonima vein due to a temporary venous access. (**b**, **c**) The stenosis was treated by two-time angioplasty. (**d**) Restoration of the normal patency of the anonymous vein

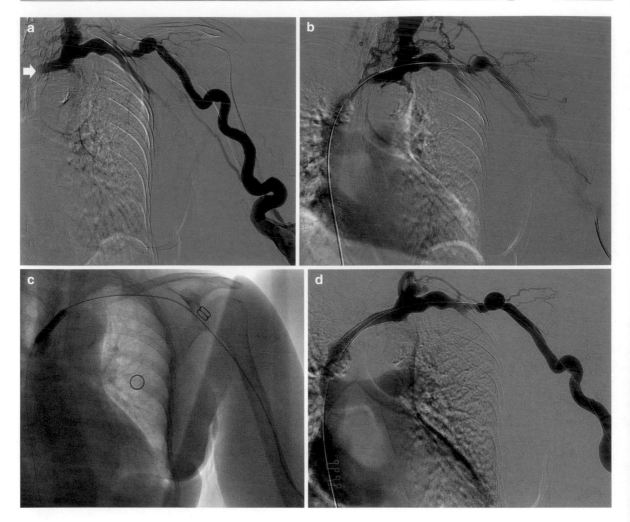

**Fig. 31.17** (**a–d**) Treatment of a thrombosis of the anonymous vein (*arrow*) preexisting to a forearm arteriovenous fistula. Patient presents with a huge swelling of the arm after arteriovenous fistula. (**a**) Digital subtraction venography shows complete thrombosis of the anonymous vein (*arrow*); (**b**, **c**) angioplasty and stenting of the anonima vein. (**d**) Restoration of the normal patency of the anonymous vein

# References

Alpers CE (2005) The kidney. In: Kumar V, Abbas AK, Fausto N (eds) Robbins and Cotran pathologic basis of disease. Elsevier Saunders, Philadelphia, pp 955–1021

Becker JA, Choyke PL, Robbin ML (1990) Dialysis and its complications. In: Pollack HM, McClennan BL, Dyer R, Kenney PJ (eds) Clinical urography. Saunders, Philadelphia, pp 3070–3083

Brouns R, De Deyn PP (2004) Neurological complications inrenal failure: a review. Clin Neurol Neurosurg 107(1):1–16

Cohen AJ, Alfred HJ (1991) Use of dialytic procedures in the intensive care units. In: Rippe JM, Irwin RS, Alpert JS, Fink MP (eds) Intensive care medicine. Little, Brown, Boston, pp 742–764

Doelman C, Duijm LE, Liem YS et al. (2005) Stenosis detection in failing hemodialysis access fistulas and grafts: comparison of color Doppler ultrasonography, contrast-enhanced magnetic resonance angiography, and digital subtraction angiography. J Vasc Surg 42(4):739–746

Dunnill MS, Millard PR, Oliver D (1977) Acquired cystic disease of the kidney: a hazard of long-term intermittent maintenance hemodialysis. J Clin Pathol 30:868–877

EBPG Expert Group on Renal Transplantation, European Renal Association-European Dialysis and Transplant Association (2000) Evaluation, selection and preparation of the potential transplant recipient. Nephrol Dial Transplant 15(suppl 7):3–38

Froger CL, Duijm LE, Liem YS et al. (2005) Stenosis detection with MR angiography and digital subtraction angiography in dysfunctional hemodialysis access fistulas and grafts. Radiology 234(1):284–291

Gardner KD (1984) Acquired renal cystic disease and renal adenocarcinoma in patients on long-term hemodialysis (letter). N Engl J Med 310:390

Heinz-Peer G, Schoder M, Rand T et al. (1995) Prevalence of acquired cystic kidney disease and tumors in native kidneys of renal transplant recipients: a prospective US study. Radiology 195:667–671

Israel GM, Bosniak MA (2005) An update of the Bosniak renal cyst classification system. Urology 66: 484 –488

Ito M, Ito M, Hayashi K et al. (1994) Evaluation of spinal bone changes in patients with chronic renal failure by CT and MR imaging with pathologic correlation. Acta Radiol 35(3): 291–295

Jevtic V (2003) Imaging of renal osteodystrophy. Eur J Radiol 46(2):85–95

Kasiske BL, Cangro CB, Hariharan S et al.; American Society of Transplantation (2001) The evaluation of renal transplant candidates: clinical practice guidelines Am J Transplant 1(suppl 2):3–95

Katz R, Makalanda L, Carmichael J et al. (2007) Musculo-skeletal manifestations of chronic renal failure and dialysis. RSNA 2007 educational exhibit

Murphey MD, Sartoris DJ, Quale JL et al. (1993) Musculoskeletal manifestations of chronic renal insufficiency. Radiographics 13:357–379

Nikeghbalian S, Bananzadeh A, Yarmohammadi H (2006) Difficult vascular access in patients with end-stage renal failure. Transplant Proc 38(5):1265–1266

Pinto C, Hickey R, Carroll TJ, et al. (2006) Time-resolved MR angiography with generalized autocalibrating partially parallel acquisition and time-resolved echo-sharing angiographic technique for hemodialysis arteriovenous fistulas and grafts. J Vasc Interv Radiol 17(6):1003–1009

Rodriguez HE, Leon L, Schalch P et al. (2005) Arteriovenous access: managing common problems. Perspect Vasc Surg Endovasc Ther 17(2):155–166

Rooijens PP, Serafino GP, Vroegindeweij D et al. (2008) Multi-slice computed tomographic angiography for stenosis detection in forearm hemodialysis arteriovenous fistulas. J Vasc Access 9(4):278–284

Salahi H, Fazelzadeh A, Mehdizadeh A et al. (2006) Complications of arteriovenous fistula in dialysis patients. Transplant Proc 38 (5):1261–1264

Scandling JD (2007) Acquired cystic kidney disease and renal cell cancer after transplantation: time to rethink screening? clin J Am Soc Nephrol 2:621–622

Scanlon MH, Karasick SR (1983) Acquired renal cystic disease and neoplasia: complications of chronic hemodialysis. Radiology 147:837–838

Schwarz A, Vatandaslar S, Merkel S et al. (2007) Renal cell carcinoma in transplant recipients with acquired cystic kidney disease. Clin J Am Soc Nephrol 2:750–756

Truong LD, Krishnan B, Cao JT et al. (1995) Renal neoplasm in acquired cystic kidney disease. Am J Kidney Dis 26(1):1–12

van der Linden J, Smits JH, Assink JH et al. (2002) Short- and long-term functional effects of percutaneous transluminal angioplasty in hemodialysis vascular access. J Am Soc Nephrol 13:715–720

Warnock DG (1992) Chronic renal failure. In: Wyngaarden JB, Smith LH, Bennett JC (eds) Cecil textbook of medicine. Saunders, Philadelphia, pp 533–541

# Imaging of the Postoperative Kidney

## 32

Emilio Quaia

## Contents

**Abstract**

> Radical nephrectomy and nephron-sparing sur-
gery represent the surgical procedures applied
in renal oncology. The resection of part of the
kidney or of the whole kidney parenchyma
determines evident change in the retroperitoneal anatomy and in the abdominal and retroperitoneal organ relationship. In this chapter,
the normal imaging findings and the fundamental complications after renal surgery detectable
by imaging are described. Moreover, the topic
of tumoral recurrence and the differential diagnosis between tumoral recurrence and normal
postsurgical findings is addressed.

## 32.1 Management of Renal Masses

Recent advances in imaging technology have led to an
increase in the number of incidentally discovered renal
masses, especially of small size, which cannot be
related to the patient's present complaint or past medical history. The small renal mass is defined as a renal
lesion 3 cm or less in diameter (Zagoria 2000), and
generally, the management of small renal masses
remains a challenging issue (Silverman et al. 2008).
The first aim of imaging is to characterize each renal
mass as cystic or solid and as benign or malignant and
to propose a likely diagnosis, and the second aim is to
suggest the correct management of the scanned renal
mass. Bosniak (1986) classification is a useful guide to
the diagnosis and management of cystic renal masses.

Solid renal masses contain little or no fluid components and usually consist predominantly of enhancing

E. Quaia
Department of Radiology, Cattinara Hospital,
University of Trieste, Strada di Fiume 447, 34149 Trieste, Italy
e-mail: quaia@univ.trieste.it

E. Quaia (ed.), *Radiological Imaging of the Kidney*,
Medical Radiology, DOI: 10.1007/978-3-540-87597-0_32, © Springer-Verlag Berlin Heidelberg 2011

tissue. However, it should also be kept in mind that not all enhancing solid renal masses represent a renal neoplasm (Israel and Bosniak 2005). Solid renal masses must be differentiated from renal pseudotumors (e.g., hypertrophied parenchyma adjacent to scar renal parenchyma, prominent column of Bertin, or lobar dysmorphism), and from inflammatory and vascular (e.g., aneurysm or arteriovenous malformation) renal lesion. Excluding inflammatory and vascular abnormalities and pseudotumors, an enhancing renal mass should be considered neoplastic. Although renal cell carcinoma (RCC) is by far the most lethal urologic malignancy, benign tumors constitute a significant proportion of incidental solid renal masses.

Different strategies have been proposed for the clinical management of nonfatty enhancing renal masses, including watchful waiting approach corresponding to the simple observation, imaging with another modality, percutaneous biopsy, ablation, or nephron-sparing surgery. The decision of the most correct management of an incidental renal mass should also include, beside tumor nature and staging, the evaluation of the patient factors such as age, life expectancy, comorbidity, and patient preference. In particular, life expectancy and comorbidity are the most important ones.

In the general population, the radical surgery is suggested for those renal solid tumors that are >1 cm in diameter (Silverman et al. 2008). When the fat is evident, the diagnosis is angiomyolipoma, while all the other imaging features may be related to the diagnosis of RCC. In asymptomatic low-risk patients, renal lesions ≤1 cm are assumed to be incidental simple renal cysts unless they are clearly solid, clearly enhance with contrast material infusion, or contain coarse calcifications or fat (Zagoria 2000). There is a direct relationship between malignancy and the size of the mass: the smaller the renal mass, the greater the percentage of benign causes (Frank et al. 2003; Silverman et al. 2008). As a general concept, the smaller the cancer, the less aggressive is the clinical behavior (Rendon et al. 2000; Frank et al. 2003) with the aggressive potential increasing dramatically beyond a tumor diameter of 3 cm (Remzi et al. 2006), while the lesion size at presentation does not predict the growth rate (Silverman et al. 2008). In indeterminate solid renal tumors ≤1 cm observation is suggested until 1 cm in diameter is achieved (Silverman et al. 2008) since a benign nature is very likely and biopsy is difficult to perform. Observation can be performed by an initial

examination by CT or MR at 3- to 6-month intervals for at least 1 year followed by yearly examinations. The lack of growth on serial scans does not exclude malignancy, even though the risk of metastases is lower in stable tumors (Kunkle et al. 2007). Evidence of lesion growth or appearance changed, assuming more aggressive features increase the likelihood of malignancy.

A watchful waiting approach is also suggested for renal masses 1.5 cm or smaller identified in the elderly (Wehle et al. 2004; Silverman et al. 2008). In patients with a limited life expectancy or comorbidities, these should be managed by observation, especially if smaller than 3 cm (Silverman et al. 2008) and biopsy can be utilized preoperatively to confirm RCC. The incidence of distant metastases is higher in renal tumors >3 cm.

Percutaneous image-guided renal mass biopsy is suggested to preoperatively characterize indeterminate renal masses and to establish definitive diagnoses (Silverman et al. 2006). The observation of small renal cancer, instead of treatment, is also supported by two fundamental retrospective observations. First, renal cancers managed with observation alone have a low risk of developing metastases during the observation period, particularly if there is no observed interval growth (Chawla et al. 2006; Silverman et al. 2008). Second, concomitant with the increasing incidence of renal cancer over the past decades, the mortality rate from renal cancer has also increased since the increased incidence of RCC is due to the increased detection of small renal cancers which are cured, while the number of large lethal renal masses has not diminished and their treatment not changed. Emerging minimally invasive procedures for renal cancer treatment such as laparoscopic nephron-sparing surgery and percutaneous ablation techniques are less invasive and carry less risk. Minimally invasive management, such as partial nephrectomy, cryotherapy (Gill et al. 2000), or radiofrequency ablation (Fotiadis et al. 2007), should also be considered for tumor removal, while conserving unaffected normal renal parenchyma.

In patients with a known extrarenal primary tumor the solid renal mass may be a renal metastases in about half of the patients, and a second primary tumor or a benign neoplasm should be considered in the differential diagnosis. If multiple solid renal masses are detected, the two most likely diagnoses are multifocal RCC or multiple oncocytomas (Silverman et al. 2008). In these cases percutaneous biopsy is suggested to plan the patient clinical management. Patients with a genetic predisposition to

RCC or with a family history of RCC and who present a solid renal mass should be examined by a 3- or 6-month imaging follow-up followed by a yearly follow-up.

## 32.2 Renal Surgery

There are different types of renal surgery interventions. Simple nephrectomy implies a posterior lumbar approach and the resection of the kidney sparing the renal fascia, the ipsilateral adrenal gland, and most of the perirenal fat, and it is employed to resect atrophic kidneys. Indications for simple nephrectomy include irreversible damage to a kidney (trauma, chronic infection, stone disease) or renovascular hypertension secondary to noncorrectable renal artery stenosis or severe parenchymal disease (nephrosclerosis, reflux nephropathy, renal dysplasia). Surgical resection is the only effective means of cure for clinically localized renal tumors (Ng et al. 2008). The two main surgical procedures in oncology are radical nephrectomy and nephron-sparing surgery. The approach to treatment of renal cancer has shifted dramatically from radical surgery to a current emphasis on nephron-sparing treatment (Linehan and Nguyen 2009). This is principally determined by the evolution of renal cancer presentation. In fact, renal cancers are increasingly being diagnosed incidentally due to the increasing utilization of abdominal imaging, and renal cancer size at presentation has decreased and fewer cases are presenting with metastasis. Moreover, mean age at diagnosis has increased slightly, and experience with active surveillance suggests that a significant percentage of small renal masses are indolent and possess a low metastatic risk (Linehan and Nguyen 2009).

Partial or "nephron-sparing" nephrectomy has been shown to be equally effective to radical nephrectomy in selected groups. Both radical and partial nephrectomies can be undertaken laparoscopically, even though the technique is still under evaluation and only mid-term outcomes are available so far (Peycelon et al. 2009). Some surgeons supplement the laparoscopic approach with direct hand assistance in the operative field. Laparoscopic approaches reduce perioperative morbidity and length of the hospital stay. However, operation times are generally longer, and morcellation of the sample leads to difficulties in pathologic staging and introduces the risk of tumor seeding.

Preoperative planning for renal surgery requires information not routinely obtained in the standard CT of the kidney, including renal arteriography and accurate depiction of the relationship between the renal mass and the pelvicaliceal system of the kidney, and arterial and venous anatomy of the portion of the renal parenchyma containing or in contract with the tumor (Zagoria 2000). Multiplanar reformations and 3D reconstructions of the CT dataset allow to obtain all these information. The assessment of the kidney immediately after surgery is usually performed by a multiphase protocol including the corticomedullary phase, nephrotomographic phase, and the excretory phase to assess lesions of the urinary tract.

### 32.2.1 Radical Nephrectomy

Radical nephrectomy implies an anterior approach, is typically undertaken via a retroperitoneal posterolateral approach, and involves the resection of the kidney, the perirenal fat, pararenal fasciae, and the ipsilateral adrenal gland. Renal hilum and paravertebral lymph nodes are also resected. The dissection involves the region from the diaphragmatic crus to the aortic bifurcation of the ipsilateral – and possibly the contralateral – aspects of the inferior vena cava or the aorta. Surgical management is not directly affected by the presence of perinephric extension of disease because a radical nephrectomy includes en bloc removal of all the contents of Gerota's fascia. To date, radical nephrectomy remains the gold standard treatment for RCC larger than 4 cm.

Laparoscopic radical nephrectomy is an alternative technique with comparable oncologic results to open nephrectomy in patients with localized pathologic stage T1 RCC (Saika et al. 2003). Ipsilateral adrenalectomy should be considered in select cases in which there are risk factors for adrenal involvement (e.g., large left-sided upper pole tumors), even though ipsilateral adrenal metastases occur in only 1–10% of patients (O'Malley et al. 2009). One of the roles of imaging is to assist in allowing adrenal-sparing nephrectomies in order to reduce the risk of future adrenal insufficiency. Surgery, although substantially more challenging, is not necessarily excluded in the presence of contiguous organ invasion, which typically involves the liver, diaphragm, psoas muscles, pancreas, and bowel (Robson stage IVA, or TNM T4 disease). Both CT and MRI may have difficulty in distinguishing abutment of tumor from invasion of adjacent organs. The main indication for a radical nephrectomy is malignant neoplasm, usually RCC.

The anatomical changes determined by nephrectomy are translated in the migration of the peritoneal content and in the overt change of the retroperitoneal anatomy. On the right side (Figs. 32.1 and 32.2), the second portion of the duodenum is shifted posteriorly, while the right flexure of the colon occupies the right side of the liver and the retroperitoneum. The pancreatic head does not present a significant position change. On the left side (Fig. 32.3), the pancreatic tail moves inferiorly and posteriorly, while the spleno-pancreatic ligament and the spleen move posteriorly. The gastric fundus may occupy the space between the spine and the pancreatic tail, and this may create some doubtful finding to be differentiated from adrenal mass or primary tumor recurrence if the stomach is incompletely opacified before scanning. The jejuneal loops occupy the space previously occupied by the kidney and agglomerate on the left of the pancreatic tail. Usually the surviving kidney becomes hypertrophic, especially in young patients.

## 32.2.2 Partial Nephrectomy: Nephron-Sparing Surgery

Partial nephrectomy – nephron-sparing surgery – entails complete excision of the renal tumor with a margin of at least 0.5 cm of normal renal tissue and preservation of the largest amount of functioning renal parenchyma. Even though partial nephrectomy corresponds to nephron-sparing surgery, the last term includes different surgical techniques, namely enucleation (nephron-sparing tumorectomy) reserved to benign tumors, polar resection or wedge resection with or without inclusion of the renal excretory tract (partial nephrectomy), or ex

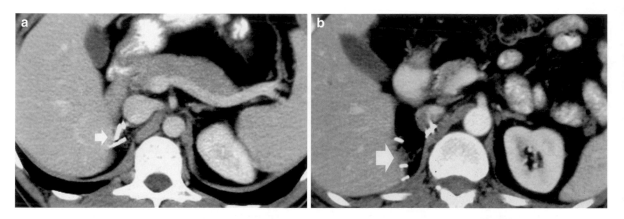

**Fig. 32.1** (**a**, **b**) Contrast-enhanced CT. Normal anatomic changes after right radical nephrectomy. Metallic surgical clips (*arrow*) are evident on the right side

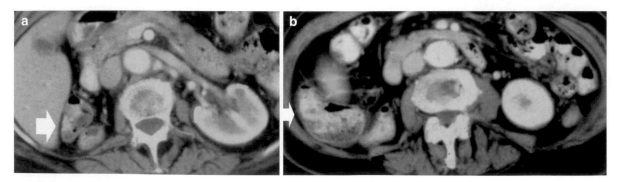

**Fig. 32.2** (**a**, **b**) Contrast-enhanced CT. Postsurgical appearance in right nephrectomy bed in 52-year-old man at follow-up. The right flexure of the colon (*arrow*) occupies the right side of the liver and the retroperitoneum. Note associated surgical vascular clips

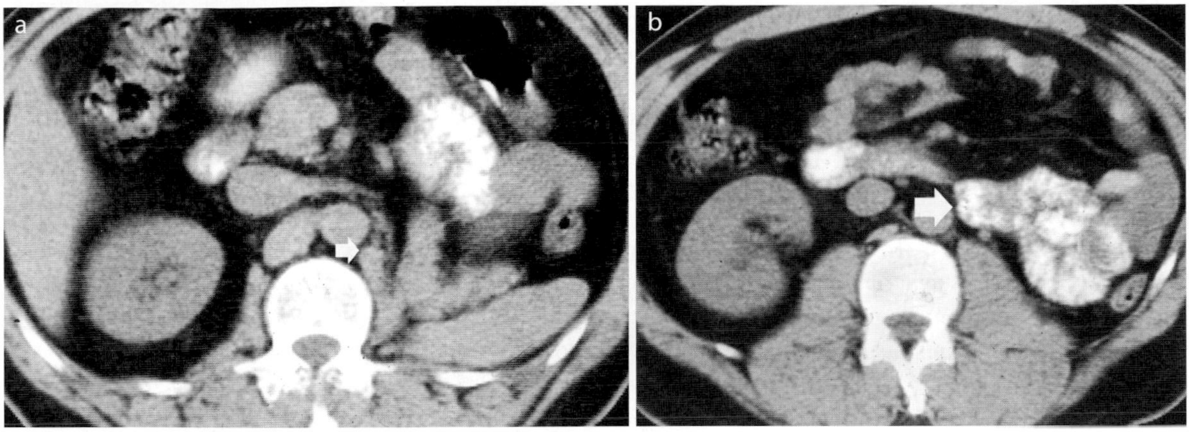

**Fig. 32.3** (**a**, **b**) Contrast-enhanced CT. Normal anatomic changes after left radical nephrectomy. The jejuneal loops (*arrow*) occupy the space previously occupied by the kidney

vivo resection. Some important changes in the manifestation of RCC have stimulated a growing trend toward nephron-sparing surgical techniques (Novic 1993). In particular, the widespread use of cross-sectional imaging techniques has led to a dramatic increase in the number of incidentally discovered small, asymptomatic renal masses. These asymptomatic tumors, which now constitute 25% to almost 50% of all surgically treated RCCs, are generally confined to the renal capsule, are generally confined to the renal capsule, are relatively small in size and associated with an excellent prognosis after surgical removal (Konnak and Grossman 1985; Smith et al. 1989).

Partial nephrectomy is now considered the treatment of choice for small renal tumors of less than 4 cm in diameter in elective indication, especially if located in the renal poles or in the renal cortex far from the renal hilum and collecting system. The tumoral invasion of the collecting system represents an absolute contraindication to partial nephrectomy. Partial nephrectomy for hilar tumors (tumors in contact with a major renal vessel on preoperative cross-sectional imaging) is a cutting edge procedure for which little data are available (Lattouf et al. 2008; Richstone et al. 2008). This surgical procedure avoids nephronic waste with an acceptable morbidity and similar oncological outcomes compared to radical surgery. Radical nephrectomy presents a significantly higher risk for proteinuria due to hyperfiltration and chronic renal insufficiency in comparison to nephron-sparing surgery (Malcolm et al. 2009; Lau et al. 2000). Laparoscopic partial nephrectomy might allow a more aggressive approach in young healthy patients with an indeterminate mass.

Although radical nephrectomy was long considered the reference standard for the treatment of RCC, the results of numerous studies have demonstrated equivalent survival rates for patients who underwent radical nephrectomy and for those who underwent partial nephrectomy for small renal neoplasms (Lerner et al. 1996; Herr 1999; Lau et al. 2000; Ghavamian et al. 2002; Israel et al. 2006), with reported controlateral recurrence rates of <2%, ipsilateral local recurrence and distant metastases of <5%, and 5-year survival rates of 87–90%, which are comparable to those from radical nephrectomy. Some authors are pushing back the limit for partial nephrectomy above the threshold of 4 cm, and more surgeons are either considering anatomical location or technical expected difficulties rather than just the tumor size. Nephron-sparing surgery leads to higher risk of bleeding, especially in case of tumors larger than 4 cm, and it is absolutely necessary to investigate thoroughly the vascularization of the tumor to avoid such complications with exhaustive and accurate preoperative imaging (Peycelon et al. 2009).

The other most important present applications of partial nephrectomy are malignant renal tumors in a solitary functioning kidney in patients with congenitally absent kidney or who had previously undergone contralateral nephrectomy for RCC, malignant tumors in patients with compromised renal function, or multicentric bilateral malignant renal tumors (Provet et al. 1991; Light and Novick 1993). Multiple RCCs can be sporadic in 4–15% cases, but are much more common in patients with von Hippel–Lindau disease and hereditary RCC (Sheth et al. 2001). In these patients, RCCs are often bilateral, multifocal, and manifest at a younger age. The challenge is to detect and delineate all lesions to ensure complete surgical excision, while preserving the maximal amount of functioning parenchyma. Nephron-sparing surgery has also been performed in young patients with bilateral synchronous Wilm's tumor (Davidoff et al. 2008). Residual applications of partial nephrectomy correspond to large benign tumors, renal traumas, renal staghorn calculosis, complicated calyceal diverticula, renal duplications with segmental hydronephrosis, and complicated renal tuberculosis.

The appearance of the postoperative kidney depends to a great extent on the size and location of the resected tumor (Israel et al. 2006), and on the imaging time delay after resection. After partial nephrectomy, the kidney presents an abnormal contour (Fig. 32.4) and presents a posterior displacement adhering to the posterior abdominal wall. This finding, especially if accompanied by reactive or fibrotic changes in the perinephric fat, is indicative of previous renal surgery (Israel et al. 2006). Evidence of surgical metallic clips, visualized on CT or MR by using in-phase and out-of-phase sequences, represents a further usual imaging feature after partial nephrectomy. Several techniques are used for partial resection, which may also include packing the postsurgical defect with fat (Baumgarten and Baumgartner 2000) to help achieve hemostasis. If

fat packing (Figs. 32.5 and 32.6) is used, the resulting appearance may mimic renal tumors by both CT (angiomyolipoma) and US (angiomyolipoma or hyperechoic RCC). Over time, the volume of fat used for surgical packing may decrease or remain unchanged, while the kidney is usually displaced posteriorly adjacent to the posterior abdominal wall (Fig. 32.6) (Israel et al. 2006). Extensive postoperative reactive changes in the retroperitoneum are also frequently visible (Figs. 32.7 and 32.8) and help in the differential diagnosis from fatty renal tumors.

Biologically absorbable hemostatic agents (Fig. 32.9) may also be used to help control intraoperative bleeding (Israel et al. 2006). Such materials may contain air pockets or bubbles (Fig. 32.10) that on early postoperative images, may resemble a focal abscess (Young et al. 1993; Israel et al. 2006). To differentiate between a collection that consists of a hemostatic agent containing air bubbles and one that consists of infected fluid containing gas bubbles, it is necessary to consider the imaging findings in combination with the patient's clinical history and symptoms (Israel et al. 2006). Anyway, some imaging findings may be important for the differential diagnosis. In most cases, the air in a hemostatic agent is rapidly resorbed during the first postsurgical week, even though air bubbles can be identified on images even 1 month after surgery (Fig. 32.10). In-phase and

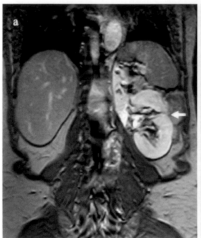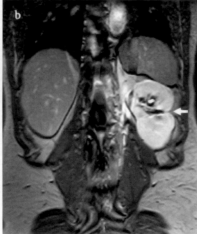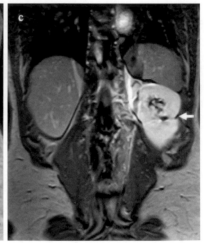

**Fig. 32.4** (**a–c**) Postoperative findings in a 60-year-old man who underwent a left partial nephrectomy for renal cell carcinoma (RCC). Coronal 3D T1-weighted fast breath-hold spoiled gradient echo sequence for dynamic imaging after intravenous injection of gadolinium (15 mL). MR image obtained 1 year after surgery demonstrates a wedge-shaped postoperative defect (*arrows*) in the lateral aspect of the kidney. At the apex of the parenchymal defect, a small signal void corresponding to surgical clips

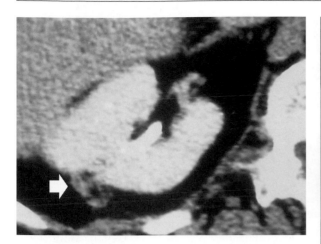

**Fig. 32.5** Right partial nephrectomy. Contrast-enhanced CT, transverse image. Fat packing with retroperitoneal fat (*arrow*) used to cover the postoperative defect (courtesy of Olivier Helenon, Paris)

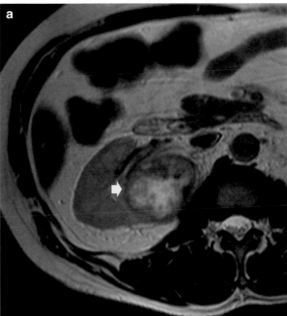

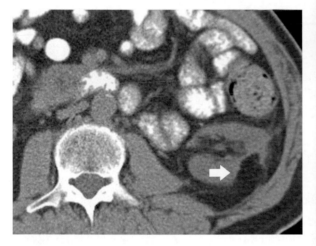

**Fig. 32.6** Postoperative findings after left partial nephrectomy for RCC. Axial unenhanced CT image demonstrates a wedge-shaped postoperative defect (*arrow*) in the lateral aspect of the left kidney. The postoperative kidney has a more posterior retroperitoneal location and adheres to the posterior abdominal wall. Extensive postoperative reactive changes in the retroperitoneum are visible as a peripheral enhancing strand surrounding the region of partial nephrectomy (courtesy of Mark Rosen, University of Pennsylvania)

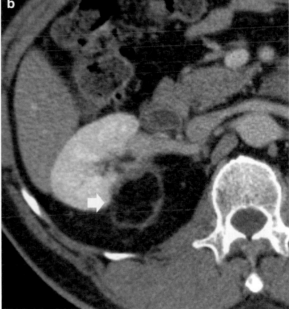

**Fig. 32.7** Postoperative findings after right partial nephrectomy for RCC. (**a**) Preoperative axial T2-weighted MR image demonstrates a solid and well-marginated right renal mass (*arrow*). (**b**) Axial contrast-enhanced CT image during nephrographic phase obtained 6 months after surgery demonstrates a wedge-shaped postoperative defect (*arrow*) in the lateral aspect of the right kidney. Reactive changes in the retroperitoneum are visible as a peripheral enhancing strand surrounding the region of partial nephrectomy (courtesy of Alfredo Blandino, Messina, Italy)

opposed-phase gradient echo MR sequences may be employed to detect the susceptibility artifact related to the surgical clips. The hemostatic agent typically reveals tightly packed gas bubbles with a geometric shape. The presence of an abscess should be suspected if a localized fluid collection that has an enhanced rim

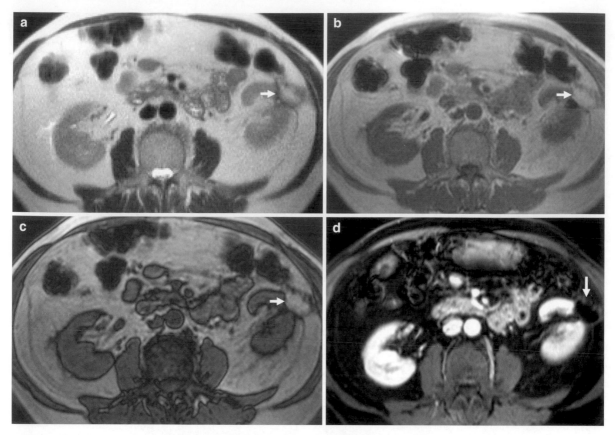

**Fig. 32.8** (**a–d**) Postoperative findings after right partial nephrectomy for RCC. (**a**) Axial T2-weighted, (**b**) in-phase and (**c**) out-of-phase T1-weighted, and fat-suppressed T1-weighted demonstrates a fat-containing mass (*arrow*) in the postoperative bed. Extensive postoperative reactive changes (*arrows*) in the retroperitoneum are also visible. At the apex of the defect, a small focal area of hypointense signal characteristic of postoperative scar tissue is visible (courtesy of Mark Rosen, University of Pennsylvania)

and contains gas bubbles or a gas–fluid level is seen. In addition, decreased intensity of the nephrogram because of edema in the surrounding renal parenchyma supports the diagnosis of an abscess.

## 32.3 Complications After Renal Surgery

Even though radical nephrectomy is a more simple surgical procedure if compared to nephron sparing surgery, both techniques may present post-operative complications after renal surgery and not related to tumoral recurrence are usually classified as early (within 30 days from surgery) and late (30 days to 1 year from surgery) complications. The most common early complications are acute or progressive renal failure and

proteinuria, even though these complications do not present typical imaging features. Other complications include pneumothorax (especially if a thoracoabdominal approach is used), trauma to adjacent structures (inferior vena cava, colon, duodenum, spleen, or pancreatic tail), lateral ernia when a flank incision is used, and postsurgical collections.

### 32.3.1 Complications After Radical Nephrectomy

After radical nephrectomy, different acute complications include formation of retroperitoneal fluid collections (hematoma – Fig. 32.11, lymphocele – Fig. 32.12, infectious collection – Fig. 32.13) and abscesses (Fig. 32.14). CT is the most reliable imaging technique

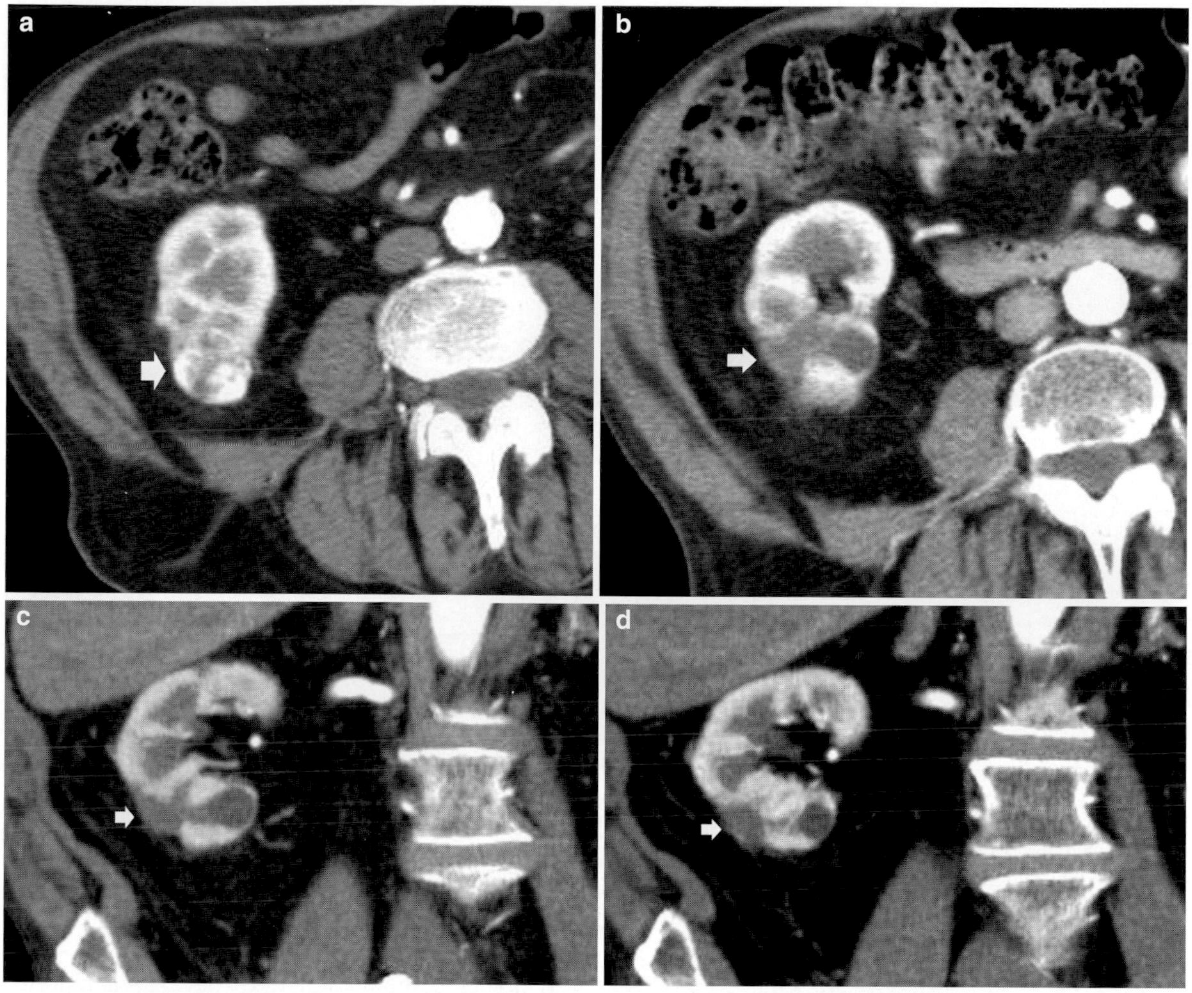

**Fig. 32.9** Biologically absorbable hemostatic agent used to help control intraoperative bleeding at CT in a 65-year-old man after an open right partial nephrectomy for clear cell-type RCC. (**a**) Axial contrast-enhanced image obtained before surgery shows a hypervascular solid renal tumor (*arrow*) on the lower pole. Axial contrast-enhanced image (**b**) and coronal reformations (**c, d**) obtained after surgery show the biologically absorbable hemostatic agent filling the surgical bed (*arrow*)

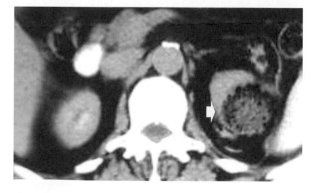

**Fig. 32.10** Tumorectomy for renal oncocytoma filled with biologically absorbable hemostatic agents. Contrast-enhanced CT, excretory phase performed 1 month after surgery. Evidence of air bubbles (*arrow*) within the hemostatic agent (courtesy of Catherine Roy, Strasburg)

to evaluate the principal complications after renal surgery. MR imaging can also be used to detect tumor recurrence, but the evaluation may be limited by artifact from metallic clips.

### 32.3.2 Complications After Partial Nephrectomy

After nephron-sparing surgery, different acute complications may occur including fat necrosis with evidence of fluid level, vascular complications, collecting system complications, and infections. The procedure can be performed by using open or laparoscopic techniques.

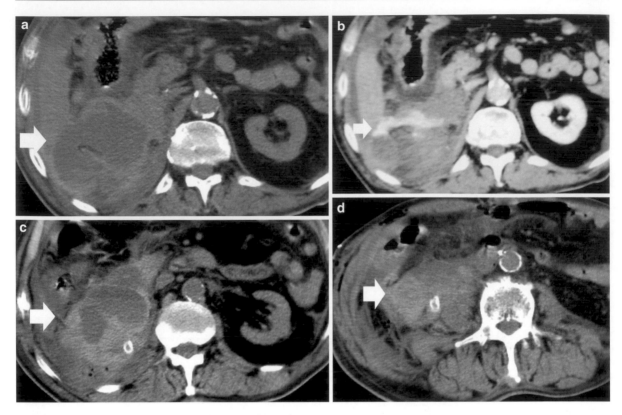

**Fig. 32.11** (**a–d**) Retroperitoneal hemorrhage after right radical nephrectomy. (**a**) Unenhanced CT. Evidence of large heterogenous collection (*arrow*) on the right retroperitoneum after right radical nephrectomy. (**b**) Contrast-enhanced CT. Arterial phase. Evidence of active blood extravasation (*arrow*). (**c, d**) Unenhanced CT performed 3 days later. CT-guided percutaneous drainage was positioned to drain the collection (*arrow*)

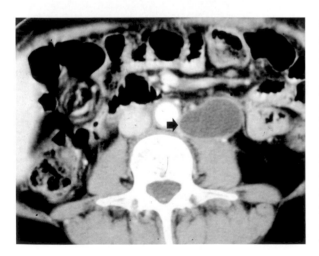

**Fig. 32.12** Contrast-enhanced CT. Retroperitoneal lymphocele (*arrow*) after left radical nephrectomy

However, nephron-sparing surgery, especially when performed with laparoscopic techniques, is a more complex operation than is traditional radical nephrectomy, and higher complication rates have been reported (Campbell et al. 1994; Israel et al. 2006). A worldwide literature review revealed a major complication rate of 10% for patients who underwent laparoscopic partial nephrectomy. An overall complication rate of 23% was reported for laparoscopic partial nephrectomy in a European multiinstitutional series (Israel et al. 2006).

Vascular complications after partial nephrectomy may be determined by a damage of the main renal artery (hilar vessels) or the intrarenal vessels. During partial nephrectomy, the renal hilar vessels must be temporarily clamped to ensure a bloodless surgical field, and clamping may injure the arterial intima and lead to thrombosis (Israel et al. 2006). If that complication is not recognized at the time of surgery or in the immediate postoperative period, renal infarction (Fig. 32.15) and atrophy will occur. Because clamping of the artery for more than 2 h may result in a complete loss of renal function and renal atrophy, urologists try to limit renal artery clamping to 30 min or less. Inadequate suture of

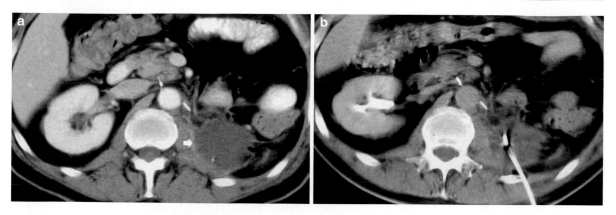

**Fig. 32.13** (**a**, **b**) Contrast-enhanced CT. Retroperitoneal inflammatory collection (*arrow*) after left radical nephrectomy (**a**) and treated by CT-guided percutaneous drainage (**b**)

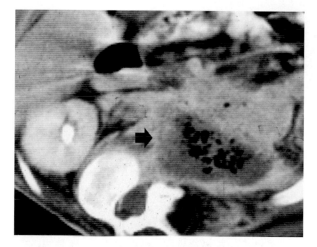

**Fig. 32.14** Contrast-enhanced CT. Excretory phase. Retroperitoneal abscess (*arrow*) with air component observed after left radical nephrectomy

transected intrarenal vessels may determine a hematoma of the postoperative bed or a true retroperitoneal hematoma. Pseudoaneurysms after partial nephrectomy may result from injury to an intrarenal artery at the surgical site or to the main renal artery or one of its major branches and represent a rare but potentially life-threatening condition. The incidence of renal artery pseudoaneurysms after partial nephrectomy has been reported to be 0.43% (Albani and Novick 2003), even though a higher incidence could be expected in the routine clinical practice. Pseudoaneurysms are easily characterized since they present the same density of the abdominal aorta after iodinated contrast agent injection (Fig. 32.16). Other less common vascular complications after partial nephrectomy are venous injury with renal vessel dilatation or rupture, or the evidence of intrarenal arteriovenous fistula.

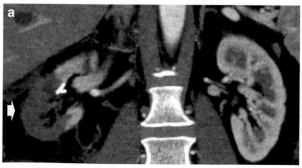
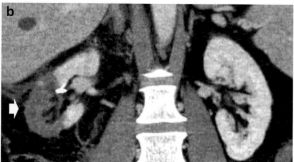

**Fig. 32.15** (**a**, **b**) Parenchymal infarct at CT in a 45-year-old man after an open left partial nephrectomy for papillary cell-type RCC. (**a**) Corticomedullary phase; (**b**) nephrographic phase. Coronal contrast-enhanced image shows an hypodense area (*arrow*) consistent with parenchymal infarct. Surgical clips are also visible, as a hypodense cystic lesion on the right liver

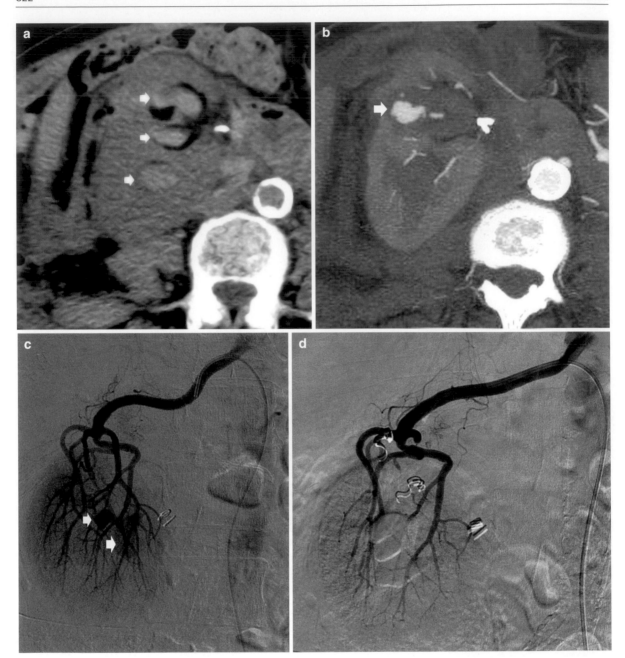

**Fig. 32.16** (**a–d**) Intrarenal pseudoaneurysms after partial nephrectomy due to injury to an intrarenal artery at the surgical site in a 48-year-old man who presented with hematuria 10 days after an open left partial nephrectomy for RCC. (**a**) Unenhanced CT. Hyperdense material (*arrows*) is evident within the intrarenal urinary tract in a malrotated kidney after partial nephrectomy; (**b**) Contrast-enhanced CT, early arterial phase. Arterial blush (*arrow*) is evident within the intrarenal urinary tract presenting almost the same density of abdominal aorta. (**c**) Digital subtraction angiography identifies two pseudoaneursysms (*arrows*) within the renal parenchyma. (**d**) Selective left renal arteriogram after transcatheter embolization of the bleeding arterial branches and placement of occluding coils

To ensure an adequate margin of resection for tumors that extend deep into renal parenchyma is often necessary to produce a deep resection close to the renal collecting system. The complications after partial nephrectomy involving the collecting system may occur if a proper calyceal repair, to avoid urinary leakage, is not performed. If the repair is not watertight, urine may leak into the surgical bed (Israel et al. 2006).

Such leakage may have the appearance of a simple fluid collection in the perirenal space or it may have a more heterogeneous appearance if it contains blood products. This complication can be diagnosed on the basis of contrast-enhanced CT and MR images acquired during the excretory phase, with the observation of contrast material leakage from the collecting system into the surgical bed or by showing a clear communication between the collection and the collecting system. In most cases, the fluid collection resolves either spontaneously or after placement of a ureteral stent or nephrostomy catheter. Less commonly, urinary leakage persists and a urinoma forms. Finally, blood clots may determine obstruction of the urinary tract.

A fluid collection (urinoma or hematoma) in the surgical bed or fat necrosis after fat packing may become infected, and an abscess may develop as a result (Fig. 32.17). With imaging alone, it may be difficult to differentiate an infected fluid collection from an uninfected one. Moreover, as mentioned earlier, the presence of air bubbles in a bioabsorbable hemostatic agent may further complicate the interpretation of imaging studies. However, patients with a postoperative

abscess are likely to manifest clinical symptoms and signs (e.g., fever and an elevated white blood cell count) suggestive of infection; in such cases, a needle aspiration is performed for laboratory analysis, followed by drainage if necessary. In addition, patients who have undergone a partial nephrectomy may present with pyelonephritis, which may appear as a striated or heterogeneous nephrogram and may be difficult to differentiate from renal infarction on images alone.

## 32.4  Tumoral Recurrence and Distant Metastases

CT is the imaging technique employed to identify the postsurgical local ipsilateral or controlateral renal tumor recurrence (Mignon and Mesurolle 2003). After nephrectomy for earlier stages of RCC, up to 50% of patients develop recurrent or metastatic disease (Janzen et al. 2003) with 85% of these recurrences occur within 3 years after initial resection (Sandock et al. 1995). Risk of relapse is stage-dependent, with a

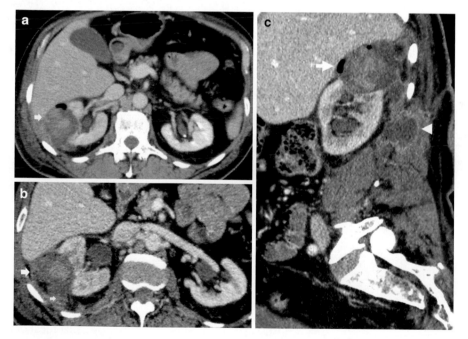

**Fig. 32.17** (**a–c**) Sixty-year-old patient who had partial nephrectomy 1 month before with fat packing of the postsurgical defect and subsequent infected fat necrosis. (**a, b**) Axial contrast-enhanced CT image, obtained 15 days after surgery, depicts a fluid and gas collection within the surgical bed at the level of the surgical packing (*arrow*), presenting a thickened wall and extension in the right kidney perinephric space (**b**; *small arrow*),

and a reduced enhancement of the involved kidney consisting in a decreased intensity of the nephrogram because of edema in the surrounding renal parenchyma supports the diagnosis of an abscess. The sagittal planar reformation of the CT data sets (**c**) shows the extension of the collection (*arrow*) up to posterior retroperitoneal space (**c**, *arrowhead*). The abscess was drained percutaneously

higher rate of relapse and shorter time to relapse in patients with pT3 and pT4 renal tumors compared with lower stages (Griffin et al. 2007). Tumor recurrence occurring after a longer disease-free interval is associated with a better prognosis (Hafez et al. 1997). Multifocality is not significantly associated with ipsilateral recurrence or death from RCC. Moreover, patients with multifocal clear cell RCC are more likely to experience a contralateral tumoral recurrence (Dimarco et al. 2004).

### 32.4.1  Tumoral Recurrence After Radical Nephrectomy

After radical nephrectomy, the tumoral recurrence very frequently involved the hilar lymph nodes, which should be completely resected on the time of primary tumor resection. Local recurrence at the nephrectomy site can be shown on CT as solid enhancing masses with central necrosis. The usual site of primary tumor local recurrence is along the psoas muscle or quadratum lomborum muscle (Figs. 32.18 and 32.19) or the perirenal fat (Figs. 32.20 and 32.21). The recurrent tumor usually presents the same histotype of the original tumor and diffuse heterogeneous contrast enhancement after iodinated contrast material injection.

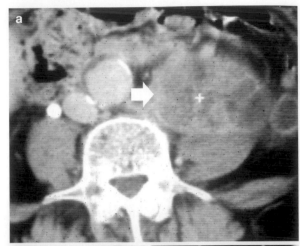

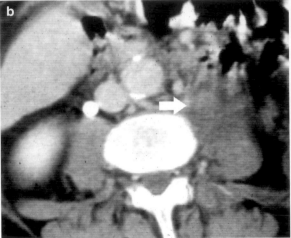

**Fig. 32.19** (**a**, **b**) Contrast-enhanced CT. Ipsilateral tumoral recurrence. Local tumoral recurrence (*arrow*) along the left psoas muscle after left radical nephrectomy

### 32.4.2  Tumoral Recurrence After Partial Nephrectomy

In those kidneys that underwent partial nephrectomy, the postsurgical scar must be differentiated from tumoral recurrence (Figs. 32.22 and 32.23). In particular, the perinephric fat may present contrast enhancement as the renal parenchyma adjacent to the resection zone due to the presence of granulomatous tissue. Recurrent renal tumor presents focal or diffuse homogeneous or heterogeneous contrast enhancement in a solid renal mass inside or adjacent to the postoperative bed. Sometimes tumoral recurrence after partial nephrectomy may be due to tumoral seeding after tumoral rupture during the surgical procedure.

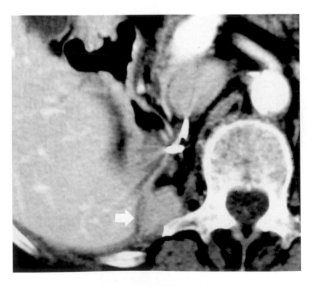

**Fig. 32.18** Contrast-enhanced CT. Ipsilateral tumoral recurrence. Local recurrence (*arrow*) along the superior region of the right psoas muscle after right radical nephrectomy

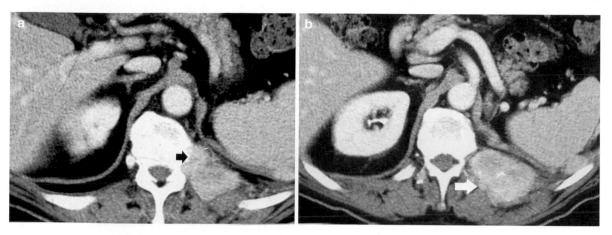

**Fig. 32.20** (**a, b**) Contrast-enhanced CT. Ipsilateral tumoral recurrence. Local tumoral recurrence (*arrows*) after left radical nephrectomy in the previous location of the perirenal fat. The tumoral recurrence shows partial lysis of the adjacent vertebral body

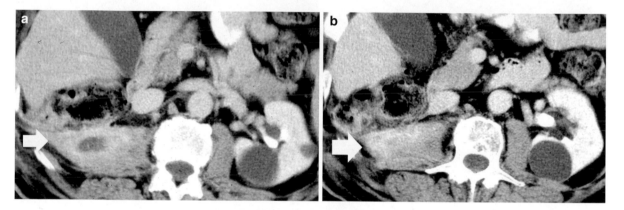

**Fig. 32.21** (**a, b**) Contrast-enhanced CT, nephrographic phase. Ipsilateral tumoral recurrence (arrow) after right radical nephrectomy

### 32.4.3 Distant Metastases

The most important risk factor for distant metastases after nephrectomy is the stage of the primary tumor (Sandock et al. 1995). The presence of metastases has been shown to give a median survival of 6–9 months if untreated, with a 2-year survival rate of only 10–20% (Flanigan et al. 2003). Metachronous metastases have a better prognosis than synchronous metastases. The following sites may show metastases, in order of decreasing frequency (Griffin et al. 2007): lung and mediastinal lymph nodes (50–60%) (Figs. 32.24 and 32.25), bone (30–40%), liver (30–40%) (Fig. 32.26), adrenal gland (Fig. 32.27), contralateral kidney (Fig. 32.28), retroperitoneum, and brain (5% each). Since RCC metastases are often hypervascular, they are difficult to detect in the enhanced liver even during the portal venous phase being frequently iso or hypervascular compared to the adjacent liver (Fig. 32.26) (Griffin et al. 2007). Liver scanning during the hepatic arterial phase of liver enhancement is therefore helpful in identifying many of these lesions. Retroperitoneal adenopathy and pancreatic involvement can occur in metastatic RCC (Griffin et al. 2007).

The risk of metastatic RCC is stage-dependent, and routine surveillance for tumor recurrence is crucial in patients who had renal surgery for RCC. According to the last WHO classification (Eble et al. 2004), T1 indicates a tumor ≤7 cm in the greatest dimension and limited to the kidney (T1a, tumors ≤4 cm; T1b, tumors >4 cm but ≤7 cm), T2 a tumor >7 cm in the greatest dimension and limited to the kidney; T3 a tumor extending into the major veins or directly invades adrenal gland or perinephric tissues but not beyond Gerota

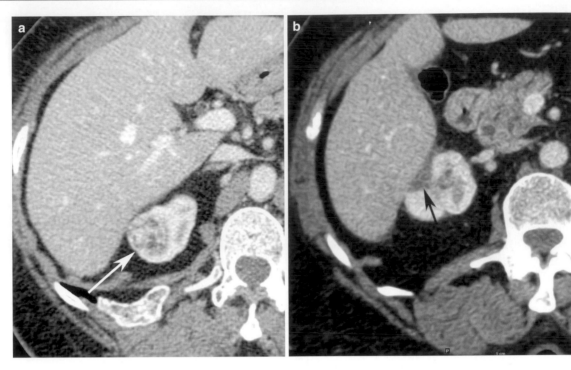

**Fig. 32.22** (**a**) Contrast-enhanced axial CT scan shows heterogeneous partially enhancing lesion (*arrow*) of the upper pole of the right
kidney representing a RCC. (**b**) Contrast-enhanced axial CT scan
1 year after the nephron-sparing surgery shows expected hypodensity
at the surgical bed (*arrow*) without evidence of tumor recurrence
(courtesy of Ali Guermazi, Boston University School of Medicine)

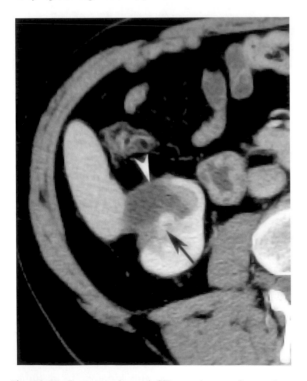

**Fig. 32.23** Contrast-enhanced CT scan 1 year after nephron-
sparing surgery shows expected hypodensity (*arrowhead*) at the
surgical bed with peripheral tissue enhancement (*arrow*) in
keeping with tumor recurrence (courtesy of Ali Guermazi,
Boston University School of Medicine)

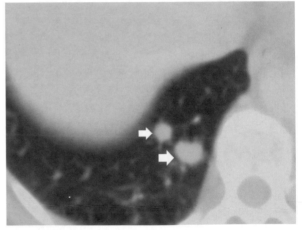

**Fig. 32.24** Contrast-enhanced CT. Lung metastases (*arrows*) from
clear cell RCC identified 4 months after radical nephrectomy

fascia; and T4 a tumor directly invading beyond Gerota
fascia. The surveillance protocols are based on the
pathological stage of the primary tumors.

Tables 32.1 and 32.2 show the suggested imaging
surveillance program, respectively, after radical and
partial nephrectomy (Levy et al. 1998; Ng et al. 2008).
CT is the most accurate technique to detect renal
tumor recurrence, while US has not been found to be

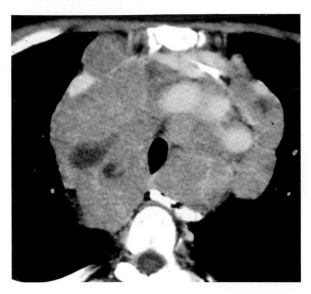

**Fig. 32.25** Contrast-enhanced CT. Mediastinal lymph node metastases from clear cell-type RCC identified 3 months after radical nephrectomy

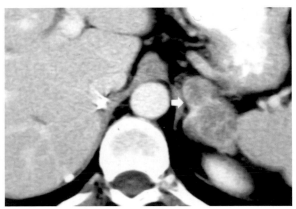

**Fig. 32.27** Contrast-enhanced CT. Left adrenal gland (*arrow*) metastasis from clear cell RCC identified 1 year after right radical nephrectomy. Metallic surgical clips are evident on the right side

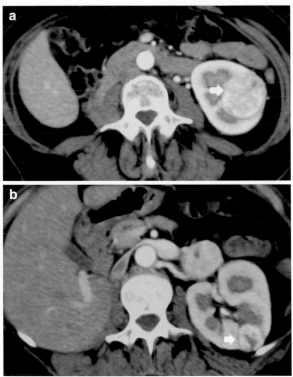

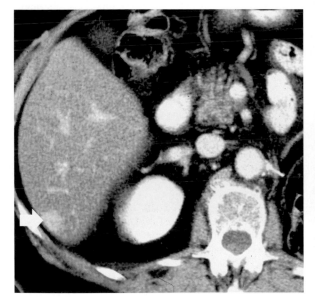

**Fig. 32.26** Contrast-enhanced CT. Portal phase in the hepatic parenchyma. Liver metastasis (*arrow*) on the sixth segment identified 6 months after left radical nephrectomy

**Fig. 32.28** (**a**, **b**) Contrast-enhanced CT, corticomedullary phase. Metachronous metastases (*arrow*) from clear cell RCC indentified in the controlateral kidney 1 year after right radical nephrectomy

reliable in assessing the nephrectomy bed (Ng et al. 2008). MR imaging can also be used to detect tumor recurrence, but the evaluation may be limited by artifact from metallic clips. Local recurrence in the nephrectomy bed occurs in approximately 20–40% of patients and typically in the first 5 years after

nephrectomy (Ng et al. 2008; Itano et al. 2000). Risk of recurrence is higher in the first 2 years after surgery (Chae et al. 2005), and for those tumors larger than 5 cm, with a higher Fuhrman grade or higher stage at the time of presentation. The risks are highest when the resection margins are incomplete (Chin et al.

**Table 32.1** Postoperative imaging surveillance after radical nephrectomy for localized RCC

| Stage | |
|---|---|
| T1 | Chest radiography yearly |
| T2 | Chest radiography every 3 and 6 months, then every 6 months for 3 years, then annually Abdominal CT at 2 and 5 years after surgery |
| T3 | Chest radiography every 3 and 6 months, then every 6 months for 3 years, then yearly Abdominal CT at 2 and 5 years after surgery |

**Table 32.2** Postoperative imaging surveillance after partial nephrectomy for localized RCC

| Stage | |
|---|---|
| T1 | Chest radiography yearly |
| T2 | Chest radiography yearly Abdominal CT every 2 years after surgery |
| T3 | Chest radiography every 6 months for 3 years, then yearly Abdominal CT every 6 months for 3 years, then yearly |

2006). Resection is difficult, but in selected patients may improve survival.

Bowel loops should be opacified before CT scanning because unopacified small-bowel loops, inevitably occupying the nephrectomy bed, may mimic local recurrence (Ng et al. 2008). During the surveillance period, potential intrathoracic disease must be identified by chest radiography, CT, or bone scanning. Brain MR should be considered only in patients with suspicious clinical symptoms or signs or increased tumoral markers. Stage-specific postoperative imaging surveillance protocol after radical nephrectomy for localized RCC is indicated in Table 32.1 as suggested by Ng et al. (2008) and Levy et al. (1998).

The follow-up strategy after nephron-sparing surgery is similar as reported in Table 32.2 (Ng et al. 2008), except that particular attention should be paid to the remnant kidney, where local recurrence rates are found in 4–6% of patients. These occur after a maximum of 6–24 months after surgery in patients with stage T3 disease and later than 48 months in stage T2

disease. Careful follow-up is also required for patients who have undergone ablation therapies including radiofrequency or cryoablation.

## References

Albani JM, Novick AC (2003) Renal artery pseudoaneurysm after partial nephrectomy: three case reports and a literature review. Urology 62(2):227–231

Baumgarten DA, Baumgartner BR (2000) Postoperative uroradiological appearances. In: Pollack HM, McClennan BL (eds) Clinical urography. Saunders, Philadelphia, pp 2928–2980

Bosniak MA (1986) The current radiological approach to renal cysts. Radiology 158:1–10

Campbell SC, Novick AC, Streem SB et al. (1994) Complications of nephron sparing surgery for renal tumors. J Urol 151: 1177–1180

Chae EJ, Kim JK, Kim SH et al. (2005) Renal cell carcinoma: analysis of postoperative recurrence patterns. Radiology 234:189–196

Chawla SN, Crispen PL, Hanlon AL et al. (2006) The natural history of observed enhancing renal masses: meta-analysis and review of the world literature. J Urol 175:425–431

Chin AI, Lam JS, Figlin RA et al. (2006) Surveillance strategies for renal cell carcinoma patients following nephrectomy. Rev Urol 8: 1–7

Davidoff AM, Giel DW, Jones DP et al. (2008) The feasibility and outcome of nephron-sparing surgery for children with bilateral Wilms tumor. The St Jude Children's Research Hospital experience: 1999–2006. Cancer 112(9):2060–2070

Dimarco DS, Lohse CM, Zincke H et al. (2004) Long-term survival of patients with unilateral sporadic multifocal renal cell carcinoma according to histologic subtype compared with patients with solitary tumors after radical nephrectomy. Urology 64(3):462–427

Eble JN, Sauter G, Epstein JI et al. (eds) (2004) World Health Organization classification of tumors: pathology and genetics of tumors of the urinary system and male genital organs. IARC, Lyon

Flanigan RC, Campbell SC, Clark JI et al. (2003) Metastatic renal cell carcinoma. Curr Treat Options Oncol 4:385–390

Fotiadis NI, Sabharwal T, Morales JP et al. (2007) Combined percutaneous radiofrequency ablation and ethanol injection of renal tumours: midterm results. Eur Urol 52:777–784

Frank I, Blute ML, Cheville JC et al. (2003) Solid renal tumors: an analysis of pathological features related to tumor size. J Urol 170:2217–2220

Ghavamian R, Cheville JC, Lohse CM et al. (2002) Renal cell carcinoma in the solitary kidney: an analysis of complications and outcome after nephron sparing surgery. J Urol 168(2):454–459

Gill IS, Novick AC, Meraney AM et al. (2000) Laparoscopic renal cryoablation in 32 patients. Urology 56:748–753

Griffin N, Gore ME, Sohaib SA (2007) Imaging in metastatic renal cell carcinoma. AJR Am J Roentgenol 189(2):360–370

Hafez KS, Novick AC, Campbell SC (1997) Patterns of tumor recurrence and guidelines for followup after nephron sparing surgery for sporadic renal cell carcinoma. J Urol 157: 2067–2070

Herr HW (1999) Partial nephrectomy for unilateral renal carcinoma and a normal contralateral kidney: 10-year followup. J Urol 161:33–35

Israel GM, Bosniak MA (2005) How I do it: evaluating renal masses. Radiology 236:441–450

Israel GM, Hecht E, Bosniak MA (2006) CT and MR imaging of complications of partial nephrectomy. Radiographics 26: 1419–1429

Itano NB, Blute ML, Spotts B et al. (2000) Outcome of isolated renal cell carcinoma fossa recurrence after nephrectomy. J Urol 164:322–325

Janzen NK, Kim HL, Figlin RA et al. (2003) Surveillance after radical or partial nephrectomy for localized renal cell carcinoma and management of recurrent disease. Urol Clin North Am 30:843–852

Konnak JW, Grossman HB (1985) Renal cell carcinoma as an incidental finding. J Urol 134:1094–1096

Kunkle DA, Crispen PL, Chen DY et al. (2007) Enhancing renal masses with zero net growth during active surveillance. J Urol 177(3):849–853

Lattouf JB, Beri A, D'Ambros OF et al. (2008) Laparoscopic partial nephrectomy for hilar tumors: technique and results. Eur Urol 54(2):409–416

Lau WK, Blute ML, Weaver AL et al. (2000) Matched comparison of radical nephrectomy vs nephron-sparing surgery in patients with unilateral renal cell carcinoma and a normal contralateral kidney. Mayo Clin Proc 75(12):1236–1242

Lerner SE, Hawkins CA, Blute ML et al. (1996) Disease outcome in patients with low stage renal cell carcinoma treated with nephron sparing or radical surgery. J Urol 155:1868–1873

Levy DA, Slaton JW, Swanson DA et al. (1998) Stage-specific guidelines for surveillance after radical nephrectomy for local renal cell carcinoma. J Urol 159:1163–1167

Light MR, Novick AC (1993) Nephron sparing surgery for renal cell carcinoma. J Urol 149:1–7

Linehan JA, Nguyen MM (2009) Kidney cancer: the new landscape. Curr Opin Urol 19(2):133–137

Malcolm JB, Bagrodia A, Derweesh III, et al (2009) Comparison of rates and risk factors for developing chronic renal insufficiency, proteinuria and metabolic acidosis after radical or partial nephrectomy. BJU Int 104(4):476–481.

Mignon F, Mesurolle B (2003) Local recurrence and metastatic dissemination of renal cell carcinoma: clinical and imaging characteristics. J Radiol 84(3):275–284

Ng CS, Wood CG, Silverman PM et al. (2008) Renal cell carcinoma: diagnosis, staging, and surveillance. AJR Am J Roentgenol 191:1220–1232

Novic AC (1993) Renal-sparing surgery for renal cell carcinoma. Urol Clin North Am 20:277–282

O'Malley RL, Godoy G, Kanofsky JA et al. (2009) The necessity of adrenalectomy at the time of radical nephrectomy: a systematic review. J Urol 181(5):2009–2017

Peycelon M, Vaessen C, Misraï V et al. (2009) Results of nephron-sparing surgery for renal cell carcinoma of more than 4 cm in diameter. Prog Urol 19(2):69–74

Provet J, Tessler A, Brown J et al. (1991) Partial nephrectomy for renal cell carcinoma: indications, results and implications. J Urol 145:472–476

Remzi M, Ozsoy M, Klinger HC et al. (2006) Are small renal tumors harmless? Analysis of histopathological features according to tumors 4 cm or less in diameter. J Urol 176(3):869–899

Rendon RA, Stanietzky N, Panzarella T et al. (2000) The natural history of small renal masses. J Urol 164:1143–1147

Richstone L, Montag S, Ost M et al. (2008) Laparoscopic partial nephrectomy for hilar tumors: evaluation of short-term oncologic outcome. Urology 71(1):36–40

Saika T, Ono Y, Hattori R et al. (2003) Long-term outcome of laparoscopic radical nephrectomy for pathologic T1 renal cell carcinoma. Urology 62(6):1018–1023

Sandock DS, Seftel AD, Resnick MI (1995) A new protocol for the follow-up of renal cell carcinoma based on pathological stage. J Urol 154:28–31

Sheth S, Scatarige JC, Horton KM et al. (2001) Current concepts in the diagnosis and management of renal cell carcinoma: role of multidetector CT and three-dimensional CT. Radiographics 21(spec issue):S237–S254

Silverman SG, Gan YU, Mortele KJ et al. (2006) Renal masses in the adult patient: the role of percutaneous biopsy. Radiology 240:6–22

Silverman SG, Israel GM, Herts BR et al. (2008) Management of the incidental renal mass. Radiology 249:16–31

Smith SJ, Bosniak MA, Megibow AJ et al. (1989) Renal cell carcinoma: earlier discovery and increased detection. Radiology 170:699–703

Wehle MJ, Thiel DD, Petrou SP et al. (2004) Conservative management of incidental contrast-enhancing renal masses as safe alternative to invasive therapy. Urology 64:49–52

Young ST, Paulson EK, McCann RL et al.(1993) Appearance of oxidized cellulose (Surgicel) on postoperative CT scans: similarity to postoperative abscess. AJR Am J Roentgenol 160:275–277

Zagoria RJ (2000) Imaging of small renal masses: a medical success story. AJR Am J Roentgenol 175:945–955

# Contrast Media-Induced Nephropathy and Nephrogenic Systemic Fibrosis

# 33

Fulvio Stacul

## Contents

**Abstract**

> Contrast-induced nephropathy (CIN) is a serious adverse event associated with the use of contrast media (CM). Patients who develop this complication can have increased morbidity, higher rates of mortality, lengthy hospital stays, and poor long-term outcomes. An important first step to reduce the chance of CIN is to identify risk factors associated with this condition. Patients with a previously elevated serum creatinine level, especially when secondary to diabetic nephropathy, are at great risk for developing CIN. Other patient-related risk factors include concurrent use of nephrotoxic medications, dehydration, congestive heart failure, age greater than 70 years. Adequate hydration is widely accepted as an important prophylactic measure for preventing CIN, but the optimal hydration regimen is still debatable. Other strategies for reducing the risk of CIN include pharmacological manipulation, hemodialysis and hemofiltration, withdrawal of nephrotoxic drugs. The risk of CIN increases with greater doses of CM, is related to the route of administration (intrarterial injection entails a greater risk) and to the choice of CM.

> Nephrogenic Systemic Fibrosis (NSF) is a rare delayed adverse reaction with gadolinium containing CM affecting patients with severe renal insufficiency or dialysis. It's a fibrosing disorder often leading to disabilities and eventually to death. Published cases received gadodiamide, gadopentetate or gadoversetamide, that is molecules with a linear structure which is considered less stable. There is increasing

F. Stacul
Department of Radiology, Ospedale Maggiore,
Piazza Ospitale, 1, 34123 Trieste, Italy
e-mail: fulvio.stacul@aots.sanita.fvg.it

E. Quaia (ed.), *Radiological Imaging of the Kidney*,
Medical Radiology, DOI: 10.1007/978-3-540-87597-0_33, © Springer-Verlag Berlin Heidelberg 2011

evidence that the risk increases with larger CM doses, either resulting from a single or multiple MR procedures. Patients referred for contrast enhanced MR should be screened for possible renal impairment by history or laboratory tests. The above agents are contraindicated in patients with CKD 4 and 5. It's recommended to use in all patients the smallest amount of contrast medium, to never deny a patient a clinically well-indicated enhanced MR procedure and to use the agent that leaves the smallest amount of gadolinium in the body.

## 33.1 Introduction

Contrast media-induced nephropathy (CIN) and nephrogenic systemic fibrosis (NSF) are topics that received large attention in the literature in the last years. The possibility of a renal function deterioration following intravascular administration of contrast media (CM) is known since decades, but apparently, the topic was revitalized following the paper by Aspelin et al. (2003), and hundreds of papers on the peer-reviewed journals were published since then, contributing to a relevant increase of our body of knowledge on this topic. On the other side, NSF is an entirely new argument, which was related to the administration of gadolinium chelates in 2006. Since then, the medical literature collected a very large number of papers dealing with this topic on journals from different subspecialties. Both arguments are still evolving, this paper representing an update and providing recommendations after consideration of the most recently published scientific data.

## 33.2 Contrast Media-Induced Nephropathy

### 33.2.1 Definition

The Contrast Media Safety Committee of the European Society of Urogenital Radiology (ESUR) suggested in 1999 the following definition of CIN: "Contrast

medium nephrotoxicity is a condition in which an impairment in renal function (an increase in serum creatinine by more than 25% or 44 μmol/L) occurs within 3 days following the intravascular administration of a contrast medium in the absence of an alternative etiology" (Morcos et al. 1999). The adoption of this definition was extremely important, as it helped in the comparison of data from different trials, but was recently challenged in the nephrologic community. Reddan et al. (2009) underscored that a relative measure is not appropriate in patients with a normal baseline serum creatinine (SCr), questioning the clinical significance of a 25% increase in these patients (i.e., from 0.6 to 0.73 mg/dL). Moreover, Waikar and Bonventre (2009) showed that the percentage changes are highly dependent on the renal function and may not perform adequately in patients with chronic kidney disease. Therefore, the absolute increase in SCr appears to be more reliable and should be preferred. Moreover, the nephrologic community suggested considering an absolute increase of SCr of 0.3 mg/dL (26.4 μmol/L) instead of 0.5 mg/dL, because such an increase relates to adverse outcomes (Mehta et al. 2007). Validation of this new criterion is expected because there is a perception that such increase could be too sensitive and introduce a large number of false positive cases.

When considering the timing of SCr, it appears that a single determination at 48 h is the most sensitive (Molitoris et al. 2007; Waikar and Bonventre 2009). A 72-h determination could eventually capture some subacute SCr rises, which appear to be rare and of doubtful clinical significance.

Lastly, it should be mentioned that alternative etiologies for renal function deterioration are often difficult to exclude, for instance, in patients concurrently receiving potentially nephrotoxic drugs or in patients who were injected intraarterially, with the possibility of a cholesterol embolization.

As a consequence, contrast-induced acute kidney injury (CIAKI) is becoming a preferred acronym instead of CIN.

### 33.2.2 Incidence

The reported incidence of CIN from different trials largely varies, depending on several factors such as different adopted definitions, different routes of contrast administration, different contrast volumes, but above all, different patient populations with variable prevalence of risk factors.

In fact, different risk factors for CIN were identified; they have different weightage and may eventually coexist, thus identifying patients at a particularly high risk. It appears that in a population referred to percutaneous coronary intervention, the incidence of CIN varies between 7 and 15% (McCullough et al. 1997; Bartholomew et al. 2004), while it is below 5% in the majority of series considering patients with impaired renal function referred to CT. However, it can be as high as 50% in patients with the coexistence of severe chronic kidney disease and diabetes referred for angiography (Manske et al. 1990).

## 33.2.3  Clinical Features

When CIN occurs, SCr usually increases within 24 h and peaks at 3–4 days after contrast administration. The renal impairment is normally nonoliguric and temporary, and it resolves in 1–2 weeks (Fig. 33.1). However, irreversible renal dysfunction can rarely occur and dialysis may be required. McCullough et al. (1997) considered a large series of patients ($n=1,826$) who underwent coronary angiography and intervention and showed that 0.7% of them experienced CIN that required dialysis. It is important to mention that although CIN requiring dialysis is relatively rare, its impact on prognosis is relevant. In

the same series, McCullough et al. (1997) showed that in-hospital mortality was 35.7% in the small group of patients who required dialysis and their 2 year survival rate was only 19%. The poor prognosis of patients who experienced CIN was underscored by a number of papers reporting in this group of patients longer hospital stays and higher rates of in-hospital and 1 year deaths showing an association between CIN and late cardiovascular events (Rihal et al. 2002; Iakovou et al. 2003; Dangas et al. 2005).

## 33.2.4  Risk Factors

Many large studies, most of them focusing on patients undergoing cardiac diagnostic and interventional procedures, considered the risk factors for CIN and contributed to enlarge our body of knowledge on this subject. We will consider risk factors that are related to the patient (most of them representing nonmodifiable patient characteristics) and those that are related to the procedure.

### 33.2.4.1  Patient-Related Risk Factors

The literature provides us a list of well-established risk factors for CIN, while some others are still questionable (Table 33.1).

There is a general agreement that chronic kidney disease (eGFR<60 mL/min) represents the most significant risk factor for CIN. Moreover, there is an association

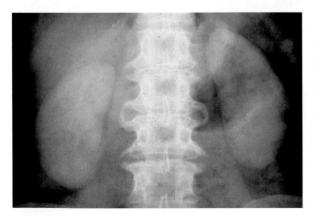

**Fig. 33.1** X-ray picture of the abdomen 24 h after an angiographic procedure showing a persistent nephrogram. The patient experienced an acute renal failure following contrast administration

**Table 33.1** Patient-related risk factors for contrast-induced nephropathy (CIN)

| Established | Questionable |
| --- | --- |
| Preexisting renal impairment with DM | DM without renal impairment |
| Preexisting renal impairment without DM | Hypertension |
| Dehydration | Hyperuricemia |
| Class III–IV congestive heart failure | Proteinuria |
| | Multiple myeloma |
| Left ventricular ejection fraction <40% | Gender |
| | Metabolic syndrome |
| Acute MI ≤24 h | |
| Periprocedural hypotension | |
| Anemia | |
| Old age | |
| Administration of nephrotoxic drugs | |

*DM* diabetes mellitus; *MI* myocardial infarction

between the severity of the renal impairment and the risk of CIN (McCullough et al. 1997; Rihal et al. 2002). Furthermore, the association of chronic kidney disease and diabetes mellitus identifies the category of patients at the highest risk for CIN.

Dehydration is normally listed among the risk factors, even if there is poor supporting evidence. Probably, dehydration was highly significant in the past when patients referred to intravenous urography experienced fluid restriction prior to the procedure. Congestive heart failure (NYHA grade 3–4) turned out to be a predictor of CIN, but only in studies considering patients undergoing cardiac catheterization. Such studies supported the significance of other risk factors, such as a left ventricular ejection fraction below 40%, an acute myocardial infarction (within the last 24 h), and the use of an intraaortic balloon pump, all features suggesting that a poor cardiac function is indeed a risk factor for CIN. The occurrence of hypotension during a vascular procedure ( resulting in reduced blood supply to the kidneys) and anemia (resulting in poor oxygen supply to the kidneys) is another recognized risk factor. Old age (usually above 70 years), appears as an independent predictor of CIN according to some authors. An additional intuitive risk factor is the assumption of nephrotoxic drugs, although the supporting evidence is limited.

Questionable risk factors include diabetes mellitus in patients without renal impairment. Probably, diabetes is indeed an independent predictor for CIN, but there is no general agreement. Insulin-dependent diabetics appear to be at a higher risk.

Hyperuricemia is common in patients with chronic kidney disease and probably is not a risk factor per se. Female gender appeared as a risk factor according to some authors, but the majority of studies did not support this result. Hypertension and metabolic syndrome were recently considered significant risk factors. On the contrary, multiple myeloma was postulated to be extremely significant in the early literature, but a retrospective review showed that this is not the case (McCarthy and Becker 1992).

### 33.2.4.2 Procedure-Related Risk Factors

The risk of CIN is related to the contrast dose, and a number of studies showed that in patients at risk, the use of doses exceeding 100 mL for coronary angiography is associated with a higher rate of CIN. However, it should be reminded that even small volumes (20–30 mL) can cause CIN in patients at very high risk.

Laskey et al. (2007) estimated the maximum contrast volume to minimize CIN which should be equal to baseline $CrCl \times 3.7$. A similar evaluation was performed by Nyman et al. (2008) who suggested limiting the contrast dose in grams of Iodine numerically to the eGFR value in milliliter per minute.

The risk of CIN appears to be lower after intravenous vs. intraarterial administration of contrast material (Katzberg and Lamba 2009). Of course, the route of administration is procedure specific, so there are no direct comparison trials, but a number of reasons may explain this difference, the main one probably being the lower volume of contrast which is usually injected in the intravenous procedures. Furthermore, lower concentration of contrast reaches the kidneys with intravenous administration; fewer patients with hemodynamic instability receive intravenous administration, and finally, the catheter used in intraarterial procedures can dislodge atheroemboli producing cholesterol embolization, with a resulting worsening of renal function that can mimic CIN.

High osmolar contrast agents turned out to be more nephrotoxic than low osmolar agents in patients with impaired renal function following intraarterial contrast administration (Barrett and Carlisle 1993). Comparative trials among low osmolar agents were limited and unable to detect significant differences with regard to renal safety. The relative nephrotoxicity of low osmolar and isoosmolar CM is a matter of debate since the publication of the NEPHRIC trial by Aspelin et al. (2003). This study showed that the isoosmolar nonionic dimer iodixanol was significantly less nephrotoxic than the low osmolar nonionic monomer iohexol in patients with renal impairment and diabetes who underwent angiography. A number of papers comparing iodixanol with different low osmolar agents were published since then. Heinrich et al. (2009) produced a meta-analysis of 25 randomized controlled trials (3,270 patients), 18 of them following intraarterial and 7 of them following intravenous contrast injection, comparing iodixanol with nonionic monomers (iohexol, iopamidol, iopromide, iomeprol, ioversol, and iobitridol). They stated that iodixanol is not associated with a reduced risk of CIN after intravenous application. In patients with intraarterial contrast application and renal insufficiency, the low osmolar agent iohexol is associated with a greater risk of CIN than is iodixanol, whereas nonsignificant difference between iodixanol and the other low osmolar agents could be found. This conclusion was additionally validated by more recent publications (Laskey et al. 2009; Wessely et al. 2009).

### 33.2.4.3 Coexistence of Multiple Risk Factors

The coexistence of multiple risk factors in a single patient can create a very high risk scenario. It is extremely important to predict the actual risk in a single patient through adequate risk stratification. In the cardiology setting, three groups considered this topic and published the risk factor analyses (Bartholomew et al. 2004; Mehran et al. 2004; Brown et al. 2008). Multiple independent risk factors were identified and weighted. These analyses allowed creating a risk score for the prediction of CIN and showed that the risk of CIN increases exponentially with increasing risk score. Such a detailed analysis is unfortunately unavailable following intravenous contrast administration, in the CT setting, and is urgently required.

## 33.2.5 Strategies for Risk Reduction

The first issue to be considered for preventing CIN is the identification of patients at risk, above all, patients with eGFR<60 mL/min/1.73 m². Measurement of eGFR (or serum creatinine) within 7 days of contrast medium administration is required in patients with known chronic kidney disease, in diabetic patients taking metformin, and in patients who will receive intraarterial contrast medium (Thomsen et al. 2005).

Otherwise, a survey may be used to identify patients at higher risk for CIN, and a history suggesting the possibility of reduced GFR has to be collected (renal disease, renal surgery, proteinuria, diabetes mellitus, hypertension, gout, recent assumption of nephrotoxic drugs).

In patients at risk for CIN, the possibility of performing another procedure not requiring the use of iodinated contrast agents (ultrasound, MRI) should be considered first. Of course, the issue of the possible onset of NSF in patients referred to contrast-enhanced MRI has to be carefully evaluated (see below). If the procedure requiring iodinated contrast is deemed necessary, a number of strategies to reduce the risk of CIN can be considered, namely hydration, use of pharmacologic agents, withdrawal of nephrotoxic drugs, hemodialysis and hemofiltration, choice of contrast material type, and dose.

### 33.2.5.1 Hydration Protocols

There is a general consensus that hydration is effective in preventing CIN, because it is effective in preventing the renal damage from other injuries even though randomized double-blind comparative trials considering hydration vs. no hydration are not available so far. It appears that intravenous hydration (more properly, volume expansion) is more effective than oral hydration (Trivedi et al. 2003), but the evidence is poor and data on the possible efficacy of oral hydration are lacking. Intravenous administration of normal (0.9%) saline is more effective than half normal (0.45%) saline (Mueller et al. 2002). Most studies in the cardiology setting suggest administering 1.0–1.5 mL/kg/h starting 12 h before the procedure, till 12 h after the procedure. The Contrast Media Safety Committee of the ESUR advocates the administration of 1 mL/kg b.w/h of normal saline for at least 6 h before and after the procedure. In hot climates the volume should be increased. However, this regimen is still impractical in the outpatient setting and trials considering the best timing for hydration are highly advisable.

It is worthwhile mentioning the possibility of performing the volume expansion using sodium bicarbonate instead of sodium chloride with the rationale of producing an urine alkalinization that could theoretically prevent the formation of oxygen free radicals with the resulting renal damage. Following the first results favoring bicarbonate (Merten et al. 2004), a large number of studies and meta-analyses were published. All the meta-analyses show a certain degree of heterogeneity and publication bias, but it seems that the evidence in favor of bicarbonate is becoming pretty strong. Additionally, it is worthwhile mentioning that administration of bicarbonate is suggested to start 1 h prior to the procedure till 6 h after, a more practical regimen for outpatients.

### 33.2.5.2 Pharmacologic Agents and Withdrawal of Nephrotoxic Drugs

A pharmacological prophylaxis for preventing CIN would be advisable and a large number of drugs were tested for this purpose. A review (Stacul et al. 2006) subdivided these drugs into three groups: potentially beneficial agents that need further evaluation, but could be considered for use in patients at risk (theophylline/aminophylline, statins, ascorbic acid, prostaglandin $E_1$), agents that have not been shown to be consistently effective in reducing the risk of CIN (N-acetylcysteine (NAC), fenoldopam/dopamine, calcium-channel blockers, atrial natriuretic peptide), and potentially detrimental agents (furosemide, mannitol, endothelin receptor antagonist). Among them, NAC is more widely used (with a standard oral regimen of 600 mg twice daily the day before and on the day of the procedure), given its low cost, safety (when administered orally), and wide availability. Nevertheless, its efficacy is still questionable despite a large number of trials and meta-analyses. The largest trial (Webb et al. 2004) failed to show a benefit of this drug, while the last published meta-analyses (Kelly et al. 2008) favors its use.

The Contrast Media Safety Committee of the ESUR, given the heterogeneous results of trials and meta-analyses, does not recommend, for the time being, any pharmacologic manipulation for routine use in the prevention of CIN (Thomsen and Morcos 2006).

It is reasonable to assume that nephrotoxic drugs increase the risk of CIN, although this topic was poorly addressed in the literature. Alamartine et al. (2003) reported a higher incidence of CIN in patients receiving anti-inflammatory drugs, aminoglycosides and amphotericin B. Other drugs, such as cyclosporine, tacrolimus, and cisplatinum appear to increase the risk. Withdrawal of nephrotoxic drugs at least 24 h before the procedure is therefore suggested, when clinically compatible.

### 33.2.5.3 Hemodialysis and Hemofiltration

Hemodialysis is actually effective in removing contrast material, but ineffective in preventing CIN even when carried out immediately after the contrast-enhanced procedure. These results are consistent with the theory that the renal damage eventually occurs very rapidly after contrast administration, probably mainly related to the contrast material-induced vasoconstriction. Therefore hemodialysis is not recommended for preventing CIN.

Marenzi et al. (2003, 2006) reported the favorable results of performing hemofiltration (started 4–8 h before percutaneous coronary intervention and continued for 18–24 h afterwards) for preventing CIN. Of course, hemofiltration itself affects SCr levels, and therefore, SCr reduction may be unrelated to renal function, but it is worthwhile mentioning that in-hospital and 1-year mortality significantly improved in the hemofiltration group. However, the high cost of the procedure and the need for intensive care unit admission limits its utility.

### 33.2.5.4 Choice of Contrast Material Type and Dose

This issue was already considered when procedure-related risk factors were discussed (see Sect. 33.2.4.2). When considering the renal safety, there are no arguments favoring the administration of one or another low or isoosmolar agent through the intravenous route. When intraarterial studies are planned, the present evidence suggests that iodixanol is less nephrotoxic than the nonionic monomer iohexol and the ionic dimer ioxaglate in patients with impaired renal function. Other comparative evaluations were unable to detect significant differences among the products.

The contrast dose to be injected should always be the lowest compatible with a diagnostic result. Recent trials (Laskey et al. 2007; Nyman et al. 2008) provided valuable information on the maximum dose of contrast to minimize the risk of CIN.

When considering contrast material injection in patients at risk for CIN, planning of multiple studies is an issue. Unfortunately, clinical trials providing suggestions on the optimal timing between two consecutive contrast-enhanced studies are not available, but waiting for 2 weeks, the expected recovery time of the kidney following an acute injury, appears reasonable, if compatible with the diagnostic requirements.

## 33.2.6 Open Questions

Despite the large number of studies that were published in the last years on this topic, many questions concerning CIN are still open and some new problems arose.

Studies by Newhouse et al. (2008) and Bruce et al. (2009) underlined that physiologic variations in SCr levels may fulfill the CIN definitions. Bruce et al. (2009) identified a high incidence of acute kidney injury among control subjects undergoing unenhanced CT and suggested that the additional risk of acute kidney injury accompanying the administration of contrast medium may be overstated and much of the creatinine elevation in these patients is attributable to the background fluctuation, underlying disease, or treatment. These results have significant implications in the planning of future trials considering CIN that should eventually consider one control arm as well.

The production of validated risk scores for patients undergoing intraarterial studies underscores the need for a similar model for predicting the risk of CIN in a single patient referred to intravenous contrast administration. Patients might be stratified according to the different risks and it appears reasonable that patients at different risks may require different prevention protocols.

An effort to produce different protocols is advisable and will favorably affect the management of at-risk patients in daily practice. Such practice will benefit from additional data on optimal timing and duration of hydration. More data on the potential benefit of sodium bicarbonate and NAC are advisable as well. Furthermore, larger multicenter trials in which clinically relevant outcomes are assessed are required to definitely resolve the issue on whether the nephrotoxicity of iodixanol is less than that of some of the low osmolar agents after intraarterial application in high-risk patients, as Heinrich et al. (2009) pointed out.

## 33.2.7 Guideline

The Contrast media Safety Committee of the ESUR produced in 1999 a guideline for preventing CIN (Morcos et al. 1999) which was updated online and is available at www.esur.org. It is interesting to realize that after 10 years and despite a huge number of studies and reviews of CIN, nothing changed substantially. Thomsen et al. (2008b) underlined that the strategies for CIN prevention are still use of the smallest possible dose of low – or isoosmolar contrast agent, volume expansion, withdrawal of nephrotoxic drugs, and avoidance of repeat contrast injections within 48 h.

## 33.3 Nephrogenic Systemic Fibrosis

### 33.3.1 Definition

NSF is a severe systemic fibrosing disorder associated with the exposure to gadolinium-containing CM. The first case was identified in 1997 and the first report in the peer-reviewed literature occurred in 2000. At the beginning, the disease was thought to involve only the skin and was termed nephrogenic fibrosing dermopathy. Later, it became apparent that multiple organs could be affected (Cowper 2005), and in 2006, a relationship between the disease and the administration of Gd-containing CM was suggested for the first time (Grobner 2006; Marckmann et al. 2006).

### 33.3.2 Clinical Features

The clinical features vary from one patient to another and over time. However, the large majority of the patients had their initial NSF symptoms within 2–3 months following Gd-containing CM exposure, although this interval is reported to vary to a large extent (range of 1–2,395 days). The early symptoms include pain, itching, erythema, and swelling. Skin changes primarily involve the lower limbs. Late symptoms include skin thickening and hardening, and the affected area may have a peau d'orange appearance and a woody texture (Fig. 33.2). The involvement of other organs is frequent (neuropathic symptoms, respiratory insufficiency caused by lung fibrosis, muscular atrophy,…). Joint contractures (Fig. 33.3), leading to disabilities and dependence on wheelchair, occur in more severe cases (Cowper 2008) and death is reported in up to 5% of the patients.

Most patients who experienced NSF are middle aged, but the age range is very large (8–87 years), without ethnicity or gender predilections.

### 33.3.3 Risk Factors

Two factors appear to coexist in the history of patients who developed NSF: the impaired renal function and the administration of Gd-containing CM (Agarwal et al. 2009; Broome et al. 2007; Sadowski et al. 2007; Van der Molen 2008). Patients with chronic kidney

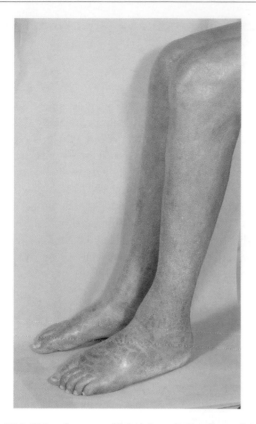

**Fig. 33.2** Thirty-five-year-old female patient on hemodialysis suffering from nephrogenic systemic fibrosis (NSF): discolored skin plaques and atrophy of the calf muscles are noticeable (Courtesy of Prof. H. Thomsen)

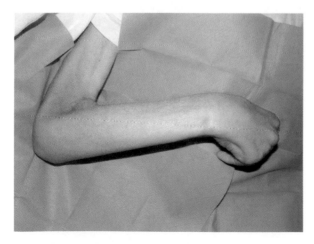

**Fig. 33.3** Forty-nine-year-old male patient with CKD 5 suffering from NSF: muscular atrophy and contractures are clearly depicted (courtesy of Prof. H. Thomsen)

disease stage 4 and 5 (GFR < 30 mL/min/1.73 m$^2$) appeared to be at high risk for NSF, the large majority of them being included in stage 5. Hemodialysis patients appear to be at risk for NSF in its most severe form, more than peritoneal dialysis patients. Patients with impaired renal function who underwent or are awaiting liver transplantation appear to be at high risk as well.

Patients with chronic kidney disease stage 3 (GFR 30–59 mL/min/1.73 m$^2$) are to be considered at risk to a lower extent, together with pediatric patients (below 1 year of age). It is extremely significant that not a single case of NSF was reported among patients with GFR >60 mL/min/1.73 m$^2$.

Almost all NSF patients received Gd-containing CM in their medical history. Actually, Broome (2008) reviewed the medical literature and reported that only five patients had NSF without previous exposure to Gd-containing CM. Deng et al. (2010) collected seven NSF patients who apparently did not receive Gd-containing agents, but in three of them, high levels of gadolinium were detected in the skin, suggesting a previous unreported exposure to the agent.

Furthermore, because NSF does not occur in all patients with impaired renal function injected with gadolinium chelates, it was suggested that other cofactors may be involved in the pathogenesis of this disease, such as proinflammatory events (surgical procedures – particularly vascular interventions and liver transplantation, severe sepsis, hypercoagulability), metabolic acidosis, high levels of erythropoietin, and immunologic disease. However, the hypothetical role of cofactors is still awaiting confirmation.

### 33.3.4 The Role of Contrast Material

Nine Gd-containing CM are approved for clinical use.

When considering the market share in the 1997–2006 period, gadopentetate dimeglumine (Magnevist®) was the leader, being used in more than 61,000,000 procedures, followed by gadodiamide (Omniscan®) in more than 33,000,000, gadoteridol (ProHance®) in more than 10,000,000, gadobenate dimeglumine (MultiHance®) and gadoversetamide (OptiMARK®).

However, when considering cases of NSF, the distribution is not the same: Broome (2008) collected 195 cases published on peer-reviewed journals and bioptically confirmed and showed that the large majority of them (157 out of 195) received gadodiamide, eight of them received gadopentetate dimeglumine, and three received gadoversetamide. The contrast agent was unknown in 18 patients, while four received multiple agents, and in five of them no Gd-containing agent was registered in the medical history. Besides the medical literature, different databases on NSF are available (International Center for NSF Research, FDA, regulatory authorities of different European countries, Contrast Media Committee of ACR, ESUR) and data can differ largely. Heinz Peer (2009) at the European Congress of Radiology reported figures on NSF mainly referring to the data provided by different companies and was able to collect 863 cases (517 after gadodiamide, 314 after gadopentetate dimeglumine, 10 after gadobenate dimeglumine (2 unconfounded), 9 after gadoteridol (1 unconfounded), 2 after gadobutrol (both confounded),and 11 after gadoterate meglumine (2 unconfounded)).

These data are clearly less reliable (some of the cases are not biopsy proven, some are confounded – that is the patient received more than one agent and it is impossible to determine with certainty which agent triggered the development of NSF), but nevertheless, they show (as any other database) that gadodiamide is by far the agent which was more frequently involved in NSF cases, followed by gadopentetate dimeglumine (Bryant et al. 2009; Kuo 2008; Rydahl et al. 2008; Thomsen et al. 2008a; Thomsen and Marckmann 2008; Van der Molen 2008). Therefore, it appears that Gd-containing CM are not related to NSF to the same extent, and moreover, this is not a reflection of the market share we mentioned. The physicochemical properties of Gd-containing agents were considered and hypotheses for the role of gadolinium chelates in the development of NSF were produced. Actually, the chemical structure (Table 33.2) is related to the contrast stability: macrocyclic agents have a rigid ring from which $Gd^{3+}$ cannot break easily, while the linear agents have an open flexible chain from which $Gd^{3+}$ can break easily (Idée et al. 2006). The stability measurements (and in particular, the kinetic stability which is considered predictive of in vivo stability) confirm the superior stability of the ionic macrocyclic chelates and the low stability of the nonionic linear chelates (Morcos 2008). In vivo data confirm that nonionic linear chelates (gadodiamide, gadoversetamide) are less stable, while no differences between ionic and nonionic macrocyclic agents were detected.

It was suggested that in less stable compounds, $Gd^{3+}$ can break free and be substituted by other cations. This is the transmetallation phenomenon which appears to be more likely when the gadolinium chelate remains for a long time in the body (i.e., in patients with impaired renal function). Free gadolinium could deposit in the tissues, gadolinium salts would be then engulfed by macrophages leading to the release of cytokines and attraction of circulating fibrocytes that can mature into fibroblasts leading to the fibrotic changes of NSF (Edward et al. 2008; Idée et al. 2009; Thakral and Abraham 2009a, b).

This theory should be validated by appropriate models, i.e., rats with renal failure, but appears to be able to explain the clinical differences that were detected among different gadolinium chelates so far (Sieber et al. 2008).

Furthermore, it was suggested that the injected contrast dose is highly significant: higher cumulative Gd dose, either from using double-dose or triple-dose injections, or a greater number of MR procedures, is associated with an increased risk of NSF (Abujudeh et al. 2009; Kallen et al. 2008; Marckmann et al. 2007). Prince et al. (2008) showed that the incidence of NSF after gadolinium-enhanced MRI was zero of 74,124 patients with the standard dose of gadolinium and 15 (0.17%) of 8,997 patients with the high dose ($p < 0.001$).

### 33.3.5 Diagnosis

A full thickness biopsy (including deep dermis and subcutaneous tissue) is essential for the diagnostic workup of suspected NSF cases (Thakral and Abraham 2009a, b). Superficial biopsies can miss the typical features of NSF, particularly in advanced cases.

However, none of the histologic features in NSF are definitive although the dual positivity of fibrocytes with CD34 and procollagen 1 is suggestive. Histological findings in skin include collagen bundles with surrounding clefts, mucin, elastic fibers, fibrocytes, histiocytes and multinucleated cells/dendritic cells, and calcification (Thakral and Abraham 2009a, b). Detection of gadolinium is relevant (High et al. 2007), but may escape if superficial biopsies are obtained.

**Table 33.2** Chemical structure of gadolinium-containing contrast media (CM)

| Open chain | |
|---|---|
| **Ionic** | |
| Gd-DTPA, Magnevist® | BOPTA, MultiHance® |
| Gd-EOB-DTPA, Primovist® | MS325, Vasovist® |
| **Nonionic** | |
| Gd-DTPA-BMA, Omniscan® | Gd-DTPA-BMEA, OptiMARK® |
| **Macrocyclic** | |
| **Ionic** | |
| Gd-DOTA, Dotarem® | |

*(continued)*

**Table 33.2** (continued)

| Nonionic | |
|---|---|
| Gd-HP-DO3A, ProHance® | Gd-BT-DO3A, Gadovist® |

## 33.3.6 Therapy

The only effective solution appears to be the correction of renal impairment, namely transplantation in patients with chronic kidney disease. Anecdotal reports actually showed a remission of NSF symptoms following kidney transplantation (Marckmann and Skov 2009). Physiotherapy and symptomatic treatments may help. Other approaches such as extracorporeal photopheresis, intravenous administration of sodium thiosulfate, plasmapheresis, and steroids administration were tried, but their efficacy is unproven.

Prevention of NSF in patients on hemodialysis could consider having a hemodialysis session immediately upon termination of the MR investigation. Actually, a greater incidence of NSF in patients in whom there was a delay between gadolinium chelates administration and hemodialysis was reported (Khurana et al. 2007; Prince et al. 2008; Wiginton et al. 2008). Nevertheless, conclusive data supporting the efficacy of an immediate hemodialysis session are not available. It is agreed that hemodialysis for NSF prevention should not be performed in patients who are not on hemodialysis or are on peritoneal dialysis.

## 33.3.7 Guideline

The Contrast media Safety Committee of the ESUR released its last version of the guideline on NSF in 2008.

The recommendations of the committee are different for different CM.

Gadodiamide, gadopentetate meglumine, and gadoversetamide are considered to be linked to the highest risk for NSF and therefore are contraindicated in patients with chronic kidney disease 4 and 5, including those on dialysis, and in patients with reduced renal function who have had or are awaiting liver transplantation. These agents should be used with caution in patients with chronic kidney disease 3 and in children less than 1 year. Serum creatinine (eGFR) measurement is deemed mandatory before their administration. Gadobenate dimeglumine, gadofosveset trisodium, and gadoxetate disodium are considered to be linked to an intermediate risk of NSF, and therefore, serum creatinine (eGFR) measurement before administration is not deemed mandatory, while the three macrocyclic agents (gadobutrol, gadoterate meglumine, and gadoteridol) are considered to be linked to the lowest risk of NSF, and again serum creatinine (eGFR) measurement before contrast administration is not mandatory. Moreover, the Committee recommends to use in all patients the smallest amount of contrast medium necessary for a diagnostic result and never to deny a patient a clinically well-indicated enhanced MR examination. Lastly, the Committee recommends to always use the agent that leaves the smallest amount of gadolinium in the body.

The adoption of this guideline and similar ones produced in the United States (Thomsen 2009) probably abruptly changed the scenario and the reported number of new NSF cases dropped down in 2008 and 2009. There is now a diffuse perception in the radiological community that though we do not fully understand NSF, we have learned to virtually eliminate it as a concern. Perez-Rodriguez et al. (2009) nicely compared the incidence of NSF before and after the implementation of an institutional policy design to assess the risk of NSF prior to gadolinium chelates use. The incidence dropped from 36.5 cases/100,000 gadolinium-enhanced MR procedures between 2003 and 2006 to 4 cases between 2007 and 2008 after the screening for NSF risk was instituted. In patients at risk, the policy included evaluation if gadolinium use was essential for diagnosis, with a maximum dose of 0.1 mmol/kg gadolinium and, if patients are on hemodialysis, two dialysis sessions separated by 1 day, the first one as soon as possible after MRI. It is interesting that the authors did not change the CM they used (gadodiamide and gadopentetate dimeglumine).

The radiological community realized that NSF is a complex issue, and information continues to be collected and the Contrast Media Safety Committee of the ESUR underscored that it may be necessary to review the guidelines as new information becomes available. No doubt caution is absolutely required in patients at risk (GFR < 30 mL/min/1.73 m$^2$), but the risk is not to be overweighted denying the enhanced MR procedure to patients who can benefit from it.

## 33.4 Conclusion

The radiologists till few years ago could easily shift a patient with impaired renal function who was at risk for CIN from CT to MRI. It has now become clear that NSF is a potential risk in these patients, and moreover, gadolinium chelates were shown to have some degree of nephrotoxicity, although lower when compared to iodinated CM. The choice between CT and MRI is no longer straightforward (Altun et al. 2009).

Patients with CKD 1 and 2 are not at increased risk of NSF, and therefore, MRI can be performed safely. Patients with CKD 3 are at extremely low risk for NSF and again MRI can be performed provided the renal function of the patient is stable and the dose of 0.1 mmol/kg of gadolinium chelate is not exceeded. The management of patients with CKD 4 and 5 and those on hemodialysis is more difficult. If the required clinical information can be equally achieved either by CT or MRI, we have to consider that the risk of CIN requiring dialysis following intravenous contrast administration is very low (although precise data are not available) and the risk of NSF following the administration of macrocyclic agents at a dose not exceeding 0.1 mmol/kg is very low as well (again precise data are not available). The author's advice would probably favor CT, but the main feature is that whatever procedure we choose, the risk is very low, provided the available guidelines are carefully considered.

## References

Abujudeh HH, Kaewlai R, Kagan A et al. (2009) Nephrogenic systemic fibrosis after gadopentetate dimeglumine exposure: case series of 36 patients. Radiology 253:81–89

Agarwal R, Brunelli SM, Williams K et al. (2009) Gadolinium-based contrast agents and nephrogenic systemic fibrosis: a systematic review and meta-analysis. Nephrol Dial Transplant 24:856–863

Alamartine E, Phayphet M, Thibaudin D et al. (2003) Contrast medium-induced acute renal failure and cholesterol embolism after radiological procedures: incidence, risk factors, and compliance with recommendations. Eur J Intern Med 14:426–431

Altun E, Semelka RC, Cakit C (2009) Nephrogenic systemic fibrosis and management of high-risk patients. Acad Radiol 16:897–905

Aspelin P, Aubry P, Fransson SG et al. (2003) Nephrotoxic effects in high-risk patients undergoing angiography. N Engl J Med 348:491–499

Barrett BJ, Carlisle EJ (1993) Metaanalysis of the relative nephrotoxicity of high and low-osmolality iodinated contrast media. Radiology 188:171–178

Bartholomew BA, Harjai KJ, Dukkipati S et al. (2004) Impact of nephropathy after percutaneous coronary intervention and a method for risk stratification. Am J Cardiol 93: 1515–1519

Broome DR (2008) Nephrogenic systemic fibrosis associated with gadolinium based contrast agents: a summary of the medical literature reporting. Eur J Radiol 66:230–234

Broome DR, Girguis MS, Baron PW et al. (2007) Gadodiamide-associated nephrogenic systemic fibrosis: why radiologists should be concerned. AJR Am J Roentgenol 188:586–592

Brown JR, DeVries JT, Piper WD et al. (2008) Serious renal dysfunction after percutaneous coronary interventions can be predicted. Am Heart J 155:260–226

Bryant BJ II, Im K, Broome DR (2009) Evaluation of the incidence of nephrogenic systemic fibrosis in patients with moderate renal insufficiency administered gadobenate dimeglumine for MRI. Clin Radiol 64:706–713

Bruce RJ, Djamali A, Shinki K et al. (2009) Background fluctuation of kidney function versus contrast-induced nephrotoxicity. AJR 192:711–718

Cowper SE (2005) Nephrogenic systemic fibrosis: the nosological and conceptual evolution of nephrogenic fibrosing dermopathy. Am J Kidney Dis 46:763–765

Cowper SE (2008) Nephrogenic systemic fibrosis: an overview. J Am Coll Radiol 5:23–28

Dangas G, Iakovou I, Nikolsky E et al. (2005) Contrast-induced nephropathy after percutaneous coronary interventions in relation to chronic kidney disease and hemodynamic variables. Am J Cardiol 95:13–19

Deng A, Bilu Martin D, Spillane J et al. (2010) Nephrogenic systemic fibrosis with a spectrum of clinical and histopathological presentation: a disorder of aberrant dermal remodeling. J Cutan Pathol 37:204–210

Edward M, Quinn JA, Mukherjee S et al. (2008) Gadodiamide contrast agent "activates" fibroblasts: a possible cause of nephrogenic systemic fibrosis. J Pathol 214:584–593

Grobner T (2006) Gadolinium-a specific trigger for the development of nephrogenic fibrosing dermopathy and nephrogenic systemic fibrosis? Nephrol Dial Transplant 21:1104–1108

Heinrich MC, Häberle L, Müller V et al. (2009) Nephrotoxicity of iso-osmolar iodixanol compared with nonionic low-osmolar contrast media: meta-analysis of randomized controlled trials. Radiology 250:68–86

Heinz Peer G (2009) Gadolinium contrast media and nephrogenic systemic fibrosis. Invited lecture at ECR 09, Vienna.

High WA, Ayers RA, Chandler J et al. (2007) Gadolinium is detectable within the tissue of patients with nephrogenic systemic fibrosis. J Am Acad Dermatol 56:21–26

Iakovou I, Dangas G, Mehran R et al. (2003) Impact of gender on the incidence and outcome of contrast-induced nephropathy after percutaneous coronary intervention. J Invasive Cardiol 15:18–22

Idée JM, Port M, Dencausse A et al. (2009) Involvement of gadolinium chelates in the mechanism of nephrogenic systemic fibrosis: an update. Radiol Clin North Am 47:855–869

Idée JM, Port M, Raynal I et al. (2006) Clinical and biological consequences of transmetallation induced by contrast agents for magnetic resonance imaging: a review. Fundam Clin Pharmacol 20:563–576

Kallen AJ, Jhung MA, Cheng S et al. (2008) Gadolinium-containing magnetic resonance imaging contrast and nephrogenic systemic fibrosis: a case control study. Am J Kidney Dis 51:966–975

Katzberg RW, Lamba R (2009) Contrast-induced nephropathy after intravenous administration: fact or fiction? Radiol Clin North Am 47:789–800

Kelly AM, Dwamena B, Cronin P et al. (2008) Meta-analysis: effectiveness of drugs for preventing contrast-induced nephropathy. Ann Intern Med 148:284–294

Khurana A, Runge VM, Narayanan M et al. (2007) Nephrogenic systemic fibrosis: a review of 6 cases temporally related to gadodiamide injection (Omniscan). Invest Radiol 42:139–145

Kuo PH (2008) Gadolinium-containing MRI contrast agents: important variations on a theme for NSF. J Am Coll Radiol 5:29–35

Laskey W, Aspelin P, Davidson C et al. (2009) Nephrotoxicity of iodixanol versus iopamidol in patients with chronic kidney disease and diabetes mellitus undergoing coronary angiographic procedures. Am Heart J 158:822–828

Laskey WK, Jenkins C, Selzer F et al. (2007) Volume-to-creatinine clearance ratio. JACC 50:584–590

Manske CL, Sprafka JM, Strony JT et al. (1990) Contrast nephropathy in azotemic diabetic patients undergoing coronary angiography. Am J Med 89:615–620

Marenzi G, Lauri G, Campodonico J et al. (2006) Comparison of two hemofiltration protocols for prevention of contrast-induced nephropathy in high-risk patients. Am J Med 119:155–162

Marenzi G, Marana I, Lauri G et al. (2003) The prevention of radiocontrast-agent-induced nephropathy by hemofiltration. N Engl J Med 349:1333–1340

Marckmann P, Skov L (2009) Nephrogenic systemic fibrosis: clinical picture and treatment. Radiol Clin North Am 47:833–840

Marckmann P, Skov L, Rossen K et al. (2006) Nephrogenic systemic fibrosis: suspected causative role of gadodiamide used for contrast-enhanced magnetic resonance imaging. J Am Soc Nephrol 17:2359–2362

Marckmann P, Skov L, Rossen K et al. (2007) Case-control study of gadodiamide-related nephrogenic systemic fibrosis. Nephrol Dial Transplant 22:3174–3178

McCarthy CS, Becker JA (1992) Multiple myeloma and contrast media. Radiology 183:519–521

McCullough PA, Wolyn R, Rocher LL et al. (1997) Acute renal failure after coronary intervention: incidence, risk factors, and relationship to mortality. Am J Med 103:368–375

Mehran R, Aymong ED, Nikolsky E et al. (2004) A simple risk score for prediction of contrast-induced nephropathy after percutaneous coronary intervention: development and initial validation. J Am Coll Cardiol 44:1393–1399

Mehta RL, Kellum JA, Shah SV et al. (2007) Acute Kidney Injury Network (AKIN): report of an initiative to improve outcomes in acute kidney injury. Crit Care 11:R31

Merten GJ, Burgess WP, Gray LV et al. (2004) Prevention of contrast-induced nephropathy with sodium bicarbonate: a randomized controlled trial. JAMA 291:2328–2334

Molitoris BA, Levin A, Warnock DG et al. (2007) Improving outcomes of acute kidney injury: report of an initiative. Nat Clin Pract Nephrol 3:439–442

Morcos SK (2008) Extracellular gadolinium contrast agents: differences in stability. Eur J Radiol 66:175–179

Morcos SK, Thomsen HS, Webb JA, Members of the Contrast Media Safety Committee of the European Society of Urogenital Radiology (ESUR) (1999) Contrast-media-induced nephrotoxicity: a consensus report. Eur Radiol 9: 1602–1613

Mueller C, Buerkle G, Buettner HJ et al. (2002) Prevention of contrast media-associated nephropathy: randomized comparison of 2 hydration regimens in 1620 patients undergoing coronary angioplasty. Arch Intern Med 162:329–336

Newhouse JH, Kho D, Rao QA et al. (2008) Frequency of serum creatinine changes in the absence of iodinated contrast material: implications for studies of contrast nephrotoxicity. AJR 191:376–382

Nyman U, Biörk J, Aspelin P et al. (2008) Contrast medium dose-to-GFR ratio: a measure of systemic exposure to predict contrast-induced nephropathy after percutaneous coronary intervention. Acta Radiol 6:658–667

Perez-Rodriguez J, Shenghan L, Ehst BD et al. (2009) Nephrogenic systemic fibrosis: incidence, associations, and effect of risk factor assessment – report of 33 cases. Radiology 250: 371–377

Prince MR, Zhang H, Morris M et al. (2008) Incidence of nephrogenic systemic fibrosis at two large medical centers. Radiology 248:807–816

Reddan D, Laville M, Garovic VD (2009) Contrast-induced nephropathy and its prevention: what do we really know from evidence-based findings? J Nephrol 22:333–351

Rihal CS, Textor SC, Grill DE et al. (2002) Incidence and prognostic importance of acute renal failure after percutaneous coronary intervention. Circulation 105:2259–2264

Rydahl C, Thomsen HS, Marckmann P (2008) High prevalence of nephrogenic systemic fibrosis in chronic renal failure patients exposed to gadodiamide, a gadolinium-containing magnetic resonance contrast agent. Invest Radiol 43: 141–144

Sadowski EA, Bennett LK, Chan MR et al. (2007) Nephrogenic systemic fibrosis: risk factors and incidence estimation. Radiology 243:148–157

Sieber MA, Lengsfeld P, Frenzel T et al. (2008) Preclinical investigation to compare different gadolinium-based contrast agents regarding their propensity to release gadolinium in vivo and to trigger nephrogenic systemic fibrosis-like lesions. Eur Radiol 18:2164–2173

Stacul F, Adam A, Becker CR et al. (2006) Strategies to reduce the risk of contrast-induced nephropathy. Am J Cardiol 98: 59K–77K

Thakral C, Abraham JL (2009) Gadolinium-induced nephrogenic systemic fibrosis is associated with insoluble Gd deposits in tissues: in vivo transmetallation confirmed by microanalysis. J Cutan Pathol 36:1244–1254

Thakral C, Abraham JL (2009) Nephrogenic systemic fibrosis: histology and gadolinium detection. Radiol Clin North Am 47:841–853

Thomsen HS (2009) How to avoid nephrogenic systemic fibrosis: current guidelines in Europe and the United States. Radiol Clin North Am 47:871–875

Thomsen HS, Marckmann P (2008) Extracellular Gd-CA: differences in prevalence of NSF. Eur J Radiol 66:180–183

Thomsen HS, Marckmann P, Logager VB (2008) Update on nephrogenic systemic fibrosis. Magn Reson Imaging Clin N Am 16:551–560

Thomsen HS, Morcos SK (2006) Contrast-medium-induced nephropathy: is there a new consensus? A review of published guidelines. Eur Radiol 16:1835–1840

Thomsen HS, Morcos SK, Barrett BJ (2008) Contrast-induced nephropathy: the wheel has turned 360 degrees. Acta Radiol 6:646–657

Thomsen HS, Morcos SK; Members of Contrast Media Safety Committee of European Society of Urogenital Radiology (ESUR) (2005) In which patients should serum creatinine be measured before iodinated contrast medium administration? Eur Radiol 15:749–754

Trivedi HS, Moore H, Nasr S et al. (2003) A randomized prospective trial to assess the role of saline hydration on the development of contrast nephrotoxicity. Nephron Clin Pract 93:C29–C34

Van der Molen AJ (2008) Nephrogenic systemic fibrosis and the role of gadolinium contrast media. J Med Imaging Radiat Oncol 52:339–350

Waikar SS, Bonventre JV (2009) Creatinine kinetics and the definition of acute kidney injury. J Am Soc Nephrol 20: 672–679

Webb JG, Pate GE, Humphries KH et al. (2004) A randomized controlled trial of intravenous N-acetylcysteine for the prevention of contrast-induced nephropathy after cardiac catheterization: lack of effect. Am Heart J 148:422–429

Wessely R, Koppara T, Bradaric C et al. (2009) Choice of contrast medium in patients with impaired renal function undergoing percutaneous coronary intervention. Circ Cardiovasc Interv 2:430–437

Wiginton CD, Kelly B, Oto A et al. (2008) Gadolinium-based contrast exposure, nephrogenic systemic fibrosis, and gadolinium detection in tissue. AJR Am J Roentgenol 190:1060–1068

# Functional Imaging of the Kidney

**34**

Nicolas Grenier

## Contents

## Abstract

> Functional imaging of the kidney, using radiological techniques, has a great potential of development because the functional parameters that can be approached noninvasively are multiple. CT can provide measurement of perfusion and glomerular filtration, but has the inconvenience of delivering irradiation and potential nephrotoxicity due to iodine agents in this context. US is able to measure perfusion only, but quantification remains problematic. Therefore, MR imaging shows the greatest flexibility in measuring glomerular filtration, tubular concentration and transit, blood volume and perfusion, diffusion, and oxygenation. Till now, its limitations in clinical applications are due to the difficulties in obtaining reproducible and reliable information in this mobile organ and, sometimes, in understanding the physiologic substrate of the signal changes observed. These approaches require either endogeneous contrast agents such as water protons (for perfusion and diffusion) or deoxyhemogobin (for oxygenation), or exogeneous contrast agents such as gadolinium (Gd) chelates (for filtration and perfusion) or iron oxide particles (for perfusion). Clinical validation of these methods and evaluation of their clinical impact are still worthwhile before diffusing them in clinical practice.

N. Grenier
Service d'Imagerie Diagnostique et Interventionelle de
l'Adulte, Groupe Hospitalier Pellegrin, Place Amélie
Raba-Léon, 33076 Bordeaux Cedex, France
e-mail: nicolas.grenier@chu-bordeaux.fr

The management of acute and chronic renal diseases requires having an access to several physiological parameters using simple and reliable tools. Unfortunately, renal

E. Quaia (ed.), *Radiological Imaging of the Kidney*,
Medical Radiology, DOI: 10.1007/978-3-540-87597-0_34, © Springer-Verlag Berlin Heidelberg 2011

physiology is complex and measurements of these parameters are either impossible or often too complex to implement on a regular basis, or not reliable enough. Renal perfusion and glomerular filtration rate (GFR) are major functional parameters which are involved in many parenchymal diseases and used to monitor the renal function. Getting an easy, reliable, and reproducible access to these data, in conjunction with precise morphological information, would significantly improve the patient care in nephrology. For example, actually, measurement of perfusion in clinics is not reliable and no reference method is available for patients. Noninvasive and accurate measurement of renal perfusion could have a major impact in understanding physiopathology of renovascular diseases and for their follow-up. Similarly, GFR is used as an index of functioning renal mass, representing the sum of filtration rates in each functioning nephron. Fall of GFR may be the earliest and only clinical sign of renal disease and its serial monitoring allows estimating the severity and following the course of kidney diseases. Its evaluation, most of the time, is only estimated, because accurate measurement requires implementing complex methods of plasma or urinary clearance. Approaches provided by imaging are promising because they are simple to implement and flexible, but many technical and theoretical limitations still preclude their diffusion in clinics.

## 34.1 Contrast Agents and Technical Issues

### 34.1.1 Sonography

Third generation of ultrasound contrast agents (USCA) is composed of microbubbles containing a gas with a low diffusibility, stabilized by a shell, with a mean diameter range between 1 and 5µm (Correas et al. 2001). Once injected into the blood circulation, these bubbles have a monocompartment distribution, purely intravascular, without interstitial diffusion or glomerular filtration. The gas is eliminated via the respiratory system. This pharmacokinetics characterizes these agents as real blood pool agents, particularly appropriate for the evaluation of renal perfusion. However, there are major constraints making quantification process difficult with US: the response of both anatomical structures and microbubbles to an ultrasound beam is complex, which requires using contrast-specific imaging modes based on the enhancement of the nonlinear response from bubbles; quantification is also mainly affected by shadowing, which results from inaccurate correction of both tissue and microbubble attenuation. Variation in attenuation across the image at a given depth is not accounted for by time-gain compensation (TGC). Several methods for automatic compensation of tissue attenuation have been proposed in vitro and, more recently in vivo, but only experimentally (Mule et al. 2008). Second, there is no linear relationship between the concentration of the agent and the intensity of received signal. Third, even if imaging protocols require a sonication with low mechanical indexes, an unpredictable part of microbubbles are destroyed within the imaging plane, in both the analyzed tissue and the feeding vessels. Some mathematical models were proposed to compensate for this effect (Lucidarme et al. 2003a, b). Finally, the last limitation is the impossibility to image both kidneys with the same acquisition. Therefore, application of functional renal US in humans is actually limited to a semiquantitative evaluation of renal perfusion.

### 34.1.2 CT

Iodine contrast agents used for X-rays can be considered as glomerular tracers, because, as [99m]Tc-DTPA or [51]Cr-EDTA used in nuclear medicine, they are freely filtered at the first pass by the glomeruli without any tubular secretion or reabsorption. The linear relation between the level of attenuation and the contrast agent concentration is a great advantage, facilitating modelisation. Axial acquisitions with CT allow including both kidneys (for comparison) and aorta to take into account the arterial input function (AIF). There are several limitations making CT poorly available for quantitative evaluation of renal function: nephrotoxicity of iodine agents in patients with decreased renal function, the induced radiation dose due to the necessary continuous irradiation during acquisition requiring the application of all dose reduction methods, and the impossibility to include the entire kidney in the volume using the axial transverse plane (4–6 cm covered). Most of developments were performed with electron beam CT (Chade et al.

2003; Daghini et al. 2007) and, more recently, with CT in animals (Liu et al. 2009). These authors demonstrated the feasibility to measure renal perfusion and glomerular filtration with a tenth of a clinical dose and low constants.

### 34.1.3 MR Imaging

Depending on the chosen method, intrinsic (as moving protons or deoxyhemoglobin) or extrinsic contrast agents are used. The former are devoted to study renal blood flow, renal perfusion, renal diffusion, and renal oxygenation. The later are devoted to study renal perfusion and renal filtration (Grenier et al. 2003).

Regular low-molecular-weight Gd-chelates are still the only extrinsic agents used in clinical imaging. As iodine contrast agents, they can also be considered as glomerular tracers. However, their role in the evaluation of renal function shows some limitations: first, as the other mentioned agents, they are also freely diffusing into the interstitium, compartment which is usually neglected in most pharmacokinetic models; second, the relationship between signal intensity (SI) and concentration is highly complex, inducing concomitant reduction of T1 and T2 (or T2*), which is not the case for radioactive agents or iodine compounds.

Concentration of agent can be calculated by the linear relationship to the $R1$ relaxation rate and the specific relaxivity of the agent ($r$):

$$C = \left(R1 - R1_0\right)/r,$$

where $R1_0$ is the bulk $R1$ in the tissue without contrast agent. In principle, this means that a precontrast measurement of $R1$ should be performed before injection of the contrast agent. To convert changes in SI into changes in $R1$, different approaches can be used. A commonly used method is based on a phantom of tubes filled with Gd solutions at various concentrations imaged with the same sequence. The acquired SI values are plotted against measured $R1$ values, and a polynomial fit is made to obtain a calibration curve. However, the relaxivity is not equivalent in solution and in tissues. Another method uses the relationship between SI and $R1$ given by the equation driven by the sequence used (Pedersen et al. 2004), which unfortunately is not straightforward.

Other types of contrast agents have appeared in the research field with different pharmacokinetic and magnetic properties: either larger Gd-chelates or iron oxide particles (Choyke and Kobayashi 2006). The first ones do not diffuse in the interstitium, but are still filtered by the glomeruli; the second are strictly confined to the vascular space, but can be captured by activated cells with a phagocytic phenotype. If their applications remain limited today, these large molecules could be useful either for functional purposes (quantification of perfusion, quantification of GFR, estimation of tubular function) or for cellular purposes (intrarenal phagocytosis in inflammatory renal diseases).

## 34.2 Measurement of Glomerular Filtration

While the level of GFR is the best index for monitoring chronic kidney diseases (CKD), measurement of glomerular filtration is difficult to obtain accurately in routine. Therefore, the kidney Disease Quality Outcome Initiative (K/DOQI) of the National kidney Foundation recommends GFR estimates for the definition, classification, and monitoring of CKD (Prigent 2008). Based on serum creatinine values, these prediction equations have limitations, especially in the normal and near-normal range of GFR, in kidney transplant recipients, and in the pediatric population. The Cockcroft and Gault formula estimates a global creatinine clearance, and the MDRD (modification of diet in renal disease study) formula estimates a GFR. Stratification of kidney diseases is based on one of these formulas in clinical practice. However, they have several limitations (Prigent 2008): variations of plasma creatinine level are around 10%; some tubular secretion may lead to overestimation of GFR, particularly in advanced renal failure; there is a reduction of creatinine excretion with age related to a decrease in skeletal muscle mass; finally, in acute or rapidly progressing renal failure, this technique provides inaccurate information when GFR is rapidly changing.

Indications of true GFR measurements in nephrology actually include systematic follow-up of renal transplants; evaluation of living donors, when measurement of creatinine clearance is not reliable (low muscle mass, obese); and during all protocols requiring a reliable and reproducible renal function estimation.

The commonest method used clinically for accurate GFR measurement is the assessment of the plasma disappearance of a substance that is excreted from the body exclusively by glomerular filtration with neither tubular reabsorption, nor tubular excretion, for example, ethylenediamine tetraacetic acid (EDTA) or iothalamate (Prigent 2008). Most of the time, these standard methods are underused because they are quite time-consuming and require several blood/urinary samplings. Therefore, a quantitative method based on a tracer intrarenal kinetics, obtained rapidly, without blood and/or urine samplings, coupled with a morphological evaluation of the kidneys and the entire excretory system, would be extremely useful in the clinical management of patients with renal disease.

Besides nuclear medicine, evaluation of the filtration function is devoted to MR imaging only (Grenier et al. 2008) because US contrast agents are not filtered by the kidneys and dynamic studies require long acquisition times, making CT not acceptable in patients yet.

### 34.2.1 Measurement of Split Renal Function

Semiquantitative evaluation of renal function as split (or differential) renal function is sufficient in urological management of most uropathies, mainly obstructive. However, it is usually not useful in the daily assessment and follow-up of renal diseases. In the nephrologic field, it can be required when a reduced renal function is associated with renal asymmetry, in renovascular diseases, before renal surgery if renal function is altered or before renal biopsy. The split renal function (given in percentage) corresponds, for each kidney, to the product:

$$RF(\%) = RF / RF_{total} \times 100,$$

where $RF_{total}$ is the sum of RFs of both kidneys. In clinical routine, the split renal function is still measured using nuclear medicine with glomerular ($^{99m}Tc$-DTPA) or tubular ($^{99m}Tc$-MAG3) agents. Two methods are promoted for that purpose: either the calculation of areas under the filtration curves or Rutland-Patlak plots.

Using dynamic contrast-enhanced MR imaging, Rohrschneider et al. (2000b) obtained calculations of the percentage of the single-kidney "activity" comparable to those derived with gamma camera scintigraphy. These studies were based on a dynamic RF-spoiled gradient-echo sequence and half of a standard clinical accepted dose of Gd-DTPA. A region of interest (ROI) was positioned around the renal parenchyma (omitting the pelvis), and calculation of the relative renal function was then based on the equation:

$$RF = AUC \, (mm^2) \times S \, (mm^2),$$

where AUC corresponds to the area under the glomerulo-tubular segment of the time-intensity curve and $S$ is the ROI area (Fig. 34.1). In both an experimental study of ureteral obstruction (Rohrschneider et al. 2000a) and in patients (Rohrschneider et al. 2002), a high correlation between MR and renal scintigraphy was found. In addition, conversion from SI to concentration of contrast agent is not necessary as recently demonstrated in rats with acute and chronic ureteral obstruction (Pedersen et al. 2004). A large multicentric trial comparing renal scintigraphy and dynamic MR imaging in adults and children presenting with unilateral obstruction is actually ongoing in France (unpublished data). The early results of this study show better concordance of MR estimation with renal scintigraphy using Rutland-Patlak plots than using AUC.

### 34.2.2 MR Quantification of Global GFR

Two methods are proposed for the measurement of global GFR using MRI and freely filtered Gd-chelates. The first one is based on the measurement of the clearance of a MR agent using blood samplings (Choyke et al. 1992). This method presents little advantage compared to other methods, because it is time-consuming and requires several blood samples. The second method is based on the measurement of the slope clearance of a freely filtered Gd-chelate from the extracellular fluid volume (ECFV) using SI changes within abdominal organs (Boss et al. 2007). GFR is calculated as the product of the ECFV (ECFV = $0.02154 \cdot weight^{0.6469} \, height^{0.3964}$) and the time constant of the second exponential phase ($\alpha_2$). The

**Fig. 34.1** Signal intensity (SI)–time curves obtained in a patient with left urinary obstruction. The anatomic image (**a**) shows dilatation of the left pyelocaliceal system. SI–time curves (**b**) obtained from regions-of-interest drawn on the entire renal parenchyma (excluding pyelocaliceal system) on each side, showing three phases: a first abrupt ascending segment followed by a first peak, corresponding to the "vascular-to-glomerular first-pass" or cortical vascular phase; a second slowly ascending segment, ended by a second peak, corresponding to the glomerulo-tubular phase; and a slowly descending segment, corresponding to the predominant excretory function and the so-called "excretory phase". Areas under the curves have been drawn to calculate split renal function

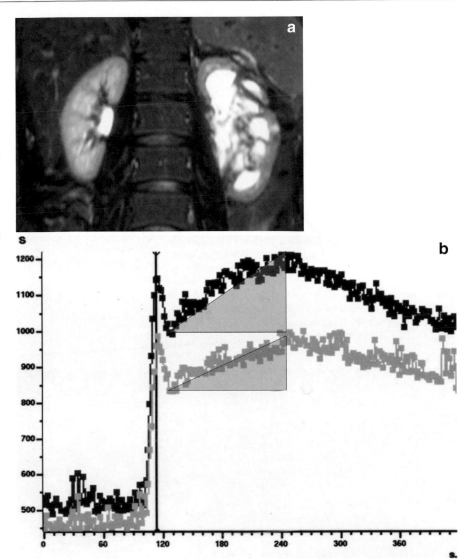

best concordance between gadobutrol clearance and iopromide clearance was observed within the liver, the exponential fit being performed between 40 and 55 min after injection (with a mean paired difference of −5.9 mL/min/1.73m² ± 14.6) (Fig. 34.2). All measurement points were within ±2 standard deviation values, but the maximum deviation from the reference GFR was 29%. With such a wide deviation, this technique can hardly be applied to an individual patient. Main drawbacks of this method are the length of MR acquisition and the sensitivity to body movements and to the selected time intervals when the analysis is performed. More experience is required with this technique.

### 34.2.3 MR Quantification of Single Kidney GFR (SKGFR)

Two methods are available for the measurement of global GFR using MRI and freely filtered Gd-chelates: (1) monitoring of tracer intrarenal kinetics; (2) measurement of the extraction fraction of the agent.

#### 34.2.3.1 Monitoring of Tracer Intrarenal Kinetics

A great heterogeneity for parameters of pulse-sequences, doses of injected Gd contrast, methods for the conversion of SI into concentration, postprocessing methods,

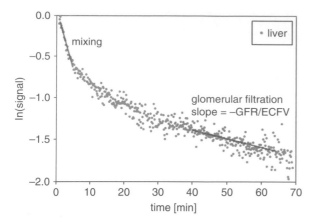

**Fig. 34.2** Measurement of renal clearance. Exponential decay on the logarithmically scaled time–SI curve (displayed for liver parenchyma) indicates linear behavior. Two exponential phases can be distinguished owing to different slopes: the fast mixing phase immediately after contrast medium injection and the more prolonged phase, in which the SI decrease is caused solely by glomerular filtration. The negative slope of this phase is equal to the GFR divided by the ECFV. (Reprinted with permission from Boss et al. 2007)

and compartment models is still noted in the literature between the different groups and no consensus exists (Mendichovszky et al. 2008).

## MR Technical Requirements

- This quantification requires an accurate sampling of the vascular phase of the enhancement with a high temporal resolution in order to measure the AIF, which is characterized by the SI changes within the suprarenal abdominal aorta. It is used for the different kinetic models in order to compensate for the noninstantaneous bolus injected into the blood (Fig. 34.3). Not taking this into account will produce an overestimation of GFR due to recirculation of the agent within the vascular space.

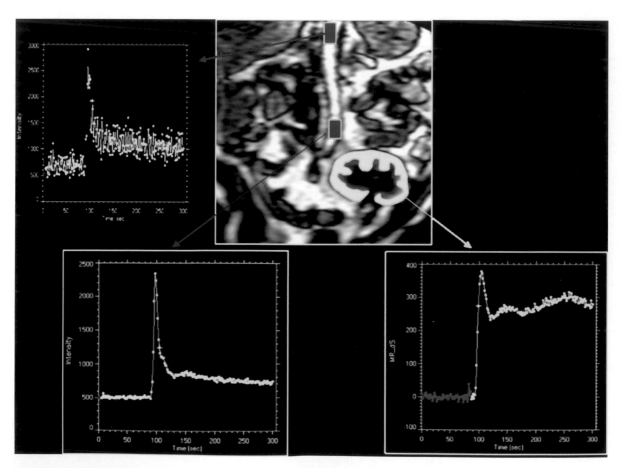

**Fig. 34.3** Dynamic acquisition to measure GFR in a renal transplant. This requires to sample SI–time curves within aorta and within renal cortex. The aortic curve, for the characterization of the arterial input function, is altered by inflow effects only when sampling of SI is done at the top of the volume. These effects disappear in the middle of imaging plane

- All pulse-sequences must have a heavy T1-weighting and be fast enough to characterize the vascular phase of the tracer kinetic which is necessary for the assessment of the AIF. Therefore, sequences with a nonselective magnetization preparation are often preferred, combining with very short TR/TE and low flip angles.
- Concentration of Gd within the kidney can be very high, due to water reabsorption in the proximal convoluted tubule and within the medulla. Therefore, to avoid T2* contribution to the signal, the injected dose must be lowered and the patient well hydrated (Rusinek et al. 2001). The choice between 0.025 mmol/kg and 0.05 mmol/kg depends on the level of signal-to-noise ratio obtained with the sequence and the system used.
- An oblique-coronal plane, passing through the long axis of the kidneys, has to be preferred to an axial plane because with the later, movement correction is impossible and the AIF can be severely impaired by inflow effects within the aorta.
- About renal coverage, some cover the entire parenchyma with several slices using a multislice or a 3D acquisition and calculate GFR by summing the GFR values of each voxel in each slice. Others acquire only one median slice, calculate a mean GFR value, and extrapolate this value to the entire renal volume to get a total GFR.

### Postprocessing

- Because dynamic MR imaging of the kidneys is performed during free breathing, the main problem is the correction of respiratory movements. Absence of correction produces artifacts in time-intensity evolution which can lead to incorrect quantification. Gated sequences would lead to severe penalties in temporal resolution. A movement correction method developed in our group (de Senneville et al. 2008) based on the estimation of a rigid transformation and correction allowed to estimate successfully small motion and provided more than 20% of reduction on GFR uncertainty on transplanted kidneys and up to 60% on native kidneys (Fig. 34.4).
- Extraction of dynamic should be ideally limited to the cortex, which requires an accurate segmentation method. In the published clinical studies, it was generally done manually. A recent review has developed and discussed extensively the principles and the difficulties on segmentation and on renal ROI generation (Michoux et al. 2006).

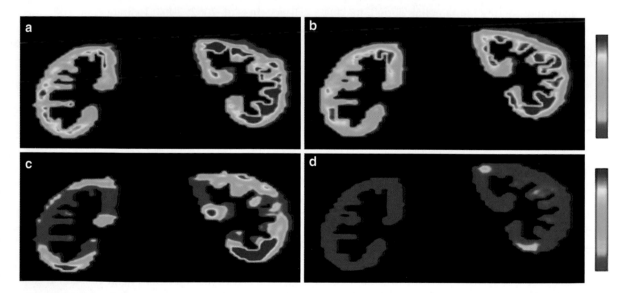

**Fig. 34.4** Example of 2D GFR (**a**, **b**) and standard deviation (**c**, **d**) maps obtained on native kidneys grenien without (**a**, **c**), and with (**b**, **d**) motion correction. Standard deviation values are lower and more homogeneously distributed with (**d**), than without (**c**) motion correction. (Reprinted with permission from de Senneville et al. 2008)

## Compartment Models

The ideal model reflecting filtration physiology remains to be worked out. Most of the reviewed MRI methods used a two-compartment model, although Lee et al. (2007) proposed a more complex compartment model.

The *Rutland-Patlak plot technique* is a graphical method based on a two-compartmental model with the assumptions that the rate of change of concentration in the kidney during the clearance phase is constant if the amount of contrast agent is taken into account during this period (Patlak et al. 1983). This method has been applied to MRI by several groups (Annet et al. 2004; Hackstein et al. 2002, 2003; Hermoye et al. 2004; Pedersen et al. 2005a). The assumption that no contrast agent leaves the ROI during the sampling period may justify theoretically the use of ROIs encompassing both cortex and medulla. The model is realized as an *x–y* plot using the ratio of the renal concentration/aortic concentration plotted against the ratio of the integral of aortic concentration/aortic concentration. When applied to the second phase of the SI–time curve (glomerulo-tubular uptake), this plot leads to a straight line, with a slope proportional to the renal clearance, and an intercept with the *y*-axis proportional to the cortical blood volume (Fig. 34.5).

The *cortical compartment model* (Annet et al. 2004; Hermoye et al. 2004) is a two-compartment model confined to the cortex, taking into account the outflow from the tubules, during the sampling period, making it possible to draw ROIs strictly limited to the cortex. Calculation of the residue function (i.e., the deconvolution of $C(t)$ with AIF(t)) then exhibits three sequential peaks (successively glomerular, proximal tubule, distal tubule) and two rate constants, $k_{in}$ and $k_{out}$, that describe the flow into and out of the proximal tubule, meaning that $k_{in}$ represents SKGFR which can be calculated according to the following equation:

$$SKGFR = maximal\ slope\ of\ proximal\ tubule\ peak/C_{(vasc)max}.$$

To calculate $C_{(vasc)max}$, the maximum of the vascular peak was divided by the RBV to take into account that the contrast agent remains in the extravascular space. This method has provided more accurate results than Rutland-Patlak model in an experimental study in rabbits, using [51]Cr-EDTA as a goldstandard (Annet et al.

2004). It is providing GFR, blood flow, and vascular volume (Fig. 34.6).

The *multicompartmental model* (Lee et al. 2007) includes three cortical compartments (glomerular, capillary, and proximal convoluted tubules, as in previous model), three medullary compartments (loops of Henle, distal convoluted tubules, collecting ducts), and the collecting system. Despite being complex, this model has the advantage of assessing some important tubular physiological parameters. Applied to the passage of Gd into the first two compartments, the model allows calculation of GFR.

## Accuracy and Reproducibility

Such studies should be accurate and reproducible when compared to a gold standard technique. But only one clinical study undertook the [99m]Tc-DTPA clearance during the Gd-MRI (Lee et al. 2007). A recent analysis of the literature emphasized the great heterogeneity of protocols (in acquisition mode, dose of contrast, postprocessing techniques etc.) and regression coefficient values, which are generally considered inadequate for replacing an accepted reference method (Mendichovszky et al. 2008). While several published papers conclude that Gd-enhanced MRI provides a reliable estimate of GFR and is suitable for use in both clinical and experimental settings (Hackstein et al. 2002, 2003; Laurent et al. 2002; Lee et al. 2003), evaluation seems still necessary at a larger scale.

### 34.2.3.2 Single Kidney Extraction Fraction

This method allows a quantification of a single kidney (SK) extraction fraction (EF), based on the measurement of T1 within flowing arterial and venous blood (Look and Locker method) during a continuous Gd infusion (Dumoulin et al. 1994; Niendorf et al. 1996, 1997, 1998):

$$EF = Ca - Cv / Ca,$$

where $Ca$ and $Cv$ are the arterial and venous Gd concentration, respectively. Because of the linear relationship between relaxation rates and concentration of Gd, EF can be expressed alternatively as:

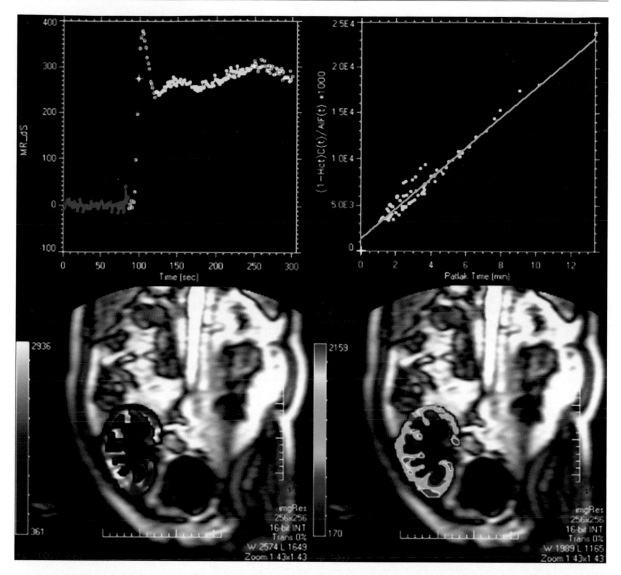

**Fig. 34.5** Patlak-Rutland method. On the SI–time curve from the cortex of a renal transplant are selected the time points corresponding to the filtration phase. The Patlak plot shows a good alignment of points. The slope corresponds to GFR. Therefore, we can draw two types of maps: the GFR map (*bottom left*) and the vascular volume map (*bottom right*)

$$EF = \left(1/T1a - 1/T1v\right)/\left(1/T1a - 1/T1_0\right),$$

where T1a is T1 in the renal artery, T1v in the vein, and $T1_0$ in the blood without Gd. Once EF is calculated for each kidney, values of SKGFR can be calculated if RBF is known:

$$SKGFR = EF \times RBF \times (1 - Hct),$$

where RBF is the renal blood flow, usually measured with the cine-phase-contrast method on the renal artery, and Hct is the level of hematocrit in the blood. Preliminary animal studies have shown concordant results with inulin clearance, but the correlation was 0.77 which is inadequate for clinical use at this stage (Fig. 34.3b) (Coulam et al. 2002). No clinical application of this method has been published till now.

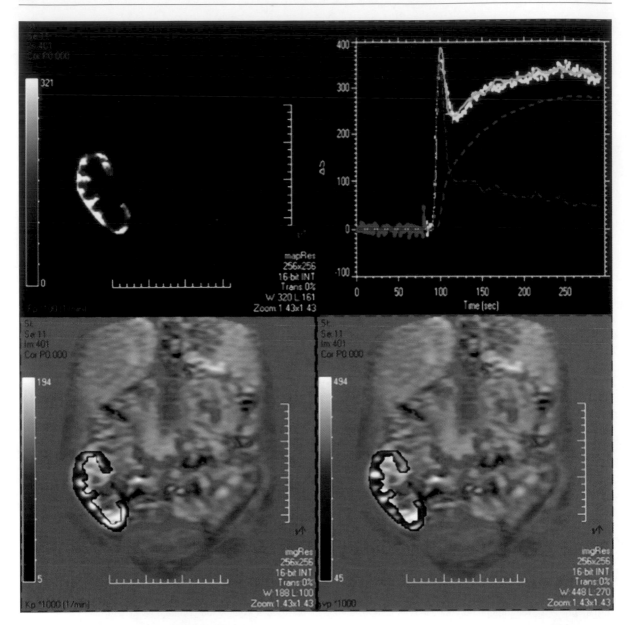

**Fig. 34.6** Two-compartment model. From the cortical SI–time curve and from the AIF, a two-compartment model can be applied on voxel-by-voxel basis. Dynamics from each compartment can be extracted: the red curve for the perfusion compo-nent and the blue one for the filtration component. We can obtain maps of perfusion (*top left*) of vascular volume (*bottom right*) and of GFR (*bottom left*)

## 34.3 Renal Flow Rate and Renal Perfusion

Renal blood flow (RBF), or flow rate, refers to the global amount of blood reaching the kidney per unit of time that is normally expressed in mL/min. This parameter is usually measured on a renal artery or a renal vein. Renal perfusion refers to the blood flow that passes through a unit mass of renal tissue (mL/min/g) in order to vascu-larize it and exchange with the extravascular space. The degree of perfusion depends on both the arterial flow rate and local factors such as regional blood volume and vasoreactivity. In clinical practice, measurement of RBF or perfusion may become important for the evaluation of renal artery stenosis or nephropathies with microvascular involvement and help in monitoring intravascular interventions.

## 34.3.1 Renal Flow Rate

Measurement of renal flow rate is based on the product of mean velocities in the renal artery and its section area. The cine-phase-contrast MR method is able to sample intraarterial velocity profile and to quantify the RBF in each renal vessel without injection of contrast agent. This technique is well-described in the literature (Debatin et al. 1994): it is based on the encoding of phase shifts of flowing spins along either one direction, perpendicular to the vessel of interest, or in all three directions. For accurate measurements in the human arteries, the imaging plane is usually positioned 10–15 mm downstream from the ostium, where respiratory movements are minimal, and perpendicularly to the renal artery (Fig. 34.7). Addition of this method to MR-angiography improved interobserver and intermodality agreement as sensitivity and specificity for the detection of significant renal artery stenosis (Schoenberg et al. 1997a, b, 2002). It was also demonstrated, in vitro, that the degree of spin dephasing was directly correlated with the transstenotic pressure gradient (Mustert et al. 1998).

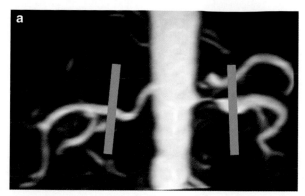

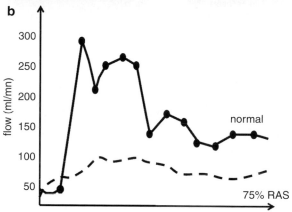

**Fig. 34.7** Technique of cine-phase-contrast on renal arteries in a patient with left renal artery stenosis. Acquisition planes are positioned after each ostium, perpendicular to the arterial lumen (**a**). Considering the surface of the arterial lumen, velocity curves can be converted into flow rate curves. The curve from the left renal artery is damped compared to the right one (**b**) (courtesy of Dr. Stephan O. Schoenberg, Heidelberg)

## 34.3.2 Renal Perfusion

### 34.3.2.1 Ultrasound

Quaia et al. (2009) applied the refilling technique to measure renal perfusion: after the blood concentration of microbubbles reached equilibrium (about 1 min after the beginning of injection), high-transmit power US pulses are sent to destroy the microbubbles filling the renal parenchyma in the imaging volume. By using a low-transmit power insonation, the progressive replenishment of the renal cortex was monitored in real time during breath-holding. A linear relation is assumed between microbubble concentration and echo–SI (Correas et al. 2000). Mathematical models previously proposed to approximate the refill kinetics of tissue after microbubble destruction present several

limitations (Potdevin et al. 2004). In this study the mathematical model used led to a piecewise linear function that has the general properties of the refill curves and took into account the laws of hydrodynamics. However, clinical applications of US-based renal perfusion studies in humans still need to be extended and validated.

### 34.3.2.2 MRI

Renal perfusion parameters, as renal blood volume (RBV) and RBF, can be assessed with MRI either by dynamic contrast-enhanced methods, using Gd-chelates or iron oxide particles, or by water spin-labeling techniques.

## Dynamic MR Imaging

Technical constraints are the same as for GFR measurement. However, acquisition time is shorter, only the first pass being necessary, and breath-holding is usually efficient. If the AIF is not taken into account, semiquantitative parameters as maximal signal change (MSC), time to MSC ($T_{MSC}$), or wash-in and wash-out slopes can be measured for comparison from right to left kidney (Fig. 34.8), from cortex to medulla or from one territory to another, or for follow-up of patients (Michaely et al. 2006, 2007a, b).

As for GFR, absolute quantification requires to take into account the AIF. Then, the calculated concentration–time curves must then be processed using specific mathematical models (Fig. 34.9). The most widely used perfusion model is derived from Peters's model (Vallee et al. 2000), developed for nuclear medicine (Peters et al. 1987). Peters et al. (1987) hypothesized that before leaving the kidney, the contrast agent behaves like microspheres that are trapped in the capillary system during a short-time interval, inferior to the minimal vascular transit time. Calculation of renal perfusion per unit of volume can be extracted from the mathematical expression:

$$RBF \,/\, vol = maxsloperenal \,/\, maxD\big(R1\big)art,$$

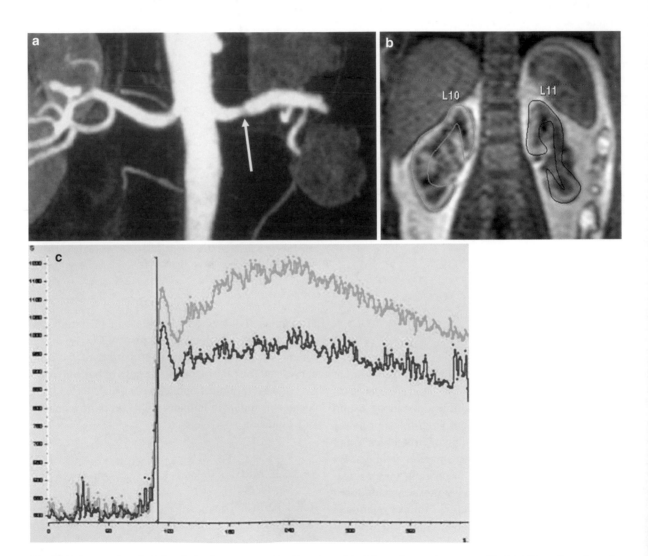

**Fig. 34.8** Asymmetry of renal perfusion in a patient with a dissection of the left renal artery (*arrow*) (**a**). The left kidney shows irregular contours (**b**) and SI–time curves show a slight asymmetry of the ascending slopes and a decreased vascular peak on the left side (**c**)

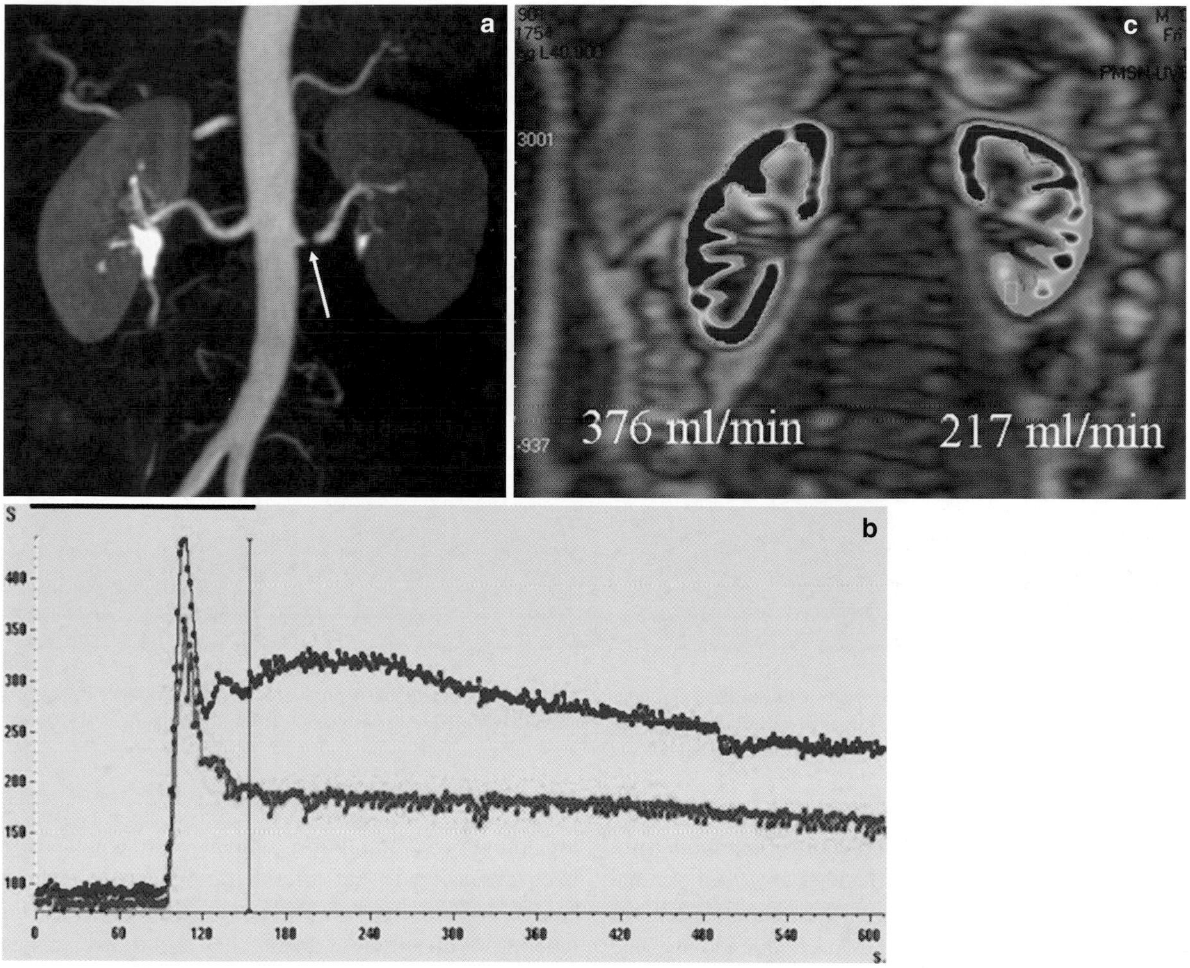

**Fig. 34.9** Quantification of renal perfusion in a patient with left renal artery stenosis (*arrow*) (**a**). SI–time curves show the asymmetry (**b**). By applying a two-compartment model and taking into account the AIF, perfusion maps can be obtained, which demonstrate the asymmetry of vascularization (**c**)

where $\Delta(R1)$art is calculated from the changes in aortic SI using a priori knowledge of the signal-vs.-$R1$ relationship that can be elucidated in vitro using a Gd-filled phantom. With a small bolus of contrast (0.025 mmol/kg) and a T1-weighted gradient-echo sequence, Vallée et al. (2000) were able to measure cortical BF in 16 normal kidneys patients (254±116 mL/min/100 g), decreasing to 109±75 mL/min/100 g in case of RAS and to 51±34 mL/min/100 g in case of renal failure. In animals, values of cortical RBF correlated linearly with reference values, but were nonetheless systematically underestimated (Montet et al. 2003).

Dujardin et al. (2005, 2009b) generalized the tracer kinetic theory from intravascular to diffusible tracers using deconvolution, which is a model-free approach.

From ROI drawn on the aorta and on the renal cortex, tissue concentration–time course has to be deconvolved pixel by pixel with the flow-corrected aortic time course, resulting in an impulse response function (IRF). This method allows getting intrarenal maps of RBF, as maximum of IRF, RBV as the time integral of the IRF over the available time interval, and MTT as the ratio RVD/RBF. They showed a significant negative correlation of RBF and RVD with patient age (Dujardin et al. 2009a).

The same approach can be applied to the measurement of perfusion using iron oxide particles which have a unicompartmental distribution within the kidney. Once injected intravenously as a bolus, they produce dynamic SI changes based on a T2* effect caused by alterations in the local magnetic susceptibility

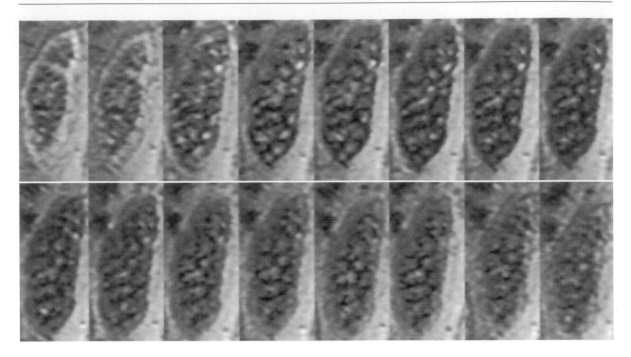

**Fig. 34.10** Perfusion imaging sequence with intravascular contrast agent. Dynamic $T*2$-weighted images of the right (*top*) and left (*bottom*) kidney demonstrate a substantially delayed and decreased enhancement with loss of corticomedullary differentiation (Reprinted with permission from Schoenberg et al. 2003)

(Fig. 34.10). Experimental applications in rabbits subjected to hydronephrosis (Trillaud et al. 1993) or renal artery stenosis (Trillaud et al. 1995) showed that the concentration–time curves of the ischemic kidneys had a lower slope and a higher area under the curve than the normal contralateral kidney. In an experimental model of RAS in dogs with four degrees of stenosis (Schoenberg et al. 2003), an increase of MTT and a decreased rRBF occurred only for severe stenosis above 90%. In patients, a decreased rRBF was noted only for severe stenosis (Fig. 34.3) or in kidney suffering from chronic damage related to other renal diseases.

## Renal Perfusion Using Spin-Labeling

Renal perfusion can alternatively be measured using pulsed arterial spin labeling (or spin-tagging) using endogenous water as a diffusible tracer. With this technique, a perfusion-weighted image can be generated by the subtraction of an image in which inflowing spins have been labeled from an image in which spin labeling has not been performed. Quantitative perfusion maps can then be calculated (in mL/min/100 g of tissue) when T1 of the tissue and efficiency of labeling are known. Several pulse sequence strategies have been described to tag arterial flowing spins, which can be divided into two groups (continuous or pulsed labeling) with different advantages and drawbacks as described in detail by Calamante et al. (1999).

Methods based on pulsed labeling are not compromised by the two major sources of errors seen with continuous labeling techniques (transit time and magnetization transfer). Pulsed labeling can be realized as an echo planar imaging sequence with signal targeting with alternating radiofrequency (EPISTAR) (Edelman et al. 1994). Using this sequence in an experimental model of renal artery stenosis in pigs, Prasad et al. (1997b) showed that a decrease of blood flow was 100% sensitive and specific for detection of 70% renal artery stenoses.

The flow-sensitive alternative inversion recovery (FAIR) (Martirosian et al. 2004) is based on two inversion recovery images, one with a slice-selective inversion (will contain flow information: T1 apparent) and one with a nonselective inversion (assuming that blood and kidney relax at the same rate, it will contain no flow information: T1). Subtraction of both images generates a value directly related to the perfusion. Recently, a technique associating a FAIR preparation and True-FISP data acquisition provided very encouraging results

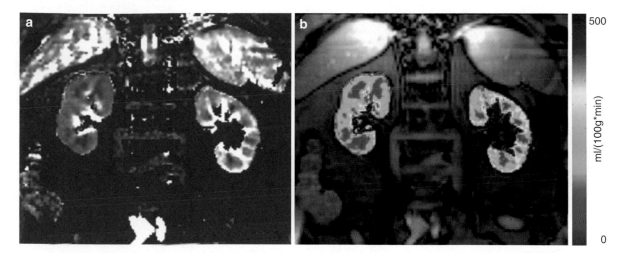

**Fig. 34.11** Mild (30%) left renal artery stenosis and severe (90%) right renal artery stenosis in 70-year-old man. FAIR True-FISP image averaged from 36 data acquisitions after section-selective inversion (**a**). (**b**) Perfusion-weighted map shows differences in perfusion between right (191 mL/100 g/min) and left (270 mL/100 g/min) kidneys. Reprinted with permission from Fenchel et al. (2006)

within the kidneys because of shorter echo time and fewer saturation effects (Fenchel et al. 2006) (Fig. 34.11). On perfusion images, severe RAS (>70% luminal narrowing) could be clearly distinguished from no or mild RAS and moderate RAS (≤70% luminal narrowing) ($p<0.005$), with significant correlations between FAIR perfusion data and grade of stenosis ($r=-0.76$).

## 34.4 Tubular Function

The tubular transit and function of concentration can be used as indirect features of renal dysfunction. Alternatively, we can evaluate either the function of concentration of diffusible Gd-chelates, based on medullary T2*-effect during water reabsorption, or the medullary transit of macromolecular Gd-chelates, based on medullary T1 effect.

### 34.4.1 Intratubular Concentration of Diffusible Gd-Chelate

When using an unspoiled gradient-echo sequence (to maintain residual transverse magnetization resulting in a T1/T2*-weighting), with a standard dose of Gd-chelate, the high concentration of Gd reached inside the kidney is responsible for a paradoxical signal drop (T2* effect), observed approximately at 30–40 s after the beginning of the cortical enhancement (Fig. 34.12). The predominant site of signal drop is in the medulla, where the tubular concentration of urine increases (by water reabsorption), thereby providing a typical medullary phase with a centripetal progression, which has been extensively described in rabbits (Carvlin et al. 1989; Choyke et al. 1989). The strength and delay of medullary signal changes depend on sequence parameters and on physiological parameters, such as hydration and renal function, but are normally symmetrical between both kidneys. In experimental nephropathies with severe renal insufficiency, the signal reversal in the medulla disappeared (Carvlin et al. 1987; Frank et al. 1989). In patients, this duration has been shown as a rough measure for SKGFR and has in fact been shown to correlate significantly with the creatinine clearance (Krestin et al. 1992). This relationship may become important in kidney diseases involving unilateral impairment, such as unilateral ureteral obstruction (Fichtner et al. 1994; Semelka et al. 1990), renal lithotripsy (Krestin et al. 1993), or renal artery stenosis (Tsushima et al. 1997).

### 34.4.2 Intratubular Transit of Macromolecular Gd-Chelate (T1 Effect)

Kobayashi et al. (2002, 2004) have developed new dendrimer-based macromolecular contrast agents

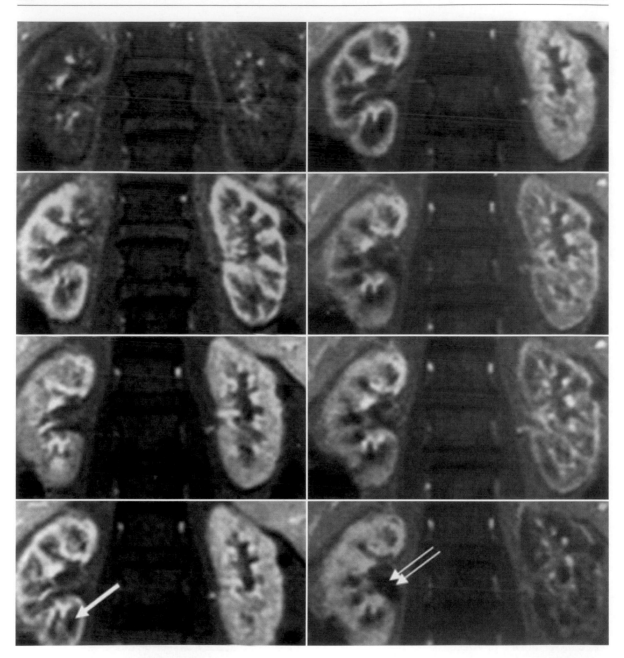

**Fig. 34.12** Dynamic Gd-enhanced MR imaging of the kidneys, with T2*w sequence, in a patient with severe left renal artery stenosis, before (**a**) and after (**b**) captopril administration (from *top-to-bottom* then *left-to-right*). (**a**) Before captopril, the tubular phase (*single arrow*) and excretion of contrast medium within renal collecting system (*double arrows*) are symmetrical. (**b**) After captopril, neither tubular phase nor excretion is visible in the left kidney (Reprinted with permission from Grenier et al. 1996)

(<8 nm in diameter and <60 kD of molecular weight), which accumulate in the renal tubules and allow visualization of structural and functional renal damage. These agents are concentrated in proximal straight tubules in the medullary rays and outer stripe of the outer medulla. The parenchyma demonstrates a layered appearance with alternating light and dark bands: (1) a bright band in the subcapsular cortex, (2) a dark band in the deep cortex, (3) a bright band in the outer stripe of the outer medulla, (4) a dark band in the

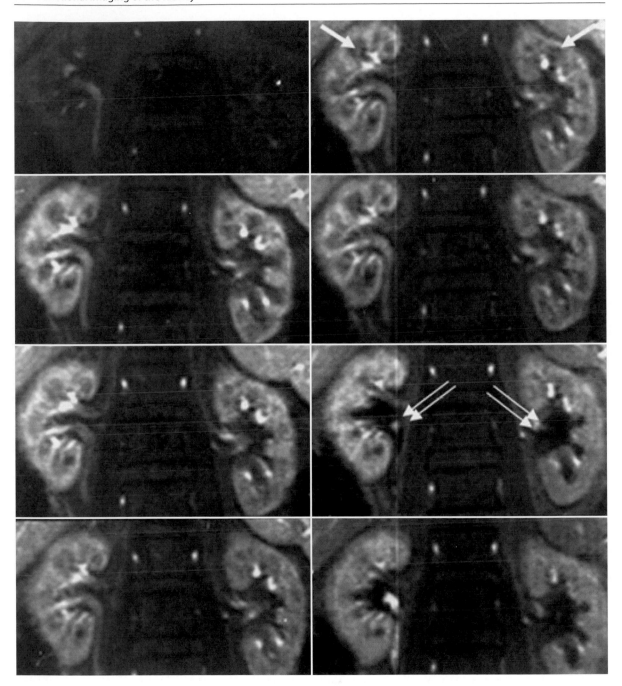

**Fig. 34.12** (continued)

inner stripe of the outer medulla, and (5) a bright inner medulla. In models of renal ischemia (cisplatin injection and ischemia-reperfusion), mildly damaged kidneys did not develop the bright band in the outer stripe and excretion was delayed, and severely damaged kidneys showed a prolonged enhancement of the superficial cortex with a low and delayed medullary enhancement. Intensity of these changes was correlated with severity or duration of ischemia and with degree of renal dysfunction. Therefore, this agent could be used in animals as a biomarker of acute tubular ischemic disorder.

## 34.5  Urinary Excretion and Renal Transit Time

In acute or chronic obstruction, functional information can estimate the severity of renal impairment and help making differentiation between nonobstructed dilated collecting system and real obstruction. Nuclear medicine techniques are routinely used for these purposes in clinical practice. MRI has the ability to associate functional data and morphological information on the renal parenchyma and collecting system. Rorhschneider et al. in an experimental model of urinary obstruction (2000a), then in patients (Rohrschneider et al. 2002, 2003), showed that, beside the split renal function estimation, classical criteria used in scintigraphy for obstruction could also be used with MRI. More recently, the renal transit time measured between the vascular enhancement of the cortex and the appearance of Gd within the ureter at the level or below the lower pole of the kidney showed good agreement with scintigraphy (Fig. 34.13).

## 34.6  Angiotensin Converting Enzyme (ACE) Inhibitor-Sensitized MR Renography

ACE inhibitors, such as captopril, decrease the synthesis of angiotensin II and block its vasoconstrictor-stimulating effect, mostly on the efferent arterioles. This block produces a decrease in hydrostatic pressure within the glomerulus and a decrease in filtration on the side of the stenosis. The principle of the test is to image the renal elimination of a tracer before and after administration of captopril to detect captopril-induced functional changes. A positive test demonstrates the diagnosis of «functional stenoses» producing renovascular hypertension. This test has been coupled with scintigraphy and, more recently, with dynamic MR.

Using the effects of tubular concentration on T1/T2* images in patients, the normal medullary phase was delayed or suppressed by captopril on the side of

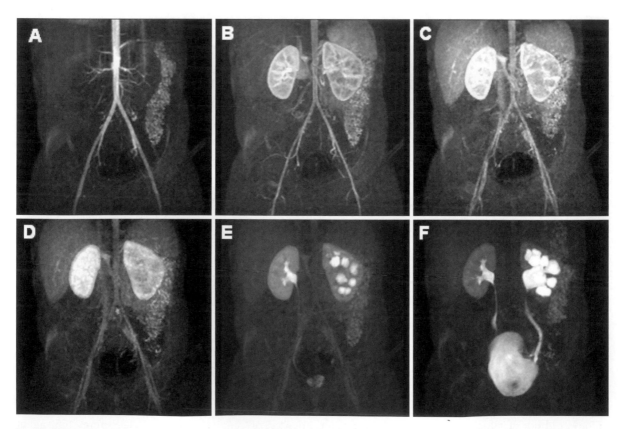

**Fig. 34.13** Renal transit time in a child with ureteral obstruction on the left side: each image is a maximum intensity projection (MIP) of dynamic volumes obtained at six time points: approximately 30 s (**a**), 1 min (**b**), 90 s (**c**), 2 min (**d**), 3 min (**e**), and 12 min (**f**) after injection. The right ureter is opacified in (**e**). The left ureter is opacified only lately (**f**). (Courtesy of Richard Jones, Emory University School of Medicine, Atlanta, USA)

significant stenosis (Grenier et al. 1996) (Fig. 34.12). These MR results were concordant with scintigraphy.

A three-compartment model with a double bolus technique (before and after ACE inhibitors) was applied recently to 18 hypertensive patients without renovascular disease and ten with significant renal artery stenosis, showing minimal systematic difference in GFR measurements in the first group and a significantly decreased GFR in stenotic kidneys (Zhang et al. 2009).

## 34.7 Intrarenal Oxygenation

Under normal conditions, the medullary partial pressure of oxygen is low (10–20 mmHg) compared to the cortex (50 mmHg) (Brezis and Rosen 1995). This medullary hypoxia is related to a low blood flow and high

oxygen consumption due to active water and sodium reabsorption by $Na^+-K^+$-ATPase pumps along the thick ascending limb of the Henle loop, which are located in the outer medulla (Brezis and Rosen 1995). An increased tubular work such as that caused by diabetes or unilateral nephrectomy or a decreased medullary perfusion such as that induced by contrast nephropathy can easily shift the balance toward hypoxia.

Gradient-echo sequences with several TE values showed a decrease in intrarenal signal within the medulla and allowed quantifying intrarenal $R2^*$ (Prasad et al. 1996, 1997a). These SI changes were related to variations in intrarenal oxygenation based on changes in the deoxyhemoglobin concentration (BOLD (blood oxygen level dependent) effect) (Fig. 34.14). $R2^*$ values are linearly correlated with $pO_2$ values, as measured with microelectrodes (Pedersen et al. 2005b). Higher fields

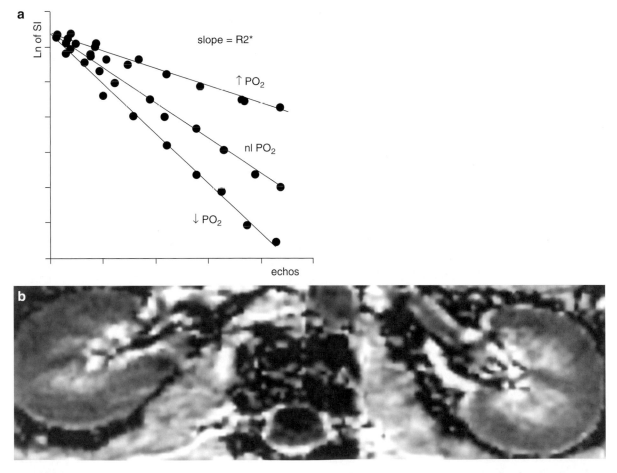

**Fig. 34.14** Principle of BOLD acquisition in the kidney. The $R2^*$ is greater when the tissue $pO_2$ is low and lower when it is high (**a**). A T2*-weighted multiecho gradient-echo sequence allows to calculate a $R2^*$ map showing a higher $R2^*$ value within medulla, here obtained at 3T (**b**) (From Li et al, 2004b)

strength, as 3 T magnets, provide a higher signal-to-noise ratio, a better spatial resolution, and a higher T2* effect (Li et al. 2004b). But, in term of reproducibility, the intrasubject coefficient of variation is 3–4% (Simon-Zoula et al. 2006), rising to 12% at long term (Li et al. 2004a).

With this method, medullary oxygenation was shown in rats to be reduced by inhibition of the synthesis of prostaglandin (Prasad and Epstein 1999), inhibition of nitric oxide, and intravenous injection of radiocontrast agents (Prasad et al. 2001). In diabetic nephropathy, the highest $R_2$* was found within the outer stripe of the outer medulla (Ries et al. 2001a). In a pig model of unilateral dynamic renal artery stenosis, Juillard et al. (2004) showed that $O_2$ consumption decreased and $R2$* increased (in cortex and medulla) proportionally to the degree of reduction of RBF.

In humans, Prasad et al. (1997a) showed that the effect was decreased by water diuresis (at least in young individuals) and by furosemide, which inhibits active reabsorptive transport in medullary tubules (Brezis et al. 1994). Diabetic patients without microalbuminuria, hypertension, or renal insufficiency presented, compared to a matched control group, no significant improvement of medullary oxygenation after water load (Epstein et al. 2002). More recently, Textor et al. (2008) reported an increase of $R2$* in normal-sized kidneys downstream of high-grade stenosis. But the prognostic value of this measurement has not been established yet. In kidney transplants, the medullary $R2$* is reported to be lower than control subjects (Thoeny et al. 2006), which could be explained by a reduced active reabsorption of sodium. In acute rejection, medullary $R2$* appears reduced when compared to normally functioning grafts and grafts with acute tubular necrosis (Han et al. 2008; Sadowski et al. 2005).

## 34.8 Renal Diffusion

Water transport is the predominant phenomenon throughout the kidney due to its role in water reabsorption and concentration-dilution function. These movements are mainly located within the tubular cells. Consequently, useful insights into the mechanisms of various renal diseases such as chronic renal failure, renal artery stenosis, and ureteral obstruction may be obtained by measuring the diffusion characteristics of the kidney. However, diffusion imaging is a challenging technique within the kidney due to the extreme sensitivity of diffusion-weighted sequences to several sources of artifacts.

The attenuation of SI observed on diffusion-weighted sequences depends on two factors. First, it depends on the molecular movements within the intra- and extracellular spaces that are determined by temperature, and biological barriers present in the tissue (cellular membranes, fibers, organelles, macromolecules etc.). Second, it depends on "external" factors like blood perfusion, magnetic susceptibility, cardiac pulsation rate, and respiratory movements (Schaefer et al. 2000). Many difficulties remain patent for abdominal applications, such as susceptibility artifacts originated from bowel gas, peristaltic and respiratory movements, and arterial pulsatility. Breath-hold or respiratory-triggered sequences significantly improves the accuracy and the reproducibility of ADC values in kidneys (Murtz et al. 2002). However, cardiac triggering is usually omitted due to the increased acquisition time. Low $b$-values (<200 s/mm$^2$) generate a higher signal-to-noise ratio and higher ADC values due to an increased contribution of factors independent of the molecular diffusion (as perfusion and flow effects). High $b$-values (>600 s/mm$^2$) decrease the signal-to-noise ratio, increase the acquisition time, but improve the precision of measurements. Therefore, it is recommended, for kidney imaging, to use several $b$-values between 0 and 800 s/mm$^2$ (Norris 2001). Normal kidneys show an oriented structure generating an anisotropic water movement (i.e., predominant in one direction), especially within medulla (Ries et al. 2001b). Therefore, it is necessary to encode at least three directions of space for each $b$-value to measure the trace of the diffusion tensor (ADC-trace) (Fig. 34.15).

In normal kidneys, ADC-trace values are higher in the cortex than in the medulla (Ries et al. 2001b). Renal ADC values are lower in neonates and increase progressively with age, with the largest increase during the first years of life (Jones and Grattan-Smith 2003). In acute renal disease, ADC values are reported to be decreased (Namimoto et al. 1999), but they are increased in the medulla in acute ureteral obstruction (Thoeny et al. 2009). In an experimental model of acute diabetic nephropathy, we showed that the regional ADC values decreased in the outer medulla, where ischemic tubular cell lesions occur (Ries et al. 2001a). A decrease of ADC is nonspecific and was

**Fig. 34.15** Diffusion imaging of a kidney transplant with encoding of 3 *b*-values in three directions. The *b*-value is 0 in (**a**), 200 in (**b**), and 500 in (**c**). The ADC-trace (**d**) shows a higher value in the cortex than in the medulla

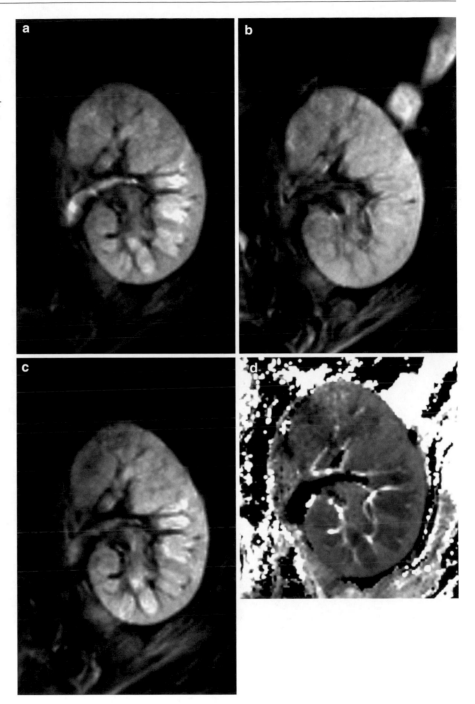

reported in CKD (Thoeny et al. 2005), renal artery stenosis (Namimoto et al. 1999; Yildirim et al. 2008), and ureteral obstruction (Muller et al. 1994; Thoeny et al. 2005). In native (Namimoto et al. 1999) and transplanted (Thoeny et al. 2006) kidneys, ADC values are highly correlated with serum creatinine levels and correlated with the split renal function (Xu et al. 2007).

Besides the measurement of ADC values, it is possible to measure the degree of anisotropy within the renal compartments by using sequences of diffusion tensor imaging (DTI). A minimum of six encoding directions are necessary for that purpose. In normal kidneys, it was shown that the value of fractional anisotropy, which is independent of the *b*-values, was higher in the medulla (0.39±11) than in the cortex (0.22±12) (Ries et al. 2001b) (Fig. 34.16). Postprocessing techniques of tractography can be applied on these data, showing a radial orientation of the diffusion tensor in the medullary compartments (Kim et al. 2008; Notohamiprodjo et al. 2008) (Fig. 34.17).

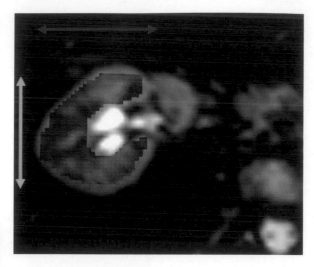

**Fig. 34.17** DTI of a kidney transplant showing, after tractography postprocessing, the main orientation of the intrarenal anisotropy around the sinus

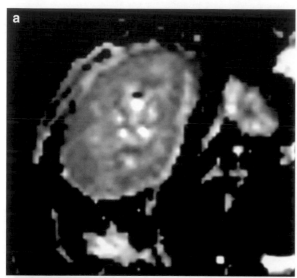

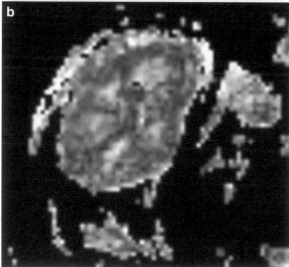

**Fig. 34.16** Diffusion tensor imaging (DTI) of a kidney transplant with encoding of 3 *b*-values in six directions. ADC-trace mapping (**a**) and corresponding map of the fractional anisotropy (FA) (**b**) with higher values in the medulla

# References

Annet L, Hermoye L, Peeters F et al. (2004) Glomerular filtration rate: assessment with dynamic contrast-enhanced MRI and a cortical-compartment model in the rabbit kidney. J Magn Reson Imaging 20:843–849

Boss A, Martirosian P, Gehrmann M et al.(2007) Quantitative assessment of glomerular filtration rate with MR gadolinium slope clearance measurements: a phase I trial. Radiology 242:783–790

Brezis M, Agmon Y, Epstein FH (1994) Determinants of intrarenal oxygenation. I. Effects of diuretics. Am J Physiol 267: F1059–F1062

Brezis M, Rosen S (1995) Hypoxia of the renal medulla–its implications for disease. N Engl J Med 332:647–655

Calamante F, Thomas DL, Pell GS et al. (1999) Measuring cerebral blood flow using magnetic resonance imaging techniques. J Cereb Blood Flow Metab 19:701–735

Carvlin MJ, Arger PH, Kundel HL et al. (1987) Acute tubular necrosis: use of gadolinium-DTPA and fast MR imaging to evaluate renal function in the rabbit. J Comput Assist Tomogr 11:488–495

Carvlin MJ, Arger PH, Kundel HL et al. (1989) Use of Gd-DTPA and fast gradient-echo and spin-echo MR imaging to demonstrate renal function in the rabbit. Radiology 170:705–711

Chade AR, Rodriguez-Porcel M, Rippentrop SJ et al. (2003) Angiotensin II AT1 receptor blockade improves renal perfusion in hypercholesterolemia. Am J Hypertens 16:111–115

Choyke PL, Austin HA, Frank JA et al. (1992) Hydrated clearance of gadolinium-DTPA as a measurement of glomerular filtration rate. Kidney Int 41:1595–1598

Choyke PL, Frank JA, Girton ME et al. (1989) Dynamic Gd-DTPA-enhanced MR imaging of the kidney:experimental results. Radiology 170:713–720

Choyke PL, Kobayashi H (2006) Functional magnetic resonance imaging of the kidney using macromolecular contrast agents. Abdom Imaging 31:224–231

Correas JM, Bridal L, Lesavre A et al. (2001) Ultrasound contrast agents: properties, principles of action, tolerance, and artifacts. Eur Radiol 11:1316–1328

Correas JM, Burns PN, Lai X et al. (2000) Infusion versus bolus of an ultrasound contrast agent: in vivo dose-response measurements of BR1. Invest Radiol 35:72–79

Coulam CH, Lee JH, Wedding KL et al. (2002) Noninvasive measurement of extraction fraction and single-kidney glomerular filtration rate with MR imaging in swine with surgically created renal arterial stenoses. Radiology 223:76–82

Daghini E, Juillard L, Haas JA et al. (2007) Comparison of mathematic models for assessment of glomerular filtration rate with electron-beam CT in pigs. Radiology 242:417–424

de Senneville BD, Mendichovszky IA, Roujol S et al. (2008) Improvement of MRI-functional measurement with automatic movement correction in native and transplanted kidneys. J Magn Reson Imaging 28:970–978

Debatin JF, Ting RH, Wegmuller H et al. (1994) Renal artery blood flow: quantitation with phase-contrast MR imaging with and without breath holding. Radiology 190:371–378

Dujardin M, Luypaert R, Sourbron S et al. (2009a) Age dependence of T1 perfusion MRI-based hemodynamic parameters in human kidneys. J Magn Reson Imaging 29:398–403

Dujardin M, Luypaert R, Vandenbroucke F et al. (2009b) Combined T1-based perfusion MRI and MR angiography in kidney: first experience in normals and pathology. Eur J Radiol 69:542–549

Dujardin M, Sourbron S, Luypaert R et al. (2005) Quantification of renal perfusion and function on a voxel-by-voxel basis: a feasibility study. Magn Reson Med 54:841–849

Dumoulin CL, Buonocore MH, Opsahl LR et al. (1994) Noninvasive measurement of renal hemodynamic functions using gadolinium enhanced magnetic resonance imaging. Magn Reson Med 32:370–378

Edelman RR, Siewert B, Darby DG et al. (1994) Qualitative mapping of cerebral blood flow and functional localization with echo-planar MR imaging and signal targeting with alternating radio frequency. Radiology 192:513–520

Epstein FH, Veves A, Prasad PV (2002) Effect of diabetes on renal medullary oxygenation during water diuresis. Diabetes Care 25:575–578

Fenchel M, Martirosian P, Langanke J et al. (2006) Perfusion MR imaging with FAIR true FISP spin labeling in patients with and without renal artery stenosis: initial experience. Radiology 238:1013–1021

Fichtner J, Spielman D, Herfkens R et al. (1994) Ultrafast contrast enhanced magnetic resonance imaging of congenital hydronephrosis in a rat model. J Urol 152:682–687

Frank JA, Choyke PL, Girton ME et al. (1989) Gadolinium-DTPA enhanced dynamic MR imaging in the evaluation of cisplatinum nephrotoxicity. J Comput Assist Tomogr 13:448–459

Grenier N, Basseau F, Ries M et al. (2003) Functional MRI of the kidney. Abdominal imaging 28:164–175

Grenier N, Mendichovszky I, de Senneville BD et al. (2008) Measurement of glomerular filtration rate with magnetic resonance imaging: principles, limitations, and expectations. Semin Nucl Med 38:47–55

Grenier N, Trillaud H, Combe C et al. (1996) Diagnosis of renovascular hypertension: feasibility of captopril-sensitized dynamic MR imaging and comparison with captopril scintigraphy. AJR Am J Roentgenol 166:835–843

Hackstein N, Cengiz H, Rau WS (2002) Contrast media clearance in a single kidney measured on multiphasic helical CT: results in 50 patients without acute renal disorder. AJR Am J Roentgenol 178:111–118

Hackstein N, Heckrodt J, Rau WS (2003) Measurement of single-kidney glomerular filtration rate using a contrast-enhanced dynamic gradient-echo sequence and the Rutland-Patlak plot technique. J Magn Reson Imaging 18:714–725

Han F, Xiao W, Xu Y et al. (2008) The significance of BOLD MRI in differentiation between renal transplant rejection and acute tubular necrosis. Nephrol Dial Transplant 23:2666–2672

Hermoye L, Annet L, Lemmerling P et al. (2004) Calculation of the renal perfusion and glomerular filtration rate from the renal impulse response obtained with MRI. Magn Reson Med 51:1017–1025

Jones RA, Grattan-Smith JD (2003) Age dependence of the renal apparent diffusion coefficient in children. Pediatr Radiol 33.850–854

Juillard L, Lerman LO, Kruger DG et al. (2004) Blood oxygen level-dependent measurement of acute intra-renal ischemia. Kidney Int 65:944–950

Kim S, Naik M, Sigmund E et al. (2008) Diffusion-weighted MR imaging of the kidneys and the urinary tract. Magnetic Reson Imaging Clin N Am 16:585–596; vii-viii

Kobayashi H, Jo SK, Kawamoto S et al. (2004) Polyamine dendrimer-based MRI contrast agents for functional kidney imaging to diagnose acute renal failure. J Magn Reson Imaging 20:512–518

Kobayashi H, Kawamoto S, Jo SK et al. (2002) Renal tubular damage detected by dynamic micro-MRI with a dendrimer-based magnetic resonance contrast agent. Kidney Int 61:1980–1985

Krestin G, Fischbach R, Vorreuther R et al. (1993) Alterations in renal morphology and function after ESWL therapy: evaluation with dynamic contrast-enhanced MRI. Eur Radiol 3:227–233

Krestin G, Schuhmann-Giampieri G, Huastein J et al. (1992) Functional dynamic MRI, pharmacokinetics and safety of Gd-DTPA in patients with impaired renal function. Eur Radiol 2:16–23

Laurent D, Poirier K, Wasvary J et al. (2002) Effect of essential hypertension on kidney function as measured in rat by dynamic MRI. Magn Reson Med 47:127–134

Lee VS, Rusinek H, Bokacheva L et al. (2007) Renal function measurements from MR renography and a simplified multicompartmental model. Am J Physiol 292:F1548–F1559

Lee VS, Rusinek H, Noz ME et al. (2003) Dynamic three-dimensional MR renography for the measurement of single kidney function: initial experience. Radiology 227:289–294

Li LP, Storey P, Pierchala L et al. (2004a) Evaluation of the reproducibility of intrarenal R2* and DeltaR2* measurements following administration of furosemide and during waterload. J Magn Reson Imaging 19:610–616

Li LP, Vu AT, Li BS et al. (2004b) Evaluation of intrarenal oxygenation by BOLD MRI at 3.0 T. J Magn Reson Imaging 20:901–904

Liu X, Primak AN, Krier JD et al. (2009) Renal perfusion and hemodynamics: accurate in vivo determination at CT with a 10-fold decrease in radiation dose and HYPR noise reduction. Radiology 253:98–105

Lucidarme O, Franchi-Abella S, Correas JM et al. (2003a) Blood flow quantification with contrast-enhanced US: "entrance in the section" phenomenon–phantom and rabbit study. Radiology 228:473–479

Lucidarme O, Kono Y, Corbeil J et al. (2003b) Validation of ultrasound contrast destruction imaging for flow quantification. Ultrasound Med Biol 29:1697–1704

Martirosian P, Klose U, Mader I et al. (2004) FAIR true-FISP perfusion imaging of the kidneys. Magn Reson Med 51:353–361

Mendichovszky I, Pedersen M, Frokiaer J et al. (2008) How accurate is dynamic contrast-enhanced MRI in the assessment of renal glomerular filtration rate? A critical appraisal. J Magn Reson Imaging 27:925–931

Michaely HJ, Kramer H, Oesingmann N et al. (2007a) Intraindividual comparison of MR-renal perfusion imaging at 1.5 T and 3.0 T. Invest Radiol 42:406–411

Michaely HJ, Kramer H, Oesingmann N et al. (2007b) Semiquantitative assessment of first-pass renal perfusion at 1.5 T: comparison of 2D saturation recovery sequences with and without parallel imaging. AJR Am J Roentgenol 188:919–926

Michaely HJ, Schoenberg SO, Oesingmann N et al. (2006) Renal artery stenosis: functional assessment with dynamic MR perfusion measurements–feasibility study. Radiology 238:586–596

Michoux N, Vallee JP, Pechere-Bertschi A et al. (2006) Analysis of contrast-enhanced MR images to assess renal function. Magma 19:167–179

Montet X, Ivancevic MK, Belenger J et al. (2003) Noninvasive measurement of absolute renal perfusion by contrast medium-enhanced magnetic resonance imaging. Invest Radiol 38:584–592

Mule S, De Cesare A, Lucidarme O et al. (2008) Regularized estimation of contrast agent attenuation to improve the imaging of microbubbles in small animal studies. Ultrasound Med Biol 34:938–948

Muller MF, Prasad PV, Bimmler D et al. (1994) Functional imaging of the kidney by means of measurement of the apparent diffusion coefficient. Radiology 193:711–715

Murtz P, Flacke S, Traber F et al. (2002) Abdomen: diffusion-weighted MR imaging with pulse-triggered single-shot sequences. Radiology 224:258–264

Mustert BR, Williams DM, Prince MR (1998) In vitro model of arterial stenosis: correlation of MR signal dephasing and trans-stenotic pressure gradients. Magn Reson Imaging 16:301–310

Namimoto T, Yamashita Y, Mitsuzaki K et al. (1999) Measurement of the apparent diffusion coefficient in diffuse renal disease by diffusion-weighted echo-planar MR imaging. J Magn Reson Imaging 9:832–837

Niendorf ER, Grist TM, Frayne R et al. (1997) Rapid measurement of Gd-DTPA extraction fraction in a dialysis system using echo-planar imaging. Med Phys 24:1907–1913

Niendorf ER, Grist TM, Lee FT Jr et al. (1998) Rapid in vivo measurement of single-kidney extraction fraction and glomerular filtration rate with MR imaging. Radiology 206:791–798

Niendorf ER, Santyr GE, Brazy PC et al. (1996) Measurement of Gd-DTPA dialysis clearance rates by using a look-locker imaging technique. Magn Reson Med 36:571–578

Norris DG (2001) Implications of bulk motion for diffusion-weighted imaging experiments: effects, mechanisms, and solutions. J Magn Reson Imaging 13:486–495

Notohamiprodjo M, Glaser C, Herrmann KA et al. (2008) Diffusion tensor imaging of the kidney with parallel imaging: initial clinical experience. Invest Radiol 43:677–685

Patlak CS, Blasberg RG, Fenstermacher JD (1983) Graphical evaluation of blood-to-brain transfer constants from multiple-time uptake data. J Cereb Blood Flow Metab 3:1–7

Pedersen M, Dissing T, Deding D et al. (2005a) MR renography based on contrast-enhanced T1-mapping. In: International Society for Magnetic Resonance in Medicine, Medicine ISfMRi (ed), Miami, USA, pp 526

Pedersen M, Dissing TH, Morkenborg J et al. (2005b) Validation of quantitative BOLD MRI measurements in kidney: application to unilateral ureteral obstruction. Kidney Int 67:2305–2312

Pedersen M, Shi Y, Anderson P et al. (2004) Quantitation of differential renal blood flow and renal function using dynamic contrast-enhanced MRI in rats. Magn Reson Med 51:510–517

Peters AM, Brown J, Hartnell GG et al. (1987) Non-invasive measurement of renal blood flow with 99mTc DTPA: comparison with radiolabelled microspheres. Cardiovasc Res 21:830–834

Potdevin TC, Fowlkes JB, Moskalik AP et al. (2004) Analysis of refill curve shape in ultrasound contrast agent studies. Med Phys 31:623–632

Prasad PV, Chen Q, Goldfarb JW et al. (1997a) Breath-hold R2* mapping with a multiple gradient-recalled echo sequence: application to the evaluation of intrarenal oxygenation. J Magn Reson Imaging 7:1163–1165

Prasad PV, Edelman RR, Epstein FH (1996) Noninvasive evaluation of intrarenal oxygenation with BOLD MRI. Circulation 94:3271–3275

Prasad PV, Epstein FH (1999) Changes in renal medullary pO2 during water diuresis as evaluated by blood oxygenation level-dependent magnetic resonance imaging: effects of aging and cyclooxygenase inhibition. Kidney Int 55:294–298

Prasad PV, Kim D, Kaiser AM et al. (1997b) Noninvasive comprehensive characterization of renal artery stenosis by combination of STAR angiography and EPISTAR perfusion imaging. Magn Reson Med 38:776–787

Prasad PV, Priatna A, Spokes K et al. (2001) Changes in intrarenal oxygenation as evaluated by BOLD MRI in a rat kidney model for radiocontrast nephropathy. J Magn Reson Imaging 13:744–747

Prigent A (2008) Monitoring renal function and limitations of renal function tests. Semin Nucl Med 38:32–46

Quaia E, Nocentini A, Torelli L (2009) Assessment of a new mathematical model for the computation of numerical parameters related to renal cortical blood flow and fractional blood volume by contrast-enhanced ultrasound. Ultrasound Med Biol 35:616–627

Ries M, Basseau F, Tyndal B et al. (2001a) Diffusion and BOLD-contrast imaging in the kidneys of diabetic rats. In: Internation Society of Magnetic Resonance in Medicine. International Society of Magnetic Resonance in Medicine, Glasgow, p 362

Ries M, Jones RA, Basseau F et al. (2001b) Diffusion tensor MRI of the human kidney. J Magn Reson Imaging 14: 42–49

Rohrschneider WK, Becker K, Hoffend J et al. (2000a) Combined static-dynamic MR urography for the simultaneous evaluation of morphology and function in urinary tract obstruction. II. Findings in experimentally induced ureteric stenosis. Pediatr Radiol 30:523–532

Rohrschneider WK, Haufe S, Clorius JH et al. (2003) MR to assess renal function in children. Eur Radiol 13:1033–1045

Rohrschneider WK, Haufe S, Wiesel M et al. (2002) Functional and morphologic evaluation of congenital urinary tract dilatation by using combined static-dynamic MR urography: findings in kidneys with a single collecting system. Radiology 224:683–694

Rohrschneider WK, Hoffend J, Becker K et al. (2000b) Combined static-dynamic MR urography for the simultaneous evaluation of morphology and function in urinary tract obstruction. I. Evaluation of the normal status in an animal model. Pediatr Radiol 30:511–522

Rusinek H, Lee VS, Johnson G (2001) Optimal dose of Gd-DTPA in dynamic MR studies. Magn Reson Med 46:312–316

Sadowski EA, Fain SB, Alford SK et al. (2005) Assessment of acute renal transplant rejection with blood oxygen level-dependent MR imaging: initial experience. Radiology 236:911–919

Schaefer PW, Grant PE, Gonzalez RG (2000) Diffusion-weighted MR imaging of the brain. Radiology 217: 331–345

Schoenberg SO, Aumann S, Just A et al. (2003) Quantification of renal perfusion abnormalities using an intravascular contrast agent (part 2): results in animals and humans with renal artery stenosis. Magn Reson Med 49:288–298

Schoenberg SO, Just A, Bock M et al. (1997a) Noninvasive analysis of renal artery blood flow dynamics with MR cine phase-contrast flow measurements. Am J Physiol 272: H2477–H2484

Schoenberg SO, Knopp MV, Bock M et al. (1997b) Renal artery stenosis: grading of hemodynamic changes with cine phase-contrast MR blood flow measurements. Radiology 203:45–53

Schoenberg SO, Knopp MV, Londy F et al. (2002) Morphologic and functional magnetic resonance imaging of renal artery stenosis: a multireader tricenter study. J Am Soc Nephrol 13:158–169

Semelka RC, Hricak H, Tomei E et al. (1990) Obstructive nephropathy: evaluation with dynamic Gd-DTPA-enhanced MR imaging. Radiology 175:797–803

Simon-Zoula SC, Hofmann L, Giger A et al. (2006) Non-invasive monitoring of renal oxygenation using BOLD-MRI: a reproducibility study. NMR Biomed 19:84–89

Textor SC, Glockner JF, Lerman LO et al. (2008) The use of magnetic resonance to evaluate tissue oxygenation in renal artery stenosis. J Am Soc Nephrol 19:780–788

Thoeny HC, Binser T, Roth B et al. (2009) Noninvasive assessment of acute ureteral obstruction with diffusion-weighted MR imaging: a prospective study. Radiology 252:721–728

Thoeny HC, De Keyzer F, Oyen RH et al. (2005) Diffusion-weighted MR imaging of kidneys in healthy volunteers and patients with parenchymal diseases: initial experience. Radiology 235:911–917

Thoeny HC, Zumstein D, Simon-Zoula S et al. (2006) Functional evaluation of transplanted kidneys with diffusion-weighted and BOLD MR imaging: initial experience. Radiology 241: 812–821

Trillaud H, Degreze P, Mesplede Y et al. (1995) Evaluation of experimentally induced renal hypoperfusion using iron oxide particles and fast magnetic resonance imaging. Acad Radiol 2:293–299

Trillaud H, Grenier N, Degreze P et al. (1993) First-pass evaluation of renal perfusion with TurboFLASH MR imaging and superparamagnetic iron oxide particles. J Magn Reson Imaging 3:83–91

Tsushima Y, Murakami T, Kuruma H et al. (1997) T2*-weighted dynamic MR imaging in renal artery or vein stenosis. AJR Am J Roentgenol 168:1041–1043

Vallee JP, Lazeyras F, Khan HG et al. (2000) Absolute renal blood flow quantification by dynamic MRI and Gd-DTPA. Eur Radiol 10:1245–1252

Xu Y, Wang X, Jiang X (2007) Relationship between the renal apparent diffusion coefficient and glomerular filtration rate: preliminary experience. J Magn Reson Imaging 26: 678–681

Yildirim E, Kirbas I, Teksam M et al. (2008) Diffusion-weighted MR imaging of kidneys in renal artery stenosis. Eur J Radiol 65:148–153

Zhang JL, Rusinek H, Bokacheva L et al. (2009) Angiotensin-converting enzyme inhibitor-enhanced MR renography: repeated measures of GFR and RPF in hypertensive patients. Am J Physiol 296:F884–F891

# Molecular Imaging and Tumoural Antigen Targeting

# 35

## Cristina Nanni and Stefano Fanti

## Contents

**Abstract**

> In vivo molecular imaging includes a range of techniques that are aimed at macroscopically and in vivo visualising molecular events at a cellular level.

> Small animal positron emission tomography (SA-PET), small animal single photon emission tomography (SA-SPET), small animal magnetic resonance imaging and optical imaging are the most interesting and are based on the use of targeted probes binding to specific molecules (receptors or ligands) or those that are included in specific metabolic processes.

> Those techniques are very expensive, but meet a wider and wider employment since they have the advantage of analysing the same subject over time.

> The application of those pre-clinical imaging techniques for the basic study of kidney diseases is still an emerging field. This chapter will approach the use of pre-clinical molecular imaging and tumoural antigen targeting in kidney diseases.

## 35.1 Pre-Clinical Molecular Imaging

The term Molecular Imaging includes a group of imaging techniques aimed at visualising molecular events at a cellular level. This can be in vivo done by injecting in a laboratory animal model or in a clinical patient a probe that is bound to a signal element, making it detectable by a specific machine in a non-invasive and repeatable procedure.

C. Nanni (✉) and S. Fanti
UO Medicina Nucleare, Azienda Ospedaliero-Universitaria di
Bologna Policlinico S. Orsola-Malpighi, Via Massarenti 9,
40141 Bologna, Italy
e-mail: cristina.nanni@aosp.bo.it

E. Quaia (ed.), *Radiological Imaging of the Kidney*,
Medical Radiology, DOI: 10.1007/978-3-540-87597-0_35, © Springer-Verlag Berlin Heidelberg 2011

The kind of probe chosen is related to the molecular event that must be detected. For example, it is possible to use "aspecific probes" (like 18F-FDG for PET imaging) aimed at the visualisation of a metabolic over-expression (18F-FDG highlights cellular glucose hyper consumption) or more "specific probes" like receptorial ligands or antibodies.

The signal element, on the other side, determines the imaging machine. The most used in vivo pre-clinical molecular imaging techniques are the small animal positron emission tomography (SA-PET), which is based on positron emitter isotopes as signal elements; the small animal magnetic resonance imaging (SA-MRI), based on paramagnetic contrast agents and atomic polarisation; the optical imaging (OI), based on fluorescence or bioluminescence and the small animal single photon emission tomography (SA-SPECT), based on gamma emitter isotopes (Levin 2005).

Besides these techniques, it is possible to image small animals also with dedicated CT tomographs and ultrasound scanners, but these are aimed to in vivo define anatomical structures rather than molecular characteristics of a tissue, providing complementary and useful data.

In recent years, pre-clinical molecular imaging is acquiring a great relevance in the research scenario, despite the high costs of the scanners. This is because molecular imaging has several advantages over the standard ex vivo studies. First of all, imaging small animals allows a longitudinal observation of the same subject over time, providing a good vision of the disease development or of the efficacy, for example, of a new therapy. Second, it is possible to significantly reduce the number of subjects evaluated, since each one is observed several times over time. Third, some of the imaging techniques are quantitative or, at least, semi-quantitative and this is very important to in vivo accurately monitor a biological process.

Another important feature to point out is the recent availability of pre-clinical hybrid scanners. This means that it is possible to buy tomographs that are able to simultaneously acquire, for example, PET image series and CT image series to be subsequently superimposed, in order to obtain as much information as possible from the same imaging procedure. The most sophisticated machines include a PET tomograph, a CT tomograph and a SPECT gamma camera, while some hybrid prototypes PET/MRI, although not yet available on the market, have been recently built. This approach increases the throughput, further reducing the time lapse to obtain final results (Schwaiger et al. 2005).

Finally, the use of imaging methods in the pre-clinical field is of much interest because it leads to the translational medicine, since the same methods that will be applied on the patients are first tried on the laboratory animal. The step between pre-clinical and clinical is, therefore, much shorter.

This chapter will focus on the basic concepts of SA-molecular imaging scanners and on the state of the art of their use in the pre-clinical evaluation of kidney diseases.

### 35.1.1 Basic Principles of Nuclear Medicine Techniques

#### 35.1.1.1 Small Animal PET (SA-PET)

Nowadays, the most sophisticated imaging techniques related to the molecular imaging field belong to nuclear medicine and are based on the use of radioactive isotopes to label several molecular probes. According to the physical characteristics of the isotope, it is possible to distinguish the positron emission tomography (PET) imaging, which is based on positron emitter isotopes, from the SPECT imaging, based on gamma emitter isotopes.

The PET imaging has some advantages over the SPECT. The most important is that it is possible to label physiological molecules (for example, glucose or aminoacids or receptorial ligands) with positron emitter isotopes without changing the molecule's shape (especially if the isotope id 11C, which is present in all the organic molecules) in order to in vivo observe its physiological kinetic, or making some specific changes in the molecule's shape in order to cause a specific block in its metabolism (for example 18F-FDG).

In recent years (Sossi and Ruth 2005; Weber and Bauer 2004), a great advance in the technological field allowed to build small PET tomographs with small gantries, significantly improving the spatial resolution, which now is below 2 mm. This is an advantage because the anatomical structures of a mouse are tiny and a standard spatial resolution of 5 mm (characteristic of clinical scanners) sometimes is not enough. Furthermore, some scanners are equipped with technical devices aimed at maintaining the spatial resolution stable over the whole field of view (i.e. the Phoswich detectors).

Another great advantage of the PET imaging applied to small animal analysis is the incredible sensitivity of this technique, which is able to in vivo detect nanograms of probe, allowing to observe even molecular events at very low concentrations.

The SA-PET can be used in several pre-clinical research fields, among which oncology, cardiology and neurology are the most important (Scott 2005; Myers and Hume 2002).

For what concerns oncology, SA-PET allows to non-invasively measure a range of tumour-relevant parameters at both the cellular and the molecular level, for example the tumour response to an experimental therapeutic intervention (Zhang et al. 2006), the tumour kinetic of growth, the tumour receptorial profile, the tumour vascularisation or hypoxia, the tumour proliferative index and so on (Herschman 2003). The most widely employed PET imaging probe is 18F-labelled deoxi-glucose, which achieves tumour-specific accumulation on the basis that tumour cells have a higher rate of glucose uptake and metabolism (glycolysis) than normal tissues. FDG is basically used in oncology to predict cancer cell engraftment (Nanni et al. 2007) and measure the response to therapy. Other important pre-clinical tracers are18F-labelled thymidine analogues (i.e. FLT or FMAU), demonstrating the proliferative index of tumour masses with high accuracy since their cellular uptake is proportional to the DNA replication.

Of minor interest for the pre-clinical applications are 11C-methionine (for the evaluation of proteic synthesis) and 11C-Choline (for the evaluation of free fatty acids metabolism), whose employment is much more important in the clinical setting.

Many other PET probes are under development to obtain more and more tumour specificity via a variety of tumour-specific mechanisms, since virtually all the biological molecules can be labelled.

Other experimental PET probes that are under evaluation are targeted to measure the tumour neo-vascularisation (RDG peptide, VEGF and $\alpha v \beta 3$ integrin), apoptosis (radio-labelled annexin V) or the presence of specific surface receptors (somatostatine, androgen, oestrogen, or epithelial growth factor receptors).

The same tracers (18F-FDG, VEGF, $\alpha v \beta 3$ integrin, radio-labelled annexin V) can be employed also in cardiology for the evaluation of the effect of anti-ischemic therapies on the myocardial viability, neo-angiogenesis, and apoptosis. Furthermore, the use of 13N-ammonia or $15OH_2O$ allows to measure the myocardial blood flow.

One SA-PET diagnostic method is the reporter-gene reporter-probe mechanism (HSV1 – 18FHBG is the most validated) (Yaghoubi and Gambhir 2006) that

allows to in vivo detect genetically labelled viable cells injected in a living animal over a long time. This is particularly useful for tracking stem cells used to re-generate areas of myocardial infarction.

Owing to the small size of rodents' brains and brain structures, SA-PET is less employed in neurology than in cardiology and oncology. Furthermore, anaesthesia tends to modify the brain and body metabolism and neurotransmitter distribution and is thus a cause of alteration in PET tracer biodistribution (Fueger et al. 2006). To obtain meaningful images of tiny structures (e.g. the basal ganglia and the nigro-striatal region), it is therefore important to use high sensitivity and high-resolution scanners, the correct anaesthesia procedure, and tracers with high specific activities (especially for receptor studies) and long acquisition times.

Several tracers are available for pre-clinical neurological studies. 18F-FDG is a metabolic tracer that is used in animal models of Alzheimer's disease or epilepsy, 18F-DOPA detects aromatic amino acid decarboxylase activity related to movement disorders, 11C-raclopride and 18F-fluoroethylspiperone are receptor tracers for dopamine D2 receptors, 11C-flumazenil binds to benzodiazepine receptors and 11C-methionine is an indicator of amino acid transporters and is mainly used for the evaluation of brain tumours.

### 35.1.1.2 Small Animal SPECT (SA-SPECT)

Similarly to PET, small SPECT tomographs feasible for the evaluation of small animals were also recently introduced in the market. Those small tomographs are characterised by a very good spatial resolution, reaching 0.7 mm or less (Walrand et al. 2005). This is possible because this technique is based on the use of single photon emitter isotopes, not presenting any intrinsic limitation to the spatial resolution (which, in the PET imaging, is caused by the range of the emitted positron after a decay) (Chatziioannou 2005).

Another advantage of SPECT imaging in the pre-clinical setting is the availability of several kits for the preparation of a number of radiopharmaceuticals, which are easy to obtain, directly reflecting the clinical imaging on patients and are cyclotron independent. It is therefore possible to acquire imaging of a bone scan, of a myocardial perfusion scan, of a thyroid scan and so on.

Despite this quite easy use and the very nice spatial resolution, SA-SPECT imaging is not really diffuse because there is a poorer versatility in the synthesis of new compounds compared to PET. In fact, the labelling technique (mainly based on the use of metal isotopes like 99mTc, 111In, 131I, or 123I) changes the molecule chemical characteristics, complicating the research of innovative tracers. Furthermore, the PET imaging will probably have a greater future development, and it is consequently more appreciated in the pre-clinical scenario as a transitional way to do research.

As described in the previous paragraphs, SA-SPECT is frequently associated to SA-CT and SA-PET, and this could be a reason why in the future a wider application of SA-SPECT could be expected.

From the published literature (Nikolaus et al. 2005), the most appealing use of this technique relies on brain studies, especially with receptorial ligands. This seems quite logical since the long half-life of SPECT tracers compared to PET tracers allows a very long acquisition time, improving the image quality and sensitivity which are very important when analysing small structures like basal ganglia.

## 35.1.2 Basic Principles of Other Molecular Imaging Techniques

### 35.1.2.1 Small Animal Magnetic Resonance Imaging (SA-MRI)

As already mentioned, molecular events at a cellular level happen at very low concentrations (up to picomolar). This requires a very high sensitivity of the detecting system, which is not an intrinsic characteristic of conventional MR imaging, in which the most favourable feature is the really good spatial resolution.

That is why it was necessary to improve the research on the applicability of MRI for molecular imaging studies to create systems aimed to increase the signal intensity.

Besides the use of Gadolinium as a contrast agent, super-paramagnetic molecules (SPIO, VSPIO, USPIO) were introduced on the market. Those agents are small particles (20–150 nm) containing a very high number of iron atoms that can be bound to ligands of specific receptors, to receptors for specific ligands (becoming targeted probes) or to in vitro label living cells that must be subsequently tracked in vivo (Hengerer and Grimm 2005).

The use of such powerful contrast agents significantly improved the possibility to employ SA-MR for

pre-clinical molecular imaging, even though the global sensitivity in detecting in vivo small amounts of probe is still lower than PET. Despite that, the applicability of new targeted probes is still limited because of their big size and the non-standardised synthesis of molecular contrast agents (Artemov et al. 2003).

MRI can be, therefore, used in pre-clinical imaging both for obtaining high-resolution morphological images and for getting "molecular images" by the injection of targeted probes (Frank et al. 2004).

### 35.1.2.2 Optical Imaging

The OI is the most widely employed molecular imaging technique in the pre-clinical setting. This is because it is much cheaper than other techniques, sensitive, fast to obtain images, simple to handle, is possible to use several different probes and does not require any particular expertise (for example, PET, SPECT and MRI which are based on ionising radiations and magnetic fields).

Despite that, it has three major drawbacks compared to the other techniques previously described: first of all, traditionally, it is not a quantitative technique but allows only a visual analysis (new quantitative scanners are coming on the market); second, being based on optical radiations that are easily absorbed by surrounding tissues, it only allows the evaluation of very superficial tissues while deep organs may not be accurately visualised; third, because of these characteristics, OI is not employed for clinical studies and therefore is not considered as a translational technique. As mentioned before, OI is based on the detection of optical radiations and the most favourable wavelength for imaging is the infrared, which can be emitted by a living body by bioluminescence or by fluorescence.

The bioluminescence (Sadikot and Blackwell 2005) is a natural phenomenon based on the production of an enzyme (Luciferase), which interacts with a protein (Luciferin) emitting light as a product of the reaction. This process happens in those cells that are genetically equipped with the specific gene encoding for Luciferase (so, genetically modified animals must be prepared), while Luciferin must be administrated to the animal intravenously (Bhaumik and Gambhir 2002).

The fluorescence is another natural phenomenon based on the fact that some molecules (called fluorophores) emit infrared light when stimulated with an external source of light. This process can be employed if, for example, a specific molecule is labelled with a fluorophore creating a probe for OI. As for PET imaging, a very wide range of probes can be created as the labelling process (especially for proteins) is easy (Mahmood and Weissleder 2003).

## 35.2 The Kidney: Molecular Imaging and Tumoural Antigen Targeting

The field of pre-clinical molecular imaging adapts very well to in vivo analyse several characteristics of a disease. The combination of different imaging modalities allows to explore many aspects of the disease behaviour like, the metabolic profile, the receptorial profile, the presence of hypoxia, the viability of tissue, the proliferation index and so on.

For what concerns renal diseases, pre-clinical molecular imaging was used for several purposes, even though the published literature is just at the beginning in this field. Most aspects related to the molecular evaluation of kidney diseases, in fact, were approached in a very traditional way based on the ex vivo demonstration of molecular processes, and in vivo pre-clinical imaging was only recently introduced (perini et al. 2008).

Despite this shortness of papers, from published literature, it is possible to divide the applications of pre-clinical molecular imaging into three main groups:

1. A-PET imaging methods to analyse the renal function.
2. SA-PET for the in vivo evaluation of renal carcinoma in animal models of cancer.
3. SA-MR for the in vivo tracking of stem cell in animal models of renal impairment.

### 35.2.1 SA-PET Imaging Methods to Analyse the Renal Function

The SA-PET can be used in a dynamic acquisition mode which is very much suitable for the evaluation of renal function (Schnöckel et al. 2008).

Furthermore, the 18F-Fluoride, a PET tracer for bone metabolism that is quite easy to produce with a cyclotron, is known to be freely filtrated through the renal glomerular capillaries with a passive tubular reabsorption attributed to diffusion. This proves that renal fluoride clearance is directly related to GFR (Figs. 35.1 and 35.2).

On this base, Schnöckel et al. validated an easy method with 18F-SA PET to quantify renal function in three groups of rats with normal renal function, acute renal failure and chronic kidney damage, comparing the TACs (time activity curves) obtained by a 60-min dynamic PET scan (list-mode acquisition) to the blood activity obtained by arterial blood withdrawal during the PET measurements, to planar renography with 99mTc-Mercaptotriglycine and to interindividual measurements as creatinine clearance and urea clearance.

The results of this experiment were satisfactory, and the accuracy of dynamic PET for the measurement of renal function turned out high. Despite this not being closely related to a molecular imaging procedure, it can be a strong base to use it in several pre-clinical scenarios.

So far, this is the only published application of pre-clinical imaging for the evaluation of renal function.

### 35.2.2 SA-PET for the In Vivo Evaluation of Renal Cell Carcinoma in Animal Models

Despite SA-imaging being mainly applied for the evaluation of animal models of cancer, renal cell carcinoma so far has not been considered for being evaluated with pre-clinical imaging.

The major paper by Zisman et al. (2003) evaluated a mouse model of renal cell carcinoma expressing the carbonic anhydrase type 9 tumour antigen. In this paper, the authors produced a SCID mouse model in which a clear cell carcinoma line of the chromophil type was implanted and was in vitro characterised from the histological point of view and from several molecular aspects, among which the expression of carbonic anhydrase type 9 was the most important, since it seems correlated to a poor prognosis. In fact, carbonic anhydrase type 9 has a role in the regulation of hypoxia-induced cell proliferation and may be involved in oncogenesis and tumour progression.

In the paper, no specific tracers were synthesised for the SA-PET imaging, but the animals were evaluated with a standard FDG-PET, showing an increased

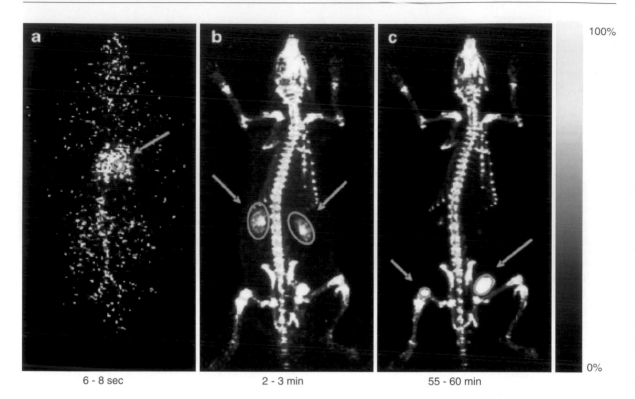

6 - 8 sec      2 - 3 min      55 - 60 min

**Fig. 35.1** Representative images of a dynamic whole body acquisition of a control rat after i.v. injection of 15 MBq 18F-fluoride (midrat coronal slice 6–8 s after injection, maximum-a-posterior projections 120–180 s after injection, and 3300–3600 s after injection. Arrows indicate ROIs drawn on the left ventricle cauity, on the renal and urinary bladder activity as well as of the osseous activity to calculate Time Activity curves

FDG uptake in the tumoural sites compared to normal kidneys. This in vivo demonstrates a high proliferative rate in renal tumours expressing carbonic anhydrase type 9. It is relevant to point out that, usually, renal clear cell carcinoma does not show any increased FDG uptake, while this human variant showed a significant FDG uptake, probably related to a poor prognosis.

### 35.2.3 SA-MRI for the In Vivo Tracking of Stem Cells in Animal Models of Renal Impairment

The issue of regenerating tissues that definitively lost their function due to a specific disease is serious and, in recent years, was approached by trying to inject in the impaired organ different types of stem cells. This technique is based on the principle that stem cells have a great differentiating capability and that they could differentiate into a viable specific and functional tissue once implanted in the impaired organ.

This approach gave controversial results, but it is well-known that one of the major problems is the difficulty to in vivo track the stem cell and to understand their homing and their in vivo differentiation.

To do this, several imaging approaches were evaluated. One of the most effective is based on the use of SA-MR, since stem cells can be in vitro labelled with SPIO particles without compromising their function and viability. SPIO particles are retained inside the cells for a long time and are aimed to increase the MR sensitivity in detecting their localization once injected in a living organism intravenously or within the arterial vessel afferent to the impaired organ.

Some papers were published in literature analysing the viability and homing of stem cells in animal models of renal impairment.

Hauger et al. (2006) produced a rat model of mesangiolysis and labelled bone-marrow stem cells by incubating them in vitro with SPIO. All the animals were evaluated with a SA-MR study before and after the injection of stem cells in the tail vein, and particular attention was put on the evaluation of the liver and

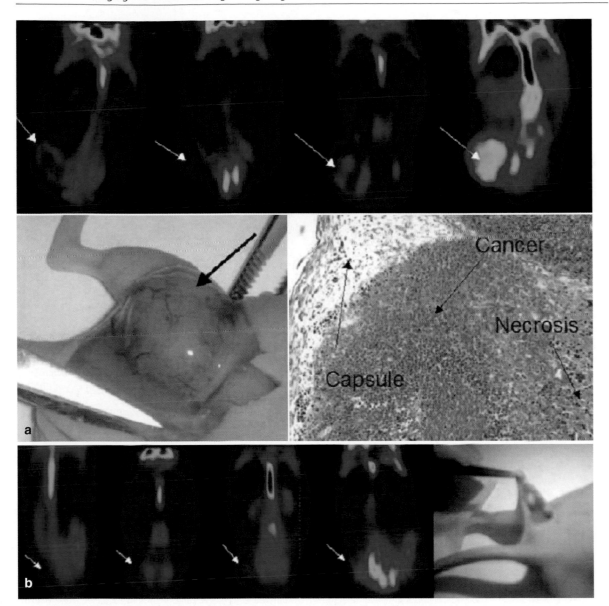

**Fig. 35.2** (**a**) Coronal slice of a positive photon emission tomography (PET) scan 2, 5, 14, and 20 days after inoculation; necropsy and histology (haematoxylin-eosin) showed a cancer mass. (**b**) Coronal slice of a negative PET scan 2, 5, 14, and 20 days after inoculation. Macroscopically, a subcutaneous mass was detectable. Histology showed a granuloma at the site of injection. Arrows indicate the site of cell injection in a and b

kidneys. Furthermore, images were acquired ex vivo after the kidneys' explant. The authors found a significant decrease in the signal intensity in the kidneys only in the ex vivo studies (demonstrating that stem cells have a specific homing in the damaged kidney), while the in vivo MR did not give satisfactory results, probably because the scanner sensitivity was not enough to demonstrate a small number of labelled cells.

Another interesting paper by Lange et al. (2005) is based on the same approach. The authors created a rat model of acute renal failure and analysed the homing of SPIO-labelled stem cells and the renal function trend. In this case they found that SA-MR was a feasible method to in vivo track labelled cells and that the signal loss in the damaged kidney (indicative of stem cells presence) was predictive of an increasing renal function.

Despite the potential opportunity to label iron particles to produce targeted MR contrast agents, no published applications are so far available for renal applications, and the in vivo stem cells tracking seems to be the major interest in this field.

# References

Artemov D et al. (2003) Molecular magnetic resonance imaging with targeted contrast agents. J Cell Biochemistry 90: 518–524

Bhaumik S, Gambhir SS (2002) Optical imaging of Renilla luciferase reporter gene expression in living mice. PNAS 99:1377–1382

Chatziioannou AF (2005) Instrumentation for molecular imaging in preclinical research micro-PET and micro-SPECT. Proc Am Thorac Soc 2(6):533–536, 510– 511

Frank JA et al. (2004) Methods for magnetically labeling stem and other cells for detection by in vivo magnetic resonance imaging. Cytotherapy 6:621–625

Fueger BJ, Czernin J, Hildebrandt I et al. (2006) Impact of animal handling on the results of 18F-FDG PET studies in mice. J Nucl Med 47(6):999–1006

Hauger O, Frost EE, van Heeswijk R et al. (2006) MR evaluation of the glomerular homing of magnetically labeled mesenchymal stem cells in a rat model of nephropathy. Radiology 238(1):200–210

Hengerer A, Grimm J (2005) Molecular magnetic resonance imaging, special edn. Medical Solutions, September 2005 Special Edition Molecular Imaging, pp 31–38

Herschman HR (2003) Micro-PET imaging and small animal models of disease. Curr Opin Immunol 15:378–384

Lange C, Tögel F, Ittrich H et al. (2005). Administered mesenchymal stem cells enhance recovery from ischemia/reperfusion-induced acute renal failure in rats. Kidney Int 68(4):1613–1617

Levin CS (2005) Primer on molecular imaging technology. Eur J Nucl Med Mol Imaging. 2005 Dec; Suppl 2:S325–S345

Mahmood U, Weissleder R (2003) Near-infrared optical imaging of proteases in cancer. Mol Cancer Ther 2:489–496

Myers R, Hume S (2002) Small animal PET. Eur Neuropsychopharmacol 12:545–555

Nanni C, Di Leo K, Tonelli R et al. (2007) FDG small animal PET permits early detection of malignant cells in a xenograft murine model. Eur J Nucl Med Mol Imaging 34(5):755–762

Nikolaus S, Larisch R, Wirrwar A et al. (2005) [123I] Iodobenzamide binding to the rat dopamine D2 receptor in competition with haloperidol and endogenous dopamine – an in vivo imaging study with a dedicated small animal SPECT. Eur J Nucl Med Mol Imaging 32:1305–1310

Perini R, Pryma D, Divgi CR (2008) Molecular imaging of renal cell carcinoma. Urol Clin North Am 35(4):605–611

Sadikot RT, Blackwell TS (2005) Bioluminescence imaging. Proc Am Thorac Soc Vol 2. pp 537–540, 2005

Schnöckel U, Reuter S, Stegger L et al (2008) Dynamic (18) F-fluoride small animal PET to noninvasively assess renal function in rats. Eur J Nucl Med Mol Imaging. 2008 Dec; 35(12): 2267–2274

Schwaiger M, Ziegler SI, Nekolla SG (2005) MR-PET: combining function, anatomy and more medical solutions special edition Molecular imaging, pp 25–30

Scott (2005) Advances in imaging mouse tumour models in vivo. J Pathol 205:194–205

Sossi V, Ruth TJ (2005) Micropet imaging: in vivo biochemistry in small animals. J Neural Transm 112:319–330

Walrand S, Jamar F, de Jong M et al. (2005) Evaluation of novel whole-body high-resolution rodent SPECT (Linoview) based on direct acquisition of linogram projections. J Nucl Med 46(11):1872–1880

Weber S, Bauer A (2004) Small animal PET: aspects of performance assessment. Eur J Nucl Med Mol Imaging. 2004 Nov; 31(11):1545–1555

Yaghoubi SS, Gambhir SS (2006) PET imaging of herpes simplex virus type 1 thymidine kinase (HSV1-tk) or mutant HSV1-sr39tk reporter gene expression in mice and humans using [18F]FHBG. Nat Protoc 1(6):3069–3075

Zhang Y, Saylor M, Wen et al. (2006) Longitudinally quantitative 2-deoxy-2-[18F]fluoro-D-glucose micro positron emission tomography imaging for efficacy of new anticancer drugs: a case study with bortezomib in prostate cancer murine model. Mol Imaging Biol 8(5):300–308

Zisman A, Pantuck AJ, Bui MH et al. (2003) A metastatic tumor model for renal cell carcinoma expressing the carbonic anhydrase type 9 tumor antigen. Cancer Res 63(16): 4952–4959

# Research Perspectives and Future Trends in Renal Imaging

# 36

## Nicolas Grenier

## Contents

**Abstract**

> Research perspectives and future trends in renal imaging will tend to characterize in vivo acute and chronic parenchymal diseases avoiding or limiting the necessity to use percutaneous biopsy for pathological examination. Such approach could have a tremendous impact on the management of patients. Identification and characterization of cellular and molecular processes in vivo are based on new molecular imaging methods using appropriate tracers. It is already possible to label the macrophages infiltrating the renal compartments and to track the labeled stem cells attracted within the kidney. Techniques of targeting overexpressed receptors and synthesized enzymes could be applied to the kidney in a close future, as a monitoring of intrarenal gene therapy. Ultrasound (US) and magnetic resonance (MR) elastographic techniques are now able to quantify structural changes that affect the extracellular matrix with the development of fibrosis.

Research perspectives and future trends in renal imaging mainly focus on better characterization of acute and chronic parenchymal diseases. Current renal imaging techniques, including ultrasound (US), computed tomography (CT), and magnetic resonance (MR) imaging does not, up to now, detect specific changes in the kidney parenchyma. In fact, each disease involves specific biological and cellular response and may produce definitive changes in the structural properties of renal tissue. Therefore, developing new imaging techniques

N. Grenier
Service d'Imagerie Diagnostique et Interventionnelle de l'Adulte, Groupe Hospitalier Pellegrin, Place Amélie Raba-Léon, 33076 Bordeaux Cedex, France
e-mail: nicolas.grenier@chu-bordeaux.fr

E. Quaia (ed.), *Radiological Imaging of the Kidney*,
Medical Radiology, DOI: 10.1007/978-3-540-87597-0_36, © Springer-Verlag Berlin Heidelberg 2011

that are able to characterize these diseases in vivo may avoid or limit the necessity to use percutaneous biopsy for pathological examination. Such approach could have a tremendous impact on the management of patients with acute or chronic nephropathy.

Identification and characterization of cellular and molecular processes in vivo are based on new molecular imaging methods using appropriate tracers. US, positron emission tomography (PET), optical imaging, and MR imaging techniques have demonstrated capabilities for such developments. Renal PET has a great potential in that field (Szabo et al. 2006). Its high sensitivity to detect a signal from a tracer at a picomolar level is a serious advantage, but it suffers from a low spatial resolution. Optical techniques are very useful for proof of concepts of new molecular imaging approaches. However, due to a high attenuation of the signal by tissues, applications to human kidney will be limited due to its depth. Chronic diseases affect the extracellular matrix (ECM) with the development of fibrosis; such structural changes can now be quantified by US and MR elastographic techniques.

macrophages produce direct renal insults or if they are a consequence of the disease in order to regulate the inflammatory response. Their role is complex, contributing to glomerular and tubulointerstitial injury through the secretion of various cytokines and proteases which induce changes in extracellular matrix and progressive fibrotic changes (glomerulosclerosis, tubulointerstitial fibrosis) (Erwig et al. 2001). The macrophagic activity may vary, depending on the type of kidney disease and its severity. It predominates within the glomeruli (i.e., within the cortex) in glomerulonephritis, or within the interstitium (i.e., diffuse, within all kidney compartments) in interstitial nephritis, or in hydronephrosis.

In current clinical practice, the degree of inflammatory response in the kidney can be approached only by renal biopsy. Therefore, identification of intrarenal macrophage infiltration with a noninvasive technique has a great potential since it could help for the characterization of kidney disease, the evaluation of its level of inflammatory activity, and for monitoring response to treatment.

## 36.1 MR Imaging of Cell Targeting

### 36.1.1 Intrarenal Macrophage Activity

Whereas only a small number of interstitial leucocytes (predominantly monocytes and differential macrophages) are present in the normal kidney, their number can be considerably increased in specific nephropathies such as acute proliferative types of human and experimental glomerulonephritides (GN) (Cattell 1994), renal graft dysfunctions (rejection and acute tubular necrosis, ATN) (Grau et al. 1998), and nonspecific kidney diseases such as hydronephrosis (Schreiner et al. 1988). This increase of the inflammatory cellular infiltration is due to both, a recruitment of circulating cells and a proliferation in situ. This macrophagic attraction is a dynamic process controlled by both chemotactic molecules (chemokines, Fc fragment of immunoglobulins, TNF-$\alpha$, etc.) and changes in the expression level of leucocyte adhesion molecules. The degree of macrophagic infiltration and proliferation is correlated with the severity of renal disease, whereas it remains unclear if

### 36.1.2 Principles of MR Targeting of Macrophages

Intravenous injection of superparamagnetic particles of iron oxide (SPIO) has been proposed for targeting phagocytic cells in several inflammatory diseases such as multiple sclerosis and atherosclerosis. For this purpose, ultrasmall superparamagnetic particles of iron oxide (USPIO) are preferred because of a longer half-life in the blood stream (2 h in rats) allowing a more effective capture by extrahepatic phagocytic cells including blood circulating monocytes and resident macrophages already present in most of the tissues (Modo et al. 2005) (Fig. 36.1). The exact mechanism of particle capture is not perfectly known and may be cell specific. Two different mechanisms might be involved: first, and most likely, the particles could be taken up directly from the vascular space of the kidney by macrophages or mesangial cells gaining endocytic activity. This cellular uptake could be mediated by fluid-phase endocytosis. Another possibility could be a cellular uptake of the particles by the circulating blood monocytes secondarily recruited into the kidney. Also, little is known about the fate of these macrophages,

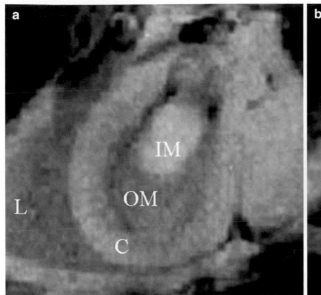
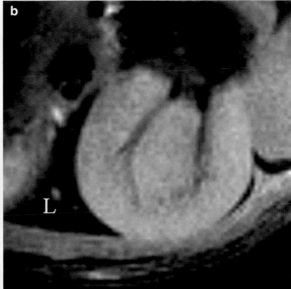

**Fig. 36.1** T2*-weighted magnetic resonance (MR) imaging of normal rat kidney at 4.7 T, before (**a**) and 24 h after (**b**) intravenous infusion of ultrasmall superparamagnetic particles of iron oxide (USPIO). Iron oxide particles are captured by the liver (*L*) but not by kidney. *C* cortex; *OM* outer medulla; *IM* inner medulla

that is, whether they die in situ or emigrate, and how long this takes. There is evidence suggesting migration of activated macrophages into the periglomerular interstitium.

### 36.1.3 Macrophage Targeting in Experimental Models

Macrophage targeting within the kidney using USPIO was first proposed for a model of nephrotic syndrome, induced by intravenous injection of puromycin aminonucleoside in rats (Hauger et al. 1999). This model induces both, lesions of glomerular epithelial cells and a glomerular and tubulointerstitial infiltration by macrophages. MR images showed a diffuse decrease of signal intensity predominantly within the outer medulla 24 h after the IV injection of Sinerem® (Guerbet Group, Aulnay-sous-Bois, France). The degree of signal decrease was correlated with the number of macrophages within each renal compartment and to the amount of iron within the tissue.

A diffuse interstitial macrophagic infiltration of renal parenchyma is a well documented feature of chronic ureteral obstruction (Schreiner et al. 1988). This cellular influx peaks the second day after the obstruction. Delayed USPIO-enhanced MR imaging demonstrated a diffuse but significant decrease of signal intensity in the three renal compartments, slightly more pronounced in the cortex (Hauger et al. 2000) (Fig. 36.2).

In acute proliferative types of GN, such as Goodpasture syndrome or vascular nephritis, macrophages also play a role in the development of glomerular inflammation (Cattell 1994). They accumulate in the Bowman space as a primary feature in the development of advanced cellular crescents which is a known as a feature of rapidly progressive GN which is associated with a poor prognosis. A model of anti-glomerular basal membrane (GBM) GN, comparable to Goodpasture syndrome in humans, was evaluated with MR imaging (Hauger et al. 2000). This model was induced in rats by IV injection of sheep anti-rat-GBM serum. The kinetics of signal intensity followed the biphasic evolution of the disease with a decrease of signal intensity within the cortex only at days 2 and 14 (Fig. 36.3a) and no change at day 21. This effect was due to endocytosis of USPIO by macrophages at day 14 and by activated mesangial cells at both phases (Fig. 36.3b). The degree of signal intensity decrease was strongly correlated with the degree of proteinuria.

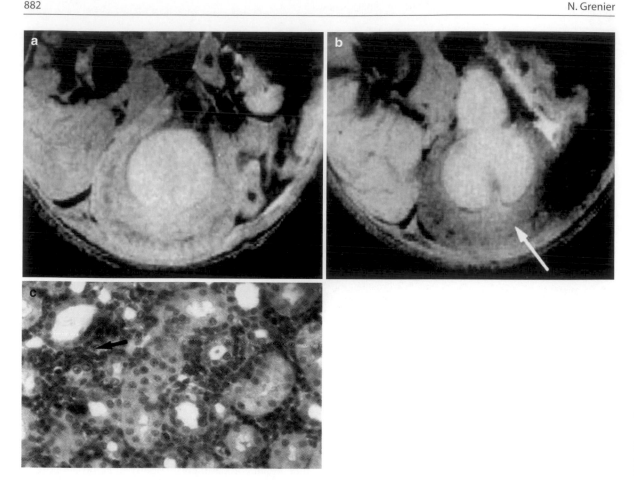

**Fig. 36.2** Obstructive hydronephrosis. T2*-weighted MR imaging of a left obstructed rat kidney at 4.7 T, before (**a**) and 24 h after (**b**) intravenous infusion of USPIO. There is a notable decrease in signal intensity (*arrow*) in all kidney compartments after the injection. Note the dilated renal collecting system. (**c**) Histological section shows a diffuse infiltration of the interstitium by macrophages. From Hauger et al. 2000, with permission

Intrinsic acute renal failure (ARF) is a multifactorial disease with concomitant ischemic, nephrotoxic, and septic components (Devarajan 2006), and ATN is its pathological counterpart. Besides alterations in hemodynamics, tubule dynamics, tubule cell metabolism and structure, the intrarenal inflammatory response plays a major role in the ischemic ARF. Neutrophils are the first leucocytes to accumulate in the postischemic kidney and macrophages are the next. Macrophages migrate into the outer medulla of rat kidneys and accumulate within peritubular capillaries, interstitial space, and even within tubules (Friedewald and Rabb 2004; Ysebaert et al. 2000). In an ischemia-reperfusion model in rats, USPIO-enhanced MR imaging demonstrated the same endocytosis pattern with a decrease of signal intensity within

the outer medulla only from 24 to 120 h after the injection of particles (Jo et al. 2003) (Fig. 36.4). Signal intensity decrease was also correlated with the level of renal function.

After renal transplantation, acute and chronic rejection episodes play a major role on long-term graft survival and involve T-cells and macrophages. Two studies evaluated a rat model of acute rejection and showed a decrease of signal intensity within the cortex and medulla, increasing with iron dosage (Ye et al. 2002) and inhibited by immunosuppressive treatments (Zhang et al. 2000). Beckmann et al. (2006) used SPIO to label macrophagic infiltration in a model of chronic rejection. They showed a dose-dependent decrease in cortical signal intensity in allografts between 8 and 16 weeks

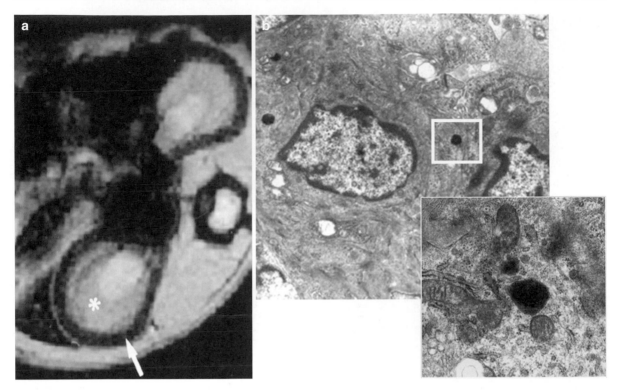

**Fig. 36.3** Nephrotoxic anti-rat-glomerular basal membrane (GBM) glomerulonephritis. (**a**) T2*-weighted MR imaging at 4.7 T, of rat kidneys in the day-2 pathologic group 24 h after the injection of USPIO. There is a notable decrease in signal intensity in the renal cortex (*arrow*) after the injection, whereas no signal intensity change is observed in any portion of the medulla (*asterisk*). (**b**) Electron microscopic image shows the presence of iron particles (see magnification) in a lysosome of a mesangial cell. (From Hauger et al. 2000, with permission)

after transplantation (Fig. 36.5). The relative cortical signal intensity in the grafts was negatively correlated to the Banff score 6 weeks after transplantation and changes in creatinine clearance occurred only after 28 weeks. Groups treated with immunosuppressive and antiproliferative drugs showed lesser degree of signal intensity change (Beckmann et al. 2003).

All these experimental results showed that USPIO-enhanced MR imaging could demonstrate intrarenal internalization of particles by macrophages or by glomerular cells gaining endocytic activity, i.e., mesangial cells, and could precisely localize this endocytic activity in the different kidney compartments. Different types of experimental renal diseases showed different patterns of signal intensity changes, but the degree of renal dysfunction always appeared correlated to the degree of endocytic activity, which may have significant implications in clinical practice.

### 36.1.4 Macrophage Targeting in Humans

These results led to the first pilot clinical study (Hauger et al. 2007), based on 12 patients exhibiting a dysfunction of either their native kidneys or their transplant. As the blood half-life of USPIO is 36 h in humans, MR imaging was performed 3 days after USPIO injection (Sinerem®, Guerbet Group) to ensure avoiding signal changes from vascular blood volume. Patients with chronic and fibrotic disease, without inflammatory component on biopsy did not show any significant change (Fig. 36.6a, b). Three patients with ATN (two transplanted kidneys and one native kidney) showed a significant decrease of signal intensity within the medulla only (Fig. 36.6c, d). All patients but one with an inflammatory component on cortical biopsy showed a significant decrease of signal intensity after USPIO injection (Fig. 36.6e, f). These preliminary clinical findings seem to corroborate the experimental results, with

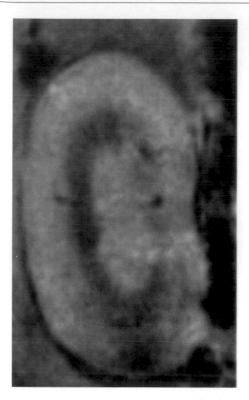

**Fig. 36.4** Ischemia-reperfusion. T2\*-weighted gradient-echo MR image 24 h after the injection of ferumodextran-10 USPIO particles in rats subjected to 60 min of bilateral ischemia. A *black band* in the outer medulla is detected 48 h after the beginning of reperfusion. (From Dagher et al. 2003, with permission)

the same topographic patterns, and call for larger multi-center clinical trials, and the evaluation of imaging at 2 days after injection to reduce delay in the diagnosis.

## 36.2 MR Imaging of Stem Cell Tracking

Recovery of renal function after acute nephrotoxic or ischemic insult is dependent on the replacement of necrotic tubular cells by functional tubular epithelium (Gupta et al. 2002). This cellular regeneration may originate from renal resident cells or from extrarenal ones. Mesenchymal stem cells (MSC) have been shown to be able to repair damaged tissues, whether genetically modified or not (Baksh et al. 2004; Pittenger and Martin 2004). They also per se have potential therapeutic effects such as those with regard to the degradation of the ECM in the experimental models of fibrosis (Fang et al. 2004) or the facilitation of the grafting of transplanted bone marrow progenitor cells by providing a competent stroma (Bacigalupo 2004). They have a well-established ability to differentiate into the mesoderm lineage, which makes them potentially useful in strategies aiming at targeting the kidney mesangium for instance.

Recently, the possibility for bone marrow-derived MSC, to differentiate into mesangial cells (Imasawa et al. 2001; Ito et al. 2001) and for hematopoietic stem cells into tubular cells was demonstrated in vivo (Lin et al. 2003), bringing great therapeutic promise for the future. Noninvasive imaging techniques allowing in vivo assessment of the location of stem cells could be of great value for experimental studies in which these cells are transplanted. It provides a tool to immediately verify if the grafted cells have reached the target organ, to estimate the number of cells that were seeded, and to assess the permanence of these cells over time with

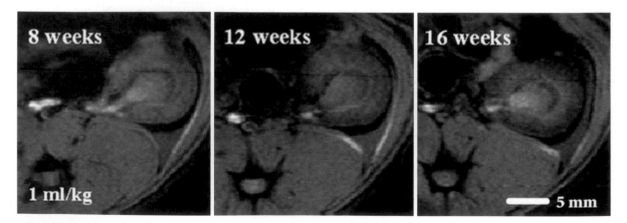

**Fig. 36.5** Gradient-echo MR images of the kidney grafts of recipient rat acquired 8, 12, and 16 weeks after transplantation, 24 h after superparamagnetic particles of iron oxide (SPIO) injection. Darkening of kidney cortex was apparent at different times after transplantation. (From Beckmann et al. 2006, with permission)

**Fig. 36.6** Examples of USPIO-enhanced MR imaging in four patients presenting with (**a, b**) a chronic glomerulohyalinosis and glomerulosclerosis (**c, d**) a drug-induced acute renal failure (ARF) (**e, f**) an extracapillary glomerulonephritis with numerous intraglomerular macrophages and (**g, h**) a type Ia acute rejection with numerous interstitial macrophages. (**a, c, e, g**) T2*-weighted MR images before the injection of USPIO. (**b, d, f, h**) T2*-weighted MR images 72 h after the injection of USPIO. (Adapted from Hauger et al. 2007, with permission)

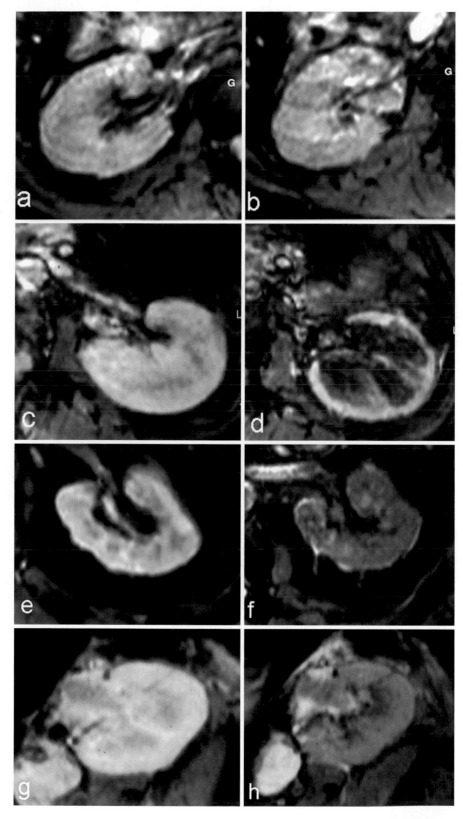

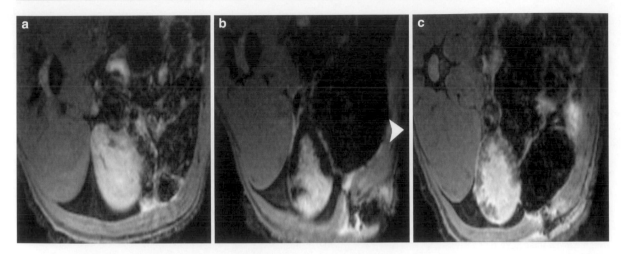

**Fig. 36.7** Renal cell therapy by intraarterial graft of mesenchymal stem cells (MSC). Transverse T2*-weighted MR images of rat kidney before (**a**), 1 h (**b**) and 7 days (**c**) after the injection of SPIO-labeled MSCs into left renal artery. *Arrowhead* indicates the ventral side of the animal. (From Bos et al. 2004, with permission)

sequential imaging. Using SPIO preparations to magnetically label the cells, several groups have demonstrated the feasibility of grafting and subsequent visualization of the progenitor of different organs (Bulte et al. 1999; Hoehn et al. 2002; Kraitchman et al. 2003). A strong R2* effect was observed in vitro after MSC labeling for 48 h with 50 μg Fe/mL and increased linearly with the iron dose (Bos et al. 2004). After intravascular administration, the renal distribution of SPIO-labeled MSC has been investigated recently. When administered into the renal artery of normal kidneys, labeled MSC could be detected in vivo within the cortex as long as 7 days after injection at 1.5 T (Fig. 36.7) and iron-loaded cells were identified in renal glomeruli using histology (Bos et al. 2004). The same experiment was repeated at 3 T (Ittrich et al. 2007) with similar results in normal kidneys. In kidneys with acute renal injury (40′ ischemia-reperfusion), the improvement of renal function was accelerated in rats treated by cell graft: lower plasma creatinine levels at days 2 and 3 (Ittrich et al. 2007). In a model of acute experimental glomerulopathy (Thy1+PAN), a homing effect was identified ex vivo, at 9.4 T, when the magnetically labeled MSC were administered intravenously. A large proportion of cells was trapped within the liver precluding their detection

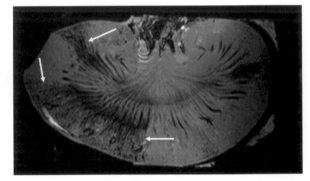

**Fig. 36.8** Renal cell therapy by intravenous graft of MSC. Ex vivo sagittal T2*-weighted 9.4-T MR image of pathologic kidney 6 days after intravenous injection of $10^7$ labeled MSCs. Distinct areas of cortical signal intensity decrease are present in the superior and superior midportion (*arrows*) poles, where labeled MSCs were homed.

in the kidneys in vivo at 1.5 T. When comparing the enhancing renal segments in ex vivo images and pathological lesions in histological sections, the areas of low signal intensity correlated well with alpha-actin and Prussian blue stains, indicating that MSCs specifically homed to injured tissues (Hauger et al. 2006) (Fig. 36.8).

## 36.3 MR Imaging and Monitoring of Gene Therapy

Up to now, MR imaging of transgene expression has been limited to the demonstration of proof-of-principle experiments, using a change of signal intensity under the control of the expression of a reporter gene. As with PET, two approaches have been proposed with MR imaging using either an enzymatic pathway or a receptor pathway. The first method is based on the expression of a reporter gene (Lac-z) coding for an enzyme (β-galactosidase), which is able to activate a Gd-chelate by giving access of water to the first coordination sphere of the Gd ions (Louie et al. 2000). The second method is based on the targeting, with iron oxide particles, of cells overexpressing the transferrin receptors on their membrane (Moore et al. 2001; Weissleder and Mahmood 2001). None of these methods has been applied in the field of urogenital diseases.

MR imaging could also play a role in controlling gene expression in space and in time. The possibility to limit the effect of a therapeutic gene to a target diseased tissue and during a predefined time window is a key challenge for the future of gene therapy. For such a purpose, expression of a transgene can be controlled by a heat-sensitive promoter, such as the promoter of the inducible heat shock protein systems, HSP70 (Rome et al. 2005). These promoters can activate gene expression several thousand-fold in response to hyperthermia (Dreano et al. 1986). Heating of the deep parts of the body can be achieved with high intensity focused ultrasound (HIFU), and temperature control is made possible by using temperature-sensitive MR sequences based on the proton resonance frequency (PRF) method (Quesson et al. 2000) and by using an automatic monitoring of the acoustic power.

This approach has been recently experimented in vivo within the rat kidney. First, modified MSC expressing the luciferase reporter gene under the control of the hsp70B promoter were administered through the left renal artery. Luciferase expression in MR-guided HIFU heated regions was first demonstrated in vitro, using immunostaining (Letavernier et al. 2007). More recently, using modified C6 cells with hsp70B-luc expression injected in the artery of superficialized rat kidneys, local luciferase expression was demonstrated for the first time in vivo, by using bioluminescence imaging (Eker et al. 2008). The optimal heating protocol was found to be 43° during 5 min to get reproducible significant expression without parenchymal deleterious effect of heating.

## 36.4 Imaging of Cell Receptors

Molecular MR imaging of cell receptors is a growing field and requires the development of specific contrast agents. The most developed strategy for targeting cells using MR imaging is to bind a contrast agent with a monoclonal antibody, an aptamer, or a peptide, able to recognize specifically a surface antigen expressed on the cell membrane surface. Up until now, the main applications focused on targeting inflammatory receptors, such as P-selectin (Chaubet et al. 2007), E-selectin (Reynolds et al. 2006), VCAM (Nahrendorf et al. 2006), ICAM (Choi et al. 2007), or tumor-specific receptors, such as HER2/neu (Daldrup-Link et al. 2005). To our knowledge, no application of these strategies involved the kidney.

Apoptosis and its regulatory mechanisms contribute to cell number regulation in ARF (Ortiz et al. 2003). Tubular cells apoptosis is promoted by both exogenous factors such as nephrotoxic drugs and bacterial products, and endogenous factors such as lethal cytokines. Conversely to necrosis, which is a nonreversible process, apoptotic pathways are potentially accessible to therapeutic modulation (Rana et al. 2001). MR imaging for the detection of apoptosis requires labeling of apoptotic cells using USPIOs as a marker and phosphatidylserine as a target. This necessitates linking the superparamagnetic nanoparticle to annexin V or synaptotagmin I both of which bind to the phosphatidylserine present on the outer leaflet of the plasma membrane of apoptotic cells (Hakumaki and Brindle 2003). Several preclinical applications using MR imaging have been reported to target apoptotic cells within the heart (Hiller et al. 2006) or within tumors during chemotherapy (Zhao et al. 2001), but, to our knowledge, this approach has never been applied to any kidney model.

## 36.5 MR Imaging of Enzyme Synthesis or Activity

Whereas enzyme activity is highly involved in renal physiopathology of many renal parenchymal diseases and urinary cancers, nothing has been done in that field using MR imaging.

### 36.5.1 MR Imaging of Matrix Metalloproteases (MMPs)

Matrix metalloproteases (MMP) are zinc-containing endopeptidases that are involved in the degradation and remodeling of the ECM, crucial for tissue development and homeostasis (Catania et al. 2007). They localize to the cell surface or extracellular compartments. Their spatial expression in the kidney is complex and has not been completely characterized. MMP activity is associated with tumor invasion and metastasis, justifying the development of MMP-inhibitors as anticancer alternatives. Within the kidney, an aberrant MMP expression is related to a number of renal pathologies, both acute and chronic. In acute renal diseases, there is strong evidence that MMPs mediate acute kidney injury and are involved in changes in the vascular endothelium, glomeruli, and tubular epithelial cells. In ischemia-reperfusion model, increased MMP-9 activity was associated with an increased vascular and tubular permeability, due to the degradation of cell adhesion molecules (Caron et al. 2005). In chronic kidney diseases (CKD), a role for MMPs has been demonstrated in several experimental models. For example, decreased MMP-9 expression was correlated with the development of tubulointerstitial fibrosis and glomerulosclerosis in rats (Bolbrinker et al. 2006). A number of studies have also demonstrated a link between aberrant MMP expression and the progression of diabetic nephropathy in animal models (McLennan et al. 2002). Overexpression of a single MMP may be a critical mediator of CKD. However, the relationship between MMP activity and inflammation remains an important component of CKD that remains to be addressed.

A Gd-chelate coupled with a MMP-inhibitor was recently developed for MR imaging of atherosclerotic plaques (Lancelot et al. 2008). The affinity of this agent in vitro was broad toward MMP-1, 2, 3, 8, 9, and 13. In vivo, its affinity and specificity allowed accurate discrimination of MMP-poor and MMP-rich plaques. Another type of MR contrast agent, specific for MMPs, was proposed by Lepage et al. (2007), based on the concept of solubility switch, from hydrophilic to hydrophobic, modifying its pharmacokinetic properties. This agent, associating Gd-DOTA and a proteinase-sensitive peptide, was designed to display a reduced solubility after cleavage by MMP-7, responsible for an increased retention, making the detection of its activity possible. Applications of such agents in the nephro-urological sphere, as acute and chronic renal diseases and urological cancers, are really attractive but must still be developed.

### 36.5.2 MR Imaging of Myeloperoxidase (MPO)

Myeloperoxidase (MPO) is one of the most abundant enzymes secreted by inflammatory mononuclear cells (neutrophils and macrophages), able to generate reactive oxygen species as hypochlorous acid/hypochlorite ($HOCl/OCl^-$) from hydrogen peroxide in the presence of chloride ions. Within the kidney, this reaction leads to a variety of chlorinated protein and lipid adducts that in turn may cause dysfunction of cells in different compartments of renal parenchyma (Malle et al. 2003). MPO is an important pathogenic factor in glomerular and tubulointerstitial diseases: for example, MPO and HOCl-modified proteins can be seen in glomerular peripheral basement membranes and podocytes in human membranous glomerulonephritis; MPO antibody complexes induce and exacerbate the inflammation in necrotizing glomerulonephritis. Antineutrophil cytoplasm antibodies with anti-MPO specificity have a key role in the pathogenesis of microscopic polyangeitis, which may damage the kidneys and other organs.

A MPO-sensitive Gd-based MR contrast agent has been developed recently (Chen et al. 2006). MPOs are able to activate this agent by inducing oligomerization and protein binding and, consequently, by increasing its relaxivity. Experiments have shown that this MPO activity could be targeted in vivo within reperfused ischemic myocardium (Nahrendorf et al. 2008) and within inflammatory demyelinating plaques in the brain (Chen et al. 2006, 2008). Applications of this technique within the kidney should be numerous in the future.

## 36.6 New Parameters of Renal Function

### 36.6.1 Imaging of Tubule Dysfunction

In ARF models, the primer site of renal injury (proximal or distal) remains uncertain (Dagher et al. 2003). Using Gd-dendrimer chelates, which are cleared by glomerular filtration, some authors could demonstrate the proximal tubule dysfunction in acute tubular damage induced by cysplatin in mice (Kobayashi et al. 2002). This contrast agent accumulates within the outer medulla, where the proximal straight tubules are located (Fig. 36.9a). In diseased kidneys, the bright SI of the outer medulla does not show and the gradation of tubular damage assessed by dynamic MR imaging correlates with renal function (Fig. 36.9b, c).

### 36.6.2 Renal pH MR Imaging

Tissue pH can be measured either by MR spectroscopy or by MRI, using intrinsic resonance changes related to pH variations or pH-sensitive Gd-complexes respectively. With the later, SI changes are dependent on both, pH value and agent concentration. Therefore, to measure tissue pH, it is necessary to inject sequentially two agents with the same pharmacokinetics: one is insensitive (allowing normalization) and the other sensitive to pH. Using this technique and a gadolinium-based pH-sensitive contrast agent, Gd-DOTA-4AmP$^{5-}$ (Zhang et al. 1999), Raghunand et al. (2003) computed pH images of the kidney before and after acetazolamide administration (Fig. 36.10). Normal kidneys showed a pH of 7.0–7.4, whereas the pixels corresponding to the papilla and calyces had a pH of 5.75–7. After administration of acetazolamide, a carbonic anhydrase inhibitor that causes systemic metabolic acidosis and alkalinization of urine, pH increased significantly within the medulla calyces and ureters (pH = 7.5–8) and decreased in the extrarenal tissues.

### 36.6.3 Renal Sodium Imaging

Intrarenal sodium distribution is characterized by a corticomedullary gradient, essential for urinary concentrating process. It is closely associated with renal function. In recent studies, Maril et al. (2004, 2005) demonstrated the three dimensional (3D) intrarenal sodium gradient (Fig. 36.11). Recording of $^{23}$Na MR signal requires specifically tuned coils. Its resonance

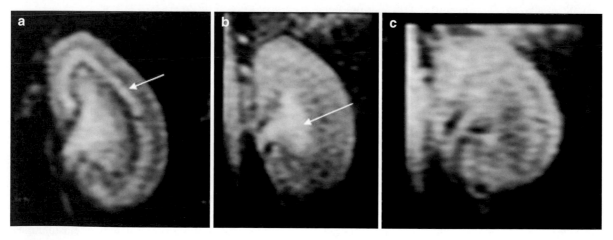

**Fig. 36.9** Renal enhancement after the injection of dendrimer-based contrast agent: in a normally functioning kidney (**a**), we note a bright band within the outer stripe of outer medulla (*arrow*) where the proximal straight tubules are located. In mildly damaged kidney (**b**), this bright band disappears and the late enhancement of inner medulla predominates (*arrow*). Severely damaged kidneys did not show the appearance of medullary enhancement (**c**) (from Kobayashi H, 2002, with permission)

**Fig. 36.10** Calculated pH images of a control female mouse (**a**), with a pH of 6.0 measured in urine, and of an acetazolamide-treated mouse (**b**), with a pH of 8.2 measured in urine. (From Raghunand et al. 2003 with permission)

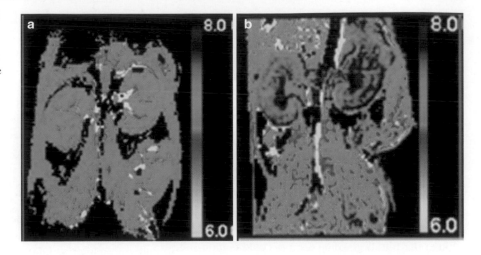

frequency is 53 MHz at 4.7 T. By measuring the sodium R1 and R2 in vivo as well as in excised kidneys, it was shown that changes in SI were directly proportional to tissue sodium concentration. In normal kidneys, sodium SI increased gradually along the corticomedullary axis, from the edge of the cortex through the outer part of the inner medulla. Conversion of intensity units to tissue sodium concentration units yielded a slope of $31 \pm 3$ mM/L/mm (from 60 mM/L in the start of the cortex to 360 mM/L in the inner medullary edge). Furosemide administration as well as urinary obstruction produced marked and distinct alterations of medullary sodium profiles. The changes in sodium gradient also correlated with the extent of damage and the residual function of the kidneys. In the ATN kidney, however, the cortico-outer medullary sodium gradient was reduced by 21% and the inner medulla to cortex sodium ratio was decreased by 40% (Maril et al. 2006a). More recently, the feasibility of sodium imaging in humans was demonstrated at 3 T (Maril et al. 2006b).

### 36.6.4 MR Imaging of Proteinuria

Localization of the origin of proteinuria may be crucial in transplanted patients to determine whether it originates in the native kidneys or in the renal allograft. To address this problem, a Gd-based albumin-bound blood pool contrast agent (MS325) was developed (Zhang et al. 2005). Nephrotic rats exhibited, after a normal peak contrast enhancement, a flattened decay curve in the cortex and medulla and a significantly prolonged excretion time, indicating reduced clearance through the kidney due to an abnormal filtration of the albumin-bound contrast agent at the glomerulus and to tubular accumulation (Fig. 36.12). However, there was no correlation between proteinuria and MS325 decay constant.

### 36.7 Imaging of Intrarenal Fibrosis

Exaggeration of ECM synthesis, with excessive fibrillar collagens, characterizes the development of fibrotic lesions in the glomerular, interstitial, and vascular compartments (Chatziantoniou et al. 2004), leading progressively to end-stage renal failure. Systems participating in these processes are increasingly identified and various therapeutic interventions have been shown to prevent or to favor the regression of fibrosis in several experimental models (Chatziantoniou et al. 2004). Therefore, the development of new noninvasive methods for identification and quantification of fibrosis would also be worthwhile. As molecular targeting of fibrosis has still not been achieved with imaging, two indirect approaches have been proposed using imaging: either MR diffusion imaging or elastography.

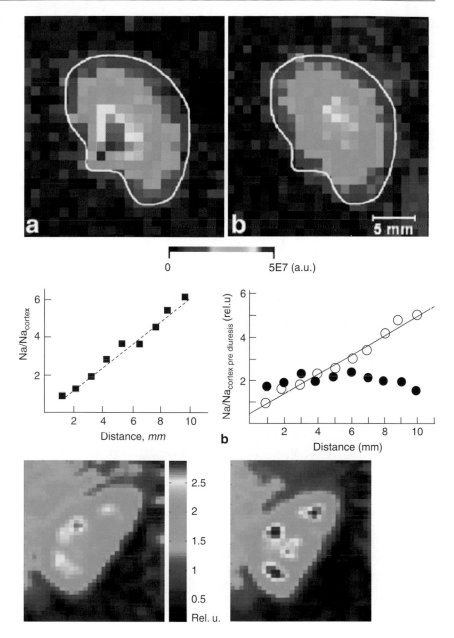

**Fig. 36.11** MR sodium imaging of the kidney. Top row: Diuretic-induced changes in sodium images and corticomedullary sodium gradients in normal rats at steady-state diuresis pre- (**a**) and postadministration (**b**) of mannitol. Middle row: Sodium profiles are shown Bottom row: Color-coded central coronal slices of the 3D sodium images of the same human kidney under normal conditions (*left*) and 12-h water deprivation (*right*) (Adapted from Maril et al. 2005 and 2006b)

Applications of diffusion imaging techniques within the kidneys are described elsewhere in this book.

Fibrotic processes altering the renal tissue structure change the biomechanical properties of the kidney. Quantification of these tissue changes is now possible with ultrasonic or MR elastography. Elastography is based on the transmission of low-frequency mechanical waves across the tissue of interest and the assessment by US or MR imaging of the wave propagation which is related to tissue elasticity (stiffness). Transient US elastography was developed first, and is actually used in clinics for staging liver fibrosis (FibroScan®,

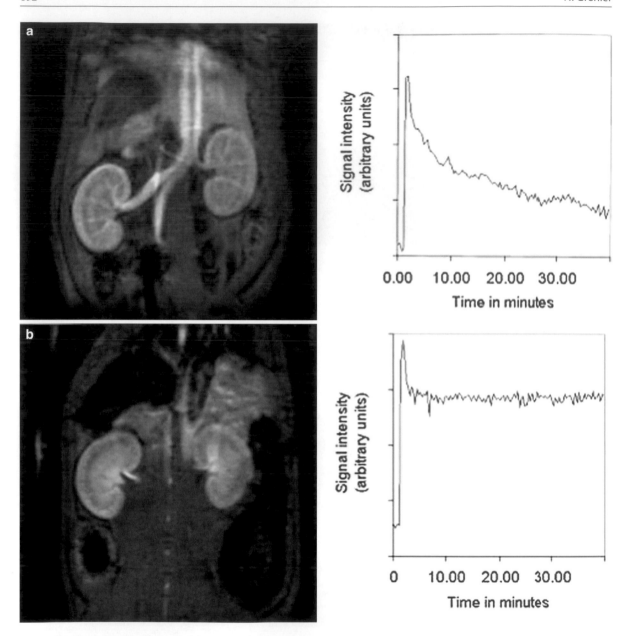

**Fig. 36.12** Contrast uptake and clearance curve in a renal cortical region of interest (ROI) after administration of MS325. (**a**) In a normal rat, the peak enhancement is seen within 2 min of contrast injection and is followed by rapid decay of signal enhancement over 40 min. (**b**) In a proteinuric rat, contrast enhancement also peaks within 2 min but then displays a remarkably flat signal decay curve, indicating impaired clearance of contrast agent from the cortex. (From Zhang et al. 2005 with permission)

Echosens, Paris, France) (Castera et al. 2008), but it cannot be applied to the kidney because the mechanical wave needs to be applied on the rigid thoracic wall to get rid of compression effects. Therefore, another approach was developed more recently, based on the US assessment of the shear wave, either on a 1D basis

(Acoustic Radiation Force Impulse, ARFI®, Siemens, Erlanghen) (Nightingale et al. 2003) or on a 2D basis (Supersonic Shear Imaging, SSI®, Supersonic Imagine, Aix-en-Provence, France) (Tanter et al. 2002) (Fig. 36.13). The first renal applications of these systems are on-going.

**Fig. 36.13** 2D elastogram of a kidney transplant using the Supersonic Shear Imaging (SSI®) system showing a higher elasticity value within the cortex (16.35 kPa) than within medulla (10.89 kPa)

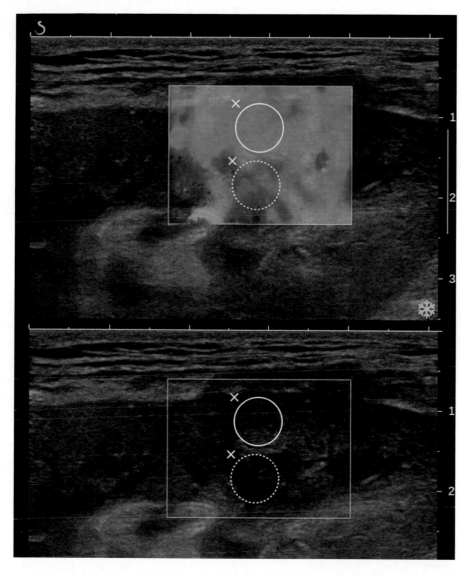

MR elastography is based on a phase contrast technique utilizing cyclic motion-sensitized gradients to image mechanically applied propagating acoustic shear waves. This method requires the application of shear waves by means of a mechanical device, producing tissue displacements in the range of nanometers to micrometers. Because propagation of these waves is dependent on the viscoelastic properties of the tissue, its elastic characteristics can be quantified and/or mapped as parametric images. In the liver, MR elastography has been validated (Huwart et al. 2007; Salameh et al. 2007). In the kidney, preliminary results have been reported on an experimental model of nephrocalcinosis in rats (Shah et al. 2004): shear stiffness of the renal cortex increased with the severity of the model. Experimental application on animal models of fibrosis is going on (Fig. 36.14).

## 36.8 Conclusion

Molecular and cellular imaging have demonstrated their great potential in characterizing diseases due to the association of high spatial resolution capabilities and the use of contrast agents specific for different

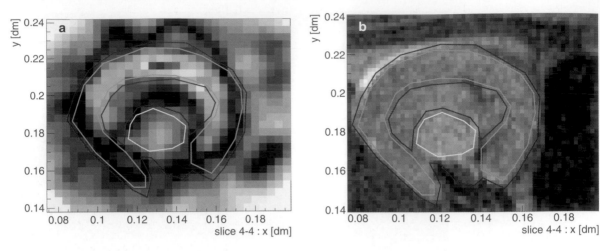

**Fig. 36.14** Example of MR-elastography of a rat kidney showing a mapping of elasticity values in each compartment (cortex, outer and inner medulla) (**a**) according to the segmentation obtained on the T2 image (**b**) (courtesy of Ralph Sinkus, Paris)

kinds of biological targets. Many parenchymal renal diseases could benefit in the future of these new imaging techniques providing a better characterization of the diseases and offering noninvasively objective prognostic criteria. Cellular targeting with superparamagnetic contrast agents already found a broad range of applications in kidney diseases and potential clinical applications will emerge soon. Elastographic techniques will probably cover renal applications in a very close future, as for liver management. However, the feasibility to apply the mentioned molecular processes to patients will require validation of specific targeted agents and will be delayed by authorization processes from regulatory agencies.

# References

Bacigalupo A (2004) Mesenchymal stem cells and haematopoietic stem cell transplantation. Best Pract Res Clin Haematol 17:387–399

Baksh D, Song L, Tuan RS (2004) Adult mesenchymal stem cells: characterization, differentiation, and application in cell and gene therapy. J Cell Mol Med 8:301–316

Beckmann N, Cannet C, Fringeli-Tanner M et al. (2003) Macrophage labeling by SPIO as an early marker of allograft chronic rejection in a rat model of kidney transplantation. Magn Reson Med 49:459–467

Beckmann N, Cannet C, Zurbruegg S et al. (2006) Macrophage infiltration detected at MR imaging in rat kidney allografts: early marker of chronic rejection? Radiology 240:717–724

Bolbrinker J, Markovic S, Wehland M et al. (2006) Expression and response to angiotensin-converting enzyme inhibition of matrix metalloproteinases 2 and 9 in renal glomerular damage in young transgenic rats with renin-dependent hypertension. J Pharmacol Exp Ther 316:8–16

Bos C, Delmas Y, Desmouliere A et al. (2004) In vivo MR imaging of intravascularly injected magnetically labeled mesenchymal stem cells in rat kidney and liver. Radiology 233:781–789

Bulte JW, Zhang S, van Gelderen P et al. (1999) Neurotransplantation of magnetically labeled oligodendrocyte progenitors: magnetic resonance tracking of cell migration and myelination. Proc Natl Acad Sci USA 96:15256–15261

Caron A, Desrosiers RR, Beliveau R (2005) Ischemia injury alters endothelial cell properties of kidney cortex: stimulation of MMP-9. Exp Cell Res 310:105–116

Castera L, Forns X, Alberti A (2008) Non-invasive evaluation of liver fibrosis using transient elastography. J Hepatol 48:835–847

Catania JM, Chen G, Parrish AR (2007) Role of matrix metalloproteinases in renal pathophysiologies. Am J Physiol Renal Physiol 292:F905–F911

Cattell V (1994) Macrophages in acute glomerular inflammation Kidney Int 45:945–952

Chatziantoniou C, Boffa JJ, Tharaux PL et al. (2004) Progression and regression in renal vascular and glomerular fibrosis. Int J Exp Pathol 85:1–11

Chaubet F, Bertholon I, Serfaty JM et al. (2007) A new macromolecular paramagnetic MR contrast agent binds to activated human platelets Contrast Media Mol Imaging 2:178–188

Chen JW, Breckwoldt MO, Aikawa E et al. (2008) Myeloperoxidase-targeted imaging of active inflammatory lesions in murine experimental autoimmune encephalomyelitis. Brain 131:1123–1133

Chen JW, Querol Sans M, Bogdanov A Jr et al. (2006) Imaging of myeloperoxidase in mice by using novel amplifiable paramagnetic substrates. Radiology 240:473–481

Choi KS, Kim SH, Cai QY et al. (2007) Inflammation-specific T1 imaging using anti-intercellular adhesion molecule 1 antibody-conjugated gadolinium diethylenetriaminepentaacetic acid. Mol Imaging 6:75–84

Dagher PC, Herget-Rosenthal S, Ruehm SG et al. (2003) Newly developed techniques to study and diagnose acute renal failure. J Am Soc Nephrol 14:2188–2198

Daldrup-Link HE, Meier R, Rudelius M et al. (2005) In vivo tracking of genetically engineered, anti-HER2/neu directed natural killer cells to HER2/neu positive mammary tumors with magnetic resonance imaging. Eur Radiol 15:4–13

Devarajan P (2006) Update on mechanisms of ischemic acute kidney injury. J Am Soc Nephrol 17:1503–1520

Dreano M, Brochot J, Myers A et al. (1986) High-level, heat-regulated synthesis of proteins in eukaryotic cells. Gene 49:1–8

Eker O, Quesson B, Rome C et al. (2010) Combination of cell delivery and thermo-inducible transcription for in vivo spatio-temporal control of gene expression: a feasibility study. Radiology In press

Erwig LP, Kluth DC, Rees AJ (2001) Macrophages in renal inflammation. Curr Opin Nephrol Hypertens 10:341–347

Fang B, Shi M, Liao L et al. (2004) Systemic infusion of FLK1(+) mesenchymal stem cells ameliorate carbon tetrachloride-induced liver fibrosis in mice. Transplantation 78:83–88

Friedewald JJ, Rabb H (2004) Inflammatory cells in ischemic acute renal failure. Kidney Int 66:486–491

Grau V, Herbst B, Steiniger B (1998) Dynamics of monocytes/macrophages and T lymphocytes in acutely rejecting rat renal allografts. Cell Tissue Res 291:117–126

Gupta S, Verfaillie C, Chmielewski D et al. (2002) A role for extrarenal cells in the regeneration following acute renal failure. Kidney Int 62:1285–1290

Hakumaki JM, Brindle KM (2003) Techniques: Visualizing apoptosis using nuclear magnetic resonance. Trends Pharmacol Sci 24:146–149

Hauger O, Delalande C, Deminiere C et al. (2000) Nephrotoxic nephritis and obstructive nephropathy: evaluation with MR imaging enhanced with ultrasmall superparamagnetic iron oxide-preliminary findings in a rat model. Radiology 217:819–826

Hauger O, Delalande C, Trillaud H et al. (1999) MR imaging of intrarenal macrophage infiltration in an experimental model of nephrotic syndrome. Magn Reson Med 41:156–162

Hauger O, Frost EE, Deminière C et al. (2006) MR evaluation of the glomerular homing of magnetically labeled mesenchymal stem cells in a rat model of nephropathy. Radiology 238:200–210

Hauger O, Grenier N, Deminere C et al. (2007) USPIO-enhanced MR imaging of macrophage infiltration in native and transplanted kidneys: initial results in humans. Eur Radiol 17:2898–2907

Hiller KH, Waller C, Nahrendorf M et al. (2006) Assessment of cardiovascular apoptosis in the isolated rat heart by magnetic resonance molecular imaging. Mol Imaging 5:115–121

Hoehn M, Kustermann E, Blunk J et al. (2002) Monitoring of implanted stem cell migration in vivo: a highly resolved in vivo magnetic resonance imaging investigation of experimental stroke in rat. Proc Natl Acad Sci USA 99:16267–16272

Huwart L, Sempoux C, Salameh N et al. (2007) Liver fibrosis: noninvasive assessment with MR elastography versus aspartate aminotransferase-to-platelet ratio index. Radiology 245:458–466

Imasawa T, Utsunomiya Y, Kawamura T et al. (2001) The potential of bone marrow-derived cells to differentiate to glomerular mesangial cells. J Am Soc Nephrol 12:1401–1409

Ito T, Suzuki A, Imai E et al. (2001) Bone marrow is a reservoir of repopulating mesangial cells during glomerular remodeling. J Am Soc Nephrol 12:2625–2635

Ittrich H, Lange C, Togel F et al. (2007) In vivo magnetic resonance imaging of iron oxide-labeled, arterially-injected mesenchymal stem cells in kidneys of rats with acute ischemic kidney injury: detection and monitoring at 3T. J Magn Reson Imaging 25:1179–1191

Jo SK, Hu X, Kobayashi H et al. (2003) Detection of inflammation following renal ischemia by magnetic resonance imaging. Kidney Int 64:43–51

Kobayashi H, Kawamoto S, Jo SK et al. (2002) Renal tubular damage detected by dynamic micro-MRI with a dendrimer-based magnetic resonance contrast agent. Kidney Int 61:1980–1985

Kraitchman DL, Heldman AW, Atalar E et al. (2003) In vivo magnetic resonance imaging of mesenchymal stem cells in myocardial infarction. Circulation 107:2290–2293

Lancelot E, Amirbekian V, Brigger I et al. (2008) Evaluation of matrix metalloproteinases in atherosclerosis using a novel noninvasive imaging approach. Arterioscler Thromb Vasc Biol 28:425–432

Lepage M, Dow WC, Melchior M et al. (2007) Noninvasive detection of matrix metalloproteinase activity in vivo using a novel magnetic resonance imaging contrast agent with a solubility switch. Mol Imaging 6:393–403

Letavernier B, Salomir R, Delmas Y et al. (2007) Ultrasound induced expression of a heat-shock promoter-driven transgene delivered in the kidney by genetically modified mesenchymal stem cells. A feasibility study. In: Hynynen K, Jolesz F (eds) MR-guided focused ultrasound surgery. Taylor & Francis, New York

Lin F, Cordes K, Li L et al. (2003) Hematopoietic stem cells contribute to the regeneration of renal tubules after renal ischemia-reperfusion injury in mice. J Am Soc Nephrol 14:1188–1199

Louie AY, Huber MM, Ahrens ET et al. (2000) In vivo visualization of gene expression using magnetic resonance imaging. Nat Biotechnol 18:321–325

Malle E, Buch T, Grone HJ (2003) Myeloperoxidase in kidney disease. Kidney Int 64:1956–1967

Maril N, Margalit R, Mispelter J et al. (2004) Functional sodium magnetic resonance imaging of the intact rat kidney. Kidney Int 65:927–935

Maril N, Margalit R, Mispelter J et al. (2005) Sodium magnetic resonance imaging of diuresis: spatial and kinetic response. Magn Reson Med 53:545–552

Maril N, Margalit R, Rosen S et al. (2006a) Detection of evolving acute tubular necrosis with renal 23Na MRI: studies in rats. Kidney Int 69:765–768

Maril N, Rosen Y, Reynolds GH et al. (2006b) Sodium MRI of the human kidney at 3 Tesla. Magn Reson Med 56:1229–1234

McLennan SV, Kelly DJ, Cox AJ et al. (2002) Decreased matrix degradation in diabetic nephropathy: effects of ACE inhibition on the expression and activities of matrix metalloproteinases. Diabetologia 45:268–275

Modo M, Hoehn M, Bulte JW (2005) Cellular MR imaging. Mol Imaging 4:143–164

Moore A, Josephson L, Bhorade RM et al. (2001) Human transferrin receptor gene as a marker gene for MR imaging.
Radiology 221:244–250

Nahrendorf M, Jaffer FA, Kelly KA et al. (2006) Noninvasive
vascular cell adhesion molecule-1 imaging identifies inflammatory activation of cells in atherosclerosis. Circulation
114:1504–1511

Nahrendorf M, Sosnovik D, Chen JW et al. (2008) Activatable
magnetic resonance imaging agent reports myeloperoxidase
activity in healing infarcts and noninvasively detects the
antiinflammatory effects of atorvastatin on ischemia-reperfusion injury. Circulation 117:1153–1160

Nightingale K, McAleavey S, Trahey G (2003) Shear-wave generation using acoustic radiation force: in vivo and ex vivo
results. Ultrasound Med Biol 29:1715–1723

Ortiz A, Justo P, Sanz A et al. (2003) Targeting apoptosis in
acute tubular injury. Biochem Pharmacol 66:1589–1594

Pittenger MF, Martin BJ (2004) Mesenchymal stem cells and
their potential as cardiac therapeutics. Circ Res 95:9–20

Quesson B, de Zwart JA, Moonen CT (2000) Magnetic resonance temperature imaging for guidance of thermotherapy.
J Magn Reson Imaging 12:525–533

Raghunand N, Howison C, Sherry AD et al. (2003) Renal and
systemic pH imaging by contrast-enhanced MRI. Magn
Reson Med 49:249–257

Rana A, Sathyanarayana P, Lieberthal W (2001) Role of apoptosis of renal tubular cells in acute renal failure: therapeutic
implications. Apoptosis 6:83–102

Reynolds PR, Larkman DJ, Haskard DO et al. (2006) Detection
of vascular expression of E-selectin in vivo with MR imaging. Radiology 241:469–476

Rome C, Couillaud F, Moonen CT (2005) Spatial and temporal
control of expression of therapeutic genes using heat shock
protein promoters. Methods 35:188–198

Salameh N, Peeters F, Sinkus R et al. (2007) Hepatic viscoelastic parameters measured with MR elastography: correlations

with quantitative analysis of liver fibrosis in the rat. J Magn
Reson Imaging 26:956–962

Schreiner GF, Harris KP, Purkerson ML et al. (1988)
Immunological aspects of acute ureteral obstruction: immune
cell infiltrate in the kidney. Kidney Int 34:487–493

Shah NS, Kruse SA, Lager DJ et al. (2004) Evaluation of renal
parenchymal disease in a rat model with magnetic resonance
elastography. Magn Reson Med 52:56–64

Szabo Z, Xia J, Mathews WB et al. (2006) Future direction of
renal positron emission tomography. Semin Nucl Med 36:
36–50

Tanter M, Bercoff J, Sandrin L et al. (2002) Ultrafast compound
imaging for 2-D motion vector estimation: application to
transient elastography. IEEE Trans Ultrason Ferroelectr Freq
Control 49:1363–1374

Weissleder R, Mahmood U (2001) Molecular imaging.
Radiology 219:316–333

Ye Q, Yang D, Williams M et al. (2002) In vivo detection of
acute rat renal allograft rejection by MRI with USPIO particles. Kidney Int 61:1124–1135

Ysebaert DK, De Greef KE, Vercauteren SR et al. (2000)
Identification and kinetics of leukocytes after severe ischae-
mia/reperfusion renal injury. Nephrol Dial Transplant 15:
1562–1574

Zhang Y, Dodd SJ, Hendrich KS et al. (2000) Magnetic resonance imaging detection of rat renal transplant rejection
by monitoring macrophage infiltration. Kidney Int 58:
1300–1310

Zhang S, Wu K, Sherry AD (1999) A novel pH-sensitive MRI
contrast agent. Angew Chem Int Ed Engl 38:3192–3194

Zhang Y, Choyke PL, Lu H et al (2005) Detection and localisation of proteinuria by dynamic contrast-enhanced MRI using
MS325. J Am Soc Nephrol 16:1752–1757

Zhao M, Beauregard DA, Loizou L et al. (2001) Non-invasive
detection of apoptosis using magnetic resonance imaging
and a targeted contrast agent. Nat Med 7:1241–1244

# Index

MONKLANDS HOSPITAL
LIBRARY
MONKSCOURT AVENUE
AIRDRIE ML60JS
☎ 01236712005